Modern Textbook of
FORENSIC MEDICINE AND TOXICOLOGY

Modern Textbook of FORENSIC MEDICINE AND TOXICOLOGY

Editor

Putul Mahanta MD FIAMLE
Associate Professor
Department of Forensic Medicine and Toxicology
Tezpur Medical College
Tezpur, Assam, India

Forewords

UC Sarma
PC Sarmah
Anil Aggrawal
RK Gorea

JAYPEE BROTHERS MEDICAL PUBLISHERS
The Health Sciences Publisher
New Delhi | London

Jaypee Brothers Medical Publishers (P) Ltd

Headquarters
EMCA House
23/23-B, Ansari Road, Daryaganj
New Delhi 110 002, India
Landline: +91-11-23272143, +91-11-23272703
+91-11-23282021, +91-11-23245672
E-mail: jaypee@jaypeebrothers.com

Corporate Office
Jaypee Brothers Medical Publishers (P) Ltd.
4838/24, Ansari Road, Daryaganj
New Delhi 110 002, India
Phone: +91-11-43574357
Fax: +91-11-43574314
E-mail: jaypee@jaypeebrothers.com

Overseas Office
JP Medical Ltd.
83, Victoria Street, London
SW1H 0HW (UK)
Phone: +44-20 3170 8910
E-mail: info@jpmedpub.com

EU GPSR Authorised Representative
Logos Europe, 9 rue Nicolas Poussin
17000, La Rochelle, France
Phone: +33 (0) 6 67 93 73 78
E-mail: Contact@logoseurope.eu

Website: www.jaypeebrothers.com
Website: www.jaypeedigital.com

Inquiries for bulk sales may be solicited at: jaypee@jaypeebrothers.com

Modern Textbook of Forensic Medicine and Toxicology

First Edition: 2014

Reprint: ***2026***

ISBN: 978-93-5152-211-9

Printed at Replika Press Pvt. Ltd.

Dedicated to

My late father Karuna Kar Mahanta, who brought me into this world,
and to my late brother Bipul Mahanta, who was my source of inspiration,
My mother Rajya Priya Mahanta and elder brother Lakheswar Mahanta, who made me a doctor,
My father-in-law, late (Prof) Birendra Nath Das, for his encouragement to do something new in life,
lastly, to my wife Manmi and my two kids Jacinth and Adriana for their sustained support
and cooperation.

CONTRIBUTORS

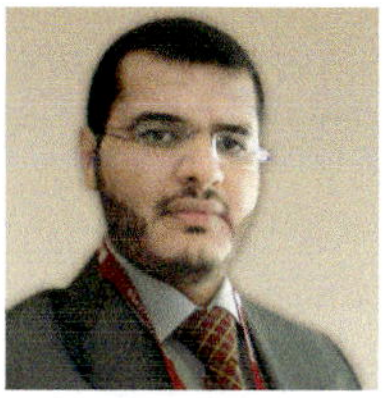

Abdulwahab Ali Abuderman MD PhD
Vice Dean
Department of Quality and Development
College of Medicine
Salman bin Abdulaziz University
Al-Kharj, Kingdom of Saudi Arabia

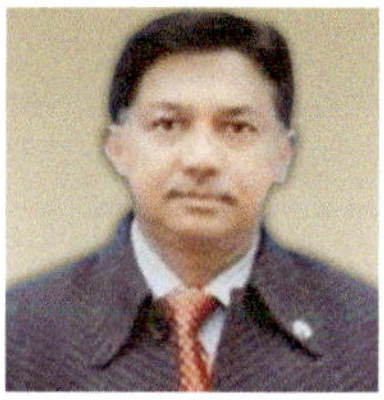

Adarsh Kumar MD PGCHM Commonwealth Fellow (UK) FRSM FIAMLE
Additional Professor
Department of Forensic Medicine and Toxicology
All India Institute of Medical Sciences
New Delhi, India

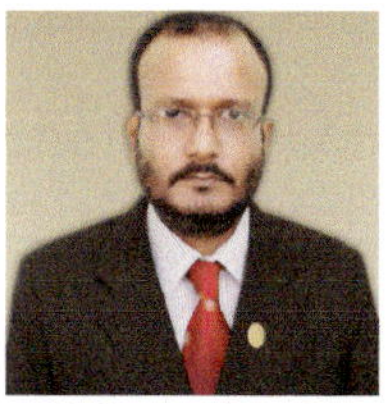

AJ Patoway MD Fellow NFCFM
Associate Professor
Department of Forensic Medicine and Toxicology
Gauhati Medical College and Hospital
Guwahati, Assam, India

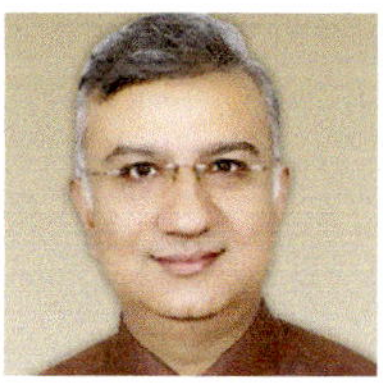

Ajay Logani BDS MDS
Associate Professor
Department of Conservative Dentistry and Endodontics
Center of Dental Education and Research
All India Institute of Medical Sciences
New Delhi, India

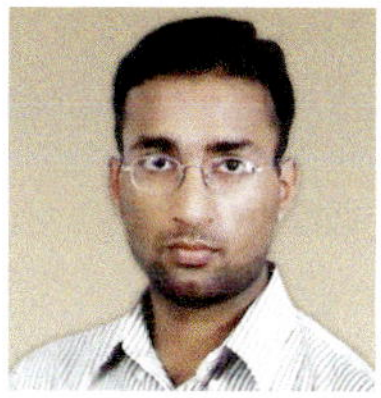

Akash Deep Aggarwal MD DNB DFM (Australia)
Associate Professor
Department of Forensic Medicine and Toxicology
Government Medical College
Patiala, Punjab, India

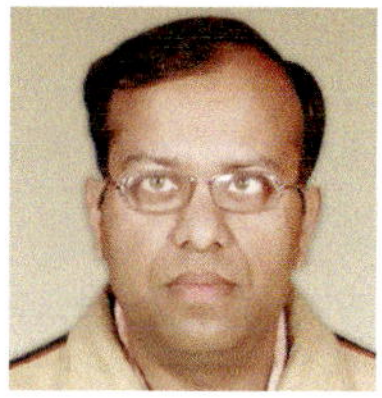

Anil Garg MD (Forensic Medicine and Toxicology)
Joint Editor
Journal of Punjab Academy of Forensic Medicine and Toxicology
Associate Professor
Department of Forensic Medicine
Gian Sagar Medical College and Hospital
Patiala, Punjab, India

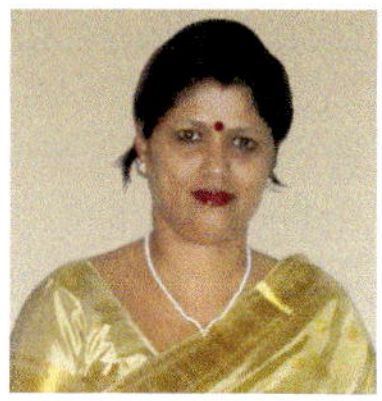

Anku Moni Saikia MD (Social and Preventive Medicine)
Associate Professor
Department of Community Medicine
Gauhati Medical College
Guwahati, Assam, India

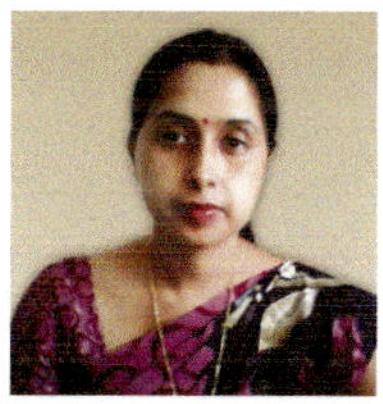

Anurupa Choudhury MD (Forensic Medicine and Toxicology)
Department of Forensic Medicine and Toxicology
Gauhati Medical College and Hospital
Guwahati, Assam, India

CB Jani MD (Patho) MD DNB (Forensic Medicine and Toxicology) LLB

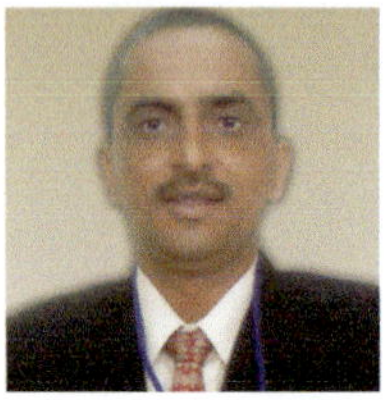

Professor and Head
Department of Forensic Medicine and Toxicology
Gujarat Cancer Society Medical College
Ahmedabad, Gujarat, India

Chaithra V BDS MDS

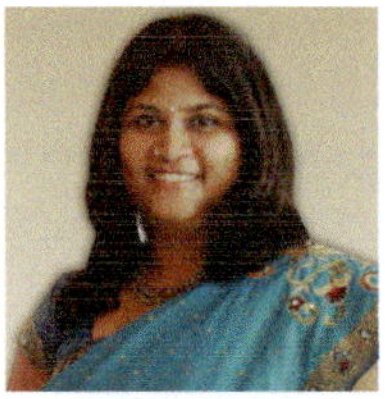

Faculty
The Oxford Dental Collage Hospital and Research Center
Bengaluru, Karnataka, India

Deepanjali Medhi MD (Psychiatry)

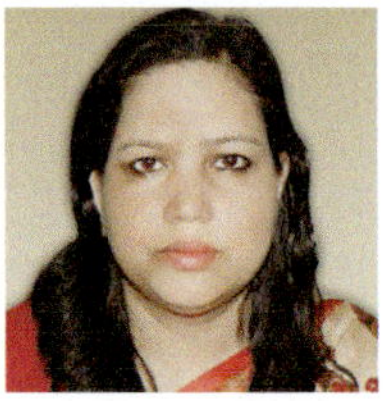

Associate Professor
Department of Psychiatry
Gauhati Medical College and Hospital
Guwahati, Assam, India

Deepjyoti Kalita MD (Microbiology)

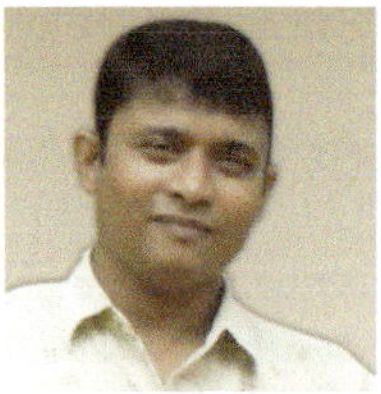

Associate Professor
Department of Microbiology
Fakhruddin Ali Ahmed Medical College
Barpeta, Assam, India

Gunajit Das MD (Forensic Medicine and Toxicology)

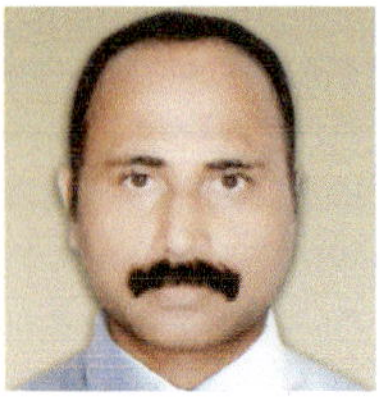

Associate Professor
Department of Forensic Medicine and Toxicology
Silchar Medical College and Hospital
Silchar, Assam, India

HK Mahanta DFM MD LLB

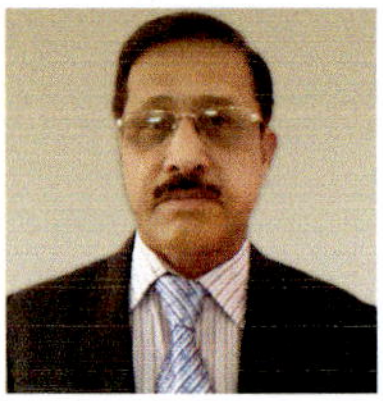

Professor and Head
Department of Forensic Medicine and Toxicology
Assam Medical College
Dibrugarh, Assam, India

Imran Sabri MD (Forensic Medicine and Toxicology)

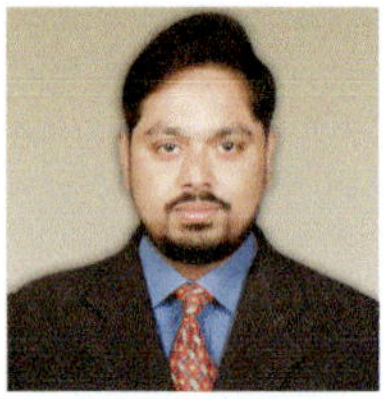

Faculty of Forensic Medicine
Department of Biomedical Sciences
College of Medicine, King Faisal University
Al-Ahsa, Kingdom of Saudi Arabia

KK Bairagi MD (Forensic Medicine and Toxicology)

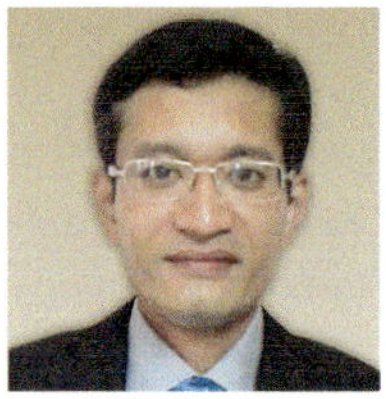

Professor and Head
Department of Forensic Medicine and Toxicology
Tagore Medical College and Hospital
Rathinamangalam
Chennai, Tamil Nadu, India

Madhab Ch Rajbongshi MS FAIS FMAS FICS

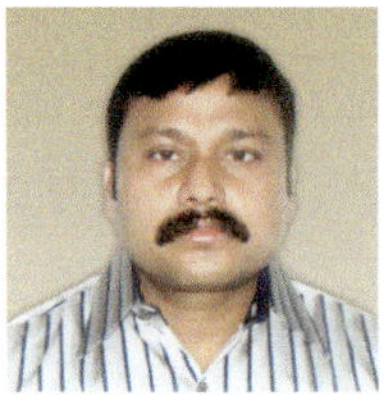

Faculty
Department of Surgery
Gauhati Medical College and Hospital
Guwahati, Assam, India

Manish Nigam MD (Forensic Medicine and Toxicology)

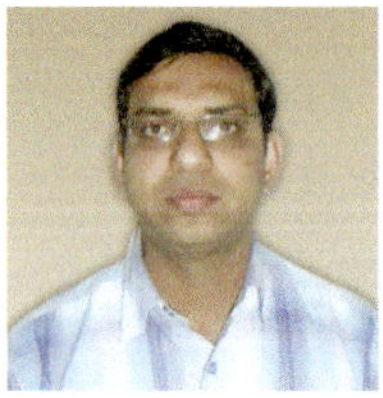

Professor and Head
Department of Forensic Medicine and Toxicology
Sri Aurobindo Medical College and PG Institute
Indore, Madhya Pradesh, India

Manjula Bai KH MD (Forensic Medicine and Toxicology)

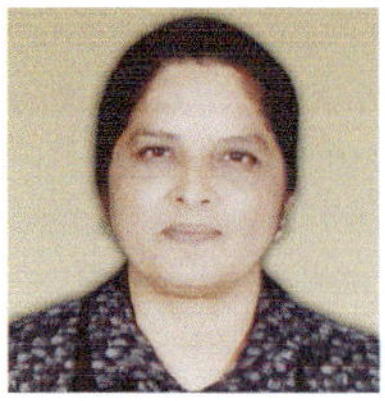

Professor and Head
Department of Forensic Medicine and Toxicology
Jawaharlal Nehru Medical College
KLE University
Belgaum, Karnataka, India

Monika Garg MD
(Pathology)

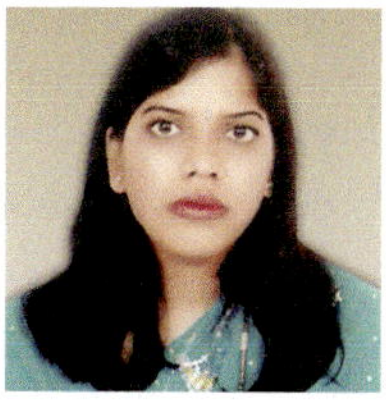

Associate Professor
Department of Pathology
MM Institute of Medical Sciences and Research
Mullana, Haryana, India

Mrinal Haloi MD
(Forensic Medicine and Toxicology)

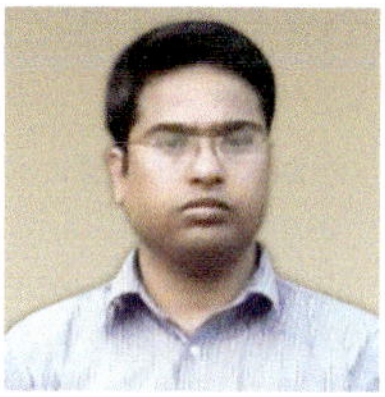

Department of Forensic Medicine and Toxicology
Gauhati Medical College,
Guwahati, Assam, India

Mukesh Yadav BSc
MD (FMT) MBA (HCA) LLB PGDHRMD

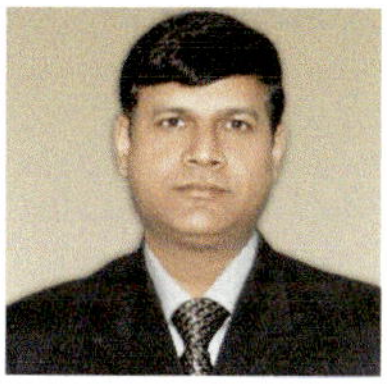

Editor
Journal of Indian Academy of Forensic Medicine
Professor and Head
Department of Forensic Medicine and Toxicology
School of Medical Sciences and Research,
Sharda University
Greater Noida, Uttar Pradesh, India

Nisha Goyal MS
(Anatomy)

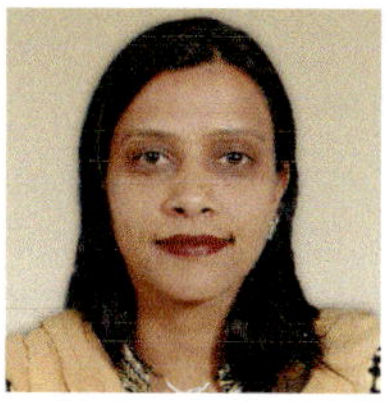

Faculty
Department of Anatomy
Adesh Institute of Medical Sciences and Research
Adesh University
Bathinda, Punjab, India

NK Aggarwal MD
WHO Fellow

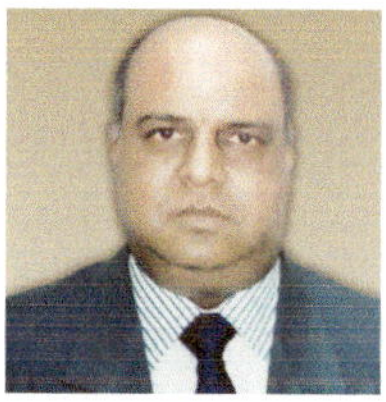

Professor and Head
Department of Forensic Medicine and Toxicology
University College of Medical Sciences and GTB Hospital
New Delhi, India

PC Sarmah DFM MD
(Forensic Medicine and Toxicology)
LLB FICFMT FIAFM

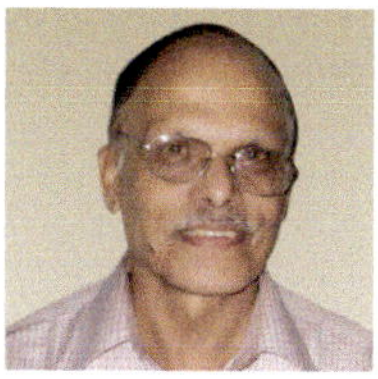

Professor and Head
Department of Forensic Medicine and Toxicology
Sikkim Manipal Institute of Medical Sciences
Gangtok, Sikkim, India
Formerly Head
Department of Forensic Medicine and Toxicology
Gauhati Medical College
Guwahati, Assam, India

Pooja Malik Puri BDS
MSc (Forensic Science)

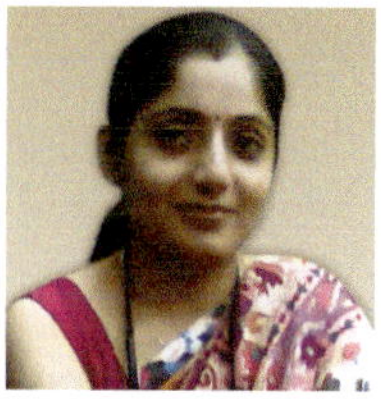

Faculty
Amity Institute of Forensic Sciences
Amity University
Noida, Uttar Pradesh, India

Prabir Kumar Dev MD
(Forensic Medicine and Toxicology)

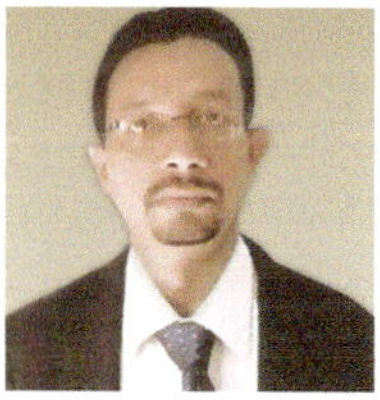

Professor
Department of Forensic Medicine and Toxicology
Nilratan Sircar Medical College
Kolkata, West Bengal, India

Pushpendra Malik

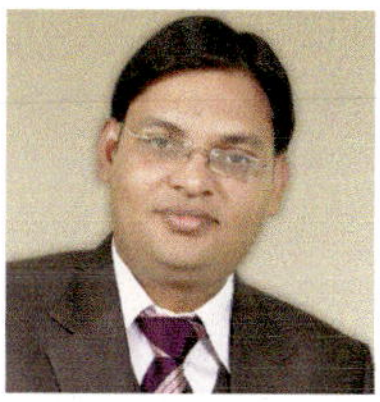

Department of Onco-surgery
Postgraduate Institute of Medical Sciences
Rohtak, Haryana, India

Putul Mahanta MD
FIAMLE

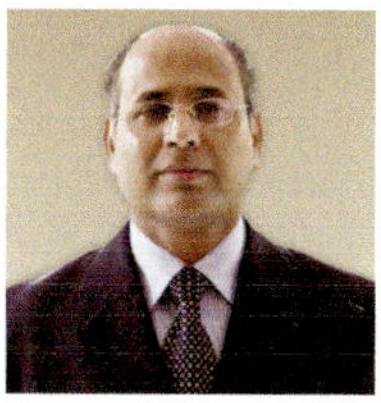

Associate Professor
Department of Forensic Medicine and Toxicology
Tezpur Medical College
Tezpur, Assam, India

Raktim Pratim Tamuli
MD (Forensic Medicine and Toxicology)

Department of Forensic Medicine and Toxicology
Tezpur Medical College
Tezpur, Assam, India

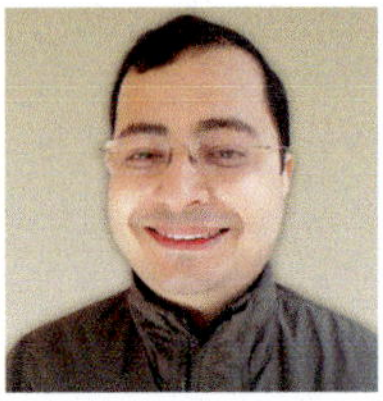

Rituraj Chaliha MD
(Forensic Medicine and Toxicology)

Professor and Head
Department of Forensic Medicine and Toxicology
Gauhati Medical College and Hospital
Guwahati, Assam, India

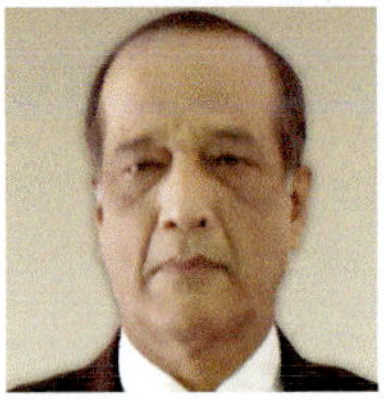

RK Gorea BSc MD PhD DNB

College of Medicine
Salman Bin Abdul Aziz University
Al Kharj, Saudi Arabia
Chief Adviser Indo-Pacific Academy of Forensic Odontology
President:Indo-Pacific Academy of Forensic Nursing Science
President:Society for Prevention of Injuries and Corporal Punishment

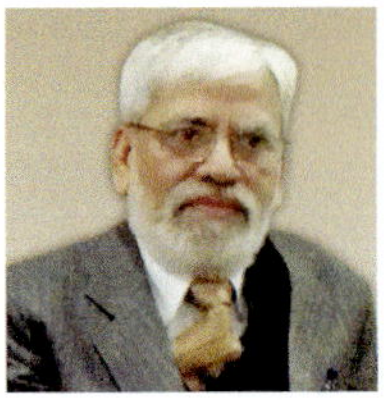

Sanjoy Das MD (Forensic Medicine and Toxicology)

Professor and Head
Department of Forensic Medicine and Toxicology
Himalayan Institute of Medical Sciences
Jolly Grant, Dehradun, Uttarakhand, India

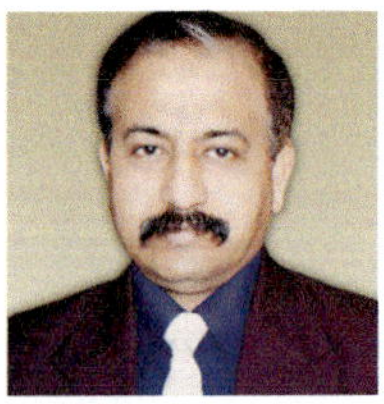

Shouvanik Adhya MD
(Forensic Medicine and Toxicology)

Faculty
Department of Forensic Medicine and Toxicology
College of Medicine and JNM Hospital
West Bengal University of Health Sciences
Kalyani, West Bengal, India

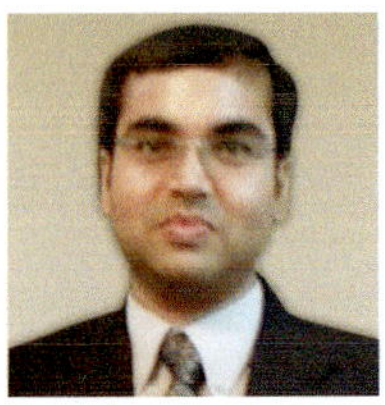

Sunit Kr Joshi MD
(Forensic Medicine and Toxicology)

Associate Professor
Department of Biomedical Sciences
KPC Medical College
Jadavpur, West Bengal, India

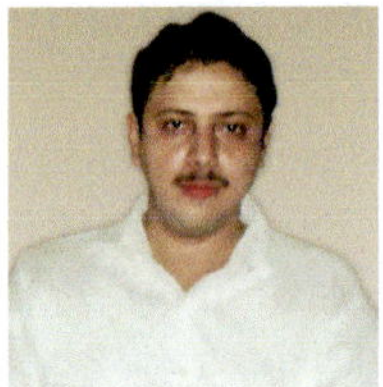

Thejaswi HT MD (Forensic Medicine and Toxicology)

Department of Forensic Medicine
All India Institute of Medical Sciences
New Delhi, India

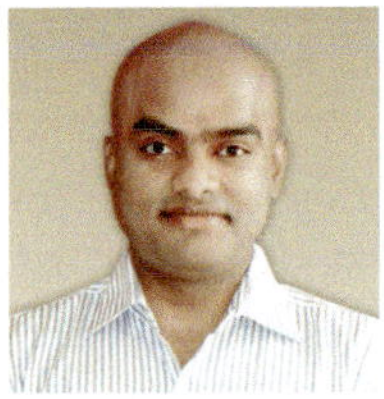

TK Bose MD DFM
(Forensic Medicine and Toxicology)

Professor and Head
Department of Forensic Medicine and Toxicology
National Medical College
West Bengal University of Health Sciences
Kolkata, West Bengal, India
Ex-Sectional President (Med Sc)
Indian Science Congress 2009-10

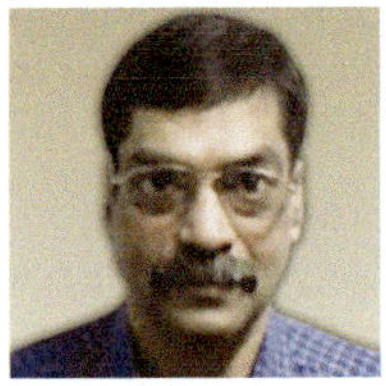

Vijayamahantesh SN
MD (Forensic Medicine and Toxicology)

Associate Professor
Department of Forensic Medicine and Toxicology
S Nijalingappa Medical College
Bagalkot, Karnataka, India

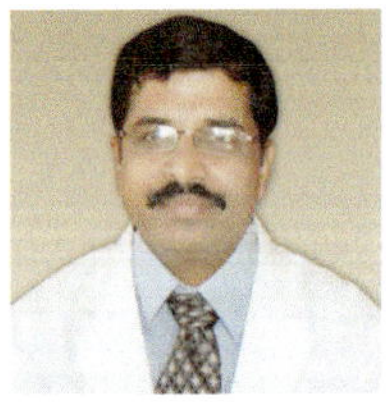

Vijayanath V MD DNB
(Forensic Medicine and Toxicology)

Professor
Department of Forensic Medicine and Toxicology
Vinayaka Mission's Kirupananda Variyar Medical College
Salem, Tamil Nadu, India

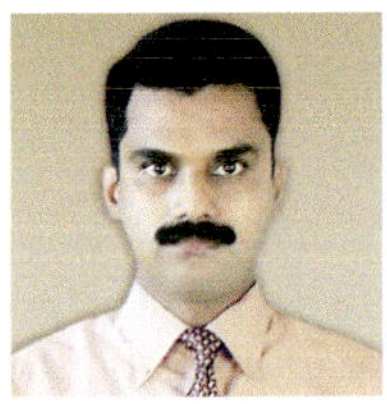

YN Singha MD (Forensic Medicine and Toxicology) RCGP FIDM

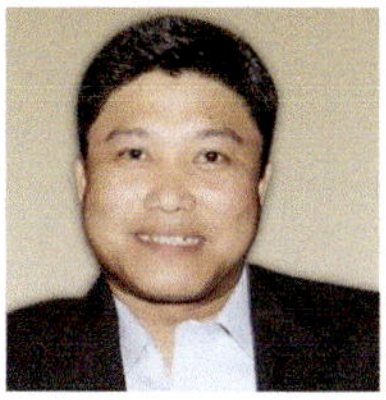

Faculty
Department of Forensic Medicine and Toxicology
Silchar Medical College
Silchar, Assam, India

Yogender Malik MD (Forensic Medicine and Toxicology)

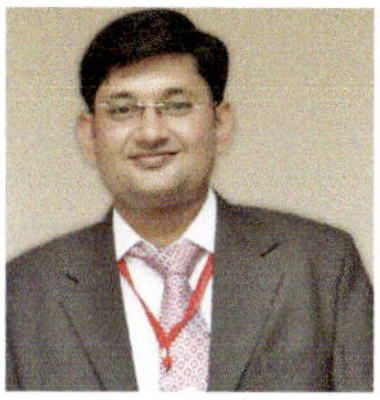

Faculty
Department of Forensic Medicine and Toxicology
Bhagat Phool Singh Government Medical College for Women
Sonepat, Haryana, India

ADVISORS

RK Sarma MD

Former Head
Department of Forensic Medicine
and Toxicology
All India Institute of Medical Sciences
New Delhi, India

TK Bose MD DFM

Professor and Head
Department of Forensic Medicine and Toxicology
National Medical College
West Bengal University of Health Sciences
Kolkata, West Bengal, India

ASSOCIATE EDITORS

Adarsh Kumar MD PGCHM Commonwealth Fellow (UK) FRSM FIAMLE

Additional Professor
Department of Forensic Medicine and Toxicology
All India Institute of Medical Sciences
New Delhi, India

AJ Patowary MD Fellow NFCFM

Associate Professor
Department of Forensic Medicine and Toxicology
Gauhati Medical College and Hospital
Guwahati, Assam, India

Akash Deep Aggarwal MD DNB DFM (Australia)

Associate Professor
Department of Forensic Medicine and Toxicology
Government Medical College
Patiala, Punjab, India

CB Jani MD (Patho) MD DNB (Forensic Medicine and Toxicology) LLB

Professor and Head
Department of Forensic Medicine and Toxicology
Gujarat Cancer Society Medical College
Ahmedabad, Gujarat, India

Gunajit Das MD (Forensic Medicine and Toxicology)

Associate Professor
Department of Forensic Medicine and Toxicology
Silchar Medical College and Hospital
Silchar, Assam, India

KK Bairagi MD (Forensic Medicine and Toxicology)

Professor and Head
Department of Forensic Medicine and Toxicology
Tagore Medical College and Hospital
Rathinamangalam
Chennai, Tamil Nadu, India

Mukesh Yadav BSc MD (FMT) MBA (HCA) LLB PGDHRMD

Editor
Journal of Indian Academy of Forensic Medicine
Professor and Head
Department of Forensic Medicine and Toxicology
School of Medical Sciences and Research
Sharda University
Greater Noida, Uttar Pradesh, India

Vijayanath V MD DNB (Forensic Medicine and Toxicology)

Professor
Department of Forensic Medicine and Toxicology
Vinayaka Mission's Kirupananda Variyar Medical College
Salem, Tamil Nadu, India

Manish Nigam MD (Forensic Medicine and Toxicology)

Professor and Head
Department of Forensic Medicine and Toxicology
Sri Aurobindo Medical College and PG Institute
Indore, Madhya Pradesh, India

FOREWORD

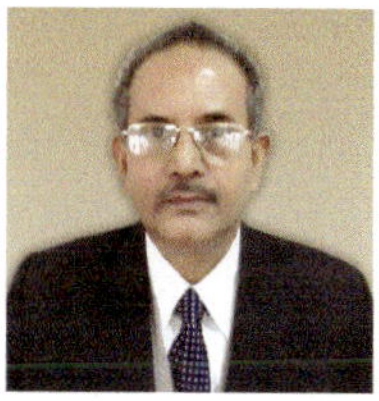

The book edited by Putul Mahanta entitled *Modern Textbook of Forensic Medicine and Toxicology* is an excellent book. The book contains 52 chapters, and eminent contributors have contributed a lot. The book also contains excellent colorful figures for easy understanding and self-learning. There was a long-felt need for a good textbook of this standard. The book deals with application of the principles and knowledge of medicine for the purpose of law, both civil and criminal. The common people believe that doctors are meant for treating patients. In addition to patient care, doctors are having the responsibilities to help the law enforcement authorities in handling legal matters. For this, medical students are to study Forensic Medicine as well as Toxicology. A doctor plays vital role in judgment delivery process as an important witness.

I hope, this book will fulfill long-felt need of both undergraduate and postgraduate students as well as teachers in the subject of Forensic Medicine and Toxicology.

UC Sarma MBBS (Gau) MD (BHU)
MSc in Epidemiology (London University)
PG Training in Epidemiology (London University)

Vice Chancellor, Srimanta Sankaradeva University of Health Sciences
Narakasur Hilltop, Bhangagarh, Guwahati, Assam, India
Former Director of Medical Education, Assam

FOREWORD

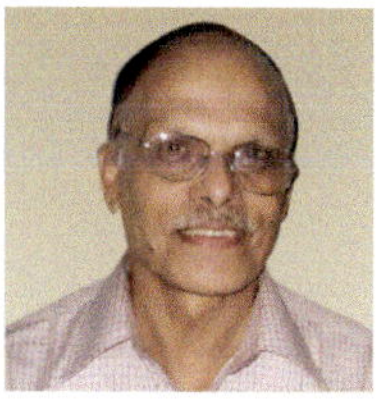

The usage of Forensic/Legal Medicine (term used in Western Countries) of medical science is by the law enforcement authorities for investigating criminal cases to identify criminals, thereby maintaining the law and order in the society. Every branch of medical science needs to be utilized for bringing out the truth and proving actual crime beyond reasonable doubt. In fact, forensic medicine serves as the link between the society and legal system.

Since time immemorial, forensic medicine has been developing to reach the present stage. In modern-day society, criminals use more sophisticated tools to commit crimes unlike the olden days' crimes committed by crude method. Apart from dealing with diseases, doctors often have to help the crime investigating authorities by providing information gathered during the treatment of victim and/or assailant and, at times have to depose in the Honorable Court about the case. Therefore, forensic medicine has been incorporated as a compulsory subject in the MBBS course.

Until *Modi's Medical Judicature and Toxicology* came out in 1920, books of forensic medicine written by foreign writers were followed in India. Subsequently, *Essentials of Forensic Medicine and Toxicology* (1973) written by Dr KS Narayan Reddy has served the purpose. At present, many standard books by Indian authors are available in the market. However, with more than 38 years of experience in the subject, I believe that it is not possible to include all possible types of medicolegal cases in one book.

That is why, I feel immense pleasure for writing this Foreword. Dr Putul Mahanta, who has been one of my beloved students and now active and dedicated teacher of the specialty of forensic medicine, has taken pain to include maximum problems in the subject. I congratulate him.

I hope, this book will provide knowledge and information on forensic medicine and toxicology to the medical students, doctors, lawyers, investigators and law enforcement authorities, apart from fulfilling the mission of the author.

PC Sarmah DFM MD (Forensic Medicine and Toxicology) LLB FICFMT FIAFM

Professor and Head
Department of Forensic Medicine and Toxicology
Sikkim Manipal Institute of Medical Sciences
Gangtok, Sikkim, India
Formerly Head
Department of Forensic Medicine and Toxicology
Gauhati Medical College
Guwahati, Assam, India

FOREWORD

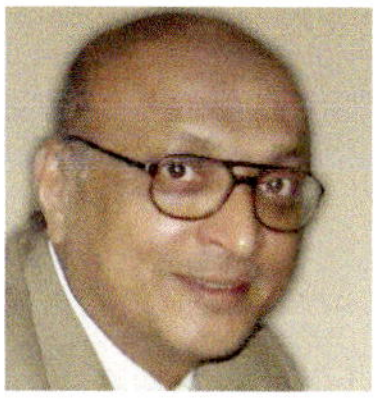

Forensic Medicine is a vast and ever-challenging subject. It is a unique subject, where undergraduates, postgraduates and faculty alike have to keep pace with developments not only in medicine but also in law. Recent changes in Transplantation of Human Organs and Tissues Act, 1994, Preconception and Prenatal Diagnostic Techniques Act, 1994, Medical Termination of Pregnancy Act 1971 and several other laws have been so wide ranging that an informed commentary is necessary on them.

Similarly, on medicine front, a number of new technologies, especially covering DNA sciences, are coming up almost on a monthly basis. So much so that there are about 20 journals, are indexed by PubMed, dedicated to forensic medicine and toxicology alone. Moreover, even all of them combined are not able to include all information, with the result that much research relevant to forensic medicine are being published in journals dedicated to other specialties. One can imagine the daunting task a postgraduate student faces in keeping pace with these latest developments.

I have always felt that this country has lacked a genuine postgraduate book in forensic medicine, which provides the latest information in law and medicine to the overburdened postgraduate student. Thankfully, Dr Putul Mahanta, a senior faculty and a highly dedicated person in our profession, has taken up this challenge and has come out with just the right type of book that was always in my mind. Dr Mahanta, whom I know for more than a decade, has worked in foreign country on an advisory basis. He regularly updates himself with the latest knowledge in forensic medicine and toxicology by reading the latest journals and has put together all the latest materials in his book.

I have gone through the contents of this book and I am quite satisfied that it contains all relevant chapters. Dr Mahanta has taken care to put on board a number of medical and legal luminaries from across the country, so that the book could be enriched by their combined experience. I wholeheartedly recommend this book to all undergraduates, postgraduates, researchers and faculty members of forensic medicine. I wish Dr Mahanta good luck in his endeavor.

Anil Aggrawal MD
Director and Professor
Department of Forensic Medicine
Maulana Azad Medical College
New Delhi, India

FOREWORD

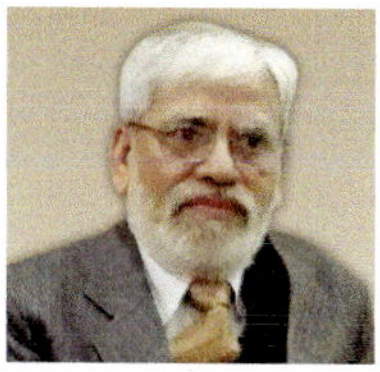

It gives me immense pleasure in writing the foreword of the *Modern Textbook of Forensic Medicine and Toxicology* edited by Dr Putul Mahanta. Dr Mahanta is known for his dedication to the field of forensic medicine, and I am overwhelmed at the hard work done by him in bringing out this book. He has been successful in inviting many renowned personalities of forensic medicine in India to write in this book and review the chapters.

I wish him all success in his endeavor and hope this book will prove very useful to undergraduate as well as postgraduate students of Forensic Medicine.

RK Gorea BSc MD PhD DNB
College of Medicine
Salman Bin Abdul Aziz University
Al Kharj, Saudi Arabia
Chief Adviser Indo-Pacific Academy of Forensic Odontology
President, Indo-Pacific Academy of Forensic Nursing Science
President, Society for Prevention of Injuries and Corporal Punishment

PREFACE

While I was pursuing my postgraduation, I felt the want of a good textbook on forensic medicine and toxicology with beautiful photographs, colorful illustrations, tables, flow charts and the valid references for faster and better comprehension. The problem prevailed when I joined the faculty as a member.

While I was abroad, I have seen many foreign books on our profession that have been written elaborately, explained with beautiful illustrations and flushed with plenty of high-resolution photographs. They also cite the references, which are essential for the readers to understand the source of the text.

Thus, the idea of writing a book, shaped in my mind, a decade ago.

This book has been aimed to cover the needs of undergraduate as well as the postgraduate students by following the whole curriculum as per Medical Council of India (MCI). I hope it would be useful not only for the students and the doctors working in rural hospitals who deal in the maximum number of medicolegal cases, but also for the faculty of our fraternity, besides students pursuing careers in Dentistry, Ayurvedic and Homeopathic professions.

The book contains 52 chapters along with a number of useful proforma as Annexures. A good number of new topics such as forensic osteology; forensic odontology; human rights, custodial torture and deaths; crime scene investigation and techniques in museum, have increased the depth and width of the book. All the text illustrations are updated with recent advancement on forensic medicine.

Special emphasis has been given to the upcoming concepts such as biomedical waste management, human experimentation, DNA profiling and related issues.

I sincerely hope this book will serve the intent and help the readers to learn the subject. All the positive critiques will be my strength for further improvement of this book.

Putul Mahanta

ACKNOWLEDGMENTS

Writing any book is a mammoth job. It would not have been possible to write this book without the help and support of the distinguished people around me.

As many as 35 experts, both national and international, have contributed materials of the book, including some illustrations. I sincerely hope that these contributions will definitely benefit the readers. I would like to take this opportunity to thank Prof PC Sarmah, Prof RK Gorea, Prof Anil Aggrawal, Prof Sanjoy Das, Prof CB Jani, Prof TK Bose, Prof Mukesh Yadav, Prof R Chaliha, Prof HK Mahanta and Prof Manjula Bai KH.

Prof SI Barbhuiyan, Prof BC Roy Medhi, Prof Kailash Bhatta, Prof KC Das, Prof Rupak Gogoi, Dr Dilip Goswami and Dr PK Thakuria were my constant source of inspiration.

Dr Adarsh Kumar, Dr AJ Patowary, Dr Vijayanath V, Dr Prabir Kr Dev, Dr Gunajit Das, Dr Deepanjali Medhi, Dr Vijayamahantesh SN, Dr Asad U Khan, Dr Anil Garg, Dr Akash Deep Aggarwal, Dr Anku Moni Saikia, Dr Deepjyoti Kalita, Dr Kaustav Bairagi, Dr Chaithra V, Dr Sunit Kr Joshi, Dr Imran Sabri, Dr YN Singha, Dr Yogender Malik, Dr Anurupa Choudhury, Dr Pooja M Puri, Dr Madhab Ch Rajbongshi, Dr Shouvanik Adhya, Dr P Malik, and Dr Raktim Pratim Tamuli deserve my deepest gratitude for providing meliorate text materials, illustrations and photographs.

I especially thank Professor Sir Alec Jeffreys, pioneer of DNA fingerprinting, for allowing me to publish his First DNA fingerprints.

Detailed chapter reviews were accredited to help me establish the necessary changes required for the book, and I am extremely grateful to Prof Ajoy Kr Gupta of KPC Medical College, West Bengal, Prof NK Hazarika, Prof KL Talukdar and Prof Joydev Sarma, from Gauhati Medical College for reviewing Medical Law, Ethics and Medical Negligence; Food Poisoning, the Forensic Osteology chapters respectively.

I had to implore and borrow some of the photographs that appear in this book from my colleagues, and I am grateful to them for their support. They are acknowledged on the respective pages. I am extremely grateful to my colleagues Dr MK Singha, Dr Kanika K Barua, Dr SJ Deka, Dr Richa Pandey, Dr NM Kakati, Dr NK Das, Dr Arnab Pratim Baruah, Dr Nayan Moni Pathak, Dr Mrinal Haloi, Dr Arpan Mazumder, Dr (Mrs) Renuka Rongpharpi and Dr Dhritiman Nath for proofreading.

Dr Khanindra Mohan Soud, Dr SMI Kabir, Dr Mamata Devi Haloi, Dr Manoj Kr Baishya, Dr Ved Prakash Gupta, Dr Biswadeep Paul, Dr Arup Kr Das, Dr Gautam Nath, Dr Braja Gopal Das, Dr Aditya Madhab Baruah, Dr Debarshee Chakraborty, Dr Noor Jahan Ahmed, Dr Sainjalee Halflongbar, Dr Dipankar Thakuria, Dr Arunav Borah and Dr Smritimala Sarmah deserve special thanks for their persistent support and encouragement.

I am especially grateful to Shri Jitendar P Vij (Group Chairman), Mr Ankit Vij (Managing Director) and Mr Tarun Duneja (Director-Publishing) of M/s Jaypee Brothers Medical Publishers (P) Ltd, New Delhi, India, for their expertise in the shaping, collation and illustration of this book. I would like to pen down my extreme gratitude to Mr Himangshu Lahkar for his valued technical support.

Since the preparation of this book, my wife Manmi Das Mahanta has reviewed the legal aspects of various chapters and typed some of the texts with our son Jacinth throughout the year. Any large endeavor of this type cannot be completed without the support of family, and my family is of no exception. My wife, son and daughter Adriana deserve special mention. I thank them for their tolerance of my absences, physically and emotionally.

CONTENTS

SECTION 1: FORENSIC MEDICINE

1. **Introduction and History of Forensic Medicine** 3
   Putul Mahanta
   - What is Forensic Medicine? 3
   - Autopsy 4
   - Phylogenesis of Forensic Medicine in India 5
   - Future of Forensic Medicine 6

2. **Legal Procedures** 8
   NK Aggarwal, HK Mahanta, Putul Mahanta
   - Legal Procedures 8
   - Inquest 9
   - Courts 10
   - Punishment (Legal Sentences) Authorized by Law in India 12
   - Medical Evidence 13
   - Witness 16
   - Offence 17
   - Duty of a Doctor as a Witness in the Court 20

3. **Medical Law and Ethics** 21
   Mukesh Yadav, Rituraj Chaliha, Putul Mahanta
   - Medical Council of India 21
   - Ethical Aspects of Medical Practice 24
   - Registered Medical Practitioner 26
   - Unethical Acts 31
   - Professional Misconduct 32
   - Legal Aspects of Medical Practice 33
   - MCI and Medical Record 34
   - Consent 34
   - Medical Negligence 42
   - Consumer Protection Act, 1986 53
   - Biomedical Waste Management 54
   - Ethics and Medical Research (Human Experimentation) 60

4. **Euthanasia (Mercy Killing)** 65
   Prabir Kumar Dev, Putul Mahanta
   - Definition 65
   - History 65
   - Physician Sentiment 66
   - Types of Euthanasia 66

- Pros and Cons 66
- Medicolegal Importance 67

5. **Identification** 69

Putul Mahanta, Vijayamahantesh SN, Vijayanath V, Imran Sabri

- Types of Identification 69
- Medicolegal Circumstances Where Identification is Needed 69
- Corpus Delicti (the Essence of Crime) 70
- Points to be Noted for the Purpose of Identification 71
- Determination of Race 72
- Religion and Caste 72
- Determination of Sex 73
- Determination of Age 78
- Stature 90
- Anthropometry (Bertillon System) 90
- Fingerprint System 91
- Footprints (Podogram) 96
- Lip Prints (Cheiloscopy) 97
- Ear Prints 97
- Nose Print 97
- Rugoscopy (Palatoprints) 97
- Superimposition 98
- Deformities and Birthmarks 99
- Scars 100
- Tattoo Marks 102
- Disease, Wounds and Stains 103
- Occupational Stigmata 104
- Complexion and Features 104
- Clothes and Ornaments 104
- Hair 105
- Fibers 105
- Miscellaneous 109

6. **Forensic Osteology** 111

Putul Mahanta, Vijayamahantesh SN, Nisha Goyal

- Examination of Skeletal Remains 111
- Growth in Individual Bones 115
- Skull 116
- Mandible 119
- Femur 122
- Tibia 126
- Fibula 127
- Scapula 128
- Clavicle 128
- Humerus 129
- Radius 131
- Ulna 131
- Sternum 132

- Hyoid Bone 133
- Pelvis and Hipbone 134
- Sacrum 138
- Vertebrae 139
- Small Bones of Hand and Feet 139

7. Forensic Odontology **142**

Adarsh Kumar, Putul Mahanta, Ajay Logani, Chaithra V

- Forensic Significance 142
- Definition 143
- Historical Events 143
- Dental Records 144
- Dentition 145
- Charting of Teeth 150
- Dental Identification 153
- Role of Forensic Odontologist 159
- Domestic Violence and Child Abuse 163
- Civil Cases in Malpractice 166
- Age and Sex Determination 166
- Organizations in the Field of Forensic Odontology 166
- Recent Advances in Forensic Odontology 166
- Limitations 168
- Diagnosis of Poisonings 168

8. Forensic DNA Typing **171**

Imran Sabri, Putul Mahanta

- Introduction to DNA 171
- Uses of DNA Typing in Forensic Investigation 175

9. Thanatology **177**

Putul Mahanta

- Types of Death 177
- What is Brain Death? 178
- Death Certificate 180
- Manner of Death 182
- Mechanism of Death 182
- Modes of Death 182
- Sudden Death 184
- Changes After Death 184
- Suspended Animation (Apparent Death) 195
- Postmortem Interval (PMI) or Time Since Death (TSD) 195

10. Autopsy **199**

AJ Patowary, Putul Mahanta

- Definition 199
- History 199
- Types of Autopsy 200
- Examination 203

- Viscera Examination Technique 210
- Fetal and Perinatal Autopsy 212
- Samples to be Preserved 212

11. Mechanical Injury 216

Putul Mahanta

- Some Terms of Medicolegal Importance 216
- Biophysics of Injury 217
- Principles of Cell Injury 218
- Types of Injury 218
- Abrasion 219
- Contusion 223
- Laceration 228
- Incised Wounds 230
- Stab or Puncture Wounds 235

12. Firearm Injuries 240

Putul Mahanta, AJ Patowary

- Terminologies 240
- General Make up of Firearm 241
- Classification of Firearms 242
- Smooth Bore Firearm Injury 247
- Rifled Firearms 252
- Rifled Firearms or Shotgun Injuries 258
- Identification of the Weapon 267
- Role of Physician in Firearm Injuries 268

13. Regional Injuries 270

Manjula Bai KH, Putul Mahanta

- Brief Anatomical Review of Head 270
- Head Injury 271
- Injury to the Bones of the Head 274
- Intracranial Hemorrhages 282
- Head Injury and Legal Responsibility 288
- Injury to Neck 290
- Injuries on the Chest 291
- Abdominal Injuries 293
- Injuries on Limbs 294
- Injuries to Private Parts 295
- Injuries to the Spinal Cord 295

14. Road Traffic Injuries 297

Putul Mahanta, Madhab Ch Rajbongshi

- Definition 297
- Brief Review of Road Traffic Accident 298
- Mechanism of Injury Production 298
- Pattern of Road Traffic Injuries 299
- Safety Devices 303

▸ Injuries of Motorcyclists 303
▸ Accident Prevention 304

15. Thermal Injuries **307**
Adarsh Kumar, Putul Mahanta
▸ Brief Review of Burns 307
▸ Classification of Thermal Injuries 307
▸ Injuries due to High Temperature (Heat) 308
▸ Scald 318
▸ Injuries due to Low Temperature (Cold) 319
▸ Electrical Injuries 320
▸ Lightning 323

16. Medicolegal Aspects of Injuries **328**
Anil Garg, Putul Mahanta
▸ Injury 328
▸ Offence 328
▸ Types of Weapon 329
▸ Legal Issues of Injuries 330
▸ Homicide 332
▸ Some Important IPC 334
▸ Manner, Mode and Mechanism of Death 336
▸ Injury Certificate/Report 337

17. Asphyxial Deaths **340**
Sanjoy Das, Putul Mahanta
▸ Definition of Asphyxia 340
▸ Gordon's Classification of Death 340
▸ Classical Signs of Asphyxia 341
▸ Classification of Asphyxia 342
▸ Hanging 343
▸ Strangulation 351
▸ Suffocation 353
▸ Drowning 356

18. Anesthetic Procedures and Death **361**
CB Jani, Putul Mahanta
▸ Brief Review 361
▸ Classification of Anesthetic Deaths 362
▸ Types of Anesthesia used in Surgical Procedure 362
▸ Causes of Death due to General Anesthesia 363

19. Starvation Death **367**
Putul Mahanta, Raktim Pratim Tamuli, Mrinal Haloi
▸ Definition 367
▸ Types of Starvation 367
▸ Clinical Features 368
▸ Causes of Starvation 369

- Postmortem Findings 369
- Medicolegal Importance 370

20. Impotence, Frigidity and Sterility **372**

Putul Mahanta

- Male Impotence 372
- Potency Test 373
- Frigidity 374
- Sterility 374
- Sterilization 375
- Artificial Insemination 376
- Surrogate Mother 376

21. Pregnancy, Delivery, Legitimacy and Paternity **378**

Putul Mahanta

- Pregnancy 378
- Diagnosis of Pregnancy in Living Women 379
- Signs of Pregnancy in the Dead 382
- Gestational Period 383
- Certain Medicolegal Term 383
- Delivery 383
- Signs of Recent Delivery in the Living 384
- Signs of Recent Delivery in the Dead 385
- Signs of Remote Delivery in the Living 385
- Signs of Remote Delivery in the Dead 385
- Legitimacy and Paternity 386

22. Abortion and MTP Act **387**

Putul Mahanta, Vijayanath V

- Definition of Abortion 387
- Incidence 387
- Classification of Abortion 388

23. Infanticide **396**

Putul Mahanta

- Definition 396
- Motive for Infanticide 396
- Medicolegal Queries 397
- Battered Baby Syndrome 404
- Shaken Baby Syndrome 405
- Munchausen's Syndrome 405
- Sudden Infant Death Syndrome 405
- Female Feticide 406

24. Virginity, Sexual Offences and Perversions **409**

Putul Mahanta, Mukesh Yadav, AJ Patowary

- Virginity 409
- Hymen 410

- Sexual Offences 412
- Indecent Assault (Molestation), Sexual Harassment and Punishment 413
- Rape 415
- Incest 432
- Adultery 433
- Unnatural Sexual Offences 433
- Sexual Perversions/Paraphilias 435
- Seminal Fluid 437

25. Forensic Psychiatry **440**

Vijayanath V, Deepanjali Medhi

- Classification of Mental Health Disorders 441
- Disturbances of Perception 442
- Disorders of Thought and Speech 443
- Commonly used Terms in Forensic Psychiatry Practice 444
- Psychiatric Disorders of Medicolegal Importance 445
- Psychosis and Neurosis 449
- Mental Health Act 1987 450
- Judicial Responsibility of Insane Offenders 454
- Criminal Responsibility 454
- Insanity in Indian Perspective 456
- Civil Responsibilities of Insane 459

26. Postmortem Artefacts **462**

Putul Mahanta, Thejaswi HT

- Definition 462
- Types of Artefact 462
- Medicolegal Importance 467

27. Forensic Serology **470**

Akash Deep Aggarwal, Putul Mahanta, Monika Garg

- Blood 470
- Semen 477
- Vaginal Fluids 480
- Saliva 480

28. Crime Scene Investigation **481**

RK Gorea, Abdulwahab Ali Abuderman, Putul Mahanta

- What is Crime Scene? 481
- Examination of the Crime Scene 482
- Must for Crime Scene Investigations 484
- Do Nots of Crime Scene Investigations 485

29. Medicolegal Importance of People Living with HIV/AIDS **487**

Putul Mahanta, KK Bairagi

- History 487
- Brief Review 487
- Modes of Transmission 488

- Rights and Privileges for Patient Living with HIV/AIDS Under Indian Legal System 488
- Some Legislations for Control of HIV 491
- Declaring HIV Status of Positive Individuals in Death Certificate 491
- Offences, Penalties as Laid Under "The Drugs and Cosmetic Act, 1940" 492
- An Approach to Medicolegal Autopsy of HIV Infected Case 492
- Universal Precautions 493

30. Human Rights, Custodial Torture and Deaths **496**

Adarsh Kumar, PC Sarmah, Thejaswi HT

- Some Important Terminologies 497
- Torture 498
- Custodial Death Investigations: NHRC Guidelines 506

31. Techniques in Museum **509**

Akash Deep Aggarwal, Putul Mahanta, Monika Garg

- Functions of a Well-Organized Museum 509
- Basic Museum Techniques 510
- Special Museum Techniques 513
- Virtual Museums 515

32. Forensic Science Laboratory **516**

Yogender Malik, Pooja Malik Puri, Pushpendra Malik

- Forensic Science in India 516
- Forensic Science Laboratory 516
- The Organizational Set up of Forensic Science Laboratory 519
- A Brief Account of Some of the Tools and Techniques used in FSL 519

SECTION 2: TOXICOLOGY

33. General Consideration of Toxicology **527**

AJ Patowary, Putul Mahanta

- What is Toxicology? 527
- Definition of Poison 527
- Nature of Poisoning in India 527
- Action of Poison 528
- Classification of Poisons 530
- Decontamination 531
- Antidote Therapy 537

34. Medicolegal Aspect of Toxicology **544**

Putul Mahanta

- Brief Statistical Review of the Poisoning Cases 544
- Role of a Doctor in Dealing with Poisoning Case 545
- Opinion on Poisoning Cases 547
- Laws Relating to Poison in India 547
- Poisons and Related Indian Penal Codes 550

35. **Corrosive Poisons** 552
Putul Mahanta
- Definition 552
- Inorganic Acids 552
- Acid Throwing 558
- Corrosive Alkalis 559
- Ammonia 560

36. **Inorganic Irritants: Non-metallic Poisons** 562
Putul Mahanta
- Inorganic Irritant Poisons 562
- Iodine 562
- Phosphorus 564

37. **Inorganic Irritants: Metallic Poisons** 567
Putul Mahanta
- Metallic Poison 567
- Arsenic (As) 567
- Lead (Pb) 573
- Mercury (Hg) 577
- Copper (Cu) 581
- Silver (Ag) 583
- Gold (Au) 584
- Thallium (Ti) 584
- Iron (Fe) 586
- Metal Fume Fever 587

38. **Organic Irritants of Plants and Vegetables Origin** 588
Putul Mahanta
- Toxic Principle in Plant 588
- Abrus 589
- Castor 590
- Croton 593
- Capsicum 594
- Calotropis 595
- Marking Nut 596
- Plumbago 597
- Colocynth 598
- Ergot on Rye 600

39. **Organic Irritants of Animal Origin** 602
TK Bose, Shouvanik Adhya, Putul Mahanta
- Organic Irritants of Animal Origin 602
- Snakes 602
- The Big Four (in India) 603
- Relevant Anatomy 604
- Identification of Poisonous and Non-Poisonous Snakes 605

- Snake Bite 608
- Management of Snake Bite 610
- Anti-Snake Venom (ASV) Serum Polyvalent 612
- Other Significant Bites and Stings in Indian Scenario 616
- Cantharides 619

40. Mechanical Irritants **620**

Sunit Kr Joshi, Putul Mahanta

- Mechanical Irritant 620

41. Somniferous Poisons **624**

Putul Mahanta

- What are Alkaloids? 624
- Opium or Afim 624
- Heroin (Diacetylmorphine) 630
- Codeine (3 Methylmorphine) 630
- Thebaine and Papaverine 630

42. Alcohol and Alcoholism **632**

Gunajit Das, Putul Mahanta

- Historical Perspective 632
- Ethyl Alcohol (Ethanol) 633
- Drunkenness 640
- Agencies Working for Curbing Alcoholism 644
- Methyl Alcohol 645

43. Agricultural Poisons **647**

Putul Mahanta, AJ Patowary, Anurupa Choudhury

- Classification 647
- Organophosphates 647
- Organochlorines 651
- Carbamates 653
- Pyrethrum, Pyrethrins and Pyrethroids 654
- Paraquat Poisoning 655
- Hazards of Pesticides 656

44. Cardiac Poisons **658**

Putul Mahanta

- Digitalis (Cardiac Glycoside) 658
- Tobacco 660
- Common Oleander 662
- Yellow Oleander 663
- Aconite 664
- Hydrocyanic Acid 666

45. **Deliriants and Psychotropic Poisons** 670
Putul Mahanta
- Datura (Anticholinergics) 670
- Cannabis 674
- Cocaine 678

46. **Spinal Poisons** 682
Putul Mahanta
- Spinal Poison 682
- Strychnine 682

47. **Peripheral Nerve Poison** 686
Putul Mahanta, KK Bairagi
- Curare 686
- *Conium maculatum* 687

48. **Asphyxiants (Toxic Gases)** 689
YN Singha, Putul Mahanta
- Classification of Asphyxiants or Toxic Gases 689
- Carbon Dioxide (CO_2) 690
- Carbon Monoxide (CO) 691
- Hydrogen Sulfide (H_2S) 693
- Phosphine 693

49. **Paracetamol and Salicylates** 695
YN Singha, Putul Mahanta
- Salicylates 695
- Paracetamol 698

50. **Food Poisoning** 701
Deepjyoti Kalita, Vijayamahantesh SN, Putul Mahanta
- What Is Food Poisoning? 701
- Bacteria 702
- Viral Agents 708
- Protozoal Agents 708
- Fungal (Mushroom Poisoning) 708
- Plants 710
- Chemicals 711
- Poisoning by Fish and Marine Organisms 711

51. **Substance Abuse** 713
Anku Moni Saikia, Putul Mahanta
- Brief Overview of Substance Abuse 713
- Definitions 714
- Some Commonly Abused Substances and Their Effects 715

52. **Weapons of Mass Destruction** 723

Raktim Pratim Tamuli, Putul Mahanta, Yogender Malik

- Weapon of Mass Destruction 723
- Chemical Warfare or Weapon 724
- Biological Weapons (Poor Man's WMD) 726
- Radiological Weapon 729
- Nuclear Weapon 729
- Mass Disaster Management (Focus on Role of Medicolegal Expert) 730

SECTION 3: ANNEXURES

1. **Proforma for Age Certification** 735
2. **Proforma for Injury Certificate** 737
3. **Proforma for Examination of a Sex Crime (Victim)** 739
4. **Proforma for Examination of an Accused of Sexual Offence** 741
5. **Proforma for Examination of a Sodomy Case** 744
6. **Requisition for Radiological Investigation** 747
7. **Letter for Permission for Analysis of Viscera, Blood, etc. at State Forensic Science Laboratory** 748
8. **Viscera Labeling Form** 749
9. **Final Opinion Form after Chemical Analysis of Viscera or Histopathological Examination of Tissue** 750
10. **Dead Body Disposal Certificate after Autopsy** 751
11. **First Information Report** 752
12. **Form for Despatching Viscera/Body Fluids for Chemical Examination** 753
13. **Examination of a Case of Drunkenness** 755
14. **Fetal and Perinatal Autopsy—A Holistic Approach** 757

    Manish Nigam

Index *761*

section 1

FORENSIC MEDICINE

Section Outline

- Introduction and History of Forensic Medicine
- Legal Procedures
- Medical Law and Ethics
- Euthanasia (Mercy Killing)
- Identification
- Forensic Osteology
- Forensic Odontology
- Forensic DNA Typing
- Thanatology
- Autopsy
- Mechanical Injury
- Firearm Injuries
- Regional Injuries
- Road Traffic Injuries
- Thermal Injuries
- Medicolegal Aspects of Injuries
- Asphyxial Deaths
- Anesthetic Procedures and Death
- Starvation Death
- Impotence, Frigidity and Sterility
- Pregnancy, Delivery, Legitimacy and Paternity
- Abortion and MTP Act
- Infanticide
- Virginity, Sexual Offences and Perversions
- Forensic Psychiatry
- Postmortem Artefacts
- Forensic Serology
- Crime Scene Investigation
- Medicolegal Importance of People Living with HIV/AIDS
- Human Rights, Custodial Torture and Deaths
- Techniques in Museum
- Forensic Science Laboratory

CHAPTER 1

Introduction and History of Forensic Medicine

Putul Mahanta

LEARNING PLAN

- Learn what forensic medicine is
- Understand about religious and public attitudes towards autopsy
- Know the phylogenesis of forensic medicine in india
- Future of forensic medicine

WHAT IS FORENSIC MEDICINE?

Forensic or Legal Medicine (Forensic: of or used in Courts of Law) deals with the application of medical knowledge to aid in the administration of justice. Earlier Medical Jurisprudence (**Juris** means law and **Prudentia** means knowledge) was used for this discipline, but now Forensic/ Legal Medicine has become more common usable (except, perhaps in Scotland!).

Forensic Medicine denotes the branch of medicine that deals with the application of the principles and knowledge of medicine for the purpose of law, both civil and criminal.[1]

The purpose of this introduction and history on Forensic Medicine and Toxicology is to introduce the fundamental concepts in these disciplines to police officers, lawyers, medical students, pathologist, residents and physicians. The history of this specialty will give some insight into how they evolved.

This is an attempt to discuss Forensic Medicine and Toxicology solely pertaining to the medicolegal investigation of the cases. The contents are intended to lead the medical students, doctors, lawyers and the police officers through the basic knowledge of the subject and the procedures that are needed in the examination of the dead body found under obscure, suspicious or in criminal circumstances. The concise but informative nature of the book is to provide maximum information in simple language, which can be easily referred to and understood.

The subject matter is chosen to cover all of the basic facts of deaths and related issues commonly witnessed during the medicolegal work. An expert of Forensic Medicine is the one who has amassed his knowledge through experience, common sense and scientific interpretation. The secrets of disease or crime are always hidden in the silent soul: "**The Dead Body**".

AUTOPSY

Antiststius, the physician, examined the body of Julius Caesar (**100–44 BC**) and opined that out of 23 injuries; only one injury in the chest was fatal. In **1374 AD,** right of holding medicolegal autopsy was given by Pope. But perhaps, the first **systemic autopsy** was held by **Dr Ambroise Pare** on the body of **King Henry II** in **1589**.

Religious and Social Attitudes of Autopsy[6]

At that time of Tertullian and Augustine, there were strong religious and social objections to the autopsy. Although in the early years of Christianity, there was no formal church prohibition, the general attitude of church leaders was still unfavorable. Both **Tertullian** (160–230) and **Augustine** (354–430) wrote strongly against dissection, apparently more on humanitarian and aesthetic grounds than on any theological basis. **Vindician**, a physician and friend of **Augustine**, is quoted in a 10th century manuscript from **Monte Cassino** as saying, "It pleased the ancient anatomists to examine the viscera of the dead to learn in what way they died, but for us humanities prohibits this".[2] **Wolf-Heidegger** and **Cetto Singer** have concluded that dissections were being done in Italy between 1266 and 1275, and that the earliest dissections were medicolegal in nature.

There were no official church decrees on the subject, but at the **Council of Tours** in **1163,** it was affirmed that "**the church abhors blood**". This was interpreted to mean that the clergy could not perform surgery on the living or the dead. Since most physicians did belong to the clergy, this effectively prevented autopsies, but did not absolutely forbid them. In **1299, Boniface VIII** forbade the cooking of bodies to separate the flesh from the bones. This had been done to bring home the bones of people who died on crusades. Although the ruling specifically referred to cooking the body, many people interpreted it to forbid any dissection.[3]

Nevertheless, it was about this time that a few physicians began to dissect and eventually the church's attitude was modified. In **1410**, **Pope Alexander** died suddenly and was autopsied by **Pietro D'Argelata. Pope Sixtus** IV (**1471–1484**) issued a bill permitting studies on human bodies by students at Bologna and Padua, and **Clement** VII (**1523–1534**) confirmed this. In **1556, Ignatius Loyola** was autopsied and stones were found in the kidneys, bladder and gallbladder.[4]

It, therefore, appears by that time autopsy was fully accepted by the Catholic Church. In fact, one autopsy had been performed in **1533** specifically for a religious reason. According to the *New World History,* compiled by **Oviedo Y Valdes**, in **1533** in **Espafiola** (now the Dominican Republic), a double monster, female twins joined from the region of the umbilicus to a point in the thorax just below the breast, were born. The infants were to be baptized, but the priest was uncertain as to whether one soul or two souls required baptism. The father reported that one would cry while the other was quiet, one might sleep while the other was awake. And so, two baptisms were performed, but the priest was still uneasy. When the infants died at the age of 8 days, an autopsy was done to settle the question. Since two complete sets of internal organs were found, it was decided that there probably were two souls. **Chavarria** and **Shipley**, who located and translated this fascinating story, commented that this was perhaps the only postmortem examination ever conducted to study the soul of the deceased.[5]

Respect for the body was an important part of the Jewish tradition, as the *Bible* taught that God created man in his image. Handling a dead body made a man unclean for several days. It was emphasized that the body must be treated respectfully and buried promptly. Even for a criminal hanged till death on a tree, "his body shall not remain all night upon the tree, but thou shall in any wise bury him that day". These laws were interpreted by the rabbis to forbid postmortem dissection, which would be a disgrace to the body. However, it is recorded that about 100 AD, the students of the Rabbi Ismael obtained the body of a young harlot who had been executed and boiled it in order to count the number of bones. They found 252.[6]

There is one passage in the *Talmud* stating that if an autopsy would save the life of an accused murderer, it would be permitted. Autopsies were otherwise not approved by Jewish authority until the **18th century,** when Rabbi Landau was asked if it were permissible to make an incision in the body of a patient who died of cancer, in order to learn the proper therapy in future cases. He replied that autopsy is a desecration of the dead and is only permissible to save the life of another patient immediately at hand, not some problematic future patient.[7] This ruling was apparently maintained by orthodox Jews until the 20th century, when the Knesset, the Israeli parliament, passed a law permitting autopsies under strictly limited conditions.[8]

Some indications of the popular objections to autopsies may be noted here. In **1538**, **Guillaume Rondelet (1507-1566)**, a scientist in Montpellier, autopsied his own infant son and later requested that autopsies be performed on his sister-in-law and his first wife. This is included in a biography, dated **1578**, by his pupil Joubert, who comments, "a cette Epoque le public avait 1'anatomie en horreur".[9]

Vesalius, who practiced medicine and performed many autopsies, died in 1564 during the return from a pilgrimage to Jerusalem. Many years later, a biographer, **Melchior Adam**, published a letter allegedly written by Hubert Languet in 1565, stating that Vesalius had been forced to make this pilgrimage as expiation for the sins of murder and impiety. O'Malley is convinced that there is no foundation of fact for this story.[10] However, he points out that it may be based on the same rumor referred to by **Ambroise Pare**, who, writing in **1573**, warned against opening a body too soon and noted that "in this century, it happened that a great anatomist ... I say great and famous ... then a resident in Spain was ordered to open the body of a woman believed to be dead of suffocation of the womb. At the second cut of the razor the woman began to move and show other signs that she still lived ... the good master had to leave the country and being exiled, soon after died of grief, which was certainly a great loss for the Republic".[11]

Jarcho has called attention to the problems of performing autopsies in Germany in **1670.** In a medical periodical of that year, there is an autopsy report with a comment, "the other structures could not be examined because a female relative changed her mind. Our people have a great horror of autopsies and very rarely allow them unless special persuasion has been used." The editor of the journal added a discussion of the difficulties of obtaining permission and some possible answers to the objections of relatives.[12]

Popular reluctance for autopsies at a slightly later period is also evident by the fact that, the **1699** ruling of the Republic of Lucca designed to limit the spread of consumption, which included the recommendation of autopsies, had to be revoked because of the citizens' objections.[13] Even today, these attitudes are encountered and further consideration would carry us too far afield.

PHYLOGENESIS OF FORENSIC MEDICINE IN INDIA

Many a genius from the pages of ancient Indian history had influenced the Rule of Law. Their word remained an integral part of the Government's functioning.

One such person was Kautilya, who wrote the ***Arthashastra***—the most comprehensive treatise of statecraft of classical times. The book covered numerous topics, e.g. the king, code of law, foreign policy, secret and occult practices and so on. Even after a lapse of more than 2000 years, the master strategist, widely known as India's Machiavelli, continues to rake up the minds of the country's modern day spiritual gurus.[14]

The **first** recorded medicolegal autopsy was performed in India by **Dr Edward Bulkley** on the afternoon of 28 August **1693**, when **Mr Wheeler**, a member of council, See a Customer and Chief Justice of Choultry in Chennai, died on 28 August, 1693.

India's **first medical school** was established in Kolkata in **1822** and was converted into a

Medical College in **1835.** In the same year, Madras Medical College was also established. In **1857**, the **first chair of professor** of medical jurisprudence was established at Madras Medical College.

The most prominent contribution of India to legal medicine during British period is modern dactylography. It was **Sir William Herschel** of the **Indian Civil Services**, who first used this method of identification in **1858.** Based on Herschel's theory, **Sir Francis Galton** of England devised the systemic study and methods of using fingerprints for personal identification in **1892.**[1]

The British government altered method from time to time till **1862**, when the **Indian Penal Code** came into existence. In fact, the foundation of our criminal laws is still Mohammedan law, but it is so altered and added to by our regulations that it ceases reflect its originality.[15]

The **police system** of crime investigation was introduced in India in **1861** and the **coroners systems** in **1871** in the presidency towns of Bombay and Calcutta.[1] The Indian Medical Council established in **1933**.

The subject of Forensic Medicine has grown from the days when it was taught as part of pathology, to being a complete specialty in itself. However, Forensic Medicine has to advance many miles to keep pace with new developments, and we need the committed efforts of all doctors in this profession to meet the expectations of society.

Presently, the teaching of Forensic Medicine has improved with the establishment and expansion of the academic departments of Forensic Medicine and Toxicology in most of the medical colleges. Postgraduate courses in Forensic Medicine and Toxicology are available in most of the universities. It is hoped that trained medicolegists will be available in India in sufficient large numbers in the districts, around the country very soon.

FUTURE OF FORENSIC MEDICINE

As history has shown, Forensic Medicine and Toxicology have made substantial contributions to society across the centuries. We have been, and will continue to be, servants to the continued development of the discipline in our pursuance to give society the very best that they have to offer. We must continue to strive for the highest standards in the practice of Forensic Medicine and Toxicology and in the application of their various subspecialties in the search for the cause and manner of death. The same principle must be applied to our participation in the Clinical Forensic Medicine. It is only through striving to attain these goals that we can best serve society.

Some Forensic Medicine and Toxicology experts argue that more autopsies are performed than necessary. However, recent studies show that autopsies can detect a person's condition that were not suspected when the person was alive, and the growing awareness of the influence of genetic factors in disease has also emphasized its importance. It is important to note that autopsies can also provide peace of mind for the bereaved family in certain cases. Therefore, an autopsy should be encouraged regardless of caste, community and religion upon all unnatural deaths. The key lies in a renewed understanding of Forensic Pathologists, clinicians and hospital administrators about the role of autopsy in health care. The autopsy room should not be seen as the place where sorrow and the specter of death come alive; rather it should be where death rejoices to aid the living.[16]

REFERENCES

1. Mathiharan K, Patnaik AK. History of forensic medicine. In: Patnaik AK, Bhanot A, Mathiharan K, Bopanna N (Eds), Modi's Medical Jurisprudence and Toxicology, 23rd ed. New Delhi: LexisNexis Butterworths India; 2005. p. 3-18.
2. Wolfe-Heidegger, Cetto p. 36

3. Proskauer C. The significance to medical history of the newly discovered fourth century Roman fresco. Bull NY Acad Med. 1938;34:672-88.
4. Ullman W.H. Obduziert wurde Ignatius von Loyola. Med Welt. 1963;35:1758-63.
5. Chavarrla AP, Shipley PG. The Siamese twins of Espafiola. Ann Med Hist. 1924;6:297-302.
6. Gordon BL. Medicine among the ancient Hebrews. Ann Med Hist (Series 3). 1942;4:219-325.
7. Rosner F. Studies in Torah Judaism, Modern Medicine and Jewish Law. New York, Department of Special Publications of Yeshiva University;1972. p. 136.
8. Kottler A. The Jewish attitude on autopsy. NY State J Med.1957;57:1649-50.
9. Pags A. Petite histoire de l'autopsie anatomo-pathoiogique. Monspeliensis Hippocrates. 1960;3(10):16-24.
10. Mahanta Putul. The medico-legal autopsy—Its religious and social attitudes. Journal of Indian Academy of Forensic Medicine. 2010;32(2):183-8.
11. Pare A. Oeuvres completes, Vol 2. Edited by JS Malgaigne, Paris, Ailliere;1840. p. 755.
12. Jarcho S. Problems of the autopsy in 1670. Bull NY Acad Med. 1971;47:792-6.
13. Castiglioni A. A History of Medicine, 2nd ed. Translated and edited by EB Krumbhaar. New York, Alfred A. Knopf, Inc;1947. p. 56.
14. Kautilya's Arthashastra comes alive for world corporate giants. [cited 2007 Jan 17]; 1(1): (2 screens). Available from: URL:http//www.c2b2bnews.com/kautilya.asp
15. Tandon MP, Tandon R. The Indian Penal Code. General Principles of Criminal Law. Allahabad: Allahabad Law Agency; 1989. p. 1-2.
16. Mahanta P. The medico-legal autopsy its religious and social attitudes. J Indian Acad Forensic Med. 2010;32(2):183-7.

CHAPTER 2

Legal Procedures

NK Aggarwal, HK Mahanta, Putul Mahanta

LEARNING PLAN

- Know the basics of legal procedures of India
- Learn about inquests, courts, summons and medical evidences
- Understand types of witness
- Know the procedures of recording of evidence

LEGAL PROCEDURES

The Indian Legal System was founded by the Colonial British by establishing various courts and enacting statutes for the administration of Justice similar to the British Legal System, which was adopted after independence by making some amendments and modification of the statutes. The administration of justice in criminal matters are mainly governed by the Indian Penal Code (IPC) 1860, Criminal Procedure Code (CrPC) 1861 and Indian Evidence Act (IEA) 1869, with amendments done on later dates.

Medical officers, in the course of their professional practice, are required to issue medical certificates to their patients for various acts and administrative purpose. They also need to examine the victims and accuse persons involved in various criminal offences and to submit reports, for which the medical officer may be summoned to appear in the court to give evidence in relation to the reports submitted by them. Therefore, they must have clear knowledge about the courts of law, and legal and criminal procedures.

Indian Penal Code 1860: It defines various offences and their punishments admissible under court of law. Jammu and Kashmir have their own panel code, known as Ranbir Panel Code.

Criminal Procedure Code 1973: It defines the procedure of investigations and trial of offences in whole of India, except the state of Jammu and Kashmir. It also deals with various types of courts and their powers.

Indian Evidence Act 1872: It relates to evidences, based on which courts come to the conclusion of the case.

INQUEST

Definition

An inquest is an enquiry into the cause of death in cases of sudden, suspicious and unnatural deaths.

It is required in cases of:

i. Sudden death in an apparently normal individual.
ii. All suspected cases of homicides, suicides and accidents, irrespective of the nature of causation.
iii. Vehicular accidents.
iv. Poisonings.
v. Deaths under anesthesia, over operation table or alleged cases of medical negligence.
vi. Dowry related deaths.
vii. Deaths under police custody or police firing.
viii. In all cases where a doctor is not in a position to issue the medical certificate into cause of death (MCCD), viz. in mass disasters, etc.

In these conditions, a doctor must not issue the cause of death certificate and police must be informed regarding the case.

Types of Inquest

Two types of inquest are followed in India now days:

a. Police inquest
b. Magistrate inquest

Police Inquest

It is practiced all over India. It is conducted by an officer-in-charge (OC) of a police station or some other police officer especially empowered by the State Government (Section 174 CrPC). The police officer who investigates the case is known as the investigating officer (IO). When the OC of a police station receives information regarding any accidental, homicidal, suicidal or any unnatural death of a person or when a dead body is found in a suspicious condition within his jurisdiction, he himself or any subordinate officer deputed by him for this purpose immediately send information to the nearest Executive Magistrate authorized to hold inquest regarding the incident. He then proceeds to the place where the dead body is lying. There, the police officer holds the inquest in the presence of two or more persons of the locality as witness (Panchas). The police officers observes the body and its surroundings and writes down about the position of the dead body, garments, presence of any stains or injury on the body, presence of any weapon or suspicious article by the side of the body. He then makes an inquiry with the people of the locality and forms an opinion regarding the cause of death of the person. The inquest report is then signed by the police officer and also by the witnesses present.

After inquiry, if no foul play is suspected and death appears to be due to natural causes, the police officer may allow the dead body to be disposed by the guardian or relative of the deceased person. But, if there is least suspicion of foul play or doubt regarding the death or if death appears to be unnatural one, then the dead body is sent to the nearest authorized government medical officer with a requisition (forwarding letter), dead body challan and copies of the inquest report for postmortem examination.

The police officer by writing may order any person, who appears to know about the facts, to answer questions for investigation purpose (Section 175 CrPC). The person so ordered is bound to appear before the police officer and answer the questions put to him, otherwise he will be liable under Section 179 IPC for not answering the questions.

The police officer may also request the medical officer conducting the postmortem examination to preserve garments, articles or visceras of the dead body for chemical tests or may request to perform such tests as may be essential for investigation of the case.

Magistrate Inquest

In some conditions, the police are not authorized to hold inquest. It is then conducted by an

Table 2.1 Differences between magistrate and police inquest

Features	Magistrate inquest	Police inquest
Investigating officer	District magistrate or SDM	Police officer
Informing magistrate	Need not inform	Need to inform
Type of cases	Can hold inquest in all cases, but usually conducts inquests in specified cases under Section 176 CrPC	All unnatural and suspicious deaths, except specified cases under Section 176 CrPC
Warrant	Can issue	Cannot issue
Exhumation	Can order	Cannot order
Value of inquest	More	Less

executive magistrate or any other magistrate specifically authorized by State Government for this purpose (Section 176 CrPC). A Magistrate's inquest is essential in the following conditions:

i. All dowry-related deaths under section 304 B of the IPC.
ii. Deaths under police custody.
iii. Death of a convict or under trial prisoner in jail.
iv. Deaths due to police firing.
v. Death in borstal school or reformatories.
vi. Death in a psychiatric hospital.
vii. Exhumation.
viii. Any other cases where government orders for the inquest to be conducted by magistrate.

In some cases of a great public interest, a magistrate can hold inquest instead of or in addition to a police inquest.

The Magistrate's inquest is superior to a police inquest as the magistrate himself hold and conduct the enquiry, records evidence like an investigating officer and can summon any person to furnish information to him. After the inquest, the magistrate sends the body to the authorized medical officer for postmortem examination.

The differences between the Magistrate inquest and police inquest are listed in **Table 2.1.**

Coroner's Inquest

This system of inquest was previously practiced only in the cities of Kolkata and Mumbai. But it is now abolished in India. It is still practiced in England and some European countries.

Coroner used to be a person with legal qualification of the rank of First-Class Magistrate, and he used to conduct inquest in all cases of unnatural and suspicious deaths.

Medical Examiner's System

This system is practiced in some states of the US. In this system, doctors having qualification in Pathology and Forensic Medicine are appointed as medical examiners. The medical examiners visit the scene of crime, prepare the inquest report and also conduct the postmortem examination. As the inquest reports and postmortem examination reports are prepared by the same medical examiner, it is far superior to the other systems of inquest, but the medical examiner does not have any judicial powers. This type of inquest is not held in India.

COURTS

Courts of Law and their Powers

The courts are mainly of two types:

i. Civil
ii. Criminal

Civil Courts

Civil courts deal with the civil matters—mainly disputes between two or more parties under provisions of the Civil Procedure Code and Indian Evidence Act relating to land and property, administrative, industrial, labor, financial and family matters. Civil courts do not award punishments, but decide the cases in favor of one or more parties on the basis of facts produced before it or award monetary compensation to an aggrieved party. Motor accident claims tribunals, consumer protection forum, administrative tribunal, industrial tribunals, labor and family courts are civil courts function under the specific Acts for limited purposes.

Criminal Courts

Criminal courts try the various criminal offences codified in the Indian Penal Code and award punishment or acquit the accused person after detailed trial proceedings. The procedure of trial, recording evidence and awarding punishments are guided by the provisions of Indian Evidence Act, Code of Criminal Procedure and Indian Penal Code.

The criminal courts are of four types:

i. Supreme Court
ii. High Court
iii. Sessions Court
iv. Magistrate's Court.

The Supreme Court and High Court are only appellate court in relation to criminal matters. They do not hold trial prima facie.

Supreme Court

It is the highest Judicial Tribunal in the country and situated at the national capital New Delhi. The judgments and decisions declare by it are binding on all courts in India. It has original, appellate, advisory and concurrent jurisdiction and decides only the cases appealed before it against the judgment of a High Court. After hearing the appellant and the opposite sides, it can enhance or reduce the quantum of punishments awarded by the lower courts or acquit the convict of charges made against him.

High Court

High Courts are the highest Judicial Tribunal in a state and situated mostly in the state capitals. Every state has a High Court. All these states are having the separate bench for their respective capitals. Exceptions are Allahabad High court, Jabalpur High Court, Cuttack High Court, etc. Guwahati High Court, which has jurisdiction over the states of Assam, Arunachal Pradesh, Nagaland and Mizoram. All High Courts have original and appellate jurisdiction. In criminal matters, they have only appellate jurisdiction and decides criminal cases on an appeal against the judgment passed by the Sessions Court. A death sentence awarded by a court of Sessions Judge has to be confirmed by a division bench of the High Court. High Courts have the power to award any sentence authorized by law and can upheld, enhance or reduce the quantum of punishment awarded by a court of Sessions Judge on an appeal or acquit the convict. If not satisfied, the convict can appeal before the Supreme Court against the judgment of the High Court.

Sessions Court

Each district has a Sessions Court and is situated at the district headquarters. A Sessions Court has two types of Judges: (1) Sessions Judge and (2) Additional Sessions Judge.

A Sessions Court is headed by a Sessions Judge, who supervises the functions of the different Judicial Courts in the district. He allocates cases to other Judges, which are committed to the Sessions Court for trial by the Magistrates.

A Sessions Judge and Additional Sessions Judge have equal judicial powers. They can pass any sentence authorized by law, including a death sentence. However, the death sentence passed by a Sessions Court must be confirmed by the High Court.

An Assistant Sessions Judge can pass any sentence authorized by law, except death sentence, life imprisonment or imprisonment exceeding 10 years. He can pass unlimited amount of fine.

It is to be noted that the Judges of the Sessions Court also hear and decide Civil Cases. When they decide the Civil Cases, the Court is known as District Court and Judges are then known as District Judge, Additional District Judge and Assistant District Judge, accordingly. That is why the court is commonly known as District and Sessions Court and Judges as District and Sessions Judge.

Magistrate's Court or Court of Magistrates

Judicial magistrates are of three types:

i. Chief Judicial Magistrate
ii. First Class Judicial Magistrate
iii. Second Class Judicial Magistrate.

Chief Judicial Magistrate: In each district, there is a Chief Judicial Magistrate who is, in general, control of all other Judicial Magistrates in the district. The Chief Judicial Magistrate commutes all Sessions triable cases to the Sessions Court for trial. A Chief Judicial Magistrate can pass a sentence of imprisonment up to 7 years and unlimited amount of fine.

First Class Judicial Magistrate or Metropolitan Magistrate can pass sentence of imprisonment up to 3 years and fine up to ₹ 10,000/- or both.

Second Class Judicial Magistrate can pass a sentence of imprisonment not exceeding 1 year and fine up to ₹ 5000/- or both.

All the Judicial Magistrates can pass both the sentences (imprisonment and fine) together.

In cases where Magistrates try cases for two or more offences in one trial, they are permitted to award twice the amount of imprisonment they are authorized normally.

In the Metropolitan Cities (cities having more than one million population), the Judicial Magistrates are known as Chief Metropolitan Magistrate, First Class Metropolitan Magistrate and Second Class Metropolitan Magistrate. First Class Judicial Magistrate posted in charge of a sub-division is known as Sub-divisional Judicial Magistrate.

Executive Magistrates (District Magistrate or Deputy Commissioner, Additional District Magistrates, Revenue Officers) are part of the State Civil Administration of the district and concerned mainly with the maintenance of law and order, like imposition of Section 144 IPC, ordering exhumation and holding inquest in some cases and other civilian matters.

In some states, Executive Magistrates are conferred with some judicial power to try some minor offences.

Juvenile Magistrates are those who preside over the Juvenile Courts meant for juvenile offenders below the age of 18 years. They are usually women of the rank of First-Class Magistrates.

PUNISHMENT (LEGAL SENTENCES) AUTHORIZED BY LAW IN INDIA

The following sentences are authorized under section 53 of Indian Penal Code to be passed by Courts in India.

i. **Death Sentence**

   It is also known as capital punishment passed by the court of Sessions Judge, which is to be confirmed by the High Court. It is awarded in cases of serious crimes like: murder, rape with murder, murder committed by a life convict, dacoity with murder, waging war against the Government of India and repeated offences under the Narcotic Drugs and Psychotropic Substances (NDPS) Act.

   Execution of capital punishment: In India, death sentence is carried out by hanging, commonly known as Judicial hanging. Other methods used to execute a convict in some other countries are: Electrocution, firing by firing squad, gas chamber, guillotine, injection of lethal dose of some sedative drugs and poisons.

ii. **Life Imprisonment**

   It is also awarded by the court of Sessions Judge. Usually, it comprises imprisonment for 20 years, which can be reduced to

14 years for good behavior by the prisoner. At present, the life imprisonment is for the rest of life of the convict.

iii. **Imprisonments:** It is of two types:
   a. **Simple Imprisonment** means imprisonment without hard labor.
   b. **Rigorous Imprisonment**: It is imprisonment with hard labor. The prisoner is to work in the prison according to his skill and physical ability.

   Solitary Imprisonment (Solitary Confinement): A prisoner may be ordered to pass a part of his period of rigorous imprisonment in solitary confinement (not more than 3 months).

iv. **Fine:** Courts can impose monetary fine only or in addition to imprisonment in some cases.

v. **Forfeiture of Property** (attachment of property): Court can order attachment of both the movable and immovable property of a person.

vi. **Detention in Reformatories**: Courts may order detention of a juvenile offender found guilty of a crime in a borstal school or reformatories till completion of 18 years of age.

MEDICAL EVIDENCE

Evidence

It is the deposition of a witness in the court of law, under oath, relating to a particular fact in issue, recorded and accepted by the court. Under Section 3 of Indian Evidence Act (IEA), evidence is defined as what a court of justice is permitted by law to take into consideration for making clear or ascertaining the truth of the fact or point in issue. Thus, evidence means and includes:

1. All statements, which the court permits or requires to be made before it by witness, in relation to matters of fact under inquiry. Such statements are called oral evidence.
2. All documents including electronic records produced for the inspection of the court. Such documents are called documentary evidence.

Types

Medical evidences are of two types:

Oral Evidence

All statements, which the court permits or requires to be made before it by witnesses in relation to the fact under enquiry.

Direct Evidence: It is the evidence given by witness from his personal knowledge, who had seen, heard or perceived directly the fact in issue. Evidence given by an eyewitness is direct evidence.

Indirect or **Circumstantial Evidence:** It is an act whereby the direct evidence of the fact in issue in relation to the circumstances and the surroundings of an event, from which interference may be drawn regarding occurrence of the principal fact under inquiry.

For example, dead body of A with multiple gunshot wounds was found in his house. C saw B, come out of the house with a gun. Circumstantial evidence requires some logical inference to the fact in issue.

Hearsay Evidence: It is the evidence given by person who had no direct knowledge regarding the incident (fact in issue), but came to know about it from somebody who had seen, heard or perceived the matter directly.

Documentary Evidence

All documents are produced for the inspection of the court.

Documents mean any matter expressed or described upon any substance by means of letters, figures or marks, which may be used for the purpose of recording that matter (Section 29 IPC). Documents may be proved either by primary evidence or by secondary evidence (Section 61 IEA).

Primary Evidence: When the original document is produced in the court for inspection (Section 62 IEA).

Secondary Evidence: When the certified copies, duplicate copies or copies made from the original by mechanical process or copies made from the original are produced in the court (Section 63 IEA). Again evidence can be direct or indirect.

Documentary Evidence in Relation to Medical Practice

A medical officer or a medical practitioner requires to issue some written documents (certificates, reports, etc.) to his patients or to the authorities relating to the health or medical aspects of the person. There are three types of documentary evidence:

i. Medical certificates
ii. Medicolegal report
iii. Dying declaration.

Medical Certificates

A medical certificate is a document of written evidence vouching for the truth of a fact as determined by a doctor issuing such a document. Common medical certificates are:

i. Sickness (ill health) and physical fitness certificates
ii. Birth and death certificates
iii. Age certificates
iv. Insanity certificate
v. Vaccination (Immunization) certificate
vi. Disability certificate
vii. Life certificate
viii. Certificate for procuring driving license and passport.

The Indian Medical Council (Professional Conduct, Etiquette and Ethics) Regulation, 2002, in Appendix 4 gives a list of 17 types of medical certificates, reports, modifications, which can be issued by a doctor for various administrative and other purposes.

The doctor should be very careful in writing these certificates, as on occasions, court may summon him to appear before it to prove the authenticity of the certificate.

Preferably, the certificates should be written in duplicate, giving one copy to the person and retaining the other for the doctor's own record. While issuing a sickness or ill-health certificate, doctor should state the exact nature of the illness and the expected period of rest or absence from duty necessary for recovery from the illness. In addition to the name, age, address of the person, it is necessary to take the signature or thumb impression of the individual at the bottom of the certificate or mention two identification marks.

In Birth Certificate

Particulars of mother, baby and the place, time and date of delivery should be given in detail.

Death Certificate

When a person dies, the doctor who had attended him in his last illness or within the fortnight, it is legally bound to issue a cause of death certificate stating the exact cause of death without charging any fee, even if he had treated the patient free of cost (Registration of Birth or Death Act 1970). It should be given to the next of kin of deceased person. The doctors must inspect the dead body to be sure that the person is dead. He should also be sure about the cause of death, and nature of death before issuing the certificate.

Death certificate should never be issued by a doctor:

i. If he is not sure of the cause of death.
ii. If he was not in attendance of the patient during his last illness or within the fortnight before his death.
iii. If he suspects any foul play.
iv. If death was due to any unnatural cause like: suicide, homicide, accident burn, drowning, poisoning, etc.

In all these cases, death certificate must not be issued, the dead body must not be handed over to the guardian or relatives for disposal, and nearest police or magistrate must be informed, who then will hold the inquest over the dead body.

Dying Declaration

It is a statement, verbal or written, made by a person who is dying as a result of some unlawful act, relating to the cause of his death or any of the circumstances of transaction that resulted in his death.

It should be recorded by a Magistrate in presence of a doctor and two witnesses. A doctor attending such a person, who is likely to die from the effect of criminal violence or act such as injury, burn or poisoning, should immediately call the nearest Magistrate to record the statement of the person. But, if the doctor feels that the condition of the person is very serious and the patient may die before arrival of the Magistrate, then the doctor should record the dying declaration in presence of two respectable witnesses. Before recording the statement, the doctor should certify that the declarant is in a sound state of mind (compos mentis) and is in a fit condition to make the statement.

Administration of oath is not necessary, as the law presumes that a dying person never tells lie (always speaks truth). The sense of impending death creates such a sanction equal to the obligation of an oath. If the person is capable to write, then it should be written by him. After recording the statement, the declarant should sign it and the doctor and the two witnesses should put their signature on it. If the declarant is unable to write, the Magistrate or the doctor should record it. The statement should be recorded in detail in the language of the person, without any correction or editing in the actual words stated by him. The declarant should be allowed to speak freely. No external prompting, insistence or undue influence should be allowed to bring to bear on the mind of the declarant. If any point needs clarification, doctor should ask him, and it should be recorded in the form of question and answer. When the recording of the declaration is complete it should be read over to the declarant who then should put his or her signature or thumb impression on it. It is then signed by the doctor recording it and also to be signed by the two witnesses present.

If the declarant becomes unconscious or dies while recording the statement, the doctor should record it and he should record as much information as he obtained. Then it should be signed by the doctor and the two witnesses.

If the declarant is unable to speak, but can only make signs in answer to questions put to him, than the questions and signs put together may properly be regarded as verbal statement made by the person.

After recording the statement, it is then sent to the Magistrate concerned, in a sealed envelope.

The dying declaration is admitted in the court as evidence after death of the person who makes it. The court gives a great importance to the dying declaration as in many cases the declarant was the only eyewitness to the whole criminal act. If the person survives, his statement is not accepted in evidence as dying declaration. It is regarded as corroborative evidence only. The person is called to appear in the court and dispose his evidence under oath.

Dying declaration is admissible in a court as evidence irrespective of (whether) the person who made it was or was not under expectation of death at the time of recording it, but it is essential that the declarant is in a sound state of mind at the time of making the statement. Therefore, the doctor should certify it before recording the statement, otherwise the declaration is not considered as evidence.

Usually, to be legal evidence, a dying declaration does not require any corroboration. But, if the circumstances surrounding the dying declaration are not clear or convincing, the court may look for corroboration or other evidences to corroborate it for its assurance.

Dying Deposition

It is a statement made by a dying person under oath and recorded by a Magistrate in presence of the accused or his lawyer, who is allowed to cross examine the person. As oath is administered, it is like a bed side court. Its practice is now abolished in India. However, the differences between dying declaration and dying deposition are narrated in **Table 2.2**.

Oral evidence is more important than documentary evidence, as it is subjected to cross examination by the opposite party. Generally, all the documentary evidences are accepted in the court of law only after oral verification and cross-examination of the person who issued the documents. There are exceptions to this general rule.

Table 2.2 Differences between dying declaration and dying deposition

Features	Dying declaration	Dying deposition
Recording of the statement	Anybody can record the statement, need not be a magistrate	Only magistrate can record
Oath	Not necessary	Must
Presence of accused or his lawyer	Not present	Always present
Cross examination	No	Yes
Legal value	Less	More

The following documents are accepted in evidence without oral testimony. They are:

i. **Dying Declaration** as the person who made the statement is dead and cannot be called to give evidence in the court (Section 32, 157 IEA).
ii. **Expert Opinion Expressed in the Treaties** (accepted textbooks) is generally accepted as evidence on production of such treaties without oral verification of the author (Section 60 IEA).
iii. **Deposition of a Medical Witness Recorded** in a lower court is accepted as evidence in a higher court, when it has been recorded and attested by a Magistrate in presence of the accused or his lawyer.
iv. **Evidence given by a Witness** in a previous judicial proceeding is accepted as evidence in a subsequent judicial proceeding when the witness is dead or untraceable, or is incapable of giving evidence (Section 33 IEA).
v. **Evidence of Mint Officers or Officer of Indian Security Press** (Section 292 CrPC).
vi. **Reports of Certain Government Scientific Experts** (Section 293 CrPC):
   a. Report of Chemical Examiner or Assistant Chemical Examiner.
   b. Report of Chief Inspector of Explosive.
   c. Report of Director, Finger Print Bureau.
   d. Report of Director, Haffkine Laboratories, Mumbai.
   e. Report of Director, Central or State Forensic Science Laboratory.
vii. **Public Records**: Birth and death certificates, marriage certificate, etc. issued by proper authority.
viii. **Hospital Records**: Routine entries like date of admission and discharge, bed head records showing blood pressure, pulse, respiration, temperature, treatment received are accepted without oral evidence. But the cause of death, nature of injuries and investigations are not accepted without oral evidence.

WITNESS

A witness is a person who gives evidence in the court of law under oath. All persons are competent to give evidence unless they are incapable of understanding the questions put to them or giving rational answer to these questions, due to tender years, extreme old age or disease.

Types of Witness

Witnesses are of two types:

Common or Ordinary Witness

Common witness or ordinary witness is one who gives evidence about a fact, which he actually saw, heard or perceived in any other manner. He is not able to draw any inference from observations made by him or express any option from observations made by other.

Expert or Skilled Witness

An expert witness is one who has acquired special knowledge, skill or experience in any science, art, trade or profession (Section 145 IEA). Such knowledge may have been acquired by practice, observation or careful studies. An expert witness is capable of drawing an inference from observations made by him or others. He may also express an opinion on hypothetical questions. Doctor, fingerprints expert, handwriting expert, ballistic expert are some examples.

Opinion of an expert is of advisors in nature and is not binding on the court in deciding a case. Court cannot pass judgment only on the basis of expert evidence deposed in the court. It is usually regarded a corroborative evidence to support the evidence of an eyewitness.

An expert witness can volunteer a statement if he feels that court has failed to understand an important issue, which may lead to miscarriage of justice.

To be an expert medical witness, a person having recognized medical degree must be registered with any of the state medical council. The Indian Medical Council Act, 1956, in Section 15(2)(b), states that no person other than a medical practitioner enrolled on a state medical register shall be entitled to give evidence at any inquest or in any court of law as an expert under Section 45 of the Indian Evidence Act 1872 on any matter relating to medicine.

A medical practitioner may act as both common and expert witness. When he describes the injuries seen on a body during medicolegal examination, he is acting as a common witness. But when he draw a conclusions or expresses an opinion stating the injury ante- or postmortem or homicidal, suicidal or accidental, he is acting as expert witness.

Hostile Witness

Hostile witness is a witness who deliberately gives false evidence in the court of law either by concealing a part or whole of the truth or making totally false statement, which he knows to be false or not true and thereby contradicts his previous statements made before the same court or in a previous judicial proceeding (Section 191 IPC). Court may declare a witness hostile when suggested by the lawyer of the party who summoned the witness. Leading questions can be asked to a hostile witness during examination in chief.

OFFENCE

Offence is an act of commission or omission made punishable by any law (Section 40 IPC and Section 2(n) CrPC).

Types of Offence

Offences are of two types:

i. **Cognizable Offence** is an offence in which a police officer can arrest a person without a warrant from a Magistrate. These are serious offence like murder, rape and dowry death, punishable with death, life imprisonment or imprisonment exceeding 2 years.
ii. **Non-cognizable Offence** is one in which a police officer cannot arrest a person without a warrant. These are less serious offences, which are punishable with fine or with imprisonment less than 2 years.

Procedure of Attendance in the Court

Medical officer or any person, whose evidence is essential in relation to a case in a court of law, is summoned to attend the court to give evidence at the time of trial.

Summons or Subpoena (Sub—Under, Poena—Penalty)

It is a written order issued by a court to a witness compelling his attendance in the court on a specific date, time and place to give evidence under penalty (Section 61 to 69 of CrPC).

It is issued in duplicate, signed by the presiding officer of the court. It also bears the seal of the court. The name of the accused person and the case number and the sections of IPC under which the person is to be prosecuted are also mentioned.

Summonses are of two types: **Subpoena Ad-testificandum**—to give evidence (testimony) in the court or **Subpoena ducistacum**—to produce some documents before the court.

The person receiving the summons must appear in the court in time. Non-compliance of summons without any lawful excuse (valid reason) may make the person liable to action for damages in a civil case, and in a criminal case, court generally issues a show cause notice under Section 350 of CrPC or a warrant of arrest may be issued to compel his attendance (Section 87, CrPC), and subsequently he may be punished with fine or imprisonment or both (Section 174 CrPC).

The summonses are served on the witness by a police officer, an officer of the court or by any public servant authorized by court. One copy of the summons is delivered to the person. The person must sign the receipt on the back of the other copy, which is then returned to the court. For government officers in service, the summonses are issued through the head of the office in which the person is working. If the person is not available, then a copy of the summons can be handed over to an adult member of his family, who then sign a receipt on the other copy. If nobody is present, the summons may be affixed on a conspicuous part of his house. Summons also can be sent by registered post.

If a person receives two summonses from two courts for his attendance, one from a criminal and other from a civil court, he should attend the criminal court first and inform the civil court of his inability to attend. If both the summons are from civil or criminal court, then he should attend the higher court informing the lower court of his inability. If both the courts are of same rank, he should attend the court from which he had received the summons first and informing the other court of his inability.

Conduct Money

It is the money offered to a witness in a civil case, at the time of serving the summons, to meet the expenses for attending the court.

If the conduct money is not paid at the time of serving the summons, the witness may ignore it. If the witness feels that the money offered to him is not sufficient to meet the expenses, he may attend the court and bring it to the notice of the presiding officer of the court before giving evidence. The presiding officer will decide the matter.

In criminal cases, no conduct money is paid at the time of serving the summons. The witness must attend the court and give evidence in the interest of the state. Court will pay him the cost as per government rules. Government servants or medical officers attending a criminal court will get a court attendance certificate from the court, and they can claim travelling allowances or other allowances from the office where he works.

Attending the Court

A doctor or any person, who receives a summons from a court for giving evidence, should go to the court on the day and time mentioned. He should report his attendance to the court and then wait in the court till he is called to the witness box. When in the witness box, the presiding officer of the court (Judge or Magistrate) will record the preliminaries like, name, age, address, qualification, designation, experience, of the witness. It is followed by oath taking.

Oath Taking

The presiding officer of the court then administers the oath to the witness. The witness takes the oath by saying—"I do swear in the name of God that the evidence I shall give to the court, shall be the truth, the whole truth and nothing but the truth. I shall not conceal anything" or if the witness desires he may solemnly affirm the oath.

An oath is a declaration to be made by a witness to speak the truth before giving evidence. It is required by law, and the witness will be liable to prosecution for perjury if he deliberately gives false evidence. A child below the age of 12 years does not require to take oath.

Perjury (Under Section 191 IPC and 344 CrPC)

It means wilfully giving false evidence in a court of law under oath. A witness who deliberately conceals a part of the truth or makes a statement, which he knows or believes to be false or not true is liable to be prosecuted for perjury (under Section 193 IPC). The punishment may be fine or imprisonment up to 7 years.

After oath, recording of evidence takes place in following steps:

1. Examination in chief
2. Cross-examination
3. Re-examination
4. Questions by the Court.

Examination in Chief

After oath taking, the witness is examined by the lawyer of the party who has summoned him to give evidence. In criminal cases, usually state government is the prosecution party and the witness is first examined by the public prosecutor. The main purpose is to place before the court all the facts and relevant matters bearing upon the case known to the witness. A medical witness usually gives evidence from the medical reports or certificates he had submitted earlier. The purpose is to elicit all relevant convincing medical facts and the conclusions and opinion, which the doctor had drawn from the facts he mentioned in the report. He is also to testify that the report submitted was prepared by him and was duly signed by him. During examination in chief, no leading questions are allowed. A ***leading question*** is one that suggest the answer by itself or where the answer lies implied in the question itself and answer to the question will be simple 'yes' or 'no.' Questions like "was the injury caused by a dagger?" or "was the injury 10 centimeter in length" are leading questions and answer suggested are "yes" or "no" (Section 141 IEA). Proper questions to the witness should be—"what was the type of weapon used?" and "what was the length of the injury?" Leading questions are allowed in examination in chief when the witness is declared ***hostile*** by the court. Both the common and expert witness may become hostile.

Cross Examination

In this stage, the witness is examined by the lawyer of the opposite partly (defense lawyer in criminal proceedings). It may be regarded as the most reliable procedure of testing the reliability and truthfulness of witness and his evidence. The defense lawyer will try to weaken the evidence given in the examination in chief by eliciting points favorable to his side. For this, he will try to establish that the evidence given was inaccurate, conflicting and contradictory, or that the opinion was ill founded and oppose to the views of well-recognized authorities. Therefore, the witness must be very careful in answering questions during cross examination.

Leading questions are allowed during cross examination. The defense lawyer may ask many irritating, vague, conflicting questions to confuse the witness and to disperse his skill, acumen and integrity.

The cross examination need not be confined to the statements to which the witness made during examination in chief. The defense lawyer may test the competency and credibility of witness by asking questions about his qualification and experience, but also the memory and power of observation of the witness. When materials are available, the defense lawyer may ask question challenging the character of the witness (Section 148, IEA). However, the court can forbid any question which appears to be insulting or annoying and offensive in form (Section 152 IEA). There is no limit for cross examination. It may last for hours to days. The witness may have to answer hypothetical questions bearing on the fact in issue, but he need not answer when he thinks that the subject is beyond his purview. If the question is not understood, the witness should ask the lawyer to explain it. The witness should be clear, direct and precise in his answer as far as possible. He should not volunteer any unrelated information.

Sometimes the cross examination may act as a double edged weapon, damaging both the prosecution and defense, if the defense lawyer is not familiar with the subject and does not put questions with care and the witness happens to be well-experienced in the subject.

Re-examination

After cross examination, the witness may be re-examined to clear any doubt or that may have arisen during cross-examination. The witness gets an opportunity to correct any mistake or explain any point, which arises during cross examination. Leading questions are not allowed at this stage. No new matter should be brought in re-examination. The opposing lawyer has the right to cross examine on the new point raised (Section 138 IEA).

Questions by the Court

The judge may ask any questions to the witness at any stage of the recording of the evidence to clear up any doubtful point or to know some more relevant matter about the fact.

The courts also have the power to recall and re-examine any witness already examined, if it appears to the court that re-examination of the witness is essential to clear some points before taking any decision in the case (Section 165 IEA and Section 311 CrPC).

Before leaving the court, the witness should read his deposition carefully, and then put his signature on bottom of each page. The witness should leave the court after getting permission from the Judge.

DUTY OF A DOCTOR AS A WITNESS IN THE COURT

i. After receiving the summon, the doctor must attend the court and should be punctual.
ii. He must be well dressed, looking modest and sober.
iii. He should carry along with him, all the records relevant to the case.
iv. Be well prepared about the case. He can discuss the case with his colleagues in the department.
v. Never discuss the case with anyone outside the court.
vi. Never lose temper in the court.
vii. Should never be nervous inside the court. He should remain calm, polite and courteous.
viii. He should never be over confident. If he does not know the answer, he can simply say, "Sir I do not know", as no one is expected to know everything.
ix. Avoid using technical terms, and always try to explain the case in simple language.
x. If a lawyer quotes a paragraph of a book. He should be asked to show the book or full chapter. Because sometimes, if we read the full chapter, the meaning totally changes.
xi. Listen to questions carefully. If it is not audible or not clear, one must ask the lawyer to repeat the question.
x. Always address the judge by "Sir" or "Your honor", giving him his due respect.
xi. Never try to memorize any fact. The law allows the doctor to refresh his memory from the records.
xii. Comments about the competency of a fellow colleague should be avoided. If, forced, one should answer in the form of no opinion or no comments.
xiii. He has to answer all the questions and does not have any professional privilege.
xiv. Limit his answer to the expertise in his field and must not volunteer any information or answer questions asked to him beyond his expertise.
xv. After conclusion of his evidence, he should read the written deposition of his evidence recorded by the court, and he should put his signature on each page, getting any corrections, if needed, done by the court under its initials. He should not leave the court until he is permitted to leave.

At the end, we can say, as the doctor is said to be a responsible and respectable person of the society, while in the court he should be well dressed, modest, polite and courteous, while giving evidence, to keep the dignity of the profession.

CHAPTER 3

Medical Law and Ethics

Mukesh Yadav, Rituraj Chaliha, Putul Mahanta

LEARNING PLAN

- Know about different attributes of Medical Council of India (MCI)
- Learn about rights and privileges of Registered Medical Practitioners (RMP)
- Know about the ethical aspects of medical practice
- Identify the different aspects of the RMP
- Identify the unethical acts
- Know about the different types of consent
- Recognize medical negligence
- Know about Consumer Protection Act
- Understand biomedical waste management
- Learn about the ethics in medical research

MEDICAL COUNCIL OF INDIA

Structure of Medical Council of India (MCI)

Medical Council is a corporate body constituted under the Indian Medical Council Act, 1956 (repealed Act 1933). Indian Medical Council's office is situated in New Delhi. It comprises a set of members of the profession elected from each state and universities, as well as nominated directly by the government of India in consultation with state governments.

Constitution and Composition of the MCI

The Central Government shall cause to be constituted a council (MCI) consisting of the following members, namely:

i. One registered medical practitioner as a member from each State other than a Union Territory to be nominated by the Central Government in consultation with the State Government concerned. Thus, the council has one member from each state nominated by government.

ii. One registered medical practitioner as a member from each University with which at least a Medical college is affiliated, to be elected from among the members of the medical faculty of the University by members of the Senate of the University or in case the University has no Senate, by members of the Court. Thus, the council has one member from each university elected.
iii. One registered medical practitioner as a member from each State in which a State Medical Register is maintained, to be elected from among themselves by persons enrolled on such register who possess the medical qualifications included in the First or the Second Schedule or in Part II of the Third Schedule. Thus, one member from each State Medical Register, representing non-Indian degrees (Part-II, III schedule) (Elected).
iv. Seven members to be elected from among themselves by persons enrolled on any of the State Medical Registers who possess the medical qualifications included in Part I of the Third Schedule of MCI. Thus, Seven members from each state medical Register representing Indian degrees (Part-I, III schedule) (Elected).
v. Eight members to be nominated by the Central Government (nominated).

Executive Committee

The above body through election among themselves forms an executive committee comprising of two officers: **President** and **Vice-President** and **20 members**. The president and vice-president of the Council shall be elected by the members of the Council among themselves. Executive committee members are elected by the General Body of Medical Council of India. The **Secretary**, who is an appointed executive of the council, is an ex-officio member. However, any number of subcommittees comprising of 7–10 members may be formed to carry out the functions of the council from the above group.

Duration of MCI

The tenure of the Medical Council of India ordinarily for a term of not more than 5 years or till formation of a new office, which could not be formed due to some technical reasons.

Functions of MCI

Maintenance of Indian Medical Register

i. An officer by name Registrar is appointed by the Council, who will maintain a register (Secretary) called Indian Medical Register. This contains the names of all medical persons who are enrolled on any of the state medical register and who possess a recognized medical qualification included in first schedule of MCI.
ii. A name once entered is erased normally on death of the doctor or as a disciplinary action. Names may also erased temporarily and then re-entered, depending on the time and condition of disciplinary actions taken.
iii. This contains the names of all medical persons who are enrolled on any of the state medical register and who possess a recognized medical qualification.

Maintenance of Quality of Medical Education

i. **Postgraduate Medical Education**: It prescribes standards of postgraduate medical education for the universities and would also offer advice to universities to maintain uniformity all over the country.
ii. **Undergraduate Medical Education**: It maintains standards at undergraduate medical education by appointing inspectors, who inspect the facilities and examinations held by university/medical institution in India, the purpose being to recommend recognition of the qualification to Central Government.

iii. To supervise the medical profession and maintain a proper standard of medical education throughout India.
iv. Recommendation to Central Government for start of new medical college/new medical courses/increase of seats for these courses.

Inspection of Medical Colleges

The MCI may arrange for an inspection of a medical college under following circumstances:

i. For every medical qualification (MBBS, MD/MS/DM/MCh/Diploma, etc.) when it is newly introduced.
ii. For every 5 years routinely, to determine the standards, equipments, training, staff pattern and other facilities. If the inspection result is unsatisfactory, the inspectors concerned can make recommendation to the Medical Council of India for withdrawing recognition accorded earlier.

Recognition of Foreign Medical Degrees

Two important sections of Indian Medical Council Act, 1956 govern this and they are:

i. **Section 12**: Empowers the council to recognize medical qualifications granted by institutions outside India and to enter in a scheme of reciprocity with Medical Councils of foreign countries in the matter of mutual recognition of medical qualifications between the two countries.
ii. **Section 13** (4) of the same Act, gives authorization to the council to recognize foreign medical qualifications, which are not included in the schedule (II), based on reciprocal recognition.

Procedure for Recognition: A person with such qualification should first send an application through Central Government. The full literature regarding the course of study, syllabi, duration of the course, etc. may also be required to be furnished. The council may consult directory of medical institutions published by World Health Organization.

Then the person should qualify the foreign medical graduate examination (FMGE), which is conducted by national board of examinations (NBE) every 6 months. Then, that foreign degree will get recognized by MCI in India and candidate would be entitled for registration with Medical Council of India and gets all the privileges of Registered Medical Practitioner except few.

Appeal against Disciplinary Action for Unethical Acts and/or **Professional Misconduct:** The Indian Medical Council can give advice to the Central Government (Health Ministry) regarding appeals preferred by a medical practitioner against the decisions taken by the State Medical Council on disciplinary matters.

Procedure of Appeal: The medical practitioner, against whom the State Medical Council has taken disciplinary action, may appeal to the Central Government in writing, stating the grounds of the appeal and be accompanied by all relevant documents including a receipt for paying the nominal fees (₹ 20/-) to Central Government. The appeal should be filed within 30 days from the date of decision appealed against.

The Final Decision: The decision of the Central Government, which is given after consulting Indian Medical Council, is final and binding on the State Government and the State Medical Council.

Issue of Warning Notice: Indian Medical Council may issue **warning notice** when unethical practice is done. This comprises of information about certain unethical practices known as infamous conduct in a professional respect.

Functions of State Medical Council

Maintenance of State Medical Register

i. The State Medical Council also maintains a State Medical Register. This Register will contain the name, address, qualifications and date of qualifying of every person who is registered under this Act on paying a prescribed fee. On registration, a Number is allotted to each person with a certificate, enabling him or her to be considered as Registered Medical Practitioner.

ii. Display of this certificate in the place of his/her practice helps the lay public to distinguish a qualified doctor from the unqualified. It is the duty of the Registrar to inform Indian Medical Council, from time to time, about the additions and deletions from the State Medical Register regularly.

Disciplinary Control

I. Disciplinary action/control over doctors registered with the council.
ii. Erasure of name and restoration of name of doctors from State Medical Register after disciplinary action and/or death of doctor.
iii. Periodic updating of State Medical Register and its information to the Medical Council of India on Annual Basis.
iv. Can issue warning notice (list of professional misconduct issued from time to time).

Procedure of Disciplinary Enquiry

Disciplinary enquiry as per the provisions of Chapter VIII of Regulations, 2002, may arise usually from two sources:

i. Accusations of professional misconduct in writing either from a member of the public or a professional colleague or a certain public officer (Point 1.7, Chapter I).
ii. An order from the court where a doctor is convicted for any criminal offense.

On receipt of such a notification or accusation of professional misconduct, the Registrar of State Medical Council submits it to the president and on scrutinizing the same, one of the following:

1. **Rejection of the case**: When false or otherwise unfounded allegations (acquittal if no *prima facie* case proved).
2. **Submission to ethical sub-committee**: The cases, which cannot be rejected, shall be referred to a special ethical sub-committee of the chairman and a few other co-opted members. The committee will examine the facts of the case and on giving an opportunity to the alleged accused physician to defend, who decides the punishment under disciplinary action. The sub-committee has to decide the disciplinary action enumerated below:
   i. **Acquittals**: The case may be either dismissed if no *prima facie* evidence against the accused.
   ii. **Warning**: If it is a case of first offense, doctor may be sent back merely with warning not to repeat the same.
   iii. **Action**: It is the eraser or suspension of the name of the doctor from the register for a specific period considering the gravity of offense, to be reinstalled at the end of the period of suspension.

Penal Erasure: This means erasure of the name of the doctor from the state medical register permanently or temporarily when the offense is proved allowing not to practice as registered medical professional. When a practitioner's name has been erased from the register, he or she may apply for restoration at various fixed intervals. He or she may also appeal to the Medical Council, which can recommend to the Union Ministry of Health and Family Welfare against the decision of the State Medical Councils.

ETHICAL ASPECTS OF MEDICAL PRACTICE

Medical Ethics

Medical ethics deals with the moral principles, which should guide members of the medical profession in their dealing with each other, their patients and the state. Ethical behavior is a self-imposed duty upon each doctor.

Medical Etiquette

It deals with the conventional laws of courtesy observed between members of the medical profession. Hippocrates, the Greek physician, introduced the concept of ethics in medicine. Chapter III of Ethical Regulations, 2002 deals with issues of etiquettes.

Duties of Doctors to Each Other (Medical Etiquette)

It is the rules of conduct growing the relationship of the medical profession and includes the following:

1. A doctor ought to behave to his or her colleagues, as he would have them behave to him.
2. A doctor must not entice patients from his colleagues.
3. A doctor must observe the principles enshrined in Chapter III of Ethical Regulations, 2002.

Declaration of Geneva

The Medical Council of India (founded in 1934) formulates the modern code of medical law and ethics in India. It is framed and worded on the same line as in the Declaration of Geneva with some modifications by the World Medical Association, which again is a restated modern version of the oldest code of medical ethics, the Hippocratic Oath: held in high esteem by every medical professional. The general principles mentioned in the **Hippocratic Oath** have been brought up to date by the **World Medical Association**.

The modernized version of the **Hippocratic Oath** is the **Declaration of Geneva and the International Code of Medical Ethics**. The Declaration of Geneva was adopted by the General Assembly of the World Medical Association at Geneva in 1948. It was amended in 1968, 1984, 1994, 2005 and 2006. It is a declaration of physician's dedication to the humanitarian goals of medicine, a declaration that was especially important in view of the medical crimes, which had just been committed by Nazi in Germany.

International Code of Medical Ethics

It was adopted in the General Assembly of the World Medical Association in London in October, 1948. It is also a modernized version of the **Hippocratic Oath**. International code of medical ethics is again solely based on Declaration of Geneva and framed as sets of duties of doctor in general, to the sick and to each other.

Duties of Doctors in General

i. A doctor must always maintain the highest standards of professional conduct.
ii. A doctor must practice his profession uninfluenced by motives of profit.
iii. Following practices are deemed unethical:
    a. Any self-advertisement except such as is expressly authorized by the national code of medical ethics.
    b. Collaboration in any form of medical service in which the doctor does not have professional independence.
    c. Receiving any money in connection with services rendered to a patient other than a proper professional fee, even with the knowledge of the patient.
iv. Any act or advice, which could weaken physical or mental resistance of a human being, may be used only in his or her interest.
v. A doctor is advised to use great caution in divulging discoveries or new techniques on treatment.
vi. A doctor should certify or testify only to that which he or she has personally verified.

Duties of Doctors to the Sick

i. A doctor must always bear in mind the obligation of preserving human life.
ii. A doctor owes to his or her patient complete loyalty and all the resources of his or her science. Whenever an examination or treatment beyond his or her capacity, he or she should summon another doctor who has the necessary ability.
iii. A doctor shall preserve absolute secrecy on all he or she knows about his or her patient because of the confidence entrusted in him.
iv. A doctor must give emergency care as a humanitarian duty unless he or she is assured that others are willing and able to give such care.

Doctors and the Media

Increasing public interest in health matters has brought doctors in closer contact with media. The British Medical Association in Handbook of Medical Ethics, 1981 has suggested guidelines for the registered medical practitioner and their dealings with media. Attending doctors should act in these situations with reference to bounden duty under professional secrecy and provisions of privileged communication so that breach of medical ethics is committed by the attending doctor.

The Indian Medical Council (Professional Conduct, Etiquette and Ethics) Regulations, 2002

Code of Medical Ethics

Declaration: Each applicant at the time of making an application for registration under the provisions of the Act shall be provided a copy of the declaration and shall submit a duly signed declaration as provided in Appendix I of the said regulation. The applicant shall also certify that he/she had read and agreed to abide by the same. The actual text of declaration of the code provided by the Medical Council of India is medical ethics in India, which may be presented as follows:

Declaration of Code of Medical Ethics in India

1. I solemnly pledge myself to consecrate my life to the service of humanity.
2. Even under threat, I will not use my medical knowledge contrary to the laws of humanity.
3. I will maintain the utmost respect for human life from time of conception.
4. I will not permit consideration of religion, nationality, race, party-politics or social standing to intervene between my duty and my patient.
5. I will practice my profession with conscience and dignities.
6. The health of my patient will be my first consideration.
7. I will respect the secrets, which are confided in me.
8. I will give to my teachers the respect and gratitude that is their due.
9. I will maintain by all means, in my power, the honor and noble traditions of the medical profession.
10. I will treat my colleagues with all respects and dignity.
11. I shall abide by the code of medical ethics as enunciated in the Medical Council Regulations, 2002 (Professional Conduct Etiquette and Ethics).
12. I make these promises solemnly, truly and upon my honor.

Place:	Signature
Date:	Name and address

REGISTERED MEDICAL PRACTITIONER

A Registered Medical Practitioner is a qualified doctor (minimum qualification MBBS degree) who has been registered in State/Indian Medical Councils.

Rights and Privileges of Registered Medical Practitioners

1. He can issue medical certificate to his patient.
2. He is entitled to receive/recover fees due to him through court of law in respect of treatment given to any person.
3. He can possess, handle and prescribe dangerous drugs if indicated to his patient.
4. He can hold office in a Government or Private job.
5. He can become an expert witness in a court of law.
6. He has right to choose patient (except in an emergency).
7. He has right to dispense medicine for his patient.
8. Right to add title, descriptions, etc., to his name.

Procedure of Getting Registered

After passing qualifying examinations (MBBS) one has to undergo a period of compulsory training of internship for minimum one year in an institution approved by the Indian Medical Council. On completion of this training he or she will have to fill in certain application forms and pay the nominal fee to the State Medical Council. The office, which will then scrutinize the contents in the application and if approved, enters the name of the doctor in the register and provides him a Registration Certificate and a code number by which he or she may be referred for all further communications.

Requirements to be fulfilled by an applicant (MBBS) at the **time of registration** with **SMC/ MCI** as follows:

1. Signed declaration from (Appendix -1).
2. Certificate that he had read and agreed to abide by the same.
3. Certificate of recognized medical qualification (MBBS).
4. Internship completion certificate.
5. Requisite fees, etc. (**Point: 1A**).

No person other than a doctor having qualification recognized by MCI and registered with MCI/SMC is allowed to practice Modern System of Medicine or Surgery (Allopathic doctors). A person obtaining qualification in any other system of medicine is not allowed to practice Modern System of Medicine in any form (**Point: 1.1.3**).

Similarly, a person, with MSc (Biochemistry, Microbiology) and PhD, but not registered with the SMC cannot practice medicine or sign any patient investigation report. Certain percentage of person with non-medical qualifications are allowed to hold teaching posts due to scarcity of qualified medical persons (like Physiology, Biochemistry, Microbiology, Pharmacology, etc.), but these degrees should also be of medical discipline, even though they cannot practice medicine as per provisions of the Indian Medical Council Act, 1956.

On getting registered, a doctor has certain merits such as achieving some special rights and privileges. He also has to perform certain duties towards the patients and the state. Both of these are discussed below.

Recognition of degree by MCI and its registration as additional qualification is necessary for the practice of that specialty, this is important especially for clinician, pathologist, radiologist, biochemist, surgeons, etc. (**Point 1.1.3, 1.4.2**). Practice without registration or without recognized degree is technically amount to negligence.

A physician shall not claim to be specialist unless he has a special qualification in that branch (**Point 7.20**). A non-medical person holding MSc and/or PhD cannot claim to be a specialist (MSc Biochemistry, etc.).

Section 15 (2) of the Indian Medical Council Act, 1956, read as "Save as provided in Section 25, **no person other than a medical practitioner enrolled on a State Medical Register**:

i. Shall hold office as physician or surgeon or any other office (by whatever designation called) in Government or in any institution maintained by a local or other authority;
ii. Shall practice medicine in any State;
iii. Shall be entitled to sign or authenticate a medical or fitness certificate or any other certificate required by any law to be signed or authenticated by a duly qualified medical practitioner;
iv. Shall be entitled to give evidence at any inquest or in any court of law as an expert under Section 45 of the Indian Evidence Act, 1872 (Act 1 of 1872) on any matter relating to medicine".

Punishment: Section 15(3), read as "any person who acts in contravention of any provision of sub-section (2) shall be punished with imprisonment for a term, which may extend to one year, or with fine, which may extend to one thousand rupees, or with both [Inserted by Act 24 of 1964, Section 7 (w.e.f., 16-06-1964)].

Court Cases: It is envisaged under section 25(4) that a person registered provisionally and if he has completed practical training referred to in sub-section (1) or such person is in the employment in resident medical capacity in any approved medical institution, shall be entitled to registration in the State Medical Register under Section 15 of the Act; [Dr Sanjeev Mittal vs. Union of India, AIR 2003 (P and H) 213].

MSc (Biochemistry) cannot be considered to be basic qualification for practicing as a Medical Practitioner; [Medical Council of India vs. State of Rajasthan, AIR 1996 sc 2073].

In view of clause (b) of sub-section (2) of Section 15 of the Act, no person who is not qualified in the system of Modern Medicine and is not registered as such, either in State Register or the Central Register, is entitled to practice modern system of Medicine; [Dr Sarwan Singh Dardi vs. State of Punjab, AIR 1987 (P and H) 81].

Section 27 of the Act does not prevent persons enrolled in the Indian Medical Register from seeking employment on such terms and conditions as they may choose to secure it nor does it prohibit agreement of service, which entail giving up of the privileges mentioned in it [Sukumar Mukherejee vs. State of West Bengal, AIR 1993 SC 2335].

Use of Generic Names of Drugs

The clause 1.5 under MCI code of medical ethics does not make it mandatory for a doctor to prescribe drugs with generic names. The clause 1.5 of MCI code of medical ethics reproduced here under:

"**Use of Generic Names of Drugs**: Every physician should, as far as possible, prescribe drugs with generic names and he/she shall ensure that there is a rational prescription and use of drugs."

The Meaning is Simple: Except in those situations where, due to certain explainable reasons, it is not possible to write generic names, the RMP should prescribe drugs with generic names. It can be reasonably expected that it should be possible to prescribe by generic names in case of majority of the drugs prescribed. If the prescriptions of a doctor show that no or only few drugs are prescribed by generic names, the onus will be upon him to explain why it was not possible to do so. If he cannot give a satisfactory explanation, he would be justifiably deemed to have broken law.

Exposure of Unethical Conduct

A physician should expose, without fear or favor, incompetent or corrupt, dishonest or unethical conduct on the part of members of the profession **(Chapter I, Point 1.7)**.

Payment of Professional Services

The physician engaged in the practice of medicine, limits the source of his income received from professional activities to service rendered to the patient. So, that maximum time can be devoted to updating his knowledge and skill in the interest of humanity. Remunerations received for such services should be in the form and amount specifically announced to the patient at the time the service is rendered. It is unethical to enter into an account of "**No cure no payment**" **(Point 1.8)**.

Physician rendering service on behalf of the state shall refrain from anticipating or accepting any consideration. NPA is paid by the government for this purpose **(Point 1.8)**.

A physician shall clearly display his fees and other charges on the board of his chamber and/or the hospital he is visiting. Prescription should also make clear if the physician himself dispensed any medicine **(Point 3.7.1)**.

Rebate and Commission (Professional Dichotomy): A physician shall not give, solicit, or receive nor shall he offer to give, solicit or receive any gift, gratuity, commission or bonus in consideration of or return for the referring or procuring of any patient for medical, surgical or other treatment. A physician shall not directly or indirectly participate in or be a party to act of division, transference, assignment, subordination, rebating, splitting or refunding of any fee for medical, surgical or other treatment **(Point 6.4.1)**.

Above provisions shall apply with equal force to the referring, recommending or procuring by a physician or any person, specimen or material for diagnostic or other study or work. Nothing shall prohibit payment of salaries by a qualified physician to other duly qualified person rendering medical care under his supervision **(Point 6.4.2)**. A physician shall not use touts or agents for procuring patients **(Point 7.19)**.

This will help in preventing exploitation of patients and unnecessary filing of suits of negligence. Commission based practice always leads to unnecessary doing of procedures and asking for unnecessary consultations and diagnostic tests.

Duties of Physicians to their Patients

1. Obligations to sick;
2. Patience, delicacy and secrecy;
3. Prognosis;
4. The patient must not be neglected;
5. Engagement for an obstetric case;
6. Unnecessary consultation should be avoided;
7. Consultation for patient benefit;
8. Punctuality in consultation;
9. Statement to patient after consultation;
10. Treatment after consultation;
11. Patient referred to specialists;
12. Fees and other charges;
13. Dependence of physician on each other;
14. Conduct in consultation;
15. Consult not to take charge of the patient;
16. Appointment of substitute;
17. Visiting another physician case;
18. He or she is entitled to sign statutory medical certificates, such as for birth, death, mental illness, etc.
19. He or she is entitled to sue for recovery of his or her fees in court of law. However, gratuitous service may be rendered to a deserving poor patient, as well as to all other physicians and his or her dependent family members;
20. He or she is entitled to perform medico-legal autopsies;
21. He or she is entitled to give evidence at any inquest or in any court of law as an expert;
22. He or she is exempted from serving on a jury and at an inquest;
23. He or she can choose his or her patient;
24. He or she can add title, description, etc., to his or her name.

Duties of Registered Medical Practitioner

1. To exercise a reasonable degree of skill and knowledge in treating a patient.
2. To attend and examine a patient as long as there is a need after commencing the treatment. However, he or she can terminate his or her services, when another physician attends his patient or using of remedies other than those prescribed by him or her.
3. To provide proper and suitable medicine to the patient either directly or by a prescription.
4. To give proper instructions to the patient or relative of the patient regarding the use of medicine, dosage schedule, diet, etc., and warn the dangers if not used properly.
5. To appoint a substitute doctor during temporary absence, with the consent of patient, especially in obstetrics and gynecology cases.
6. To warn the possibilities of cross-infecting the others in case the patient is suffering from communicable disease.
7. To take proper care of children and adult patient who are unable to take care of themselves.
8. To inform all the risks involved in treatment plan. However, under the **Doctrine of Therapeutic Privileges**, doctor need not disclose everything.
9. To handle poisons carefully and give proper treatment to a poisoning case and also co-operate with law enforcement authorities in deciding the case whether it is a suicide, homicide or accident.
10. To inform health authorities on a communicable disease reported to you under the **Doctrine of Privileged Communication** forgoing the professional secrecy principles of ethical code.
11. To exercise all duties with regard to surgery, i.e. taking consent, operate under proper anesthesia, aseptic measures, pre and postoperative care, etc.
12. To treat war prisoners, civilians of any country, etc., under the duties proposed in Geneva Convention.

13. To refer the patient to a specialist/consultant as and when needed after taking prior consent.
14. To take an X-ray of injured part (unless trivial) for ruling out fractures.
15. To maintain professional secrecy.

Professional Secrecy and Privileged Communications

i. Confidence concerning individual or domestic life entrusted by patients to a physician and defects in the disposition or character of patients observed during medical attendance should never be revealed unless their revelation is required by the **laws of the state.** Sometimes, however, a physician must determine whether his **duty to society requires** him to employ knowledge, obtained through confidences to him as a physician, **to protect a healthy person** against a communicable disease to which he is about to be exposed. In such instances, the physician should act as he would desire another to act toward one of his own family in like circumstances **(Point 2.2).** For example, HIV positive case.
ii. Disclosing patient's secrets amount to professional misconduct: the RMP shall not disclose the secrets of a patient that have been learnt in the exercise of his profession except:
   a. In a court of law under orders of the presiding judge;
   b. In circumstances where there is a serious and identifiable risk to a specific person and/or community; and
   c. Notifiable diseases.
iii. In case of communicable/notifiable diseases, concerned public health authorities should be informed immediately **(Point 7.14).**

Duties of Physician in Case of Consultation

A physician always thinks of risk-benefit involved with the patient first and also keeps in mind other factors like cost-effectiveness, patient's economic status (Government or Private Hospital) except in cases of **serious illness** and in **doubtful** or **difficult conditions.** All these constitutes **emergency situation (Point 3.1.1).**

Rights and Duties of Attending Physician in Consultation

1. Justifiable consultation.
2. Benefit of the patient.
3. Frank with the patient and his attendants.
4. Announcement of the opinion to the patient or his relatives after consultation.
5. Continue with the treatment even with subsequent variations in the treatment, but reasons should be recorded in writing and explained to the consultant at the next consultation.
6. May prescribe medicine any time to his patient **(Point 3.1.1–3.5).**

Rights of Consultant during Consultation

1. Utmost punctuality.
2. Consultant may prescribe medicine only in emergency during the absence of the attending physician.
3. No criticism or adverse comment against attending physician **(Point 3.1.1–3.5, 4.3).**
4. Normally not take charge of the case, especially on the solicitation of the patient or friends **(Point 4.3).**
5. He should discuss the diagnosis /treatment plan only with the referring physician not with the patient or attendants **(Point 4.3).**

Procedure of Referral of Patient

When a patient is referred to a specialist by the attending physician, a case summary should be given to the specialist.

Duty of the Consultant when a Patient is referred for Consultation: Specialist should always communicate his opinion in writing to the attending physician **(Point 3.6)**.

Duties towards Patient in Case of Difference of Opinion after Consultation: Differences of opinion should not be divulged unnecessarily; but when there is irreconcilable difference of opinion, the circumstances should be frankly and impartially explained to the patient or his relatives either by the attending physician himself or in the presence of all consultants as agreed. It would be open to the patient or his relatives to seek further advice, should they so desire **(Point 3.4.2)**.

Pharmacists/Nurses: Physician should recognize and promote the practice of different paramedical services such as, pharmacy and nursing as professions and should seek their co-operation wherever required.

Display of Registration Number

1. **Regulation 1.4.1 of the MCI Code of Ethics Regulations, 2002, reads:** "1.4.1 every physician shall display the registration number accorded to him/her by the State Medical Council/Medical Council of India in his clinic and in all his prescriptions, certificates, money receipts given to his patients". It is obvious that the above direction is mandatory.
2. **Regulation 7.3 provides that it is professional misconduct:** "If he/she does not display the registration number accorded to him/her by the State Medical Council or the Medical Council of India in his/her clinic, prescriptions and certificates, etc. issued by him or her, violates the provisions of Regulation 1.4.2."

UNETHICAL ACTS

Patent and Copyrights

A physician may patent surgical instruments, appliances and medicine or copyright applications methods and procedure. However, it shall be unethical if the benefits of such patents or copyrights are not made available in situations where the interest of the large population is involved.

Running an Open Pharmacy Shop (Dispensing of Drugs and Appliances by Physician)

A physician should not run an open shop for sale of medicine for dispensing prescriptions prescribed by doctors other than him or for sale of medical or surgical appliances. It is not unethical for a Physician to prescribe or supply drugs, remedies or appliances as long as there is no exploitation of the patient. Drugs prescribed by a physician or brought from the market for a patient should explicitly state the proprietary formulae as well as generic name of the drug.

Rebates and Commission

See page no 28 (Professional Dichotomy)

Secret Remedies

The prescribing or dispensing by a physician of secret remedial agents of which he does not know the composition, or the manufacture or promotion of their use is unethical and as such prohibited. All the drugs prescribed by an Allopathic physician should always carry a proprietary formula and clear name as per Indian, British and United States Pharmacopoeia.

Human Rights

The physician shall not aid or abet torture on any human being nor shall be a party to either infliction of mental or physical trauma or concealment of torture inflicted by some other person or agency in clear violation of human rights.

Euthanasia

Practicing euthanasia shall constitute unethical conduct, however on specific occasion, the question of withdrawing supporting devices to sustain cardiopulmonary function even after brain death, shall be decided only by a team of doctors and not merely by the treating physician alone. There is no legal sanction for euthanasia in India.

Organ Transplantation

A team of doctors shall declare withdrawal of support system. Such team shall consist of the doctor in charge of the patient, Chief Medical Officer/Medical Officer in charge of the hospital and a doctor nominated by the in-charge of the hospital from the hospital staff or in accordance with the provisions of the Transplantation of Human Organ Act, 1994.

PROFESSIONAL MISCONDUCT

Regulations of MCI nowhere defined it, but professional misconduct can be defined as something done by a doctor during professional medical practice, which is considered as disgraceful and dishonorable by his or her professional brethren of good repute and competence after enquiry by the State Medical Council/Medical Council of India.

The following **acts of commission** or **omission** on the part of a physician shall constitute professional misconduct rendering him/her liable for disciplinary action:

1. Violation of the Regulations 2002.
2. If he/she does not maintain the medical record and refuses to provide the same within 72 hours.
3. If he/she does not display the registration number.
4. Adultery or improper conduct.
5. Conviction by court of law.
6. Sex determination tests with the intent to terminate the life of a female fetus developing in her mother womb, unless there are other absolute indications for termination of pregnancy as specified in the Medical Termination of Pregnancy Act, 1971.
7. Selling Schedule "H" and "L" drugs and poisons to the public except his patients; contravention of the above provisions shall constitute gross professional misconduct on the part of the physician.
8. Performing or enabling unqualified person to perform an abortion or any illegal operation for which there is no medical, surgical or psychological indication.
9. A registered medical practitioner shall not issue certificates of efficiency in modern medicine to unqualified or non-medical person.
10. A physician should not contribute to the lay press articles and give interviews regarding diseases and treatments, which may have the effect of advertising himself of soliciting practices; but is open to write to the lay press under his own name on matters of public health, hygienic living or to deliver public lectures, give talks on the radio/TV/internet chat for the same purpose and send announcement of the same to lay press.
11. An institution run by a physician for a particular purpose such as maternity home, private hospital, rehabilitation center or any type of training institution, etc. may be advertised in the lay press, but such advertisement should not contain anything more than the name of the institution, type of patient admitted, type of training and other facilities offered and the fees.
12. It is improper for a physician to use an unusually large sign board and write on it anything other than his name, qualifications obtained from a University or a statutory body, titles and name of his specialty, registration number including the name of the State Medical Council under which registered. The same should be the contents of his prescription papers. It is improper to affix a sign-board on a chemist shop or in places where he does not reside or work.

A medical practitioner is, however, permitted to make a formal announcement in press regarding the followings:
- On starting practice
- On change of type of practice
- On changing address
- On temporary absence from duty
- On resumption of another practice
- On succeeding to another practice
- Public declaration of charges.

13. The registered medical practitioner shall not disclose the secrets of a patient that have been learnt in the exercise of his/her profession except when in a court of law under orders of the presiding judge, in circumstances where there is a serious and identified risk to a specific person and/or community, notifiable diseases. In case of communicable/notifiable diseases, concerned public health authorities should be infirmed immediately.
14. The registered medical practitioner shall not refuse on religious grounds alone to give assistance in or conduct of sterility, birth control, circumcision and medical termination of pregnancy when there is medical indication, unless the medical practitioner feels himself/herself incompetent to do so.
15. Before performing an operation, the physician should obtain in writing the consent from the husband or wife, parent or guardian in case of minor, or the patient himself as the case may be. In an operation, which may result in sterility, the consent of both husband and wife is needed.
16. A registered medical practitioner shall not publish photographs or case reports of his/her patients without their permission, in any medical or other journal in a manner by which their identity could be made out. If the identity is not to be disclosed, the consent is not needed.
17. In the case of running of a nursing home by a physician and employing assistance to help him/her, the ultimate responsibility rests on the physician.
18. A physician shall not use touts or agents for procuring patients.
19. A physician shall not claim to be specialist unless he has a special qualification in that branch.
20. No act of in vitro fertilization or artificial insemination shall be undertaken without the informed consent of the female patient and her spouse as well as the donor. Such consent shall be obtained in writing only after the patient is provided, at her own level comprehension, with sufficient information about the purpose, methods, risks and inconveniences, disappointments of the procedure and possible risk and hazards.
21. **Research**: Clinical drug trial or other research involving patients or volunteers as per the guidelines of ICMR can be undertaken, provided ethical consideration are born in mind. Violation of existing ICMR guidelines in this regard shall constitute misconduct. Consent taken from the patient for trial of drug or therapy which is not as per guidelines shall also be construed as misconduct.

Punishment and Disciplinary Action: It must be clearly understood that the instances of offences and of professional misconduct, which are given above do not constitute and are not intended to constitute a complete list of the infamous acts, which call for disciplinary action and that, by issuing this notice, the Medical Council of India and State Medical Council are in no way excluding other form of professional misconduct on the part of a registered practitioner.

LEGAL ASPECTS OF MEDICAL PRACTICE

Different Acts (Evasion of Legal Restrictions)

A physician should observe the provisions of the state Acts like:

1. Drugs and Cosmetics Act, 1940.
2. Pharmacy Act, 1948.
3. Narcotic Drugs and Psychotropic Substance Act, 1985.

4. Medical Termination of Pregnancy Act, 1971.
5. Transplantation of Human Organ Act, 1994.
6. Mental Health Act, 1987.
7. Environmental Protection Act, 1986.
8. Pre-natal Sex Determination Test Act, 1994.
9. Drugs and Magic Remedies (Objectionable Advertisement) Act, 1954.
10. Bio-Medical Waste (Management and Handling) Rules, 1998.

Physicians are obliged to follow and cooperate in enforcement of such other Acts, Rules and Regulations made by the Central/State Governments or Local Administrative Bodies or any other Act relating to the protection and promotion of public health in addition to above list.

MCI AND MEDICAL RECORD

As per the provisions of MCI provisions under Regulations, 2002, every physician shall maintain the medical records pertaining to his/her indoor patients for a period of 3 years from the date of commencement of treatment in a standard Performa laid down by it. If any request is made for medical records either by the patients/authorized attendants or legal authorities involved, the same may be duly acknowledged and documents shall be issued within the period of 72 hours.

A registered medical practitioner shall maintain a Register of Medical Certificates giving full details of certificates issued. When issuing a medical certificate, he/she shall always enter the identification marks of the patient and keep a copy of the certificate. He/she shall not omit signature and/or thumb marks, address and at least one identification mark of the patient on the medical certificate or report. Efforts shall be made to computerize medical records for quick retrieval. If physician does not maintain the medical record and refuses to provide the same within 72 hours, it will amount to professional misconduct, for which State Medical Council and/or MCI can start disciplinary proceedings and punishment accordingly.

CONSENT

Consent means "Voluntary agreement, compliance or permission". Section 13 of The Indian Contract Act lays down that "Two or more persons are said to consent when they agree upon the same thing in the same sense".

Sir James Stephen defines consent in criminal law to mean "a consent freely given by a rational opinion upon the matter to which he consents". He further adds that, "consent is said to be given freely, what is not procured by force, fraud or threats of whatever nature".

Importance of Consent

Explaining the 'right to privacy' in R Raj Gopal vs. State of Tamil Nadu (1994), the Supreme Court has held that it is the right to be let alone and a citizen has the "right to safeguard the privacy of his own", his family, marriage, motherhood, child bearing and education among other matters. No one can publish anything concerning the above matters without his consent, whether truthful or otherwise and whether laudatory or critical. Exception may be made if a person voluntarily thrusts himself into controversy or any of these matters becomes part of public record or relates to an action of a public official duty.

An HIV positive person does not have the right to privacy against the doctor not to disclose his status. Nor does such a patient has, an absolute right to marry under **Article 21** of the Constitution of the India. '**Right of others to healthy life**' justifies a '**breach of confidentiality**' in such cases '**X**' vs. **Hospital** '**Z**' (1998).

Thus, subject of consent involves the confrontation between '**rights to privacy**', and '**right to autonomy**' of the patients, '**Right of others to healthy life'** on one hand and **medicolegal**, **ethical** and **moral duties of the doctors** on the other hand as well as their duty to safeguard the interests of patients, public and themselves.

Types of Consent

1. Implied consent
2. Oral consent
3. Written consent
4. Express or informed consent

Implied Consent

The conduct of the greater part of medical practice is on the basis of '**Implied Consent**', although entirely correct, is apt **to lead medical practitioners to overlook the fact that medical examination is a subject of consent**, which is necessary **in the appropriate form**. Moreover, it is easily forgotten that any step beyond routine physical examination calls for '**Express Consent**' or '**Informed Consent**', **oral** or **written**, according to the circumstances.

The circumstances of medical practice do not ordinarily call for 'formal written consent' to medical examination because the patient conducts himself in a manner, which implies consent. When he attends a surgery, consulting room or outpatient's department, or when he agrees to be admitted to a hospital or nursing home, he thereby implies that he will submit to routine physical examination.

Informed Consent

Concept of 'informed consent' developed by American Courts: The concept of 'informed consent' developed by American courts, while retaining the basic requirements consent, shifts the emphasis to the doctor's duty to disclose the necessary information to the patient to secure his consent.

'**Informed consent**' is defined in Taber's *Cyclopedic* medical dictionary as: "Consent that is given by a person after receipt of the following information: the nature and purpose of the proposed procedure or treatment; the expected outcome and the likelihood of success; the risks; the alternatives to the procedure and supporting information regarding those alternatives; and the effect of no treatment or procedure, including the effect on the prognosis and the material risks associated with no treatment. Also included are instructions concerning what should be done if the procedure turns out to be harmful or unsuccessful."

Informed consent is an **ongoing process**, **a two-way** or **mutual conversation** extending over time, rather than a form of signed document once and for all, which is never again to be discussed.

Every person has the right to do what he likes with his body in order to protect and preserve his health. To examine/treat a person without his consent is therefore a violation of that right and can lead to legal action. **Consent is a must.** Usually, **doctor is legally bound to divulge all information** regarding condition of the patient/ treatment/prognosis, etc., to patient/guardian **before obtaining consent.**

Exception to Informed Consent

There may be some exceptions to doctor's duty to make prior disclosure of material risks:

i. A doctor may conclude that the disclosure of a risk may pose such a serious psychological threat or detriment to the patient as to be medically contraindicated. However, it is not to be based upon the view that the doctor may remain silent because divulgence might prompt the patient to forego needed therapy. This is known as "**Therapeutic Privilege**" or "**Professional Discretion**". Depending upon the circumstances, the doctor may make the revelations to the next of the kin.
ii. This privilege applies only when a patient is unusually sensitive, anxious or emotional. A general policy of not disclosing information because of the presumed hypersensitivity of patient is not an acceptable basis for this privilege.
iii. A physician relying on 'therapeutic privilege' should document carefully why the information ordinarily required by patient should be withheld from the particular patient.
iv. When the physician's use of 'therapeutic privilege; is challenged, it must be determined whether the physician followed

sound medical judgment in withholding information.

v. A competent patient may specifically ask not to be informed, i.e. a patient may waive of his or her right to make an informed consent. The patient may reject disclosure out of a desire to remain ignorant or the patient may have already had a similar medical experience.

vi. A doctor is privileged not to advise the patient of the matters that are of common knowledge or of the matters of which the patient has actual knowledge, particularly on the basis of his/her experience.

vii. No duty to inform arises in an emergency in which the patient is unconscious or otherwise incapable of giving valid consent and harm of failure to treat is imminent and outweighs any harm threatened by the proposed treatment.

Other Exceptions

If a matter becomes a matter of public record, the 'right to privacy' no longer exists and a legitimate subject for comment by press and media among others.

Again, an exception must be carved out of this rule in the interest of decency under Act 19 (2) in the following cases, viz. a female who is the victim of a sexual assault, kidnapping, addiction or a like offence should not further be subjected to the indignity of her name and the incident being published in press or media.

The second exception is that 'the' 'right to privacy' or the remedy of action for damage is simply not available to public officials as long as the criticism concerns the discharge of their 'public duties'.

Emergency Cases: In case where a patient is:

1. Unconscious/of unsound mind.
2. Relative/guardian not available.
3. No time to contact them.
4. Urgency of situation to save the life or avoid further damage.

In these circumstances, law presumes that consent has been given in 'Good Faith'. Doctor is **immune** to proceedings for '**damages**', '**assault**' or '**negligence**'.

As per **Section 92**, IPC: "Nothing is an offence by reason of any harm, which it may cause to a person for whose benefit it is done in good faith, even without that person's consent, if the circumstances are such that it is impossible for that person to signify consent, or if that person is incapable of giving consent, and has no guardian or other person in lawful charge of him from whom it is possible to obtain consent in time for the thing to be done with benefit, provided":

This exception shall not extend to the intentional causing/attempting to cause death. This exception shall not extend to "doing of anything likely to cause death or for any purpose other than preventing of death or of grievous hurt or curing of any grievous disease or infirmity".

Components of Consent: Consent should be free, voluntary, informed, clear and direct, and wherever possible, taken in writing.

Voluntariness of Consent: The patient's consent must be 'voluntary' and must be free from any coercion or unfair persuasion (use of touts or advertisement). In other words, after providing adequate information, leave it to the patient or his guardian, as the case may be, whether he is willing to give his consent or not.

Criteria for Consent

Consent and Age

Most **confusing aspect** of 'consent' among medical fraternity is the issue of '**age of giving legally valid consent**' for medical purposes. There are '**three schools of thought**' among medical jurist. According to one school of thought, it is **12 years**, for routine medical examination other than operations and other invasive medical procedures (relay on Sections 87 and 88, IPC), another school of thought considers it as 12 years for all practical purposes irrespective of invasive or non-invasive medical procedures, and **third school of thought** considers it as 18 years, for operations or invasive medical procedures, and 12 years for routine medical procedures. This confusion is also evident among our legislatures, when we go through different statutory provisions like organ transplantation, blood donation, abortion, etc.

Reasons for this confusion, according to our opinion, could be many, like lack of awareness and illiteracy of most of India's population, leading to no dispute on this issue with medical fraternity. No sincere efforts are made by medical jurist to seek clarification from Honorable **Supreme Court** on this issue.

In England, regarding the issue of 'age of consent', Section, 8 of The Family Law Reform Act, 1960, which provides that the consent to medical, surgical or dental treatment of a 'minor' who has attained the age of 16 years shall be effective consent and that in such cases, it is not necessary to obtain the consent of the parent or guardian.

In **USA**, age of giving consent is different in different States varies between **18** and **19 years.** (NMS series) I have made an attempt so that this confusion can be removed from the minds of concerned persons. First, I would like to discuss legal provisions related to this issue.

Emancipated Minors: This class of minors (who have not attained age of 18 years) include minors who are married, live away from their parent's home or are financially independent and are regarded as having an adult capacity to consent to health care.

Some States in the USA, by statute, have fixed **a lower age of consent** for health care, especially regarding the diagnosis and treatment of sexual and reproductive problems (contraception, abortion, pregnancy, venereal diseases) and drug or alcohol abuse.

Mature Minor Exception: Some States in the USA, by case law, recognize a 'mature minor exception', allowing minors to give consent to health care under certain circumstances, such as when there is a pressing need for care, when the consent of a patient or guardian cannot be obtained easily and when the minor patient has sufficient mental ability to understand the implications of the treatment.

As per **Section 87 IPC**: A person above 18 years of age can give valid consent for an "act not intended and not known to be likely to cause death or grievous hurt".

As per **Section 88 IPC**: A person can give valid consent for an "act not intended to cause death, done in good faith for person's benefit. **Section 88, IPC** is ambiguous and are not specific for medical treatment. The implication is that consent of parents or guardians is necessary for surgical or medical procedures if the patient is a minor.

Section 88 sanctions the infliction of any harm if it is for the benefit of the person to whom it is caused. If a person gives a free and intelligent consent to take the risk of an operation, which in a large proportion of cases has proved fatal, the surgeon who operates cannot be punished even if death ensues. Section **88** differs from the Section **87** in **two aspects**:

1. Under this Section, any harm except death may be inflicted.
2. The age of the person consenting is not mentioned.

Persons not qualified as medical practitioners cannot claim the benefit of this section as they can hardly be deemed to act in '**good faith**' as that expression is defined in Section 52, IPC.

As per **Section 89 IPC**: A child under 12 years of age and an insane person cannot give valid consent for an "act done in good faith for its benefit. The consent of the guardian is necessary."

As per **Section 90 IPC**: Consent known to be given under fear of injury or due to misconception of the fact is not valid.

As per **Section 92 IPC**: "Act done in good faith for benefit of the person without consent".

Competency for Giving Consent

It is perhaps the most **important legal ingredient** and may be best considered as a '**capacity**', i.e. '**soundness of mind**' and '**maturity of the mind**' to understand the nature and consequences to which he is going to give consent. In India, a child above 7 years of age and under 12 years, is presumed to be capable of committing an offence, if he has attained 'sufficient maturity of understanding' to judge the nature and consequences of his conduct on that occasion. According to English law, the maturity is presumed between 8–14 years, until the contrary is proved.

In USA, The President's Commission for the Study of Ethical Problems in Medicine and Biomedical and Behavioral Research (1983) defined competency as "the patient's capability to understand information relevant to the decision and to reason about relevant alternatives against a background of reasonably stable personal values and life goals".

According to **Section 118**, IEA, every person is competent to testify as witness, unless the court considers that he is prevented from understanding the questions put to him, or from giving rational answers to those questions due to tender age, whether of body or mind, or any other cause of same kind. Under the **Indian Oath Amendment Act, 1939**, the unsworn evidence of a child under 12 years of age is admissible.

Concept of Adult, Majority or Minority

Under the **Indian Majority Act, 1875**, a person is deemed to attain his '**majority**' on the completion of 18 years, when he assumes full civil rights and responsibilities. Where a minor is under the guardianship of the **Court of Wards** (a guardian appointed by the Court) he is not deemed to attain his '**majority**' until he is 21 years of age.

Under The **Bombay Prevention of Hindu Bigamous Marriages Act**, 1946, a '**minor**' means any person who is under 16 years of age. The **Bombay Children Act, 1948**, provides that a 'child' means a boy or a girl who has not attained the age of 16 years.

Under The **Factories Act, 1948**, an 'adult' is defined as a person who has **completed his 18th year**, an '**adolescent**' is defined as a person who has completed his 15 years, but has not completed 18 years, and a '**child**' is defined as a person who has not completed his 15th year (Sections 2, 51, 54, 55, 67, 70, and 71).

Scope of Consent

When a patient gives his consent to a surgical procedure or for a specific type of treatment, the performance of that particular procedure or treatment, the legal validity, the scope and extent of consent is limited to whatever contents were expressed to the patient at the time of obtaining the consent; however, in exceptional circumstances, an extension of the scope of the consent would be permissible.

The general rule, however, dictates that a doctor commits assault or battery if he exceeds the scope of the consent given by the patient. Thus, if a doctor who performed a non-emergency hysterectomy when he found infected fallopian tubes during the surgery in a patient who had consented only to a repair of a lacerated uterus, it would exceed the scope of consent.

Consent of Female Patients

Examination of a gynecology/obstetrics case should be made after obtaining a written, informed consent and in presence of a witness (female nurse/relative of a patient). Similar guidelines applied for examination of private parts of a male patient.

As per The **MTP Act, 1971**, consent for termination of pregnancy of the pregnant woman alone is sufficient, provided she is:

i. Not of unsound mind.
ii. Understands the nature, purpose and consequences of what she is consenting to.
iii. Consent of spouse is not necessary.
iv. Above 18 years of age. It is enough if she says that "she is above 18 years of age, no documentary proof is needed". In England, the age is 16 years.

Consent is Not Required

Statutory Provisions: When an operation has been made compulsory by law (vaccination, polio drops, etc.), no consent is necessary.

Unconscious Patient: Findings can be divulged to the police only after the patient regains consciousness and gives his valid consent.

Consent of Spouse: Not necessary in cases of procedures involving no genital organs or reproductive functions. It is advisable to take consent of spouse if the act involves danger to life, impairment of sexual functions or destruction of an unborn child.

Consent for Sterilization

In 1973, in the UK, the Minister of State, Department of Health and Social Security, was asked in the House of Lords whether 'it is a fact that under either English or Scottish law, a woman must obtain her husband's permission for a ligation of tube, but a man can have a vasectomy performed without the permission of his wife?'. He replied that he had been advised that there was no statutory requirement under either English or Scottish law that the consent of a spouse must be obtained to the sterilization of the partner. It is detained, however, whether in common law, a man has a legal right to the opportunity of having children by his wife and whether, if deprived of that right without his agreement, he could claim damages against a surgeon. Accordingly, doctors would be wise to continue to obtain the signatures of both spouses whenever possible until an actual Court case arises, which would set a precedence under either English or Scottish law.

If the operation is to be carried out on therapeutic grounds, it would not be necessary in law to obtain the consent of the spouse. If the patient is not living with his or her spouse, the consent of the patient is all that is necessary.

Consent for Abortion

For sterilization operations, consent of both the spouses is necessary—for 'tubectomy' take consent of husband; and for 'vasectomy' take consent of wife.

The written consent of the patient who is to undergo a termination of pregnancy should always be obtained. If the patient is married and living with her husband, the proposed operation should be discussed with him if time and circumstances permit. Every endeavor should be made to obtain his consent to the termination of the pregnancy unless the patient expressly forbids it.

If the patient is single, no consent is required from the putative father. Prudence dictates, however, that the doctor should endeavor to obtain the consent of the parents of such a girl, if she is living with them. The practitioner must obtain the girl's authority before he seeks the consent of her parents as her wishes must always be respected. If the girl is under 16, her parents should always be consulted even if she herself forbids the doctor to do so. In such cases, written consent of the parents should be obtained, but their refusal should not be allowed to prevent a lawful termination to which the patient herself consents and which, in the doctor's opinion, is clinically necessary. A termination should never be carried out in opposition to the girl's wishes even if the parents demand it.

Doctrine of Loco Parentis

As per **Section 92 IPC**, emergency situation involving children, when parents/local guardians are not available, consent can be taken from people at the spot, like teachers/hostel wardens/guides/medical superintendent/principal or court of law, etc.

'S', a surgeon, sees a child suffer an accident, which is likely to prove fatal unless an operation be immediately performed. There is no time to appeal to the child's guardian. 'S' performs the operation in spite of the enteritis of the child, intending, in good faith, the child benefit. 'S' has committed no offence.

In another illustration, 'A' is thrown from his horse, and is **insensible**. 'S' a surgeon, finds that 'A' requires to be trepanned. 'S', not intending 'A's death, but in good faith, for 'A's benefit, performs the trepan before 'A' recovers his power of judging for himself. 'S' has committed no offence.

This Section is designed to meet those cases, which do not come under either Section 88 or Section 89. The main objective is protection of the medical practitioners. In above illustrations, it is impossible to obtain consent from the patients.

The Authors of the Code Observe: "There yet remains a kindred class of cases which are by no means of rare occurrence. For example, a person falls down in an apoplectic fit. Bleeding can alone save him, and he is unable to signify his consent to be bled. The surgeon who bleeds him commits an act falling under the definition of an offence. The surgeon is not the patient's guardian, and has no authority from any such guardian, yet it is evident that the surgeon ought not to be punished."

"In these examples, there is what may be called a '**temporary guardianship**' justified by the exigency of the case and by the humanity of the motive. This 'temporary guardianship' bears a considerable analogy to that of 'temporary magistracy' with which the law invests every person who present when a great is committed, or when the public peace is concerned. To acts done in the exercise of this '**temporary guardianship**', we extend a protection very similar to that, which we have given to the acts of regular guardians".

Law and Consent

As per Section 90, IPC: '**Consent**' is **not valid** if it is given by the **person under**:

1. Fear of an injury.
2. Misconception of fact.
3. Unsoundness of mind.
4. Intoxication.

- And the person obtaining the consent knows or has reason to believe this.
- And who is unable to understand the nature and consequences of that to which he gives his consent.

If consent is refused, it is an absolute bar for examination/treatment. If a doctor fails to give correct information regarding the procedure before obtaining consent, he may be **sued for Negligence** (**U/S 304**) or **punished by the MCI/SMC**, for unethical act or professional misconduct.

If he does not take consent at all, he **may be charged with** assault (Section **351**, **IPC** Tress pass of Privacy). Thus, consent is a legal requirement also for medical examination and treatment both surgical and conservative. The nature of the consent varies according to circumstances and needs of the patient.

Consent and Medicolegal Cases

In medicolegal cases, as practiced in the North India (States of Punjab, Haryana, Union Territory of Chandigarh and Himachal Pradesh), where the doctor usually obtains the consent in the following manner:

1. That "I am willing for my medicolegal examination".
2. That "I have not been examined before by any other doctor".
3. That "There are no other injuries except those describe".
4. That "The address given by me is correct".
5. That "I have been informed about the nature and consequences of the examination".

Consent may be obtained in following wordings

I Mr/Mrs ____________________
S/O, W/O, D/O ____________________
hereby give my full, free and voluntary consent for myself/my ward's ____________
complete medical examination along with all relevant investigations for preparing a medicolegal report, the consequences of which have been fully explained to me by doctor ____________________

Signature (relation with patient if minor)

Written, informed consent is absolutely essential before commencing to examine the patient (**victim/accused**). Patient has to be explained by the examining doctor about the

- **Nature**: Medicolegal examination (detailed procedure)
- **Purpose**: To make a medicolegal report
- **Consequences**: Findings may go against the patient under the examination.

Only after obtaining his **free**, **voluntary** and **written consent**, doctor can proceed with the examination. In these cases, consent should be taken after informing the person that he has the right to refuse examination and that the report may go in his favor or against him. Consent of the legal heir of the deceased is not necessary for medicolegal postmortem examination of the body of the deceased. But, consent of the legal heir of the deceased is necessary for pathological postmortem examination to be conducted on the body of the deceased or for removal of organs or organ.

This is Every Man's Fundamental Right

In cases where **a person has been arrested on charge of committing an offence** of such a nature and alleged to have been committed under such circumstances that there are reasonable grounds for believing that an examination of his person will yield evidence as to commission of an offence, it shall be lawful for a medical practitioner, acting at request of a police officer **not below the rank of a sub-inspector**, and for any person acting **in good faith** in aid and under his direction, to make such an examination of the arrested person as is reasonably necessary in order to ascertain the facts, which may afford such evidence, and to use such force as is reasonably necessary for that purpose [Section 53 (1), CrPC].

Section 53 (2) CrPC: "Whenever the person is a female she is to be examined under this section, the examination shall be done only by or under the supervision of a female registered medical practitioner".

Cases of Drunkenness

A patient should not be examined in such cases for the purpose of making a medicolegal report without his valid consent. If the person is not in a state of sound mind or he is unconscious, then the same may be taken from his relative who may act as temporary guardian, so for his examination and treatment is concerned.

But if he is not accompanied by anybody, then, for his benefit, his examination and treatment can be carried out without consent. A medicolegal report may be prepared without his consent, but it should be submitted only with his consent when he becomes conscious. But, if he is involved in an offence and arrested, then the same may be furnished and submitted even without his consent, if needed by the court of law or investigating police officer (Section 53 CrPC).

As per **Section 90 IPC**, consent of a person who is under the influence of alcohol/any other inebriant/stupefying agent at the time of giving, is not a valid consent. The physical examination and any relevant investigations for the purpose of treating alone may be carried out. The purpose of the examination/investigations can be divulged to the police only after the patient regains consciousness and gives his valid consent.

Such a patient loses this right if he has been arrested by the police for causing nuisance under influence of alcohol in **Public Interest** [(Section 53 (1) CrPC].

Right to Refuse Consent

When a patient or his guardian rejects or refuse a treatment, he should be advised in a discreet, ethical, moral and professional manner about the consequences of not taking treatment. After that it is open to the patient or his guardian whether they want to continue the treatment or not. If not, the same may be noted down in the records of the patients as "**leave against medical advice**" (**LAMA**) and patient may be discharged. This is what may be termed by some authors as "Informed Refusal" of the patient.

Only Competent Patient has a 'Right to Refuse Treatment'

It is generally agreed that in the absence of an emergency, only a competent patient can refuse surgical or medical treatment. However, 'right to refuse' life-saving treatment is not absolute. There may be situations where certain refusal to medical treatment may conflict with the compelling state-interests. A patient's right to refuse life-saving treatment is balanced by the

State's right in human life under Article 21 of The Constitution of India.

The following are '**Compelling State's Rights**', recognized by the law:

1. Preservation of human life is a paramount State's duty.
2. The State has a compelling interest to override a person's right to refuse life-saving treatment to protect innocent third parties (minor children, spouse and incompetent adults).
3. The state has a duty to prevent suicide.
4. Allowing forcible feeding to a patient sitting on hunger strike, if his condition becomes critical.
5. The State has a duty in maintaining the ethical integrity of the medical profession.

Discharge from Hospital: It is unlawful to detain a patient (adult and of a sound mind) in a hospital against his wishes. If he demands discharge against medical advice (**DAMA**), the same is to be recorded in his case.

MEDICAL NEGLIGENCE

Negligence involves not "neglect" or "carelessness" but failure to take such care as the circumstances demand. Negligence was first defined by Justice Baron Alderson in 1856 as "The omission to do something which a reasonable man could do or doing something which a prudent and a reasonable man would not do".

Professional negligence is defined as want of reasonable care and skill or wilful negligence on the part of the medical practitioner while treating a patient resulting in bodily injury, ill health or death.

Definition and Explanation

The definition of negligence as given in *Law of Torts*, Ratanlal and Dhirajlal (edited by Justice GP Singh), referred to hereinabove, holds good. Honorable Supreme Court in "Mahadev Prasad Kaushik vs. State of UP and Anr (2009)" in paragraph 31 states:

"Though the term 'negligence' has not been defined in the Code, it may be stated that **negligence is the omission to do something which a reasonable man, guided upon those considerations, which ordinarily regulate the conduct of human affairs would do**, or **doing something, which a reasonable and prudent man would not do**."

The essential components of negligence are three: "**duty**", "**breach**" and "**resulting damage**".

Negligence in the context of the medical profession necessarily calls for a treatment with a difference. To infer rashness or negligence on the part of a professional, in particular a doctor, additional considerations apply. A case of occupational negligence is different from one of professional negligence.

Classification of Medical Negligence

1. Civil Negligence
2. Criminal Negligence
4. Contributory Negligence
5. Corporate Negligence
6. Negligence per se

Civil Negligence

Civil negligence (malpraxis) is a form of negligence in which a patient brings an action for damages in a civil court against his medical attendant, who owned him a duty in tort of care, if he had suffered injury in consequence of negligence or unskilled treatment. This question arises:

i. When a patient or, in the event of his death, his relatives, sue a doctor in a civil court for compensation for the injury or death of the patient as the cause may be, due to negligence of the doctor, or
ii. When the doctor brings a civil suit for realization of his professional fees from the patient or his relatives who refuse to pay the same on ground of malpractice.

The differences between civil and criminal negligence are listed in **Table 3.1**.

Table 3.1 Differences between criminal and civil negligence

Features	Criminal negligence	Civil negligence
Type of wrong	Public wrong	Civil wrong
Law applicability	Indian Penal Code	Common law/law of tort
Breach of duty	Against public/community/state	Against individual
Affected party	Public/Community/Society	Individual/family
Violation of duty/right	Clear violation of defined duty or rights of public, e.g. 304-A, 320, 336, 337, 338 IPC	Need not clear violation
Degree of proof	Proved beyond reasonable doubt	Prove of mere preponderance of probability is enough
Contributory negligence	Not a defense	A good defense
Consent	Not a defense	A good defense
Petitioner	State prosecuting agent or agency	Individual/legal heir
Award	Punishment (imprisonment and/or fine)	Damages (monetary compensation)
Trial-court of law	Criminal court	Civil court/consumer court
Trial	Exhaustive trial	Exhaustive/summary trial in case of consumer court

Essential Elements of Negligence

Liability of negligence arises if the following conditions are satisfied:

1. **Duty of care:** Existence of duty of care by a doctor.
2. **Dereliction of duty:** The failure on the part of the doctor to maintain applicable standard of care and skill.
3. **Direct causation:** The failure to exercise a duty of care must lead to damage.
4. **Damage:** The damage should be of a type that would have been foreseen by a reasonable physician.

It needs no emphasis that in the medical negligence actions, the burden is on the claimant to prove breach of duty, injury and causation. The injury must be sufficiently proximate to the medical practitioner's breach of duty. In the absence of evidence to the contrary adduced by the opposite party, an inference of causation may be drawn even though positive or scientific proof is lacking. Any absence of proper skill or care that causes the patient's death, diminishes his chances of recovery, prolongs his illness or increases his sufferings, constitutes injury in a legal sense. Some examples are:

- Loss of earnings
- Expenses incurred
- Reduction in expectation of life
- Reduced enjoyment of life
- Pain and sufferings
- Loss of potency
- Aggravation of a pre-existing condition
- Death.

Standard of Judgment

Any task, which is required to be performed with a special skill, would generally be admitted or undertaken to be performed only if the person possesses the requisite skill for performing that task. Judged by this standard, a professional may be held liable for negligence on one of two findings:

1. Either he does not possess the requisite skill which he professes to have possessed, or,
2. He did not exercise, with reasonable competence in the given case, the skill, which he did possess.

The standard to be applied for judging, whether the person charged has been negligent or not, would be that of an ordinary competent person exercising ordinary skill in that profession. It is not necessary for every professional to possess the highest level of expertise in the branch he practices.

In a case, CA Sedley LJ said that where a profession embraces a range of views as to what is an acceptable standard of conduct, the competence of the defendant is to be judged by the lowest standard that would be regarded as acceptable.

What is 'Bolam Test'?

The quoted passage defining negligence by professionals, generally and not necessarily confined to doctors, is to be found, in the opinion of McNair J, in a Bolam case in the following words:

"Where you get a situation which involves the use of some special skill or competence, then the test as to whether there has been negligence or not, is not the test of the man on the top of a Clapham omnibus, because he has not got this special skill. The test is the standard of the ordinary skilled man exercising and professing to have that special skill... A man need not possess the highest expert skill; it is well-established law that it is sufficient if he exercises the ordinary skill of an ordinary competent man exercising that particular art".

The water of Bolam test has ever since flown and passed under several bridges, having been cited and dealt with in several judicial pronouncements, one after the other and has continued to be well-received by every shore, it has touched as neat, clean and well-condensed one. After a review of various authorities, Bingham LJ, in his speech in a case, summarized the Bolam test in the following words:

"From these general statements, it follows that a professional man should command the corpus of knowledge, which forms part of the professional equipment of the ordinary member of his profession. He should not lag behind other ordinary assiduous and intelligent members of his profession in knowledge of new advances, discoveries and developments in his field. He should have such awareness as an ordinarily competent practitioner would have of the deficiencies in his knowledge and the limitations on his skill. He should be alert to the hazards and risks in any professional task he undertakes to the extent that other ordinarily competent members of the profession would be alert. He must bring to any professional task he undertakes no less expertise, skill and care than other ordinarily competent members of his profession would bring, but needs bring no more. The standard is that of the reasonable average. The law does not require of a professional man that he be a paragon combining the qualities of polymath and prophet".

Degree of Skill and Care Required by a Medical Practitioner

Deviation from normal practice is not necessarily evidence of negligence. To establish liability on that basis it must be shown:

1. That there is a usual and normal practice;
2. That the defendant has not adopted it; and
3. That the course adopted is one no professional man of ordinary skill would have taken had he been acting with ordinary care.

Aforementioned three tests have also been stated as determinative of negligence in professional practice by Charles Worth and Percy in their celebrated work on Negligence.

Instances of Medical Negligence

1. Refusal to admit patients requiring urgent hospitalization.
2. Failure to obtain informed consent.
3. Failure to examine patient himself.
4. Failure to inform the patient of the risk of refusal for treatment.
5. Failure to immunize and to perform sensitivity tests when indicated.
6. Not ordering X-ray examination where the history suggests the possibility of a fracture or dislocation or presence of a foreign body in a wound.

7. Not reading the X-ray film correctly or in failing to get it read by a competent person.
8. Failure to attend the patient in time.
9. Making a wrong diagnosis due to absence of skill or care.
10. Negligent management of procedures.
11. Failure to provide a substitute during his absence.
12. To delegate his duty of treating or operating upon a patient to another doctor without the consent of the patient.
13. Failure to give proper postoperative care.
14. Failure to give proper instructions.
15. Failure to keep well-informed of advances in medical sciences.
16. Failure to warn the patient of side effects.
17. Failure to obtain consultation where appropriate.
18. Experimenting on patient without consent.
19. Giving overdose of medicine and giving poisonous medicines carelessly.
20. Continue to practice regarding which several warnings as to its dangers have been given.
21. Iatrogenic medical complications during diagnosis or treatment.
22. Prematurely discharging the patient.

Doctrine of Res Ipsa Loquitur

It means "**the facts** or **things speak for itself**"; the patient need not prove the negligence. This doctrine is applied to both civil and criminal negligence. It cannot be applied against several defendants. *Res Ipsa Loquitur* is a rule of evidence, which in reality belongs to the law of torts. Inference as to negligence may be drawn from proved circumstances by applying the rule, if the cause of the accident is unknown and no reasonable explanation as to the cause is coming forth from the defendant. In criminal proceedings, the burden of proving negligence as an essential ingredient of the offence lies on to prosecution. Such ingredient cannot be said to have been proved or made out by resorting to the said rule.

Incidentally, it may be noted that in another case, the court has observed that there may be a case where the proved facts would themselves speak of sharing of common intention and while making such observation one of the learned judges constituting the Bench has in his concurring opinion merely stated "*Res Ipsa Loquitur*". Nowhere, it has been stated that the rule has applicability in a criminal case and an inference as to an essential ingredient of an offence can be found proved by resorting to the said rule. In our opinion, a case under Section 304A IPC cannot be decided solely by applying the rule of *Res Ipsa Loquitur*.

Even in civil jurisdiction, the rule of *Res Ipsa Loquitur* is not of universal application and has to be applied with extreme care and caution to the cases of professional negligence and in particular that of the doctors. Else, it would be counterproductive. Simply because a patient has not favorably responded to a treatment given by a physician or a surgery has failed, the doctor cannot be held liable per se by applying the doctrine of *Res Ipsa Loquitur*.

Examples of Res Ipsa Loquitur

The doctrine means that things speak for themselves. Where there is such a situation, the negligence on the part of the surgeon is taken for granted without any further evidence. In the case of Spring Meadows Hospital vs Ahluwalia, the Supreme Court has observed that gross medical mistakes will always result in a finding of negligence. Use of wrong drug or wrong gas during the course of anesthetic administration will frequently lead to the imposition of liability and, in some situations, even the principle of *Res Ipsa Loquitur* can be applied.

In another case, the Supreme Court made somewhat similar observations. In this case, one Chandrika Bai was admitted to the Government Hospital where she delivered a child on 10.07.1963. She had a sterilization operation on 13.07.1963. This operation is not known to be serious in nature and, in fact, was performed under local anesthesia. Complications arose thereafter, which resulted in second operation being performed on her on 19.07.1963. She did not survive the operation and died on 24.07.1963.

Both Dr Divan and Dr Purandave stated that the cause of death was peritonitis. It was held that in a case like this, the doctrine of *Res Ipsa Loquitur* clearly applies because a mop (towel) was left inside her peritoneal cavity. The State was made to pay the damages. The doctor was found negligent.

The Karnataka State Commission, while commenting on the doctrine of *Res Ipsa Loquitur*, observed as under:

"The Court also took note that the law recognizes the dangers, which are inherent in surgical operations and that mistakes will occur on occasions despite the exercise of reasonable skill and care. The Court further quoted Street on Tort, wherein it was stated that the doctrine of *Res Ipsa Loquitur* was attracted.

"Where an unexplained accident occurs from a thing under the control of defendant, and medical or other expert evidence shows that such accident would not happen if proper care were used, there is at least evidence of negligence for a jury."

Criminal Negligence and Res Ipsa Loquitur

In a case from Bihar, the complainant was operated for retinal detachment in right eye. He lost his eyesight. Though neither side could produce any clear or credible explanation for damage, the Commission observed that the maxim *Res Ipsa Loquitur* would be attracted. The complainant had vitreous hemorrhage, and it should have invited serious attention of doctor to have treated it effectively.

Non-applicability in Certain Other Cases

It may, however, be mentioned that if according to medical science, there are chances of failure of any surgical operation, then the maxim of *Res Ipsa Loquitur* shall not apply. The Gujarat High Court in a case observed in First Appeal Nos. 145 to 150 (decided on 5.7.1995) that in case of failure of family planning operation, the doctrine of *Res Ispa Loquitur* shall not apply because 1–4% of the operations for removal of tissues in the region of prostate could cause incontinence.

A similar observation was made in the case Gray vs. Wehetar to the effect that the maxim of *Res Ipsa Loquitur* would not apply in the case of failure of sterilization by means of tubal ligation.

Respondent Superior (Vicarious Liability)

The employer is responsible for the wrongful deeds of his employees. Doctrine of common knowledge is based on the assumption that the issue of negligence in a particular case is not related to the technical matters, which are within the knowledge of medical profession. Here the patient must prove the causative factors that had resulted in the negligence, but he need not produce the evidences to establish the standard of care.

Court's Views in Favor of Doctors

A medical practitioner faced with an emergency, ordinarily tries his best to redeem the patient out of his suffering. He does not gain anything by acting with negligence or by omitting to do an act. Obviously, therefore, it will be for the complainant to clearly make out a case of negligence before a medical practitioner is charged with or proceeded against criminally. A surgeon with shaky hands under fear of legal action cannot perform a successful operation, and a quivering physician cannot administer the end-dose of medicine to his patient.

Loss to Society

"If the hands be trembling with the dangling fear of facing a criminal prosecution in the event of failure for whatever reason, whether attributable to himself or not, neither a surgeon can successfully wield his life-saving scalper to perform an essential surgery nor a physician can successfully administer the life-saving dose of medicine. Discretion being better part of valor, a medical professional would feel better advised to leave a terminal patient to his own fate in the case of emergency where the chance of success may be 10% (or so), rather than taking the risk of making a last ditch effort towards saving the subject and facing a criminal prosecution if his effort fails. Such timidity forced upon a doctor would be a disservice to the society."

What is the Purpose of Law for Holding a Doctor Negligent?

The purpose of holding a professional liable for his act or omission, if negligent, is to make the life safer and to eliminate the possibility of recurrence of negligence in future. Human body and medical science both are too complex to be easily understood. To hold in favor of existence of negligence, associated with the action or inaction of a medical professional, requires an in-depth understanding of the working of a professional as also the nature of the job and of errors committed by chance, which do not necessarily involve the element of culpability.

Negligence by Medical Professionals Calls for Treatment with a Difference

The subject of negligence in the context of medical profession necessarily calls for treatment with a difference. Several relevant considerations in this regard are found mentioned in the literature.

Human Attitude

There is a marked tendency to look for a human actor to blame for an untoward event: a tendency, which is closely linked with the desire to punish. Things have gone wrong and, therefore, somebody must be found to answer for it. To draw a distinction between the blameworthy and the blameless, the notion of *mens rea* has to be elaborately understood. An empirical study would reveal that the background to a mishap is frequently far more complex than may generally be assumed. It can be demonstrated that actual blame for the outcome has to be attributed with great caution.

Need for a Deeper Understanding of the Practical Side of Medicine

For a medical accident or failure, the responsibility may lie with the medical practitioner and, equally, it may not. The inadequacies of the system, the specific circumstances of the case, the nature of human psychology itself and sheer chance may have combined to produce a result in which the doctor's contribution is either relatively or completely blameless.

Human body and its working is nothing less than a highly complex machine. Coupled with the complexities of medical science, the scope for misimpressions, misgivings and misplaced allegations against the operator, i.e. the doctor, cannot be ruled out. One may have notions of best or ideal practice, which are different from the reality of how medical practice is carried on or how in real life the doctor functions. The factors of pressing need and limited resources cannot be ruled out from consideration. Dealing with a case of medical negligence needs a deeper understanding of the practical side of medicine.

Need for Careful Consideration by the Judiciary

At least three weighty considerations can be pointed out that, any forum trying the issue of medical negligence in any jurisdiction, must keep in mind:

1. That legal and disciplinary procedure should be properly founded on firm, moral and scientific grounds;
2. That patients will be better served if the real causes of harm are properly identified and appropriately acted upon; and
3. That many incidents involve a contribution from more than one person and the tendency is to blame the last identifiable element in the chain of causation: the person holding the 'smoking gun.'

Medical Professionals in Criminal Law Treated on Different Footings

The criminal law has invariably placed the medical professionals on a pedestal different from ordinary mortals. Act in 'good faith,' 'not intended to cause death' even 'without consent' for the 'benefit of sufferer' is not negligence. Section 88 IPC provides exemption for act not intended to cause death, done by consent in good faith for person's benefit.

No Security of Human Life

"To punish as a murderer, every man who, while committing a heinous offence, causes death by pure misadventure, is a course which evidently adds nothing to the security of human life. No man can so conduct himself as to make it absolutely certain that he shall not be so unfortunate as to cause the death of a fellow-creature. The utmost that he can do is to abstain from everything, which is likely to cause death. No fear of punishment can make him do more than this; and therefore, to punish a man who has done this can add nothing to the security of human life. The only good effect, which such punishment can produce, will be to deter people from committing any of those offences, which turn into murders what are in themselves mere accidents. It is in fact an addition to the punishment of those offences, and it is an addition made in the very worst way".

The following statement of law on criminal negligence in reference to surgeons, doctors, etc., and unskillful treatment is classic:

"Where a person, acting as a medical man, he be, whether licensed or unlicensed, is so negligent in his treatment of a patient that death results, it is manslaughter if the negligence was so great as to amount to a crime, and whether or not there was such a degree of negligence is a question in each case for the jury. In explaining to juries the test which they should apply to determine whether the negligence in the particular case amounted or did not amount to a crime, judges have used many epithets, such as 'culpable', 'criminal', 'gross', 'wicked', 'clear', 'complete'. But whatever epithet be used and whether an epithet be used or not, in order to establish criminal liability the facts must be such that, in the opinion of the jury, the negligence of the accused went beyond a mere matter of compensation between subjects and showed such disregard for the life and safety of others as to amount to a crime against the State and conduct deserving punishment".

"Whether he be licensed or unlicensed, if he display gross ignorance, or gross inattention, or gross rashness, in his treatment he is criminally responsible. Where a person who, though not educated as an accoucheur, had been in the habit of acting as a man midwife and had unskillfully treated a woman, who died in childbirth, was indicted for the murder, L Ellenborough said that there was no evidence of murder, but the jury might convict of man-slaughter. "To substantiate that charge the prisoner must have been guilty of criminal misconduct, arising either from the grossest ignorance or the [most?] criminal inattention. One or other of these is necessary to make him guilty of that criminal negligence and misconduct, which is essential to make out a case of manslaughter".

Examples of Criminal Negligence

There is no role for morally delinquent doctor who shows violent indifference, deliberate omission and having associated ego in dealing with patient leading to aggravation of patient's sufferings. Court deals with such cases with strictness. In a case, patient suffered fistula as a result of operational hazards, where patient was operated where there was no indication and complete disregard to patient wishes and suffering. Honorable Bombay High Court refused to acquit punishment awarded by the lower court as an exemplary punishment for social impact it leave on such behavior in a noble profession.

i. The judgment in the matter of "Jacob Mathew vs. State of Punjab and Anr." or "Dr Suresh Gupta vs. Govt. of NCT of Delhi and Anr." cannot be applied with the same scale as the facts in both the matters are distinct. It is well settled, "each case depends on its own facts and projects different shades to assess." One cannot apply same colors of reported case to the facts of the present case. The texture of the present case has cumulative effect of Dr Desai disowning the patient, opining for operation, neglecting to operate and then neglecting to take postoperational care. Present case certainly conceives effects of Section 320 of IPC and 338 thereof.

ii. Dr Suresh Gupta's case was for quashing the proceedings; however, in the present case such exercise carried by Dr Desai up to Supreme Court in Special Leave to Appeal (Cri) No. 959 of 1996 has been negated by the Honorable Supreme Court. He was directed to face trial. He knew, patient's condition was too advanced as he had access to her medical papers, still opted for operation. Dr Hegde, another expert examined as defense accepts, "It is correct that the surgeon will not propose "**exploratory laparotomy**", if the patient's condition is too advanced or there is lot of fluid in the abdomen.

When and Where Criminal Negligence Happens?

The criminality lies in running the risk of decision of operating, then perpetuated by recklessness or indifference as to the consequences. Dr Desai failed to exercise reasonable and proper care and avoided operating the patient himself in spite of risky decision taken by him. This involves moral delinquency. Social impact of such crime cannot be lost sight of warranting exemplary condemnation. The violent indifference, deliberate omission, associated ego demonstrated by Dr Desai has put the life of the patient in a miserable situation. Patient ultimately succumbed due to abscess and operational hazards.

Doctrine of Error of Judgment

The classical statement of law in Bolam's case has been widely accepted as decisive of the standard of care required both of professional men generally and medical practitioners in particular. It has been invariably cited with approval before courts in India and applied as touchstone to test the pleas of medical negligence. In tort, it is enough for the defendant to show that the standard of care and the skill attained was that of the ordinary competent medical practitioner exercising an ordinary degree of professional skill. The fact that a defendant, charged with negligence acted in accord with the general and approved practice is enough to clear him of the charge. Two things are pertinent to be noted:

1. Firstly, the standard of care, when assessing the practice as adapted, is judged in the light of knowledge available at the time (of the incident), and not at the date of trial.
2. Secondly, when the charge of negligence arises out of failure to use same particular equipment, the charge would fail if the equipment were not generally available at that point of time on which it is suggested as should have been used.

A mere deviation from normal professional practice is not necessarily evidence of negligence. Let it also be noted that a mere accident is not violence of negligence. So also an error of judgment on the part of a professional is not negligence per se. Higher the acuteness in emergency and higher the complication, more are the chances of error of judgment. At times, the professional is confronted with making a choice between the devil and the deep sea and he has to choose the lesser evil. The medical professional is often called upon to adapt a procedure, which involves higher element of risk, but which he honestly believes as providing greater chances of success for the patient rather than a procedure involving lesser risk but higher chances of failure. Which cause is more appropriate to follow, would depend on the facts and circumstances of a given case. The usual practice prevalent nowadays is to obtain the consent of the patient or of the person in charge of the patient if the patient is not be in a position to give consent before adopting a given procedure.

So long as it can be found that the procedure, which was adopted was one that was acceptable to medical science as on that date, the medical practitioner cannot be held negligent merely because he chose to follow one procedure and not another and the result was a failure.

Doctrine of Calculated Risk

1. The doctrine is that, *Res Ipsa Loquitur* should not be applied when the injury

complained is of type that may occur even though reasonable care has been taken.
2. It is an important defense to any doctor.
3. Doctor has to produce evidence/statistics that the accepted method of treatment he employed had unavoidable risks.

Doctrine of Common Knowledge

1. It is based on the assumption that the issue of negligence in the particular case is not related to specialized knowledge or technical matters of the medical profession, but an act involving application of common knowledge.
2. It is a variant of *Res Ipsa Loquitur*.
3. Here, the patient must prove the act of commission or omission, but he need not produce evidence to establish the standard of care.

Novus Actus Interveniens

1. *Novus actus interveniens* means an unrelated action intervening, and it is accepted rarely as a plea in the courts when an element of negligence is there, e.g. like leaving a swab, gauge piece, any surgical instrument inside the abdomen after an operation.
2. If doctor is negligent, which results in deviation from the logical sequence of events, then the responsibility for the subsequent disability of death may pass from original incident to the negligent act of doctor.
3. For a plea of *novus actus interveniens*, an element of negligence is essential. It usually applies to cases of accidents and assaults.
4. Plea is rarely accepted by the courts.

Medical Maloccurrence

1. Medical maloccurrence is the legal term, which defines a less than ideal outcome of medical care and it is often unrelated to the reasonable risks of quality of care that was provided.
2. In some cases, in spite of good medical attention and care, an individual fails to respond properly, e.g. idiosyncratic response to drugs in some patients of damage to recurrent laryngeal nerve during thyroidectomy, leading to vocal paralysis.

Therapeutic Misadventure

It is a case in which an individual has been injured or had died due to some unintentional/inadvertent act by doctor or his agent or hospital (somewhat similar to medical maloccurrence). Such mishap does not provide ground for negligence. For example,

1. Hypersensitivity reactions caused by penicillin, tetracycline, aspirin and new antibiotics.
2. Radiological procedures for diagnostic purposes, e.g. poisoning by barium enema, traumatic rupture of rectum of chemical peritonitis during barium enema, injection of dye.
3. Thyroid cancer with Iodine therapy.
4. Fatal complications from hemolytic reactions with blood transfusion.
5. Prolonged use of diethylstilbestrol, a synthetic form of estrogens, may cause breast cancer.
6. Misadventure is mischance, accident of disaster.

It is three types:

- **Therapeutic**: When treatment is being given.
- **Diagnostic**: When diagnosis is the only objective at that time, e.g. injection of radiopaque dye in radiological investigation, bronchoscopy and angiography.
- **Experimental**: Where patient has agreed to serve as a subject in an experimental study (drug/operative procedure).

Mischance or 'Misadventure' or an 'Error of Judgment' Not Negligence

In the opinion of Lord Denning, "a medical practitioner was not to be held liable simply because things went wrong from mischance or misadventure or through an error of judgment in choosing one reasonable course of treatment in preference of another. A medical practitioner would be liable only where his conduct fell below that of the standards of a reasonably competent practitioner in his field".

The decision of House of Lords in a case by a Bench consisting of five Law Lords has been accepted as having settled the law on the point by holding that it is not enough to show that there is a body of competent professional opinion, which considers that decision of the defendant professional was wrong, if there also exists a body of professional opinion, equally competent, which supports the decision as reasonable under the circumstances. It is not enough to show that subsequent events show that the operation need never have been performed, if at the time the decision was taken, it was reasonable in the sense that a responsible body of medical opinion would have accepted it as proper. Lord Scarman, who recorded the leading speech with which, at her four Lords agreed, quoted the following wards of Lord President (Clyde) in another case, observing that the words cannot be bettered: "In the realm of diagnosis and treatment there is ample scope for genuine difference of opinion and one man clearly is not negligent merely because his conclusion differs from that of at her professional men.... The true test for establishing negligence in diagnosis or treatment on the part of a doctor is whether he has been proved to be guilty of such failure as no doctor of ordinary skill would be guilty of it acting with ordinary care ......" .

Lord Scarman added, "A doctor who professes to exercise a special skill must exercise the ordinary skill of his specialty. Differences of opinion and practice exist, and will always exist, in the medical as in other professions. There is seldom any one answer exclusive of all others problems of professional judgment. A court may prefer a one body of opinion to another but that is no basis for a conclusion of negligence. His Lordship further added that a judge's 'preference' for one body of distinguished professional opinion to another also professionally distinguished is not sufficient to establish negligence in a practitioner whose actions have received the seal of approval of those whose opinions, truthfully expressed, honestly held, were not preferred".

Meaning of Accident

Accident during the course of medical or surgical treatment has a wider meaning. Ordinarily, an accident means:

1. An unintended and unforeseen injurious occurrence;
2. Something that does not occur in the usual course of events; or
3. That could not be reasonably anticipated.

Care has to be taken to see that the result of an accident, which is exculpatory, may not persuade the human mind to confuse it with the consequence of negligence.

Doctrine of Respondent Superior

An employer is responsible for the negligent act of his employees by the principle of *respondent superior* (Latin, let the master answer) if these following conditions are satisfied:

1. There must be an employer-employee relationship.
2. The employee's conduct must occur within the scope of his employment.
3. Incident must occur while on the job.
4. It also called the Master-Servant Rule.
5. In medical practice, usually, the principal doctor becomes responsible for any negligence of his assistants (both medical and paramedical). Both may be sued by the patient even though the principal has no part in the negligent act.
6. A doctor may be associated temporarily with another doctor with the establishment of an employee-employer relationship between them. Thus, if one doctor assists another in the operating room for a fee the assistant is considered as an employee of the principal surgeon.

7. When two doctors practice as partners, each is liable for negligence of the other even though one may have no part in the negligent act.
8. If a swab, sponge instrument, is left in the patient's body after the operation the surgeon is liable for damages. A surgeon is not liable for the negligence of anesthetist and the anesthetist is not liable for the negligence of the operating surgeon.
9. **Borrowed servant doctrine**: An employee may serve more than one employer, e.g. the nurse employed as servant of the operations will be the borrowed servant of the operating surgeon during the operation and the servant of the hospital for all other purposes.
10. Physicians and surgeons are not responsible for the negligent acts of competent nurse or other hospital personnel unless such acts are carried out under their direct supervision and control.
11. A hospital as an employer is responsible for negligence of its employees who are acting under its supervision and control.
12. Hospital management cannot be held responsible for the negligent acts of members of the senior medical staff in the treatment of patients, if it can be proved that the management exercised due care and skill in selecting properly qualified and experienced staff.
13. Hospital management is held responsible for the mistakes of resident physicians and interns in training who are considered employee when performing their normal duties. A physician is responsible for the acts of the interns and residents carried out under his direct supervision and control.
14. Both the employer and employee are sued by the patient because the employee may lack funds for paying the damages. Usually, liability will be fixed upon those actually at fault and those whose control over the negligence is demonstrable.

To avoid vicarious liability, an employer must demonstrate either that the employee was not negligent or the employee was reasonably careful or that the employee had gone on a detour wherein the employee was acting in his own right rather than on the employer's business.

Contributory Negligence

Any unreasonable conduct or absence of ordinary care on part of the patient or his attendant, which combined with doctor's negligence contributed to the injury complained of, as a direct cause and without which the injury would not have occurred. Absence of reasonable care on the part of the patient or his attendant that combines with the negligent action of the doctor resulting in the damage completed off directly and without which, damage should not have occurred.

Advantages of Contributory Negligence

1. Good defense of the doctor in civil cases, but not in criminal cases.
2. Doctor has to prove patient's negligence. But doctor is expected to foresee that the patient may harm himself and to warn accordingly, e.g. patient did not give proper history, failure to follow doctor's instructions, drugs tests and diet, or leaving the hospital against doctor's advice.
3. Damages awarded by the court may reduce.
4. Not to provide proper history to the doctor (acute abdomen, female unmarried patient, history of sexual contact), but it is the duty of the doctor to take all possible history significant in a particular case.
5. Failure to follow the line of treatment.
6. Refusal to take up the suggested advice (hot water bottle).
7. Leaving the hospital against the doctor's advice (LAMA).
8. Failure to seek further medical treatment if the signs and symptoms persists (follow-up treatment/advice).

Composite Negligence

Injury is caused to the person without any negligence on his part, but as a result of the combined effect of the negligence of some other persons (two or more) and the persons responsible for such damage is known as **composite tortfeasors.**

Corporate Negligence

It is the failure of those in hospital administration who are responsible for providing the treatment, accommodation and facilities necessary to carry out the purpose of the institution to follow the established standard of conduct. It occurs when hospital:

i. Provides defective equipment or drugs.
ii. Selects or retains incompetent employee including doctors.
iii. Fails in some other manner to meet the accepted standard of care and such failure results in injury to a patient to whom the hospital owes a duty.

Product Liability

It refers to the physical agent that caused the injury or death of the patient during treatment.

i. The plaintiff must prove that:
   a. Manufacturer departed from standards of due care, with respect to design, manufacture assembly, packing failure to test and inspect for defects or failure to warn or give adequate instructions.
   b. Defect was the proximate to cause injury/death.
ii. If it is proved, the manufacturer becomes responsible for injury or death.
iii. The burden of proving the safety and effectiveness of a new drug/device/instrument lies with the manufacturer.

Defenses Available in Case of Medical Negligence

i. No duty owed to the plaintiff by the physician.
ii. The duty was discharged according to the prevailing standards of practice of medicine.
iii. The damage caused could be due to other person who was concerned in providing the treatment.
iv. The damage was the result of third party intervention without his or her knowledge.
v. The case is contributory negligence.
vi. The damage suffering is an expected outcome of the disease of the patient suffered from.
vii. It was a therapeutic misadventure. Therapeutic misadventure is an accident or unexpected damage to the patient when the doctor is attending the patient during the treatment.
viii. It was error in judgment, but all errors of judgments are not defense against negligence.
ix. The case should be filed within 2 years from the date of alleged negligence.
x. *Res Judicata*—(law a matter already decided upon that cannot be raised again).
xi. The case is therapeutic or diagnostic misadventure.
xii. Doctrine of limitation.
xiii. Even free treatment of patient does not absolve a doctor from his or her responsibility towards his patient and does not give him defense against negligence.

CONSUMER PROTECTION ACT, 1986

It came in to force on 1st July, 1987, and subsequently quasi-judicial machineries known as Consumer Disputes Redressal Agencies were established at the district, state and central levels. It extends to whole of India except the state of Jammu and Kashmir.

Consumer Redressal Forum

Consumer Redressal Forum is shown diagrammatically in **Figure 3.1**.

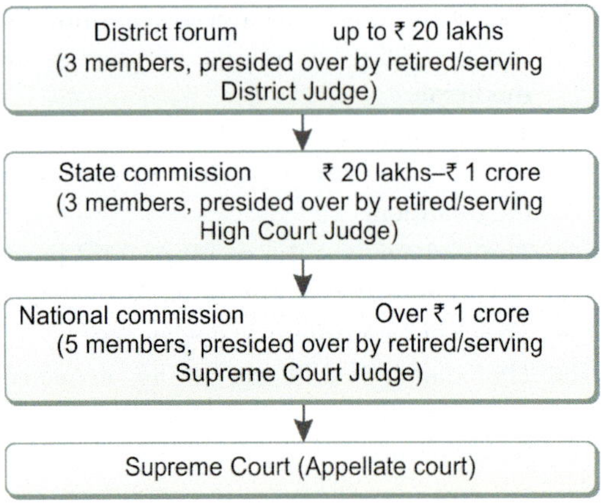

Figure 3.1 Consumer redressal forums

Salient Features of Consumer Protection Act (CPA)

1. A serving or retired judge or a High Court judge or Supreme Court judge will be the president with 2 more persons (4 persons in National Commission) as members.
2. The accused party should reply within a period of 30 days or such extended period not exceeding 15 days.
3. The opinion of majority is the order of Consumer Forum/Commission.
4. The consumer disputes redressal agencies are conferred with the power of the First-Class Judicial Magistrate.
5. The consumer disputes redressal agencies can issue interim orders.
6. The consumer disputes redressal agencies have provisions for recovery of amounts ordered to be paid as arrears of land revenue.
7. A complaint filed in the Consumer Forum/Commission should be adjudicated, within a period of 90 days from the date of notice received by opposite party and within 150 days, if it requires analysis or testing of commodities.
8. The maximum time limit for a claim to be filed under CPA is 2 years from the date of occurrence of the cause of action.
9. A complainant/respondent can represent his case on his own without the help of lawyer.
10. Every complaint filed shall be accompanied with the prescribed amount of fees.
11. CPA has provisions to award costs not exceeding ₹ 10,000 to the respondent when the complaint is found to be vexatious or frivolous and imprisonment up to 3 years.
12. Any person who is aggrieved by an order has a right to appeal to the appellate court within a period of 30 days from the date of order.
13. At present, CPA exempts only those hospitals and practitioners of such hospitals which offer free service to all patients at all times. All government hospitals except PHCs come under the purview of CPA.

A good medical practice involves not only medications and therapeutic interventions but also judicious use of legal and ethical guidelines. In the recent times, it has been observed that many cases of litigations have brought forward against the healers because either of lack of associated legal knowledge or inappropriate record keeping. Every physician must be familiar with medical and ethical guidelines laid down by law of the nation, for the benefit of both the doctor and the patient.

BIOMEDICAL WASTE MANAGEMENT

Importance

Management of biomedical waste is a global humanitarian issue today. With the introduction of Biomedical Waste (Management and Handling) Rules from 20th July, 1998, medical fraternity find themselves in a difficult situation in view of their busy schedule and technicality of legal words.

The World Health Organization Regional office for Europe convened a meeting of concerned personal at **Bergen, Norway** in 1983, which was the first time when this issue was discussed. The seriousness of improper biomedical waste management was brought to the limelight during the "**beach wash-ups**" during summer 1998; which was investigated by the Environment Protection Agency (EPA) of the USA; and it culminated in the passing of **Medical Waste Tracking Act** (MWTA) **November 1988.** This made USA the pioneer as far as waste management is concerned.

The issue of indiscriminate biomedical waste management in India has attracted the attention of the highest judicial body at the level of **Honorable Supreme Court of India**; and Apex Court has, from time to time, issued instructions regarding management of biomedical waste.

Under background, in persuasion to the directive of the Court, the **Ministry of Environment and Forests, Government of India** notified the **Biomedical Waste** (Management and Handling) **Rules** on **27th July 1998;** under the provision of **Environment Protection Act, 1986.** Accordingly all the hospitals in the public and private sector are now bound to follow these rules to evade legal actions.

There are many examples and ample evidences that indiscriminate management of biomedical waste could cause serious hazards to health and environment as follows:

There are many harmful agents in the biomedical waste. The most important are **biological agents**, which pollute water and food and cause alimentary infections like cholera, typhoid, dysentery, infective hepatitis, polio and ascariasis and hookworm diseases, etc.

The blood borne pathogens have gained significant attention after the attack of HIV and HBV, HCV, which can lead to AIDS and hepatitis B, C, etc., in addition to other viral and bacterial infections. The hepatitis B virus (HBV) carries the greatest risk of transmission as about 25% of HBV infected persons develop acute hepatitis with the possible complications of cirrhosis of liver and liver cancer. The HBV transmission is quite similar to HIV as it only occurs through direct contact between an open wound, non-intact skin or mucous membrane, contaminated blood and body fluids, sexual contact, transplacental route. The needle prick injuries and broken injection foils may cause the transmission of HBV. Similarly, HIV is the most critical infection with no cure.

Why Biomedical Waste Needs Management?

It is needed due to health, environmental, legal and aesthetic reasons in addition to ethical reasons.

Ethical Aspect

The ethical aspect related to the social responsibilities. The health professionals have, as a result of their status, knowledge and skills and an obligation to alert those who are at risk. This is reflected by the compulsory notification of infectious and notifiable diseases as a measure of public welfare. As far as biomedical waste management is concerned, health professionals bear a responsibility to act in such a way to prevent exposure to various health hazards and exposures to dioxins.

Reasons for Indiscriminate Management and Handling of Biomedical Waste

1. Lack of priority in policy on biomedical waste management and funds on the issue.
2. Lack of managerial skill and training of biomedical waste management.
3. Lack of appropriate technologies for treatment and disposal of biomedical waste.
4. Lack of strict implementation of infection control measures like sterilization and disinfectant techniques.
5. Lack of awareness among medical personnel, patients, attendants and people in large.
6. Lack of coordination between municipality, pollution control board and hospital authorities.
7. Lack of accountability of persons involved in the management of biomedical waste.

The working group on Hospital Waste Management, constituted by **WHO** in **1983,** was unanimously agreed upon that health care establishments should be held legally accountable for their waste management practices, based on the universal principle that the "**generator is responsible**". As far as possible the "**cradle to grave**" system of notification should be followed, which implies that all stages of waste disposal are systematically controlled.

What is Biomedical Waste?

The biomedical waste means any solid, fluid or liquid waste, including the containers and any intermediate products, which is generated during the diagnosis, treatment or immunization of human beings or animals. In other words, the rubbish containing human tissues, body fluids, excreta, unused drugs, swabs, disposable syringes and sticky bandages, etc. constitutes biomedical waste.

Classification of Biomedical Waste: This schedule of classification should be displayed at strategic locations like inside the dressing rooms, nursing stations, OT, pharmaceutical units so that doctors and nurses are made aware, preferably in local language so that patients and attendants also benefit from it.

Who are the Generators of the Biomedical Waste?

Definition

"**Generator**" means any person nominated on behalf of a hospital, nursing home, clinic, dispensary, laboratory, animal house, slaughter house, veterinary institutions, including those established by or under the control of Government, which generates or cause to be generated, handles or cause to be handled any biomedical waste or where no such person is nominated the person in charge thereof.

Thus, all the hospitals, nursing homes, veterinary hospitals, clinics, dispensaries, diagnostic laboratories, pathological laboratories, blood banks, mortuary and any other healthcare establishments are the potential generators of Biomedical Waste.

To ensure a clean and healthy environment, we require, segregated collection, safe transportation and storage, environmentally sound treatment and disposal of biomedical waste in eco-friendly manner. There are following stages of management of these wastes:

Segregation of Biomedical Waste

Definition

Segregation means "separation of different types of wastes by sorting or the systematic separation of biomedical waste into designated categories".

Significance

It is the most important step in the entire process of biomedical waste management, as it needs special attention to be given to the relatively small quantities of infectious and hazardous waste, thereby reducing not only the risks but the cost of handling, treatment and disposal. For example, if general waste gets mixed with infectious waste, the whole waste has to be incinerated, which may prove to be costly.

Responsibility for Segregation

It is universally accepted fact that segregation of biomedical waste is and should be the responsibility of the generator of the waste. The generators of the waste are those persons in any healthcare establishment who generate or produce wastes, viz. doctors, nurses, paramedical staff, patients and their attendants. These medical persons, who are educated and trained, surprisingly, are least bothered about the amount, quantity and type of waste they generate and the way it is disposed.

Emphasis on Sharps

During segregation, special emphasis should be given to infectious, hazardous and sharp wastes. From among all categories of waste, the "**sharps**", which include syringes, needles, trocar, cannula, guide wires, broken glasswares, scalpels, blades, etc., have the highest disease transmission potential. Almost 85% of sharp injuries are caused between their usage and subsequent disposal, and more than 20% of those handle them encounter "**stick**" injuries. The emphasis should be on safe handling, rather than on the various treatment and disposal options. However, use of needle cutter or needle malter is of great help.

Solution

Till the doctors do not wake up to this problem, the ground reality will not improve in any way. Thus, it can very well said that "**sensitizing**" the generators of waste to properly segregate the waste at the source of generation is the "**key**" to the successful implementation of **Biomedical Waste** (Management and Handling) **Rules 1998.**

Collection of Biomedical Waste

Biomedical waste should be segregated at source of generation and collected in prescribed color-coded bins according to classification.

Containers

1. The dustbin should be light with a cover and size enough to be carried by a person.
2. Inner plastic bag is also used to facilitate the lifting of waste content for transferring.
3. Colored bags/dustbins should be placed in different parts of the hospital.

Segregation and collection both can be considered as being complementary to each other.

Labeling

If containers are transported inside the premises for treatment, then it shall be labeled according to **schedule III**, but if a container is transported outside the premises, where Biomedical waste treatment facility is not present, the containers shall, apart from the label prescribed in **schedule III**, also carry information prescribed in **schedule IV**.

Storage of Biomedical Waste

Definition

Storage means "the holding of biomedical waste for such period of time, at the end of which waste is treated and disposed of".

The container in which such wastes are stored shall display promptly "**International biohazards symbol label in red color**" with details of biomedical wastes as specified in **schedule III**. The packaging of all such wastes is done in sturdy, leak-proof containers conforming to specifications **mentioned in schedule II**.

Duration

No such waste shall be stored in any place where it is generated beyond a **period of 48 hours**, provided that, if for any reasons, it is necessary to store any such wastes beyond a period of 48 hours. The authorized person shall take necessary permission of appropriate authority and shall take such measures so that waste does not decay or putrefy so as to cause hazard to human or animals or environment.

Transportation of Biomedical Waste

Definition

It means "movement of biomedical waste from the point of generation or collection to the final disposal".

Type of Vehicle

No such waste shall be transported on site or off site in any vehicle other than those specially designed and recommended for the purpose. The appropriate authority shall evolve a protocol of safe transportation of such wastes taking into account various local factors and make available a copy of the same to every authorized person.

Timing of Transportation

It should not clash with peak working hours, visiting hours and meal distribution timing.

Documentation System

There should be proper documentation system in which should be recorded the type of biomedical waste, taken by whom, for which type of disposal on a specific date/shift. This is to ensure that all such wastes are actually disposed of, as per guidelines.

Treatment of Biomedical Waste

Definition

Treatment means "any method, technique or process for altering the biological, chemical or physical characteristics of waste to reduce the hazards it presents and facilitate, or reduce the costs of disposals".

Objectives

The basic treatment objectives of biomedical waste include volume reduction, disinfections, neutralization or other change of composition to reduce hazards to health and environment. After such treatment, the residues can be handled safely, transported, stored and disposed of.

Site

As prescribed by the competent authority.

Technology Options for Treatment: There are mainly five technology options available for the treatment of biomedical waste, which are as follows:

i. **Chemical treatment**
ii. **Thermal treatment**
   a. Autoclaving
   b. Hydroclaving
   c. Incineration
   d. Pyrolysis
   e. Plasma and plasma pyrolysis systems
   f. Microwave
iii. **Mechanical treatment**
   a. Compaction
   b. Pulverization
   c. Grinding and shredding
iv. **Irradiation**
v. **Biological method.**

Disposal of Biomedical Waste

Definition

It means "**burial, deposit, discharge, dumping,** or **release of any biomedical waste into or on air, land** or **water**". After treatment of the biomedical waste, it becomes non-infectious or non-hazardous and, depending upon the quantity of the solid waste generated, the following disposal options are available:

Site

As prescribed by competent authority.

Disposal of Solid Waste

- Land fill
- Use of pills
- Composting
- Biogas.

Disposal of Liquid Waste

- Discharge into sewers
- Soakage pits
- Waste stabilizing pond.

Duties of Biomedical Waste Management Facility Operator

Definition

Operator of a biomedical waste facility means an "authorized person or an institution owing or providing the biomedical waste facility".

Authorization

If you are a generator of biomedical waste and **treating more than one thousand patients**

per month, it is mandatory to register with State Pollution Control Board/Committee before specified date. You are required to submit the following with the appropriate application form:

1. Duly filled application form with prescribed fee payable for 3 years.
2. Affidavit regarding proof of beds.
3. Copy of the agreement if any with operator of facility/transporters of biomedical waste.

The occupier (owner) of a biomedical waste management facility shall be responsible for proper collection, reception, treatment, storage and disposal of biomedical waste due to following reasons:

Legal Obligation

1. To manage biomedical waste according to the standard prescribed, failing which legal action can be initiated.
2. To prevent health hazards associated with indiscriminate biomedical waste management.
3. To prevent environmental hazards especially due to inadequate treatment and faulty disposal methods.
4. To provide necessary information to the concerned person, make arrangements of training for creating awareness.

Maintenance of Records

1. Every authorized person shall maintain record related to the generation, segregation, collection, storage, transportation, treatment, disposal and/or any form of handling of biomedical waste in accordance with these rules and guidelines issued in appropriate **Form V**.
2. All records shall be subject to inspection and verification by the prescribed authority at any time.

Submission of Annual Report: Every occupier/operator shall submit an annual report to the prescribed authority, in prescribed **Form I** by **31st January every year**, to include information about the categories and quantities of bio-medical waste **handled during the preceding year**. The **prescribed authority** (SPCB) shall send this information in a compiled form to the **central pollution control board** by **31st March** every year.

Accident Reporting

When any accident occurs during handling at any site where biomedical waste is handled or during transportation of such waste, the authorized person shall report the accident in **Form VI** to the prescribed authority forthwith.

Legal Implications

As per law, it is mandatory for all types of medical services provider to ensure proper implementation of **Biomedical Waste** (Management and Handling) **Rules, 1998.** Installation of incinerator is mandatory for hospitals with more than 50 beds.

It may be kept in mind that any person can report any alleged negligence in management and handling of biomedical waste to the appropriate authority. The state pollution control board/committees have been asked to take action against the defaulting hospitals or nursing homes under **Section 15 (1) of the Environment** (Protection) **Act, 1996,** which reads as "Whoever fails to comply with or contravenes any of this act, or the rules made or orders or directions issued hereunder, shall, in respect of each such failure or contravention, be punishable with imprisonment for a term, which may extend to 5 years or with fine which may extend to one lakh rupees, or with both, and in case of failure or contravention continues, with additional fine, which may extend to five thousand rupees for every day during which such failure or contravention continues after the conviction for the first such failure or contravention."

Statutory warning to all hospitals for installation of biomedical waste treatment and disposal systems is already issued by appropriate authority.

Appeal against Punishment

Any person aggrieved by an order made by the prescribed authority under these rules may within 30 days from the date from which the order is communicated to him, prefer an appeal to such authority as the government of State/ Union Territory may think fit to constitute; provided that the authority may entertain the appeal after the expiry of the said period of 30 days if it is satisfied that the appellant was prevented by sufficient cause from filing the appeal in time. The appropriate authority shall dispose of such appeal within a period of 6 months from the date of its receipt.

Biomedical waste management program cannot be successfully implemented without the willingness, devotion, self-motivation, co-operation and participation of all sections of employees of any healthcare establishment. If we want to protect our environment and health of community, we must sanitize ourselves to this important issue not only in the interest of health managers, but also in the interest of community.

ETHICS AND MEDICAL RESEARCH (HUMAN EXPERIMENTATION)

Indian Medical Council (Professional Conduct, Etiquette, and Ethics) Regulations, 2002

Research

Clinical drug trial or other research involving patients or volunteers as per the guidelines of ICMR can be undertaken, provided ethical consideration are born in mind. Violation of existing ICMR guidelines in this regard shall constitute misconduct. Consent taken from the patient for trial of drug or therapy which is not as per guidelines shall also be construed as misconduct **(Chapter VII, Point 7.22)**.

Human Experimentation

All research involving human subjects should be conducted in accordance with **three basic ethical principles**, which have **equal moral force** and guide the conscientious preparation of proposals for scientific studies. These are:

i. **Respect for persons**: This incorporates at least two fundamental ethical considerations:
   a. **Respect for autonomy**: This requires that those who are capable of deliberation about their personal choices should be treated with respect for their capacity for self-determination.
   b. **Protection of persons with impaired** or **diminished autonomy**: This requires that those who are dependent or vulnerable be afforded security against harm or abuse.

ii. **Beneficence**: This refers to ethical obligation to maximize benefit and minimize harms and wrongs. This principle gives rise to norms requiring that the risks of research be reasonable in the light of the expected benefits and that the research design is sounds enough to safeguard the welfare of the research project.

iii. **Justice**: This refers to the ethical obligation to treat each person in accordance with what is morally right and proper to him/her.

Types of Human Experimentations

Human experimentation may be:

i. **Therapeutic experimentation**: It is concerned primarily with improving the condition of a particular patient under treatment.

ii. **Research experimentation**: It is concerned primarily with using a human subject as a means of expending scientific knowledge for the benefit of humanity.

iii. **Innovative experimentation**: These are therapeutic procedures that have not yet earned a place in medical practice.

The Declaration of Geneva: The Declaration of Geneva of the World Medical Association binds the doctor with the words, "the health of my patient will be my first consideration".

International Code of Medical Ethics: It declares, "Any act or advice, which could weaken physical or mental resistance of a human being may be used only in his interest".

Helsinki Code

The code of ethics for biomedical research, known as Declaration of Helsinki, was drawn in 1964 and revised in 1975 as follows:

Basic Principles

1. Biomedical research involving human subjects must confirm to the generally accepted scientific principles and should be based on adequately performed laboratory and animal experimentation.
2. It should be based on a thorough knowledge of scientific literatures.
3. Design and the performance of each experimental procedure involving human subjects should be clearly formulated in an experimental protocol, which should be transmitted to a specially appointed independent committee for consideration, comment and guidance.
4. Biomedical research involving human subjects should be conducted only by scientifically qualified person and under the supervision of a clinically competent medical person.
5. Responsibility for the human subject must always be with medically qualified person and never rest on the subject of the research, even though the subject has given his/her consent.
6. Biomedical research involving human subjects cannot legitimately be carried out unless the importance of the objective is in proportion to the inherent risk to the subject.
7. Every biomedical research project involving human subjects should be preceded by careful assessment of predictable risks in comparison with foreseeable benefits to the subject or to the others.
8. Concern for the interest of the subject must always prevail over the interest of science and society.
9. Right of the research subject to safeguard his/her integrity must always be respected.
10. Every precaution should be taken to respect the privacy of the subject, to minimize the impact of the study on the subject's physical and mental integrity and on the personality of subjects.
11. Doctors should abstain from engaging in research projects involving human subjects unless they are satisfied that the hazards involved are believed to be predictable.
12. Doctors should cease any investigation if the hazards outweigh the potential benefits.
13. In publication of results of his/her research, the doctor is obliged to preserve the accuracy of his results.
14. Reports of experimentation that are not in accordance with the principles laid down in this declaration should not be accepted for publication.
15. In any research on human beings, the subject must be adequately informed of the aims, methods, analytical benefits, potential hazards of the study and discomfort it may entail and that he/she is at liberty to abstain from participation in the study and is also free to withdraw consent to participation at any time.
16. Doctor should then obtain the subject's freely given informed consent in writing.
17. Doctor should be particularly cautious if the subject is in a dependent relationship to him/her or may consent under duress. In that case, an independent doctor who is not engaged in the investigation and is completely independent of his official relationship should take informed consent.
18. In case of legal incompetence, informed consent should be obtained from a legal guardian in accordance with national legislation.
19. If the person is physically or mentally incapacitated and cannot give informed consent or when the subject is minor, permission from the responsible relative replaces that of the subject in accordance with national legislation.

20. Research protocol should always contain a statement of ethical considerations involved and should indicate that the principles encountered in the present declaration are complied with.

Medical Research Combined with Professional Care (Clinical Research)

1. In the treatment of the sick person, the doctor must be free to use a new diagnostic and therapeutic measure if in his/her judgment it offers hope of saving life, re-establishing health or alleviate suffering.
2. Potential benefits, hazards and discomfort of a new method should be weighed against the advantages of the best current diagnostic and therapeutic methods.
3. In any medical study, every patient, including those of a control group, if any should be assured of the best-proven diagnostic and therapeutic methods.
4. Refusal of the patient to participate in a study must never interfere with the doctor-patient relationship.
5. If the doctor considers it not essential to obtain informed consent, the specific reasons for this proposal should be stated in the experimental protocol for transmission to the independent committee.
6. Doctor can combine medical research with professional care, the objective being the acquisition of new medical knowledge only to the extent that medical research is justified by its potential diagnostic or therapeutic value of the patient.

Non-therapeutic Biomedical Research Involving Human Subjects (Non-clinical Biomedical Research)

1. In the purely scientific application of medical research carried out on a human being, it is the duty of the doctor to remain protector of the life and health of that person on whom biomedical research is being carried out.
2. Subjects should be volunteers, either healthy persons or patients for whom the experimental design is not related to the patient's illness.
3. Investigator and the investigating team should discontinue the research if in his/her or their judgment it may, if continued, be harmful to the individual.
4. In research on man, the interest of science and society should never take precedence over consideration related to the well-being of the subjects.

Salient Features of Helsinki Declaration

1. Extensive **animal research is an absolute prerequisite** to the use of an innovative technique in the treatment of human beings.
2. Most difficult innovative cases will be those, in which prior animal research is impossible or would be uninformative.
3. Treatment should be given cautiously and its after effects noted and appreciated.
4. Experiment on volunteers can only be justified if they do not cause significant harm to the subject and the results are likely to be beneficial.
5. It would be unethical to do something merely by way of experimentation that is which is not strictly related to cure patient's illness.
6. There must also be no great risk in proposed examination even if the patient consents to run the great risk.
7. In considering whether a new treatment is as effective as an old one, side effects of the two treatments and their costs should be considered.

ICMR Guidelines for Human Research, 1995

The ICMR has laid down certain ethical guidelines for biomedical research on human subjects.

It states that medical and related research using human beings should necessarily ensure that:

1. **Purpose** of such research is directed towards the increase of knowledge about human conditions in relation to its social and natural environment.
2. Research is **conducted** under such conditions that the subjects are dealt with in a manner conducive to and consistent with their dignity and well being.
3. Research must be subjected to a regimen of evaluation at all stages.

General Principles

1. **Principle of essentiality**: Whereby the research is considered absolutely essential after a due consideration of all factors and options involved.
2. **Principle of voluntariness, informed consent and community agreement**: Whereby, the subjects are fully apprised of the research and the impact and risks on him and others; and he retains the right to abstain from further participation in the research irrespective of any obligation they may have entered, subject to only minimal recitative obligations of any advance consideration received.
3. **Principle of non-exploitation**: Whereby as a general rule, the research subjects are remunerated for their involvement in the research or experiment.
4. **Principle of privacy and confidentiality**: Whereby, the identity and records of the subjects are kept confidential as far as possible.
5. **Principle of precaution and risk minimization:** Whereby, due care and caution is taken at all stages of a research to ensure that the subjects are put to minimum risk and generally benefit from the experiment.
6. **Principle of professional competence**: Whereby, the research is conducted at all times by competent and qualified persons who act with total integrity and impartiality and who have been made aware of the ethical considerations.
7. **Principle of accountability and Transparency**: Whereby, the research experiment will be conducted in a fair, honest, impartial and transparent manner after full disclose of all aspects of their interest.
8. **Principle of maximization of public interest and of distributive justice**: Whereby, the research or experiment and its subsequent applicative use are conducted and used to benefit all human kind.
9. **Principle of institutional arrangement**: Whereby, there shall be a duty on all persons connected with the research to ensure that all institutional arrangements required to be complied with and all institutional arrangements required to be made in respect of the research and its subsequent use or application are duly made in a transparent manner.
10. **Principle of public domain**: Whereby, the research is brought into public domain so that its results are generally made known through scientific and other publications.
11. **Principle of totality of responsibility**: Whereby, the professional and moral responsibility, for the due observance of all the principles, guidelines and prescriptions rests with all those involved in conducting the experiment.
12. **Principle of compliance**: Whereby, there is a general and positive duty on all persons, conducting with any research entailing the use of a human subject to ensure that these guidelines are adhered in letter and spirit.

SUGGESTED READING

1. Knight B. Legal Aspects of Medical Practice. 2nd ed. 1976. pp. 24-9.
2. Mukherjee JB. Forensic Medicine and Toxicology. 1st ed. Delhi: Academic Publishers; 1981. pp. 59-63.
3. Pillay VV. Handbook of Forensic Medicine and Toxicology. 13th ed. Hyderabad; Paras Publication; 2003. pp. 24-5.
4. Rao GN. Textbook of Forensic Medicine and Toxicology. 1st ed. New Delhi: Jaypee Brother's Medical Publishers (P) Ltd; 2000. pp. 47-52.
5. Rao NKG. Practical Forensic Medicine. 2nd ed. 1998. p. 14, 17, 19, 31, 35-6, 114.
6. Ratanlal and Dhirajlal's The Indian Penal Code. 28th ed. Bharat Law House;1997 (Reprint-2000).pp. 100-5.
7. Reddy KSN. The Essentials of Forensic Medicine and Toxicology. 19th ed. 2000. pp. 40-3.
8. Subrahmanyam BV. Modi's Medical Jurisprudence and Toxicology. 22nd ed. Butterworth's Tripathi Publication; 1999. pp. 60-6.
9. Taylor AS. Taylor's Principles and Practice of Medical Jurisprudence. 13th ed. Indian Edition; 1994. pp. 48-51.
10. The Indian Contract Act, 1972.
11. Waste characterization and quantification. "Parivesh" Newsletter on Hospital Waste; Vol.4 (iv) March 1998, CPCB. Ministry of Environment and Forest, Govt. of India, New Delhi: 3-4.

CHAPTER 4

Euthanasia (Mercy Killing)

Prabir Kumar Dev, Putul Mahanta

LEARNING PLAN

- Know the definition of euthanasia and its types
- Learn about the historical background
- Know about the physicians' sentiment
- Learn the pros and cons
- Identify the medicolegal issues about it

Euthanasia is a Greek word meaning easy death where **eu** means 'good' and **thanasia** means 'death'. It is a practice of producing painless death of a person suffering from incurable disease or a permanent damage to the brain.

Francis Bacon first used the word **euthanasia** in a medical context in the 17th century, to refer to an easy, painless and happy death, during which it was a physician's responsibility to alleviate the 'physical sufferings' of the body.[1] The first apparent use of the term 'euthanasia' belongs to the historian Suetonius, who described how the emperor Augustus, "dying quickly and without suffering in the arm of his wife, Livia", experienced the euthanasia he had wished for.[2]

DEFINITION

It can be defined as producing painless death of a person suffering from hopelessly incurable and painful disease or permanent damage to the brain.

A committee on Medical Ethics selected House of Lords defined Euthanasia as "a deliberate intervention undertaken with the express intention of ending a life, to relieve intractable suffering".[3]

HISTORY

Euthanasia was practiced in ancient Greece and Rome; for example, Hemlock was employed as a means of hastening death on the Island of Kea. Euthanasia in the sense of deliberate hastening of a person's death was supported by Socrates, Plato and Seneca the Elder in the ancient world, although Hippocrates appears to have spoken against the practice, writing "I will not prescribe a deadly drug to please someone or give advice that may cause his death".[4-6]

In 1870, Samuel Williams, a school teacher, initiated the contemporary euthanasia debate through a speech given at Birmingham speculative club, which was subsequently published in a one-off publication entitled 'Essay of the Birmingham speculative club.' William's proposal was to use chloroform to deliberately hasten the death of terminally ill patients.[7]

America saw the first attempt to legalize euthanasia, when Henry Hunt introduced legislation into the 'General assembly of Ohio' in 1906. But the bill failed to pass.[8]

On 24th July, 1939, killing of severely disabled infant in Nazi, Germany was described in a BBC "Genocide under the Nazis Timeline" as the first 'State-Sponsored Euthanasia.'[9]

PHYSICIAN SENTIMENT

i. A survey in the United States of more than 10,000 physician case to the result that approximately 16% of physicians would consider halting life-sustaining therapy because the family demands it, even if they believed that it was premature. Approximately, 55% would not, and for the remaining 29%, it would depend on circumstances.
   This study also stated that 46% of physicians agree that physicians-assisted suicide should be allowed in some cases, 41% do not, and the remaining 14% think it depends.[10]
ii. Dignity of dying is a United Kingdom's nationwide campaigning organization. Dignity of dying points out that in 2010 British Social Attitudes survey, 82% of general public believed that a doctor should probably or definitely be allowed to end the life of a patient with a painful incurable disease at the patient's request. That was further analyzed to show 71% of religious people supported this statement.[11]
   At this present juncture, the practice of euthanasia is not permissible in most of the countries of the world; however, the same has been legalized in some countries like Belgium, Switzerland, America (Washington and Oregon) and the Netherlands on certain grounds after family consent.

TYPES OF EUTHANASIA

Voluntary Active Euthanasia

Intentionally administering medicines or other interventions to cause patient's death at the patients request and with full informed consent.

Involuntary Active Euthanasia

Intentionally administering medicines or other interventions to cause patient's death when patient was competent but without patient's request and or full consent, e.g. patient may not have been asked.

Non-voluntary Active Euthanasia

Intentionally administering medicines or other interventions to cause patient's death when patient was incompetent and mentally incapable of requesting, e.g. patient in coma.

Passive Euthanasia

Withdrawing life-sustaining measures and letting him die.

Physician Assisted Suicide

A physician providing medications or other interventions to a patient with an understanding that the patient intends to use them to commit suicide. A doctor provides a medical treatment intended to cause death of a terminally ill patient without the patient or family members consent that may be charged with murder or culpable homicide.

PROS AND CONS

Is mercy killing humane? Do we have the right to assess whether a life is worth living? Should euthanasia be practiced only in the terminally ill people or for the debilitated and mentally ill too? Few of the pros and cons of euthanasia are:

i. An individual should have the liberty to choose induced death, if he is suffering from an incurable disease, where even the best treatment does not improve his quality of life.
ii. Legalizing euthanasia would help to alleviate suffering in terminally ill patients. It would be inhuman and unfair to make them endure the unbearable pain.
iii. Maintaining life-support system against patient's wish is considered unethical by law.
iv. Family heirs who would misuse euthanasia as a tool for wealth inheritance does not hold true. Reason being, the relatives can withdraw life-support leading to early death of the said individual even in the absence of legalized euthanasia. Here, they are not actually causing death, but passively waiting for it without patients consent. This is passive involuntary euthanasia.
v. Healthcare expenditure is and will be a concern for the family irrespective of the euthanasia laws and only those who can afford a prolonged unproductive treatment will continue to do so.

MEDICOLEGAL IMPORTANCE

Many of us support the right of a terminally ill patient to die, but what if the right becomes an obligation? What of the potential for abuse by impatient heirs?

Should dying patients have the right to order their doctors not to start or continue their medical treatment? Should the doctors be protected from prosecution if they shorten a patient's life-expectancy with pain-killing drugs?

Many people would answer yes to both the questions. But, does this mean we need a 'right to die' law? There are more to the issue of euthanasia than first meets the eye.

In India, active euthanasia is not legalized. On request, nothing can be done to assist the patient to end his life. It will be an offense by the patient of suicide covered under Section 309 IPC and the medical man who causes death of such person are abetting the act and is covered under Section 306 IPC (abetment of suicide).

Passive euthanasia is legal in India.[13] On 7th March, 2011, the Supreme Court of India legalized passive euthanasia by means of the withdrawal of life-support to patients in a permanent vegetative state. The decision was made as part of the verdict in a case involving Aruna Shanbaug, who had been in a vegetative state for 37 years at King Edward Memorial Hospital. The High Court rejected active euthanasia by means of lethal injection. In the absence of a law regulating euthanasia in India, the court stated that its decision becomes law of the land until the Indian Parliament enacts a suitable law.[14]

As per Indian Medical Council (Professional conduct, etiquette and ethics) regulations, practicing voluntary euthanasia shall constitute unethical conduct.[12]

REFERENCES

1. Bacon F. The major work by Francis Bacon, Brian Vickers. p. 630.
2. Letellier P. History and definition of word. In: Euthanasia: Ethical and Human Aspects by council of Europe.
3. Harris NM. The euthanasia debate. JR Army Med Corps. 2011;147(3):367-70. PMID 11766225.
4. Mystakidou K, Parpa E, Tsilika E, Katsouda E, Vlahos L.The evolution of euthanasia and its perceptions in Greek culture and civilization. Perspect Biol Med. 2005;48(1):97-8.
5. Stolberg M. Active euthanasia in pre-modern society, 1500–1800: Learned debates and popular practices. Social History of Medicine. 2007;20(2):206-7.
6. Gesundheit B, Steinberg A, Glick S, Or R, Jotkovitz A.Euthanasia: An overview and the Jewish perspective. Cancer Invest. 2006;24(6):621-9.
7. Emanueel EJ. The history of euthanasia debate in the United States and Britain. Ann Intern Med. 1994;121(10):793-802.

8. Appel JM. A duty to kill? A duty to die? Rethinking the euthanasia controversy of 1906. Bull Hist Med. 2004;78(3):610-34.
9. Genocide under the Nazis Timeline. 24 July, 1939; BBC.
10. Kane L. Doctors Struggle with Tougher-than-ever Dilemmas: other Ethical issues. Exclusive Ethics Survey Results. 2010.
11. British Social Attitudes Survey: 2009-10.
12. Indian Medical Council (Professional conduct, etiquette and ethics) Regulations, 2002.
13. The Hindu. "India joins select nations in legalizing "passive euthanasia". 2011 March 7th. [cited 2011 march 8th]. Available from: URL:http://www.thehindu.com/news/national/article1516973.ece
14. The Hindu. Supreme Court disallows friend's plea for mercy killing of vegetative Aruna. 2011 March 7th [cited 2011 March 7th]. Available from: URL:http://www.thehindu.com/news/national/article1516644.ece

CHAPTER 5

Identification

Putul Mahanta, Vijayamahantesh SN, Vijayanath V, Imran Sabri

LEARNING PLAN

- Learn about circumstances where identification is required
- Know the commonly used data for identification
- Learn about differences in male and female identification
- Learn about determination of age from available methods
- Understand the usefulness of the methods in different situations

Identification means fixing the exact personality of an individual. It is the determination of the individuality of a person based on certain physical characteristic. Identification of the person is usually carried out by the police. However, a medical person, in certain situations, has to confirm the identity of an individual based on his medical knowledge. It is done in a living person or dead by recognizing certain specific features that are unique to that person.

TYPES OF IDENTIFICATION

Identification may be of two types:

a. Complete identification
b. Incomplete or partial identification

Complete (absolute) identification refers when all the features of a person are known and we can fix the individuality of a person absolutely. Incomplete (partial) identification means when only certain features of an individual are known.

MEDICOLEGAL CIRCUMSTANCES WHERE IDENTIFICATION IS NEEDED

The methods of identification vary with: (i) circumstances of death, (ii) time elapsed since death and (iii) antemortem data available for comparison. Identification may become difficult in cases of fire, explosions, advanced decomposition mutilation, mass disasters like earthquakes, aircraft accidents (**Figure 5.1**), etc. Medicolegal circumstances where identification is required are narrated in **Table 5.1**.

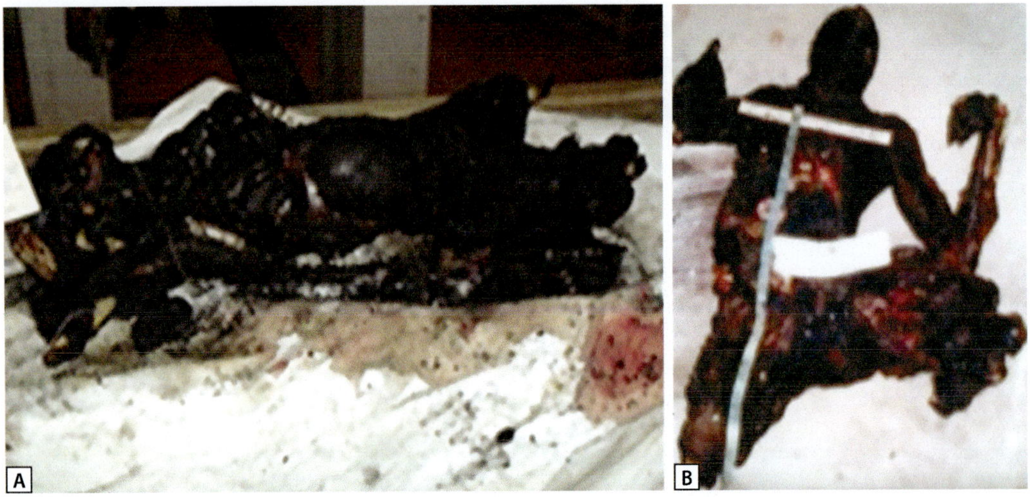

Figures 5.1A and B Burnt bodies of an aircraft accident

Table 5.1 Medicolegal circumstances where identification is required

With Living Person		
Medical purposes	**Civil purposes**	**Criminal purposes**
a. Unconscious patient b. Patient with true amnesia c. Mental confusion	a. Problems of inheritance b. Marriage c. Employment or immigration d. Call for military service e. Disputed paternity or maternity f. Pension, life insurance, voting right g. Disputed sex h. Missing person, etc.	a. Sexual offences b. Kidnapping c. Determine the criminal personality d. Criminal abortion e. Accused of criminal offences
With Dead Person		
a. A missing and presumed dead person b. Issuing death certificate c. Accidental death d. Accused in criminal offenses e. Mass disaster f. Exhumation, etc.		

CORPUS DELICTI (THE ESSENCE OF CRIME)

It means the facts of any criminal offence or the body of the crime. The main part of corpus delicti is the establishment of identity of the person, in a case of murder. The corpus delicti includes the body of the victim and other facts, which are indications of foul play like a bullet or a part of the knife found in the body and responsible for death. Photograph of the person depicting injuries, cloths with defects or blood stains and scratches are all included in this. It becomes difficult for the police to solve the crime if the identity of the victim is not known. The identification of the dead body and proof of corpus delicti is essential before a sentence is passed in a murder trial, because to support false charges, unclaimed decomposed bodies or parts of the bodies may be produced.

It is one of the most important concepts in a murder investigation. When a person disappears and cannot be contacted, many police agencies initiate a missing person case.

If, during the course of the investigation, detectives believe that he/she has been murdered, then a "body" of evidentiary items, including physical, demonstrative and testimonial evidence, must be obtained to establish that the missing individual has indeed been murdered before a suspect can be charged with homicide.[1] However, there were cases where the body was not found or was not identified as in the case of King Emperor vs. Ramnath alias Natha, where the learned judges were of the opinion that however, the body of the murdered man was not found, but this was not a sufficient reason for not awarding capital punishment.

POINTS TO BE NOTED FOR THE PURPOSE OF IDENTIFICATION

Commonly Recorded Data for both Living and Dead

1. **Name** (in full)
2. Name of father, family members, relatives
3. Address for correspondence
4. General **appearance**: Weight, height, skin color and hair (color, texture, pattern)
5. **Features:** Face, eyebrows, iris, chin, nose, configuration of ear, Portrait Parle, etc.
6. **Clothing:** Refer the occupation and social status
7. Age
8. Sex
9. Blood groups (A, B, AB, O)
10. Prints
11. **Congenital abnormality:** Asymmetry, harelip, cleft palate, polydactyl, etc.
12. Birthmarks
13. **Occupational** marks
14. **Scars** and Moles
15. Tattoos
16. Photographs
17. **Anthropometry** not used nowadays: Span of outstretched hands, chest circumference, length of foot, forearm, fingers; ear measurements, shape ofthe chin or nose, etc.
18. **Race** (Negro, Caucasians, Mongoloids).

Methods of Identification of Living Person

1. **Personal characters:** Voice, speech, mental power, education, occupation, handwriting, gait, etc.
2. Signature or thumb impression.
3. Identification marks (two).
4. **Nationality:** Country of birth.
5. **Religion** and caste.

Methods of Identification of Dead Person

1. **Documents:** Personal papers, photographs, ID card, credit cards, etc.
2. **Jewellery:** Rings, bracelets, earrings, watches, lighters, pens, keys.
3. **Contact traces:** Give occupational data, e.g. paint, grease, flour, dyes.
4. **Height:** From the skeleton.
5. **Teeth** examination.
6. **Internal physical examination** and medical appliances: (a) Underlying disease, (b) X-ray of the whole body may reveal the old fracture, prosthesis like plates or nail, etc., (c) Pacemakers and (d) Artificial valve.
7. **Data from the skull** (if previous X-ray is available): (a) Frontal sinus, (b) Skull suture pattern and (c) Vascular grooves in the skull.
8. The time that the body or bones have been buried.

Identification Based on Advanced Laboratory Test

- DNA profile or DNA fingerprinting
- Videograph
- Voice identification
- Superimposition technique
- Facial reconstruction (Plastic/2D/3D)
- Digital signature
- Retina and iris scan.

Identification: Special Techniques

- Dactylography (fingerprints)
- Poroscopy (study of pores)
- Footprints or foot-marks (podogram)
- Cheiloscopy (lip prints)
- Rugoscopy (palatal rugae prints).

DETERMINATION OF RACE

Race can be determined by:

i. **Complexion**: It is of little value. Generally, the skin is brown in Indians, fair in Europeans and black in Negroes. Color of skin is changed in burns and when the body is decomposed.

ii. **Eye color**: This is also unreliable. Usually, Indians have black eyes and few have brown eyes. Europeans have blue or gray eyes and Negros have black eyes (iris color).

iii. **Hair**: Generally speaking, Indians have black thin hair. Europeans have fair or light brown hair. Negroes have their hair arranged in spirals.

iv. **Clothing**: Identifying the race by clothes can be misleading due to changes in the cultural trends.

v. **Teeth**: The incisors, as well, differ in their basic shape. The incisors fall into two basic categories, based on the shape of the lingual (tongue) surface of the tooth. These two categories are: **Shovel-shaped** and **spatulate** or **spatula-shaped** (**Figure 5.2**). As there is more than one race with spatulate incisors, other indicators are necessary to positively identify race, although this single feature can be used to eliminate one of the possibilities. Each of the following three races has their own shaped incisor, viz., **African** and **European** have spatulate, and **Asian** has shovel-shaped incisor.

vi. Skeletal features and indices (**Discussed in Chapter 6—Forensic osteology**).

vii. Genetic DNA identification will revolutionize this aspect in near future.

viii. **Physical features**: Various physical features of the skull like shape of the orbit (**Figure 5.3**), shape of the nasal aperture (**Figure 5.4**) and shape of the hard palate (**Figure 5.5**) are also useful to determine the race (**Table 5.2**).

RELIGION AND CASTE

Hindu males are not circumcised. Other features like cast marks on the forehead, sacred thread, necklace of wooden beads and tufts of hair on the back of head if present is useful to ascertain the religion.

Hindu females may have vermilion on the head and forehead, silver toe ornaments, Mangal sutra, tattoo marks, nose ring in left nostril with few openings for ear rings along the helix.

Muslim females may have a nose ring aperture in the septum, several openings in the ears along the helix and usually no tattoo marks are found.

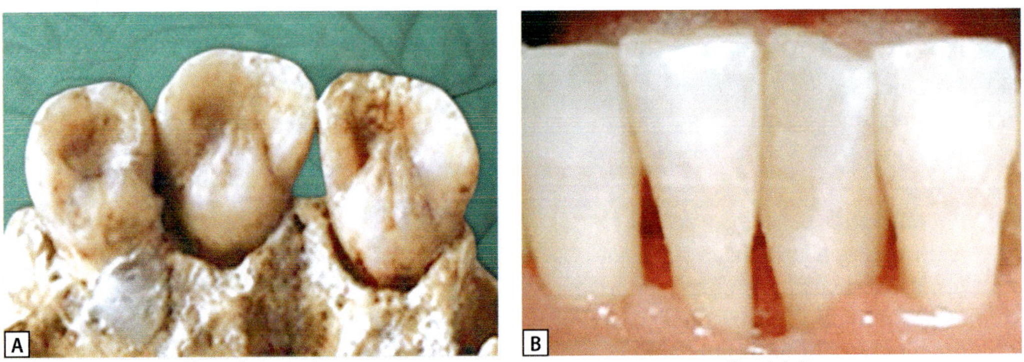

Shovel-shaped   Spatulate

Figures 5.2A and B Different shaped incisors

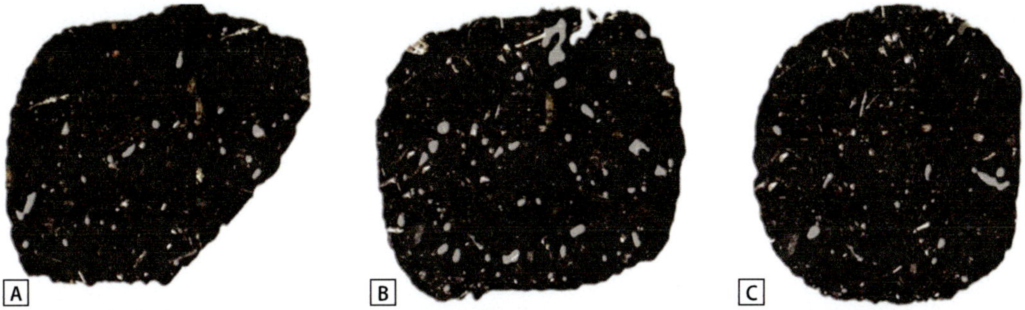

Figures 5.3A to C Shape of orbits, (A) Caucasoid; (B) Negroid; (C) Mongoloid

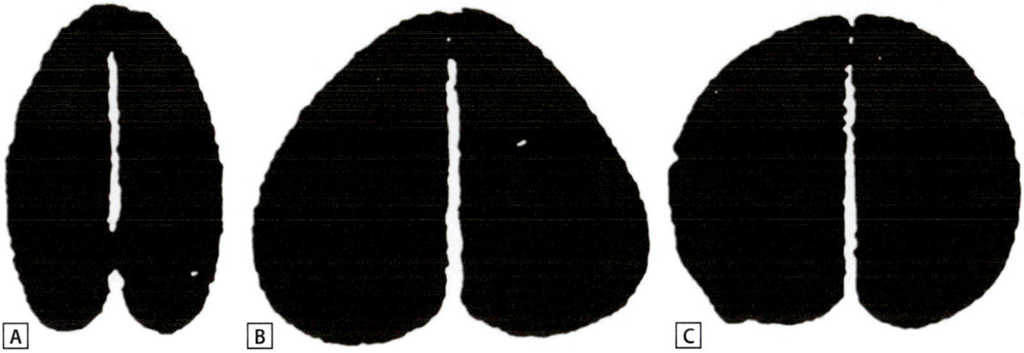

Figures 5.4A to C Shape of nasal aperture, (A) Caucasoid; (B) Negroid; (C) Mongoloid

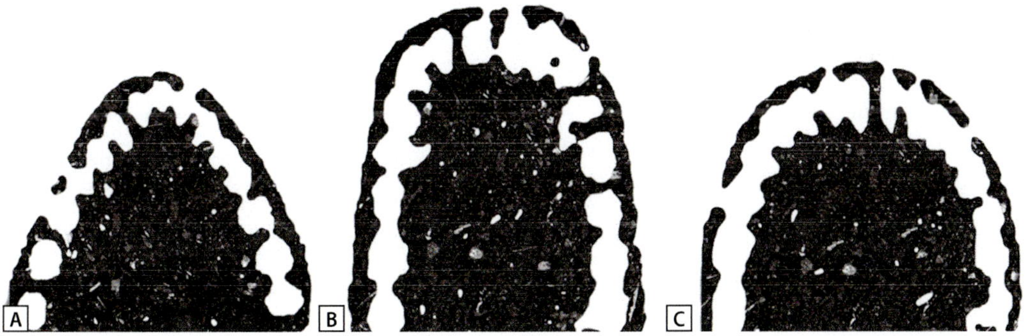

Figures 5.5A to C Upper jaw showing hard palate, (A) Caucasoid; (B) Negroid; (C) Mongoloid

Muslim males are circumcised and callosities may be found on the forehead, knee and ankle due to special attitude adopted during the prayers.

DETERMINATION OF SEX

Why Sex Determination is Important?

It is important in cases (i) relating to heirship, disposal of property, marriage, education, impotence, rape, divorce, etc.; (ii) identification in living or in dead (mainly in advance decomposition cases) bodies and (iii) when sex appears ambiguous.

Identification of Sex

1. **Presumptive evidence about sex:** (i) Outward appearance of the person, the physical features; (ii) General contours of the face, moustache and beard, evidence of shaving, length of head hair; and (iii) Clothes, figure, habits and voice, etc.

Table 5.2 Differentiating points between races from physical features

Features	Caucasian	Mongolian	Negro
Complexion	Fair	Yellowish	Black
Eyes: Iris color	Gray or blue	Black	Black
Skull	Rounded with raised forehead	Square, forehead inclined backward	Narrow and elongated with small compressed forehead
Orbit	Triangular	Rounded	Square
Nasal aperture	Elongated	Rounded	Broad
Nose	Sharp	Flattened	Blunt
Face	Small	Large and flattened	Protruding jaw, prominent molar bone with oblique teeth set
Hard palate	Triangular	Rounded	Rectangular
Upper limbs	Proportionate to body	Smaller than trunk	Larger than trunk, forearm larger in comparison to arm, small hand
Lower limbs	Proportionate to body	Smaller than trunk	Leg larger in comparison to thigh, feet wide and flat, heel bone projecting backward

2. **Highly probable signs**: External sexual structures like: (i) Developed breasts; (ii) Appropriate muscular development; (iii) The female distribution of body hair and subcutaneous fat; and (iv) The vagina in the female.
   Absence of breast tissue, male distribution of hair, appropriate physical development and penis in the male are the most probable signs for the male sex.
3. **Most certain signs**: Presence of ovaries (menstruation after puberty) in female and testes (seminal emission after puberty) in male is the most certain signs of sex. Before this period, in doubtful cases nuclear sexing and the study of sex chromosomes will be helpful.

Determination of Sex of an Individual

A normal person has 46 chromosomes. The chromatin pattern in males is XY, and in females it is XX. The difficulty arises when there is ambiguity of the external genitalia and the secondary sexual characters are unable to confirm the sex. The sex of a person can be determined from:

1. Morphological examination
2. Microscopic examination
3. Hormone assay
4. Gonadal biopsy
5. DNA profiling
6. Radiological investigation.

In the dead, determination of sex is done by demonstration of the specific sex organs.

Highly probable and presumptive evidence is useful in, (i) Highly decomposed bodies where the sex organs have disappeared, (ii) Grossly mutilated bodies, (iii) Portions of the body and (iv) Deliberate destruction of the sex organs.

Morphological Examination

If the external genitalia are normal, then mere external examination is enough to determine the sex of the individual, and after puberty, the secondary sexual characters help to differentiate and confirm the sex. The various morphological differentiating physical features of human sex are mentioned in **Table 5.3**.

Determination of sex from bones is discussed in Chapter 6 (**Forensic Osteology**).

Microscopic Examination

Sex chromatin test (nuclear sexing) for sex determination can be done by demonstrating Barr body and Davidson body, which are more with the female cells as a collection of chromatin

Table 5.3 Differentiating points between male and female

Features	Male	Female
Built	Muscular, stronger	Less muscular, delicate
Height and weight	More	Less
Scalp hairs	Shorter, coarse	Longer and finer
Eyebrow	Coarse and thicker	Fine and thin
Voice	Hoarse after puberty	Soft
Moustache and beard	Present	Absent or rudimentary
Hair on pinna	Present	Absent
Body hairs grow over	Chest, abdomen and limb	May be seen over limbs
Pubic hairs	Thicker, coarse, extend upwards up to the navel rudimentary	Horizontal, covering only mons pubis, triangular in distribution
Breast	Rudimentary	Well development
Thyroid cartilage angle	Prominent, angle <90°	Less prominent, angle >120°
Shoulder and hip	Broader than hip	Hip broader than shoulder
Chest and abdomen	Chest dimension is more	Abdomen dimension is more
Gluteal region	Flat	Full and roundish
Forearm	Anteroposteriorly flat	Roundish
Thigh	Cylindrical	Conical
Wrist and ankle	Coarse and rough	Smooth and delicate
External genitalia	Scrotum, testis and penis	Labia, clitoris and vagina
Internal genitalia	Vas deferens, prostate, seminal vesicle, ejaculatory ducts	Ovaries, uterine tube and uterus

material as shown in **Figure 5.6** can be of helpful. In the buccal smear, the percentage of nuclei having a chromatin body (Barr body) ranges from zero to four in males and 20–80 in females. Details discussed in the Chapter of **Forensic Serology**.

The Chromosomal Study: The Y chromosome of the male cells can be visualized by using a fluorescent microscope and quinacrine hydrochloride stain in the cells of hair sheaths, nerve cells and dental pulp.

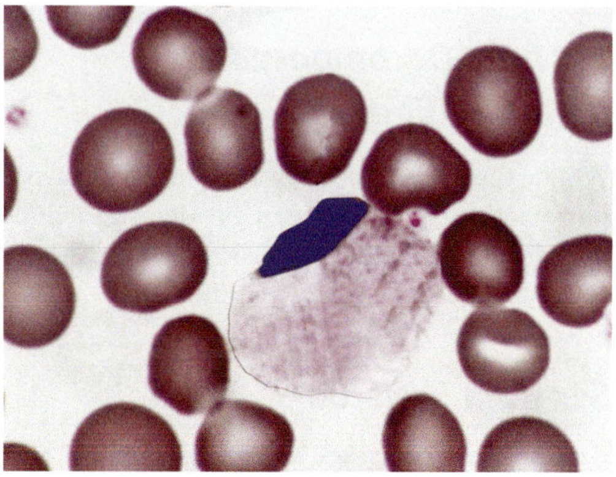

Figure 5.6 Barr body

Hormonal Analysis

Hormonal imbalance will alter the secondary sexual characters and will confuse the determination of sex. Hormones are responsible for body contour, hairiness, fat distribution and genital morphology.

Gonadal Biopsy

The gonadal biopsy provides essential information for the identification, besides classification and early detection of neoplasias in patients with disorders of sex development. A biopsy from the gonads, if indicates testis in male and ovary in female, is the definite identity of the sex of the person.

DNA Profiling

DNA profiling can determine the sex of a person from blood stains or even from fragmentary remains.[2] Details discussed in Chapter 8 (**Forensic DNA Typing**).

Troubles in Sex Determination

- Concealed sex
- Decomposed or mutilated bodies
- Skeleton
- Intersex state.

Concealed Sex

Concealed or hidden sex is the lack of distinctive signaling that an individual may show to hide his or her sex for some criminal motives or some other objects, etc. Criminals may conceal their sex to avoid detection by changing dress or other methods. This can be detected by proper physical examination.

Sex from Decomposed or Mutilated Bodies

When the body is found in the advanced putrefaction state, sex can be determined by the presence of either uterus or prostate, which resist putrefaction for a long time.

Sex from Skeleton

It is not possible to determine from skeleton with the full amount of certainty till puberty, since the sexual characteristics of the bone begin to manifest only after attainment of puberty. Only exception is the pelvis where the greater sciatic notch can be utilized for sex determination in children. Details are discussed in Chapter 6 (**Forensic Osteology**).

Intersex State

Types of Intersex: It is mixing of characters of both sexes in one individual in varying degrees, including physical form, reproductive organs and sexual behavior as a result of some defect in the embryonic development. It can be categorized into four groups:

i. Gonadal agenesis
ii. Gonadal dysgenesis
iii. True hermaphroditism
iv. Pseudohermaphroditism

Gonadal Agenesis

In this condition, the testes or the ovaries have never developed and nuclear sexing is negative.

Gonadal Dysgenesis

Here, the external sexual structures are present, but they fail to develop at puberty and have no gonads. The examples are: Klinefelter's Syndrome and Turner's syndrome.

Klinefelter's Syndrome (Figure 5.7): In this condition, anatomical structure is male, but the nuclear sexing is female. The study reveals the

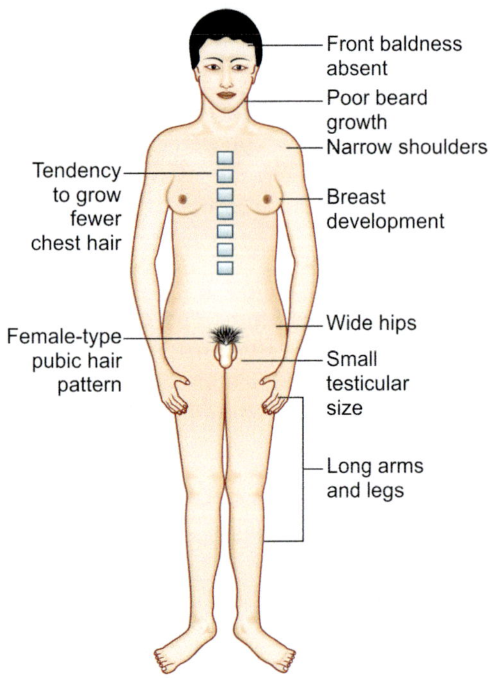

Figure 5.7 Klinefelter's syndrome

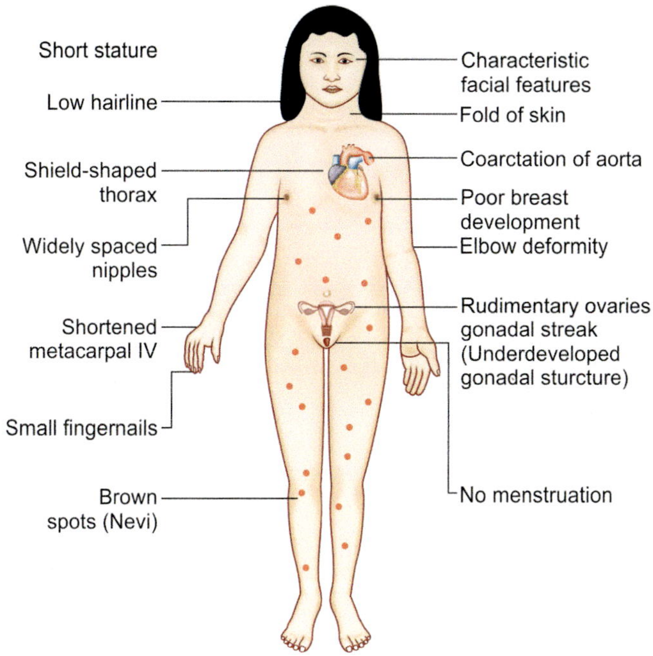

Figure 5.8 Turner's syndrome

presence of two X chromosomes in combination with one Y chromosome, the sex chromosome pattern is XXY (47 chromosomes). The incidence of this syndrome is 1:500, and it increases with advancing maternal age. It is diagnosed when there is delayed onset of puberty, behavioral disorders and mental retardation. Hair on the chest and chin are reduced with absence of axillary and pubic hair. Gynecomastia, azoospermia, low levels of testosterone, sterility, increased urinary gonadotropin and increased height are commonly seen. Histologically, there is atrophy of the testicles with hyalinization of seminiferous tubules.

Turner's Syndrome (Figure 5.8): In this condition, the anatomical structure is female, but nuclear sexing is male. The cytogenetic study shows monosomy X, the sex chromosome pattern is XO. It can be diagnosed at birth by the presence of edema of hand and feet, loose skin folds at the nape of the neck, low birth weight and short stature.

It is characterized by primary amenorrhea, sterility, lack of development of primary and secondary sexual characteristics, infantile streak ovaries, increased urinary gonadotropin excretion, short fourth metatarsal, webbed neck, shield-chest, wide straight nipples, high arched palate, low set ears, slow growth, learning problems. It is also associated with other congenital malformations like color blindness, spina bifida, coarctation of the aorta, septal defects, renal defects like horseshoe kidney, endocrinological defects like Cushing's syndrome and high incidence of diabetes mellitus.

True Hermaphroditism (Figure 5.9)

It has both gonadal organs, i.e. +ve test. It is a very rare condition. The person will be having internal and external gonads of both sexes and be able to function as either a male or a female, depending on how he or she has been brought up initially.

The gonads may be abdominal, inguinal, labioscrotal in position. The phallus may be penile or clitoral; labia may be bifid as in female or fused resembling the scrotum of the male.

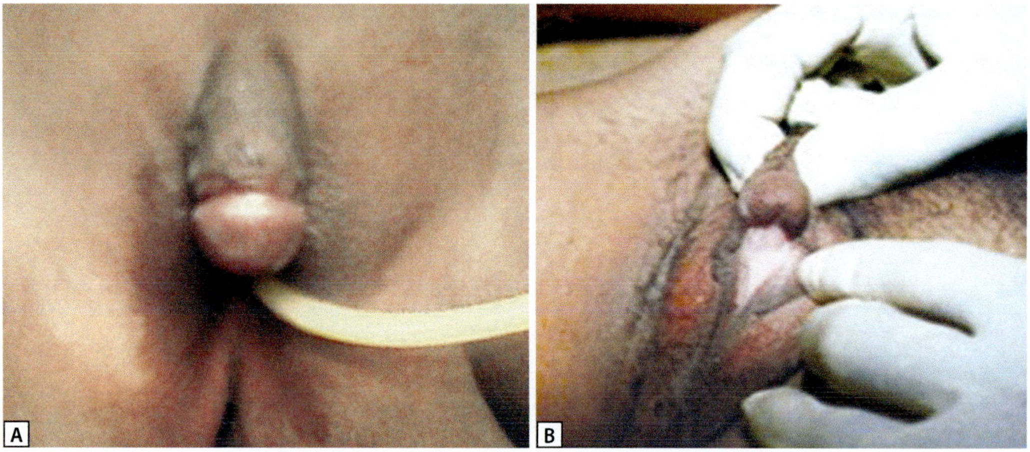

Figures 5.9A and B Example of true hermaphroditism

Neither gonad is functional; histology reveals both testicular and ovarian tissues.

Pseudohermaphroditism

Sex determined from the gonads, nuclear sex gives true sex. In this condition, the presence of gonadal tissue of only one sex is seen internally, while the external appearance is of the opposite sex. It is of two types male and female:

a. Male pseudohermaphroditism
b. Female pseudohermaphroditism

Male Pseudohermaphroditism: Nuclear sexing is XY, but sex organs and sexual characteristics deviate towards female form because of testicular feminization. There is the inability to convert testosterone into active form dihydro-testosterone. Organs and sexual characteristics towards male are seen due to adrenal hyperplasia.

Female Pseudohermaphroditism: Female pseudohermaphrodites are chromo-somally and gonadally female, but have male or ambiguous external genitalia. There is a variable degree of clitoral hypertrophy and labial fusion. The ovaries are sometimes cystic. Secondary sexual characteristics may also show virilization or poor feminization. Female pseudohermaphroditism is caused by excess of androgens, e.g. testosterone of extragonadal origin. It is an uncommon condition and found with ratio of <1:10,000.

DETERMINATION OF AGE

Age estimation is an important activity that is frequently required to be carried out by a medicolegal expert. An individual is often referred to a medical man by the court or investigating authority in criminal as well as in civil cases to give the opinion regarding his or her age. Forensic age estimation in living subjects has gained increasing significance in recent years. Determination of age is required in the fetus, children and adult and even in dead bodies including skeletal remains.

The following data are utilized for determination of age:

i. Psychological data
ii. Physical data
iii. Dental data
iv. Radiological data
v. Other senile changes.

First 7 to 10 days after conception, i.e. until the implantation occurs the term developing ovum is used. It is called an 'embryo' from one week to the end of the second month, and later it is called a fetus. It becomes an infant when it is completely born. The different period in regards to an infant are shown in **Table 5.4**.

Table 5.4 Different periods of infant
Prenatal period: Ovum or zygote – from zero day to 14 days; Embryo – from 14 days to 8 weeks; Fetus – from 9 weeks to birth
Perinatal period: It is the time period pertaining to the period immediately before and after birth. The perinatal period is an interval extending approximately from the 28th week of gestation to the 28th day after birth
Postnatal period: Postnatal a Latin word means after birth (from post, meaning after and Natalis, means birth) is the period beginning immediately after the birth of a child and extending for about 6 weeks. The term postpartum period, refers to the mother, whereas postnatal refers to the infant

Age of the Fetus

Age of a fetus can be assessed as follows:

- Crown-heel length
- Crown-rump length
- Weight
- Physical features
- Appearances of epiphyseal centers.

Length and Weight

The male infants weigh about 100 g more than the female. The circumference of the head is 33–36 cm. At full term, the head of a child is nearly one-fourth of the whole length of the body. The surface of the brain shows convolutions, and the gray matter begins to form.

The scalp hair is dark, 3 to 5 cm long. The face is not wrinkled. Lanugo is absent except on the shoulders. The skin is pale and covered with vernix caseosa. The nails project beyond the end of fingers, but reach only the tip of the toes. The cartilages are formed in the nose and ears. The testes are present in the scrotum; vulva is closed and labia minora are covered by fully developed labia majora. The rectum contains dark brownish, green or black meconium.

The placenta is 22 cm in diameter, one and half cm thick at the center, and weight about 500 g. The umbilicus is situated midway between the pubis and xiphoid cartilage. The umbilical cord is 50–55 cm long and one cm thick. The center of ossification is found in the lower end of the femur and sometimes in the cuboids and in the upper end of the tibia. Six fontanelles are usually present in the neonatal skull.

Rule of Haase

This is a rough method of calculating the age of the fetus. The length of the fetus is measured from the crown to the heel in cm. During the first 5 months of pregnancy, the square root of the length gives the approximate age of the fetus in months, e.g. a fetus of 16 cm is of 4 months duration. Until the fetus reaches the length of 25 cm, the square root of the crown-heel length is taken to arrive at the age.

When the length of the fetus is more than 25 cm, it is divided by five. Hence, for the last 5 months, the length in cm divided by five give the age in months, e.g. fetus of 35 cm is 7 months.

Physical Features

End of First Month: Length 1 cm; weight 2.5 g. The eyes are seen as two dark spots and the mouth as a cleft. Nucleated red cells begin to form in the placenta.

End of the Second Month: Length is 4 cm; weight 10 g. The hands and feet are webbed. The placenta begins to form. The anus is seen as a dark spot. First ossification center in a fetus appears in clavicle (4 to 5 weeks), followed by maxilla (6 weeks).

End of Third Month: Length 9 cm; weight 30–35 g. The eyes are closed, the pupillary membrane appears. Nails appear in membranous form and the neck is formed.

End of Fourth Month: Length 16 cm; weight 120–130 g. At this stage sex can be recognized. Lanugo hair is seen on the body. Convolutions begin to develop in the brain. Meconium is found in the duodenum.

End of Fifth Month: Length 25 cm; weight 400 g. Nails are distinct and soft and up to a proximity to the tips of fingers. Light hair appears on the head. Skin is covered with vernix caseosa. Meconium is seen at the beginning of the large intestine. Center for manubrium, 1st segment of sternum are seen.

End of Sixth Month: Length 30 cm; weight 700 g. Eyebrows, eyelashes appear and adherent. Skin is red and wrinkled and subcutaneous fat begins to be deposited. The testes are seen close to the kidneys. Sylvian fissure of brain is formed. Meconium is in transverse colon.

End of Seventh Month: Length 35 cm; crown-rump length 23 cm; foot length 8 cm; weight 900–1200 g. Nails are up to tips of fingers. Eyelids open and pupillary membrane disappears. Skin is dusky red, thick and fibrous. Meconium is found in the entire large intestine. Testes are found at the external inguinal ring. Gallbladder contains bile and cecum is seen in the right iliac fossa. Ossification center for talus appears.

End of Eighth Month: Length 40 cm; weight 1.5 kg. Nails reach the tips of fingers. Scalp hair is thicker. Skin is not wrinkled. Left testis is present in the scrotum. Placenta weighs 500 g.

End of Ninth Month: Length 45 cm; weight 2.5–3 kg. Scalp hair is dark and 4 cm long. Meconium is seen at the end of large intestine. Scrotum is wrinkled and contains both testes. Placenta weighs 500 g. Ossification centers are usually present in the lower end of the femur.

End of Tenth Month (full term child): Length 50–53 cm; crown-rump length 30–33 cm; weight 2.5–5 kg; the length is much less variable than the weight.

The different age-related changes in the fetus are briefed in **Table 5.5**.

Appearances of Ossification Centers

i. **Sternum**: It is placed flat on a wooden board and cut with the cartilage knife in its long axis in midline, which exposes the ossification centers (**Figure 5.10**).
ii. **Lower end of the femur and upper end of the tibia**: The leg is flexed against the thigh and a transverse or vertical incision is made into the knee joint. The patella is removed. The end of the femur is pushed forward through the wound, and a number of parallel cross-sections are made through the epiphysis starting from its articular surface and continuing until the largest part of ossification center is reached.
The center is seen as a brownish red nucleus surrounded by bluish white cartilage above it until the diaphyseal center is reached (**Figure 5.11**). The center appears in about the 36th week. Its diameter is about 4–5 mm at 37–38 weeks and 6–8 mm at full term. The upper end of tibia is similarly examined.
iii. **Bones of the foot**: The foot if grasped in the left hand behind the heel, the toes pointing

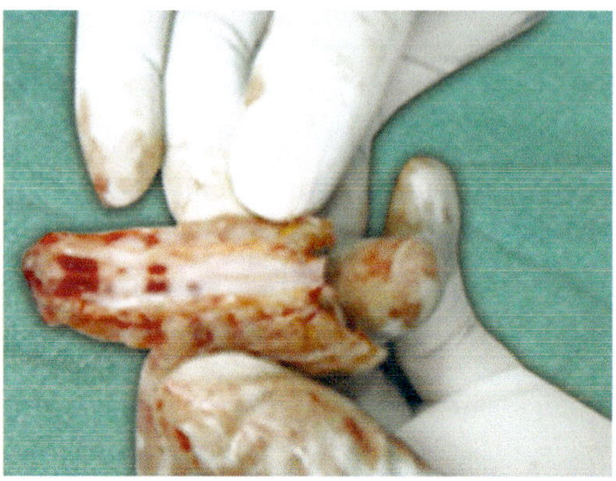

Figure 5.10 Ossification centers of sternum

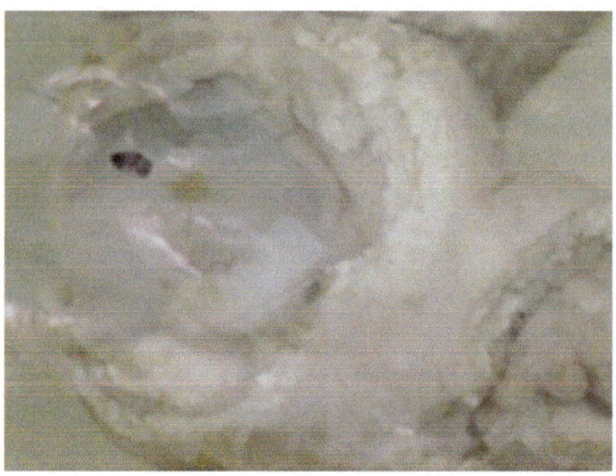

Figure 5.11 Ossification centers at lower end of femur

Table 5.5 Age-related changes in the fetus

Month (IUL)	Three months	Four months	Five months	Six months	Seven months	Eight months	Nine months
Length (cm)	9	16	25	30	35	40	45
Weight	30–35 g	120–130 g	400 g	700 g	900–1200 g	1.5 kg	2–2.25 kg
Nails	Present in membranous form	-	Up to proximity of tip of finger	-	Up to tip of finger	-	Beyond the tip of finger
Hairs	-	Lanugos appears	Scalp hairs appear	-	Scalp hair 1 cm long	Scalp hair 1.5 cm	Scalp hair 2 cm
Sex	-	Distinguishable	-	Well distinguished	-	-	-
Eyelids	-	-	-	Adherent and eye lash present	Non-adherent and eye lashes present	Well formed	-
Brain	-	-	-	Sylvian fissure formed	-	-	-
Intestine	-	Meconium in upper part of small intestine	Meconium up to ascending colon	Meconium in transverse colon	Meconium in descending pelvic colon	-	Meconium in rectum
Scrotum	-	-	-	Empty	-	Corrugated	Occupied by testes
Testes	-	-	-	On psoas muscle	Near the internal inguinal ring	In canal (L>R)	Inside scrotum (L>R)
Centers of ossification	-	-	Manubrium, 1st segment of sternum	-	Talus and 2nd and 3rd segments of sternum	-	Lower end of femur and cuboid

towards the dissector. An incision is made between the interspaces of third and fourth toes with a long knife, backwards through the sole of the foot and heel. If center in calcaneum and talus are not exposed, thin slices of cartilage of these bones should be cut until the presence or absence has been shown. Center in the calcaneum appears at the end of the fifth and in talus at the end of the seventh month of intrauterine life. A center may be present in cuboid at birth, or it may appear shortly afterwards.

Age from Birth till 25 Years

Physical Examination for Age Estimation

An approximate age of a person can be estimated from height and weight. Development of secondary sexual characteristics like axillary and pubic hair, growth of beard and moustache, development of sexual organs and menstrual history, etc., can be of added help. Feature of graying hair, balding, decrease in stature, changes in the skin, arcus senilis, corneal opacity, cataract, etc., give an idea of advancing age.

Secondary Sexual Characters

These develop at the time of puberty due to the influence of hormones and are useful for the determination of age at that period.

The voice becomes deep due to elongation of the vocal cords. This change is more prominently seen in boys than in girls. Fine hair begins to appear on the penis. The development of pubic hair and genital organs can be assessed by **Tanner staging**, which divides it into five stages as follows:

In Boys

Stage 1: No pubic hairs and penis and testicles are in the same proportions as in childhood.

Stage 2: Sparse growth of long, slightly darkened, pubic hair at the base of the penis is seen. The testicles begin to get larger, and the scrotum begins to get a reddened and altered texture. The penis may grow slightly.

Stage 3: Pubic hair gets darker, coarser and curlier. It begins to spread over the pubic bone. The testicles continue to enlarge and the scrotum texture becomes more like that of an adult. The penis gets longer.

Stage 4: Pubic hair grows to cover the base of penis and begins to grow on the upper part of scrotum. The hair gets darker, coarser and curlier. The scrotal skin gets darker as the testicles continue to grow. The penis continues to grow longer and gets wider. The Glans or head, of the penis becomes much more prominent.

Stage 5: Pubic hair has spread to inside of the thighs. The scrotum, testicles and penis grow to their final adult size and shape.

Development of axillary hair, beard and moustache and body hair takes place subsequently.

In Girls

Stage 1: No pubic hair.

Stage 2: There is sparse growth of long, slightly darkened, downy hair mostly along the labia. This hair is usually straight or slightly curled.

Stage 3: Hair becomes darker, coarser and curlier. It now grows sparsely over the Mons Veneris area.

Stage 4: Hair growths are seen more densely. It becomes as coarse and curly as in the adult, but does not extend onto the inner thighs.

Stage 5: Classic, coarse and curly pubic hair that extends up to inner thighs.

Tanner staging of breast development is as follows:

Stage 1: Small elevated nipple with no significant underlying breast tissue.

Stage 2: Elevation of breast and nipple as small mound; the areola begins to enlarge.

Stage 3: Further enlargement and elevation of the breast and areola (with no separation of their contours) takes place. The areola begins to darken in color.

Stage 4: Projection of the areola and nipple to form a secondary mound.

Stage 5: Mature adult breast, there is a projection of nipple only.

Development of axillary hair and body hair takes place subsequently.

Dental Examination for Age Estimation

In dental age estimation, tooth eruption is a parameter of developmental morphology that can be analyzed by either clinical examination or by evaluation of dental X-ray.[3]

The three stages of human dentition, viz. deciduous or temporary, mixed and permanent follow a periodic sequence that can be utilized for estimation of age of different accuracy and have discussed thoroughly in Chapter 7 (**Forensic Odontology**).

Radiological Examination for Age Estimation

This procedure is used to know:

- Appearance and fusion of ossification centers
- Study of diaphyseal length
- Calcification of root of teeth.

Appearance and Fusion of Ossification Centers

Radiological data are accepted to be the most reliable. The appearance and union of ossification centers follow a definite time sequence, which can be utilized for the age estimation. However, following common features should be remembered while opining the age from radiological finding of a bone:

Common Features

i. Radiological data can easily be determined by studying appearances of ossification centers and their fusion with the adjacent centers by radiological examination of the bones.
ii. The bones of the whole skeleton develop from the preformed hyaline cartilage by the process of "**Osteogenesis**".
iii. Large numbers of ossification centers appear in the preformed cartilage at different periods of life. At 11–12th week of intrauterine life, there are 806 ossification centers, at birth, they are about 450 and an adult skeleton contains only 206 bones.
iv. Usually in epiphyses, ossification starts centrally and then spreads to the periphery.
v. At the start with, the centers are small, rounded, size of a pinhead, as it grows it takes the shape of the bone.
vi. Small bones like, carpal, tarsal bones grow from a single center, where as long bones grow from multiple centers.
vii. Shaft or diaphysis of most of the long bones develops from one center, while the ends or the epiphysis are developed from separate centers. These epiphyseal centers are secondary centers.
viii. Increase in length of long bones occurs in the layered cartilage persisting in between the diaphysis and epiphysis, until it attains the adult shape and size.
ix. Both the terminal ends of the long bones of the limbs develop from separate ossification centers, while the ends of the bones like clavicle, rib and metacarpal, metatarsal develop from one epiphysis at one end only.
x. Epiphyseal union occurs 1 to 2 years earlier in females than males.
xi. Epiphyseal union is earlier in tropical countries than in temperate zones.

The time of bony epiphyseal union is not same throughout India. It differs even up to 2–3 years from south to north, east to west. The centers of ossification as per **Galstaun** are mentioned in **Table 5.6**.

In young children, radiological examination of hand and foot alone can give an accurate estimation of age, but in adult two or three joints, viz. wrist, elbow, shoulder, hip, knee and ankle joint and skull (anteroposterior and lateral view) are to be radiographed, depending upon the person's age. Chest with sternoclavicular joints in anteroposterior and chest with sternum and vertebrae is to be X-rayed in a lateral view position for the purpose of age estimation.

Table 5.6 Centers of ossification as observed by Galstaun in Indian subjects

Bone/Joint (A-Appearance, F-Fusion)		Female		Male	
Clavicle (sternal end)		A F	14–16 years 20 years	A F	15– 19 years 22 years
Scapula	Base of coracoid of scapula	A F	2.5 months 2.5 years	A F	2.5 months 2.5 years
	Coracoid tip	A F	10–11 years 16 years	A F	10–11 years 16 years
	Angle of coracoid	A F	8–10 years 16 years	A F	10–14 years 17–18 years
	Acromion	A F	12–14 years 13–16 years	A F	14–17 years 14–19 years
Humerus	Head of humerus	A F	1 year 14–16 years	A F	1 year 14–18 years
	Greater tubercle (fusion to head)	A F	7 months 2–4 years	A F	7 months 2–4 years
	Greater tubercle (fusion to lesser tubercle)	A F	7 months 5–7 years	A F	7 months 5–7 years
	Trochlea Fusion to Capitulum	A F	10 years 9–13 years	A F	11 years 11–15 years
	Lateral epicondyle Fusion to capitulum	A F	10 years 10–12 years	A F	11 years 11–16 years
	Medial epicondyle Fusion to shaft distal humeral epiphysis	A F	5 years 14 years	A F	7 years 16 years
Radius	Head	A F	6 years 14 years	A F	8 years 16 years
	Distal end	A F	1 year 16.5 years	A F	1 years 16–17 years
Ulna	Olecranon	A F	9–12 years 15 years	A F	11–13 years 17 years
	Distal end of ulna	A F	8–10 years 17 years	A F	10–11 years 18 years
Hip bone	Iliac crest	A F	14 years 17–19 years	A F	17 years 19–20 years
	Ischium and pubis	A F	... 8.5 years	A F	.... 8.5 years
	Acetabulum: Disappearance of triradiate cartilage		14 years		15–16 years
	Ischial tuberosity	A F	14–16 years 20 years	A F	16–18 years 20 years
Femur	Head of femur	A F	1 year 14–15 years	A F	1 year 16–17 years
	Greater trochanter	A F	3 years 14 years	A F	3 years 17 years
	Lesser trochanter	A F	l year 15–17 years	A F	1 year 15–17 years
	Distal end of femur	A F	Before birth 14–17 years	A F	Before birth 14–17 years

Contd...

Contd...

Tibia	Proximal end of tibia	A F	Shortly before or after birth 14–15 years	A F	Shortly before or after birth 15–17 years
	Distal end of tibia	A F	… 14.1–14.4 years	A F	… 16 years
Fibula	Proximal end of fibula	A F	… 14–16 years	A F	… 11–16 years
	Distal end of fibula	A F	… 13–15 years	A F	… 14–16 years
Patella	–	A	4 years	A	3–7 years
Carpal bones	Capitate	A	½ years	A	½ years
	Hamate	A	8–14 months	A	8–14 months
	Triquetral	A	2–3 years	A	3–4 years
	Lunate	A	5 years	A	5 years
	Trapezium	A	5–6 years	A	7 years
	Trapezoid	A	5–6 years	A	4–7 years
	Scaphoid	A	6 years	A	7–11 years
	Pisiform	A	9–12 years	A	12–17 years
Metacarpals	First metacarpal bone	A F	3 years 14–15 years	A F	4 years 16–18 years
	2nd, 3rd, 4th and 5th metacarpal bones	A F	2–3 years 14–15 years	A F	3–4 years 16–18 years
Phalanges of hand	Proximal row	A F	1.5 years 14–15 years	A F	2–4 years 17–18 years
	Middle row	A F	2–3 years 14–16 years	A F	3 years 16–18 years
	Terminal row	A F	3 years 15 years	A F	3–5 years 17–18 years
Tarsal bones	Calcaneum and talus	A	At birth		At birth
	Cuboid	A	At birth	A	At birth
	Internal cuneiform	A	1–3 years	A	1–4 years
	Middle cuneiform	A	1–3 years	A	2–4 years
	External cuneiform	A	1–3 years	A	1–4 years
	Navicular	A	1–3 years	A	1–4 years
Metatarsals	1st metatarsal bone	A F	3 years 14–15 years	A F	4–5 years 16–18 years
	2nd, 3rd, 4th and 5th metatarsal	A F	3 years 14–15 years	A F	4–5 years 16–18 years
Tarsal phalanges	Proximal row	A F	1–3 years 14–15 years	A F	3–4 years 16–18 years
	Middle row	A F	3–4 years 14–15 years	A F	3–4 years 16–18 years
	Terminal row	A F	4–6 years 13–14 years	A F	4–6 years 15–17 years

As a rule, the aging of bones is more accurate with the appearance of ossification centers than the union of same. In the long bones of upper limbs, the union is earlier at the elbow joint and later at the wrist joint. Head of the humerus is the last long bone epiphysis to unite in the upper limb. In lower limb, union occurs earlier at the hip and ankle joints and later at the knee joint.

The **epiphyseal plate** is a hyaline cartilage plate in the metaphysis at each end of a long bone. The plate is found in children and adolescents; in adults, who have stopped growing, the plate is replaced by an **epiphyseal line**. The epiphyseal lines on the long bones of a young individual appear as circular grooves around the ends of the bones, and on X-rays, it appears as irregular lines resembling a fracture. When bones are dried, the epiphyses may be separated in a young child from the shaft, which should not be mistaken for fractures. Skeletal age is based on appearance and union of epiphyseal centers, which should be expressed as plus or minus some years, e.g. 10 ± 1.

The process of fusion of epiphysis with diaphysis is called "**Union**". Union may be interpreted as (a) not united (b) uniting, all on the basis of stage of union. The radiological bony union is 2–3 years earlier than anatomical bony union. This is due to the fact, that towards the end of the growth period, the epiphyseal plate of the hyaline cartilage becomes thin and irregular in outlines called epiphyseal line, which may not be detected on X-ray. In X-ray plate, persistent scar is neither the evidence of incomplete union nor the recent union.

Disturbance in Skeletal Growth and Maturation

The relationship of the endocrine glands to skeletal growth and maturation is very important. Roentgen examination of the growing skeleton may give valuable information concerning thyroid, pituitary and gonadal disturbances. They all cause generalized skeletal age abnormality. Delay in appearance or fusion or retardation of epiphyseal centers may result from deficient secretion of one or more of these glands. Hypersecretion may accelerate this process.

Graham CB[4] in his study indicates a number of glandular disturbances and their effect on skeletal maturation. Focal increases in maturation may occur following infection, burns, frostbites, radiation therapy or trauma, particularly epiphyseal separations. These all impair the growth potential either by destroying the resting cells or by disrupting the blood supply and growth may cease. Premature closure of the epiphysis may occur as the result of bone infarcts, particularly in sickle cell disease. Some important X-ray plates are shown in **Figure 5.12** from **A** to **L** commonly used for the purpose of age estimation.

Apart from X-rays, computed tomography of head for suture closure ectocranially can also be done. The most reliable estimation of age is from ectocranial union of suture and the order of accuracy is: sagittal, lambdoid and then coronal.

Ages from **skeletal** changes and **histological age** estimation from bone are discussed in the Chapter 6 (**Forensic Osteology**).

Medicolegal Importance of Age

1. **Above seven months of intrauterine**: Viability is attained. Under section 302 of IPC, charge of infanticide is leveled.
2. **Five years of age**: (i) According to Section 6 (a) of "The Hindu Minority and Guardianship Act, 1956", a minor who has not completed the age of 5 years shall ordinarily be in the custody of the mother; (ii) Half fare in railway; (iii) Child is held responsible for any wreckage caused to train (as per Railway Act).
3. **Criminal responsibility**: Any act done by a child under 7 years of age is not an offence (Section 82 IPC). A child between 7 and 12 years is presumed to be capable of committing an offence, if he has attained sufficient maturity of understanding to judge the nature and consequences of his

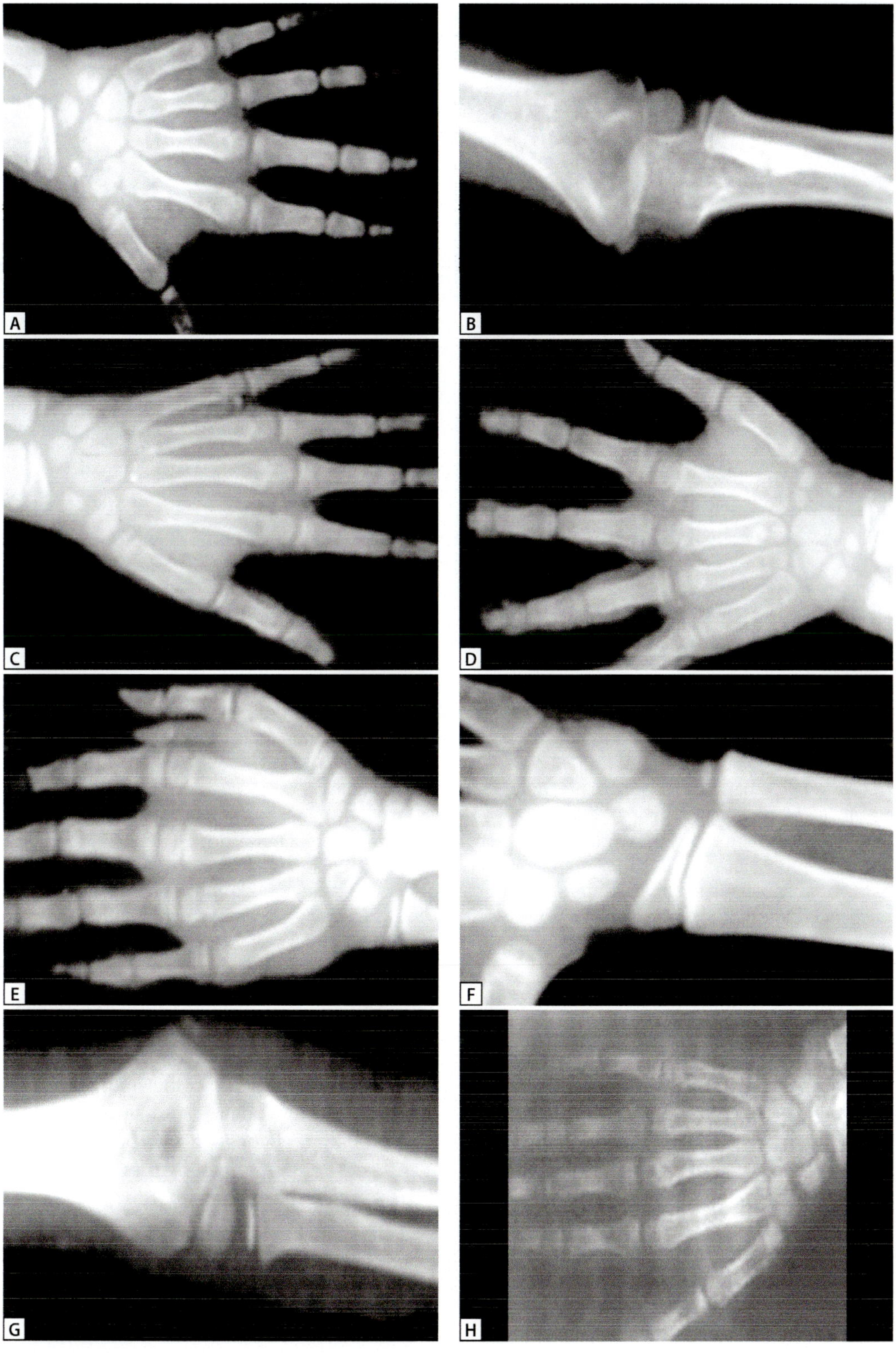
A
B
C
D
E
F
G
H

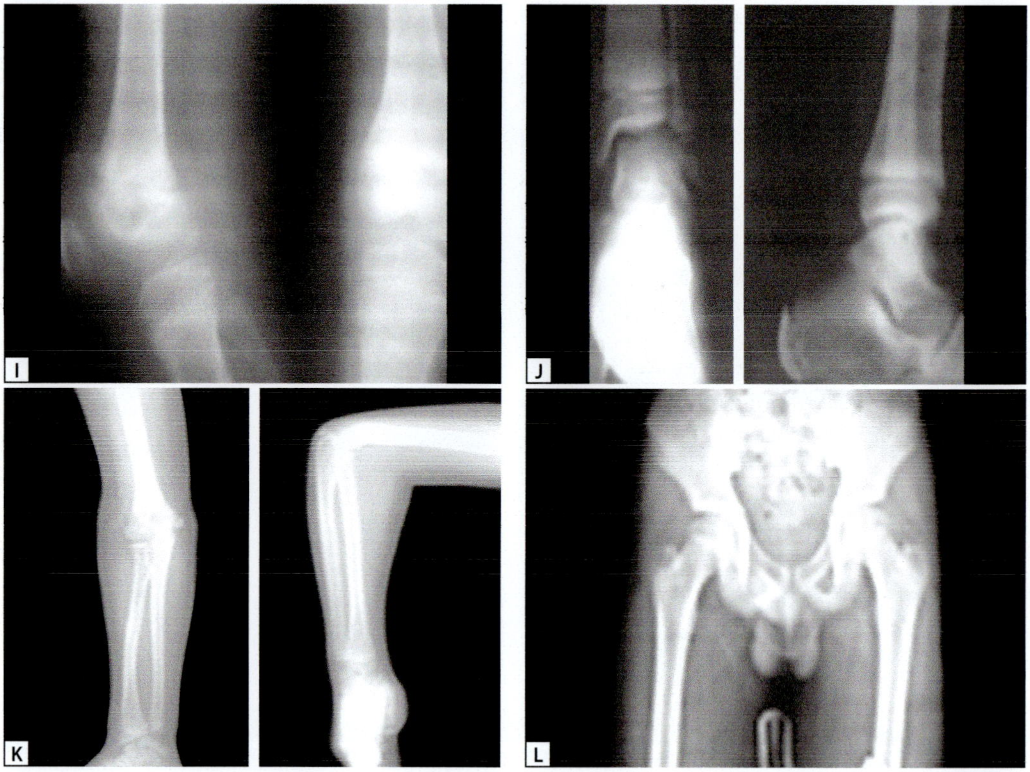

Figures 5.12A to L X-ray showing, (A) Ossification center of lunate, minimum age: 5 years (both sex); (B) Ossification center of medial epicondyle, minimum age: 5 (Female) and 7 (male) years; (C) Wrist and hand showing ossification center of trapezium, trapezoid and scaphoid, minimum age: 6 years; (D) Center of trapezium and trapezoid, minimum age: 7 years; (E) Wrist and hand showing lower epiphysis of first metacarpal not united with shaft, age: 12-15 years; (F) Hand showing ossification center of trapezium and distal ulna, age: 6 years; (G) Elbow joint shows ossification center of medial epicondyle, minimum age: 5 (Female) and 7 (male) years; (H) Wrist joint showing non-union of epiphysis of the metacarpal bone around the joint, age below 18 years; (I) Knee joint non-union of epiphysis of lower end of femur and upper ends of tibia and fibula, age below 17 years; (J) Ankle showing non-union of epiphyses of lower ends of tibia and fibula with appearance of secondary center for calcaneum, age bellow 16 years; (K) Elbow and wrist joints of 14 years old boy; (L) Hip joint of 14 years old boy

conduct on that occasion (Section 83 IPC). This maturity is presumed in a child unless otherwise proved by defense. A child under 12 years of age cannot give valid consent to suffer any harm, which may occur from an act done in good faith and for its benefit (Section 89 IPC). A person above 18 years can give valid consent to suffer any harm, which may result from an act not known to cause death or grievous hurt (Section 87 IPC).

4. **Judicial punishment**: According to the **Juvenile Justice** (Care and protection of children) **Act 2000**, 'Juvenile or boy' mean a person who has not completed 18 years of age. The Juvenile Justice Board may advise or admonish the juvenile or order to participate in group counseling or perform community service or to be released on probation of conduct or to pay a fine or to make an order directing the juvenile to be sent to a special home for the period until he becomes a major. No juvenile found guilty by law shall be sentenced to death or life imprisonment or committed to prison.
5. **Rape**: Sexual intercourse by a man with a girl under 15 years, even if she is his own

wife (by a local amendment this age has been reduced to 13 years for the state of Manipur), or with any other girl under 16 years even with her consent is rape (Section 375 IPC).

However, anti-rape bill has been passed in Lok Sabha on **19th March, 2013**, which provides that the age of consent for sex would be 18 years. Details of it are discussed in the chapter of "Virginity, Sexual Offences and Perversions".

6. **Employment:** A child below 14 years of age cannot be employed to work in a factory or mine or in many other risky employments. A child between 14 and 15 years of age can be engaged in non-hazardous factory-jobs for a limited period during the day hours. A person who has completed 15 years is allowed to work in a factory as an adult if a fitness certificate is issued to him by a certifying surgeon.
7. **Kidnapping:** In criminal law, **kidnapping** is the taking away or transportation of a person against the person's will, usually to hold the person in false imprisonment (a confinement without legal authority). It is an offence to kidnap a (i) child with the intension of taking dishonestly any movable property, if the age is under 10 years (Section 369, IPC); (ii) minor from lawful guardianship if the age of a boy is under 16 years and that of a girl under 18 years (Section 366, IPC); (iii) girl for prostitution, if her age is below 18 years (Section 366-A, IPC) and (iv) girl to import into India from a foreign country for purposes of eliciting intercourse, if her age is less than 21 years (Section 366-B, IPC).
8. **Attainment of majority:** As per Section 3 of the Indian Majority Act, 1875, a person attains majority on the completion of 18th years, but if a person is under a guardianship of the Court of Wards (under a guardian appointed by the Court), he attains majority on the completion of 21 years.
9. **Evidence:** Competency for giving evidence depends upon understanding, but not on age. Section 118 of IEA states that a person of any age can give evidence if the court is satisfied that the child is truthful.
10. **Marriage contract:** As per Child Marriage Restraint Act 1978, the minimum age of marriage for females is 18 years and that for males is 21 years.
11. **Criminal abortion:** One cannot charge a woman for procuring criminal abortion for a woman who has passed childbearing age.
12. **Infanticide:** If the infant is under the age of 7 months of intrauterine life, then the charge of infanticide cannot be supported.
13. **Identification:** An approximate age is important in any identification data.
14. **Impotence and sterility:** A boy is sterile before puberty, though not impotent. Women become sterile after menopause.
15. **Importance of 25 years of age:**
    i. According to Article 84(b) of The Constitution of India, minimum age for contesting for the membership of parliament is 25 years.
    ii. According to Article 173 (b) of the Constitution, minimum age for contesting for the membership of any State Legislative Assembly is 25 years.
    iii. This is the maximum age for entry into some government services.
    iv. According to Punjab Excise Act 1914, a person below this age cannot buy and consume liquor.
16. **Importance of 30 years of age:**
    i. According to Article 84(b) of The Constitution of India, this is the minimum age for election to the Council of States (Rajya Sabha).
    ii. According to Article 173(b) this is the minimum age for election to the State Legislative Council.
17. **Importance of 35 years of age:**
    i. According to Article 58(1)(b) of The Constitution of India, this is the minimum age for appointment as the President of India.
    ii. According to Article 66(3)(b), this is the minimum age for appointment as the Vice-President of India.

iii. According to Article 157, this is the minimum age for appointment as the Governor of any State.
iv. According to Section 4(3)(i) of the Prenatal Diagnostic Techniques (Regulation and Prevention of Misuse) Act 1994, no prenatal diagnostic technique shall be used or conducted unless the age of the woman is above 35 years.

18. **Importance of 60 years of age**: This is the age of retirement from government service.
19. **Importance of 65 years of age**: According to Section 10 (2) of the Consumer Protection Act 1986, every member of the District Forum shall hold office for a term of 5 years or up to the age of 65 years, whichever is earlier, and shall not be eligible for reappointment. District Forum is a kind of civil court, which delivers judgments in cases of consumer grievances. Similarly, the State Commission and the National Commission (mentioned below) are also akin to civil courts, which are higher in rank to District Forum.
20. **Importance of 67 years of age**: According to Section 16 (3) of the Consumer Protection Act 1986, every member of the State Commission shall be below 67 years of age.
21. **Importance of 70 years of age**: According to Section 20 (3) of the Consumer Protection Act 1986, every member of the National Commission shall be below 70 years of age. This is the age prescribed by some State Governments, which qualifies a person to get pension from "Old Age Pension Scheme".

STATURE

Stature means body height of a person. It shows a **diurnal variation** by half to two cm. It is less in the afternoon and evening due to the reduced elasticity of the intervertebral discs and the longitudinal vertebral muscles. Both malnutrition and advancing years reduce stature. After the age of 30, the natural processes of senile degeneration cause gradual decrease in stature by about 0.6 mm per year on an average. The stature is greater by 1–3 cm on lying. Due to complete loss of muscle tone, relaxation of large joints and loss of tensioning effect of para-spinal muscles on intervertebral discs, the body shows lengthening after death by about two cm.

Stature of Dismembered Body

In case of **dismembered body**, the approximate **stature** is **determined** as follows:

1. The length from the tip of the middle finger to the tip of the opposite middle finger, when arms are fully extended, approximately equals the height.
2. Twice the length of one arm, with 30 cm added for two clavicles and four cm for the sternum, is equal to the height.
3. The length from the vertex to the symphysis pubis is roughly half of stature.
4. The length from the sternal notch to symphysis pubis multiplied by 3.3 gives the stature.
5. The length of forearm measured from tip of olecranon process to tip of the middle finger is equal to 5/19 of the stature.
6. The height of head measured by the vertical distance from the top of the head to the tip of the chin is about one-seventh of the total height.
7. The length of vertebral column is 35/100 of the height.
8. To the length of entire skeleton add two-and-half cm to four cm for the thickness of the soft parts.
9. Maximum foot length divided by 0.15 gives stature.

Statures from individual bones are discussed in Chapter 6 (**Forensic Osteology**).

ANTHROPOMETRY (BERTILLON SYSTEM)

The science of measuring the body parts constitutes Bertillon system or anthropometry.

Principle

After the age of 21 years, the skeleton stops growing, hence the dimensions of the skeleton remain unchanged and that the ratio in size of different parts to one another varies considerably in different individuals. As such, this can be applied only to adults.

This system includes recording of:

i. **Descriptive data**: Such as color of hair, eyes, complexion, shape of nose.
ii. **Body marks**: Such as moles, scars, tattoo marks.
iii. **Body measurements**: Such as height, anteroposterior diameter of head and trunk, the span of outstretched arms, the length of left middle finger, left little finger, left forearm, left foot, length and breadth of right ear and color of left iris. The photographs of a front view of the head, a profile view of the right side of head are also taken. Though photographs are very useful means of identification, they are not free from errors. This system has now been replaced by dactylography.

FINGERPRINT SYSTEM

This is also known as dactylography or dermatoglyphics or Galton system.

Definition

Fingerprints are impressions of patterns formed by the papillary or epidermal ridges of the fingertips. At birth, a fine pattern of ridges is seen on the skin of the bulbs of the fingers and thumbs, parts of the palms and the soles of the feet.

Principle of Use

The skin of the fingertips is covered with ridges on which the sweat pores open in certain characters that are specific for each person. The pattern is absolutely individual, as it develops at the 16th weeks of intrauterine life and remains constant for life. No two person's fingerprints are exactly alike, not even those of identical twins.

Fingerprints are present in both epidermis and dermis, and so, they are not destructed by the peeling of the superficial epithelium that may occur in early submersion under water or putrefaction. Fingerprints are transiently lost in exposure to ionizing radiation, but permanently lost in surgical removal, chemical destruction, chronic skin diseases, e.g. leprosy and by LASER leaving no scar for identification.

Historical Background

i. Clay tablets from ancient Babylonia indicate the first civilizations to have attempted to identify criminals by their fingerprints. As early as 200 BC, the Chinese used fingerprints as a personal signature. The use of finger print in record in official documents of China dates back to 3000 BC.
ii. It is stated that the first scientific study on fingerprint was done by **Professor Melphige** in 1680.
iii. **Sir William Herschel**, working in the Hooghly district of Bengal, used palm prints of Indian people for identifying them legally. Herschel, a British officer in India in the 1850's, is credited with the first systematic use of fingerprints for identification. Fingerprint Bureau was first established in Kolkata.
iv. The first system that allowed fingerprints to be matched against each other in an efficient manner was devised by Sir Francis Galton, an English scientist, in 1892. He also published his work in the form of a book 'Fingerprint'.
v. His system was modified and implemented in criminal investigations by **Sir Edward Henry**, a commissioner of Scotland Yard in London, in 1901. The Henry system is used in most countries today. Some South American countries, however, use a system devised by Juan Vucetich, an Argentine.

Fingerprints were first used in the US in 1903 in New York State prisons. The Federal Bureau of Investigation (FBI) has maintained its central file since 1924. FBI holds the largest collection of fingerprints.

Classification

Sir Galton classified fingerprints into four major or primary types based on the arrangement of papillary ridges:

i. **Arches**: Comprising 6–7% of all prints. The ridges go from one side of the finger to the other (**Figure 5.13**).
ii. **Loops** (**Figure 5.14A**): About 67%. The ridges make a backward turn in their course from one side of the finger to the other. This turn may be radial (3%) or ulnar (65%).
iii. **Composites** (**Figure 5.14 B**): A combination of one or more of the previous types. It comprises 1–2% of all prints. It is further subdivided into (a) Central pocket loops, (b) Lateral pocket loops, (c) Twinned loops, (d) Accidentals.
iv. **Whorls** (**Figure 5.15**): The ridges make one or more than complete turn. It comprises 25% of all prints. It is further categorized into (a) Concentric, (b) Spiral, (c) Double spiral, (d) Almond-shaped.

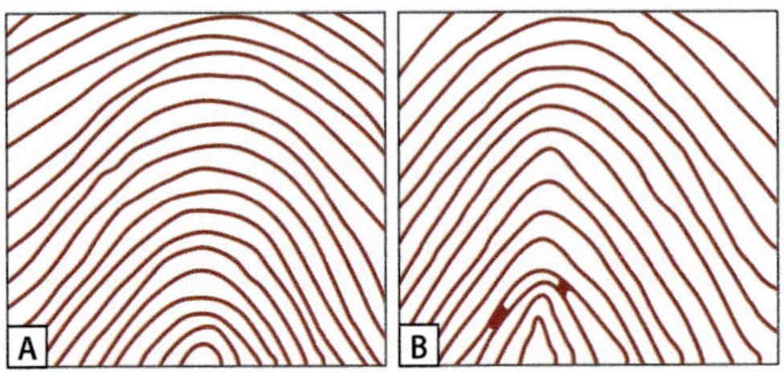

Figures 5.13A and B (A) Plain arch; (B) Tented arch

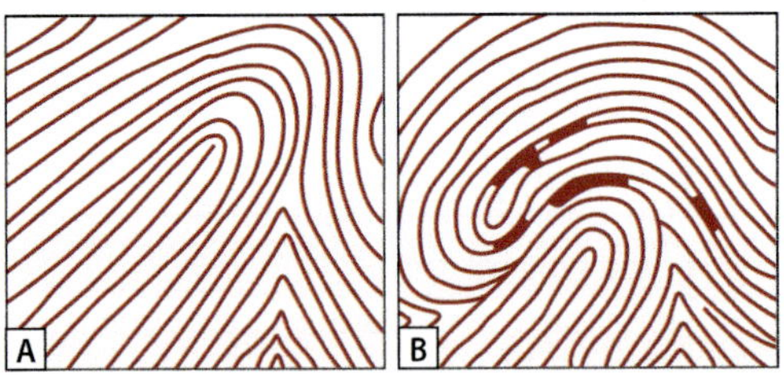

Figures 5.14A and B (A) Loop; (B) Composite

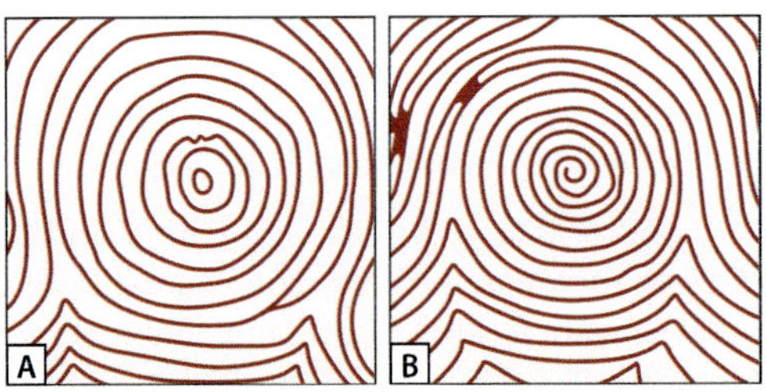

Figures 5.15A and B Whorls

Loops usually begin on side of the finger and end on the same side and can be further of radial or ulnar subtypes. In a whorl, the ridges form a series of circles or spirals around the core. Whorl can be concentric, spiral, double spiral or almond-shaped. Arches are wave like pattern from one side to the other side and may have subtypes like plain, tented and exceptional. In a composite, there are combinations of two or more of the type. Composite variety may include the central pocket loops, lateral pocket loops, twinned loops or accidentals.

Identification of any fingerprint is made by comparison of many details of characteristics, which occur throughout the ridge areas and by the sequence in which these characteristics occur, but not by comparing the patterns. The characteristics may take the form of ridge endings, bifurcations, lake formations or island formations. In practice, 16–20 points of fine comparison are accepted as proof of identity. The patterns are not inherited and paternity cannot be proved through fingerprint patterns. The details of these can be accurately teleprinted. Palm and footprints also provide similar material.

Exemplar Prints: An exemplar print, or known as prints, is the name given to fingerprints deliberately collected from a subject, whether for purposes of enrolment in a system or when under arrest for a suspected criminal offense. During criminal arrests, a set of exemplar prints will normally include one print taken from each finger that has been rolled from one edge of the nail to the other, plain (or slap) impressions of each of the four fingers of each hand, and plain impressions of each thumb. Exemplar prints can be collected using live scan or by using ink on paper cards.

Latent Prints

Although the word latent means hidden or invisible, in modern usage for forensic science, the term latent prints means any chance or accidental impression left by friction of epidermal ridges of skin on a surface, regardless of whether it is visible or invisible at the time of deposition. Electronic, chemical and physical processing techniques permit visualization of invisible latent print residues, whether they are from natural sweat of the skin or from a contaminant, such as motor oil, blood, ink, paint or some other form of dirt.

Latent prints may exhibit only a small portion of the surface of a finger, and this may be smudged, distorted, overlapped by other prints from the same or from different individuals or any or all of these in combination. For this reason, latent prints usually present an "inevitable source of error in making comparisons", as they generally "contain less clarity, less content, and less undistorted information than a fingerprint taken under controlled conditions, and much less detail compared to the actual patterns of ridges and grooves of a finger".

Patent Prints

Patent prints are chance friction ridge impressions, which are obvious to the human eye and which have been caused by the transfer of foreign material from a finger onto a surface. Some obvious examples would be impressions from flour and wet clay. Because they are already visible and have no need for enhancement, they are generally photographed rather than being lifted in the way that latent prints are. An attempt to preserve the actual print is always made for later presentation in court, and there are many techniques used to do this. Patent prints can be left on a surface by materials such as ink, dirt or blood.

Plastic Prints

The plastic print is an impression made on a soft surface, such as soap, cheese, etc. A plastic print is a friction ridge impression left in a material that retains the shape of the ridge detail. Although very few criminals would be careless enough to leave their prints in a lump of wet clay, this would make a perfect plastic print. Commonly encountered examples are melted candle wax; putty removed from the perimeter of windowpanes and thick grease deposits on car parts. Such prints are already visible and need no enhancement, but investigators must not overlook the potential that invisible latent prints deposited by accomplices may also be on such surfaces. After photographically recording such prints, attempts should be made to develop other non-plastic impressions deposited from sweat or other contaminates.

The Individuality of Fingerprints

The fingerprint patterns are distinctive and permanent in individuals. The fingerprint system is the only guide to identity, which is unfailing in practice. The pattern is different even in identical twins and exhibit endless variation so that it has been speculated that there is one in 64 billion chances of two persons having identical fingerprints.

Mode of Production

Skin is covered by stream of sweat, and when the person is excited, the output of sweat increases. Sweat contains about 99% water and 1% solids, which include salt, urea, fatty acids, formic acid, acetic acid, butyric acid and, sometimes, a little albumin. The fingerprint may also contain oil exuded by the sebaceous glands, which is present on the fingertips through touching the face, neck hair, scalp, etc. If any part of finger is applied to a smooth surface, a greasy impression of its pattern is made on it.

Techniques of Fingerprints

The hands are washed, cleaned and dried, as otherwise the print will be blurred. Fingerprints are recorded on unglazed white paper using printer's ink as follows: (i) A plain print is taken by applying ink to the tips of the fingers and placing the fingers directly on paper, (ii) The rolled fingerprint is taken by rolling the fingers on paper from outward to inward in such a way as to obtain an impression of the whole tip (**Figure 5.16**).

Burnt skin of the fingers, on healing shows its original pattern. In manual laborers working with lime, sand and cement, the ridges on the bulbs get unduly rubbed and become broken and indistinct. Ridge impressions get malformed if the quality of ink is poor, when the ink is too liquid and spreads into the depressions, if the digit is rolled often or pulled and when paper is placed upon an uneven or rough surface.

Fingerprints may be taken from almost any surface with which the finger comes in contact, including certain fabrics and human skin. A latent print may be developed by dusting the area with colored powders to provide a contrast, and its pattern is recorded by photography. It can also be examined by oblique lighting. The commonly used powder is **gray powder** (**aluminum dust**), but **white powders** (**lead carbonate** or **French chalk**) are used for dusting dark surfaces. Iodine vapors, Ninhydrin solution and Silicon nitrate solution are also used for developing fingerprints. Fingerprints on paper, wood and fabrics are developed by treating them with 5% silver nitrate solution and then fixing them with sodium thiosulfate. Fingerprints on paper can also be developed by exposing it to the vapors of iodine or osmium tetroxide. Electron autoradiography method uses a high-energy beam of X-rays to irradiate the lead dust on finger marks. The scanning electron microscope visualizes latent fingerprints on metal and glass.

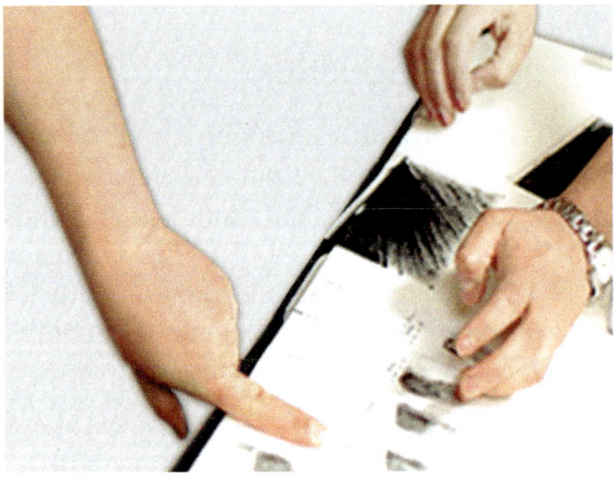

Figure 5.16 Development of fingerprint

Lifting of Fingerprints

Fingerprints on a large immovable hard surface is usually first developed, photographed and then adhesive surface of cellophane tape is pressed on the print, taken out gently and then it is pasted against a cardboard sheet for permanent preservation (**Figure 5.17**).

Fingerprints in Decomposed Bodies

Ridges are present in both dermis and epidermis. In advanced putrefaction and in cases of drowning, the skin is frequently found loose like a glove. This should be removed, preserved in formalin and used for impressions. Prints can be obtained from the dermis after epidermis is lost. Histological sections up to a depth of 0.6 mm from the surface of the skin give satisfactory fingerprints. In dead bodies, the palmar skin of the terminal phalanx of each

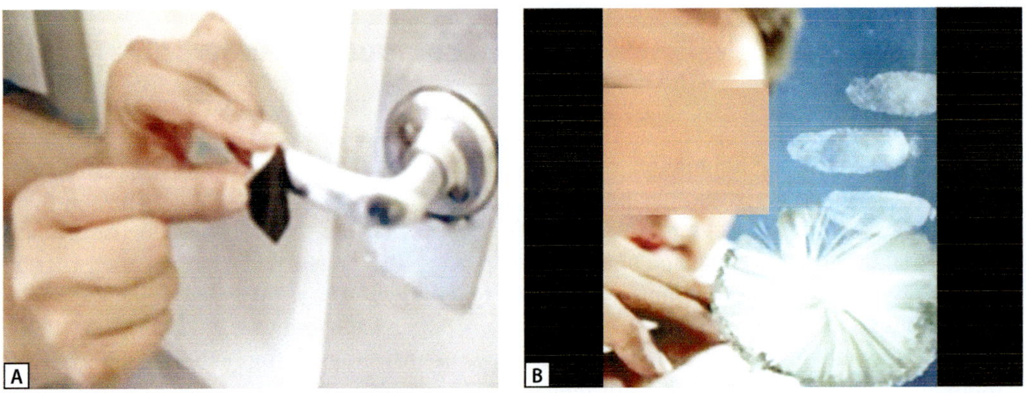

Figures 5.17A and B Lifting of fingerprints

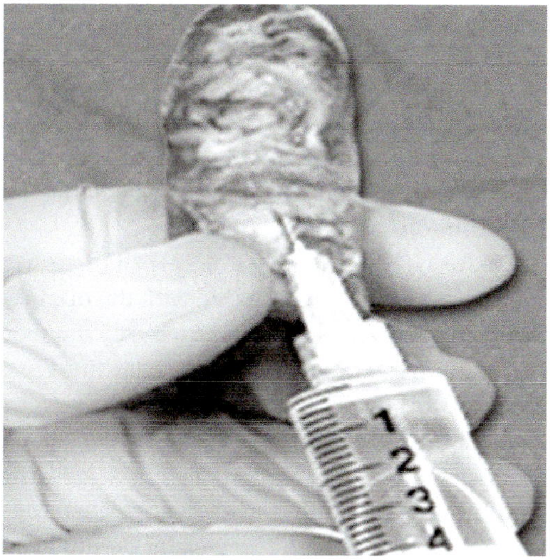

Figure 5.18 Injection of liquid paraffin into terminal phalanx

finger should be removed separately from both hands, and after labeling, placed in separate containers containing 10% formalin, and sent to the fingerprint bureau, if it is not possible to take the prints. If the fingers are shriveled, they should be immersed in 20% acetic acid for 24–48 hours.

If the fingers are sodden, wrinkled or mummified, their outline can be made level by injecting liquid paraffin, or even formalin, within the tissues of the palmar aspects of the terminal phalanx of each finger (**Figure 5.18**).

Persistence of Impression at Scene of Crime: Impressions may persist for years, if undisturbed by cleaning. Even outside the house, they may persist for weeks. On glazed paper, they persist for more than 3 years.

Mutilation of Fingerprints

Criminals sometimes attempt to mutilate the pattern by self-inflicted wounds or burns, application of corrosives or erosion against hard surface, but the prints are not destroyed unless the true skin is completely destroyed. They produce additional characteristics. In most cases of celiac disease, there is moderate epidermal ridge atrophy and even loss of pattern. Incomplete atrophy of the ridges is usually seen in dermatitis. Permanent impairment of the fingerprint pattern occurs in leprosy, electric injury and after exposure to radiation. In infantile paralysis, rickets and acromegaly, though the pattern is not altered; but the distance between the ridges can be changed. Fingerprints are better protected than other parts of the body, e.g. in case of burns, they are bent inwards against the palm of the hand.

Computerization: Fingerprint reader (FINDER) is a computerized automatic fingerprint reading system, which can record each fingerprint datum in half a second. Prints of eight fingers are recorded, excluding little fingers. The light reflected from a fingerprint can be measured and converted to digital data, which is classified, codified and stored in the computer.

Medicolegal Importance

1. The recognition of impressions left at a scene of crime, e.g. on weapons, furniture, doors, utensils, clothes, etc., establish the identity of the criminal.
2. The identification of suicides, deserters, persons suffering from loss of memory or those dead or unconscious after being involved in an accident and decomposing bodies can be made by this technique.
3. Identification in case of accidental exchange of newborn infants.
4. The prevention of impersonation.
5. To maintain identity records.

In criminals, impressions of all the 10 fingers are taken, but for civil purposes, only the left thumb impression is taken.

Poroscopy (Figure 5.19)

The method was discovered and developed by Edmond Locard in 1912. The ridges on fingers and hands are studded with microscopic pores, formed by mouths of ducts of subepidermal sweat glands. Each mm of a ridge contains 9–18 pores.

These pores are permanent and unchanged during life and vary in size, shape, position, extent and number over a given length of ridge in each individual. This method of examining pores is called poroscopy and is useful when only fragments of fingerprints are available.

Palm Prints

It may identify a person, if his hands were moist with blood or fluids. A palm print refers to an image acquired of the palm region of the hand. It can be either an online image, i.e. taken by a scanner, or CCD device or offline image where the image is taken with ink and paper. It is an extension of the fingerprint system, which records and matches images of the entire palm.

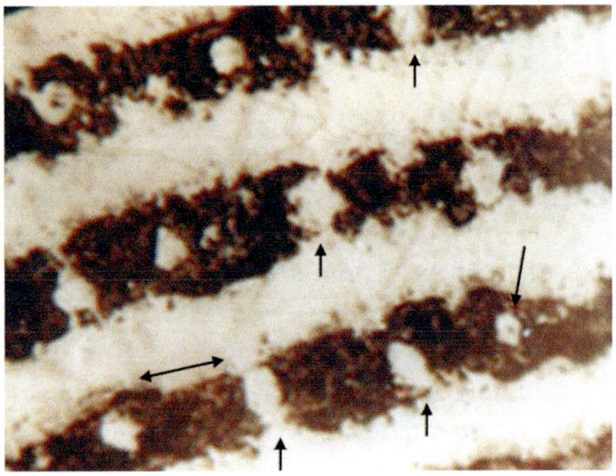

Figure 5.19 Poroscopy: A method of personal identification

FOOTPRINTS (PODOGRAM)

The skin patterns of toes and heels are as distinct and permanent as those of the fingers. Footprints of newborn infants are used in some maternity hospitals to prevent exchange or substitution of infants.

A fresh footprint (**Figure 5.20**) of a suspected person is taken and compared with the original. Any peculiarities in the foot, such as a flat foot, supernumerary toes, scars or callosities are likely to be found in the footprint. In case of bookmark, the pattern and arrangement of nails or holes in the sole may be useful. A footprint produced by walking is usually larger than one produced by standing. The imprint on soft loose material like sand is smaller than the foot, and the imprint produced on mud or clay is larger.

A footmark expert may identify a shoe with a mark made at the scene of crime and by general examination may find out the number of persons involve there and their actual movements at the scene and their point of entry. Individual impressions, especially in yielding soil, will indicate the shoe size and approximate weight of the person and any peculiarity of gait. A partial footmark may be quite sufficient to positively identify a shoe. Footmarks are recorded by photography, casts or lifting or by a combination. Casts can only be taken when there is a footmark in depth. As they are three-dimensional, they can easily be compared with the suspect's shoes even by lay persons.

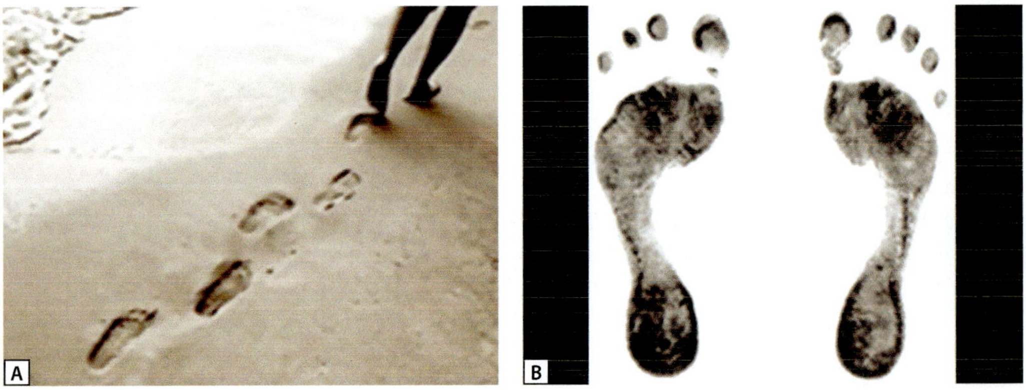

Figures 5.20A and B Different types of footprint

LIP PRINTS (CHEILOSCOPY)

Definition

It is the study of wrinkles and cracks of lips that has specific individual characters. They are useful in personal identification.

History

Identification using lip prints was first performed in the 1950s and was the subject of much research in the 1960s and 70s, leading to the acceptance of this technique as evidence in the criminal justice system.

Features

Previous research has focused on identifying lip print types or on methods of obtaining hidden lip prints left at the crime scene. Lip prints are divided into **six different patterns (Figure 5.21)**: vertical, partial straight, branched, intersected, and reticular, and undifferentiated patterns. Minor differences can be noted between the right and the left and upper and lower lips.

EAR PRINTS

The shapes of ear lobes and the tips of ears are of various types. The suspected person is asked to press the ear on a glass pane in a door. The print made visible as in the case of fingerprints and a photograph of the print is taken. The same process is applied to the ear prints from the scene. Photocopies of both known and unknown ear prints are produced on plain and transparency overlays. The transparency overlay is put on the top of the unknown print and taped to the top of a light box. If the tragus point, crus of the helix points and antitragus point fit, look at the lower and upper crura of the antihelix and the helix rim. If all details coincide, then they are from the same source.

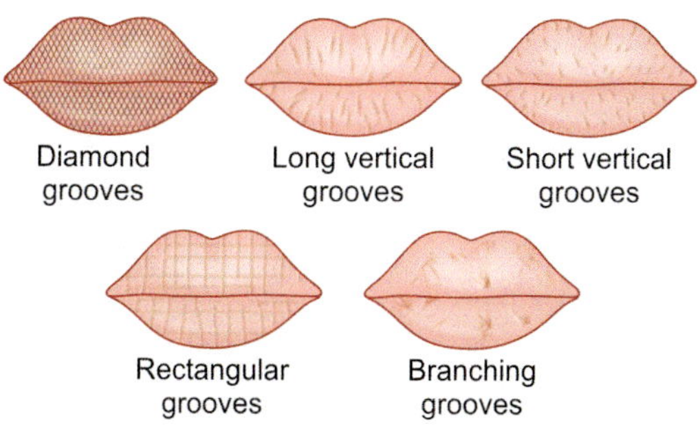

Figure 5.21 Lip print

NOSE PRINT

The lines on the nose and the shape of the nose are helpful in identification.

RUGOSCOPY (PALATOPRINTS)

In the anterior part of the palate, the structural details like the rugae are specific to individual and permanent. The palatoprints can be used in the same way as fingerprints. They are well protected from trauma and are insulated from heat by the tongue and buccal fat.

Rugoscopy is the observation and study of the patterns of the grooves, wrinkles and ridges (rugae) of the palate to identify individual patterns. Harrison Allen suggested palatal rugae, as a method of identification, as early as 1889. The shape of the rugae may be curved, wavy, straight or circular.

The advantages of palatal rugae as an ideal method of postmortem identification include:

i. They are protected from trauma by their position.
ii. No two palates are alike in their configuration. Study of the rugae pattern of twins showed that they are similar, but not identical.
iii. They do not change during growth.

Thomas and **Kotze** have classified rugae into three types as follows:

i. Primary rugae: 5–10 mm or more
ii. Secondary rugae: 3–5 mm
iii. Fragmented rugae: Less than 3 mm.

Srinivasan Method of Identity: An ECG tracing of every individual is unique. By comparing the ECG tracings, it can be possible to decide whether they belong to the same individual or not.

SUPERIMPOSITION (FIGURE 5.22)

Superimposition is the technique applied to determine whether the skull is that of the person in the photograph. A recent photograph is better. The photograph of lateral and semi-lateral view of face can also be used.

Technique

If the negative of the photograph is not available, negative of the available photograph is prepared by recopying it. The photograph is enlarged to natural size from the presence of some standard thing in the photograph of the missing person to indicate the scale. The negative is placed under the ground glass of camera and salient features of the face are marked out carefully on the glass. The soft parts are removed from the skull. A comparison can be made even in the absence of the lower jaw. The skull is mounted on an appropriate skull rest to align it as accurately as possible with the outline of the head on the ground glass in the corresponding portrait, making due allowance for the tissues covering the bone. The distance of the camera is adjusted so that the one-inch scale on the ground glass of the camera is exactly equal to the scale on the skull. This, when photographed, gives a life-sized negative of the skull. The negatives of the photographs and the skull are superimposed by aligning the characteristic points in the negatives.

Comparison Points

- The eyes within the orbital plates, with the two pairs of canthuses properly aligned
- The nasion
- The prosthion in the central line
- The nasal spine in the center which is a little above the tip of the nose
- The lower border of the nose
- The lower border of the upper jaw, i.e. below the tip of the nose
- The zygomas below the eyes
- Supraorbital ridges
- Angle of the jaw
- External auditory meatus
- Teeth.

The two superimposed negatives are then photographed on bromide paper. The resulting photograph brings out the points of similarity or dissimilarity between the photograph and the skull. The superimposition is correct if the outlines and the size of the skull accurately correspond to the face in the photograph. A clear effect of the superimposed area can be obtained by combining the negative of the skull with the positive of the portrait. For this, positive and negative of the skull are rephotographed on X-ray film, thus producing a transparent positive of the skull. Finally, the two films are bound together in register and thus superimposed; they are then re-photographed on X-ray film by transmitted light.

Opinion: This test is of a more negative value because it can definitely be stated that the

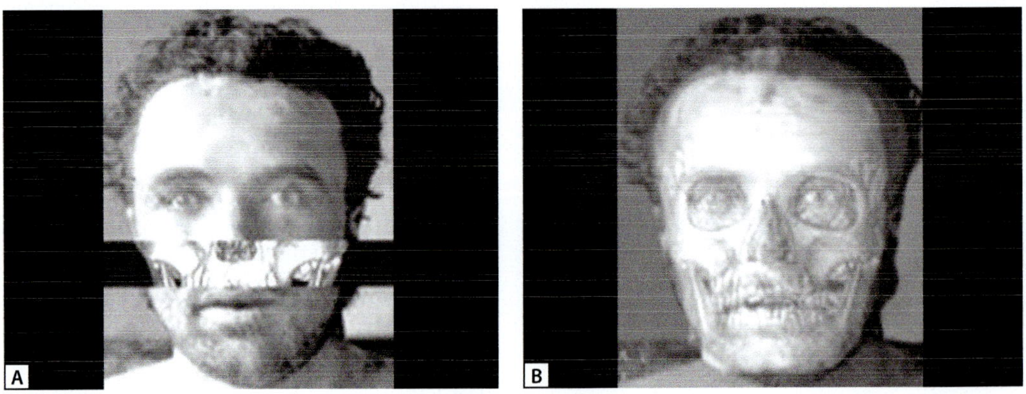

Figures 5.22A and B Superimposition

skull and the photograph are not those of the same person. If they tally, it can only be stated that the skull could be that of the person in the photograph, because of the possibility that another skull of that size and contour may tally with the photograph.

Disadvantages: Even a slight variation in the magnification of the photograph or change in angulations of skull can lead to major differences resulting in mismatch. The process is laborious and time consuming.

Computer-assisted Skull Identification Using Video Superimposition

The skull is mounted on an adjustable support allowing movement in three planes. The photograph is also mounted similarly. A colored video camera is aligned at right angles to the photograph and a second camera is aligned to the skull. The individual video signals from each camera are fed into a vision mixer. By this, superimposition and negative simulation can be done. In cases where sufficient anterior teeth remain on the cranium and a photograph showing suspected deceased smiling is available, image superimposition can be done. Digital image manipulation technique is better.

This system consists of two main units, namely a video superimposition system and a computer-assisted skull identification system. The video superimposition system is comprised of the following five parts: a skull-positioning box having a monochrome CCD camera, a photo-stand having a color CCD camera, a video image mixing device, a TV monitor and a videotape recorder. The computer-assisted skull identification system is composed of a host computer including original application software, a film recorder and a color printer. After the determination of the orientation and size of the skull to those of the facial photograph using the video superimposition system, the skull and facial photograph images are digitized and stored within the computer, and then both digitized images are superimposed on the monitor.

For the assessment of anatomical consistency between the digitized skull and face, the distance between the landmarks and the thickness of soft tissue of the anthropometrical points are semi-automatically measured on the monitor. The wipe images facilitate the comparison of positional relationships between the digitized skull and face.

The software includes the polynomial functions and Fourier harmonic analysis for evaluating the match of the outline such as the forehead and mandibular line in both the digitized images.

DEFORMITIES AND BIRTHMARKS

They may be congenital or acquired. Congenital deformities, such as talipes, polydactylism (**Figure 5.23**), web-fingers or toes, undescended testicles, harelip, cleft palate (**Figure 5.24**), etc., are frequently treated surgically and are, therefore, losing some of their past importance. Old amputations, spinal defects, old fractures and deformities of the bones and nails, either from injuries or disease and surgical prostheses, such as implanted artificial heart valves, plates in the skull, etc., should be described.

Birthmarks

A birthmark is a skin marking that is present at birth. Birthmarks include cafe-au-lait spots, moles (caused by excess skin pigment cells) and Mongolian spots. Birthmarks are usually caused by overgrowth of blood vessels, melanocytes, smooth muscle, fat, fibroblasts, or keratinocytes.

Moles are usually round, brown or black, raised or flat with or without hair. The size and exact anatomical position should be noted. A Mongolian spot (congenital marks) appears as dark blue or violet, single or multiple maculae in the lumbosacral region in some young children of Asiatic and African origin (**Figure 5.25**).

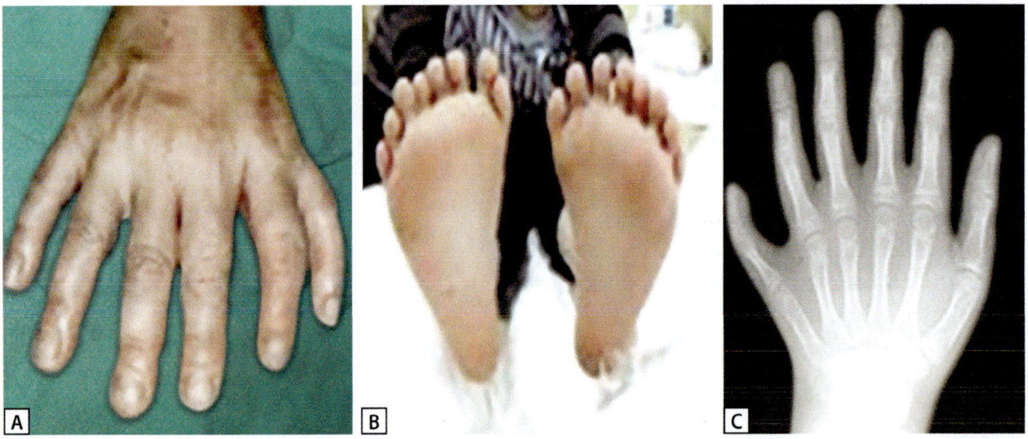

Figures 5.23A to C Different polydactyl types

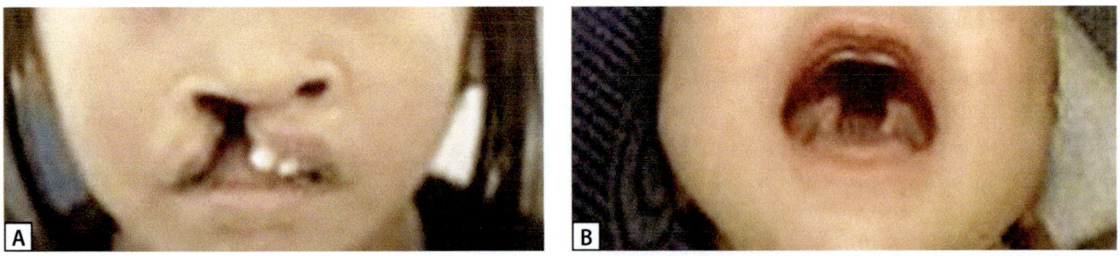

Figures 5.24A and B (A) Harelip; (B) Cleft palate

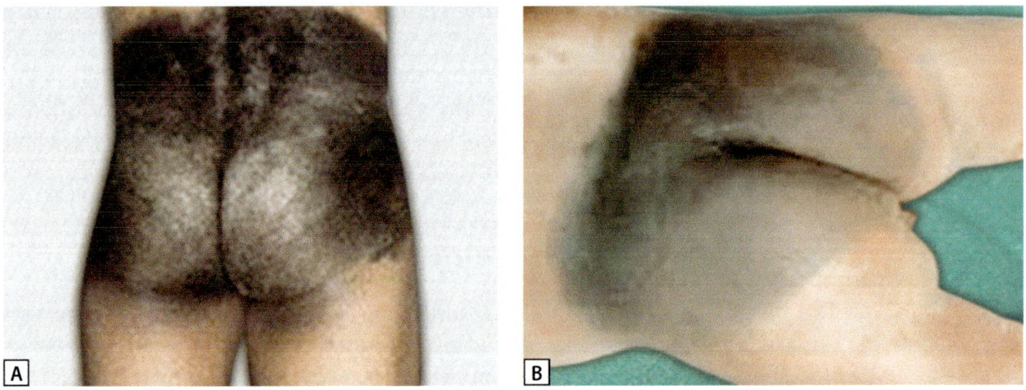

Figures 5.25A and B Mongolian spot (birthmark)

SCARS

A scar is the result of a repair mechanism to an injury involving the dermis of the skin. These are simply the fibrous tissues covered by epithelium without hair follicles, pigments or sweat glands, produced from the healing of a wound. Injury to the dermis produces a scar, while superficial injuries involving only the epidermis do not produce a scar. Scars are permanent.

Examination

Examination of scar is done in good light and description should include their number, site, size and shape, the level it bears to the body surface, fixed or free, smoothness or irregularity of the surface, color and the presence or absence of the glistening and tenderness. The condition of the ends, whether tapering or not, and the probable direction of original wound should be determined. The application of heat, filtered ultraviolet light or surface friction, marks faint scars readily visible. A magnifying glass is very useful. Suspected scars in the dead body can be proved by microscopy, by a section stained to show the elastic tissue, which is absent in a scar. Elastic tissue is present in striae gravidarum.

Characters

The shape of the scars may indicate the type of injury which produced them.

i. Incised wounds produce linear scars. If healing is secondary, the scar is wider and thicker in the center than in the periphery.
ii. Scars from lacerated wounds are firmer, irregular, more prominent and are attached to the deeper tissues.
iii. Stab wound due to a knife-blade produces oval, elliptical, triangular or irregular scars, which are depressed but may be elevated due to keloid formation.
iv. A bullet wound causes a circular depressed scar.
v. Scars from scalds are spotted in appearance, tend to be continuous, often run downwards and show evidence of splashing about the main injury.
vi. Scars due to corrosive acids, burns or radiation are irregular and keloid may develop in the scar tissue.
vii. Vaccination scars are circular or oval flat or slightly depressed (**Figure 5.26**).
viii. Many skin diseases, like smallpox and syphilis, cause multiple scars on the skin.

Growth

A scar produced in childhood, grows in size with the natural development of the individual, especially if situated on the chest or limbs.

A **keloid**, also known as **keloidal scar**, is a type of scar, which depending on its maturity, is composed mainly of collagen. It results of an overgrowth of granulation tissue (collagen type III) at the site of a healed skin injury, which is then slowly replaced by collagen type 1. Keloids are firm, rubbery lesions or shiny, fibrous nodules and can vary in color from pink to flesh-colored or red to dark brown (**Figure 5.27**).

Age of Scars

Freshly formed scar appears reddish or bluish and is tender and soft. These features are appreciated for about a couple of weeks. Due to gradual decrease in the vascularity, it is pale but is still tender and soft up to a couple of months. Then the scars contracts, but still is little tender and soft. The age of such scar is between 2 to 6 months. As the scar contracts further, it becomes tough, white and glistening. Such scar is probably not less than 6 months old. After this, there is no further change.

Erasure: The scar can be erased by excision and skin grafting or suture of the edges of the excised area. This results in a scar, which is less clearly seen.

Medicolegal Importance

1. They form important marks for identification of a person.
2. The age of the scar is important in a criminal offence. If the age of a wound corresponds with the date of the attack, it may have value as circumstantial evidence.
3. The shape of the scar may indicate the nature of weapon or agent that caused the injury.
4. A person may be disfigured due to scars, or contracture around a joint produced by scar may restrict the movement and function of the joint, making it a grievous hurt.
5. Linea albicantes may indicate previous pregnancy.
6. The accused may attribute scars of wounds to disease or therapeutic procedures.
7. To charge an enemy with assault, a person may claim that scars due to disease are those of wounds.

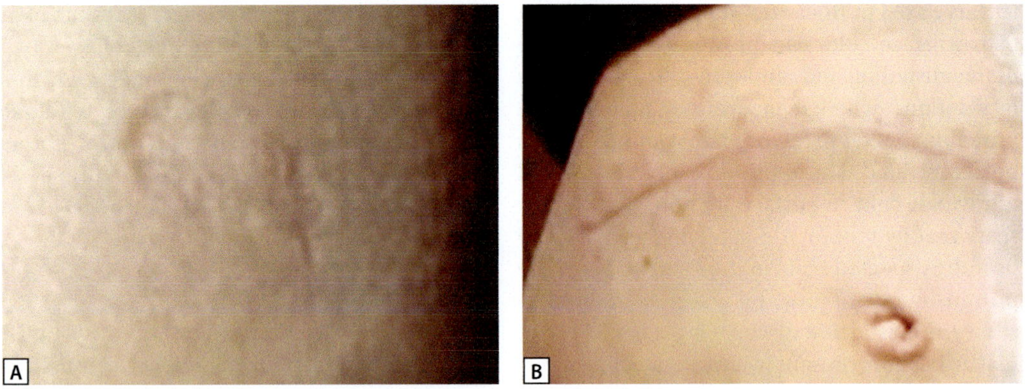

Figures 5.26A and B Different scars, (A) Vaccination scar; (B) Surgical scar

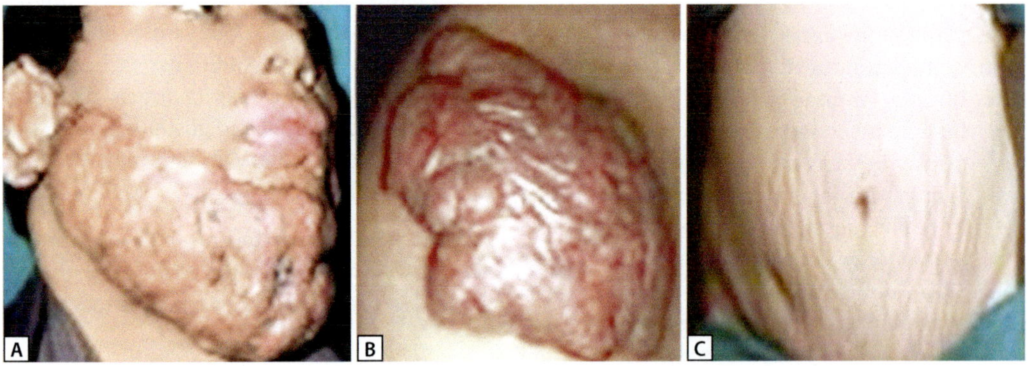

Figures 5.27A to C Different types of scars, (A) and (B) Keloid; (C) Linea albicantes

TATTOO MARKS

The word 'tattoo' comes from Polynesian '**tatau**' meaning '**to mark**'. Tattoo marks are a good identification marks for both living and dead, and provide a wide range of information about the person having them. Tattoo marks are designs (**Figure 5.28**) made by multiple small puncture wounds in the skin through needles or similar penetrating tools dipped in a coloring dye. The permanency of tattoo marks depends upon the type of dye used, the depth of its penetration and the part of body tattooed.

The dyes commonly used are Indian ink, carbon (black) cinnabar or vermilion (red), chromium (green), indigo, cobalt, Prussian blue and ultramarine (blue). Techniques and dyes vary from country to country. Tattooing may be done mechanically or by electric device.

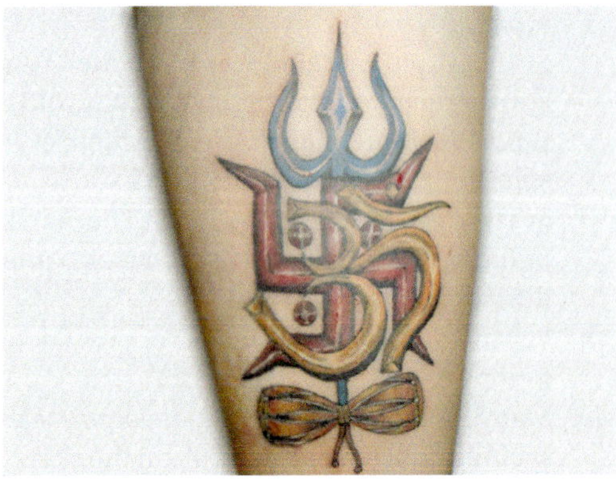

Figure 5.28 Tattoo mark

Most of the marks are found on the arms, forearms and chest, but may be present on any part of the body. The most permanent pictures are made when the dye penetrates the dermis. If the dye is deposited into deeper layers of the dermis, it will be removed by phagocytes. Tattoos slowly become fainter and certain pigments, such as vermilion and ultramarine may disappear after about 10 years. The rate of fading depends not only on the composition of the pigment but also on the depth to which it penetrates the skin and the site, which is tattooed: parts protected by clothing retain the design for longer period than the exposed parts of the body.

Due to constant friction, tattoos on the hands disappear early. A faded tattoo mark becomes visible by the use of ultraviolet lamp or rubbing the part and examining with magnifying lens. Infrared photography marks old tattoos readily visible. The marks are recognized even in decomposed bodies when the epidermis is removed. Lymph nodes near a tattoo mark show a deposit of a pigment.

Complications

Tattooing can lead to septic inflammation, erysipelas, abscess and gangrene. Syphilis, AIDS, leprosy and tuberculosis may occur due to sharing of the needle.

Erasures

i. Surgical methods: (a) complete excision and skin grafting, (b) production of burn by means of red hot iron, (c) scarification and (d) carbon dioxide snow.
ii. Electrolysis.
iii. Caustic substances remove pigment by producing inflammatory reaction and a superficial scar, e.g. mixture of papain in glycerin, zinc chloride and tannic acid.
iv. Laser beam: By exposure to laser beams, the particles of the dye get vaporized and are expelled from the tissues in gaseous form.
v. Confluent smallpox and, sometimes, chronic eczema in children can obliterate tattoo marks.

Medicolegal Importance

i. Positive identification can be made by tattoos alone, if there is a large number of tattoos, initials and dates, regimental details, identity numerals, one's own name, etc.
ii. Religion designs of Cross or Christ (in Christians) and Hanuman, Lord Krishna (in Hindus) may provide religion.
iii. Tattoos may also represent someone's social status.
iv. The distribution of tattooing and the nature of designs and figures may indicate a particular country or region.
v. The presence of indecent figure points to definite perversion in the individual.
vi. They reflect travel, history, war, occupation, sex interest, etc.
vii. Drug addicts may tattoo front of elbow or wrist to conceal needle puncture marks.
viii. Race: Extensive tattooing of the chest and limbs is common among the Japanese.
ix. Profession, some criminal gangs have certain specific emblems of tattoo marks. Some occupations, e.g. coal miners leave visible tattoo marks on the hands and face from the material handled by the workers.
x. Political convictions like sword and sickle, cow and calf.
xi. Behavioral characteristics like erotic tattoos of the sexual fanatic, blue bird design on the extensor surface of the web of thumb of homosexuals, number 13 inside the lower lip of drug pushers, addict type of tattoo marks to conceal injection sites, etc.

DISEASE, WOUNDS AND STAINS

Disease

The finding of a disease, e.g. gallstones, renal stones, calcified leiomyoma, silicosis, asbestosis, and congenital anomalies, like horseshoe kidney, is helpful in identification of an individual. The unidentified body should be checked for amputations, body deformities, pace makers, implanted heart valves, enlarged joints of the fingers due to arthritis, immovable joints due to disease, bowed-legs and curvature of the spine. X-rays will show the presence of healed fractures, metal pins, plates or screw used in treating fractures. Commonly found missing organs at autopsy are tonsils, appendix, gallbladder, kidney, prostate, uterus and ovaries.

Surgical scars may indicate hernia repair, circumcision or an operation upon the thyroid gland.

Wounds

Sometimes, the presence of wounds on the body may assist in connecting a suspected criminal with a given crime, e.g. a piece of skin adherent to a window glass may correspond with the wound on the thief or rupture of frenum of penis may be present in a person accused of rape. Dust, sand, etc., may be recovered from wounds and identified.

Stains

Stains found on body or clothing of the accused and the victim may be the same and may be derived from the walls, doors, furniture, etc., at the scene of crime.

OCCUPATIONAL STIGMATA

Occupational marks are the characteristics that result from adaptation to work. Distinctive marks of occupation have decreased in incidence and importance but still some of these can be useful for identification. They may be recent and temporary, and permanent marks.

Recent and Temporary

They include paint spots on painters, grease on engineers and mechanics, flour on bakers and millers and dyes on dye workers. The microscopic examination of dust and debris on clothing in the pockets, under the fingernails and in the ear wax is important in identification of unknown bodies. They may also connect the body with a specific place where a crime was committed.

Permanent

A callosity is seen on the outer side of the distal phalanx of the middle finger of the right hand of a clerk. This is rarely seen these days. Thickening of the palmar skin of fingers are seen on the right hands of butchers. Manual laborer show horny and rough hands. Tailors have marks of needle punctures on their left index finger. Certain occupations may change the color of the hair, e.g. hair of copper smelters may be greenish, while that of indigo workers and cobalt miners are bluish. Coal miners have multiple 'blue scars' on the face and arms due to coal-dust contamination of small lacerations. Steel workers usually have multiple small scars from metal burns. Workers in chemicals and photography usually have discolored, distorted fingernails. Carpenters have callosities on the thumb and index finger, on the palms, and one shoulder is usually higher than the other. The violinist has hardened tips on the fingers of the left hand.

COMPLEXION AND FEATURES

Complexion may be fair, white colored, dark-brown, pale-brown or pale-yellow. Details of the features regarding eyes, hair, nose, ears, eyebrows, lips, chin and teeth should be noted. The features may change considerably from disease or even from worries over a long duration.

Shape of mouth, nose, ear, eyebrows, beard and moustache are the important points, which help in identity establishment. Any irregularities of teeth, artificial teeth, etc., are also helpful in this event. Few persons can cleverly alter their features by changing the expression of their face. Expression is altered after death.

CLOTHES AND ORNAMENTS

The clothing, from the texture and value, may indicate the social status to a certain extent. Any variety of uniform is very valuable for identification. Clothing may also indicate the occupation. The examination of clothing and personal effects is helpful in the identification of victims in mass disasters, such as fires, explosions and aircraft crashes. A detailed description of the size, color, condition and type of each garment and a record of laundry marks, name tags and labels of tailors should be given. Photograph and examination for invisible laundry marks by ultraviolet light are useful. The clothing may contain keys, letters, bank books, visiting cards, licenses or other documents, which may give a clue to the name and address of the individual.

Other personal effects like watches, rings, keys, belt buckles, etc., may be engraved with initials, names or dates. Eyeglasses may also be helpful. A criminal may interchange his identity with that of another person by clothing and personal effects. Bullet holes, tears, cuts or tyre marks found on clothing may give information regarding the cause and manner of death. The design of the ornaments varies from region to region.

General cleanliness of the person and the state of the teeth, hands and feet give some idea of social status. If shoes are worn, the epidermis of the soles of the feet is thin and smooth without any fissures and cracks.

HAIR

Human Hair

Study of hair is known as trichology. In most of the human hair, there are three well-defined layers as follows:

a. **Cuticle**: This is the outer layer and consists of thin non-pigmented scales.
b. **Cortex**: This is the middle layers comprising of longitudinally arranged, elongated cells without nuclei.
c. **Medulla**: Within these cells, there will be granules of pigment. This is the innermost layer composed of keratinized remains of the cells. Medulla may be narrow. It may be absent, fragmented or discontinuous (**Figure 5.29**).

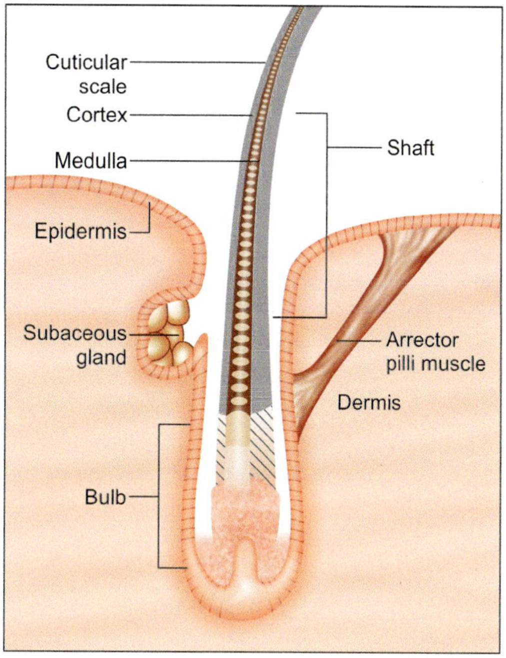

Figure 5.29 Anatomy of human hair

FIBERS

Cloth fibers are often found at the scene of the crime or on a suspect. In some cases, a small piece of cloth may be found. The police may even find a matching piece of cloth whose torn edge will fit the torn edge of the first piece. Such a match is called a jigsaw fit. Most cloth is made of fibers woven or intertwined in some way. There are some simple tests, which help greatly in distinguishing fabrics, the most common being the burning test and chemical tests.

The fibers may be of cotton, linen, jute, silk, etc. They may resemble hair. Each of this fiber has different morphological features.

Linen Fibers: Linen is a textile made from the fibers of the flax plant, Linum usitatissimum. The fiber is linear, jointed, segmented with swelling, like bamboo. Fibers are usually run in bundles (**Figure 5.30 A**).

Silk Fibers: Silk is a natural protein fiber, some forms of which can be woven into textiles. The shimmering appearance of silk is due to the triangular prism-like structure of the silk fiber, which allows silk cloth to refract incoming light at different angles, thus producing different colors. The fibers are long, clear, regular, cylindrical, retractile threads without any cell with any twisting or joints or swelling (**Figure 5.30 B**).

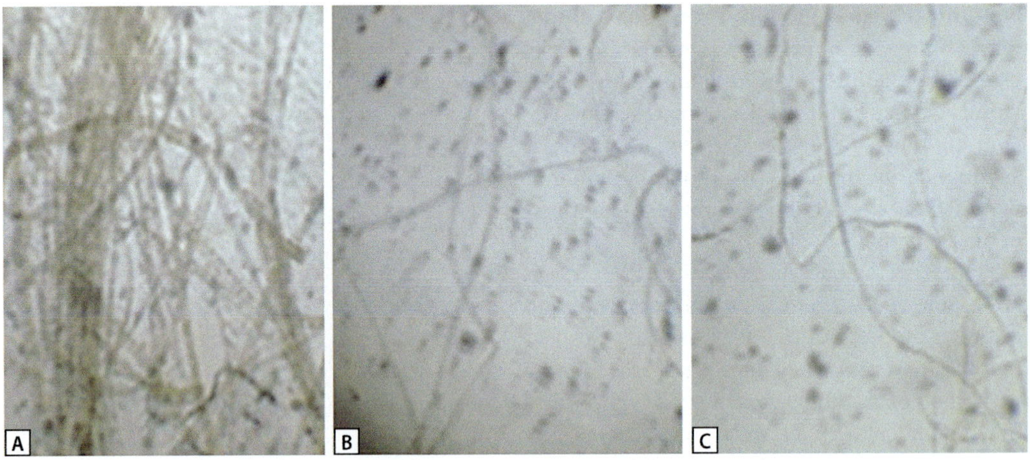

Figures 5.30A to C Microscopic pictures of (A) Linen; (B) Silk; and (C) Cotton fibers

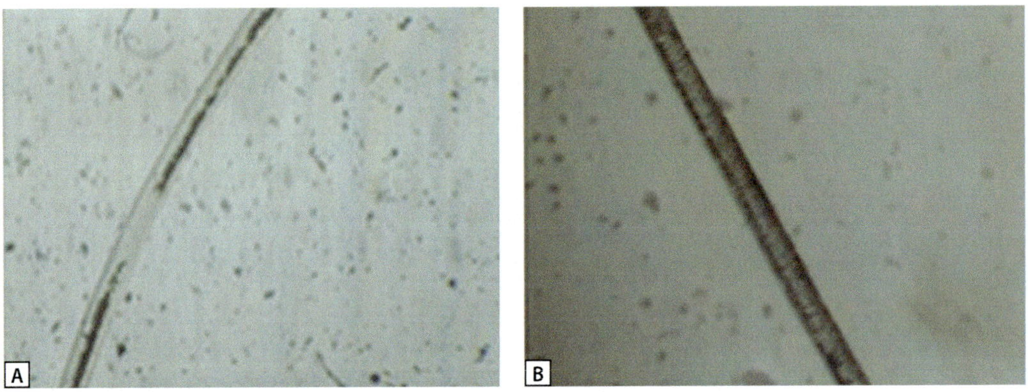

Figures 5.31A and B Cross section of (A) Human; and (B) Animal hair

Cotton Fibers: Cotton is a soft, fluffy staple fiber. It is fairly uniform in width, flattened, twisted, tubes like bands (twisted ribbons) with thickened edges and blunt pointed end (**Figure 5.30 C**). Resiliency is low and resistant to alkali, but damaged and weakened by acid.

Difference between Human and Animal Hair

Human and animal hair may be differentiated by features shown in **Table 5.7**. The cross section of human and animal hair is shown in **Figure 5.31**.

Medullary Index of Hair: It is the ratio of diameter of medulla to the diameter of whole shaft of hair. In humans, it is less than 0.3, and in case of animals it is more than 0.5. The value also varies in hair from different parts of the body. This is useful to determine the part of the body from which it is derived.

i. **From what part of the body is it derived?** Scalp hair is usually soft and taper gradually from the root to the tip. The beard and moustache are thicker than hair from other parts of the body. The hair on chest, axilla and pubic region is short, stout and curly. There may be split ends in hair from axillary and pubic region. Hair of eyebrow, eyelash and nostril is stiff, thick and taper to a point. The hair from other parts of the body is fine, short and does not show pigment cells in the cortex.

Table 5.7 Differences between human and animal hair

Trait	Human hair	Animal hair
General	Fine and thin	Coarse and thick
Cuticle	Scales short, broad thin, irregularly annular	Scales large and has step like wavy projection
Cortex	Thick, 4–10 times as broad as medulla	Thin, twice as broad as medulla
Medulla	Narrow non-continuous, fragmented	Continuous and wider
Pigment	Evenly distributed	Mostly near medulla
Precipitin test	Specific for human	Specific for animal
Medullary index	<0.3	>0.5

ii. **Sex**: Male hair is usually thicker, coarser and darker. In human scalp hair, the barr bodies are found in the hair follicles in about 30% in females and 6% in males. Presence of certain hair like that from beard and moustache makes the sex determination easier.

Atebrin-stained human hair roots under the fluorescent microscope is an easy, quick and efficient method for accurate counting of Barr bodies in females, Y bodies in males and, simultaneously, both types of bodies in Klinefelter patients.[5] Refractive index appears to be one of the most significant criteria for sex determination, as there is significant difference between male and female hair.

iii. **Age**: The age can be determined from hair with vary wide limits. Root of hair from children will dissolve rapidly in a solution of caustic potash, but in elder people, roots will resist the treatment. Fetus and newborn child have fine, soft, non-pigmented and non-medullated hair called as lanugo hair. This lanugo hair is replaced by coarser, pigmented and medullated hair, which has more complex scale pattern.

The diameter of hair increases from childhood to adult age group: 0.024 mm in new-born child, 0.053 mm at 15 years and 0.07 mm in adults. At puberty, the axillary and pubic hair grow, which is fine, soft and curly and later becomes coarse and pigmented. Maximum pigmentation is seen in adult hair. Gray hair usually appears after 40 years.

iv. Hair is altered by dyeing, bleaching and diseases. Bleached hair is brittle, dry and straw yellow. Colored hair is rough, brittle and lusterless and color is not uniformly seen. Color of head hair is different from other parts of the body. The time of color last applied can be known by measuring the uncolored part at the base which has grown after color application. The scalp hair grows at a rate of 2–3 mm a week. Any metal present in the paint can be found out by chemical examination of the hair. Dyed hair shows fluorescence with ultraviolet light.

If the hair bulb is present, ABO blood group can be determined from single hair from any part of the body by modified absorption elution method. The distribution and concentration of trace elements along shaft of the hair varies as the hair grows. The color of hair may vary with diseases. It is lighter in malnutrition, ulcerative colitis and kwashiorkor. This may become normal with restoration of health. Color of hair becomes green from copper, yellow from picric acid and blue from cobalt poisoning.

Medicolegal Questions

Is the hair identical to that of suspect?

It can be said that the hair could have come from a particular person by careful examination of the debris, grease, etc., adherent to hair. Factors, which help in individualization: (a) ABO blood grouping can be done in a single hair from any part of the body by a modified absorption elution technique with 100% accuracy; (b) Isozyme typing, i.e. PGM, RGD, AK, GLO, etc.; (c) Identification of trace elements by neuron activation analysis; (d) Evidence of

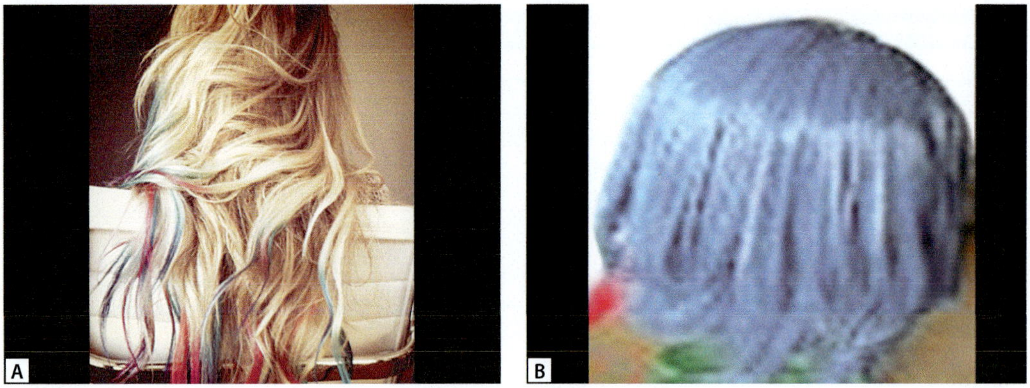

Figures 5.32A and B Dyed hairs

disease and (e) Evidence of application of dyes (**Figure 5.32**), henna, etc.

Did the hair fall naturally or it was forcibly removed?

The base must be examined for the presence of the root. In a naturally fallen hair, the root will be distorted and atrophied without sheath (**Figure 5.33**).

If the hair is forcibly pulled out, the hair bulb will be larger, irregular and the sheath will be ruptured as shown in **Figure 5.34**.

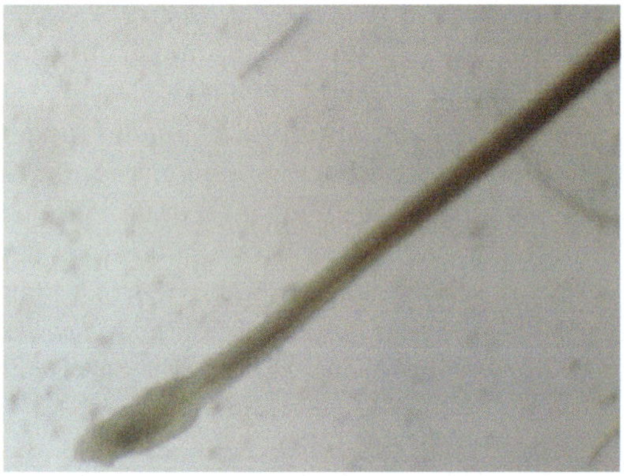

Figure 5.33 Degenerated atrophied root without sheath fallen by itself

What is the cause of the injury?

The tip of the hair is pointed and non-medullated if hair has not been cut, but repeated injury to tip damages the cuticle resulting in splitting and fraying of the cortex. A sharp weapon produces a uniform cut surface while a blow with blunt object crushes the shaft with flattening and splitting as shown in **Figure 5.34**. Hair may get singed due to burns or firearm injury, where the hair is swollen, black, fragile, twisted or curled has a peculiar odor and may show deposition of carbon.

Medicolegal Importance of Hair and Fiber

i. Hair is a valuable trace element in crime investigation as it remains on clothes, body and on weapons for a long time. It can be a connecting link between the weapon or even the accused and the victim of an assault. In sexual offences like rape and sodomy, the pubic hair of the accused may be found on the victim and vice versa. In bestiality, animal hair may be found on the body or clothing of the accused or his hair may be found on the genitals of animal. The vehicle responsible for producing injuries in accidents can be identified by presence of hair on the vehicle. Examination of the stains on the hair can be useful to indicate the nature of assault like seminal stains in sexual offences, mud stains in struggle and blood stains in injuries.
ii. By observing the injuries to hair and hair bulb, the nature of weapon can be made out.
iii. Hair becomes useful in identification in the presence of some peculiarity like dying and bleaching.

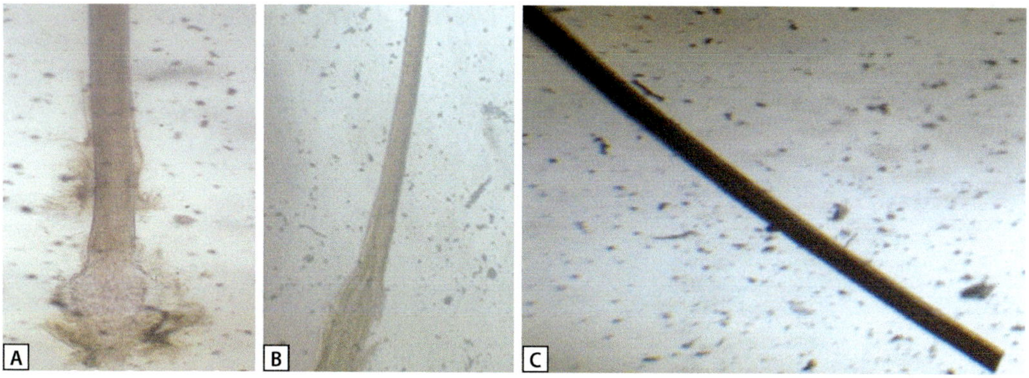

Figures 5.34A to C Human hair, (A) Pulled by force; (B) Crushed end indicative of blunt force impact; (C) Cut by sharp cutting weapon

iv. By growth of hair on different parts of the body, age of a person may be determined.
v. By distribution, texture and barr bodies, sex of a person may be made out.
vi. Singeing of hair indicates burns or close range firearm injury.
vii. Hair is useful in differentiating burns from scalds.
viii. The absorbent property of hair makes its examination important in cases of arsenic poisoning. Hair picks up the poisons from the bloodstream, and it is possible to work out the approximate strength and frequency of the dosage by analysis.
ix. Time since death may be determined from length of hair on face. Head hair grows at an average weekly rate of about 2.5 mm, beard grows faster and body hair slower. Growth ceases at death, but as the skin shrinks, hair, especially the beard, becomes more prominent, giving rise to the murder myth that hair grows after death.
x. Hair can be used in helping to reconstruct events. Collection of hair and fibers can indicate contact with surfaces or individuals and so where individuals have been.
xi. Examination of the root structure can indicate whether hair has fallen out or been forcefully removed, indicating a struggle.
xii. Hair can also be used to assist identification through DNA analysis. If some root structure is present, standard DNA profiling can be used. Even if you only have the shaft, mitochondrial DNA testing can be tried.

MISCELLANEOUS

Handwriting (Calligraphy)

Handwriting of every individual is characteristic, especially if it is written rapidly, but it may be disguised or of forged. Mental and nervous disease and rheumatism may alter the character of handwriting. Evidence of handwriting experts is opinion evidence, but it is not conclusive.

Speech and Voice

Certain peculiarities of speech, e.g. stammering, stuttering, lisping and nasal twang, become more evident when the individual is talking excitedly should be noted. Speech is also affected by nervous disease. It is too risky to recognize a person from the voice alone. It is possible for a person to alter his voice at will. No two voices are really alike. Acoustic "**spectrogram**" characteristic of the speaker can be produced by utterance of a single syllable plotted on a time baseline. This can be utilized in trapping anonymous telephone callers.

Gait

Any identification based on recollection of physical characteristics of a person in question by friends and relatives is unreliable. The gait may be altered by an accident or by design.

Tricks of Manner and Habit

They are frequently hereditary, e.g. left-handedness. Jerky movement of shoulders or muscles of face is an individual characteristic.

Memory and Education

They are sometimes useful, especially in cases of impostor.

REFERENCES

1. Press M. A Scream on the Water: A True Story of Murder in Salem.
2. Fukushima H, Hasekura H, Nagai K. Identification of male bloodstains by dot hybridization of human Y chromosome-specific deoxyribonucleic acid (DNA) probe. J Forensic Sci. 1988;33:621-7.
3. Olze A, Peschke C, Schulz R, Schmeling A. Studies of the chronological course of wisdom tooth eruption in a German population. J Forensic and Legal Med. 2008;15(7):426-9.
4. Graham CB. Assessment of bone maturation methods and pitfalls. Radiol Clin North Am. 1972;10: 185-202.
5. Francois J, Matton-Van Leuven MT, Acosta J. Male and female sex determination in hair roots. Clinical Genetics. 1971;2(2):73-7.

CHAPTER 6

Forensic Osteology

Putul Mahanta, Vijayamahantesh SN, Nisha Goyal

LEARNING PLAN

- Learn the ways of examination of skeletal remains
- Know about the information that can be gathered from bone
- Identify the importance of bones in forensic application

Forensic osteology is a sub-specialty of forensic medicine that deals with examination of human bones. Whereas a forensic pathologist is experienced in dealing with bodies that still retain soft tissues, the field of forensic osteology deals almost exclusively with skeletal material and the manner in which the skeletonization occurred. **Forensic anthropology** adds to the field of osteology by combining archeological field techniques with the area of skeletal anatomy. **Carbon dating** can conclude the archeological age of human skeleton recovered during excavation.

EXAMINATION OF SKELETAL REMAINS

Examination of unknown skeletal remains, which carries lots of medicolegal importance, requires knowledge and discipline. Before examination, care should be taken to note the condition of the bones, whether they are dried or moist, or about the periosteum whether it is adherent to it or not. Careful assessment should be made whether soft tissues or ligaments are attached to it or not and about its condition of decomposition. If any garments and apparels are found adhering to the skeleton, it should be noted.

After this, the bones should be arranged in proper anatomical order and then listed and examined carefully.

After a thorough examination of human skeleton (**Figure 6.1**), opinion on the following medicolegal points can be given.

Bone or Not

It is really important to examine the given samples and opine whether it is a bone or not, as many objects like wood pieces, mistaken for bone, are produced before the doctor for examination by the police.

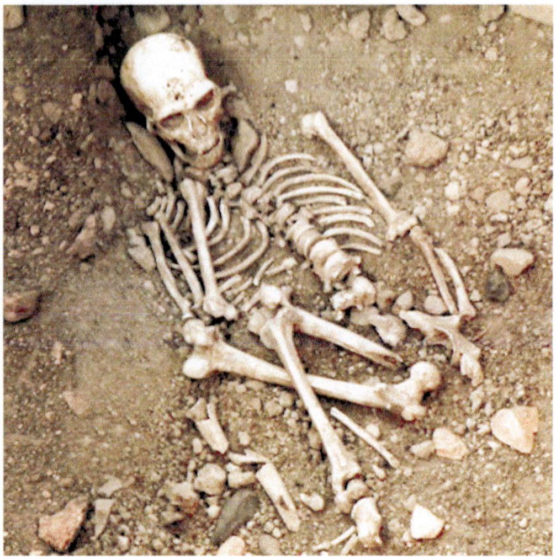

Figure 6.1 Human skeleton recovered on the bank of river

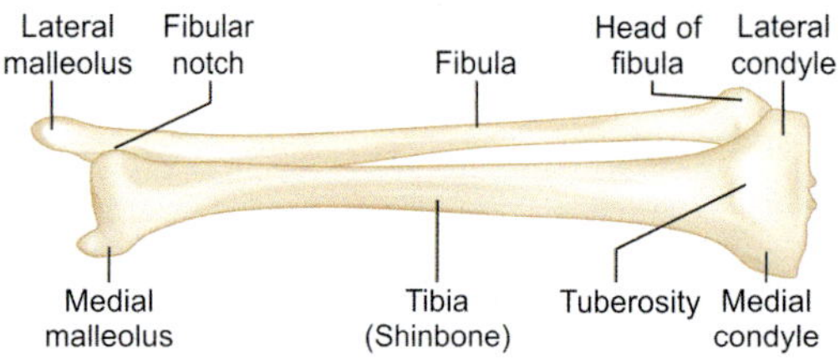

Figure 6.2 Tibia with fibula showing gross features

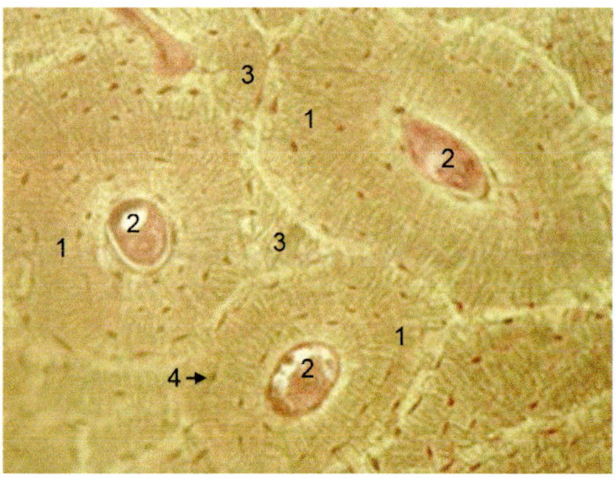

Figure 6.3 Microscopic findings of cortical bone

Gross Examination: Naked-eye examination of the bone in respect to shape, size, texture, weight and anatomical landmark will reveal whether the specimen is a bone or not (**Figure 6.2**).

Microscopic Examination: Microscopic examination of bone shows: Haversian system (osteons), Haversian canal, interstitial system (older, partially resorbed, Haversian system) and osteocytes which are confirmatory.

The different histological structures, viz (1) Haversian system (osteons); (2) Haversian canal; (3) Interstitial system (older, partially resorbed, Haversian system); (4) Osteocytes are shown in **Figure 6.3**.

Human or Animal

Whether the bones are human or not? Difficulty arises when there is marked fragmentation, pieces of burnt bones or smaller bones of animal are received as specimen. The differentiation is done by:

i. **Anatomical Knowledge**
ii. **Microscopic Examination**: The Haversian system is different in animals from human. In human, Haversian systems and canals are of larger diameter than animals.
iii. **Serological Technique**: Precipitin test is done by extracting species specific protein from bone into solution that can be tested against specific antisera of human. The electrophoresis or gel diffusion technique can also identify the human tissues.

Single or Multiple Individual

If human, whether it belongs to one or more than one individual is to be ascertained. This can be done by reconstructing the skeleton in an anatomical position. If there is no disparity in the size of various bones or reduplication, etc. and if the age, sex and race of all bones are same, they belong to one individual.

Age from Bone

The age can be determined from:

- Dental findings
- Appearance and fusion of epiphyseal centers of available bones
- X-rays of bones

- **Histological Examination:** It is observed that the size and shape of osteons increases with age.[1] Rai B, Anand SC and Dhattarwal SK have stated a regression equation of age. The equation: Age = number of osteons + 8.3. The relation between osteons and age is given in **Table 6.1**.

Studies were conducted to quantitate histological age changes in human bone cortex. Ground (un-decalcified) and decalcified cross sections of mandible, femur and tibia were measured for: (i) Number of osteons in two fields, (ii) Average number of lamellae per osteon and (iii) Average Haversian canal diameter. Multiple regression techniques were then utilized to estimate the age at death from several combinations of these measurements. With age, the number of osteons per unit area of bone and the number of lamellae per osteon increased, but Haversian canal diameter decreased. The number of lamellae per osteon had the least significant correlation with age. Histological measurements of the mandible provided estimates that were consistently more accurate than those based on the other two long bones.[2] Thus, age can be studied by histological analysis of long bones from 18–85 years.

Sex from Bone

The determinations of sex from bones play an important role in identifying unknown bodies, parts of bodies or skeletal remains. Sex can be well determined from the secondary sexual characters of the bone as follows:
- Anatomical knowledge
- Multivariate discrimination function analysis
- Y-chromosome demonstration and DNA profiling if soft part is available with the bone.

Two factors influence the accuracy of sex determination from skeletal remains:
- Age at the time of death
- Completeness of the skeleton.

In general, the skeleton shows a marked lack of sexual dimorphism until puberty, when the structural constraints associated with childbirth for females and the bony landmarks associated with the increased muscle mass of adult males begin to be manifest. **Krogman** ranked accuracy of sex determination using different bones, which are given in **Table 6.2**.

Sex differences in the morphology of skull, mandible and pelvis with hip bones are considered quite reliable, hence used extensively for medicolegal purpose. While the female skull retains the gracile attributes seen in prepubertal skull, the male cranium becomes markedly rougher in adulthood at the site of muscle attachments.

The pelvis is generally agreed to be the part of the skeleton, best studied for sex determination as it is associated with female structural capability to bear children.

Sex determination is only really possible with adult skeletons because there is not much sexual dimorphism in pre-adolescence children, again towards old age, there occurs blurring of sexually dimorphic traits; hence determination of sex from bones should ideally be limited to 15–55 years of age. The only exception is greater sciatic, where the sex differences can be appreciated even during fetal life.

Table 6.1 Relation between osteons and age

Number of the osteons in each microscopic field	Age (in years)
12	20
15	23
30	38
40	48
50	58

Table 6.2 Krogman accuracy of sexing from bones

Sexing of bones	Percentage of accuracy
Whole skeleton	100%
Skull and pelvis	98%
Pelvis	95%
Skull	92%
Long bones	80%

Although long bones have also been investigated for their accuracy and reliability in determination of sex (80% accuracy as per Krogman), they are only used when the skull and pelvis are not available.

Race from Bone

There are several features that can be used to ascertain the race of an individual. Unfortunately, a true examination of racial characteristics is not possible on a piece of paper. However, the following features may be of great help to know about the race of an individual:

i. In terms of the skull, a great place to start with the maxillary bone. The left and right maxillary bones extend from the roof of the mouth, containing the upper 16 teeth in the adult (upper 10 teeth in the child), and form the outline of the nasal cavity (the nasal cavity itself involves several other bones: ethmoid, inferior nasal conchae, lacrimal, nasal, sphenoid and vomer).
The arch of the maxilla can be found in three basic shapes: hyperbolic, parabolic and rounded (**Figure 6.4**). Each of the following three races has their own shape, viz. **African**-hyperbolic, **European**-parabolic and **Asian**-rounded.
ii. From the shape of the teeth which differ in different races, the race of a person can be ascertained, which has discussed in the Chapter 5 (**Identification**).
iii. There are features of the skull that can be used to determine the race of an individual. Many of these features are quite subtle and require detailed examination of the skull. A couple of features, however, are more easily seen, viz in people of African ancestry, the nasal opening is more flared. Another example is that of the zygomatic arch (or cheek bone), which is angled more forward in people of Asian ancestry, thus giving the person a slightly more flattened face.
iv. **Cephalic index** is of great value in determination of race which is discussed later.

Stature from Bone

Determination of stature from bone means estimation of body height of the person. Long bones are widely selected and also are more reliable than flat or irregular bones. The length of a bone is taken with the help of **Hepburn osteometric board** shown in **Figure 6.5**.

The stature or height of an individual is useful information for making forensic identification. They are not exact and should always be expressed with a range of error. Stature estimates are usually calculated in centimeters.

While taking measurements of bones, their maximum length is to be considered. To get the maximum length of the bone, it is placed length wise in between the two vertical planes of the board. Maximum length is the distance between these two planes. For example, in case of femur, overall maximum length is from head to medial epicondyle. Wet bones are slightly longer than dry bones. To maintain uniform standards, some authors recommend the use of right side bones only. However, right sided bones may not always be available. Hence, to get a correct result, all the available long bones should be included in the

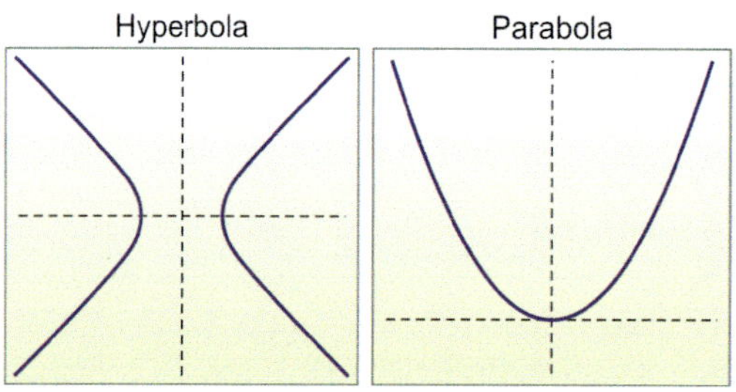

Figure 6.4 Arch of maxilla

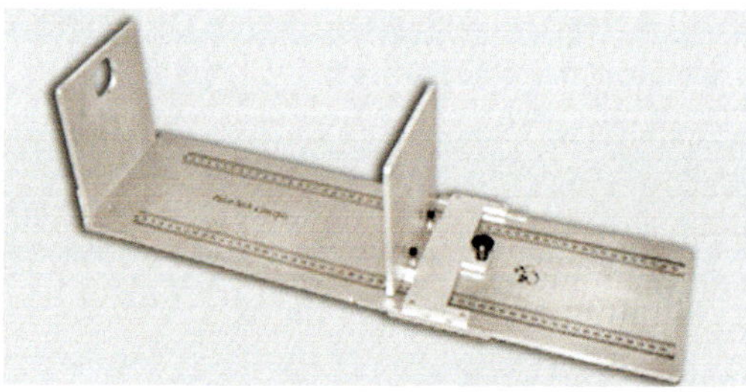

Figure 6.5 Osteometric board

examination and an average of all is to be taken for stature estimation of long bones.

When stature is estimated from a bone, 2.5-4 cm is added to the estimated stature in order to compensate the loss of soft tissue. Following formulae are used to estimate stature:

- Glessor and Trotter
- Karl Pearson
- Dupertuis and Hadden
- Pan
- Nat
- Shah and Siddiqui
- Singh and Shoha
- Mehta and Thomas.

For fragmented long bones, stature can be estimated by following formulae: (i) Muller, (ii) Steele and (iii) Steele and Mckern.

Personal Identity

Personal identity can be ascertained by the following methods:

i. From the skull (superimposition technique).
ii. Dental examination:
   Accurate charting of teeth, various dental works like number of teeth present or missing, restorations or prostheses, dental caries, malposition and malrotation, peculiar shapes of teeth, root canal therapy or endodontics, fillings, etc. are the important findings to compare with dental records of missing persons, which often leads to a positive identification.
iii. Blood grouping from bone marrow or teeth.
iv. DNA profiling.

Time since Death

From the condition of bones, like presence or absence of soft tissues, wetness or dryness of bone, time passed since death may be calculated roughly. The local condition of the weather, place of occurrence and manipulation by animal, etc. should be considered. If the bones appear to be very old, radio-carbon dating by using neutron activation analysis technique may be tried. However, radio-carbon dating is not useful for medicolegal purposes.

Cause of Death

Opinion as to the cause of death can be ascertained with varying amount of certainty based on the following features:

- Presence of any injury or fractures during life.
- Presence of foreign body like bullet inside the body.
- Toxicological analysis for poison.
- Radiological examination for any pathology, etc.

Nature of Death

From the circumstances, pattern of injuries or fractures and its distribution, it is possible to give opinion regarding the nature of death.

Manner of Separation

Absence of any cut marks, complete presence of bone with intact articular cartilage suggests natural separation. If available, the state of soft tissues should be noted and recorded.

GROWTH IN INDIVIDUAL BONES

Most of the bones of the human skeleton are performed in the hyaline cartilage. This is gradually converted into hard osseous tissue by the development of osteogenesis. The appearance of centers of ossification is spread over a long period of time from embryonic time till few years after the birth. The earliest center of ossification appears at the end of second month of pregnancy. At 11-12 weeks of intrauterine life, there are 806 centers of ossification, at birth there are about 450. The adult skeleton has 206 bones. This indicates that 600 centers of bone growth have united with adjacent centers to form adult bone.

The process of appearance and union has a sequence and a time. As a rule, ossification begins centrally in an epiphysis and spreads peripherally as it gets bigger. In the beginning it is amorphous, rounded and pinhead sized. As it grows, it takes on the osteological details of the bone. Some bones are ossified by single centers, like the carpals and tarsals, while most of the bones are ossified by multiple centers, one of which appears near the middle of the future bone. This center is concerned with progressive ossification towards the bone ends. Their ends are cartilaginous at birth and are ossified by separate centers called as secondary centers.

There may be countable differences in the appearance and fusion activities of ossification centers depending upon the race, sex and geographical distribution. The ossification process may also be influenced by food habit, nutritional status and presence of some disease, physical activities, hormonal and metabolic disorders. Generally speaking, the ossification activities occur early in Indian population compared with the western population and earlier in females than in males.

The union of epiphysis, as seen in radiographs, appears approximately about six months earlier than the periods of fusion indicated by anatomical evidence. This can be explained by the fact that towards the end of the growth period, the epiphyseal end of cartilages become very thin and may not be visible in radiograph. Sometimes one or more transverse lines are observed at the diaphyseal ends in radiographs, called **scars of arrested growth** due to growth disturbance.

SKULL

Sex

Sex differences in the morphology of skull and mandible are considered quite reliable, hence used extensively for medicolegal purpose. While the female skull retains the gracile attributes seen in pre-pubescent skull, the male cranium becomes markedly rougher in adulthood at the site of muscle attachments. Determination of sex is based on two methodological approaches:

Morphological (based on shape): Adult males and females differ in both general size and shape, and this variation is reflected in the skeletal anatomy. **Table 6.3** provides the morphological differences between male's and female's skull including mandible.

Osteometric (based on bone dimensions): Males are longer or larger than females. Sex can be determined from skull by morphological examination and by doing craniometry.

Stature

Stature correlation to skull and jaw dimensions is frequently reported among various populations. Stature reconstruction is important as it provides a forensic anthropological estimate of

Table 6.3 Sex differences in the skull and mandible[3]

Trait	Male	Female
General size	Large	Small
Architecture	Rugged, ridges more marked	Smooth
Supraorbital ridges	Medium to large	Small to medium
Mastoid processes	Medium to large	Small to medium
Frontal and parietal eminences	Small	Large
Orbits	Square, lower, smaller with rounded margins	Rounded, higher, larger with sharp margins
Forehead	Steeper, less rounded	Rounded, full, infantile
Check bones	Heavier, more laterally arched	Lighter, more compressed
Mandible	Larger, higher symphysis, broader ascending ramus	Small
Palate	Larger, broader, U shaped	Small parabola
Occipital condyles	Large	Small
Teeth	Large, lower M1 often five cusped	Small molars, often four cusped

the height of a person in the living state; playing a vital role in the identification of individuals from their skeletal remains.

Since long bones are not always available for forensic analysis, it became necessary to use other bones such as the skull for stature estimation. Somatometry of the skull is performed on diameter (distance between glabella and external occipital protuberance) and circumference (length around the skull through two points: The glabella and the external occipital protuberance). Various formulae for estimation of stature from skull:

i. **Stature = Height of skull × 8**

   Eight times the height of skull is equal to approximate height of an individual. Height of skull is measured from basion (a point where the anterior margin of foramen magnum meets the mid-sagittal plane) to the bregma.

ii. The regression equations:[4]

   Stature in males = (diameter + circumference) × 1.35 + 70.6 (standard error of estimate (SE) = 6.96 cm)

   Stature in females = Circumference × 1.28 + 87.8 (SE = 6.59 cm)

   Stature in both sexes = (diameter + circumference) × 1.95 + 25.2 (SE = 7.95 cm)

   This SEs appears to be larger than those obtained for other parts of the body.

Race

Race of an individual is determined from morphological features and cephalic index.

Morphological Features

Various morphological features of the skull are also useful to determine the race as follows:

Caucasian (White): Skull is rounded, orbits are triangular, nasal aperture is elongated, palate is triangular and limbs are in proportion to body.

Mongoloid (Yellow): Skull square, orbits, nasal aperture and palate are rounded. Limbs are smaller than trunk.

Negro (Black): Skull narrow and elongated, orbits square, nasal aperture is broad, palate is rectangular, and limbs are longer than trunk.

Cephalic Index

Cephalic index or **Cranial index** (CI) = Maximum breadth of the skull ÷ maximum length × 100 (i.e. in the horizontal plane, or front to back). **Table 6.4** present cephalic indices found in various races.

The index was widely used by anthropologists in the early 20th century to categorize human populations. Today, it is mainly used to describe individuals' appearances and for estimating the age of fetuses for legal and obstetrical reasons.

A cephalic index of 80 or more is called brachycephalic or broad or short headed; a measurement between 75 and 80 is mesaticephalic; below 75 is considered dolicocephalic or long. The cranial index is the same ratio taken on a skull. The cephalic index of Indian population is between: 75–80 as the Indian skull is Caucasian like (with few Negroid characters), we take the value for Europeans, i.e. 75–79.9 and remember that Caucasians are Europeans.

Age

Age from the skull can be determined by studying the following:

- Closure of fontanelles
- Fusion of bone
- Suture closure
- Secondary changes in the skull.

Table 6.4 Cephalic index in various races

Type of skull	Cephalic index	Race
Dolicocephalic or long headed	70–75	Pure Aryans, Aborigines, Negroes
Mesaticephalic or medium-headed	75–80	European, Chinese
Brachycephalic or short-headed	80–85	Mongolian

Closure of Fontanelles (Figures 6.6 and 6.7)

i. Posterior fontanelle closes at 6 to 8 months after birth
ii. Anterior fontanelles, along with two half of mandible unite at the second year
iii. Two posterolateral fontanelles close within short time after birth
iv. Two anterolateral fontanelles close within six months after birth.

Fusion of Bone

i. By the end of the 2nd year of life, squamous part of occipital bone unites with condylar part
ii. Squamous part of occipital bone unites with the basilar part in the 6th year.

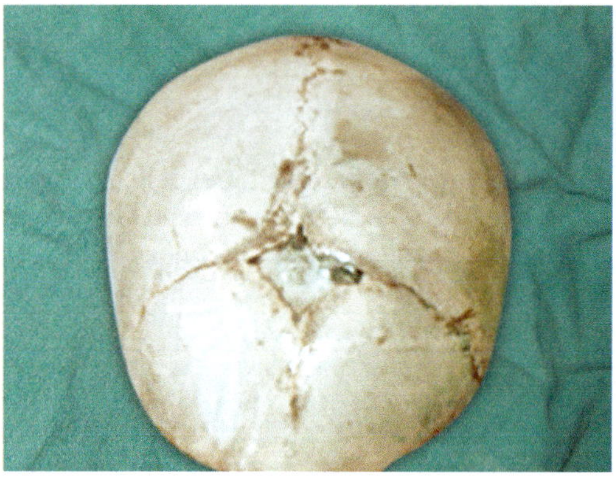

Figure 6.6 Non-closure of anterior fontanelle

Suture Closure

A suture is a type of fibrous joint which only occurs in the skull. They are bound together by Sharpey's fibers. It is normal for many of the bones of the skull to remain unfused at birth.

Lapsed Union: When fusions of sutures of skull at the ectocranial surface are incomplete, it is called 'lapsed union' and occurs most often in the sagittal suture.

Precocious Closure: It is the closure of suture before the age of seven years. At this age, the cranial growth is about 95% completed. The union of the cranial sutures can follow a somewhat erratic course.

Premature Closure: It is the closure after the age of seven years, but considerably before the usual or normal age of closure.

Vault Sutures: They are sagittal, coronal and lambdoid suture.

Circummeatal Suture: They are spheno-temporal, parietomastoid, masto-occipital and squamous suture.

Basal Suture: It is spheno-occipital.

Age of Fusion

The use of cranial sutures for age estimation has always been a matter of considerable debate, and its reliability within the parameter has not been demonstrated conclusively. Age can only be calculated in decades on adult, hence it is

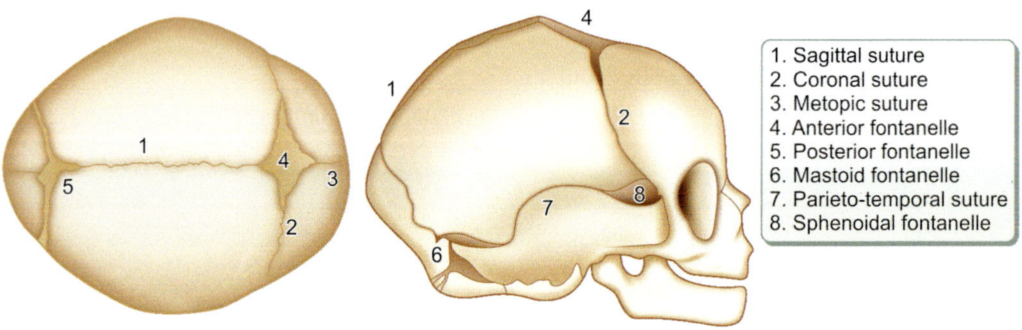

Figure 6.7 Diagrammatic representation of suture closure of vault of skull

not reliable. Due to process of lapsed union, found frequently on ectocranially, more reliability of union is found on endocranial closure. X-rays are commonly carried out to see the fusion, but computed tomography of head for suture closure ectocranially can also be done. Following are the approximate age of fusion of skull suture.

i. The **metopic suture** begins at the nose and continues superiorly to meet the sagittal **suture.** It closes at two to four years, but in 5–10% of the cases, it may persist. This is called as metopism.

ii. The **frontal suture** is a dense connective tissue structure that divides the two halves of the frontal bone of the skull in infants and children. It usually disappears by the age of 6 years, with the two halves of the frontal bone getting fused together. If it does not disappear, it may be called a "**sutura frontalis persistens**".

iii. The condylar portions of occipital bone fuse with the squama in the third year and with the basi-occipital at the fifth year.

iv. The basi-occiput fuses with the basi-sphenoid in about 18–21 years.

v. **Cranial Sutures**

   a. In the vault of the skull, the closure of sutures begins on the inner side 5–10 years earlier than on the outer side.
   b. Most reliable estimation of age is from ectocranial union of sutures which start to close at about 25 years and the order of accuracy is: sagittal, lambdoid and then coronal sutures.
   c. Sagittal suture unites from back to front.
   d. Both left and right half of the skull fuses evenly with no variation.
   e. The union of cranial sutures is earlier in male than in female.
   f. As per Krogman, vault suture fuses between 17 and 50 years, whereas circummeatal suture closes above 50 years.

On the ectocranium, the union of sutures occurs in the following order: Posterior 1/3rd of the sagittal suture at about 30–40 years, anterior 1/3rd of the sagittal and lower half of the coronal at about 40–50 years and middle third of sagittal and upper half of the coronal at about 50–60 years. Lambdoid suture starts uniting close to the lambda and union is usually completed by 40–50 years (**Figure 6.8**). Squamous suture united at above 80 years. Basal suture fuses by 18–20 years.

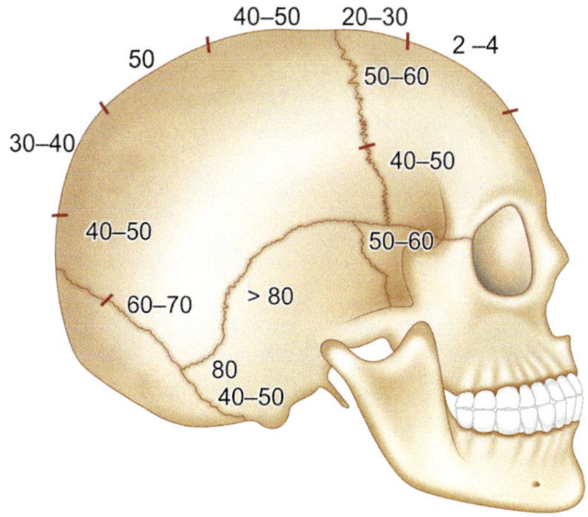

Figure 6.8 Union of cranial sutures

MANDIBLE

Sex

The human mandible can be analyzed to determine gender and is commonly used in forensic medicine for this purpose.

It has several distinctive characteristics that provide reliable information to determine gender. Teeth, bone shape and distance measurements (**Table 6.5**) can all distinguish between a male and female mandible (**Figure 6.9**). Observations for gender indication in children are less accurate.

Stature

Stature of mandible = Distance from symphysis menti to angle of mandible × 16

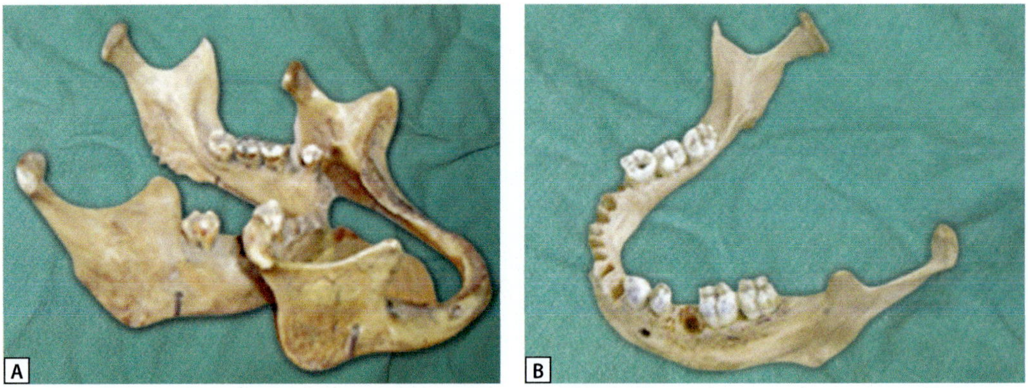

Figures 6.9A and B Mandibles, (A) Old male; (B) Female

Table 6.5 Male and female differences in mandible

Trait	Male	Female
General size	Large, thicker	Small, thinner
Architecture	Rugged	Smooth
Muscular attachment	Prominent	Smooth
Mandibular angle	Everted	Inverted
Chin	Square	Round
Shape of mandible	V shaped	U shaped
Mental tubercle	Large and prominent	Insignificant
Myelohyoid line	Prominent and deep	Shallow
Height at symphysis menti	More	Less
Ascending ramus	Broad	Narrow
Condylar process	Large	Small
Mental tubercle	Large, prominent	Insignificant
Teeth	Large, lower M_1 often five cusped	Small molars, often four cusped

Race

As per Schultz (1933), mandible in white people has:

- Larger breadth
- Higher and narrower ramus
- Greater gonial angle
- Ramal surface more parallel to the median sagittal plane
- Protrusive chin
- Mental tubercles placed more lateral in position.

As per Schultz (1933), the mandible of black people has:

- Lower, wider and more vertical ramus
- Greater dental arch length, i.e. a long 'U' shaped dental arch
- Small breadth
- Less prominent chin
- Mental tubercles are placed more medial in position and smaller.

Age from Mandible

The various age related changes with the mandible (**Table 6.6**).

Table 6.6 Age-related changes of mandible

Trait	Infancy	Adult	Old age
Body	Shallow	Thick and long	Shallow
Ramus	Obtuse angle with body	Less obtuse angle with body	Obtuse angle with body and about 140°
Mental Foramen	Opens near lower margin	Opens midway between upper and lower margins	Opens near alveolar margin
Condyloid Process	Lower than coronoid process	Projects above coronoid process	Lower than coronoid process

At Birth (Figure 6.10)

- Two halves of mandible are united by fibrous symphysis menti
- Body is shell like, with imperfectly separated sockets of deciduous teeth
- Mandibular canal is of large size and run near the lower border of the bone
- Mental foramen is directed forwards and opens beneath the socket of first deciduous molar tooth
- Coronoid process is of large size and projects above the level of the condyle.

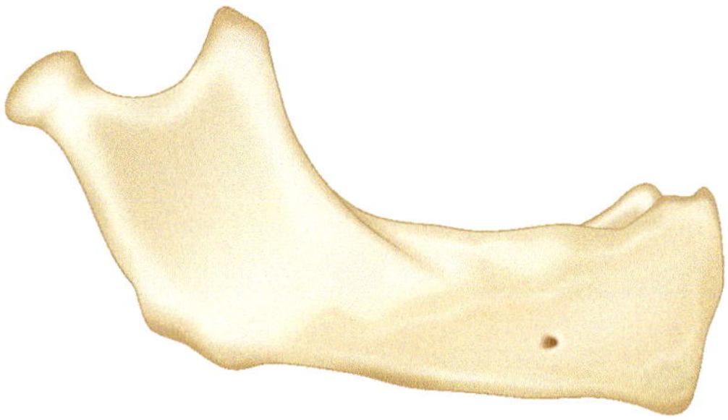

Figure 6.10 Mandible at birth

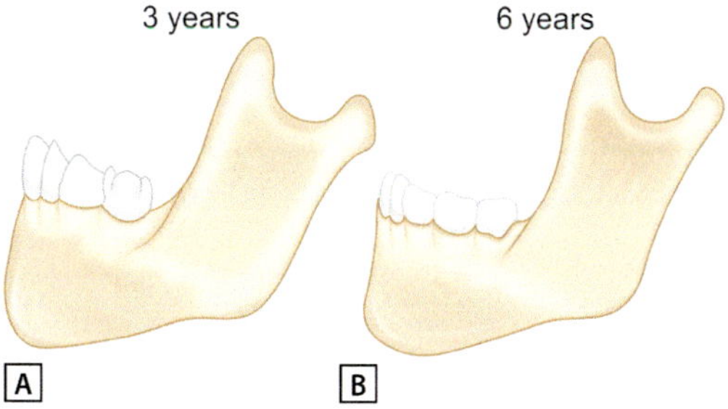

Figures 6.11A and B Mandible of, (A) Three; and (B) Six years old

At 1–3 Years (Figure 6.11A)

- Two halves join at symphysis from below upwards with separation at alveolar margin that may persist into second year
- Body of mandible elongates behind mental foramen
- Chin develops during first and second year
- Condylar cartilage is covered on articular aspect by fibrous tissue
- Body height increases, alveolar growth make place for root of teeth
- The sub-alveolar area becomes thicker and deeper.

At 6 Years (Figure 6.11B)

- Mandible increase in size
- Remodeling continuous with bone added at posterior border of ramus.

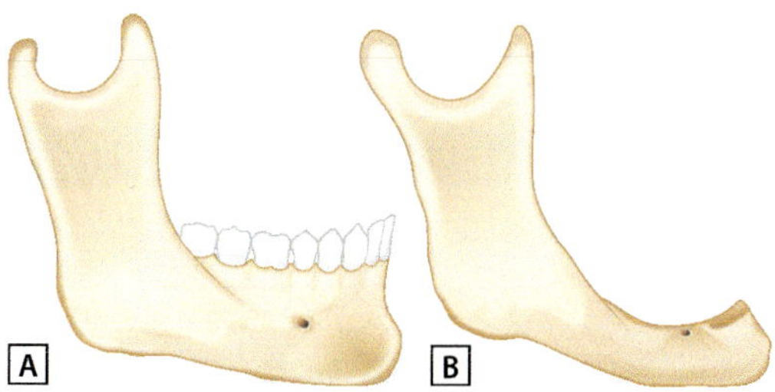

Figures 6.12A and B Mandible, (A) Adult; (B) Old-aged person

Adults (Figure 6.12A)

- The alveolar and sub-alveolar areas of the bone are usually of equal depth
- The mental foramen opens midway between the upper and lower borders of the bone
- Mandibular canal runs nearly parallel with the mylohyoid line

- The ramus is almost vertical in direction, the angle measuring from 110° to 120°
- Condyle is higher than the coronoid process and the sigmoid notch becomes deeper.

Old Age

- Bone is reduced in size (**Figure 6.12B**)
- Alveolar region is absorbed that mainly affects the thinner alveolar part
- Mandibular canal near to upper border
- Mental foramen near to upper border
- Ramus becomes oblique, the angle is 140°
- Neck is inclined backwards.

FEMUR

Sex

The sex differences between male and female femur are narrated in **Table 6.7** and **Figure 6.13**.

Age

Age estimation from the femur can be done by:
- Examination of ossification centers
- Radiographic changes

Examination of Ossification Centers

The femur is ossified from five centers: One for the body, one for the head, one each for each trochanter and one for the lower extremity. Of all the long bones, except the clavicle, it is the first to show traces of ossification; this commences in the middle of the body, at about the seventh week of fetal life and rapidly extends upward and downward (**Table 6.8 and Figure 6.15**).

Radiographic Changes

The **medullary cavity** is the central cavity of bone shafts where red bone marrow or yellow

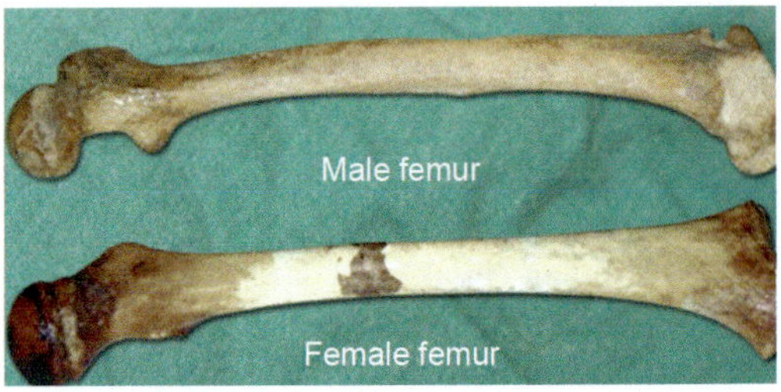

Figure 6.13 Femur of both sex

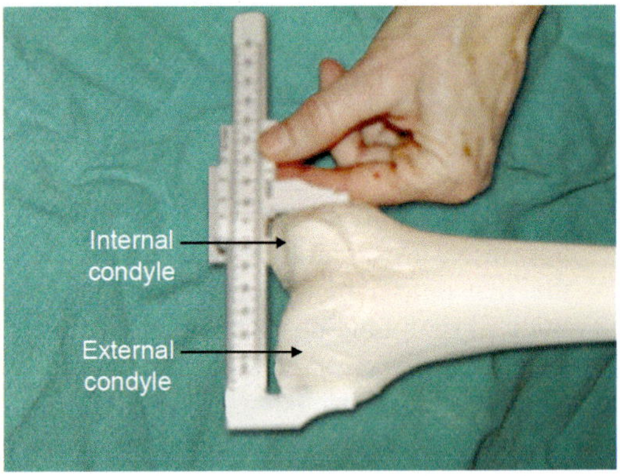

Figure 6.14 Bicondylar width of femur

Table 6.7 Differences between male and female femur

Trait	Male	Female
General	Heavier, rough	Light and smooth
Head	Articular surface is more than 2/3rd of a sphere	Articular surface is less than 2/3rd of a sphere
Muscular attachment	Prominent	Smooth
Collodiaphyseal angle	45°	46°
Angulation of shaft with condyles	Around 80°	Around 76°
Head diameter horizontal	44.1 mm	39.8 mm
Head diameter, vertical	>48 mm	44 mm
Bicondylar breadth **(Figure 6.14)**	77.9 mm	71.1 mm
Popliteal Length	135–145 mm	106–114 mm

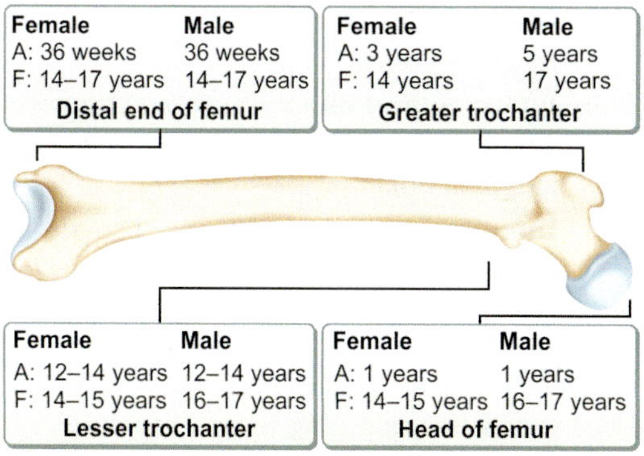

Figure 6.15 Ossification centers of femur, (A-appearance, F-fusion)

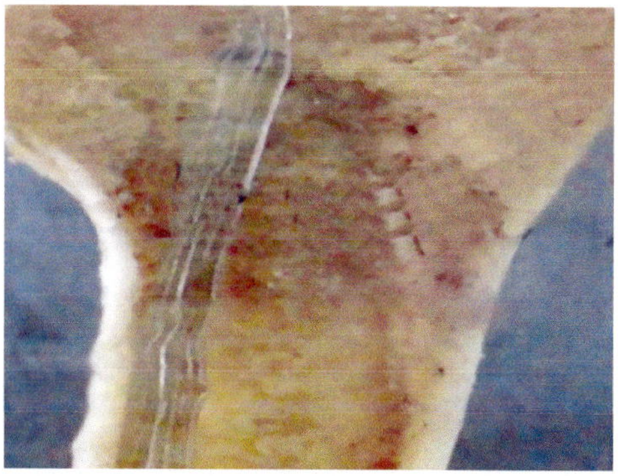

Figure 6.16 Medullary cavity reaches the anatomical neck

Table 6.8 Ossification of femur (Galstaun)

Ossification centers	Female	Male
Head		
Appearance Fusion	One year 14–15 years	One year 16–17 years
Greater trochanter		
Appearance Fusion	3 years 14 years	3 years 17 years
Lesser trochanter		
Appearance Fusion	12–14 years 15–17 years	12–14 years 15–17 years
Lower end of femur		
Appearance Fusion	36 weeks 14–17 years	36 weeks 14–17 years

Table 6.9 Correlation of various phases and age (in years)

Phase	Mean age (Years)
1	31.4
2	44
3	52.6
4	56
5	63
6	67.8

bone marrow is stored; hence, the medullary cavity is also known as the marrow cavity. The changes with age in the medullary cavity of femur are becoming of increasing clinical interest in forensic investigation. It is based on measurements of medial-lateral and posterior-anterior radiographs of the proximal one-third of the femur below the greater trochanter. There is proximal extension of medullary cavity as age advances and the features are more prominent in the age group of 31–70 years.

Acsadi and **Nemeskeri**[5] (1970) divided the changes into five or six phases. The phases are described below and the correlation with age is presented in **Table 6.9**.

Phase 1: Apex of the medullary cavity below the lesser trochanter. Texture of trabeculae is thick.

Phase 2: Apex of the medullary cavity reaches or surpasses the lower limit of lesser trochanter.

Phase 3: Apex of the medullary cavity reaches the upper limit of lesser trochanter.

Phase 4: Apex of the medullary cavity extends above the upper limit of lesser trochanter.

Phase 5: Apex of the medullary cavity extends beyond the upper limit of lesser trochanter. A cavity of 3 mm diameter is formed in the greater trochanter. Cavity appears in the head beneath fovea capitis and at the medial and lateral border.

Phase 6: Cavities in medial part of neck merges with the medullary cavity. Cavities formed in the neck and greater trochanter gets enlarged.

In **Figure 6.16**, a cut section of head of femur is shown where medullary cavity has reached the anatomical neck, i.e. above the upper limit of lesser trochanter.

Race

There are several features of femur that can be used to determine the race of an individual. These features can be obtained from:

- Structural appearance
- Bone length
- Index.

Structural Appearances

Examination of anterior curvature of femur was carried out by different individual. Stewart (1962) and Walensky (1965), who studied the same, have noted that:

- In Negroid (Black people) race femur is much straighter (**Figure 6.17**)
- In White people it is bowed forward
- In American Indians, femur has more anterior curvature and a more distal positioning of the point of maximum curvature.

Bone Length

The male bones are longer than female bones. It is also slightly longer in Blacks than in Whites.

Index

Table 6.10 has shown the value of indices amongst different races. To determine the race, following are the indices frequently used:

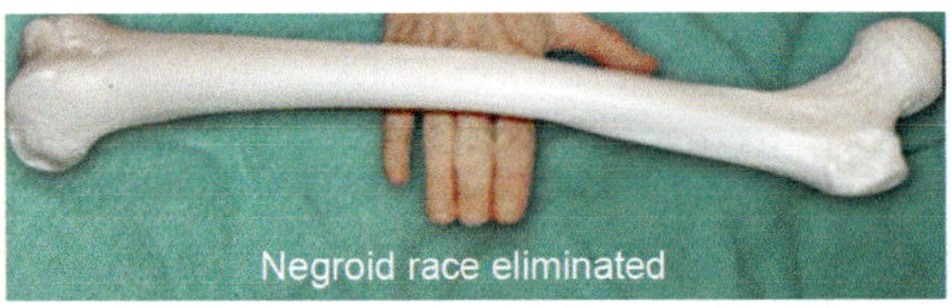

Figure 6.17 Race determinations using a femur: Hands fit under femur

Table 6.10 Indices in various races			
Different indices	**Indian**	**European**	**Black**
Crural Index	86.49	89.3	86.2
Intermembral Index	67.27	70.4	70.3
Humerofemoral Index	71.11	69	72.4

i. **Crural Index** = Length of tibia × 100 ÷ length of femur

ii. **Intermembral Index** = Length of humerus + length of radius × 100 ÷ length of femur + length of tibia

iii. **Humoro-femoral Index** = Length of humerus × 100 ÷ length of femur

Stature

The weight bearing long bones, especially the lower-limb bones, are supposed to provide more reliable estimates of stature as compared to the other bones. The length of a bone is measured and multiplied by multiplication factor, e.g. **Stature** = Length of femur × multiplication factor. There are different formulae and multiplication factors that are available as mentioned bellow:

Rollet conducted the first serious research on this subject of stature determination by measuring the length of all the long bones of both the limbs for 50 males and 50 females as early as 1888. Different sets of data were documented for fresh bones as well as for dry bones.

Karl Pearson (1899) developed regression formulae based on the data provided by Rollet, which become popular in the UK and other parts of the Western world. This formula was in use for a long time. It gives different calculating factors for bones from males and females of European people, depending on whether the bones are wet with intact cartilages or are dried and devoid of cartilages. The stature calculated is usually less than the actual stature by 2.5–4 cm and that should be added to the resulted figure. The multiplying factor is different for different bone. The formula for male and female against long bones of European individual are mentioned in **Table 6.11**.

Dupertuis and **Hadden** suggested using more than one long bone in the calculation of stature and felt that the tibia and femur provided better estimates than radius and humerus. Dupertuis and Hadden's formulae for stature from dry long bones are mentioned in **Table 6.12**.

Trotter and **Gleser** studied the racial differences in stature calculation and evolved regression formulae for the three major races, as well as the Mexican and Puerto Rican groups.[6]

Table 6.11 Karl Pearson formula for adult long bones of European origin

Bone	Male	Female
For dry bones (length in cm)		
Femur	81.306 + 1.880 × length of femur	72.884 + 1.945 × length of femur
Tibia	78.664 + 2.376 × length of tibia	74.774 + 2.352 × length of tibia
Humerus	70.641 + 2.891 × length of humerus	71.475 + 2.754 × length of humerus
Radius	89.925 + 2.271 × length of radius	81.224 + 3.343 × length of radius
For wet bones (length in cm)		
Femur	81.231 + 1.880 × (length of femur – 7 cm)	73.163 + 1.945 × length of femur
Tibia	78.807 + 2.376 × (length of tibia – 5 cm)	75.369 + 2.352 × length of tibia
Humerus	70.714 + 2.894 × (length of humerus – 5 cm)	72.046 + 2.754 × length of humerus
Radius	86.465 + 3.271 × (length of radius – 3 cm)	82.189 + 3.343 × length of radius

Table 6.12 Dupertuis and Hadden's formulae for stature from long bones

Sex		Centimeters	Inches
Male	2.238 F (F-Femur)	+69.089	27.200
	2.392 T (T-Tibia)	+81.688	32.161
	2.970 H (H-Humerus)	+73.570	28.965
	3.650 R (R-Radius)	+80.405	31.655
	1.255 (F+T)	+69.294	27.281
	1.728 (H+R)	+71.429	28.122
	1.422 F + 1.062 T (F-Fibula)	+66.544	26.198
	1.789 H + 1.841 R	+66.400	26.142
	1.928 F + 0.568 H	+64.505	25.396
	1.422 F + 0.931 T + 0.083 H + 0.420 R	+56.006	22.050
Female	2.317 F	+61.412	24.178
	2.533 T	+72.572	28.572
	3.144 H	+64.977	25.581
	3.876 R	+73.502	28.938
	1.233 (F+T)	+65.213	25.674
	1.984 (H+R)	+55.729	21.941
	1.657 F + 0.879 T	+59.259	23.330
	2.164 H + 1.525 R	+60.344	23.757
	2.009 F + 0.566 H	+57.600	22.677
	1.544 F + 0.764 T + 0.126 H + 0.295 R	+57.495	22.636

Steele devised formulae to estimate stature from fragmented bones.[7] He deduced the ratio of various segments of long bones in relation to their entire length, so that the length of a bone could first be estimated from its fragments, which can then be applied to regression formulae to arrive at the stature. This formula is basically considered for White and Negro origin, only between 28 and 30 years of age. Therefore, due consideration should be given for elderly people in whom there occurs some decrease in the stature.

These formulae also cannot be satisfactorily used for Indian individuals. Further, people from different regions of India bear different morphological characteristics depending on their geographical distribution.

Pan, **Nat**, **Jit** and **Singh** have worked out data for the calculation of stature of Asian Indians from the length of the long bones. Of all the formulae used for deducing stature from long bones, those devised by **Dupertuis** and **Hadden** are generally considered the most reliable one. The bones must be measured in a dry state without cartilage, using a Hepburn osteometric board. The maximum length should be taken for all bones except femur and tibia, which are to be measured obliquely (**Figure 6.18**).

Best results are obtained from lower limb bones, mainly from femur and tibia. Different formulae available for different parts of India are narrated in **Table 6.13**.

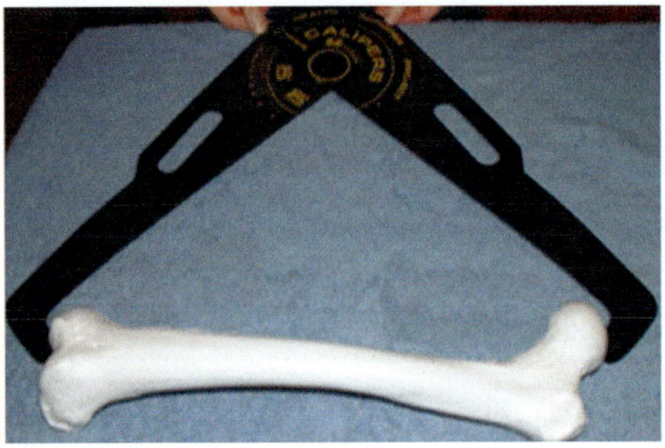

Figure 6.18 Length of femur

TIBIA

Sex

Sexual differentiation of the tibia is not clearly defined until adolescence. The brief sex differentiations from tibia are shown in **Table 6.14**.

Stature

Stature can be determined from tibia by using Karl Pearson formula for adult long bones of European origin and Dupertuis and Hadden's formulae as shown in **Tables 6.11** and **6.12**, respectively. It can also be calculated from the multiplication formula as shown in **Table 6.15**.

Race

By using Crural and Intermembral index, race from tibia can be determined.

Age

From the appearances and fusion of ossification centers of tibia as shown in **Table 6.16**, the age of a person can ascertained.

Table 6.13 Multiplication factors for different bones for calculation of stature of Indian

Femur	Shah and Siddiqui	PAN (Bengal, Bihar and Odisha)		NAT (UP)	Singh and Shoha Punjab	Mehta and Thomas (Mysore)	
Sex	Male	Male	Female	Male	Male	Male	Female
Multiplication factor	3.6	3.82	3.8	3.7	3.57	3.6	3.75

Table 6.14 Sex differences from tibia

Traits	Male	Female
General	Heavier, rough	Lighter, smooth
Muscle markings	Prominent	Not prominent
Length[8]	373 mm	341.5 mm
Mid-shaft circumference[8]	76.4 mm	65.7 mm
Proximal breadth[8]	73.3 mm	64.4 mm
Distal breath[8]	47.7 mm	42.6 mm
Direction	Vertical, and parallel with the bone of the opposite side	Slightly oblique direction downward and laterally

Table 6.15 Multiplication factors by different methods for calculation of stature from tibia

Tibia	Shah and Siddiqui	PAN (Bengal, Bihar and Odisha)		NAT	Singh and Shoha	Mehta and Thomas	
Sex	Male	Male	Female	Male	Male	Male	Female
Multiplication factor	4.2	4.49	4.46	4.48	4.18	4.2	4.39

Table 6.16 Ossification of tibia (Galstaun)

Ossification centers	Female	Male
Proximal end		
Appearance Fusion	Shortly before or after birth 14–15 years	Shortly before or after birth 15–17 years
Distal end		
Appearance Fusion	1 year 14.1–14.4 years	1 year 16 years

Table 6.17 Sex differences from fibula

Traits	Male	Female
General	Heavier, rough	Lighter, smooth
Muscle markings	Prominent	Not prominent
Length[9]	>362 mm	<236 mm
Mid-shaft circumference[9]	40.3 mm	34.9 mm
Distal end breath[9]	24.5 mm	21.8 mm

Table 6.18 Multiplication factors for calculation of stature from fibula

Fibula	Shah and Siddiqui	PAN (Bengal, Bihar and Odisha)		NAT	Singh and Shoha	Mehta and Thomas	
Sex	Male	Male	Female	Male	Male	Male	Female
Multiplication factor	4.4	4.46	4.43	4.48	4.35	4.44	4.55

FIBULA

Sex

The sexual dimorphism is seen in fibula and is mentioned in **Table 6.17**.

Stature

Stature can be determined from fibula by using Dupertuis and Hadden's formulae as shown in **Table 6.12**. The multiplication factors used for determination of stature from fibula is shown in **Table 6.18**.

Table 6.19 Centers of ossification for fibula (Galstaun)

Ossification centers	Female	Male
Proximal end		
Appearance Fusion	One year 14–16 years	One year 11–16 years
Distal end		
Appearance Fusion	One year 13–15 years	Two years 14–16 years

Age

From the appearances and fusion of ossification centers of fibula, the age of a person can be ascertained (**Table 6.19**).

SCAPULA

Age

The cartilaginous scapula is ossified from eight or more centers. One for the body, two for each for the coracoid process and the acromion, one each for the medial border, inferior angle and lower glenoid rim.

The center for the body appears in the 8 intrauterine weeks. Ossification begins centrally in the coracoid process in the first year (2.5 months as per Galstaun), rarely before birth.

Soon after puberty (during 14–15 years), centers appear in the lower glenoid rim, inferior angle and in the medial border. All they are fused by 17-18 years, i.e. Before the 20th year. The various centers of ossification of scapula are mentioned in **Table 6.20** and **Figure 6.19**.

CLAVICLE

Sex

The sex differences between male and female from clavicle are shown in **Table 6.21**.

Age

The clavicle is considered to be a long bone, as it has a medullary cavity and an epiphysis at either end to permit growth. The clavicle is the first fetal bone to undergo primary ossification, and its medial epiphysis is the last to fuse.[15,16]

The appearance and fusion of ossification centers[17] for clavicle are mentioned in **Figure 6.20** and **Table 6.22**.

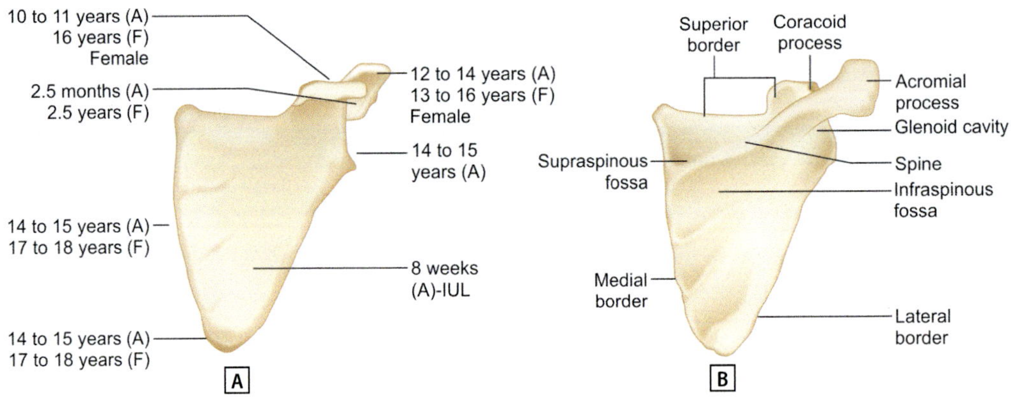

Figures 6.19A and B Appearance and fusion of ossification center of scapula

Table 6.20 Centers of ossification for scapula (Galstaun)

Scapula (A- Appearance, F- Fusion)		Female		Male
Base of coracoid of scapula	A F	2.5 months 2.5 years	A F	2.5 months 2.5 years
Coracoid tip	A F	10–11 years 16 years	A F	10–11 years 16 years
Angle of coracoid	A F	8–10 years 16 years	A F	10–14 years 17–18 years
Acromion	A F	12–14 years 13–16 years	A F	14–17 years 14–19 years

Table 6.21 Sex differences from clavicle

Traits	Male	Female
General	Heavier, longer, rough and more curved	Lighter, shorter, smooth and less curved
Muscle markings	Prominent	Not prominent
Length (mean)[14]	147.6 mm	129.8 mm
Weight	> 20.10 g	< 7.82 g
Mid clavicular circumference[14]	35.7 mm	29.5 mm

Stature

Singh and Sohel[15] have estimated the stature from clavicle in the following manner:
Stature = Length of clavicle × multiplication factor
Multiplication factor = 11.1

HUMERUS

Sex

Sex determination of adolescent skeletons using the humerus is shown in **Table 6.23**. The male and female humerus is shown in **Figure 6.21**.

Stature

The stature from the humerus can be determined by using Dupertuis and Hadden's and multiplication formulae as shown in **Tables 6.12** and **6.24** respectively.

Race

Race from humerus is determined from:

i. Bone length
ii. Index.

Bone Length

Male humerus is longer than female one and little longer in blacks than in whites. The racial variation from humerus between American Blacks and Whites are shown in **Table 6.25**.

Index

There are several features of humerus that can be used to determine the race of an individual.

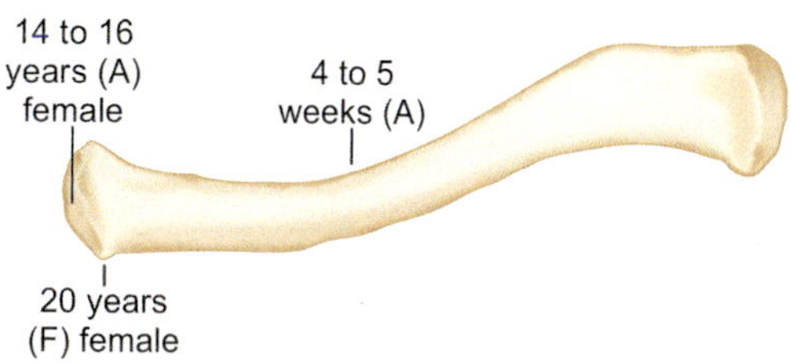

Figure 6.20 Appearance and fusion of ossification centers of clavicle

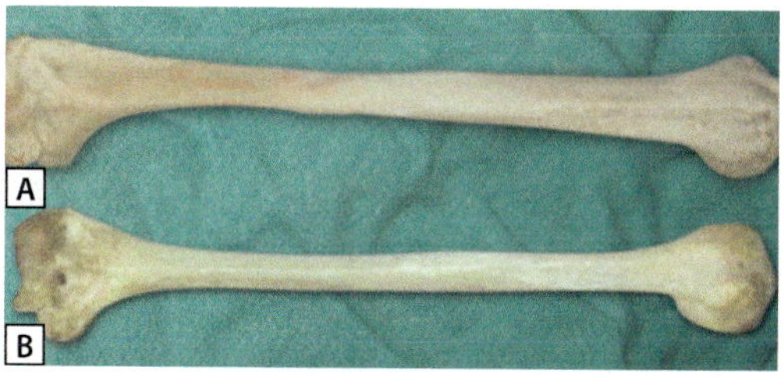

Figures 6.21A and B (A) Male and; (B) female humerus

Table 6.22 Ossification of clavicle (Galstaun)

Ossification centers	Female	Male
Sternal end		
Appearance Fusion	14–16 years 20 years	15–19 years 22 years

Table 6.23 Sex differences from humerus

Traits	Male	Female
General	Heavier, rough	Lighter, smooth
Muscle markings	Prominent	Not prominent
Length[10]	31.1 cm	27.9 cm
Vertical diameter of head	48 mm	40.5 mm
Transverse diameter of head	44.6 mm	38.9 mm
Mid-shaft circumference[10]	58.5 mm	49.1 mm
Epicondylar breadth[10]	60.4 mm	52.4 mm

Table 6.24 Multiplication factors for calculation of stature from humerus

Humerus	Shah and Siddiqui	PAN (Bengal, Bihar and Odisha)		NAT	Singh and Shoha	Mehta and Thomas	
Sex	Male	Male	Female	Male	Male	Male	Female
Multiplying factor	5	5.31	5.31	5.3	4.97	5.08	5.31

Table 6.25 Variation in humerus length against different races

Length variability	White		Black	
	Male	Female	Male	Female
Maximal humerus length	321 mm	292 mm	329 mm	303 mm
Humerus length (in range)	276–371 mm	240–328 mm	278–364 mm	265–348 mm

Table 6.26 Indices from humerus in various races

Index	Indian	European	Black
Brachial	76.49	75.5	78.5
Intermembral	67.27	70.4	70.3
Humerofemoral	71.11	69	72.4

Table 6.27 Ossification of humerus (Galstaun)

Ossification centers (A-appearance, F-fusion)	Female		Male	
Head of humerus	A F	1 year 14–16 years	A F	1 year 14–18 years
Greater tubercle (fusion to head)	A F	7 months 2–4 years	A F	7 months 2–4 years
Greater tubercle (fusion to lesser tubercle)	A F	7 months 5–7 years	A F	7 months 5–7 years
Trochlea Fusion to capitulum	A F	10 years 9–13 years	A F	11 years 11–15 years
Lateral epicondyle Fusion to capitulum	A F	10 years 10–12 years	A F	12 years 11–16 years
Medial epicondyle Fusion to shaft distal humeral epiphysis	A F	5 years 14 years	A F	7 years 16 years

The indices frequently used to determine races are mentioned in **Table 6.26**.

i. **Brachial Index:** Length of radius × 100 ÷ length of humerus
ii. **Intermembral Index:** Length of humerus ÷ length of radius × 100 ÷ length of femur ÷ length of tibia
iii. **Humerofemoral Index:** Length of humerus × 100 ÷ length of femur

Age

The age of a person can be determined from humerus by examination of the following features: (i) Ossification centers and (ii) Radiographic alterations.

Ossification Centers: From the appearance and fusion of ossification centers for humerus, the age can be determined (**Table 6.27**).

Radiographic Alterations: The gradual proximal extension of medullary cavity with due progression of age can be a method for age estimation (range 41–61.1 years).

RADIUS

Sex

Sex determination of adolescent skeletons using the radius is shown in **Figure 6.22** and **Table 6.28**.

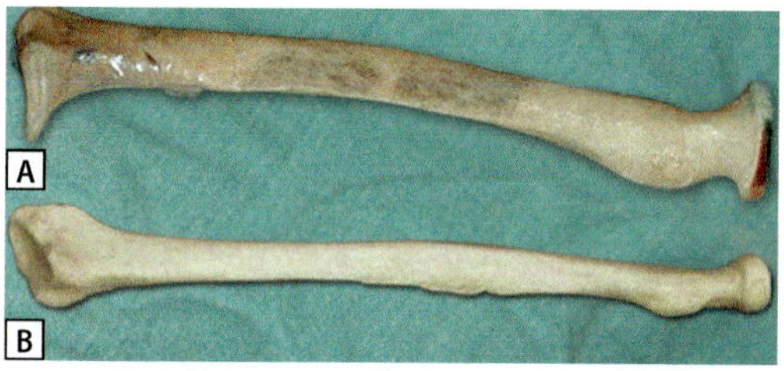

Figures 6.22A and B (A) Male and; (B) Female radius

Age

The appearance and fusion of ossification center of radius is mentioned in **Table 6.29**.

ULNA

Sex

The sex differences between male and female from ulna are shown in **Table 6.30**.

Stature

Stature from ulna can be determined by multiplication formulae as shown in **Table 6.31**.

Age

The appearance and fusion of ossification center of ulna is mentioned in **Table 6.32**.

Table 6.28 Sex differences from radius

Traits	Male	Female
General	Heavier, rough	Lighter, smooth
Muscle markings	Prominent	Not prominent
Diameter of the head	22.50 mm	21.50 mm
Head circumference[11]	67.8 mm	59.5 mm
Tuberosity circumference[11]	48.5 mm	42.2 mm
Mid-shaft circumference[11]	67.8 mm	59.5 mm
Distal end breadth[11]	32.7 mm	28.5 mm

Table 6.29 Ossification centers of radius (Galstaun)

Ossification centers	Female	Male
Appearance (Upper end) Fusion	6 years 14 years	8 years 16 years
Appearance (Lower end) Fusion	1 year 16.5 years	1 year 16–17 years

Table 6.30 Sex differences from ulna

Traits	Male	Female
General	Heavier, rough	Lighter, smooth
Muscle markings	Prominent	Not prominent
Mid-shaft circumference[12]	43 mm	37.1 mm
Distal end breadth[12]	19 mm	16.7 mm

Table 6.32 Ossification of ulna (Galstaun)

Ossification centers	Female	Male
Proximal end olecranon		
Appearance Fusion	9–12 years 15 years	11–13 years 17 years
Distal end		
Appearance Fusion	8–10 years 17 years	10–11 years 18 years

Table 6.31 Multiplication factors for calculation of stature from ulna

Ulna	Shah and Siddiqui	PAN (Bengal, Bihar and Odisha)		NAT	Singh and Shoha	Mehta and Thomas	
Sex	Male	Male	Female	Male	Male	Male	Female
Multiplying factor	6	6	6	6.3	5.93	6.4	6.85

STERNUM

Sex

From Morphological Changes: The male sternum is longer and broader in size (**Figure 6.23**); the body is more than double the length of the manubrium. The female sternum is shorter and narrower in size, and its body is less than double the length of the manubrium (**Table 6.33**).

Sternal Index: Although the sternal index is found to be significantly higher in females, various analyses suggest that sex determination can't be made conclusively from the sternal index. The sternal index is derived by dividing the length of manubrium by the length of body and multiplying it by 100. **Sternal index** as a discriminator of sex:

$$\frac{\text{Manubrial length (mm)}}{\text{Body length (mm)}} \times 100$$

Male: 46.2

Female: 54.3

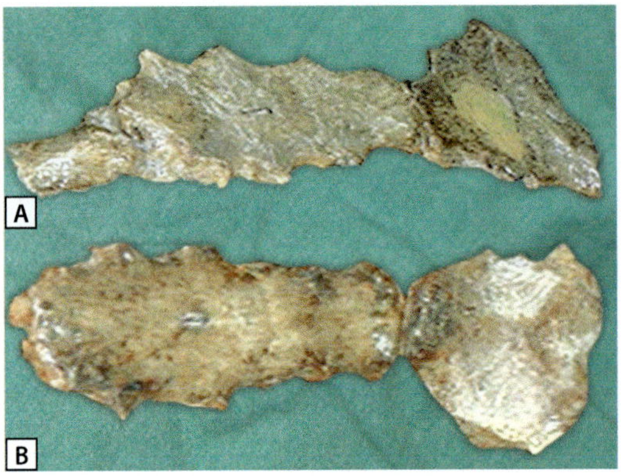

Figures 6.23A and B (A) Male; and (B) Female sternum

Age

The sternum consists of two cartilaginous sternal plates, situated one on either side of the median plane and connected with the cartilages of the upper nine ribs of their own side. These two blocks fuse with each other along the middle line to form the cartilaginous sternum which is ossified from six centers: five primary and one secondary center.

One primary center is for the manubrium and four for the body, i.e. for sternal segments respectively. The secondary center is for the xiphoid process.

The primary centers appear in intervals between the articular depressions for the costal cartilages, in the following order:

i. Manubrium ossified from one to three centers appearing in the fifth fetal month
ii. The **first** and **second** sternebrae usually from single center about fifth fetal month.

Table 6.33 Sex differences from sternum		
Traits	**Male**	**Female**
General	Heavier, rough	Lighter, smooth
Muscle markings	Prominent	Not prominent
Length	Body is more than double the length of the manubrium	Body is less than double the length of the manubrium
Manubrial length[13]	51.7 mm	48.4 mm
Body length[13]	95.4 mm	78.6 mm
Length	>149 mm	<149 mm
Width of first segment of sternum (sternebra)[13]	27.5 mm	24.3 mm
Width of third segment of sternum (sternebra)[13]	32.6 mm	29.2 mm
Sternal index	46.2	54.3
Relative width index[13]	85.2	84.3

Table 6.34 Appearance and fusion of ossification of sternum			
Ossification centers	**Segment**	**Appearance**	**Fusion**
Manubrium	-	5th fetal month	Usually remain un-united. Rarely united in old age (> 60 years)
Body	1st and 2nd sternebrae	5th fetal month	Between puberty (14th) and 25th years, they all are united from below upwards
	3rd and 4th sternebrae	5th to 6th fetal month	
Xiphoid Process		3 years	After 40 years

iii. **Third** and **fourth** sternebrae are commonly paired and appear in the fifth and sixth months, respectively, but one of either pair may be delayed until the 7th or even or 8th month

iv. The xiphoid process begins to ossify in the third year or later.

Union of the various centers of the body begins about puberty and proceeds from below upward by the age of 25 years, they are all united.

The xiphoid process may become joined to the body before the age of 30, but this occurs more frequently after 40; on the other hand, it sometimes remains un-united till old age. In advanced life, usually above 60 years, the manubrium is occasionally joined to the body by bone. Appearance and fusion of ossification centers of sternum are shown in **Table 6.34** and **Figure 6.24**.

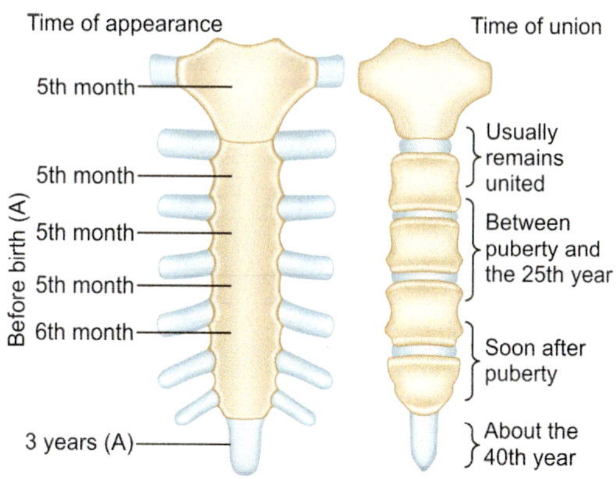

Figure 6.24 Ossification centers for sternum

HYOID BONE

Age of fusion of hyoid bone can help in determining the age of an individual, especially of unknown dead bodies where only skeletal remains are available. A victim of compression of neck will more likely have fracture of hyoid bone if his hyoid bone is fused. Indian authors have reported that the fusion of greater cornu of the hyoid bone with the body occurs between 40 and 60 years of age. Studies done by foreign workers observed that hyoid bone fused at an earlier age (30–40 years).

PELVIS AND HIPBONE

Sex

The pelvis is generally agreed to be the part of the skeleton best studied for sex determination as it is associated with female structural capability to bear children.

Sex determination is only really possible with adult skeletons because there is not much sexual dimorphism in pre-adolescence children. Again towards old age, there occurs blurring of sexually dimorphic traits. Hence, determination of sex from bones should ideally be limited to 15–55 years of age. Important differentiating features between male and female are given in **Table 6.35** and **Figure 6.25**.

Age

The age from hipbone can be estimated from:
- Ossification centers
- Pubic symphysis phases
- Pubic symphysis component.

Ossification Centers

Hipbone ossifies from eight centers; three primary one each for the ilium, ischium and pubis; and five secondary one each for the crest of the ilium, the anterior inferior spine, the tuberosity of the ischium, the pubic symphysis and one or more for the Y-shaped piece at the bottom of the acetabulum:

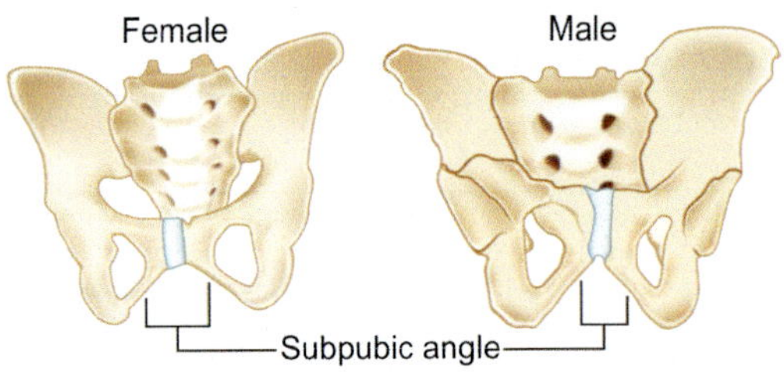

Figure 6.25 Male and female pelvic bones

Table 6.35 Sex differences in pelvis[3]

Trait	Male	Female
General	Heavier, rugged with marked muscle markings	Lighter, gracile, smoother with less prominent muscle markings
Symphysis	Higher	Lower
Sub-pubic angle	Narrow - V shaped	U shaped, obtuse angle
Obturator foramen	Large, often ovoid	Small, triangular
Acetabulum	Large, directed laterally	Small, directed anterolaterally
Greater sciatic notch	Smaller, narrower, deeper	Larger, wider, shallower
Ischiopubic rami	Slightly everted	Strongly everted
Sacroiliac joint	Large	Wide
Pre and postauricular sulcus	Not frequent	More frequent, better developed
Ischial tuberosity	Not everted	Everted
Sacrum	Longer, narrower and curved; well marked promontory; sacroiliac joint reaches 3rd sacral vertebra; body of the first sacral vertebra is larger	Shorter, wider and straight; less well marked promontory; sacroiliac joint reaches 2nd sacral vertebra; body of the first sacral vertebra is smaller
Pelvic brim (inlet)	Heart shaped	Circular, elliptical
True pelvis or cavity	Relatively smaller	Oblique, shallow, spacious

Table 6.36 Ossification of hipbone (Galstaun)		
Ossification centers	**Female**	**Male**
Iliac crest		
Appearance Fusion	14 years 17–19 years	17 years 19–20 years
Triradiate cartilage (fusion)	13–14 years	15–16 years
Ischial tuberosity		
Appearance Fusion	14–16 years 20 years	16–18 years 20 years
Ischio-pubic rami (fusion)	8½ years	8½ years

i. Ilium, immediately above the greater sciatic notch, about the eighth or ninth week of fetal life
ii. Superior ramus of the ischium, about the third month
iii. Superior ramus of the pubis, between the fourth and fifth months.

The secondary centers, its appearance and fusion are mentioned in **Table 6.36.**

About in the 13th-14th year, the three primary centers have extended their growth into the bottom of the acetabulum and are separated from each other by a Y-shaped portion of cartilage, which now presents traces of ossification, often by two or more centers.

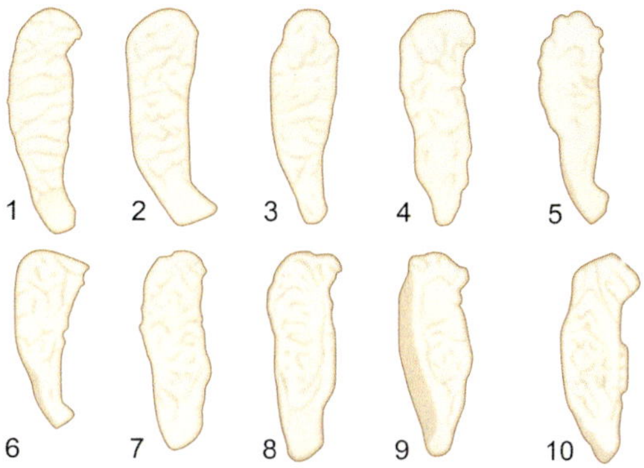

Figure 6.26 Different stages of pubic symphysis

Pubic Symphysis Phase

At the time of birth, the symphysis pubis is 9–10 mm in width, with thick cartilaginous end-plates. By mid-adolescence, the adult size is achieved. During adulthood the end-plates decrease in width to a thinner layer. Degeneration of the symphysis pubis accompanies aging and postpartum. The pubic symphysis can be used to estimate the age of adult skeletons. Throughout life, the surfaces of the pubic symphysis are worn at a more-or-less predictable rate. By examining the wear of the pubic symphysis, it is possible to estimate the age of the person from 30 to 50 years.

A morphological change of the articular surfaces of the innominate provides an excellent postcranial age indicators for adult remains. Variation in the face of the pubic symphysis, the anterior-most point of articulation between the two innominates in the pelvic girdle, is a common region analyzed for age determination. **Todd** (1920) outlined a 10-stage method for assessing this surface, based on a large sample of male innominates (**Figure 6.26**).[18] According to Todd, the pubic symphysis has usually oval outline and has five main features as follows:

- Surface
- Ventral border or rampart
- Dorsal border or plateau
- Superior extremity
- Inferior extremity.

Phase 1: Symphyseal face rugged, traversed by horizontal ridges separated by well-marked grooves, there being no distinction in size between the upper and lower ridges. None of the following structures are present: Nodules fusing with the surface, a delimiting margin or definition of extremities (Age: 18–19 years).

Phase 2: Symphyseal surface still rugged. Horizontal grooves are becoming filled near their dorsal limit with new, finely textured bone. Bony nodules may be present, fusing with upper symphyseal face. Dorsal delimiting margin begins to develop. No delimitation of the extremities. Ventral bevel commences (Age: 20–21 years).

Phase 3: Symphyseal face shows progressive obliteration of ridge and furrow system. Commencing formation of a dorsal platform is seen. Bony nodules may be present. Definition of dorsal margin, with sharp lipping is present. Ventral bevel is more pronounced. Extremities not delimited (Age: 22–24 years).

Phase 4: Great increase of ventral bevelled area. Corresponding diminution of ridge and furrow formation is present. Complete definition of dorsal margin through the formation of the dorsal platform. Commencing delimitation of lower extremity is present (Age: 25–26 years).

Phase 5: Little change in symphyseal face and dorsal platform. Margin more clearly defined and more sharply lipped. Lower extremity is better defined. Upper extremity forming with or without the intervention of a bony nodule is present (Age: 27–30 years).

Phase 6: Increasing definition of extremities. Development and practical completion of ventral rampart present. Retention of some granular appearance of symphyseal face indicating that activity has not yet ceased. Failure of ventral aspect of pubis adjacent to ventral rampart to become transformed into a compact surface is seen. The rampart may therefore be somewhat undermined. Retention of the pectinate outline of the dorsal margin and slight ridge and furrow system are seen. No lipping of ventral margin and no increased lipping of dorsal margin (Age: 30–35 years).

Phase 7: Face and ventral aspect change from granular to fine-grained or dense bone. Slight changes in symphyseal face and marked changes in ventral aspect from diminishing activity are present. No formation of symphyseal rim. No ossification of tendinous and ligamentous attachments. (Age: 35–39 years).

Phase 8: Symphyseal face and ventral aspect of pubic bone generally smooth and inactive. Oval outline is completed. Extremities clearly defined. No distinct 'rim' to symphyseal face. No marked lipping of ventral or dorsal margin. Development of ossification in tendinous and ligamentous attachments, especially those of sacro-tuberous ligament and gracilis muscle is present (Age: 40–45 years).

Phase 9: Symphyseal face presents a more or less marked rim. Dorsal margin uniformly lipped; ventral margin irregularly lipped (Age: 45–49 years).

Phase 10: Ventral margin eroded at a greater or lesser extent of its length, continuing somewhat onto the symphyseal face. Rarefaction of face and irregular ossification is present. Disfigurement increases with age (Age: 50 years+).

Analysis has shown the Todd method to be the most accurate of the pubic symphyseal methods available. It should be noted, however, that a tendency to over age individuals has been found after age 40 years by some, while others claim under aging of the 45+ year old individuals is problematic.

Pubic Symphysis Component

Mckern and **Stewart** in 1957 made the revision of Todd method. They divided surface of pubic symphysis into three components by a vertical grove into dorsal and ventral halves. These components are termed as dorsal demi-face and ventral demi-face. The third component consists of whole surface. Each of the components had been allotted scores ranging from 0 to 5. The three components are as follows:

Component I: Dorsal plateau (dorsal demi-face). Details in **Table 6.37**.

Component II: Ventral Rampart (ventral demi-face). Details in **Table 6.38**.

Component III: Symphyseal rim (symphyseal surface). Details in **Table 6.39**.

Race

Race can be determined from:

- Morphology (**Table 6.40**)
- Interspinous and bi-iliac diameter (**Table 6.41**).

Table 6.37 Component I-dorsal plateau (dorsal demi-face)

Score	Age range (years)	Description
0	17–18	Dorsal margin absent
1	18–21	A slight margin formation first appears in the middle third of the border
2	18–21	The dorsal margin extends along entire dorsal border
3	18–24	Filling-in of grooves and resorption of ridges to form a beginning plateau in the middle third of dorsal demi-face
4	19–29	The plateau, still exhibiting vestiges of billowing, extends over most of the dorsal demi-face
5	23+	Billowing disappears completely and the surface of the entire demi-face becomes flat and slightly granulated in texture

Table 6.38 Component II-ventral rampart (ventral demi-face)

Score	Age range (years)	Description
0	17–22	Ventral beveling absent
1	19–23	Ventral beveling is present only at superior extremity of ventral border
2	19–24	Bevel extends inferiorly along ventral border
3	21–28	The ventral rampart begins by means of bony extension from either or both of the extremities
4	22–33	The rampart is extensive, but gaps are still evident along the earlier ventral border, most evident in the upper two-thirds
5	24+	The rampart is complete

Table 6.39 Component III-symphyseal rim (symphyseal surface)

Score	Age range (years)	Description
0	17–24	The symphyseal rim is absent
1	21–28	A partial dorsal rim is present, usually at the superior end of the dorsal margin, it is round and smooth in texture and elevated above the symphyseal surface
2	24–32	The dorsal rim is complete and ventral rim is beginning to form. There is no particular beginning site
3	24–39	The symphyseal rim is complete. The enclosed symphyseal surface is finely grained in texture and irregular or undulating in appearance
4	29+	The rim begins to break down. The face becomes smooth and flat and the rim is no longer round but sharply defined. There is some evidence of lipping on the ventral edge
5	38+	Further breakdown of the rim (especially along superior ventral edge) and rarefaction of the symphyseal face. There is also disintegration and erratic ossification along the ventral rim

Table 6.40 Racial variation from morphological changes

	White people	Black people
Ilium	Flare outwards and upwards	Ilium is more vertical
Pelvis	Broader	Not broader
Symphysis	Placed low	Placed high

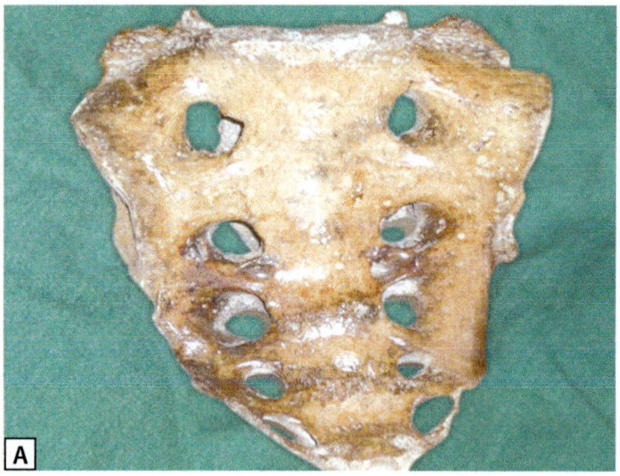

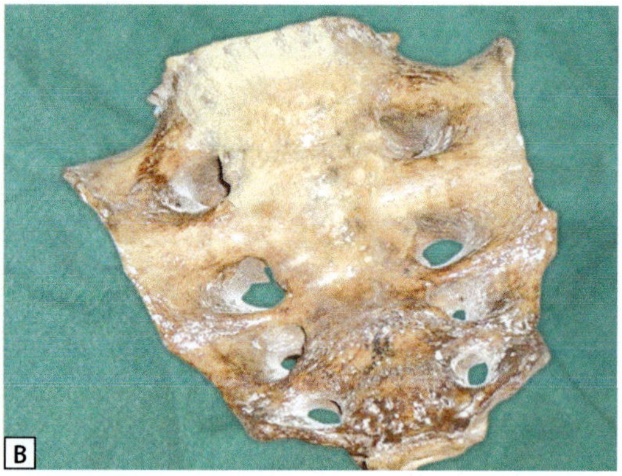

Figures 6.27A and B (A) Male; and (B) Female sacrum

Table 6.41 Racial variation from interspinous and bi-iliac diameter (**Adair 1921**)

Population	Interspinous diameter	Bi-iliac diameter
American (Indian)	226 mm	257 mm
Chinese	205–226 mm	220–252 mm
European	222 mm	266 mm
Aryan	260 mm	270 mm
Bengalese (Indian)	179 mm	216 mm

SACRUM

The **sacrum** is a large, triangular bone at the base of the spine and at the upper and back part of the pelvic cavity, where it is inserted like a wedge between the two hip bones. Its upper part connects with the last lumbar vertebra and bottom part with the coccyx.

Sex

As a rule, the female sacrum is wider and flatter than that of the male, a morphology again permitting a greater outlet for the birth canal (**Figure 6.27**). In the St. Stephenas collection, 97% of the sacrum showed the narrowness and curvature of males. Though sacrum is often consider to be an important bone while dealing with sex differences in skeletal material, there is dearth of metrical data available for this bone (**Table 6.42**).

Measured study about the sacrum has been done by various authors. **Jit** and **Singh** (1966) advocated the demarking point which identifies the sex with 100% accuracy.

Corporo-Basal Sacral Index as a Discriminator of Sex

$$\frac{\text{Breadth of 1st sacral vertebra (mm)}}{\text{Breadth of base of sacrum (mm)}} \times 100$$

Male : 45

Female : 40.5

Sacral index = Breadth of base of sacrum × 100 ÷ anterior length of sacrum

Age

i. Sacrum ossifies from 35 centers, consisting of 21 primary and 14 secondary centers.
ii. Primary centers for 1st, 2nd and 3rd segment appears at three month of IUL whereas for 4th and 5th segments appears between 5 and 8 months of IUL. A primary center for costal elements appears between 5 and 6 months of IUL.
iii. A secondary center appears at puberty. There are two secondary centers for upper and lower surface of body of each vertebra (5 × 2 = 10). Amongst two secondary centers, one appears for articular surface and other for narrow edge below it.

Table 6.42 Sex differences from sacrum

Traits	Male	Female
General	Heavier, rough and larger	Lighter, smooth and smaller
Muscle markings	Prominent	Not prominent
Breadth of body of first sacral vertebra	More than breadth of one side ala	Less than breadth of one side ala
Sacral promontory	More projected ventrally	Less projected ventrally and less prominent
Inner curvature	Uniformly curved anteriorly	Abruptly curved at last two segments
Sacro-iliac joint	Extends up to 3rd segment	Extends up to 2nd segment
Number of sacral segments	May be 5 or 6	Always 5
Corporo-basal sacral index	>42	<42
Sacral index	<114	>114

Table 6.43 Determination of race from sacrum

Dimensions	Japanese	White	Black
Width of base in mm (Mean)			
Male	50	48.9	48.8
Female	45.1	43.6	43.6
Width of wing in mm (mean)			
Male	32.7	37	32.3
Female	35.7	40	37.5
Base-wing index (Mean)			
Male	65.8	76.2	66.7
Female	79.7	92.2	86.4

iv. In children, it consists of usually five unfused vertebrae, which begin to fuse from below upwards between ages 16 and 18 and are usually completely fused into a single bone by age 25 year. A gap may persist between S_1 and S_2, until 32 years due to '**lapsed union**.'

Race

In 1982, Kimura had evolved base-wing index for determination of race. The features are mentioned in **Table 6.43.** Here, width of base is the transverse length of sacral vertebra, width of wing is the transverse width of wing (ala). **Base-wing index** = Width of wing ÷ Width of base × 100.

VERTEBRAE

The immature vertebral body has a series of deep radial furrows both on the upper and lower surfaces. The features increases in prominence up to the age of 10, and then gradually fades from 21 to 25 years.

After 45 years, osteoarthritis changes in the form of lipping of the vertebrae are seen. Atrophic changes in the intervertebral discs start around 50–60 years.

SMALL BONES OF HAND AND FEET

Age from Small Bones of Hand

Phalanges are ossified from a primary center for the shaft and a proximal epiphyseal center. Ossification begins prenatally in shafts as follows: Distal phalanges in the 8 or 9 weeks, proximal phalanges in the tenth, middle phalanges in the eleventh week or later. Epiphyseal centers appear in proximal phalanges early in the second year (females) and in its later months (males); in middle and distal phalanges in the second year (females) or third or fourth year (males). All epiphyses unite about the 15th–16th year in females, 17th–18th in males.[19] Details are shown in **Figure 6.28.**

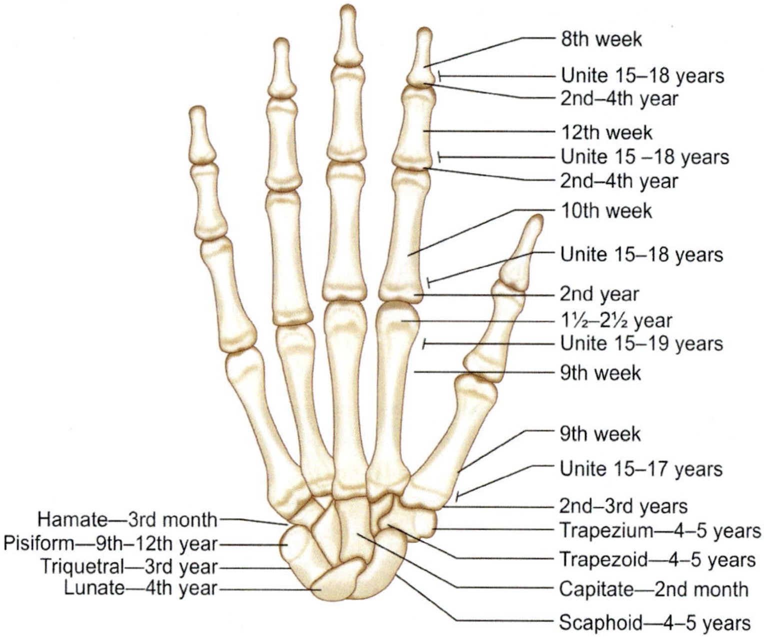

Figure 6.28 Ossification of small bones of hand

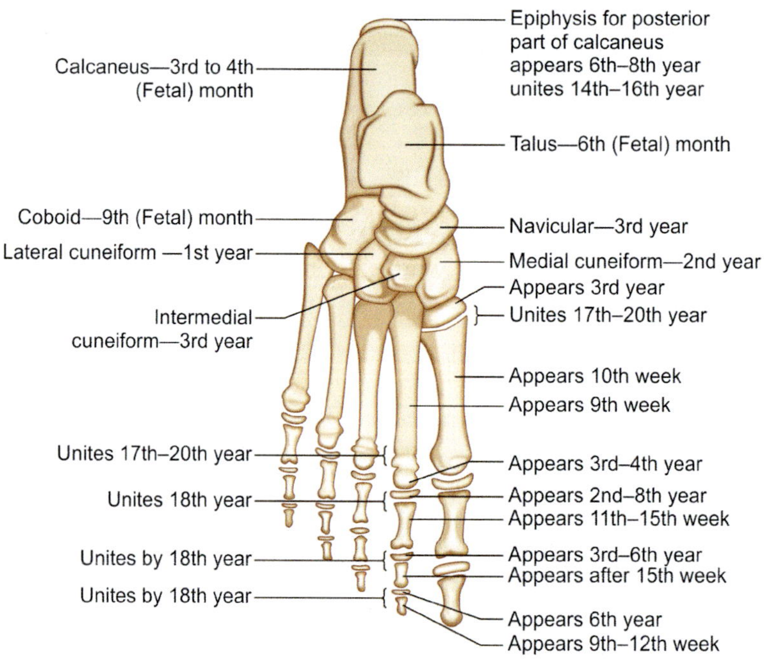

Figure 6.29 Ossification of the bones of the foot

Age from Small Bones of Foot

The metatarsal ossify from a primary center for the shaft and a secondary epiphysis for the base of the first and for the head in the other four. In the second to fourth ossification begins in the midshaft in the ninth prenatal week, in the first and fifth about the tenth week; all unite between the 17th and 20th years.[19] Details are shown in **Figure 6.29**.

REFERENCES

1. Press M. A Scream on the Water: A True Story of Murder in Salem. St. Martin's Paperbacks; 1997. ISBN 0312962991 (ISBN13: 9780312962999).
2. Singh IJ, Gunberg DL. Estimation of age at death in human males from quantitative histology of bone fragments. Am J Phy Anthropol. 1970;33(3):373-82.
3. Krogman WM, Iscan MY. The Human Skeleton in Forensic Medicine. 2nd ed. Springfield, Illinois, US: Charles C. Thomas Pub Ltd; 1986.
4. Chiba M, Terazawa K. Estimation os stature from somatometry of skull. Forensic Sci Int. 1998;97:87-92.
5. Rajesh B. Principles of Forensic Medicine and Toxicology. 1st ed. New Delhi: Jaypee Brothers Medical Publishers (P) Ltd. 2011. p. 96.
6. Trotter M, Gleser GC. Estimation of stature from long limb bones from American whites and Negroes. Am J Phys Anthropo. 1977;47:255-56.
7. Steele DG. Estimation of stature from fragments of long limb bones. In: Stewart TD (ed). Personal Identification in Mass Disasters. National museum of national History; Washington DC: 1970. pp. 85-97.
8. Singh G, Singh S, Singh SP. Identification of sex from tibia. J Anat Soc India. 1975;24:20-4.
9. Singh G, Singh SP. Identification of sex from fibula. J Indian Acad Forensic Sci. 1976;15:29-34.
10. Singh S, Singh SP. Identification of sex from humerus. Indian J Med Res. 1972;60:1061-7.
11. Singh G, Singh SP, Singh S. Identification of sex from radius. J Indian Acad Forensic Sci. 1974;13:10-6.
12. Singh S, Singh G, Singh SP. Identification of sex from ulna. Indian J Med Res. 1974;62:731-5.
13. Jit I, Jhingan V, Kulkarni M. Sexing the human sternum. Am J Phys Anthropol. 1980;53:217-24.
14. Jit I, Singh S. The sexing of adult clavicle. Indian J Med Res. 1966;54:551-71.
15. Humphrey L. Growth patterns in the modern human skeleton. Am J Phys Anthropol. 1998;105(1):57-72.
16. Scheuer L, Black S. Developmental Juvenile Osteology. New York: Academic Press. 2000.
17. Galstaun G. A study of ossification as observed in Indian subjects. Indian J Med Res. 1937;25:267-323.
18. Todd T. Age changes in the pubic bones I: The white male pubis. Am J Phys Anthropol. 1920;3:285-334.
19. Bannister LH, Berry MM, Collins P, Dyson M, Dussek JE, Ferguson MWJ. Gray's Anatomy. 38th ed. Edinburgh: Churchill Livingstone; 2000. p. 658.

CHAPTER 7

Forensic Odontology

Adarsh Kumar, Putul Mahanta, Ajay Logani, Chaithra V

LEARNING PLAN

- Know about forensic significance of odontology
- Understand the usefulness of dental records in forensic investigation
- Learn about the information gathered from teeth

Health profession has been considered as the 'noble profession' since time immemorial. The doctors or the dentists, in many instances, save lives and create an impact by improving the standards of health and well-being in the society.[1] The professional obligation of the dental surgeon to mankind is not only to serve in examination, investigation, diagnosis and treatment of oral and oro-facial conditions, but also serve in other community services and legal matters as well through forensic science.[2] Forensic odontology is a branch of dentistry which, in the interests of justice, deals with the proper handling and examination of dental evidence and proper evaluation and presentation of dental findings.[3]

FORENSIC SIGNIFICANCE

The probable reason for this expanded interest is that a vast number of forensic and legal professionals, law enforcement personnels and insurance companies rely on the dental evidence for their operations. Forensic odontology has played a key role in identification of persons in mass disasters (aviation, earthquakes, tsunamis), crime investigation, ethnic studies and identification of decomposed and disfigured bodies like that of drowned persons, fire victims and victims of motor vehicle accidents (**Figure 7.1**).

Forensic odontologist helps in identification of bite marks on the victims of attack or in other substances such as wood, leather and foodstuffs and to compare with the teeth of a suspect and presentation of this evidence in court of law as an expert witness. They help in identification of unknown bodies through dental records, estimation of age, and contribute even in the absence of dental records through profiling the deceased using features related to teeth. Teeth, with their physiologic variations, pathos and effect of therapy record information that remains

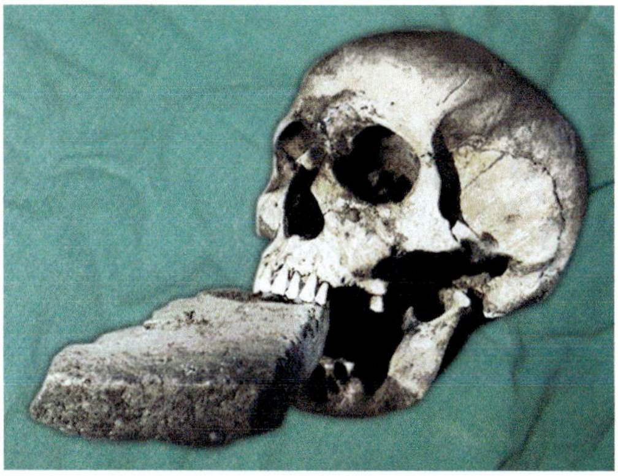

Figure 7.1 Recovered skull with a piece of stone between teeth of both jaws

throughout the life and beyond. This chapter explores an insight into forensic odontology and outlines some of its medicolegal applications.

DEFINITION

Forensic odontology, also known as forensic dentistry, is the area of dentistry concerned with the correct management, examination, evaluation and presentation of dental evidence in criminal or civil legal proceedings in the interest of justice. Classically, forensic dentistry can be considered a subspecialty of oral and maxillofacial pathology.[4]

Forensic odontology is a vital and integral part of forensic science that is most widely used for identification of the living and deceased persons. Over time, forensic odontology has been evolved as a new ray of hope in assisting forensic medicine.[5]

HISTORICAL EVENTS

Although great attention was not paid to dental identification until recent times, the process has been used for more than 2000 years (**Barsley RE 1993**). There are historical reports of identification by recognizing specific dental features as early as 45 AD. However, forensic odontology, as a science, did not appear before 1897, when Dr Oscar Amoedo wrote his doctoral thesis entitled "**L'art dentaire en medecine legale**" describing the utility of dentistry in forensic medicine with particular emphasis on identification. Few of the historical milestones in this field include:

i. **45 AD**: The Roman Emperor Nero used dental impressions to identify slaves; this practice continued throughout Europe and the US during the slave trade.[6]

ii. **66 AD**: The earliest recorded incident of use of teeth for identification is that of Agrippina, the wife of Roman emperor Claudius, who demanded the disembodied head of her husband's mistress, Lollia Paulina. The severe malocclusion and a discolored tooth confirmed her identity.[7]

iii. **1453**: The first formally reported case of dental identification was that of the 80 years old warrior John Talbot, Earl of Shrews Bury, who fell in the battle of Castillon.[8]

iv. **1776**: Dr Paul Revere, first forensic odontologist in the US, identified the body of his friend and patient Dr Joseph Warren, who was killed during the US revolutionary war, with the help of the bridge work (prosthesis).[9]

v. **1837**: Examination of teeth, official method of age determination for employment in the textile industry in the UK.[10]

vi. **1849**: Dental evidence was first accepted in the US court in the Webster-Parkman case. Dr JW Webster allegedly stabbed and dismembered Dr George Parkman. It was Dr Nathan Keep's dental identification of Dr Parkman's dental remains, which led to the conviction of Dr Webster.[11]

vii. **1867**: Oscar Amoedo, an Italian dentist, helped identify hundreds of victims of the 'Great Fire of Paris.' Techniques and protocols developed during that fire are still in use today.[12]

viii. **1897**: First dental mass identification in Paris after a fire broke out at charity bazaar resulting in 126 deaths.[12]

ix. **1898**: Dr Oscar Amoedo wrote the first textbook on forensic dentistry "**L'art Dentaine en Medicine Legale**" and is rightly called as "Father of Forensic Odontology".[12]

x. **1937**: In Chantilly, a murderer was convicted on the evidence of the bite marks that the victim inflicted during her struggle for life.[13]

xi. **1945**: Norway established the first forensic odontology identification committee to investigate crime scenes with multiple victims. Each committee consisted of a police officer, a dentist and a doctor working together to identify the deceased.[14]

xii. **1946**: Welty and Glasgow devised a system in which as many as 500 cards with dental data could be sorted in one minute by a computer.[13]

xiii. **1950**: Le Moyne Snyder, a forensic expert from California, introduced a concept that the wrinkles and cracks of the lips could be used as a method of identification.[15]

xiv. **1972**: The first criminal conviction in North America to feature evidence in the form of forensic odontology was that of Wayne Boden. Boden's trial featured evidence from orthodontist Gordon Swann who was able to link bite marks on the victims to Boden's teeth.[14]

xv. **1977**: Bagi BS mentioned that the bodies of Hitler and his mistress Eva Brauma were identified by his dentist.[16]

xvi. **1978**: Ted Bundy, an American serial killer who murdered numerous young women between 1974 and 1978, confessed to 30 murders. He was proven guilty on the basis of bite marks, which he inflicted on the victim before raping and strangling them to death.[17]

xvii. **1991**: Dr Mark Skinner and Professor Gail Anderson of Simon Fraser University, Canada, reported the case of a Native-American child whose cranium was discovered in British Columbia, Canada. The child's age was determined through examination of the tooth enamel as well as stress markers in the teeth, which were correlated to incidents of stress in the child's life.[17]

xviii. **1995**: General Zia-Ul-Haq, late president of Pakistan, died in 1988 in a plane crash. His body was identified using his dentition.

xix. The first case of dental identification in India was reported by Sansare K and Dayal PK in their review. Raja Jayachandra Rathore of Kannouj died on the battlefield in 1191. His body was identified by using his false anterior teeth.[18]

xx. **2001**: Thousands of people who lost their life in the World Trade Center disaster in the US were identified on the basis of DNA extracts from the tooth brushes of the victims.[19]

xxi. **2004**: Forensic odontologists, as a team of international disaster victim identification, identified about 4280 bodies of tsunami victims in Phuket, Thailand.[20]

xxii. Recently the identities of the two sons of Saddam Husain were confirmed by dental identification (CNN News).

DENTAL RECORDS

A dental record is the detailed document of the history of present illness, clinical examination, diagnosis, treatment done, prognosis and management of a patient. The dental professionals are compelled by law to produce and maintain adequate patient dental records.[21]

Patient Record

Good record-keeping is fundamental for good clinical practice and is an essential skill for practitioners. The primary purpose of maintaining dental record is to deliver quality patient care and follow-up. A patient's dental record consists primarily of a patient's registration form with all the basic personal information. All the information in the dental records should be clearly written, and the person responsible for entering new information should sign and date the entry.[22]

The written notes in the patient record should include:

i. The demographic details: Name, date of birth, phone numbers to be contacted during emergencies.
ii. Medical and dental history.

iii. Clinical examination with accurate charting.
iv. Diagnosis.
v. Treatment plan.
vi. Obtaining and documenting of the informed consent.[23,24]

Maintenance of Dental Records

Mostly notes on paper are used for the dental records. However, with the advancing technology, paper notes are getting replaced by the computerized filing systems. Patients' records or files are arranged in a way for easy retrieval in open or lateral shelving system by methods like; color coding, active and inactive patient files.[25]

Management and Storage of Dental Records

Accurate recording of patient's details that documents all diagnostic information, clinical notes, treatment given, instructions given to the patient for home care and consent to treatment is essential. This helps in defense of allegations of malpractice and in medicolegal cases.

Management of the dental records can aid in identification of a dead or missing person in cases of various crimes and mass disasters. The common element of forensic dentistry that a general practitioner is likely to encounter is to supply antemortem records to a forensic odontologist.[26]

The radiographs needs to be documented and stored in small envelops with patients' details, type of radiographs and date written on front. The films should be properly developed, fixed and rinsed to avoid any degradation of films. The National Health Service (NHS), UK's, Terms of Service states that dental records should be kept for a period of 2 years, while the defense organizations suggest that records to be kept permanently. But due to space constraints it may not be possible; hence it has been advised as follows:

i. Treatment records, X-rays, study models and correspondence is to be retained for 11 years after completion of treatment.
ii. For children, retention until the patient is 25 years old.[14]

Forensic Uses of Patient Records

a. Supply of antemortem records to aid in identification of person.
b. In the process of death certification.
c. Investigation of homicides or other suspicious deaths.
d. Medicolegal cases.
e. Professional misconduct.
f. Crime scenes and mass disasters.[27,28]

DENTITION

The diversity of dental characteristics is wide, making each dentition unique. The dental enamel is the hardest tissue in the body, and would thus withstand peri- and postmortem damages, and so, would dental materials adjoined to teeth. Being diverse and resistant to environmental challenges, teeth are considered excellent postmortem material for identification with enough concordant points to make a meaningful comparison.[29]

About Dentition

i. Dentition means set of teeth.
ii. Human dentition is diphyodont (only two sets of teeth, i.e. deciduous and permanent) acrodont (teeth attached to the jaw by a connective tissue) and heterodont (different types of teeth like incisors, canines, premolars and molars).
iii. A few animals like chimpanzee, gibbon, gorilla and orangutans have similar dentition as in humans.
iv. The three stage of human dentition, viz. deciduous or temporary, mixed and permanent, follow a periodic sequence that can be utilized for estimation of age of different accuracy.

Anatomy of the Tooth

i. The anatomy of the tooth is divided into two parts: the visible part is called crown and the hidden part embedded in the bony socket with connective tissue is the root (acrodont), as shown in **Figure 7.2.**

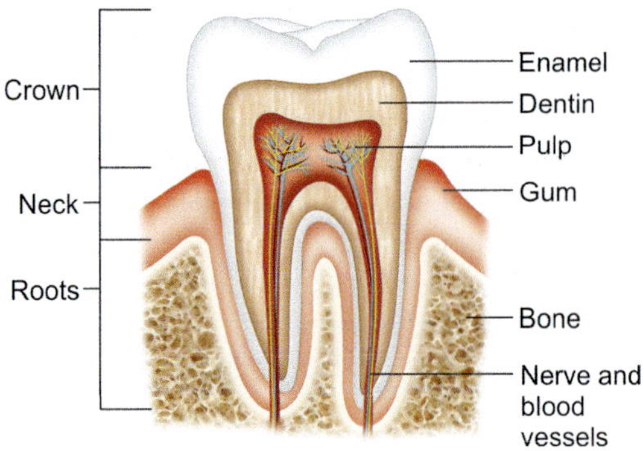

Figure 7.2 Diagrammatic representation of tooth

ii. Both the crown and the root consist of hard and soft tissues.
iii. The crown portion of the tooth is made of enamel (hardest substance in the body), dentine (bulk of the tooth is made up of this material) and pulp tissue, which is housed in a hollow cavity.
iv. The pulp tissue supplies the blood and nerve supply to the tooth.
v. The outer-most portion of the root is called the cementum. Dentine and pulp tissue form the other two layers of the root.
vi. The root portion of the tooth may be single with one apex or terminal end, as usually found in anterior teeth and some of the premolars, or multiple with bifurcation or trifurcation, dividing the root portion in two or more extension or roots with their apices or terminal ends, as found in all molars and in some premolars.
vii. The portion of jaw serving as support for the tooth is called the alveolar process. The bone of the tooth socket is called alveolus.
viii. The crown portion is never covered by bony tissue after full eruption in humans, but it is partly covered at cervical third in young adults by soft tissue of the mouth known as gingival tissue or gums.

Tooth Development

The alveolar cavity, which contain the teeth, are formed around third or fourth month of intrauterine life. Tooth development begins with the formation of cellular tooth germ within alveolar bone in the shape of a crown. Apposition and calcification of enamel and dentine takes place within this germ.

Rudiments of all temporary teeth and of the first molar teeth may be found at birth. Root formation begins after the completion of the crown, and as the root becomes longer, the crown erupts through the bone and comes out of the jaw. The teeth calcify from crown to neck to roots. During the eruption of permanent teeth, the overlying root of its deciduous teeth undergoes absorption simultaneously until crown remains. The unsupported crown then falls off.

Chronology of Eruption/ Emergence of the Temporary Teeth

It is the process where a tooth moves from within the crypts, erupts through the alveolar bone and occludes with the opposing teeth in the mouth (**Hillson 1996**).

i. Calcification, eruption and resorption of root of temporary teeth are shown in **Table 7.1**.
ii. Lower deciduous teeth erupt first, thus initiating the deciduous dentition.
iii. The appearance of the deciduous second molars completes the deciduous dentition by 2–2.5 years of age.
iv. Eruption dates are variable.
v. Deciduous teeth shed and permanent teeth erupt earlier in girls.
vi. The root of a deciduous tooth is completely formed in just about one year after eruption of that tooth into the mouth.
vii. The intact root is short lived, and then it begins to reabsorb at the apex or depending upon the position of the permanent teeth.
viii. Upper molars have three roots; lowers have two roots.
ix. Upper and lower second deciduous molars resemble first permanent molars in the same quadrant.
x. Upper first deciduous molars vaguely resemble upper premolars. Lower first deciduous molars are odd and unique unto themselves.

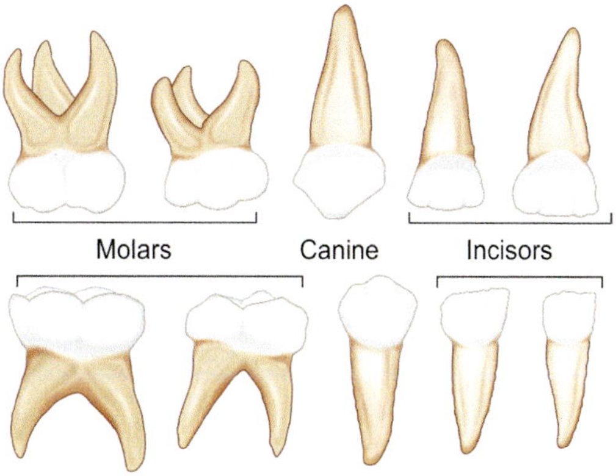

Figure 7.3 Set of temporary teeth in each jaw

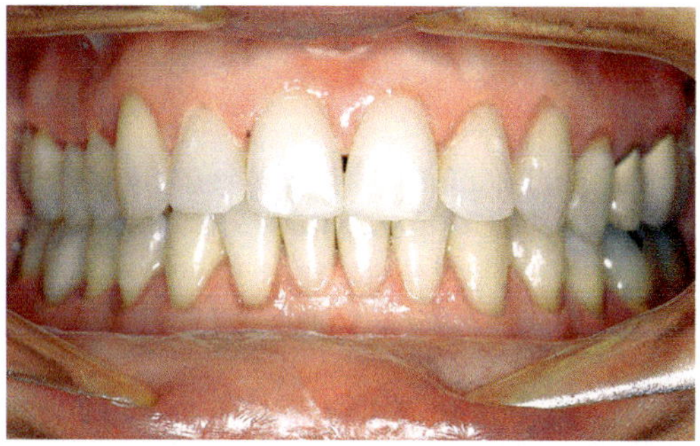

Figure 7.4 Mixed dentition

Table 7.1 Calcification and eruption of deciduous teeth

Tooth	Calcification begins	Eruption	Calcification completed	Resorption root begins
Central incisor (Lower)	5–6 months IUL	6–8 months	1.5–2 years	4th year
Central incisor (Upper)	5–6 months IUL	7–9 months	1.5–2 years	5th year
Lateral incisor (Upper)	5–6 months IUL	7–9 months	1.5–2 years	5th year
Lateral incisor (Lower)	5–6 months IUL	10–12 months	1.5–2 years	5th year
First molar	5–6 months IUL	12–14 months	2–2.5 years	6th year
Canine	5–6 months IUL	17–18 months	2.5–3 years	8th year
Second molar	5–6 months IUL	20–30 months	3 years	7th year

Abbreviation: IUL, Intrauterine life

Temporary Teeth

They are also called as deciduous or milk teeth. They are 20 in number, comprising of four incisors, two canines and four molars in each jaw (**Figure 7.3**).

The dentition may be delayed in ill-nourished children, rickets and hypothyroidism, whereas dentition may be premature or teeth may be present at birth in certain diseases like syphilis. At about 6th or 7th year, first permanent molar teeth erupt behind the second temporary molars. After this, the temporary teeth begin to fall off.

If there is doubt whether any particular teeth is temporary or permanent, X-ray can be taken for confirmation, in which germ of the permanent teeth can be seen underneath if it is a temporary teeth.

Mixed Dentition (5–13 Years)

The mixed dentition refers to the presence of primary and permanent teeth together in the oral cavity (**Figure 7.4**).

In this photograph of mixed teeth, the upper incisors are permanent and lower incisors are temporary. Note the difference in the size and color of the teeth. This usually occurs between the ages of 5 and 13 years as primary teeth are exfoliated and permanent teeth erupt. It is during the time of mixed dentition that dental abnormalities become apparent. Dental conditions, such as missing permanent teeth or malformed teeth become visible. It is at this time of mixed dentition that skeletal and dental malformations will come into view.

The eruption of deciduous and permanent teeth occurs early in the lower jaw, except for the

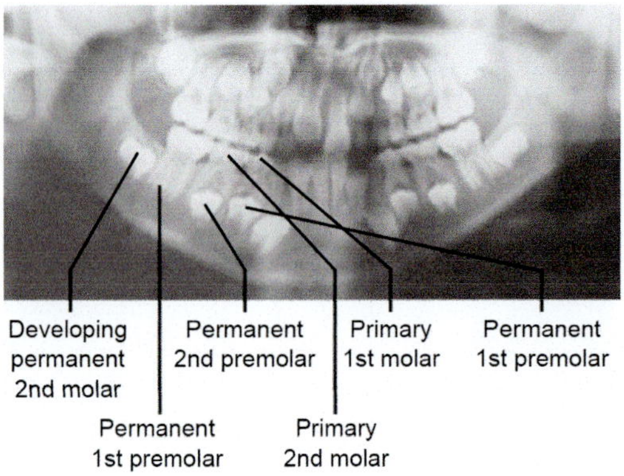

Figure 7.5 Dental X-ray (Orthopantomograph showing mixed dentition)

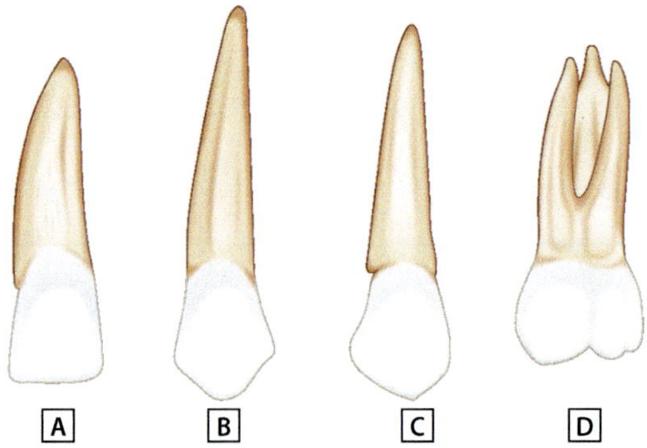

Figures 7.6A to D (A) Incisor; (B) Canine; (C) Premolar; (D) Molar

Table 7.2 Differences between temporary and permanent teeth

Trait	Temporary teeth	Permanent teeth
Size	Smaller, lighter except molar	Big except molar
Direction	Vertical	Forward
Crown	China white	Ivory white
Neck	More constricted	Less
Root	Small and divergent	Large and less
Ridge	Present at junction of crown and fangs	Absent
Regularity in eruption	More regular	Irregular

lateral incisors, which erupt earlier in upper jaw. The eruption of deciduous teeth is more regular than that of permanent teeth. The differences between temporary and permanent teeth are narrated in **Table 7.2**.

The eruption is not always bilaterally symmetrical and occurs about one year early in females than in males. Various factors like hereditary, environment, endocrine and nutrition play a role in the eruption and calcification of teeth. The eruption of teeth tends to occur earlier in warmer climates and in urban areas.

Dental X-rays (**Figure 7.5**) can be utilized to know the developmental status of un-erupted teeth and to know the degree of root completion in erupted teeth. The degree of formation of root and crown structures, stage of eruption and intermixture of temporary and permanent teeth are useful in the estimation of age from birth till 14 years of age.

Two Sets of Teeth

i. **Superadded Permanent Teeth** are those which do not have deciduous predecessors. They erupt behind temporary teeth. All the permanent molars belong to this group and are six in each jaw.
ii. **Successional Permanent Teeth** are those which erupt in the place of deciduous teeth. Permanent premolars erupt in place of temporary molars. There are 10 successional teeth in each jaw.

Permanent Teeth

They are 32 in number comprising of four incisors, two canines, four premolars and six molars in each jaw (**Figures 7.6** and **7.7**).

Incisors: The crown is of the shape of chisel and is convex on its labial surface and concave on its lingual surface. It has a constricted neck with a single root.

Canines: They are larger than incisors. Crown is large and conical, concave on its labial surface and slightly concave on its lingual surface. Its masticatory edge is pointed and projects beyond the level of other teeth. The root is single.

Premolars or **Bicuspids**: They are smaller and shorter than canines. Crown is circular in cross section and slightly compressed mesiodistally. It has two cups on the chewing surface, and root is usually single but may be double.

Molars: They are the largest teeth with broad cubicle crown, which is convex on its labial and lingual surfaces and flattened on its mesial and distal surfaces. The cusps may vary from three to five. The upper molars have three roots and lower molars have two.

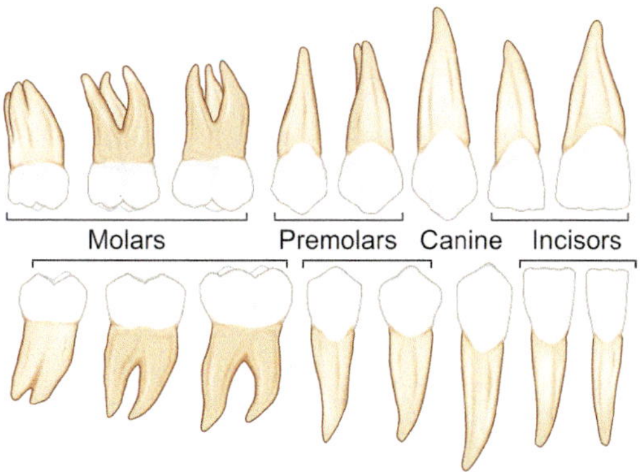

Figure 7.7 Set of permanent teeth in each jaw

Chronology of Eruption/ Emergence of the Permanent Teeth

From the **14th** to **20th year**, dental age estimation is based upon the stage of development of the third molar, which is highly variable. The body of the jaw grows posteriorly and the ramus is elongated after eruption of the second molar teeth. If the third molars are absent, it should be noted whether there is space in the jaw behind second molar teeth. Eruption of third molar is indicative that age is more than 17 years. In some individuals, the third molar may not erupt due to inadequate jaw space, particularly the mandibular ones. Such trapped teeth are called as **impacted teeth**. The calcification and eruption of permanent teeth are mentioned in **Table 7.3**.

Estimation of age from dental examinations, especially from the eruption of 3rd molar, are implemented in forensic age assessments to discriminate between juveniles and adults, considering the judgment of young unaccompanied asylum seekers. The third molar is very variable in eruption, often it is found impacted and even absent because of agenesis. X-ray of the jawbone will reveal impacted teeth, while in cases of agenesis, it will be completely absent on X-ray. As per a recent Indian study, impaction may be seen in a significant number of individuals, while agenesis can occur in up to 20% of individuals.[30]

Even in the absence of the third molar eruption, X-ray of the jaw must be undertaken

Table 7.3 Calcification and eruption of permanent teeth

Tooth	Calcification begins	Eruption	Calcification complete
First molar	At birth	6–7 years	9–10 years
Central incisor	3–4 months	6–8 years	10 years
Lateral incisor	1 year	7–9 years	11 years
First bicuspid	1.5 years	9–11 years	12–13 years
Second bicuspid	2 years	10–12 years	12–14 years
Canine	4–5 months	11–12 years	12–13 years
Second molar	2.5–3 years	12–14 years	14–16 years
Third molar	8–10 years	17–25 years	18–25 years

for assessing calcification of third molar, if space is present behind the second molar. If calcification is complete even without eruption of third molar, age can be considered to be more than 25 years.

Abnormalities of Size and Number

Abnormality in Number

i. **Anodontia**: It is the total lack of tooth development in human.
ii. **Hyperdontia**: It is the presence of more than normal number of teeth.
iii. **Hypodontia**: It is the lack of some teeth. Usually, it refers to the lack of development of one or more teeth and the term Oligodontia may be used to describe the absence of 6 or more teeth.

Abnormality in Size

i. **Microdontia:** It is a condition where teeth are smaller than the usual size and more likely to occur in a maxillary lateral incisor.
ii. **Macrodontia:** It is where teeth are larger than the usual size. Macrodontia of all the teeth is known to occur in pituitary gigantism and pineal hyperplasia.

Laboratory Methods of Approximation of Age

Boyde's Method: Cross striations in the enamel of teeth represent daily incremental lines. The age of an individual can be calculated by counting the number of lines from the neonatal line onwards. This method is applicable mainly on infants. The age so calculated is accurate with an error of around 20 days.[31]

Stack's Method: In this method, weight and height of a tooth is taken and from this, Stack estimated the age of a child.

It is known that chronology of dental development is less variable than bone development and the method applied for this particular period of life is a reliable indicator of age. Though eruption of teeth may be effected by dietary, climatic, racial and geographical variation, the eruption time for deciduous and permanent teeth are fairly constant. Eruption of teeth is one of the changes observed easily among the various dynamic changes that occur from formation of teeth to the final shedding of the teeth.[32]

CHARTING OF TEETH

There are more than 150 different methods of identifying, numbering and charting of teeth. Some of them are discussed below:

Universal System

According to Universal System, each tooth is given a number, i.e. 1–16 for upper jaw from right to left and 17–32 for lower jaw from left to right (for permanent). Similarly 1–10 for upper jaw from right to left and 11–20 for lower jaw from left to right (for temporary).

Palmer Notation

According to palmer notation, numbering is done from 1–8 from medial to lateral both for upper and lower jaw (for permanent) and 1–5 from medial to lateral for both upper and lower jaw (for temporary).

Haderup System

It is a modified form of palmer notation. In this '+' and '–' signs are added to the numbers to indicate the upper and lower jaws, respectively. Position of these signs before or after the number of the teeth will indicate the side, e.g. 1+/1-/+1/-1, etc.

Federation Dentaire Internationale (FDI) Two Digit System

It bears slight resemblance to palmer system in that both utilize the same numbers, but the FDI system substitutes a number for the quadrant side and that number is placed before the tooth number. Thus, the lower right canine will be numbered 43 in this system.

Modified FDI System

According to modified FDI system, quadrant number is modified as follows: Even numbers, (i.e. 2, 4) denotes the left side and odd numbers, (i.e. 1, 3) denotes the right side.

Diagrammatic or Anatomical Chart

In this, each tooth is represented by a pictorial symbol that gives the same number of teeth surfaces as those in the same teeth on the mouth. The incisors and canines are represented by four surfaces and the premolars and molars by five (due to occlusal surface). The positions of the crowns, caries, fillings or other abnormalities are marked on these diagrams. The diagram also includes deciduous teeth.

Features of three important system of numbering the teeth are mentioned in the **Table 7.4** and shown diagrammatically in **Figure 7.8.**

Gustafson's Method

The age estimation in an adult over 21 years depends on the physiological changes in the dental tissues.

i. **Attrition:** Occlusal surface of the teeth is destroyed gradually due to wear and tear from mastication. This firstly involves the enamel, then dentin and at last the pulp is exposed in old age. It depends upon the hardness of the enamel and the functional use of teeth.
ii. **Periodontosis:** Regression of the gums and periodontal tissues takes place in advancing age, gradually exposing the neck and adjacent parts of roots because of which the teeth become loose and fall off.
iii. **Secondary Dentine:** It is deposited at the pulp chamber and gradually extends downwards to the apex decreasing the size of the pulp cavity. This may occur not only due to aging but also due to pathological conditions like caries and paradentosis.
iv. **Cementum Apposition:** Cementum is the calcified tissue that surrounds the dentine and forms the attachment site for the periodontal fibers that link the tooth to the alveolar bone.[33] Cementum is formed as a result of a continuous process throughout life, and it has been shown to triple in thickness between the ages of 20 and 60 years. The thickness varies, with the

Table 7.4 Different systems of numbering teeth

	Zsigmondy Palmer system	**ADA system (Universal system)**	**FDI system**
	Quadrant system	The Universal Numbering System is a simplified method of identifying teeth that is approved and adopted by the American Dental Association	Two digit system
Permanent dentition	The mouth is divided into four quadrants Each tooth in the quadrant is denoted by the numbers 1–8, where the numbering runs from central incisor to the third molar	The tooth numbering starts from the right upper third molar (1) and continues along the upper teeth towards the front and across to the left upper third molar (16). The numbers continue by dropping down to the lower jaw left (17) and again continues along the lower teeth towards the front and across to the lower third molar on right (32)	Each quadrant is assigned a number (1–4 in the clockwise direction) and the teeth within each quadrant are assigned numbers from 1–8 with 1 being central incisor and 8 being the third molar
Deciduous dentition	The mouth is divided into four quadrants Each tooth in the quadrant is denoted by the alphabets A-E where the numbering runs from central incisor to the second molar.	The tooth numbering starts from the right upper third molar (A) and continues along the upper teeth towards the front and across to the left upper third molar (J). The numbers continue by dropping down to the lower jaw (K) and again continues along the lower teeth towards the front and across to the left lower third molar (T)	Each quadrant is assigned a number (5–8 in the clockwise direction) and the teeth within each quadrant are assigned numbers from 1–5 with 1 being central incisor and 5 being the second molar

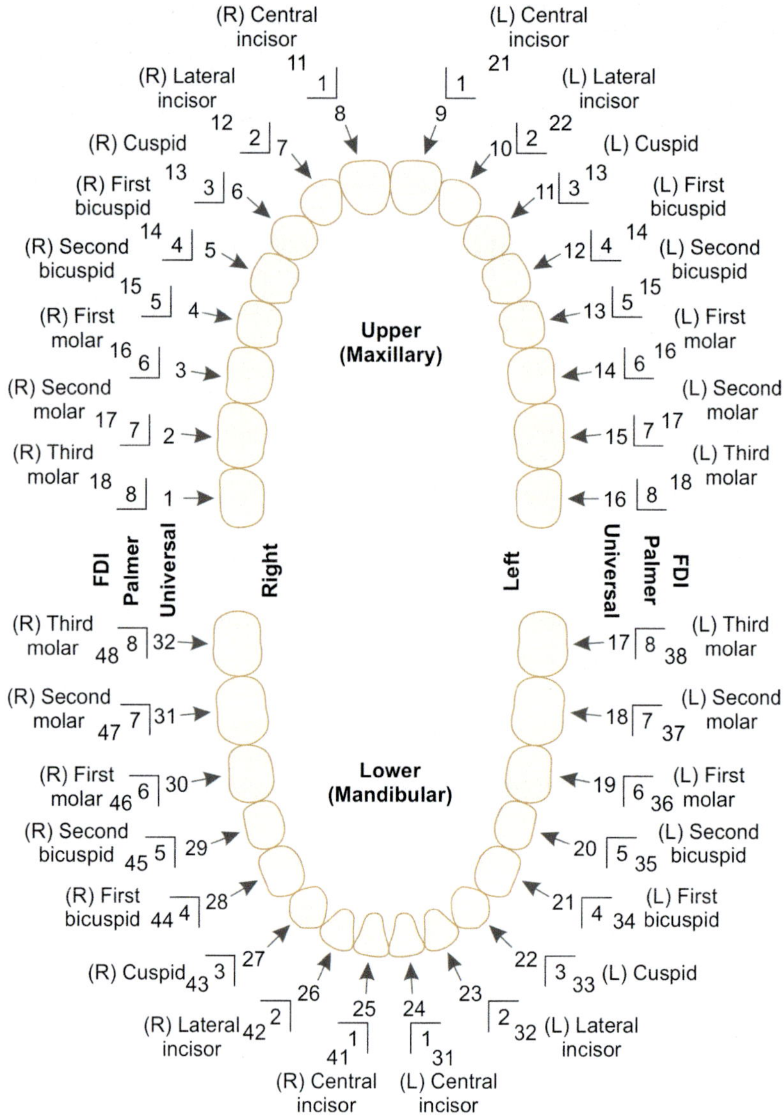

Figure 7.8 Different systems of numbering the permanent teeth

maximum at the apex and the minimum near the cementoenamel junction.[34] The continuous apposition of cementum may be influenced by function, occlusion, and pathologic processes. Further, functional teeth are furnished with less cementum than non-occluding teeth, while impacted teeth seem to have less cementum than functional teeth.[34] It was hypothesized that since cementum apposition have been observed in all mammalian genera studied, they may also be found in humans and may be used to determine age in that genus. The ability to accurately estimate the ages of victims of natural or manmade disasters would be a valuable tool in forensic dentistry.[35]

v. **Root Resorption:** Absorption of the root starts first at the apex and extends upwards, involves both cementum and dentin. This can also be appreciated microscopically.

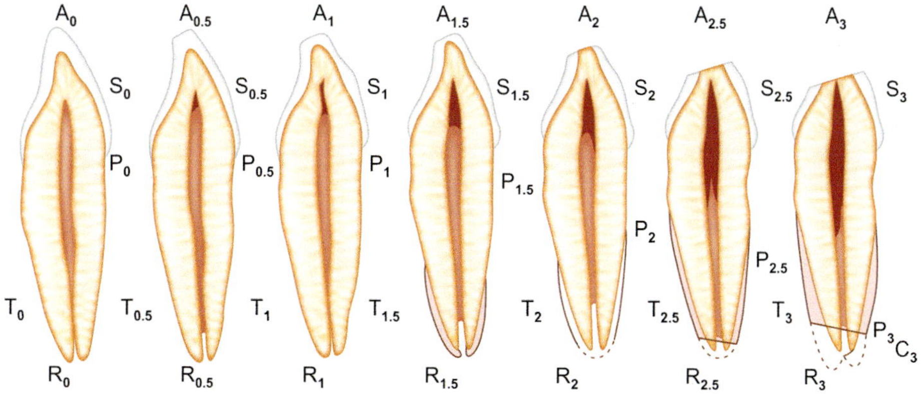

Figure 7.9 Six stages of changes in teeth (Gustafson method): attrition (A), secondary dentine (S), cementum apposition (C), paradentosis (P), root resorption (R) and root translucency (T)

vi. **Translucency of the Root**: Not seen till the age of 30 years. The canals in the dentin are at first wide. With age, they are filled by minerals so that they become invisible and dentin becomes transparent. This change is best seen on ground section of the tooth. It is the most reliable of all the criteria.

All the changes mentioned above are absent at 15 years of age. Arbitrarily, 0–3 points are allotted to indicate the degree of any of these changes. Stage '0' indicates no change; 1 the beginning of the change; 2 obvious change and stage 3 maximum change. There is + 4–7 years of error in calculation of the age. The physiological changes as per Gustafson's method are shown in **Figure 7.9**.

Radiographic Estimation of Dental Age

A study of radiographs of the teeth is a non-destructive, simple method to obtain information.[36] Inspection of radiographs and subsequent comparison with radiographic images, drawings and descriptions in charts yields 'maturity scores' that help us to assess the age of an individual.[37] Alternative approaches based on digitalization of panoramic radiographs and their computerized storage has recently become available. These procedures exploit image analysis to obtain non-destructive metric measurements of both pulp chambers and teeth, which can be used to assess the age of an individual. Forensic odontologists can utilize these techniques that are relatively precise and accurate and avoid the bias inherent in observer subjectivity.[38]

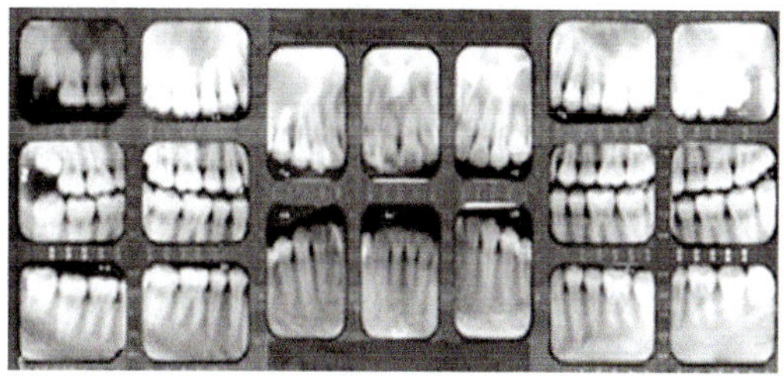

Figure 7.10 Dental records

DENTAL IDENTIFICATION

In cases of mass disasters where physical features are destroyed beyond recognition, teeth can be used since these are heavily calcified, resist fire well and are strong enough to resist severe trauma. Identification is made by comparison of the postmortem data with any available clinical or radiological antemortem data.

For successful dental identification, antemortem data need to be available. This relies heavily on dental professionals recording and keeping dental notes, radiographs, study models, clinical photographs, etc. The availability of dental records will allow comparing the dental characteristics of the person during life with those retrieved from the person after death (**Figure 7.10**).

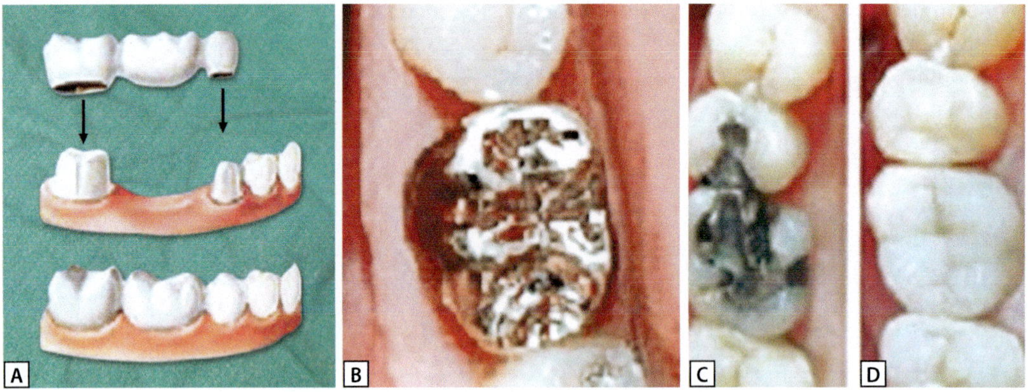

Figures 7.11A to D Various dental works

The American Board of Forensic Odontology recommends four conclusions while reporting for the dental identification:

i. **Positive Identification**: The antemortem and postmortem data match in sufficient detail, with no unexplainable discrepancies, to establish that they are from the same individual.
ii. **Possible Identification**: The antemortem and postmortem data have consistent features but, because of the quality of either the postmortem remains or the antemortem evidence, it is not possible to establish identity positively.
iii. **Insufficient Evidence**: The available information is insufficient to form the basis for a conclusion.
iv. **Exclusion**: The antemortem and postmortem data are clearly inconsistent.

The discretion of identification lies with the odontologist who must be prepared to justify the conclusions in court.[29] Number of teeth, restorations or prostheses, dental caries, malposition and malrotation, peculiar shapes of teeth, root canal therapy or endodontics, bone patterns, complete dentures, relationship of the bite, occupational changes and socioeconomic pattern of the dentition and lip prints are of great value.[39]

Some of the dental works are shown in **Figure 7.11.**

The adult teeth comprises of 32 teeth, each teeth having five surfaces. The infinite combination of missing, filling material, carious lesions, crowns and prosthesis involved in this 160 surfaces form the basis for dental identification. The characterization is further enhanced by the specific morphological patterns of the individual restorations, prosthesis (crowns, removable dentures, fixed prosthesis), additional features incorporated in the root canals, periapical and surrounding soft tissues (**Figure 7.12**). Hence, the basic concept that no two dentitions are alike is the basis of dental identification.

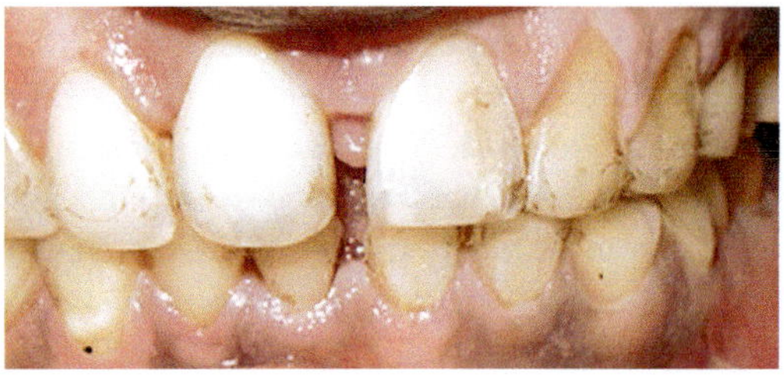

Figure 7.12 Special features like diastema of the teeth or anteriorly proclined upper teeth

Factors of Dental Identification

Dental identification depends on the following factors:

Number of Teeth

The assessment of teeth in the mouth should include those that are present and missing.

The number of possibilities that exist for the combination of teeth missing or present may well be enough to obtain a positive identification. It is important to establish whether the teeth were lost antemortem or postmortem or around the time of death (perimortem). This will help establish the pattern of treatment undertaken with regard to any exodontia, and closer examination of any tooth sockets may give an indication as to the time elapsed since this treatment.

Tooth Loss

It is important to determine the period when the teeth were lost from the arch. In postmortem loss, the bone surrounding the socket margins would be unresorbed and have a sharp profile whereas in antemortem loss, due to the evidence of the healing process taking place within the socket; varying degrees of bone remodeling around the rim and complete fill-in of the socket with secondary bone formation is seen.

Restorations (Figure 7.13)

A tooth is restored when there is loss of tooth substance due to dental caries, fracture of tooth, any abnormal wearing away of teeth or for an aesthetic reason. Restorations frequently involve multiple surfaces of the teeth. A full description of the restoration must be included in the post-mortem records, and this must include the material used and the surfaces restored.

Restorations on the anterior teeth involve four surfaces (mesial, distal, labial, lingual/palatal) and posterior teeth involve five surfaces (buccal, lingual, mesial, distal and occlusal). The types of filling materials used range from silver amalgam, tooth colored material (composite, glass ionomer cement), precious and non-precious metal used for inlays, crowns of gold or porcelain or porcelain fused to metal and precious and non-precious metal bridgework with fused porcelain. Temporary dressings or fillings (Zinc oxide eugenol) may also be used. It is important to be able to recognize the areas of dislodged restorations, untreated dental caries, malpositioned and rotated teeth, anomalous tooth, endodontically treated tooth, teeth with attrition and abrasion. Dental radiographs may substantiate the findings.

Dental Prosthesis

Like a full denture, removable partial dentures, bridges and orthodontic appliances is very helpful if known (**Figure 7.14**).

Bony Pattern

The medullary bone of the jaws possesses a characteristic trabecular pattern, which can be duplicated on the postmortem radiograph. Tooth angulation, root morphology, bone loss, specific changes in pulp chambers and pulpal outlines may also be assessed. Examination of the supporting alveolar bone may give some indication of periodontal diseases during life. The position of the maxillary sinus and its relation to the roots of the upper posterior teeth should be taken into account during comparison of dental data.

Occlusion

Occlusion and malocclusion (**Figure 7.15**) have been described according to whether the jaws have a normal relationship when closed and the teeth may be misplaced or whether the relationship of the maxilla and mandible is disturbed. The amount of overjet and overbite should also be noted as well as the first lower molar relationship.

Oral Pathology

Deviation from the normal anatomic configuration of the oral cavity like mandibular and maxillary tori, geographic tongue, dilantin-induced gingival hyperplasia, enamel hypoplasia and pre-existing bone pathologies (cysts) are some examples. The presence of healed or healing fractures and the establishment of an approximate time of injury could be of help in the identification process.

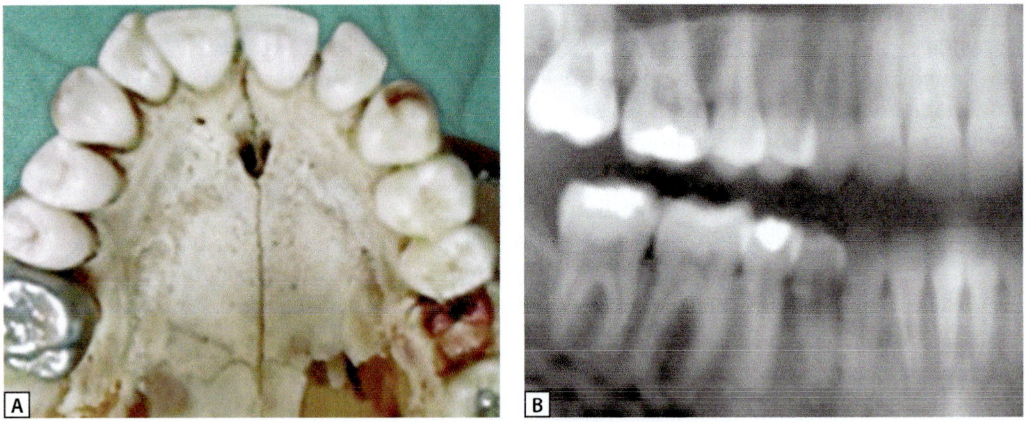

Figures 7.13A and B (A) Dental restorations; (B) Radiographic view of dental restorations

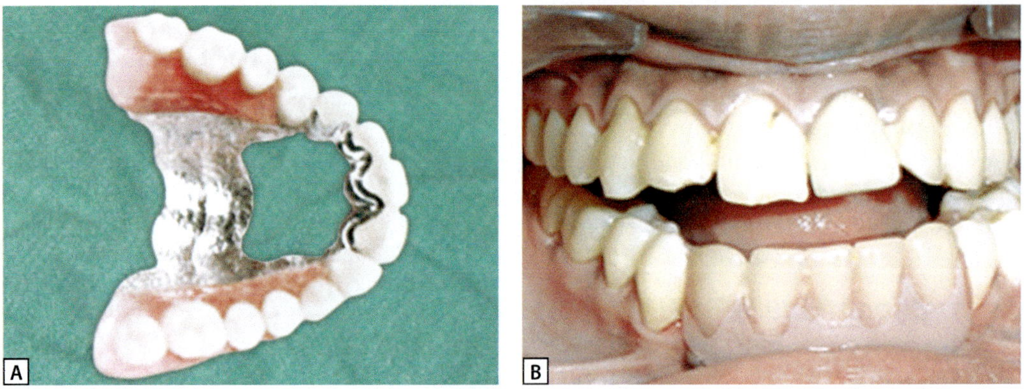

Figures 7.14A and B Dental prosthesis

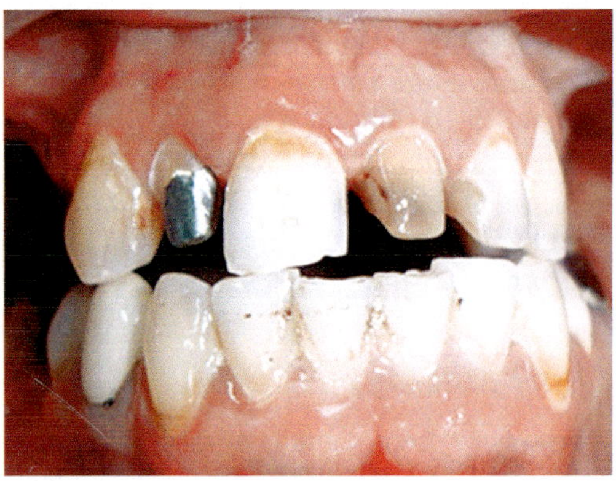

Figure 7.15 Malocclusion

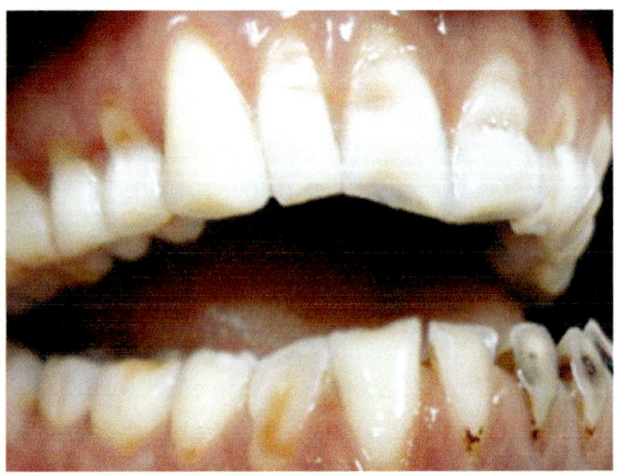

Figure 7.16 Severely attrited teeth

Occupation, Habits and Social Position

The trained dentist can derive a great deal of information from the teeth and mouth with regard to occupation, habits and social position, e.g. severe generalized tooth attrition is common among workers continually exposed to atmospheres containing abrasive dust (**Figure 7.16**). Certain habits may also leave permanent vestiges that may help develop a profile of the individual like chronic pipe smoking or

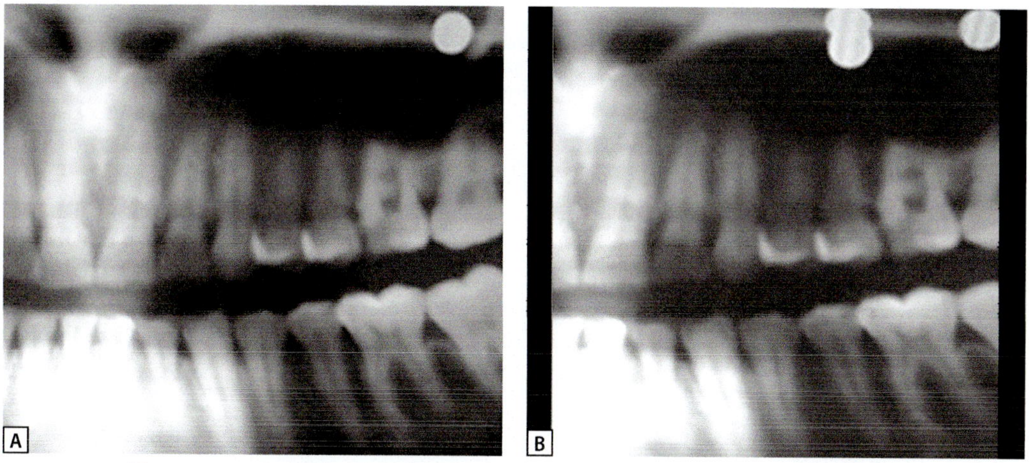

Figures 7.17A and B (A) Antemortem radiograph; (B) Postmortem radiographs

Table 7.5 Comparison between antemortem and postmortem data

Antemortem data	Postmortem data
The dental data like written dental records, dental radiographs, study models, prosthetic appliances and photographs (especially those that shows a prominent anterior teeth)	The postmortem dental data may be recorded by using diagrammatic dental chartings, FDI international type forms, tape recordings, radiographs, photographs and/or models. The most common parameters which have features of specificity and should be included are: Number of teeth, tooth loss, restorations, dental prostheses, dental caries, malposed and rotated teeth, anomalous tooth formation, endodontic treatment, bony pattern, occlusion, oral pathology, unusual wear

longterm bagpipe playing may result in obvious unilateral bimaxillary wear pattern. Notching of the upper incisors has been frequently noted in hair dressers due to their habit of holding the hair pin in their teeth before placing it in a client's hair.

Dental Identification Methods

Dental identification of an individual can be made mainly by two methods namely:

1. Comparative method of dental identification.
2. Postmortem dental profiling.

Comparative Method of Dental Identification

1. The postmortem dental remains can be compared with antemortem dental records to confirm identity.
2. Individuals with numerous and complex dental treatments are often easier to identify than those individuals with little or no restorative treatment.
3. The postmortem record by carefully charted and written descriptions of the dental structures and radiographs are made.
4. This postmortem record is compared with antemortem data, radiographs or any other record (**Table 7.5**).

Radiographs should be marked with a rubber-dam punch to indicate antemortem or postmortem to prevent confusion, one hole for antemortem films and two holes for postmortem X-ray films (**Figure 7.17**).

Postmortem Dental Profiling

The role of the forensic dentist is to narrow down the identification process by giving information about the sex, race, age, socio-economic status, occupation, dietary habits, dental and some systemic diseases as well, by careful examination of the deceased or the left over human remains at the site of disaster.

Table 7.6 Determinant of race from teeth

Race	• Careful examination of the skull and its form and shape		
	• Shovel-shaped incisor		
	• Multi-cusped premolars		
	• Talon's cusp		
	• Taurodonts		
	• Cusp of Carabelli		
Gender	Root length of cuspids — longer in males approximately (3 mm)		
	Dorion's method		
	Y-chromatin and DNA analyses from the microscopic examination of teeth		
	Edges of the teeth		
Occupation or dietary habit	Erosion	Alcohol, substance abuse, working in an industry with use of acids, excessive consumption of carbonated beverages or disorders like anorexia nervosa, other eating disorders like hiatus hernia	
	Stains	Smoking, ingestion of tetracycline, chewing betel nut and smokeless tobacco, dental fluorosis (**Figures 7.18** to **7.20**)	
	Unusual wear pattern		
	• Notching of incisors	Habitual placement of nails between the teeth, opening bobby pins, cutting of threads, placement of pipe stems, cigarette holders, hair pins	
	• Previous orthodontic treatment	Gives information on: i. Dental attitude and awareness of the individual. ii. Quality and quantity of dental treatment (**Figures 7.21** and **7.22**)	Some clues on the socio-economic status
Age	Below 18 years		• Calcification of enamel • Formation of root • Eruption sequence
	Between 18 and 25 years		Assessment of third molars • Crown formation • Root formation • Eruption sequences
	Above 25 years		• Occlusion • Amino acid racemization • Gustafson's method

These characteristics are complemented by various secondary characteristics like features, personal belongings (pocket contents, clothes including any mark, defect, stitching, jewellery, etc.), hair, scars, tattoos, external peculiarities including deformities (whether natural or due to disease, occupational stigmata), race, religion or nationality. The race of the deceased is identified to some extent by the examination of the skull for its shape and form (**Table 7.6**).

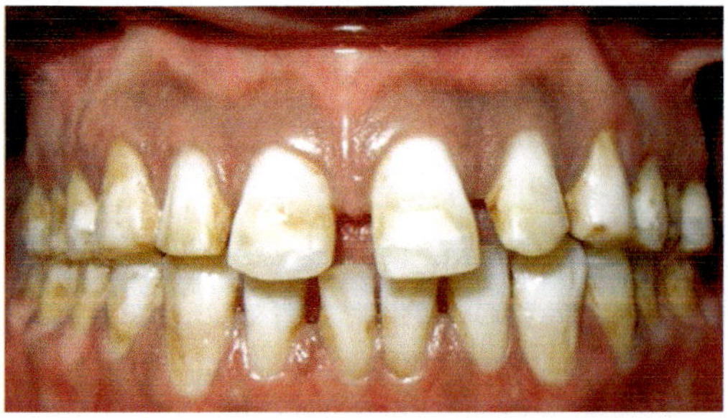

Figure 7.18 Stains on teeth

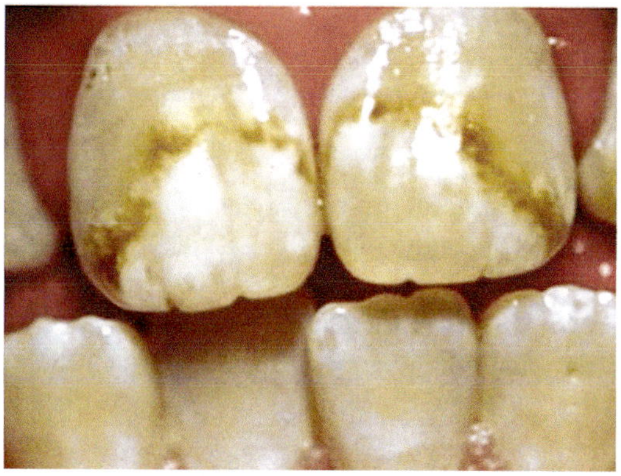

Figure 7.19 Fluorosis stains

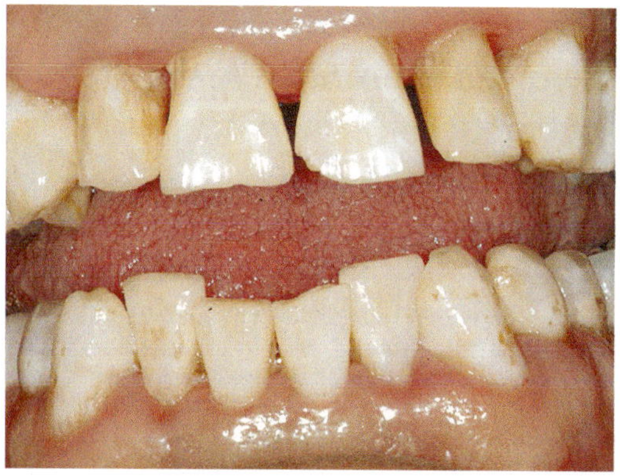

Figure 7.20 Tobacco stains

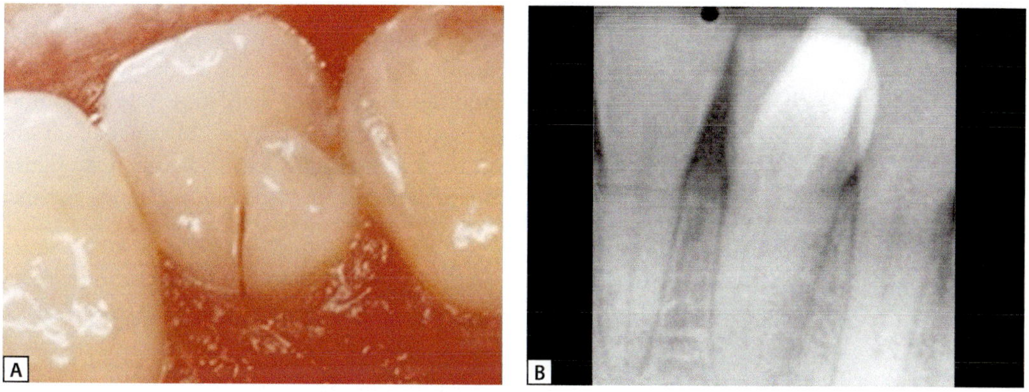

Figures 7.21A and B (A) Talons cusp; (B) Talons cusp X-ray

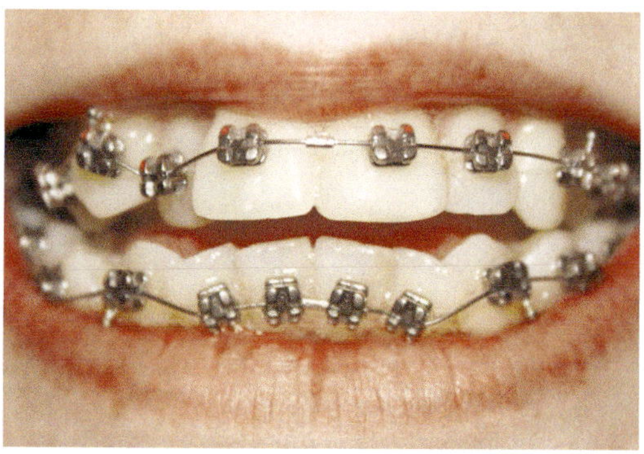

Figure 7.22 Orthodontic brackets

ROLE OF FORENSIC ODONTOLOGIST

Forensic odontology is a specialization within the field of dentistry. Forensic odontologists identify human corpses through their teeth or dental records, if there is no other available method for identifying the body. Forensic odontologists also use teeth marks to identify assailants in court cases or to estimate the age of a deceased party through examining their teeth, and they are usually required to testify in open court about their discoveries.[40]

They are responsible for examining the teeth of corpses and bite marks on bodies. There are four primary roles for a forensic odontologist: consulting services, expert opinions, teaching and research. In absence of obvious ways to identify an unknown person, a forensic odontologist is called. They are responsible for taking a cast or mould of the teeth and jaw from the remains and using this to accurately identify the person according to the dental records. This identity is used to ascertain the next of kin and to initiate the investigation into the cause of death.

Forensic Odontologists are Involved in Six Main Areas of Practice

i. Identification of found human remains.
ii. Identification in mass fatalities.
iii. Assessment of bite mark injuries.
iv. Assessment of cases of abuse (child, spousal, elder).
v. Civil cases involving malpractice.
vi. Age estimation and sex determination.[41]

Identification of Human Remains

Unidentified bodies come to light frequently, having drowned, burned, been murdered, having committed suicide or dead from natural causes. Usually, sufficient evidence is apparent to be able to positively identify the body, but from time to time, this identification will rely on dental evidence. Most accurate will be the charting of the teeth, fillings present to compare with dental records of missing persons, which often leads to a positive identification[23] as shown in **Figure 7.23**.

Methods of Identification

a. Visual identification.
b. Medical records and anthropological methods.
c. Fingerprints analysis.
d. DNA analysis.
e. Craniofacial techniques.

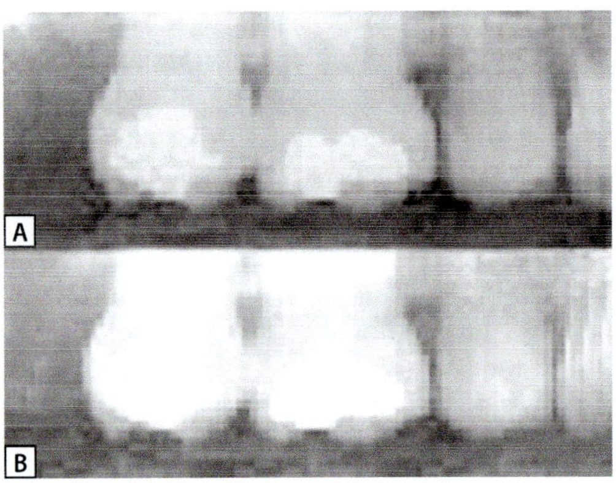

Figures 7.23A and B (A) Antemortem radiograph; (B) Postmortem radiograph

In Mass Fatality Incidences

Dental identification can be confirmed in a case of mass disaster, where identity is a challenge as shown in **Figures 7.24** and **7.25**.

Routine identification tasks are a simple one-to-one matching process. This is not the case in disasters. Mass fatality incidences represent a big challenge to local authorities. Another challenge is the damage inflicted on infrastructure that includes hospitals, transportation, and communications, which impede recovery.[41]

Forensic odontologists have contributed to the resolution of many mass disasters. The 2004 Indian Ocean tsunami is probably the most eminent example on the success of forensic odontologists in identifying large number of victims in short time. Nearly half of the victims in Thailand were identified by dental characteristics method alone, and forensic

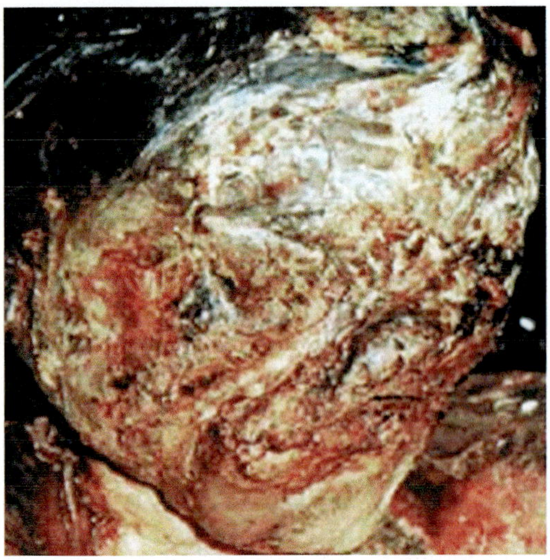

Figure 7.24 Case of mass disaster

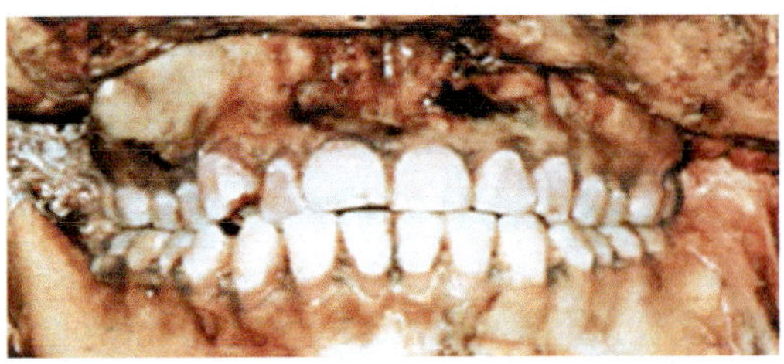

Figure 7.25 Dental identification in mass disaster

odontologists contributed to the identification of the remaining half by assisting the fingerprint, DNA and physical characteristics teams.[23,41]

Bite Mark Analysis

Injuries induced by teeth and left on objects, such as skin, have a distinctive pattern as shown in **Figures 7.26** to **7.28**. Those patterned injuries (bite marks) are useful to judicial authorities because they help in reconstructing past events that surrounded the biting process. For example, bite marks indicate a violent interaction between the perpetrator and the victim, and they might tell us something about the criminal intentions of the perpetrator, whether sexual, child abuse or other forms of assaults.[41]

A representative human bite is described as an elliptical or circular injury that records the specific characteristics of the teeth. Human bite marks are found when teeth are used as weapons of anger, passion, control or destruction.

The injuries caused by teeth can appear as bruises, abrasions, lacerations and even avulsion of the tissue, depending on the intensity and duration of the biting force applied. Skin is elastic and distortable, which makes forensic bite mark analysis complicated; and the human jaw grows and changes over time, which makes teeth marks left by a suspect a few years before, not always easy to match accurately to his/her teeth. However, often, saliva is found on bite marks, which can assist law enforcement with DNA profiles for identification.

Human bite marks are most often found on the skin of victims. Women are most often bitten on the breasts, buttocks and leg during sexual attacks, whereas bites on men are commonly seen on the arms and shoulders. Bite marks generally present as superficial abrasion, and/or sub-surface hemorrhage or bruising of the skin.

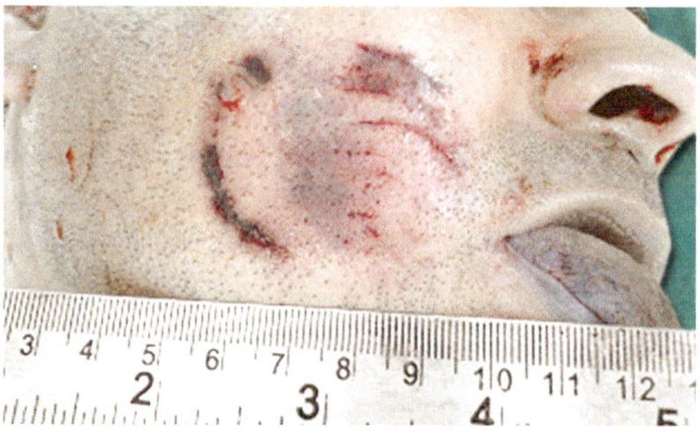

Figure 7.26 Bite mark over cheek
(*Courtesy:* Dr Mrinal Haloi, GMC)

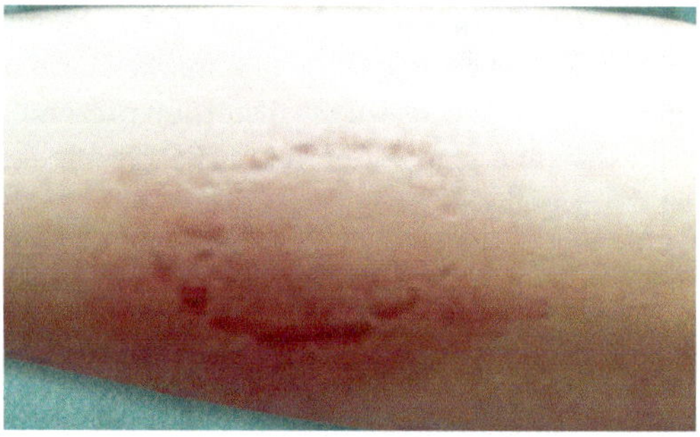

Figure 7.27 Bite mark over human leg

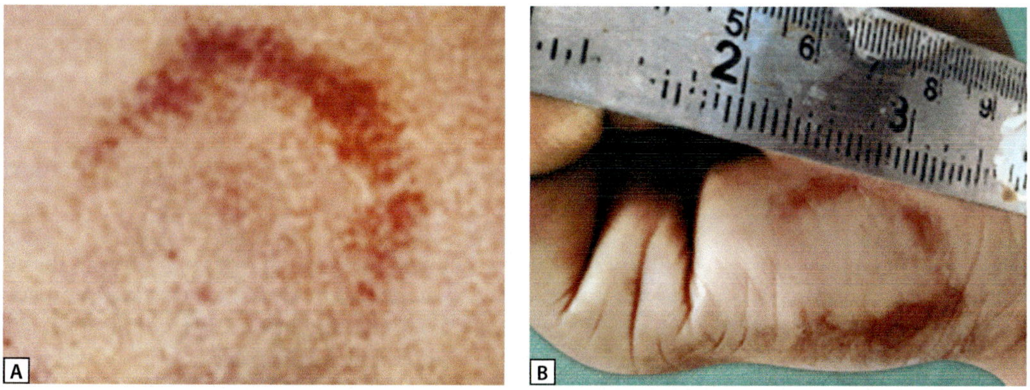

Figures 7.28A and B Bite marks, (A) Over leg; and (B) Palmer aspect of hand

Bite Mark Evidence

Bite-mark pattern may be deposited within foodstuffs, other objects or upon the victim of an assault or homicide. Bite mark analysis, in a forensic investigation, can elucidate the kind of violence and the elapsed time between its production and the examination. Bite mark evidence inflicted by a deceased victim may also be seen on a living assailant. For children, in cases other than those of domestic violence or physical or sexual abuse, biting can represent a form of expression that occurs when verbal communication fails.

Bite marks, in general, are circular, ovoid or horseshoe-shape patches. Moreover, human adult dentition consists of 32 teeth and each one of them has its own size, shape and features. The action of the dental arch on the skin may produce many kinds of lesions, as the dental elements act as incisive instruments. The evidence of a bite mark is usually crucial to establish that two subjects have been involved in a violent contact in a crime scene. The greatest challenge to Forensic Dentistry is the bite marks found in human skin, because of the distortion presented and the time elapsed between the production and the analysis.

Description of Bite Mark

i. A representative human bite is described as an elliptical or circular injury that records the specific characteristics of the teeth.
ii. The injury may be shaped like a doughnut with characteristics recorded around the perimeter of the mark. The injury can be two 'U' shaped arches separated by an open space.
iii. Generally, bite mark consists of superficial abrasion and/or sub-surface hemorrhage or bruising of the skin.[3]
iv. Specific teeth are identified by their class characteristics, i.e. incisors produce rectangular injuries and canines produce triangular injuries.
v. Factors like fracture, rotation, attrition, wear, congenital malformation.

Moreover, bite marks are the only patterned injuries that can indicate (with different levels of certainty) who the biter was. By comparing the locations and measurements of teeth marks, which are matched with the dental cast (**Figures 7.29** and **7.30**) of the suspect(s), forensic odontologists can exclude or include persons suspected of causing the bite marks.

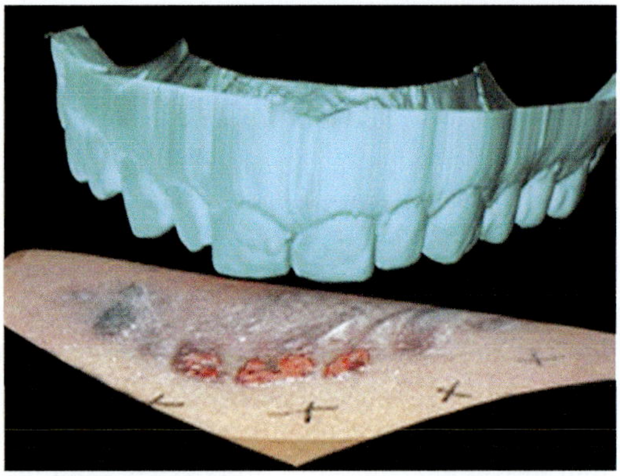

Figure 7.29 Bite marks matched with the dental cast of the suspect

Details of Evidence Collection Techniques

i. Often the bite marks are clear, but at times they are faint or even not visible to the naked eye and are only picked up when the ultraviolet (UV) light detects saliva. A saliva sample can be taken from the bite from which DNA analysis and blood typing can be done.
ii. Then linear scales, one for width and one for height, are placed near the mark and the bite marks or suspected bite marks are photographed.

Principles of Writing: Description of Bite Marks

i. Both in the case of a living victim or deceased individual, the odontologist should determine and record certain vital information.
ii. The demographic detail including name of the examiners should be recorded.
iii. The anatomical location, surface contour (flat, curved or irregular) and tissue characteristics (bone, cartilage, muscle and fat) and the skin (mobile or fixed) should be noted.
iv. The shape of the bite mark should be described.

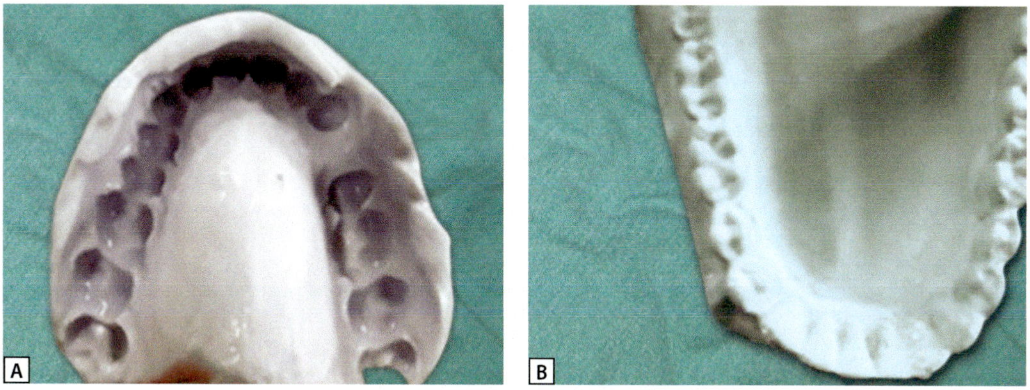

Figures 7.30A and B (A) Dental impression; (B) Dental cast

v. The color should be noted.
vi. Vertical and horizontal dimensions of the bite mark should be noted, preferably in the metric system (**Figure 7.31**).
vii. It should also be noted whether the skin surface is indented or smooth.

The odontologist will evaluate the evidence to determine such things as position of maxillary and mandibular arches, location and position of individual teeth and intradental characteristics.

However, several erroneous bite mark analysis, mainly from the US courts, rendered this type of evidence questionable. The validity of bite mark analysis has undergone decent review in the last 10 years aiming at boosting the scientific weight and improving the technique in a manner that is reproducible. New research is underway to allow digital comparison of teeth and bite marks at a 3-dimensional level. This novel technique is aimed to overcome perspective distortion, a significant morbid factor in bite mark analysis that results from reducing 3-dimensional objects to 2-dimensional images.[41]

Collection of Evidence from Victim

1. The evidence gathering from bite mark victims should be done with authorization from the appropriate authorities.
2. It should first be determined whether the bite mark has been affected by washing, contamination, lividity, embalming, decomposition, change of position, etc.

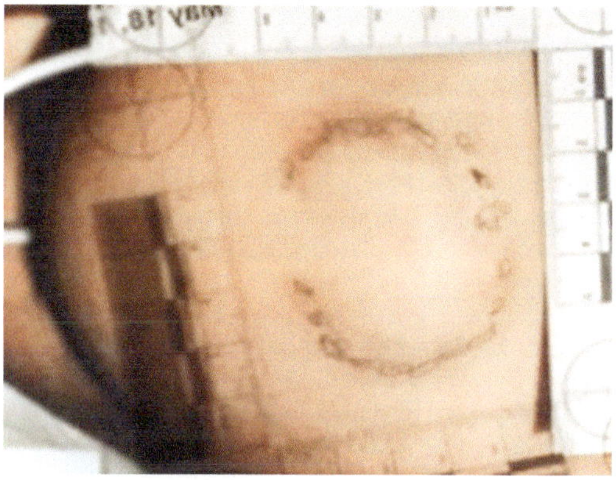

Figure 7.31 Measurement of bite mark

3. Collection of evidence should involve the following steps given in **Table 7.7**.

DOMESTIC VIOLENCE AND CHILD ABUSE

The World Health Organization (WHO) has declared that violence is a major and growing public health problem across the world. This landmark declaration meant that healthcare providers are involved in detecting and managing cases of violence, including abuse to vulnerable populations, i.e. children, elderly and women.[42]

Child abuse is a non-accidental trauma or abuse inflicted on a child by a caretaker that is beyond the acceptable norm of child care. Non-accidental injuries may manifest

Table 7.7 Collection of evidence

Victim	Accused
Photography: A variety of types of photographic equipment and films may be used as described below: • Orientation and close-up photographs should be taken • Photographic resolution should be of high quality • If color film is used, accuracy of color balance should be assured • Photographs of the mark should be taken with and without a scale in place • When the scale is used, it should be on the same plane and adjacent to the bite-mark. It is desirable to include a circular reference in addition to a linear scale • The most critical photographs should be taken in a manner that will eliminate distortion • In the case of a living victim, it may be beneficial to obtain serial photographs of the bite-mark • Whenever possible, salivary trace evidence should be collected according to recommendations of the testing laboratory **Impressions:** Impressions should be taken of the surface of the bite mark whenever it appears that this may provide useful information The impression materials used should meet American Dental Association specifications and should be identified by name in the report	**History:** Obtain history of any dental treatment subsequent to, or in proximity to, the date of bite-marks **Photography:** Whenever possible, good quality extra oral photographs should be taken, both full face and profile. Intraoral photographs preferably would include frontal view, two lateral views, occlusal view of each arch, and any additional photographs that may provide useful information. It is also useful to photograph the maximum interincisal opening with scale in place. If inanimate materials, such as foodstuffs, are used for test bites, the results should be preserved photographically **Extra-oral examination:** (i) The extra-oral examination should include observation and recording of significant soft and hard tissue factors that may influence biting dynamics, such as temporo-mandibular joint status, facial asymmetry, muscle tone and balance. (ii) Measurement of maximal opening of the mouth should be taken, noting any deviations in opening or closing, as well as any significant occlusal disharmonies. (iii) The presence of facial scars or evidence of surgery should be noted, as well as the presence of facial hair **Intraoral examination:** (i) The cases in which saliva evidence has been taken from the victim, saliva evidence should also be taken from the suspect in accordance with the specifications of the testing laboratory. (ii) The tongue should be examined in reference to size and function. Any abnormality such as ankyloglossia should be noted. (iii) The periodontal condition should be observed with particular reference to mobility and areas of inflammation or hypertrophy. (iv) Also, if anterior teeth are missing or badly broken down it should be determined how long these conditions have existed. (v) It is recommended that, when feasible, a dental chart of the suspect's teeth be prepared, in order to encourage thorough study of the dentition
Suitable support should be provided for the impression material to accurately reproduce body contour The material used to produce the case should accurately represent the area of impression and should be prepared according to the manufacturer's instructions **Tissue samples:** Tissue specimens of the bite mark should be retained whenever it appears, this may provide useful information	**Impressions:** Whenever feasible, at least two impressions should be taken of each arch using accepted dental impression techniques. The interocclusal relationship should be recorded **Sample bites:** Whenever feasible, sample bites should be made into an appropriate material, simulating the type of bite under study **Study casts:** (i) Master casts should be prepared using American Dental Association approved Type II stone prepared according to manufacturer's specifications, using accepted dental techniques. (ii) Additional casts may be fabricated in appropriate materials for special studies. When additional models are required, they should be duplicated from master casts using accepted duplication procedures. Labeling should make it clear which master cast was utilized to produce a duplicate. (iii) The teeth and adjacent soft tissue areas of the master casts should not be altered by carving, trimming, marking or other alterations

as cutaneous injury, skeletal trauma or head injury. Measurement of child abuse is inherently difficult since it is rarely seen directly by people outside the immediate family and is often unreported. Child maltreatment happens in all countries and in families of all racial and religious groups.

The WHO further distinguishes four types of violence: physical, sexual, psychological and neglect. All forms of violence can manifest in the oro-facial region and hence should be of concern to dentists. Prevalence of physical violence, as a cause of maxillofacial injuries, ranges from 3.3% to 41% in various countries.[43] This wide range is

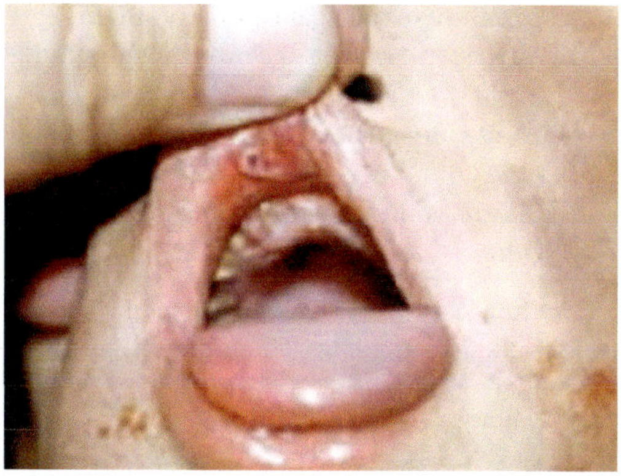

Figure 7.32 Child having lip lacerations depicting abusive injuries

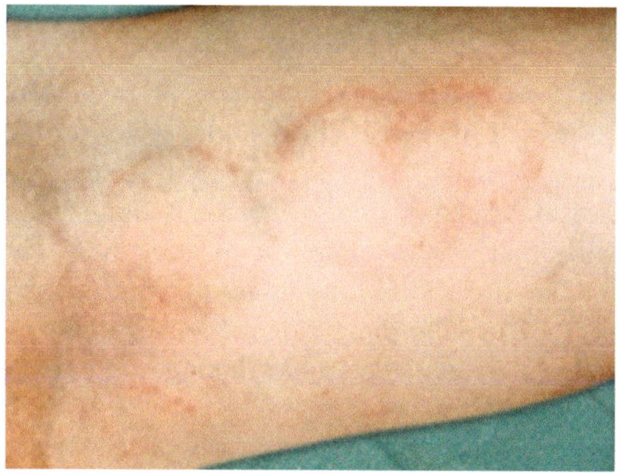

Figure 7.33 Love bite or hickey

Table 7.8 Features of non-accidental (abusive) injuries
• The history of the injury is vague and inconsistent with the clinical findings
• Injuries appear in places away from the bony prominences
• Injuries are inconsistent with the child's age-dependent activities, such as crawling, walking or playing sports
• Unexplainable delay in seeking health care
• Injury occurred in the absence of witness or a sibling is blamed for causing injury
• Evidence of neglect, such as malnutrition, head lice and poor hygiene
• Presence of other injuries or repeated attendance to healthcare facilities with similar complaints
• Injuries appear in groups and of different ages

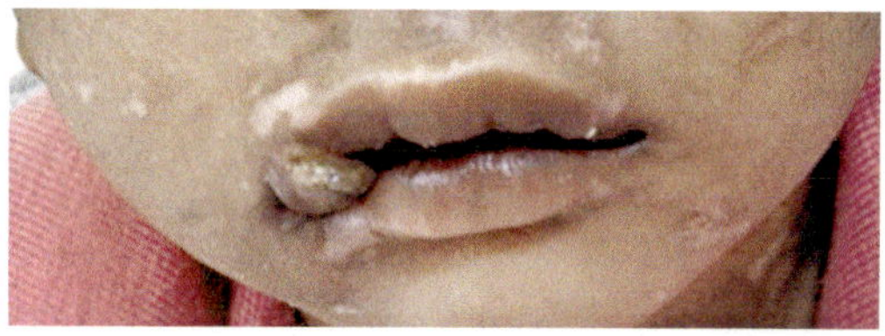

Figure 7.34 Typical case of child abuse: Multiple injuries over oro-facial region of different durations

probably due to different reporting thresholds in different communities. The true prevalence of violence is thus difficult to establish because of not or under-reporting this problem.[44]

Injuries due to abuse can manifest in the oro-facial region in various forms, including fractured anterior teeth, fractured alveolar bone, lacerations of the labial and buccal mucosa, lacerations to the frenum and bruises to the lips, face and neck (**Figure 7.32**).

Non-accidental injuries have certain characteristics, which help in their recognition as shown in **Table 7.8**.

The most common site to be non-accidentally traumatized is the head. Therefore, injuries to the oro-facial region should raise reasonable suspicion to the treating dentist. Suspicion should lead to investigation and reporting, but the reporting must be well thought of. On one hand, there is a necessity to report those cases to authorities. But, on the other hand, reporting false cases is stigmatizing and is an unacceptable interference in the victim's personal affairs.[44]

In various countries, there are laws that govern reporting of violence. Some laws penalize healthcare workers by imprisonment and/or fines for not reporting violence manifested on their patients. However, due to the sensitivity of this matter, reporting has to follow a sound mechanism and be addressed to a proper authority with specifically trained personnel. Readers are advised to search for the proper reporting authority in their respective countries.[45,46]

Forensic odontologists may be called to confirm and identify the signs of abuse (violence) appearing on their patients, which may be a bite marks as shown in **Figures 7.33** and **7.34**, besides others.

CIVIL CASES IN MALPRACTICE

In law, **malpractice** is a type of negligence in which the professional under a duty to act fails to follow generally accepted professional standards, and where breach of duty is the proximate cause of injury to a plaintiff who suffers harm. It is committed by a professional or her/his subordinates or agents on behalf of a client or patient that causes damage to the client or patient.[47]

The health professionals have been viewed as providers of service for consideration. The Consumer Protection Act (CPA) was enacted in 1986 for better protection of the consumers as well as to provide quick redressing consumer grievances. Since 1995, health professionals have been included in this act, empowering patients to file lawsuits. Professional negligence in dental practice is liable in the court for civil or criminal negligence and to pay compensation.[1]

AGE AND SEX DETERMINATION

The estimation of age at time of death is often an important step in the identification of human remains. If this age can be accurately estimated, it will significantly narrow the field of possible identities that will have to be compared to the remains in order to establish a positive identification. Some of the more accurate methods of age estimation, in the juvenile and younger adult, have been based on the assessment of the degree of dental development as it relates to chronological age. Details of age estimation using teeth are discussed in the chapter of identification.

Sex determination from teeth can be done from anatomical landmarks using tooth dimensions and by nuclear sexing from DNA sample like dental pulp, etc.

ORGANIZATIONS IN THE FIELD OF FORENSIC ODONTOLOGY

Four organizations are dedicated to the field of forensic odontology in the USA. They are:

a. The Bureau of Legal Dentistry (**BOLD**).
b. American Society of Forensic Odontology (**ASFO**).
c. The American Board of Forensic Odontology (**ABFO**).
d. International Organization for Forensic Odonto-stomatology (**IOFOS**).

Other countries have their own forensic odontological societies, including the British Association for Forensic Odontology (**BAFO**) and the Australian Society of Forensic Odontology (**AuSFO**). In 1996, BOLD was created at the University of British Columbia to develop new technology and techniques in forensic odontology. The University of British Columbia program is the only one in North America that provides graduate training in forensic odontology. This organization also supports the creation of a database of dental records, which could help in verifying dental uniqueness. This database could be created using criminal records or possibly all dental patients.

The Bureau of Legal Dentistry encourages the use of multiple dental impressions to create a "dental line-up", similar to a suspect line-up used to identify alleged perpetrators of crime. Currently, dental impressions collected as evidence are compared only to those collected from a given suspect, which may bias the resulting outcome. Using multiple dental impressions in a line-up may enable forensic odontologists to significantly decrease the current bias in matching bite marks to the teeth of a suspect.

RECENT ADVANCES IN FORENSIC ODONTOLOGY

In some instances, more novel and innovative techniques have been applied. For instance, denture labeling, dental profiling, DNA identification, digital forensics in dentistry and identification of latent lip prints.

Denture Labeling

There has been number of requests from individuals and dental organizations over the years to insist that dental prostheses are labeled with the patient's name or a unique number as shown in **Figure 7.35**.

The National Health Service (NHS) provides a fee for dentists who label their patient's dentures, although this is often only used in instances where the wearer is a resident in a care home.[48]

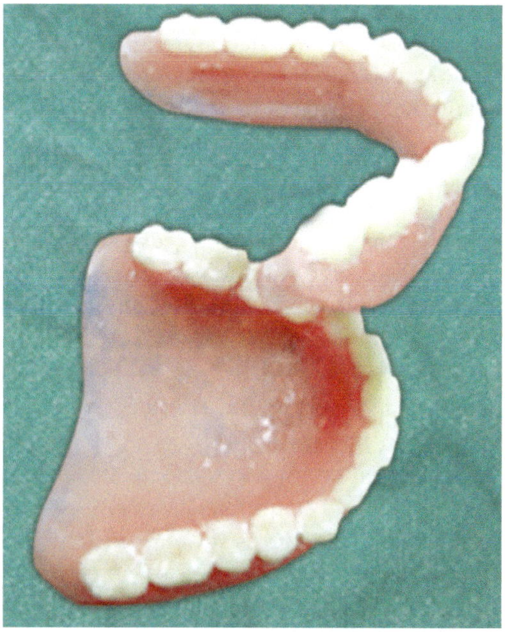

Figure 7.35 Labeled dentures

Dental Profiling

When the dental records are unavailable and other methods of identification are not possible, the forensic dentist can often produce a "picture" of the general features of the individual. A dental profile will typically provide information on the deceased age, ancestry background, sex and socioeconomic status, in some instances additional information regarding occupation, dietary habits and habitual behaviors and occasionally on dental and systemic diseases.

The use of reconstructive postmortem dental profiling may be helpful in giving the odontologists clues to the profile of the deceased and can narrow the search parameters for investigators. In collaboration with forensic anthropologists, forensic odontologists can help to determine the race (Caucasoid, Mongoloid and Negroid) and sex of the deceased using indicators like skull make up and the presence of a Y chromosome.[49] By studying characteristics like tooth development, corrosion and stains present on tooth artefacts, factors like alcohol use, substance abuse, smoking habits and age can be determined or approximated.[50]

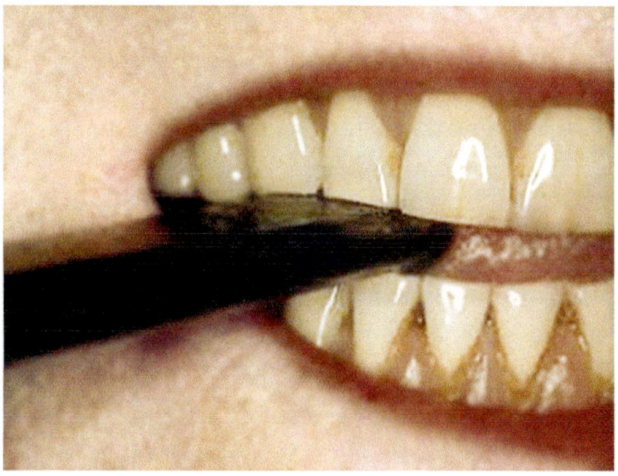

Figure 7.36 Case of dental profiling

Figure 7.36 shows the tooth wear associated with pipe smoking. Individuals found with wear of this sort are likely to have smoked a pipe, and this information could be useful to the police in narrowing the search for antemortem records.[51]

DNA Identification

Dental structures are relatively more resistant to higher temperatures. Techniques involving DNA in forensic dentistry offers a new tool when traditional identification methods fail due to the effects of heat, traumatism or autolytic processes, as well as in distortions and difficulties in analysis. They can provide a source of DNA for easy identification. Due to this abundance of material, the use of the technique based on polymerized chain reaction (PCR) has acquired great importance in DNA postmortem analysis in forensic cases. PCR is an enzymatic amplification of a specific DNA, aiming millions of copies production from this sequence in a test tube (first described by Kary Mullis, in late 1980's) and enabling a new strategy of gene analysis through a simple and fast method, excusing all the laborious stages of genic cloning. It is necessary to broaden the pertinent studies to establish protocols to allow additional tools in criminal investigation.[52]

Digital Forensics

With advanced technology, computers have taken a leap into the forensic world and the digital revolution has impacted all aspects of forensic odontology. The digital forensic process encompasses the seizure, forensic imaging and analysis of digital media and the production of a report into collected evidence of a crime. This also can be used to attribute evidence to specific suspects, confirm statements, determine intent, identify sources or authenticate the documents.[53]

Digital forensics involves several sub-branches, such as computer forensics, mobile device forensics, network forensics and database forensics, and is related to the investigation of various types of devices, media or artefacts. Digital forensics is a maturing science that needs to be continuously held to higher standards.

Latent Lip Prints

The last few decades have seen the development of the exaggerated importance of lip prints as another skin impression. Cheiloscopy deals with the examination of system of furrows on the red part of human lips and is an important tool in forensic science. Traditional lipstick produces a print that is easily identifiable. However, lip prints made without lipstick is invisible, known as latent lip prints, requiring reagents that are more sensitive than conventional materials to locate and develop the invisible prints. There are unusual techniques of cheiloscopy used in detection and development of latent lip prints that aids in identification of suspects in criminal offences, sex determination and person identification.[2]

LIMITATIONS

Forensic odontology has played a key role in identification of persons in mass disasters (aviation, earthquakes, tsunamis), in crime investigations, in ethnic studies and victims of motor vehicle accidents. All the methods described above have some or the other shortcomings. The discrepancies associated with them are to be weighed cautiously to make forensic odontology a more accurate, reliable and reproducible investigatory science. As dental features change over time, changes can occur after obtaining antemortem records. Extraction, trauma, exfoliation, periodontal disease, caries and prosthesis work can change the configuration of teeth.

The judges and the jury usually do not have enough knowledge to assess the scientific merit of the new methods and must rely on experts within the approved judicial guidelines. Errors may develop in sample collection, processing and interpretation. Though forensic odontology has achieved giant strides in recent times, various techniques that have been utilized are abided by limitations, and this should be kept in mind while prosecuting the accused and answering queries in the court of law.[54]

Forensic dentistry is the overlap of the dental and legal professions. The most common element of forensic dentistry that a general practitioner is likely to encounter is to supply antemortem (before death) records to aid in personal identification. The identification is normally carried out by the comparison of the antemortem and postmortem records. The identification of the deceased individual is an essential element in the process of death certification and is a crucial component in the investigation of homicides or other suspicious deaths.

DIAGNOSIS OF POISONINGS

The appearance of colored lines on the teeth and gum due to certain chronic poisoning give the clue of a poison as shown in **Table 7.9**.

Table 7.9 Colored line on teeth and gum following chronic toxicity

Poisonous substances	Diagnosis
Lead	Blue line along the gum, with bluish black edging in the teeth
Mercury	Gray line on the gums
Copper	Green line on the gums
Cadmium	Yellow line on the gums
Bismuth	Black line on the gums
Arsenic	Detected on chemical analysis (as it is deposited in teeth enamel)
Phosphorus poisoning	Phossy jaw
Repeated tetracycline injection in child	Dirty yellow coloration of the teeth

REFERENCES

1. Acharya AB, Savitha JK, Suresh VN. Professional negligence in dental practice: Potential for civil and criminal liability in India. J Forensic Dental Sci. 2009;1(1):2-7.
2. Sharma P, Saxena S, Rathod V. Cheiloscopy: The study of lip prints in sex identification. J Forensic Dental Sci. 2009;1(1):24-7.
3. Keiser-Neilsen S. Person Identification by Means of Teeth. John Wright and Sons, Bristol, 1980.
4. Edward EH. Forensic Dentistry: Oral and Maxillofacial Pathology, 2nd ed. Elsevier; 2005. p. 763.
5. Bagi BS. Role of forensic odontology in medicine. J Indian Dental Assoc. 1977;49:359-63.
6. Luntz LL. History of forensic dentistry. Dent Clin N Am. 1977;7:21.
7. Cottone JA, Standish SM. Outline of Forensic Dentistry. Yearbook Medical Publishers, Chicago, 1982.
8. Swanson HA. Forensic dentistry. J Am Coll Dent. 1967;34:174.
9. Harvey W. Dental Identification and Forensic Odontology. Henry Kimpton Publishers, London, 1976.
10. Miles AEW. Dentition in the estimation of age. J Dent Res. 1963;42:255.
11. Luntz LL, Luntz P. Handbook for Dental Identification: Techniques in Forensic Dentistry. JB Lippincott, Philadelphia, 1973.
12. Bernstein M. Forensic odontology. In: Eckert WG (Ed). Introduction to Forensic Sciences. 2nd ed. Boca Raton, FL:CRS Press; 1997. pp. 304-51.
13. History behind Forensic odontology. [cited 2013 Feb 10; Available from: URL:http://www.biology-online.org/articles/forensic-odontology/history-behind-forensic-odontology.html
14. History behind Forensic Odontology. [cited 2013 Feb 10; Available from: URL:http://www.ehow.com/about_6526606_history-forensic-dentistry.html
15. Gustafson G. Forensic Odontology, American Elsevier, Inc., New York, 1966.
16. Devore DT. Radiology and photography in forensic dentistry. Dent Clin North Am. 1977;21:69-84.
17. Barsley RE. Forensic and legal issues in oral diagnosis. Dent Clin North Am. 1993;37:133-56.
18. Dayal PK. Textbook of Forensic Odontology. 1st ed. Paras Medical Publisher; 1998.
19. Budimlija ZM, Prinz MK, Zelson-Mundorff A, Wiersema J, Bartelink E, MacKinnon G, et al. World trade centre human identification project: Experiences with individual body identification cases. Croatian Med J. 2003;44(3):259-63.
20. Sweet D, Dizinno JA. Personal identification through dental evidence— tooth fragments to DNA. J Calif Dent Assoc. 1996;24:35-42.
21. Lawney M. For the record: Understanding patient record keeping. N Y State Dent J. 1998;64:34-43.
22. Charangowda BK. Dental records: An overview. J Forensic Dental Sci. 2010;2(1):5-10.
23. Sobel MN. Forensic Odontology, 2012 Feb [cited 2012 Jun 25]; Available from: URL:http://www.forensicdentistryonline.com
24. Collins D. What a dentist should know oral health record. Northwest Dent. 1996;75:35-9.

25. ADA Principles of Ethics and code of professional conduct, council on ethics, Bylaws and judicial affairs, American Dental Association [cited on 28 July 2012]; Available from: URL:http://www.ada.org
26. Platt M, Yewe-Dyer M. How accurate is your charting? Dent Update. 1995;22:374.
27. American Board of Forensic Odontology. Body identification guidelines. J Am Dent Assoc. 1994;125: 1244-54.
28. Nelson GV. Guidelines to the prevention of problems in record-keeping. Part 1. Pediatr Dent. 1989;11: 174-7.
29. Chandrashekhar BR, Reddy CVK. Role of dentist in person identification. Indian J Dent Res. 2009;20(3): 356-60.
30. Metzger Z, Buchner A, Gorsky M. Gustafson's method for age determination from teeth- a modification for the use of dentists in identification terms. J Forensic Sci. 1980;25(4):742-9.
31. Pillay VV. The deductive art of Sherlock Holmes. Police professional. 1988;27:19-22.
32. Reddy V. (Ed). Dental Anthropology-Application and Methods, Inter India Publication. 1985. pp. 368-9.
33. Backofen UW, Gampe J, Vaupel JW. Tooth cementum annulations for age estimation: results from a large known age validation study. Am J Phys Anthropol. 2004;123:119-29.
34. Solheim T. Dental cementum apposition as an indicator of age. Scand J Dent Res. 1990; 98:510-9.
35. Stott GG, Sis RF, Levy BM. Cementum annulations as an age criterion in forensic dentistry. J Dent Res. 1982;61:814-7.
36. Bosmans N, Ann P, Aly M, Williams G. The application of Kvaal's dental age calculation technique on panoramic dental radiographs. Forensic Sci Int. 2005;153:208-12.
37. Kvaal SI, Kolltveit KM, Thomsen IO, Solheim T. Age estimation of adults from dental radiographs. Forensic Sci Int. 1995;74:175-85.
38. Cameriere R, Ferrante L, Cingolani M. Variations in pulp/tooth area ratio as an indicator of age: A preliminary study. J Forensic Sci. 2004;49:317-9.
39. Neville Damm. Oral and Maxillofacial Pathology: Forensic Dentistry,2nd ed. 2005. pp. 763-82.
40. Forensic Odontologist Requirements 15 Oct. 2012, Available from: URL:http//:www.ehow.com/list_6028160_forensic-odontologist-requirements.html
41. Suhail Hani Al-Amad. Forensic dentistry. Smile dental J. 2009;4(1):22-4.
42. Borrman HI, Dizinno JA, Wasen J, Rene N. On denture marking. J Forensic Odontostomatol. 1999;17:20-6.
43. Marella GL, Rossi P. An approach to identification by means of dental prostheses in a burnt corpse. J Forensic Odontostomatol. 1999;17:16-9.
44. Whittaker DK. A Colour Atlas of Forensic Dentistry. Saint-Louis: Harcourt; 1989.
45. Schwartz TR, Schwartz EA, Mieszerski L, McNally L, Kobilinsky L. Characterization of deoxyribonucleic acid (DNA) obtained from teeth subjected to various environmental conditions. J Forensic Sci. 1991;36: 979-90.
46. Sweet D, Hildebrand D. Recovery of DNA from human teeth by cryogenic grinding. J Forensic Sci. 1998;43:1199-202.
47. Dental malpractice, [cited on 30 June 2012]; Available from: URL:http://www.en.wikipedia.org/wiki/employee
48. Hutchison CA, Newbold JE, Potter SS, Edgell MH. Maternal inheritance of mammalian mitochondrial DNA. Nature. 1980;251:536-8.
49. Sweet D, DiZinno JA. Personal identification through dental evidence-tooth fragments to DNA. J Calif Dent Assoc. 1996;24:35-42.
50. Whittaker DK, Rawle LW. The effect of conditions of putrefaction on species determination in human and animal teeth. Forensic Sci Int. 1987;35:209-12.
51. Pretty IA, Addy LD. Associated post-mortem dental findings as an aid to personal identification. Sci Justice. 2002;22(2):1-10.
52. Potsch L, Meyer U, Rothschild S, Schneider PM, Rittner C. Application of DNA techniques for identification using human dental pulp as source of DNA. Int J Leg Med. 1992;105:139-43.
53. Digital Forensics. [cited on Feb 2013]; Available from: URL:http://www.digitalforensics/wikipedia.com
54. Kavita B, Einstein A, Sivapathasundaram B. Limitations in forensic odontology. J Forensic Dental Sci. 2009;1(1):8-10.

CHAPTER 8

Forensic DNA Typing

Imran Sabri, Putul Mahanta

LEARNING PLAN

- Know the definition and related issues about DNA
- Learn the methods of DNA typing
- Solving criminal and civil cases with the help of DNA
- Understand the ways of collection and preservation of DNA samples
- Know the uses of DNA typing in medicolegal practice

Synonyms: DNA analysis, DNA profiling, DNA studies, genetic typing, DNA testing, genetic fingerprinting, genetic profile.

> DNA fingerprinting is the technique applied to prepare a profile of an individual containing Deoxyribo-Nucleic Acid (DNA) in their cell nucleus. More specifically, this technique is applied to human beings, although DNA fingerprinting is also done in bacteria, fungus, plants, etc. In this chapter, we are focusing with only human DNA fingerprinting.

In simpler terms, DNA fingerprinting means "**taking photograph** or **auto-radiograph of DNA**", which is very similar to that of taking photograph of human being; but since DNA is a very small molecule, we need some sophisticated technique to do so: that is DNA fingerprinting. The photograph or auto-radiograph is taken in ultraviolet light with specific DNA sequence emitting radioactive waves by a radioactive dye (ethidium bromide, etc.). The photograph so produced is in the form of light and dark band and sequence of bands will tell us about the genetic makeup of a particular repeated sequence.

DNA fingerprinting is a technique employed to assist in the identification of individuals by their respective DNA profiles. DNA profiling technique was first reported in 1985 by Professor **Alec Jeffreys** at the University of Leicester in England (**Figure 8.1**).

INTRODUCTION TO DNA

Deoxyribo-Nucleic acid (DNA) is a long chain of base pairs, adenine, thiamine, cytosine and guanine, usually represented by A, T, C and G, respectively. Two chains of base pairs join

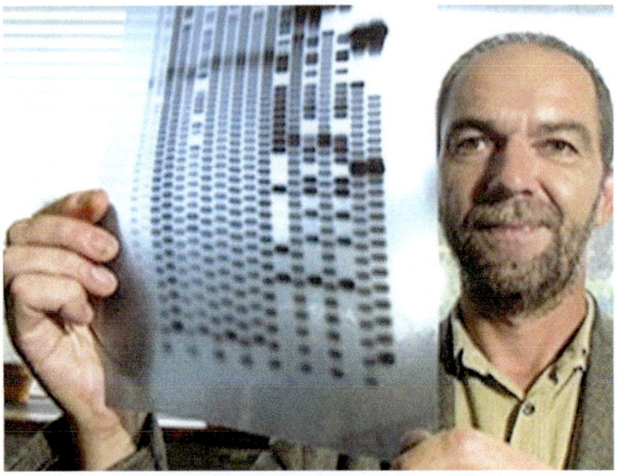

Figure 8.1 Professor Alec Jeffreys, DNA fingerprinting pioneer

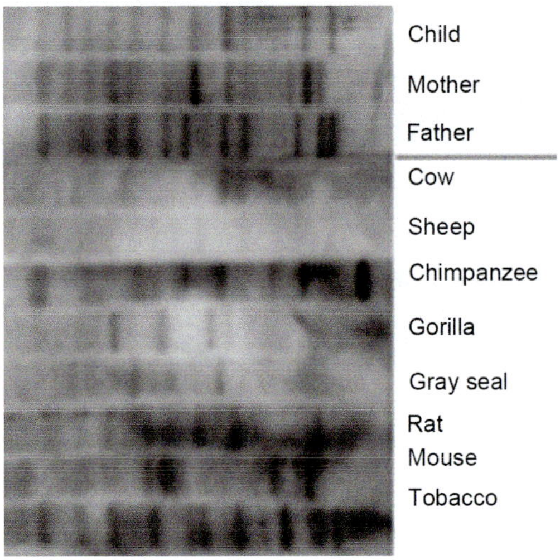

Figure 8.2 First DNA fingerprints
(*Courtesy:* Professor Sir Alec Jeffreys)

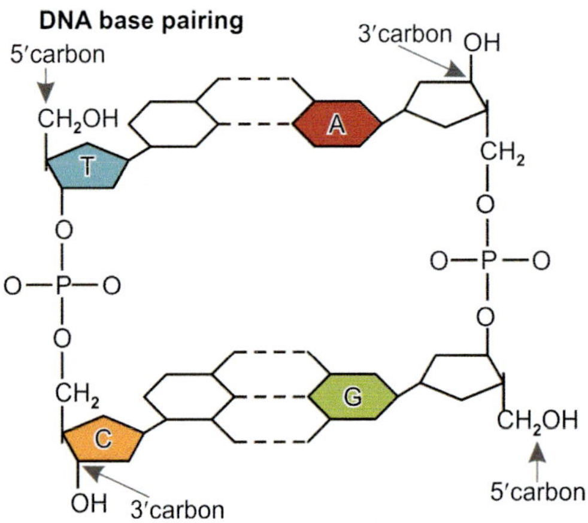

Figure 8.3 DNA structure: Adenine paired thiamine while cytosine bonded with guanine

with each other in a reverse pattern to form complete DNA molecule. These double helical chains are attached on histone protein to form a chromosome responsible for the characteristic features in living organism. Gene is a small portion of this DNA, responsible for a particular character or trait or is responsible to code for a particular protein. Adenine and thiamine connect with each other by two bonds, while cytosine and guanine bonded with each other with three bonds.

Although 99.9% of human DNA sequences are the same in every person, enough of the DNA is different to distinguish one individual from another. The very first DNA fingerprint by Professor Alec Jeffreys is shown in **Figure 8.2**.

Base Pair Sequence in DNA (Figure 8.3)

A-C-C-T-G-A-T-A-G-G-T-C-T-A-A

The opposite base pair strands will be

T-G-G-A-C-T-A-T-C-C-A-G-A-T-T

DNA strands are read in a particular direction from the top to bottom (5′ or "five prime" end to 3′ or "three prime" end) as seen below:

5′ A-C-C-T-G-A-T-A-G-G-T-C-T-A-A 3′
3′ T-G-G-A-C-T-A-T-C-C-A-G-A-T-T 5′

The chemical structure of DNA is the same for all organisms containing DNA. The difference between organisms is the sequence of the base pairs.

Constituents of DNA

i. Phosphates.
ii. Deoxyribose sugar.
iii. Organic nitrogenous base: Adenine, thymine, guanine, cytosine.
iv. Single DNA molecules consist of 50–500 million base pairs.

Chromosome: It is a rod-like structure of tightly coiled DNA on histone proteins, found in the cell nucleus of plants and animals. In human beings, there are 23 pairs of chromosomes. Out of these, 22 pairs are common in both male and female. The 23rd pair is different for both sexes and is responsible for determination of the sex of an individual.

Restriction Enzyme: An enzyme, which cuts DNA at specific sites always acts upon DNA in the same manner.

Procedure included for DNA fingerprinting is:

i. Take biological sample as per protocol.
ii. Extract whole DNA by standard method.
iii. Cut DNA in small pieces with the help of restriction enzymes.
iv. Mix DNA sample with radioactive dye like ethidium bromide.
v. Load sample in well of gel documentation.
vi. Run samples on gel documentation system under influence of voltage (**Figure 8.4**).
Vii. Take photograph/autograph at different time and voltage.

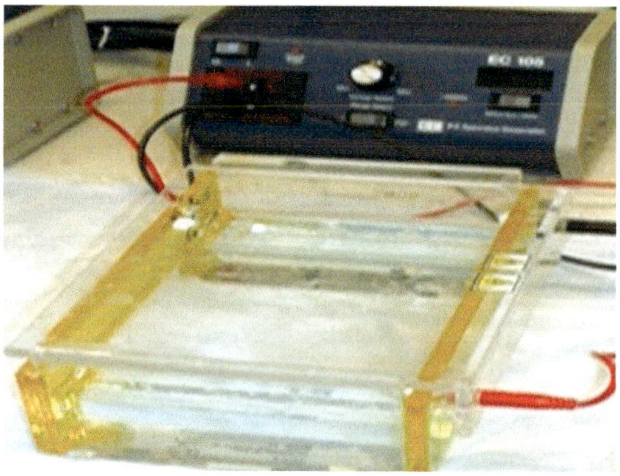

Figure 8.4 Gel documentation

Methods of DNA Fingerprinting for Forensic Purpose

Methods Applied in DNA Fingerprinting

I. **Restriction Fragments Length Polymorphism (RFLP) Method**

In this method, biological samples like blood, semen, tissues, muscles, bones, are collected and DNA is extracted with the help of standard phenol-chloroform method or with the help of commercially available DNA extraction kits. The extracted DNA is mixed with restriction enzymes which breaks the DNA into smaller pieces. The fragmented DNA is run on gel electrophoresis under the influence of electric field. The smaller fragments move faster compared with large fragments (**Figure 8.5**).

The distribution of DNA band pattern is transferred to a nylon sheet by placing the sheet on the gel and soaking them overnight by a technique known as Southern blotting. A radioactive DNA probe is prepared which binds with specific DNA sequences to produce a fluorescent image. It is known as hybridization. Hybridized probe fragments are visualized by auto-radiography. The bands on the X-ray film appears corresponding to hybridized fragments. This is DNA fingerprint.

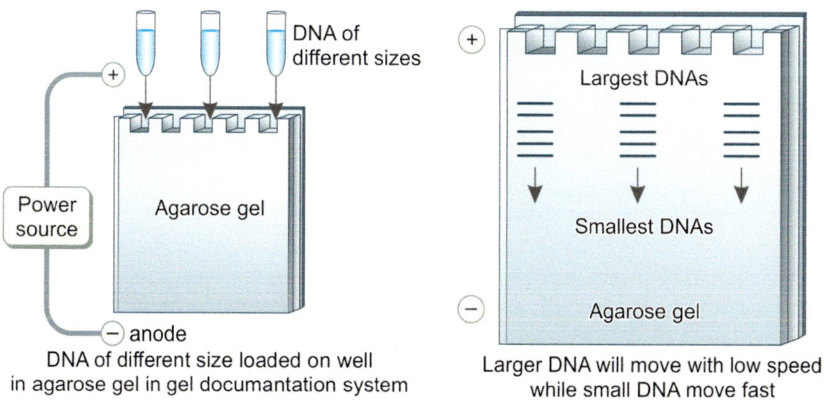

Figure 8.5 DNA extractions from sample

ii. **Variable Number Tandem Repeat and Short Tandem Repeat**

Variable number tandem repeats (VNTRs) represent specific locations on a chromosome in which tandem repeats of 9-80 or more bases repeat a different number of times between individuals. These regions of DNA are readily analyzed using the RFLP approach and a probe specific to a VNTR locus. The fragments are a little shorter than RFLPs (about 1-2 kilo base pairs), but are created through the exact same process. Unlike VNTRs, which analyze minisatellites that have repeat sequences of 9-80 base pairs, short tandem repeats (STRs) use microsatellites which have repeat sequences of only 2-5 base pairs—introducing the "less is more" philosophy to the world of DNA fingerprinting. This was a big step forward in forensic science since the length of DNA fragment being analyzed is short enough to be amplified by polymerase chain reaction.

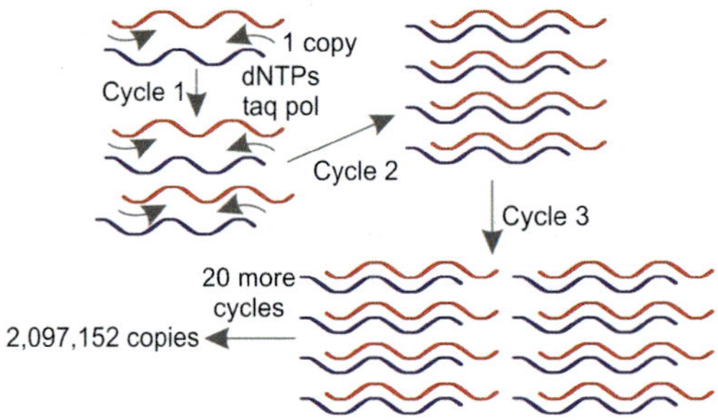

Figure 8.6 Cycles of amplification in polymerase chain reaction

iii. **Polymerase Chain Reaction (PCR) (Figures 8.6 and 8.7)**

PCR is done when the amount of recoverable DNA is small. The smaller amount of DNA is amplified with this process. It is like doing photocopy of a small DNA fragments. In this method, the two strands of DNA are separated and allowed to regrow their own fragment under controlled temperature and availability of raw material (oligonucleotide primers, deoxynucleotide) and catalysts (magnesium chloride).

Factors that Influence the Applicability of DNA Technique

i. Non-human DNA sample.
ii. Decomposition or degradation of DNA sample.
iii. Mix-up of many samples.
iv. Multiple contributors to the sample.

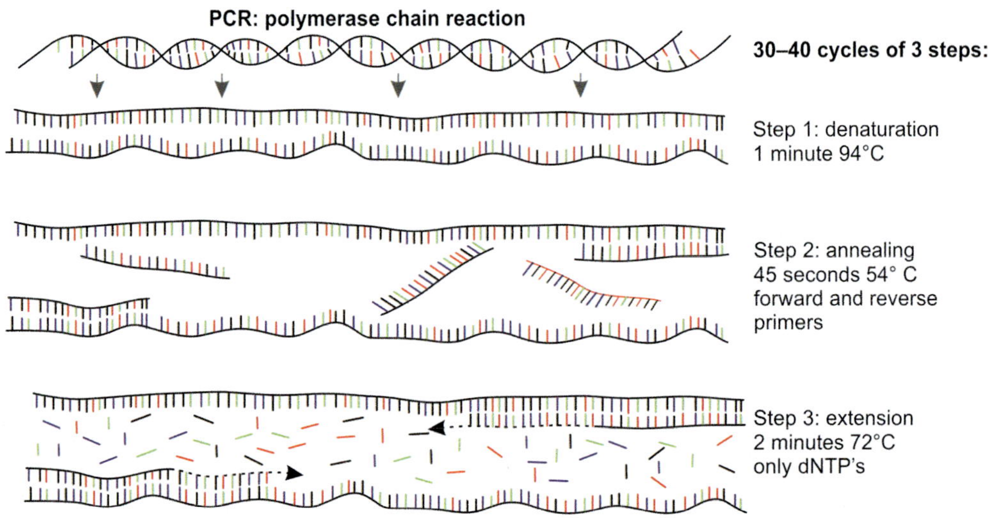

Figure 8.7 Steps of polymerase chain reaction like denaturation, annealing and extension

Collection of Samples for DNA Extraction

Blood

i. **Whole Liquid Blood:** About 5 mL of whole liquid blood is taken in EDTA vial (in elective live cases, collection of blood in EDTA vial is a must).
ii. **Blood Clot:** Whole blood clot is taken if size is small.
iii. **Wet Blood Stains:** Blood is taken on sterile cotton swab and air dried and then sent to laboratory in zip-locked polybags.
iv. **Dried Blood Stains:** Whole dried blood is sealed in zip-locked polybags.

Other Biological Samples

i. Dried seminal stain similarly as blood.
ii. Wet seminal stains are taken in a test tube.
iii. Hair root is taken for DNA sampling.
iv. Saliva and salivary stains taken in glass tube.
v. Body tissue cells: taken in clean sterile container.
vi. Fingernail scraping taken in polybags.
vii. Postmortem samples like muscle, spleen, bone marrow, organs, and vascular pulp of tooth are taken in clean sterile plastic tube without any preservative. If delay is there, then freeze at -20°C.

USES OF DNA TYPING IN FORENSIC INVESTIGATION

The applications of DNA profiling in various forensic investigations are shown in **Table 8.1**.

Paternity Disputes

i. The VNTR patterns can be used to establish paternity and maternity. The patterns are so specific that a parental VNTR pattern can be reconstructed even if only the children's VNTR patterns are known.
ii. Parent-child VNTR pattern analysis has been used to solve standard father-identification cases as well as more complicated cases of confirming legal nationality and, in instances of adoption, biological parenthood.

In **Figure 8.8**, D1 bands matches with mom and dad hence true parents. D2 bands matches only with mom means D2 have separate father. S1 bands matches with both mom and dad hence real parents. S2 do not match with either mom or dad hence both are not real parent of S2 (may be adopted son).

Usefulness of DNA Profiling

The advantage and disadvantages of DNA profiling are mentioned in **Table 8.2**.

Table 8.1 Various application of DNA profiling

Identification	Parenthood	Others Uses
• Mass disaster including several casualties which need to be identified as separate entity • Bomb blast cases in which all sort of samples are recovered • Fragment remains which may be accidentally recovered • Unidentified bodies or mutilated remains • Mass casualties: Train, road and air accidents • Doubtful identification cases • Missing soldiers • Missing foreigners or travelers • Wildlife identification • Exhumation cases	• Disputed maternity and paternity • Exchange of child in hospitals • Exchange of child in early stage • Finding missing child after long time • Transfer of property cases • Citizenship disputes • Rape cases	• Diagnosis of inherited disorders • Biological relationship for transplant • Detection of bacteria and other organisms • Hit and run cases of road traffic accidents • Disputed diagnosis in case of histopathological examination on doubtful cases relating to patient with particular sample

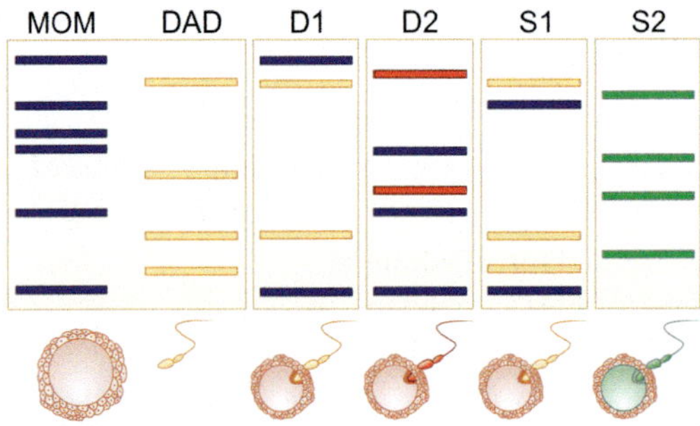

Figure 8.8 Pattern of DNA bands to solve paternity or maternity disputes

Abbreviations: MOM= Mother, DAD= Father, D1= First daughter, D2= Second daughter, S1= First son, S2= Second son

Explanation: D1: Two bands match [blue color] with MOM and two bands match with DAD [yellow color]. Result D1 belongs to MOM and DAD as real mother and father.

D2: Three bands match with MOM [blue color]. Two band did not match with DAD [red color]. MOM is mother of D2 but DAD is not father of D2.

S1: Three bands match with DAD [yellow color]. Two band did not match with MOM [blue color]. Result S1 belongs to MOM and DAD as real mother and father.

S2: No band mathes with MOM and DAD. S2 belongs to different parents or MOM and DAD are not real mother and Father of S2 (may be adopted son).

Table 8.2 Usefulness of DNA profiling

Advantages	Disadvantages
• DNA is very stable molecule, can sustain in adverse conditions • Small Quantity of sample is needed • Reliable technique • Permanent record can be kept • Easy availability of DNA samples • Repetition of same results with same or different samples • Lack of awareness or knowledge by the Criminal	• Identical twins: The profile is same, cannot differentiate between identical twins • Expensive and sophisticated method • Expert knowledge is needed • Intermixing of samples of culprit with others available at crime scene • Lack of police training in sample collection • Require more time and hence accused can run away • Chances of error are there • Lack of availability of DNA Laboratories • Chances of deliberate samples exchanges

CHAPTER 9

Thanatology

Putul Mahanta

LEARNING PLAN

- Know about death, its types and related issues
- Understand the diagnosis of brainstem death
- Learn about the death certificate
- Understand manner and modes of death
- Identify the changes after death
- Know the ways of estimation of time since death

Thanatology (Greek, **Thanatos**—death, **Logus**—science) is the branch of medical science that studies death with all its aspects. The term death is commonly employed to denote 'the cessation of life in the body as a whole'. As per registration of **birth** and **deaths act 1969**, Section 2(b), death is the permanent disappearance of all the evidence of life at any time after live birth has taken place.

A person who has sustained either: (i) Irreversible cessation of circulatory and respiratory functions, or (ii) Irreversible cessation of all the functions of the entire brain, including the brainstem, is dead. Determination of death, which has tremendous social and legal importance, must be made in accordance with accepted medical standards.

TYPES OF DEATH

Death is of two types.

Somatic or Clinical or Systemic Death

It is the complete and irreversible stoppage of the "**tripod of life**", i.e. circulation, respiration and brain functions. But there is no legal definition of death. The question of death is important in resuscitation and organ transplantation[1] besides many others medico legal implications.

Somatic death indicates demise of a person, and it entitles Registered Medical Practitioner to certify that death has occurred.[2]

Molecular or Cellular Death (Few Minutes to Hours)

Molecular or cellular death is the death at the cellular level and takes place sometime after the clinical death. The molecular death is responsible for cooling of the body, and the temperature of the body becomes that of its environments in due course of time.

It takes place one to two hours after the stoppage of vital functions. Nervous tissues die rapidly, the vital centers of the brain in about five minutes, but the muscles live up to 1–2 hours. As long as circulation of oxygenated blood is maintained to the brainstem, life exists. Whether the person is alive or dead can only be tested by withdrawal of artificial maintenance. A person who cannot survive upon withdrawal of artificial maintenance is dead.[1]

WHAT IS BRAIN DEATH?

Brain death is the irreversible end of all brain function, including involuntary activity necessary to sustain life, due to total necrosis of the cerebral neurons following stoppage of brain oxygenation. It should not be confused with a persistent vegetative state. Patients classified as brain dead can have their organs surgically removed for organ donation.

Brain death is of three types and is used as a legal indicator of death in many jurisdictions. The types of brain death are:

a. Cortical brain death.
b. Brainstem death.
c. Whole brain death.

In regard to understand these three types of brain death, a schematic diagram of brain (**Figure 9.1**) showing different parts of brain.

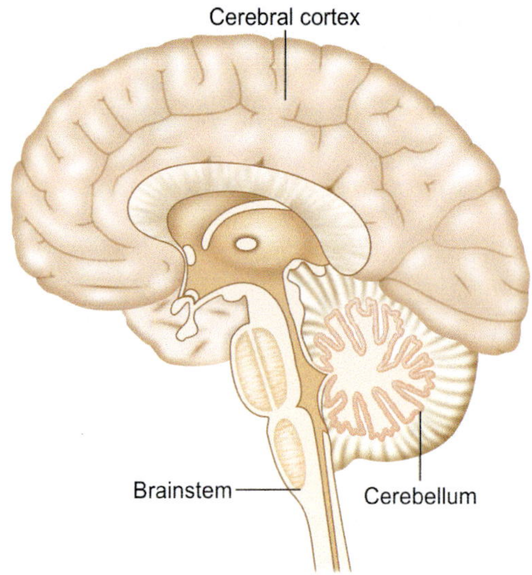

Figure 9.1 Different parts of brain

Cortical Brain Death

In cortical brain death, the cortex is destroyed. Often the brainstem is still intact, e.g. persistent vegetative state, wherein the patient can survive indefinitely with sufficient nutrition. For this condition to be diagnosed there must be a demonstration of no perfusion of the cortex via cerebral angiography. It is not sufficient to just show no electroencephalogram (EEG) activity.

Cortical death is a state of unconsciousness and loss of awareness, in which the patient can open the eyes, swallow and produce tears without any stimulus. Such vegetative people cannot be considered dead, but as the coma is irreversible, they sometimes are called **'living cadavers'**. As the brainstem is intact, they maintain respiration and cardiac activity.

Brainstem Death

Brainstem death of an individual is considered death which is permanent and cannot be repealed. While an individual dies, the heart stops beating and no blood gets circulated to the brain normally, therefore the death of brain occurs. However, if a patient has suffered an insult to the brain due to disease or injury and they are put on a ventilator, brainstem death may occur before the heart stops.

It is a clinical syndrome that can be defined by the absence of brainstem reflexes with pathways through the brainstem, the 'stalk' of the brain, which connects the spinal cord to the mid-brain, cerebellum and cerebral hemispheres, in a profoundly comatose, ventilator dependent patient.

Identification of this state of brainstem death carries a very grave prognosis for survival, cessation of heartbeat often occurring within a few days, although it may continue for weeks or even months if intensive support is maintained.[3]

The brainstem relays the information to and from the brain to the rest of the body, therefore it plays a key role in the brain's core operation, such as consciousness, awareness and movement. Possibility for consciousness or maintaining breathing or bodily functions is not possible in event of brain death of the individual.

The concept of brainstem death is also accepted for legal purposes in India[4] and Trinidad and Tobago.[5] Elsewhere in the world, the concept upon which the certification of death on neurological grounds is based is that of permanent cessation of all function in all parts of the brain—whole brain death—with which the reductionist United Kingdom concept should not be confused.[6]

Whole Brain Death

It is also called mixed brain death, which is a combination of both cortical and brainstem death. The process of brain death occurs in steps and the cells die because of hypoxia. The first part of the brain to die is the cerebral cortex, then midbrain and finally brainstem.

Diagnosis of Brainstem Death

For the diagnosis of brainstem death as per the Transplantation of Human Organ Act of 1994, requires a panel of four doctors that consist the doctor in charge of the patient, the doctor in charge of the hospital where the patient was treated, an independent specialist of unspecified specialty and a neurologist or a neurosurgeon. The burden of proof rests with the specialist of the neurosciences, with the other members confirming the diagnosis.

British Code (or Harvard Criteria) for Diagnosis of Brainstem Death

Preconditions

i. Comatose patient on a ventilator.
ii. Positive diagnosis of cause of coma (irremediable structural damage).

Exclusions

i. Primary hypothermia must be excluded as the cause of unconsciousness, and the patient's core temperature should be over 34°C.
ii. Drugs intoxication. This refers to narcotics, hypnotics and tranquillizers as well as neuromuscular blocking drugs.
iii. Severe metabolic or endocrine disturbances.

Brainstem Death Tests

Apnea Test: This test aims at providing that the patient is incapable of breathing. In doing this test, one disconnects the patient from ventilator and allows carbon dioxide to build up to a point where it would trigger off respiration if there were any cells alive in the respiratory center of the brainstem.

Brainstem death tests will include the following:

i. Blink reflex
ii. Pupil reaction to light
iii. Gag or cough reflex
iv. Vestibulo-ocular reflex
v. No response to physical stimulation
vi. Whether the patient can breathe.

Only when doctors are certain that all these reflexes are absent on both occasions will the diagnosis of brainstem death be made.

The time of death is the time at which brainstem death is established, and not some time later when the ventilator is switched off or the heart beat ceases. Clinicians should emphasize this when explaining the situation to the relatives, and they should make it clear that ventilation is not being withdrawn to let the patient die, but because continued ventilation is immaterial for a patient who is already dead. The only justification for maintaining ventilation for a short time is to preserve the condition of the organs when it has been agreed they are to be made available for transplantation.[1]

Medicolegal Issues of Brain Death

Why Death Diagnosis in Time is Important?

It is very important to confirm the time of death for many reason as mentioned below:

i. Resuscitation of a dying person
ii. Organ transplantation
iii. Withdrawal of ventilator
iv. Homografting
v. Forensic age estimation
vi. Inheritance of property
vii. Insurance claim
viii. Successor-chief.

Organ Transplantation

Success of homograft mainly depends upon the type of tissue involved and the rapidity of its removal after circulation has stopped in the donor.[1]

i. Viable skin graft can be obtained for 24 hours.
ii. Bone graft for 48 hours.
iii. Arterial graft for 72 hours.
iv. Cornea, skin, bone, blood vessels and blood can be removed from the body six hours or more after death for transplantation.
v. Kidneys, heart, lungs and liver must be obtained soon after circulation has stopped as they deteriorate rapidly.

Persistent Vegetative State

There is a difference between brain death and a persistent vegetative state (PVS), which can occur after extensive damage to the brain. Someone in a PVS can show signs of wakefulness (they may open their eyes, for example) but have no response to their surroundings.

In rare cases, some patients may demonstrate some sense of response that can be detected using a brain scan, but not be able to interact with their surroundings.

However, the important difference between PVS and brain death is that a patient with PVS still has a functioning brainstem, therefore:

i. Some form of consciousness may exist in a PVS.
ii. A person in a PVS can still breathe unaided.
iii. A person in a PVS has a slim chance of recovering because the core functions of the brainstem are often unaffected, whereas a person with brain death has no chance of recovery as the body cannot survive without artificial support.

Stupor

The patient appears to be asleep and shows little or no spontaneous activity, responding only to vigorous stimulation and then lapsing back to somnolence.

Beating Heart Donor

In this condition, even after brainstem death has been established, ventilator is continued to make cadaver fully oxygenated to facilitate organ transplantation.

Suspended Animation

In this condition, signs of life are not found as the functions are interrupted for some time or reduced to minimum. However, life continues and resuscitation is successful in such cases.

Agonal Period

It is the time between lethal occurrence and death. This period is variable and various activities have been reportedly performed by the victim.

DEATH CERTIFICATE

What is Death Certificate and why is it Needed?

A death certificate is a documentary evidence issued by the Government to the closest relatives of the deceased, stating the date, fact and cause of death. It is essential to register death to prove the time and date of death, to establish the fact of death for relieving the individual from social, legal and official obligations, to enable settlement of property inheritance and to authorize the family to collect insurance and other benefits.

Cause of Death

A cause of death is a disease, abnormality, injury or poisoning that contributed directly or indirectly to death. It may often result from the combined effect of two or more conditions responsible for the sequence of events, which may be brief or prolonged and which produces death.

Form for Medical Certificate

It consists of two parts. First parts includes framed in the following order:

i. Immediate cause
ii. Antecedent cause
iii. Other significant conditions.

Immediate Cause

It does not mean the modes of dying, i.e. heart failure, respiratory failure, asthenia, etc. These words should not appear on the certificate at all, since they are modes of dying, not the cause of death. It is the disease, injury or complication that directly preceded death of a person. For example, in a case of violent death, enter the result of the external cause, viz. fracture of vault of skull, crushed chest.

Antecedent Cause

This condition must be antecedent to the immediate cause of death, both with respect to time and etiological or pathological relationship. For example, in case of injury, the form of external violence of accident is antecedent to an injury entered on immediate cause and should be entered on here, although the two events are almost simultaneous, e.g. road traffic accident (RTA), fall from tree.

Other Significant Conditions

The other conditions contributing to the death, but not related to the diseases or conditions causing it should be here.

Format of the Certificate

i. The certificate should always be filled up by the attending doctors.
ii. The certificate of cause of death has two parts I and II.
iii. Part I is again divided into three parts, lines (a), (b), (c).
iv. If a single morbid condition fully explains the death, it should be written on the line (a) of part I. Nothing more need to be written on rest of part I or part II, e.g. lobar pneumonia, smallpox, etc.
v. If a death is followed by a number of morbid causes, the doctor is to complete the certificate properly.
vi. First fill the part I (a) the immediate cause of death.
vii. Next look whether the immediate cause is a complication or delayed result of some other cause. If present fill the antecedent cause in part I (b).
viii. If there is third stage which leads to death, put it in part I line (c).
ix. Other significant conditions contributing to the death but not related to the disease or conditions causing it should be in part II.

Death Certification and its Significance

Data on cause of death certificate serve many purposes

i. Help in assessing the effectiveness of public health programs.
ii. Provide a feedback for future policy and implementation.
iii. Essential for better health planning and management.
iv. For deciding priorities of health and medical research programs.

Declaration of death is one of the foremost challenges on ethical and legal ground. Death certification is a huge demand as the death of undocumented people are changing magnitude, viz., in mass disaster, etc. and involves the need to protect the rights of people recognized in national and international treaties.

Physician's Responsibility

i. The primary responsibility of a physician is to complete the medical part of the certificate regarding all diseases, morbid conditions or injuries, which either resulted in or contributed to death.

ii. In case of violent deaths and other medico-legal cases usually brought to the notice of a medical examiner at the postmortem stage, the certificate may be filled by the medical examiner on the basis of evidence noticed by him. The fact of death in such cases should, however, be communicated to the local registrar in the prescribed format pending the final filling up and transmission of the medical certificate to the registrar concerned.

iii. Section 10 (3) in the Registration of Births and Deaths Act (RBD), 1969, a medical practitioner shall, after the death of the person last attained, forthwith, issue without charging any fee, a certificate in the prescribed form stating to best of his knowledge and belief the cause of death.

MANNER OF DEATH

Manner of death refers to the way (design or fashion) in which the cause of death was produced, whether natural or unnatural, i.e. accidental, suicidal and homicidal.

i. Deaths not due to external cause should be identified as 'natural'.

ii. If it is not known whether the manner is suicidal, homicidal or accidental and is subject to further investigation, the cause of death should invariably be filled in and manner of death should be shown as 'pending investigation'.

MECHANISM OF DEATH

It is the physiological or biochemical disturbances, produced by the cause of death which is incompatible with life, e.g. shock, sepsis, metabolic acidosis and alkalosis.

MODES OF DEATH

There are three modes of death according to Bichat, depending on whether death begins in one or other of the three systems, irrespective of what the remote causes of death may be. These modes are: syncope, asphyxia and coma.

Table 9.1 Clinical features and autopsy findings of syncope

Clinical features
• Pallor of face or lips • Skin cold, clammy • Sense of sinking • Restlessness • Pulse—slow and weak • Giddiness, dimness of vision, vomiting • Convulsion (rare)
Autopsy findings
• Anemia from hemorrhage: Chambers of heart empty, heart muscle contracted • Asthenia: Chambers of heart may be full on immediate examination • The other organs are pale

Syncope

In this, it is the heart which stops functioning first. The term "syncope" is often used for transient unconsciousness, e.g. in cardiac arrest. The clinical features and autopsy findings in syncope are mentioned in **Table 9.1**.

Causes of Syncope

i. **Hemorrhage:** Excessive loss of blood as a result of injury to a large blood vessel or blood vessel of internal organs resulting in severe anemia may cause syncope.

ii. **Vasovagal Shock**: There is excessive stimulation of the vagus nerve resulting in stoppage of heart. This is brought about by severe head injuries, sudden evacuation of natural or pathological fluids of the body.

iii. **Asthenia**: This is because of lack of the heart muscle power to function in its normal way. The commonest cause being the coronary artery disease (**Figure 9.2**) where there is reduced blood supply to the heart muscle.

Asphyxia

It is the respiratory system of the body which stops functioning first. The causes of asphyxial deaths are:

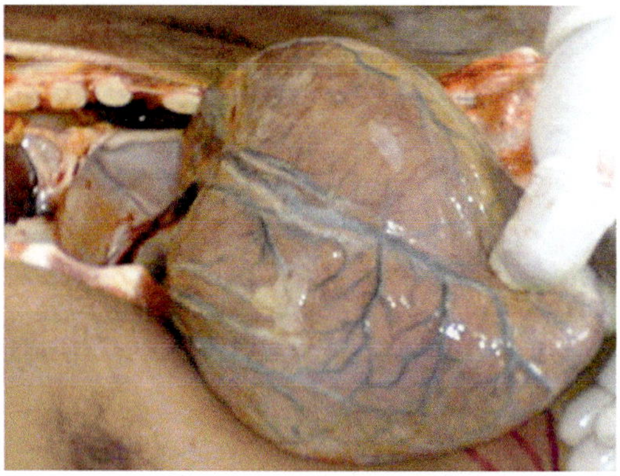

Figure 9.2 Thickened coronaries

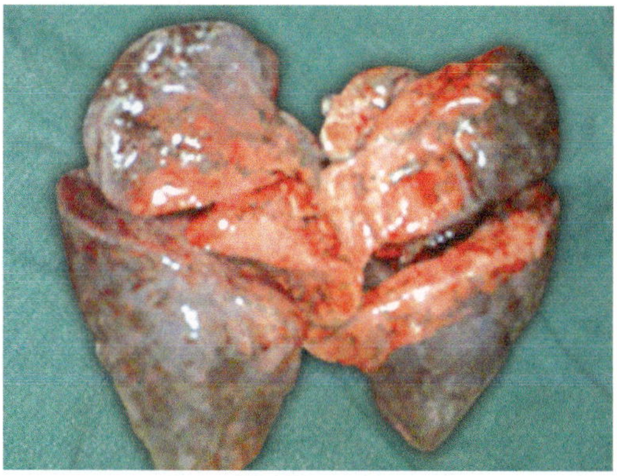

Figure 9.3 Congested lungs

i. Mechanical obstruction to the passage of respiratory tract as in: (a) Mechanical pressure from outside, i.e. in hanging, strangulation, etc., (b) Foreign body, (c) Inward blockage of the respiratory passage from structures such as tumors of the lungs compressing the main bronchus and spasmodic edemas of the glottis.
ii. Disease leading to respiratory depression as in diphtheria, laryngeal or pulmonary edema, pneumonias, etc.
iii. Respiratory paralysis because of depression of higher centers due to poisonings such as by barbiturates, opium, etc.
iv. Collapse of the lung because of penetrating injuries of the lungs, pleural effusions, etc.
v. Obstruction of the blood flow to the lungs by an embolus.

Postmortem Findings

External: Postmortem lividity is more marked because of the excess of CO_2 in the blood. Face is cyanosed. Tongue is bugged out. Froth may be at the mouth. Since the sphincters are relaxed, there may be escape of feces, urine or seminal fluid. Pupil may be dilated. **Tardieu's** spots present. These are petechial hemorrhage seen under the skin all over the body or conjunctiva.

Internal: The mucosa of the respiratory tract may be inflamed and congested. The right-side circulation is full whereas the left side circulation is empty. The lungs are congested and edematous (**Figure 9.3**). Petechial hemorrhage may be seen under the mucous membranes of the various organs.

Coma

It is the brain which loses its functioning first. It is a stage of unconsciousness resembling deep sleep and involves the stoppage of the action of brain. The important causes of coma are listed in **Table 9.2**.

Clinical Features

Initially the patient is in a condition of stupor; a condition from where the patient can be aroused, the reflexes are exaggerated. The next condition is the coma. This condition is characterized by the absence of reflexes. The sphincters are relaxed resulting in the incontinence of urine and feces.

Postmortem Findings

External: There may be evidence of external injuries on the scalp or fractures of the skull.

Table 9.2 Causes of coma
Head injury: Concussion, subarachnoid hemorrhage, skull fractures, brain tumor, cerebral thrombosis or embolism, etc.
Exogenous toxins: Barbiturates, opium, alcohol, etc.
Endogenous toxicant: Produced due to hepatic disease, renal disease, etc.

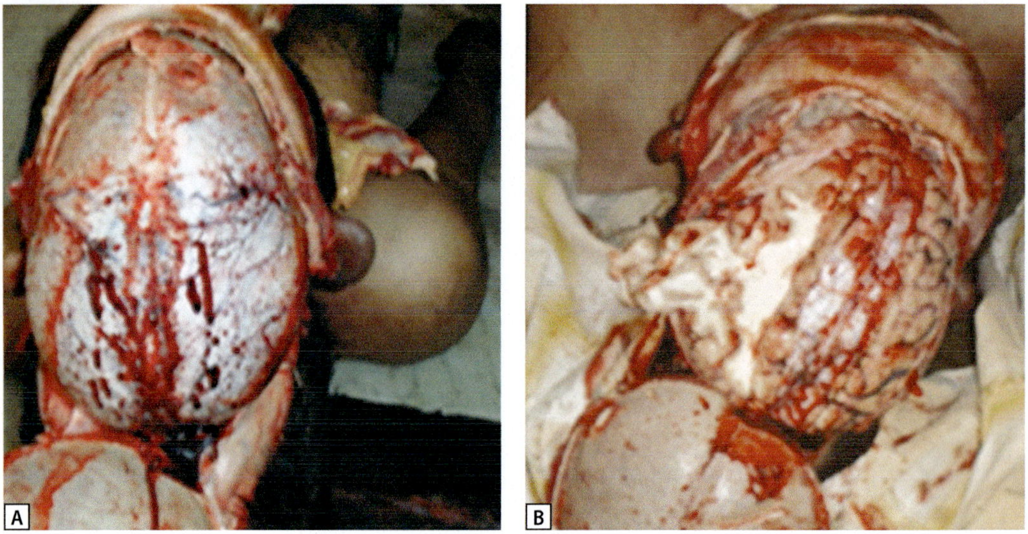

Figures 9.4A and B Congested membrane

In addition to this, there may be extravagation of blood.

Internal: Brain membranes may be congested and inflamed (**Figures 9.4A and B**). The right side of the heart is full and the left usually empty. Other organs may be congested.

SUDDEN DEATH

Death is said to be sudden or unexpected when a person not known to have been suffering from any disease, injury or poisoning is found dead or dies within 24 hours after the onset of terminal illness. Out of all only, 10% of the deaths reported are sudden.

Causes of Sudden Death

Sudden death does not mean instantaneous death. A sudden death may be various origins that are listed in **Table 9.3**.

Cardiac Tamponade

Cardiac tamponade, as a complication of myocarditis, MI, trauma, etc. can also be the cause of sudden death. Cardiac tamponade is pressure on the heart that occur when blood or fluid builds up in the space between the heart muscle (myocardium) and the outer covering sac of the heart (pericardium) as shown in **Figure 9.5**.

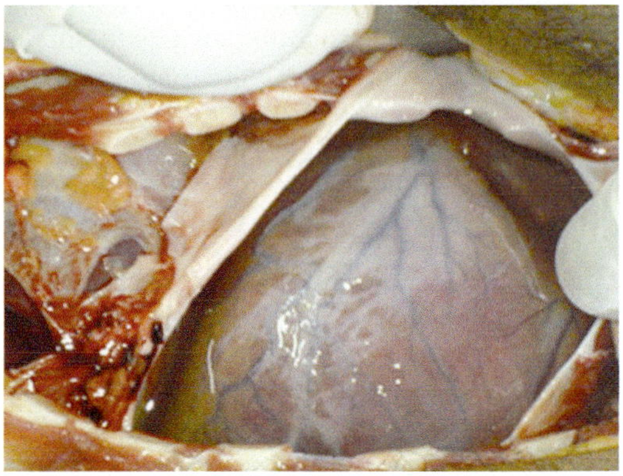

Figure 9.5 Cardiac tamponade

CHANGES AFTER DEATH

The stoppage of the functioning of the heart was taken previously as the time of death. The present concept of death includes the stoppage of respiration, heart and brain functions. In fact, the loss of functioning of brain should be called the time of death. It is at this time the electroencephalogram (EEG) becomes flat. The signs of death henceforth can be listed in **Table 9.4**.

Table 9.3 Causes of sudden death
Diseases of cardiovascular system (45–50%)
Acute myocarditis (e.g. diphtheritic, enteric or non-specific infections), myocardial infarction, left ventricular failure as a result of valvular disease or hypertension, rupture of an aneurysm or any major blood vessel closely associated with the heart, mural thrombosis or embolism and pulmonary embolism, etc.
Congenital heart diseases of newborn
Diseases of respiratory system (15–23%)
Lobar pneumonia, bronchopneumonia, foreign body impaction in respiratory tract, pulmonary edema, pulmonary tuberculosis, acute edema of glottis, carcinoma of lungs, diphtheritic laryngitis, air embolism, aspiration pneumonia, massive collapse of a lung, etc.
Diseases of gastrointestinal system (6–8%)
Bleeding from peptic ulcer, cancer of stomach, esophageal varices, intestinal obstruction, acute pancreatitis, acute cholecystitis, rupture of spleen, perforation of an ulcer of GIT, viz. peptic ulcer, enteric ulcer, carcinomatous ulcer, tuberculous ulcer, rupture of hernia because of strangulation and bursting of a liver abscess, etc.
Disease of central nervous system (10–18%)
Cerebral hemorrhage, cerebral embolism, cerebral atherosclerosis and thrombosis, subarachnoid hemorrhage, meningitis, brain abscess, acute encephalitis, brain tumor, epilepsy, etc.
Disease of genitourinary system (3–5%)
Rupture of ectopic pregnancy, rupture of obstructed part of the genitourinary tract by any cause, toxemia of pregnancy, profuse uterine bleeding from various causes, twisting of an ovarian cyst, tumor, acute renal failure due to stones, infection, etc.
Miscellaneous causes (5–10%)
Vagal inhibition, diabetic coma, blood dyscrasias and mismatched blood transfusion, Addison disease, idiosyncratic reaction, e.g. anaphylactic shock of penicillin, cerebral malaria, etc.

Table 9.4 Signs of death

Immediate signs (Somatic death)	Early signs (Cellular death)	Late signs (Decay and decomposition)
• Permanent cessation of brain function • Entire and permanent cessation of respiratory function • Complete cessation of circulatory function	• Changes in the skin • Changes in the eye • Primary flaccidity of muscles • Cooling of the body • Cadaveric lividity • Rigor mortis	• Putrefaction • Saponification or adipocere • Mummification

Immediate (Somatic Death) Signs

Permanent Cessation of Brain Function

This can be tested by:

i. Loss of sensations, viz. touch, pain and temperature.
ii. Loss of reflexes.
iii. Total loss of EEG rhythm that follows immediately after brain death.

Insensibility and loss of voluntary power and reflexes are the earliest manifestation of death, but it can lead to error if precautions are not taken. They are found in cases of prolonged fainting attack, vagal inhibitory phenomenon, epilepsy, trance, catalepsy, narcosis, electrocution, etc. Hence, confirmation of brainstem death is necessary.

Entire and Permanent Cessation of Respiratory Function

The respiration ceases after death. This is evident by the absence of breath sounds in the chest. In majority of the cases, it is sufficient to auscultate the chest to confirm the complete cessation of the respiratory functioning of the body. However, the following tests may be done to confirm it.

Mirror Test: A cool bright mirror is placed in front of the nostril of a man. A deposit of moisture will be found if the man is living.

Winslow's Test: A basin of mercury or water is placed on the chest or abdomen. A living man with a functioning process of respiration will show a movement of the reflected spot of light.

Complete Cessation of Circulatory Function

The heart stops beating, as a result of which there is no pumping of blood into the arteries. The pulses of the body fail to be perceptible. On auscultation of the heart, there is absence of heart sounds.

The following are the tests done to detect the stoppage of circulation:

i. **Magnus**: A ligature is tied at the base of the finger sufficient enough to cut off the venous circulation without any obstruction to the arterial circulation. The finger will remain white if circulation of blood has ceased.
ii. **Diaphanous Test**: In a living person, the webs of finger have a scarlet red glow. This is evident when the hand is held against a strong light. After death, it becomes dull yellow.
iii. **Icard's Test**: If fluorescein is injected hypodermally in a living person, the neighboring skin becomes yellowish green. In a dead person, where the circulation has ceased, there is no such reaction.
iv. In a living person when an artery is cut, there is a jerky flow of the blood. This response is absent in a dead person, where there is complete cessation of circulation.
v. In response to an injury like a burning matchstick, the skin will show a true blister with a red line of demarcation. This indicates that there is circulation of blood.
vi. **ECG**: After five minutes of death, the ECG show no electrical activity.

Cessation of respiration and circulation cannot be taken as the definite sign of death in certain cases. Cases have been reported where circulation and respiration ceases for sometime (from a few seconds to about half hour), and the person was alive with complete and proper refunctioning of the body process.

Early (Cellular Death) Signs

Changes in the Skin

Skin becomes pale and ashy white and loses elasticity within a few minutes of death. The lips appear brownish, dry and hard due to drying.

Changes in the Eye

i. **Loss of Corneal Reflex**: This is found in all cases of deep insensibility, and therefore, not a reliable sign of death.
ii. **Opacity of the Cornea**: This may occur in certain diseases like cholera and wasting diseases, before death. The opacity is due to drying, and delayed if the lids are closed after death.
iii. **Flaccidity of the Eyeball**: The eye looks sunken and becomes softer within minutes due to reduction of intraocular pressure (IOP). During life, the IOP varies between 14–25 g; soon after death it is less than 12 g; within half an hour, it is less than 3 g, and becomes nil at the end of 2 hours.
iv. **Pupils**: Become dilated and do not react to even strong solution of atropine and serine.
v. **Retinal Vessels**: Fragmentation or segmentation (trucking or shunting) of blood columns in the retinal vessels appear within minutes after death and persist for about an hour. This is known as **Kevorkian** sign.
vi. **Biochemical Changes**: A steady rise in the potassium values occur in the vitreous humor after death.

The normal antemortem concentration of potassium in vitreous humor in human eye is 2.6–4.2 mEq per liter. There is linear rise in vitreous potassium with advancing time since death.[7] Vitreous transaminase (SGOT) estimation shows steady rise in the vitreous fluid as the postmortem interval increase.[8]

Primary Flaccidity of Muscles

This is the stage which immediately follows death. Its usual duration is 1–2 hours. All the muscles of the body become completely relaxed. They can be moved in any direction. Muscular irritability is present, but there is loss of normal tone of the muscles. In a case of a person in lying down position, the lower jaw falls down and the eyelids start falling down and become loose.

Cooling of the Body

Synonym: Algor Mortis (algor—coldness, mortis—after death), chill of death.

The cooling of the body after death is a complex process, which does not occur at the same rate throughout the body. The body tries to assume the temperature of the surroundings. It loses heat by conduction, convection and radiation and cools down.

The rate of cooling depends mainly on the difference between the atmospheric temperature and body temperature. In colder climates, the rate is very fast. In hot climates, the rate is -16.3°C (or 2.5°F) per hour in the first six hours. In the next six hours, it is -16.94°C (or 1.5°F) per hour. In 12–24 hours, the body assumes the temperature of the surrounding atmosphere.[1]

Number of hours after death

$$\frac{\text{Normal body temperature (37°C or 98.4°F)} - \text{Rectal temperature of body}}{\text{1.5 (where 1.5 is taken as the average rate of temperature fall per hour)}}$$

The clinical thermometer is used to record the temperature. This thermometer is about 25 cm in length, with graduation ranging from 0°C to 50°C. In cadaver, the temperature is recorded at rectum (4 inches above the anus), sub-hepatic region, etc.

Factors Modifying the Rate of Cooling

i. **Age:** Cooling is faster in children and old people than younger people.
ii. **Sex:** Female have a slow rate of cooling as they have more fat than the males.
iii. **Manner of Death:** In chronic wasting diseases the loss of heat is faster.
iv. **Surrounding of the Body:** If the body is kept in a small room with no ventilation, the rate of cooling will be slow in comparison to when the body is placed in an open space with sufficient ventilation. A naked body cools faster than a clothed body.

Postmortem Caloricity

This is a condition where body temperature is increased for the first two hours after death. The postmortem caloricity occurs in the following conditions:

a. When the heat regulation system is disturbed before death, as in sunstroke
b. Due to excessive bacterial activity as in septicemias
c. Convulsive condition where heat production is increased before death like in tetanus, strychnine poisoning, etc.

Few of the important conditions and mechanism of production of caloricity are mentioned in **Table 9.5**.

Cadaveric Lividity

Synonyms: Hypostasis, postmortem staining, livor mortis, vibices, suggillations and darkening of death.

Table 9.5 Conditions and their mechanism of production

Cause of death	Mechanism
Sunstroke	Heat regulation system is disturbed
Septicemia or infectious disease	Increased production of heat
Pontine hemorrhage	Heat regulation center disturbed
Tetanus or strychnine poisoning	Heat production due to muscular activity

Definition

It is the bluish purple or purplish red discoloration which appears under the skin in the most superficial layers of the dermis (**rete mucosum**) of the dependent parts of the body after death, due to capillo-venous congestion.

Mechanism of Production

a. After death, the body is like that of an inanimate object, hence the collection of blood is in accordance of gravitational laws, i.e. to sink by force of gravity.
b. It starts appearing in patches. After 6 hours, the patches merge to completely discolor its back.
It begins in 2–3 hours after death, fixed at 6–8 hours and disappears with onset of putrefaction.[9] Apurba Nandy has mentioned that it appear in end of one hour, completely develops in 5–6 hours, fixed in 10–12 hours. Spitz and Fisher reported that it appear in end of 2 hours, completely formed in 8–10 hours, Fixed after 8–10 hours.[10] In Northern India, it begins within an hour of death, well marked in 4–12 hours and fixed in 6–12 hours.[11]
c. The blood coagulation occurs 6–10 hours after death. The postmortem staining changes in site and position according to the position of the body. Henceforth, it is significant to make sure that the body has not been touched by anybody. The position is often helpful in determining whether the death has been homicidal or suicidal.

Medicolegal Importance

i. It is a reliable sign of death.
ii. Help to know the position of the body and consequent cause of death. In the body lying on its back, postmortem staining is first seen on its neck and shoulders and then spreads to the back (**Figure 9.6**). In typical hanging, where the body is suspended, it is seen in legs and hands.
iii. In certain cases there is a change in the normal coloration like:
   a. In asphyxial deaths, it is cherry red
   b. In carbon monoxide and hydrocyanic acid poisoning, it is bright red or pink

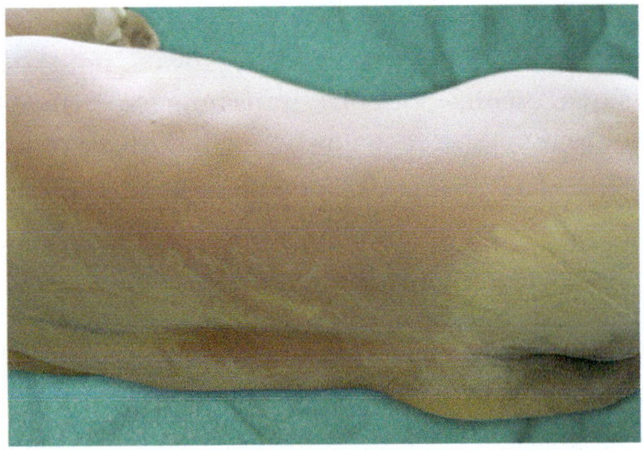

Figure 9.6 Postmortem lividity on the back

   c. In potassium chlorate poisoning, it is chocolate in color
   d. In phosphorous poisoning, it is deep blue in coloration.
iv. Its extent is a means of estimating the time of death.
v. The postmortem lividity sometime may be confused with antemortem bruise. Differences with antemortem bruises are listed in **Table 9.6**.
vi. It is also confused sometimes with congestion. The important differentiating points with congestion are mentioned in **Table 9.7**.

Rigor Mortis

Synonyms: Cadaveric rigidity. Latin word: Rigor —rigidity, mortis—of death.

Definition

Rigor mortis is one of the recognizable signs of death, caused by chemical changes in the muscles after death, causing the dead body to become stiff with some degree of shortening and difficult to move or manipulate that follows the period of primary flaccidity (**Figure 9.7**).

This is supposed to be after the cellular death. The electrical activity of the muscle is lost. The muscle becomes rigid. This phenomenon of rigor mortis first involves the muscles of eye, back of neck, lower jaw, face and front of the neck, chest, upper limb, upper abdomen and finally, lower limb. The impact of rigor mortis is that the whole body becomes stiff, muscles

Table 9.6 Differences between postmortem lividity and antemortem bruise

Trait	Postmortem lividity	Antemortem bruise
Position	Epidermal, due to capillo-venous congestion seen through the skin	Subepidermal due to ruptured vessels which may be deep also
Cuticle	Cuticle is not injured	Cuticle may be injured
Site	Over extensive area of most dependent parts	At the site and surrounding the injury, circumscribed and may appear anywhere on the body
Appearance	No elevation of the involved area	Often swollen because of extravasated blood and edema
Edges	Clearly defined	Merge with the surrounding area
Color	Uniform in color	Varies as per the time of injury. Fresh bruises may be more intense than the adjacent hypostatic area
Cut-section	Blood is seen in blood vessels, which can be easily washed away, subcutaneous tissues pale	Extravasations of blood into surrounding tissues which is firmly clotted and cannot be washed by running water. Subcutaneous tissues are deep reddish to black
Effects of pressure	Absent in areas of the body which are even under slight pressure	Little lighter over the area of pressure or support

Table 9.7 Differences between postmortem lividity and congestion

Trait	Postmortem lividity	Congestion
Redness	Irregular, more on a dependent part	Uniform all over
Mucous membrane	Dull and lusterless	Normal
Exudates	No inflammatory exudates	Exudates may be seen
Hollow viscus	Stomach and intestine when stretched show alternative stained and unstained areas according to the position of coils	Uniform staining

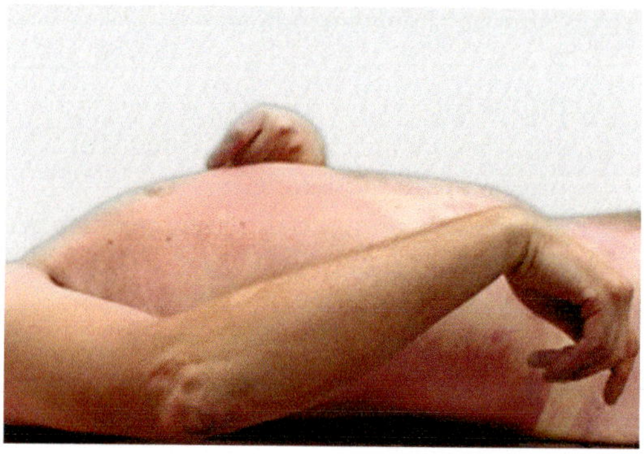

Figure 9.7 A dead victim in a state of rigor mortis

become short and hard and joints of the body are slightly in a flexed state.

In humans, it commences after about three to four hours of death, reaches maximum stiffness after 12 hours and gradually dissipates until approximately 48-60 hours after death.[12] The state lasts for a period of 24–48 hours in winter, and 18–36 hours in summer.

In **summer**, it follows the sequences as follows: End of first hour: Eyelid; 3 hours: Face, neck, jaw, trunk, upper limb; 12–18 hours: Passes off. In **winter**, it appears in 2–3 hours, develops in all over body in 4–6 hours and retained for 24–48 hours.[10]

Mechanism of Rigor Mortis

Adenosine triphosphate (ATP) keeps the muscle in hydrated form. When there is no oxygen, the ATP breaks down and finally disappears leading to the accumulation of lactic acid and the actinomyosin (muscle protein) combine.

Cellular respiration in organisms ceases to occur after death, depleting the corpse of oxygen used in the production of ATP. ATP is no longer provided to operate the **SERCA** pumps in the membrane of the sarcoplasmic reticulum, which pump calcium ions into the terminal cisternae.

This causes calcium ions to diffuse from the area of higher concentration (in the terminal cisternae and extracellular fluid) to an area of lower concentration (in the sarcomere), binding with troponin and allowing for cross bridging occurring between myosin and actin proteins.[13]

Unlike in normal muscular contraction, after death, the body is unable to complete the cycle and release the coupling between the myosin and actin, creating a state of muscular contraction (**Figure 9.8**), until the breakdown of muscle tissue by enzymes (endogenous or bacterial) during decomposition. As part of the process of decomposition, the myosin heads are degraded by the enzymes, allowing the muscle contraction to release and the body to relax.[14]

Factors Affecting Rigor Mortis

i. **Atmospheric Condition**: It commences slowly and lasts for a longer duration in dry and cool air than in warm and moist climates, where the rigor mortis commences fast, but is short lasting. In case where the body is immersed in cold water, it appears rapidly and last for a longer period.
ii. **Age**: In extreme age, it appears early and is short lasting. In premature births, usually, rigor mortis is not seen. It is observed in full term stillbirths.
iii. **Manner of Death**: In patients with chronic illness, diseases and in emaciation the onset is quick and the duration is less. In patients where a sudden death is reported, the onset is quick and the duration is more.
iv. **Muscular Condition**: The onset of rigor mortis is slower and duration is increased in cases where the muscles are in a healthy condition before death than in those cases where the muscle has been feeble and exhausted.

Medicolegal Importance

i. It is an early sign of death.
ii. Time since death can be estimated.
iii. It indicates position of the body.
iv. Sometimes rigor mortis may be confused with cadaveric spasm, heat, cold and gas stiffening.
v. Rigor mortis is not functionally related with the nervous system, and therefore it is also developed in paralyzed limb.[15]

Differential Diagnosis

Heat stiffening

This state of stiffening is seen after being exposed to a temperature higher than 75°C or when the body is exposed to a high voltage electric current. Both the events lead to coagulation of the muscle protein causing stiffening of muscles. In burns, a special posture is attained known as **pugilistic attitude**, an attitude of flexion of all joints of the body with clinched hands which may be regarded as defensive attitude. It can be differentiated from rigor mortis by following points:

i. Presence of evidences of burn injuries on the body.
ii. Muscles usually lacerate when tried to breaks in heat stiffening.
iii. Till putrefaction, the stiffening persists in a case of heat stiffening.

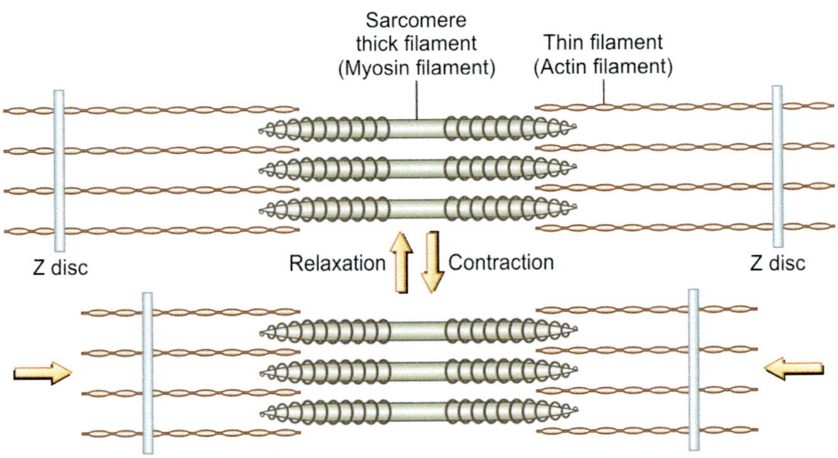

Figure 9.8 Schematic diagram of muscular contraction in rigor mortis

Cold stiffening

When human being is exposed to a freezing temperature, fats and tissues of muscle gets solidified and disappears on replacement by hot temperature. It sets quickly and disappears very rapidly.

Cadaveric spasm

Synonyms: Instantaneous rigor, instant rigor, cataleptic rigidity.

Cadaveric spasm, also known as postmortem spasm, is a rare form of muscular stiffening that occurs at the moment of death, persists into the period of rigor mortis[16] and can be mistaken for rigor mortis. The cause is unknown, but is usually associated with violent deaths happening under extremely physical circumstances with intense emotion.[17]

The muscles, which were contracted during life, become stiff soon after death. There is absence of the first stage, viz. the stage of flaccidity. This usually takes place when there has been a mental excitement immediately before death. The posture is held of the last few seconds of life, so it also called the '**last act of life**'. The differences between rigor mortis and cadaveric spasm are shown in **Table 9.8**.

Gas stiffening

This occurs in dead bodies showing signs of decomposition. Because of decomposition, false rigidity may be produced because of production of gas in the tissues.

Period of Secondary Relaxation

The muscle becomes flaccid soon after rigor mortis. This is due to the disintegration of the protein matter caused by the action of the alkaline liquids produced by putrefaction. The enzymes developed in dead muscle dissolve myosin, which is called auto digestion. They do not react physically or chemically. Putrefaction is present along with. In certain cases, rigor mortis passes off quickly and it is difficult to differentiate primary relaxation from secondary relaxation.

Late (Decomposition and Decay) Signs

Decomposition is the disintegration of body tissues after death. Decomposition often refers to bacteria decomposing tissues. It is the last stage in the resolution of the body, from the organic to the inorganic state and is a certain sign of death. Decaying often refers to radioactive atoms. It means that something breaks down over time on its own accord. Bacteria and fungi are the main groups of decomposer. They release enzymes to break down tissues, so that they can absorb the nutrients, a process known as autolysis characterized by:

i. Rise of enzyme levels in the tissue cells after death.
ii. Softening and liquefying of the body tissue.
iii. Starts 3–4 hours after death and continues for 2–3 days.

Table 9.8 Differences between rigor mortis and cadaveric spasm

Trait	Rigor mortis	Cadaveric spasm
Time of onset	1–2 hours after death	Instantaneous
Predisposing factor	Nothing particular	Sudden death, excitement, fear, exhaustion, nervous, etc.
Muscle involved	All the muscles of the body both voluntary and involuntary	Usually restricted to a single group of voluntary muscles
Muscle stiffening	Not so marked; moderate force can overtake it	So marked that required strong force to overtake
Electrical stimuli	Muscles do not respond	Muscles respond to stimuli
Body temperature	Cold	Warm
Molecular death	Occurs	Does not occur
Medicolegal importance	Time since death, position of the body can be known	Manner of death, whether suicidal, homicidal or accidental

What Factors Affect Decomposition and Decay?

There are many factors that affect decomposition and decay. The three most important factors are mentioned in the **Table 9.9**.

Speeding up Decomposition

Decomposers such as bacteria and fungi causes decay at **microscopic** level. Other larger organisms help speed up decay by feeding on dead matter and breaking it down into smaller pieces, thereby increasing the surface area for the bacteria and fungi.

These larger organisms include earthworms that help break down dead tissues, and maggots that feed on animal tissue. These larger organisms are detritivores.

Putrefaction

This phenomenon is the result of the action of enzymes derived from the body itself after death. It may also be caused by the action of bacteria and fungi. Bacteria, mainly *Streptococcus, Staphylococcus, Clostridia welchii, E. coli,* present in the gastrointestinal tract during life disseminate into the whole body through the blood within a very short time after death. The main devastating bacteria is *Cl. welchii* that causes marked hemolysis, liquefaction of postmortem clots, fresh thrombi and emboli, disintegration of tissues and gas formation in vessels and tissue spaces.

External Changes

i. **Color changes**: The color change is first observed in the region of cecum, which is fairly superficial, where there is greenish yellowish discoloration due to the conversion of hemoglobin into sulfmethemoglobin. This discoloration can be seen virtually over the whole abdomen, front of the external genitalia, chest and neck in course of time (**Figure 9.9**).
As the time passes, it turns into a purplish one. The usual duration of onset is 6–12 hours in summers and 1–3 days in winters. This is accompanied by swelling of the body. The sphincters are relaxed and urine and feces comes out. The eyes are forced out of the sockets, tongue protruded, lips are swollen and reddish froth start coming out (**Figure 9.10**). The body becomes offensive because of the formation of decomposing gases. The body is distorted because of collection of gases inside the cavities, which further leads to formation of blisters.

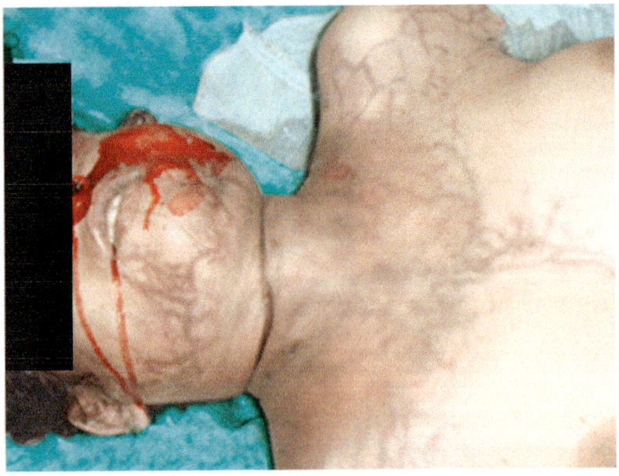

Figure 9.9 Marbling on the chest

Table 9.9 Factors affecting decomposition and decay

Factor	Effect	Explanation
Temperature	High temperatures prevent decay and decomposition, low temperatures slow it	High temperatures destroy enzymes and proteins, killing the organisms responsible for it. Low temperatures slow the rate of reaction of enzymes and will prevent growth and reproduction
Oxygen	Lack of oxygen will slow or prevent most forms of decay and decomposition	Oxygen is needed for respiration by organisms. Some bacteria can survive without oxygen, such as those used in biogas generators
Water	Lack of water will slow or prevent decay	Water is needed for transport and to support reactions inside organisms. Decay organisms need water to digest their food

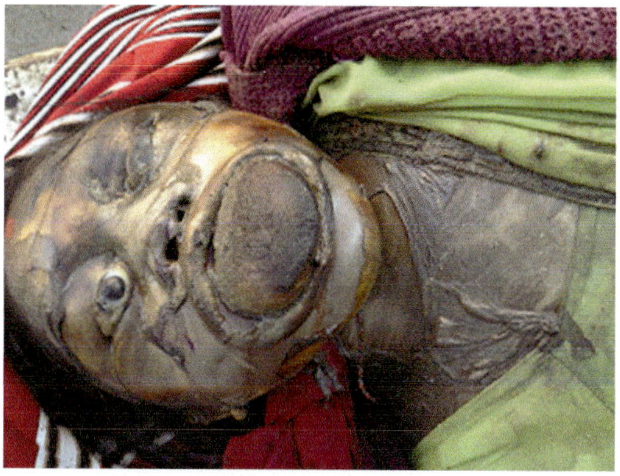

Figure 9.10 Bloated features in decomposition

Table 9.10 Sequence of putrefaction of internal organs

Organs which putrefy early	Organs which putrefy late
• Mucosa of trachea • Mucosa of larynx • Brain, especially of children • Stomach • Intestine • Liver • Spleen	• Esophagus • Diaphragm • Heart • Lungs • Kidneys • Urinary bladder • Prostate (in male) • Non-gravid uterus (in female)

Time sequences:

12–24 hours: Greenish discolorations of right iliac fossae.

36–48 hours: Marbling appears, ballooning effect, dispersion of lividity, unpleasant smell with postmortem blister. Evolution of gases appears as early as in 18 hours, fully developed in 48–72 hours. Colliquative putrefaction appears in 3–5 days. Nail and hair become loose and pulled off with ease. Teeth loose and pulled out from socket, Abdomen and thorax burst open.

5–10 days: Tissues and organs converted into soft thick black pultaceous mass.[9]

ii. **Blisters**: Appear after 36 hours of death. The skin cuticle, which contains a reddish colored fluid, poor in albumin, can be peeled off easily.

iii. **Maggots**: At the time of putrefaction, flies are attracted by the smell of the body. They lay their eggs which hatch in 8–24 hours to form larvae, also called maggots. In 4–5 days, maggots hatch into pupa which takes another 4–5 days to form an adult fly. At this stage, the sutures of the skull give way and liquefied material runs out. The rectum and uterus protrude out completely and gravid uterus may easily expel out the contents. The hair and nails can be pulled out easily. The abdomen and chest may burst out due to excessive amount of gas. If putrefaction continues, the tissues becomes soft, loose and dark brown.

Internal Changes

The internal organs of the body also undergo putrefactive changes. The changes are of the same nature. The tissues changes into a brown mass. However, some organs putrefy early and some late (**Table 9.10**).

Putrefaction in Water

It is much slower than in ordinary environment. Once the body is taken out from the water, rate of putrefaction becomes 16 times faster. Therefore, autopsy should be conducted as soon as possible in cases of drowning. In deep and dirty water, it is still speedily putrefied. The drown body takes 24 hours to float.

Floatation Depends on

i. **Age**: Adult float earlier than children and old people.

ii. **Built**: Strong and fatty people float early. The weak and thinly built people float late.

iii. **Sex**: Female float quicker than male.

iv. **Surrounding water**: In clear water, floatation takes more time in comparison to dirty water.

v. **Weather**: In summer, floatation is three times earlier than in winter.

Factors Modifying the Rate of Putrefaction

i. **Temperature**: Most favored temperatures for putrefaction are "between 70°F and 100°F". It slows down above 100°F and below 70°F. It is arrested below 32°F and above 212°F.

ii. **Access of air**: Free access of air promotes putrefaction. The rate of putrefaction is slow in water and slower in earth than in air.
iii. **Moisture**: Presence of moisture promotes putrefaction.
iv. **Age and condition of the body**: Body of children putrefies more rapidly than adults. It is delayed in cases of the aged and emaciated.
v. **Cause of the death**: Injured parts usually putrefy more rapidly.

Certain poisons delay putrefaction, e.g. arsenic, antimony and zinc. Bodies of individuals who die of chronic illnesses putrefy early than those of healthy individual.

Adipocere

Synonym: Saponification, corpse, grave or mortuary wax.

Definition

It is a phenomenon where the ordinary putrefactive processes after death do not take place and are replaced by the formation of adipocere—formation of soft, waxy material in the dead body.

Adipocere was first described by Sir Thomas Browne in his discourse Hydriotaphia, Urn Burial (1658).

Features

Adipocere is a wax-like organic substance which is soft, greasy to touch and varies in color from a dull white to dark brown and formed by the anaerobic bacterial hydrolysis of fat in tissues, such as body fat (**Figure 9.11**).

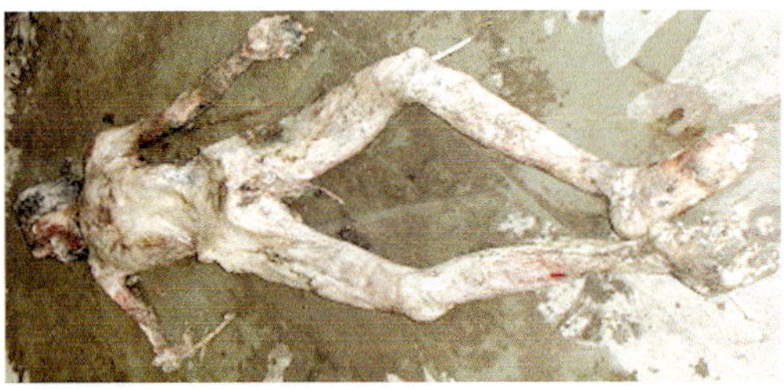

Figure 9.11 Saponification or adipocere seen all over the body

Adipocere is a crumbly, waxy, water-insoluble material consisting mostly of saturated fatty acids. Depending on whether it was formed from white or brown body fat, adipocere is greyish white or tan in color.[18]

These are formed by postmortem hydrolysis and hydrogenation. The presence of bacterial enzymes and water is most essential for the said changes. Hence, adipocere formation takes place in bodies submerged in water or in clayey soils or cesspools. The time required for the formation of adipocere is variable from 1 to 10 weeks.

Mummification

Definition

Mummification is a modified form of decomposition by which a dead body is preserved either in a wet or frozen or in a dried condition. It can be a natural process, or it may be deliberately achieved.

The word of mummy was first used to describe the bandaged bodies of ancient Egyptians. The Egyptians are considered as the 'fathers of the process of mummification'. However, mummies are found in many places of the world. Some of the world's best-known mummies were created accidentally, when a body's final resting place happened to prevent the natural process of decay.

Features

A mummy is the body of a human being or an animal preserved for a durable period. It is the desiccation of dead body resulting in drying and shriveling of the parts of the body. The skin becomes dry, leathery and closely adheres to the skeleton as shown in **Figures 9.12** and **9.13.**

The features of the individual are retained to a great extent. The phenomenon takes place naturally in hot and dry climates like that in Egypt, where the body is buried in shallow graves and hot winds keep blowing resulting in rapid evaporation of the body fluids. The time taken for mummification to set on from 4 months to few years.

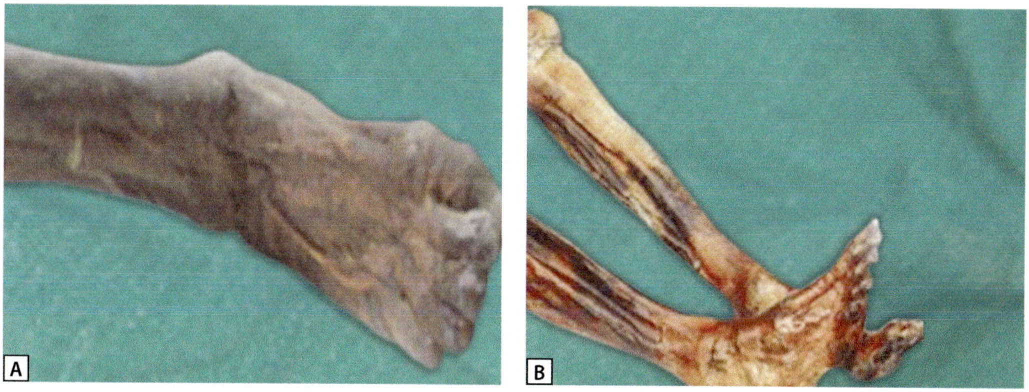

Figures 9.12A and B Mummified human legs

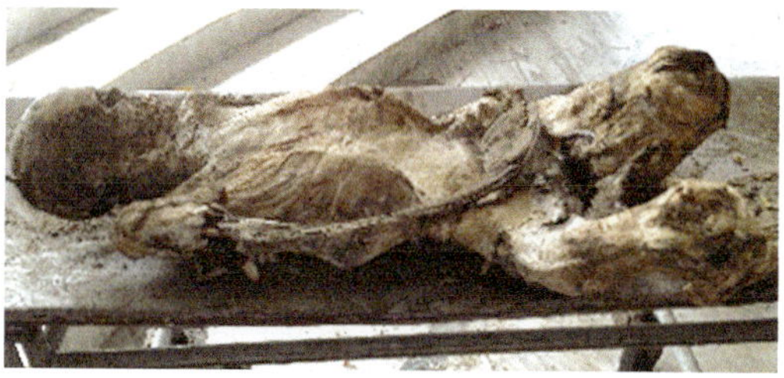

Figure 9.13 Mummified body

SUSPENDED ANIMATION (APPARENT DEATH)

Suspended animation is also called apparent death. In this condition, signs of life are not found as the functions are interrupted for some time or are reduced to minimum. It is a temporary cessation of vital functions with loss of consciousness resembling death; usually seen with asphyxia. This condition can be voluntarily induced by virtue of experienced practice of *yoga*. There have been studies where a *yogi* went into self-induced trance for 3 days and his pulse become imperceptible and the slightest heartbeat could not be heard with the stethoscope. The *yogi* continued to live for several years.

Voluntary conditions resembling the state of suspended animation:

i. Severe shock following accidents
ii. Electric shock
iii. Barbiturate or narcotic poisoning, etc.

In such cases where doubt exists, the following test should be done to avoid the embarrassment:

i. Demonstration of rectal temperature at or below 23.88°C or 75°F.
ii. Ophthalmoscopy should be done routinely and death confirmed by detecting segmentation and fragmentation of retinal blood vessels.
iii. ECG and EEG.

POSTMORTEM INTERVAL (PMI) OR TIME SINCE DEATH (TSD)

Postmortem Interval (PMI) is the time interval between the time of examination and time of death, i.e. the time that has elapsed since a person had died.

Estimating the PMI can be vitally important in a decomposed human remains case. A carefully constructed PMI estimate can reduce the potential pool of decedents that the remains could belong to and, thus, can contribute to the eventual identification of the individual. In homicide cases, law enforcement personnel can use the PMI to exclude possible assailants and to corroborate witness testimony. Knowing the PMI can also help to establish the range of natural events and environmental forces that were likely to have affected the remains with the passing of the seasons, permitting a more thorough pathognomic analysis.[19]

Table 9.11 Changes after death to ascertain PMI
Algor mortis or cooling of the body
Eye changes
Livor mortis or postmortem lividity
Rigor mortis
State of decomposition: Autolysis and progress of decomposition like putrefaction, adipocere and mummification
Forensic entomology
Condition of the gastrointestinal and urinary tract
Changes in the cerebrospinal fluid (CSF)
Changes in blood profile
Changes in bone marrow
Changes in hair growth
Personal effects on the cadaver

If time is not known, a number of medical or scientific techniques can be used to determine it. Many changes occur in the body after death. Some of those can be used to determine the PMI are listed in **Table 9.11**.

Forensic Entomology

If the lice are present on the person during life, they usually die within 3 to 6 days of the death of the individual. Therefore, if lices were seen on the dead body, it would indicate that death has occurred within 3–6 days. Maggots or larvae crawl into the body within a period of 8–24 hours in summers. The maggots develop into pupa in 4–5 days and into adults in 7–10 days.

Condition of the Gastrointestinal and Urinary Tract

The coarse particle remains in the stomach for about two hours, after this and before the emptying time the food becomes pulpy, soft and chime.

Changes in the CSF

The lactic acid concentration increases from 15 mg% (normal) to more than 200 mg% in about 15 hours. Amino acid concentration rises from 1 mg% to 12 mg% in 15 hours.

Changes in Blood Profile

There is rise of levels of non-protein nitrogen, free amino acid nitrogen, creatinine, magnesium and potassium after death. The rise is inconsistent.

Changes in Bone Marrow

In life, about 40% of the cells are neutrophils. Within an hour after death, the nuclei begin to swell, and after four hours it becomes round. Vacuoles form in the cytoplasm and the cell outlines become obscure, and in about 10 hours, the cell fuse into a syncytial mass.

Changes in Hair Growth

The growth of hair on the face is one of the important factors. Generally, men shave in the morning, in case the face is found shaven, death may have occurred after morning. The rate of growth of hair is approximately 0.4 mm/day. It stops after death. After the haircut, minimum 2 weeks are needed to have the pointed end of the hair.

Personal Effects on the Cadaver

Some personal effects, such as wristwatch, newspapers, letters which are dated, personal shares, dress all may be helpful in estimating the time since death.

Table 9.12 Gross effects on cadaver in due course of time

PMI	Effects
End of 1st hour	Rigor mortis at the eyelid (summer)[10]
2–3 hours	Early lividity[9] (draining of blood into the dependent part of the body, patchy blotches); rigor mortis at summer over face, neck, jaw, trunk, upper limb, but in winter it just start appearing[10]
4–6 hours	Rigor mortis developed in all over body (winter)[10]
5–6 hours	Lividity completely developed throughout the body[10]
6–12 hours	Lividity ends with onset of putrefaction
10–12 hours	Lividity fixed[10]
12 hours	Maximum stiffness from rigor mortis
12–18 hours	Rigor mortis passes off (summer)[10]
21 (3 weeks) days	Adipocere is fully developed (winter)[10]
20–24 hours	Body reaches ambient temperature
24 hours	Body has ambient temperature, decomposition begins, discoloration of body started
24–36 hours	Marbling appears
24–48 hours	Rigor mortis retained (winter)[10]
2–4 days	PM blister appear
3–7 days	Colliquative putrefaction, rigor mortis relaxes completely. Bacteria begin to decomposes intestines
7 days	Adipocere is appears (hot and moist climate)[10]
5–10 days	Teeth loose, pulled out from socket, abdomen and thorax burst open[20] with bad smell
10–20 days	Black putrefaction—liquids seep out into surroundings, very bad smell, black patches on flesh, flesh is creamy, gas has left the body
21 days	Adipocere appears (winter)[10]
20–50 days	Butyric fermentation: body is flat, flesh is removed, and body dried out, mold forms where contacts ground, cheesy smell. Grave wax starts at 30 days in absence of insects
1–3 months	Skeletonization (if body kept in open)[10]
90 days	Adipocere completed (winter)[10]
2–6 months	Skeletonization (if body buried)[10]
3–6 months	Mummification[9]
50–365 days	Dry decomposition hairs gradually disappear, bone remains
100 years	Grave wax still present in coffin

If the body has been lying over the green grass, the grass becomes pale in about 5 days' time due to the loss of chlorophyll owing to non-exposure to the sun. Studies have been done to know the changes appearing in the structure of the cells after death in due course of time after death.

The gross effects on cadaver as time lapses, which help with estimation of PMI, are shown in **Table 9.12**.

REFERENCES

1. Reddy NKS. Death and its causes. In: The Essentials of Forensic Medicine and Toxicology by Narayan KS, 22nd ed. Hyderabad: K. Suguna Devi; 1999. pp. 108-21.
2. Gordon I, Shapiro HA. The diagnosis and the early signs of death: the phenomenon that occurs after death. In: Forensic Medicine—A Guide to Principles, 2nd ed. Churchill Livingstone: Edinburgh; 1982. pp. 1-63.
3. A Code of Practice for the Diagnosis and Confirmation of Death. Academy of Medical Royal Colleges: 70 Wimpole Street, London; 2008.

4. The Transplantation of Human Organs Act, 1994. Act No.42 of 1994. s. 2.
5. Human Tissue Transplant Act 2000. S. 19(1).
6. Controversies in the determination of death. A White Paper by the President's Council on Bioethics, Washington, DC. p. 66.
7. Singh D, Prashad R, Prakash C, Bansal YS, Sharma SK, Pandey AN. Determination of time since death from vitreous potassium concentration in subjects of Chandigarh Zone of North-West India. Int J Medical Toxicol Legal Med. 2001;4:12-7.
8. Behera A, Das S, Das GS. Eye is the spy of forensic medicine. Medico legal Update. 2005;5:43-5.
9. Pillay VV. Textbook of Forensic Medicine and Toxicology, 16th ed. Hyderabad (New Delhi): Paras Medical Publisher; 2011.pp. 119-25.
10. Nandy A. Principles of Forensic Medicine including Toxicology, 3rd ed. Kolkata: New Central Book Agency; 2012.pp. 250-64.
11. Mathiharan K, Patnaik AK. Modi's Medical Jurisprudence and Toxicology, 23rd ed. Haryana: LexisNexus; 2009. pp. 428-37.
12. Saladin KS. Anatomy and Physiology, 6th ed. McGraw-Hill; 2010.
13. Freudenrich Craig. How muscle work. p. 1, [cited 2012 Dec 4]; Available from: URL:http://www.howstuffworks.com/muscle.htm
14. William MR. Rigor mortis. [cited 2012 Dec 4]; Available from: URL:http://www.newton.dep.anl.gov/askasci/zoo00/zoo00248.htm
15. Pillay VV. Thanatology. In: Textbook of Forensic Medicine and Toxicology, 14th ed. Paras Publishing: Hyderabad; 2004. pp. 95-112.
16. "Postmortem Changes and Time of Death". Dundee.ac.uk. Retrieved 2012-08-22.
17. Lyle DP. Forensics for Dummies. Indianapolis, Indiana: Wiley Publishing; 2004. p. 165. ISBN 0-7645-5580-4.
18. Murad TA. Adipocere. In: Ayn Embar-seddon, Allan D. Pass (Eds.). Forensic Science. Salem Press; 2008. p. 11. ISBN 978-1-58765-423-7.
19. Megyesi MS, Nawrocki SP, Haskell NH. ADD Postmortem Interval. J Forensic Sci. 2005;50(3). [cited 2012 Dec 4]; Available from: URL:http://www.astm.org
20. Krishan V. Textbook of Forensic Medicine and Toxicology, 5th ed. New Delhi: Elsevier; 2011. pp. 95-8.

CHAPTER 10

Autopsy

AJ Patowary, Putul Mahanta

LEARNING PLAN

- Know about autopsy, its type and related IPCs
- Understand the procedures in autopsy and different incisions
- Learn about the viscera/materials to be preserved routinely
- Understand different preservatives and their uses

DEFINITION

The term autopsy came from the Greek word 'autopsia', which means seeing with one's own eyes (auto + opsis). An autopsy is the scientific examination of the body after death.

Postmortem examination, autopsy and necropsy; these all terms are used as synonyms, but the most appropriate term is the necropsy, which means investigative dissection of dead body.[1] So, from the literal meaning, the term necropsy is the appropriate term.

In autopsy, it is the duty of the surgeon to examine each and every detail in the cadaver so as to find out the truth. Each autopsy must be a meticulous one with careful external examination as well as exploration and examination of all the body cavities to provide all the information as per the requirement of the law enforcing agencies in relation to the case. On the basis of these findings only, many a times the law enforcing agencies prosecute criminals as well as help some innocents to free themselves from any allegations. But a carelessly performed autopsy not only fails to help them but, at times, misleads the law enforcing agencies. So, we should adopt the best possible method so as to detect all the possible evidences and injuries and at the same time also to note some important negative findings which may help with the administration of justice. An autopsy surgeon should be able to serve as a link between the investigative agencies and the corpse; he should know the art of interacting with the corpse.

HISTORY

The earliest known forensic dissections were recorded in the middle of the 13th century in Italy at the University of Bologna.[1]

Antistius, the physician, examined the body of Julius Caesar (100-44 BC) and opined that out of 23 injuries; only one injury in the chest was fatal. In **1374** AD, right of holding medicolegal autopsy was given by the Pope. But, perhaps, the first systemic **autopsy** was held by **Dr Ambroise Pare** on the body of **King Henry II** in **1589**.

In India, the first modern autopsy was performed by Dr Buckley on August 1693 at Madras on a case of alleged arsenic poisoning.[2]

TYPES OF AUTOPSY[1,3-6]

There are various types of autopsies described by different authors. The most commonly used types are described below.

Academic or Clinical Autopsy

It is the type of autopsy conducted with the consent of the relatives of the diseased, to arrive at the exact cause of death, the nature and extent of disease, etc.

Medicolegal Autopsy

It is the type of autopsy carried out in cases of sudden, unexpected or unexplained or any suspicious or unnatural deaths. In such a case, the medical officer performs the autopsy on receiving the requisition from the concerned authority, which may be a police officer, a magistrate, judge or coroner, depending upon the prevailing judicial setup of the particular country. In such conditions, the body belongs to the state for protection of public interest and justice, till all the investigations into the circumstances leading to the death of the person are completed. During this time, any portion of the body or even the whole body may be kept for detailed investigation and also can be preserved for the interest of justice; the consent of the relatives of the deceased is not required for this purpose. One can make any incision on any body part or explore any body cavity for collection of evidences. In India, it is done by a registered medical practitioner authorized by the government for this purpose, upon receiving the requisition from the investigation officer of police.

Psychological Autopsy

This is a retrospective study of the events of death, especially in cases of suicidal deaths, to find out whether the person was at high risk for death by suicide or for accidental death. Interviewing the close associates of the deceased, such as his family members, friend or any other persons who knew the deceased can lead to the vital information in this regard and help in the reconstruction of the events leading to the death of the person. This process not only help in solving the mystery of the death, but also help in counseling the bereaved family and relieving the guilt feelings of them and also in finding out many unanswered questions associated with the death.

Objectives of Medicolegal Autopsy

The approach of the **forensic pathologist** to the investigation of a death is different from that of the **hospital pathologist**. Several health care areas are dependent on people's willingness to dispose of their body or parts thereof after death, and the issue of procedures involving corpse's entails important and, to some extent, growing problems. At this time, there were still strong religious and social objections to the autopsy. Autopsy is only one part of death investigation; body, history and scene are equally important (**diagnostic triangle**). It is like a three legged tool, which will fall over if one leg is removed or even shortened).[7] The different objectives of the medicolegal autopsy are shown in **Table 10.1**.

Prerequisites: (Indian CrPC)

All medicolegal autopsies are conducted in India by a registered medical practitioner on police requisition. The police officers as well as the magistrates responsible for the investigation of the cases perform their job as per the provision laid down under the CrPC 174 and CrPC 176, respectively.

Table 10.1 Objectives of medicolegal autopsy
First and foremost duty of an autopsy surgeon is to find out the cause of death. This includes whether the death was due to any violence, poisoning or natural disease
To find out the approximate time since death
To note all the internal as well as external injuries present in the body
To find out any external or internal malformation, deformities or disease present in the body
To find the position of the body after death as far as possible
To collect relevant information or samples of tissues or body fluid for examination and analysis, the result of which will assist the investigating officer to arrive at a conclusion as to whether the death was accidental, suicidal or homicidal
To establish the identity in case of an unidentified dead body
In case of infants, to ascertain whether it has attained the age of viability or not and was live born, still born or dead born and if live born to find out the period of survival and cause of death

CrPC 174

i. When the officer in charge of a police station or some other police officer especially empowered by the State Government in that behalf receives information that a person has committed suicide or has been killed by another or by an animal or by machinery or by an accident, or has died under circumstances raising a reasonable suspicion that some other person has committed an offence, he shall immediately give intimation thereof to the nearest Executive Magistrate empowered to hold inquests, and, unless otherwise directed by any rule prescribed by the State Government, or by any general or special order of the District or Sub-divisional Magistrate, shall proceed to the place where the body of such deceased person is, and there, in the presence of two or more respectable inhabitants of the neighborhood shall make an investigation, and draw up a report of the apparent cause of death, describing such wounds, fractures, bruises, and other marks of inquiry as may be found on the body, and stating in what manner, or by what weapon or instrument (if any), such marks appear to have been inflicted.

ii. The report shall be signed by such police officer and other persons, or by so many of them as concur and shall be forthwith forwarded to the District Magistrate or the Sub-divisional Magistrate.

iii. When
   a. The case involves suicide by a woman within 7 years of her marriage; or
   b. The case relates to the death of a woman within 7 years of her marriage in any circumstances raising a reasonable suspicion that some other person committed an offence in relation to such woman; or
   c. The case relates to the death of a woman within 7 years of her marriage and any case relative of the woman has made a request in this behalf; or
   d. There is any doubt regarding the cause of death; or
   e. The police officer for any other reason considers it expedient so to do, he shall, subject to such rules as the State Government may prescribe in this behalf, forward the body, with a view to its being examined, to the nearest Civil Surgeon, or other qualified medical man appointed in this behalf by the State Government, if the state of the weather and the distance admit of its being so forwarded without risk of such putrefaction on the road as would render such examination useless.

iv. The following Magistrates are empowered to hold inquests, namely, any District Magistrate or Sub-divisional Magistrate and any other Executive Magistrate especially empowered in this behalf by the State Government or the District Magistrate.

CrPC 176 (inquiry by magistrate into cause of death)

1. When any person dies while in the custody of the police or when the case is of the nature referred to in clause (i) or clause (ii) of sub-Section (3) of Section 174, the nearest Magistrate empowered to hold inquests shall, and in any other case mentioned in sub-Section (1) of Section 174, any Magistrate so empowered may hold an inquiry into the cause of death either instead of, or in additional to, the investigation held by the police officer; and if he does so, he shall have all the powers in conducting it which he would have in holding an inquiry into an offence.
2. The Magistrate holding such inquiry shall record the evidence taken by him in connection therewith in any manner hereinafter prescribed according to the circumstances of the case.
3. Whenever such Magistrate considers it expedient to make an examination of the dead body of any person who has been already interred, in order to discover the causes of his death, the Magistrate may cause the body to be disinterred and examined.
4. Where an inquiry is to be held under this Section, the Magistrate shall, wherever practicable, inform the relatives of the deceased whose names and addresses are known, and shall allow them to remain present at the inquiry.

Explanation

In this Section, the expression "relative" means parents, children brothers, sisters and spouse.

After completion of the inquest, the police officer will send the body to the mortuary along with other relevant papers escorted by the police personals and relatives of the deceased. All the medicolegal autopsies are conducted in an approved place specially designed for that purpose in natural light; if at all an autopsy is to be performed during the night, then adequate arrangements for proper lighting resembling the day light should be there for conducting the autopsy with prior order from the District Magistrate, citing the reason for the night autopsy, unless the center is pre-approved by the authority for night autopsy.

There should not be unnecessary delay in conducting the autopsy, the Medical Officer or autopsy surgeon is to perform the autopsy as soon as he receives the corpse as well as the relevant papers which include the following:

i. **Command Certificate**: Commanding the police person accompanying the corpse to report before the autopsy surgeon and do the other things as per rule, i.e. the command regarding his duty.
ii. **Forwarding Report**: Letter requesting the Medical Officer or autopsy surgeon to perform the autopsy. It also contains the name and address of the deceased along with a brief history of the case.
iii. **Inquest Report**: As prepared by the investigating police officer or the Magistrate after preliminary investigation.
iv. **Dead Body Challan**: Containing the relevant information, including the time of sending the corpse, distance to the mortuary from the scene as well as the names of the Police Officer or person and the relative of the deceased accompanying the corpse.

Before conducting the autopsy, the corpse must be identified by the escorting police person whose name is mentioned in the list of the escort in the dead body challan; a written note regarding the identification should be taken along with the signature and date from the police person.

No unauthorized person should be allowed in the autopsy hall during the procedure.

All the materials including the cloth are to be examined properly; all the body cavities must be opened, all the materials that are preserved for forensic investigations, like the toxicological investigations, are to be sealed and labelled properly and are to be handed over to the escorting police person. The tissues which are preserved for histopathological or other laboratory investigations are also to be sealed and labeled properly and sent to the respective laboratories immediately.

EXAMINATION[1,3-12]

After the identification by the escorting police person and the relative of the deceased if accompanying the body, the dead body is taken to the autopsy table. The body is then examined to note the external findings.

External Examination

The body should be examined first along with the wearing garments and after examination and noting the findings, the garment should be removed with minimal disturbance to the body as well as the garments.

Clothing

All the garments are to be examined properly, which include the description of the garments, their condition, any stain, tear or any other peculiarity are to be noted. If any tear cut is present, then it should be noted in regards of number of tears or cuts, its dimension and position and whether, these tears correspond with the injuries (if present) on the body or not. In presence of any stain, the same should be preserved for further tests for identification of the stain as well as personal identification. All such stains should be cut along with a normal cloth, dried, initialed and then packed in sealed and labeled paper envelops so that the moisture that may be in the stain do not decompose the stain, as it happens when packed in polyethylene or plastic bags.

After completion of the examination, the garments should be dried, packed, sealed and labeled and then handed over to the escorting police person.

The body is then subjected to the external examination, under the flowing headings:

1. **Weight**, **length**, **built** and **complexion** of the body.
2. **Scalp Hairs:** For length, color, distribution, whether any recent shaving or cuts, singeing or presence of any foreign materials in it as well as for presence of any dyes, injury mark, etc. The beards and moustaches should be examined in the same manner in case of male.
3. **Natural Orifices**: All the natural orifices are to be examined for any discharge, foreign body or any other material. Samples of the material are to be preserved where and when necessary. The vaginal and anal or oral swabs are to be collected in case of suspicion of any foul play.
   In male, the condition of the scrotum and penis should be noted along with whether penis is circumcised or not.
   Oral cavity should be examined for the position of the tongue along with for any injury, examination of the teeth for its number and condition, any stain or any other peculiarity. Apart from these, the cavity should be examined for any discharge or any foreign body in it.
4. **Eyes:** Should be examined for its condition, whether open or closed, condition of the cornea whether hazy or clear; presence of cataract, size and shape of the pupil, any stains or injury in the conjunctiva.
5. **Body Surface**: The whole body surface should be examined for any stain, color change or any injury. In presence of any stain, the same should be preserved.
   For dry stains, it can be scrapped off from the surface of the body and preserved. In cases of wet stains, swabs can be taken which is then dried, and preserved in paper envelop as mentioned above. The condition of the skin should be noted for any pallor, cutis anserina or any other findings.
   i. **Bluish discolorations** particularly in the finger nails, tip of nose, ear lobules.
   ii. **Petechial hemorrhages** may be found in the conjunctivae, the face and also in other part of the body depending up on the case.
   iii. **Postmortem color changes** if present should be noted for its color and distribution. Postmortem hypostasis if present should be noted for its distribution, color and whether it is fixed or not.

iv. **Rigor mortis**: Should be checked for its appearance and distribution. Cadaveric spasm if present should be noted with the content in the grasping hand.
v. **State of decomposition**: Should be noted along with adipocere or mummification if present. Maggots if present should be preserved separately in a bottle containing formalin and another bottle containing a piece of muscle from the same environment so as to study the life cycle.

6. **Female breast** should be examined for signs of previous or present pregnancy along with bite marks or any nail scratches.
7. **Neck** should be examined for any ligature mark or any other injuries such as bruises, nail scratches, etc. Ligature mark around the neck, if present, should be noted for its position, dimension, direction and number of turns, type, appearance and whether continuous or not, along with the position of the knot if any.
   Ligature material if present should be preserved without disturbing the knot; for this, the ligature should be removed by cutting away from the knot and the two ends should be tied by a thread. In presence of a slip knot, the knot should be stabilized first by tying with a thread.
8. **Injuries**: All the external injuries should be noted with their type, size, shape and site. While noting the site, it should be noted in reference to two anatomical landmarks.
   While examining, look for the signs of vital reaction which will differentiate the antemortem and postmortem injuries.

While noting the pattern of injury, one should note the probable weapon of offence, mode of infliction as well as the direction of application of force apart from the data for estimation of time since injury. In homicidal cases, look for the defense injuries as well as the mark of resistance.

Apart from these, one should scan the whole body for any needle prick mark which may be due to some injection in therapeutic procedure as well as deliberate attempt to end one's life and also for any concealed punctured wound which are homicidal in nature.

Internal Examination

For examination of the internal organs, all the three body cavities, namely cranial, thoracic and the abdominal cavities, are to be opened using the suitable incision depending upon the case.

Head should be opened first in cases of suspected head injury and cases with findings in the cranial cavity. In case of suspected poisoning, head should be opened first so that smell of poison can be appreciated before contamination by the abdominal visceral smell as well as in cases where there may be findings in the neck so that all the blood in the vessels of the neck are drained out and we get a clear field of vision while dissecting the neck structures.

The abdominal should be opened first particularly in the fetus or newborns so that one can note the actual position of the diaphragm which is one of vital data to opine the live birth or stillbirth.

Incisions[1,3-5,8-10]

There are different incisions for opening the body cavities; they are:

"I" Shaped Incision

It is the most widely used incision all over the world. It is carried out by placing the body in supine position with a wooden block under the shoulder. The incision extends from the symphysis menti to the symphysis pubis with deviation at the umbilicus, preferably towards the left. Both the skin flaps including the subcutaneous tissues and portion of the muscles are reflected laterally to expose the deeper structures (**Figure 10.1**).

It is the most convenient method, completed within a very short time, though the exposure of the neck structure, particularly the most lateral aspect, is very restricted; also there is no exposure of the back of the body, i.e. the back of neck, chest and abdomen, so chances of missing the deeper injury at the back of the body is there. Again, for examination of the spinal cord, another incision is to be made at the back. Moreover, there is incision mark in the front of the neck which remains visible.

"Y" Shaped Incision

It is used for the cosmetic purpose only. For carrying out this incision, the body is placed in supine position with a wooden block under the shoulder. Incision is stared from the tip of the Acromion processes bilaterally, passing below the breasts up to the xiphoid process. From there, the incision passes up to the symphysis pubis with deviation at the umbilicus. The upper flap is reflected upward and the lower two flaps are reflected laterally to expose the deeper structures (**Figure 10.2**).

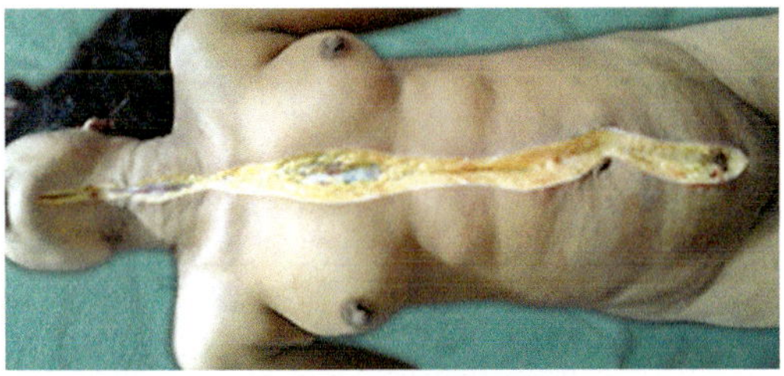

Figure 10.1 "I" shaped incision

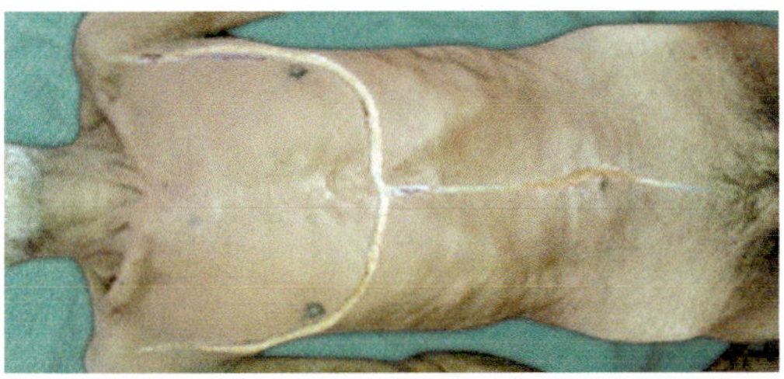

Figure 10.2 "Y" Shaped incision

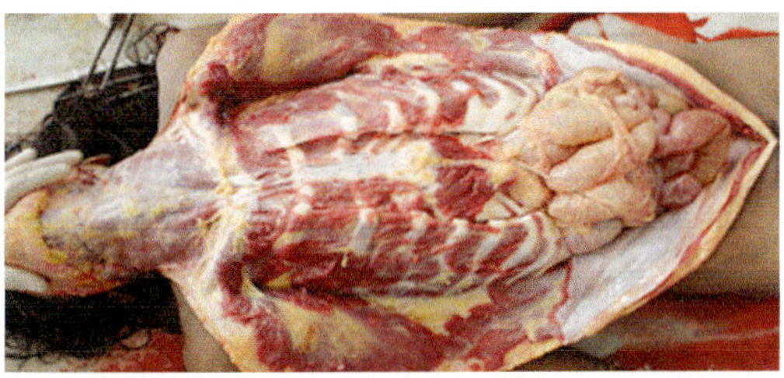

Figure 10.3 Modified "Y" shaped incision

As already mentioned, it is used for the cosmetic purpose only, as the incision mark is not visible in the front of the neck. The main disadvantage of the incision is that, it does not give proper exposure to the structures of the neck as well as no exposure to the back of the body.

Modified "Y" Shaped Incision

As before, the body is placed in supine position, with a wooden block under the shoulder. The incision starts from mastoid process up to the mid clavicular point bilaterally, and then continued over the clavicle up to the suprasternal notch from where a straight incision is made downward up to the symphysis pubis with deviation at the umbilicus. The flap of skin in the neck is reflected up ward and the lower two flaps are reflected laterally (**Figure 10.3**).

It is the most commonly used incision when injury or any other findings in the neck structures is suspected; as visualization of the neck structures in the front of the neck and to some extent, also the sides of the neck is achieved. But as in the other two incisions, the back of the neck, chest and abdomen is not visualized.

Opening the Abdominal Cavity

The peritoneum is first lifted and a nick is made in it near to the xiphoid process. Then the peritoneal cavity is opened by making an incision using an enterotome or blunt scissors, with index and the middle fingers using as guard, up to the symphysis pubis.

Opening the Thoracic Cavity

The sternum is removed by cutting at the costochondral junction first and then separating at the sterno-clavicular joints.

Opening the Cranium

The scalp incision is made from the mastoid of one side to the mastoid of the other side in coronal plane through the vertex and the flaps are reflected to expose the skull. The vault of the skull is removed by using an autopsy saw and chisels.

Cosmetic Incision or Dr AJ Patowary's Incision (The Fourth Incision)[4,8,9]

It is the procedure of examination of the body where the problems faced in the above mentioned incisions are minimized. Here, incision is made both anteriorly as well as from the posterior aspect. Following are the steps of the incision:

Exposure of the Posterior Aspect

Positioning the body

Body is placed in prone position with a wooden block under the shoulder, so that the neck is flexed anteriorly (**Figure 10.4**).

i. A scalp incision is made from the mastoid of one side to the mastoid of the other side in coronal plane through the vertex as in the conventional methods (**Figure 10.5**).
ii. From the mastoid process, the incision is extended to the posterior aspect of acromion process through the posterior border of the sternocleidomastoid and then through the posterior border of the trapezium bilaterally (**Figure 10.6**)
iii. A curved incision is made bilaterally from the tip of acromion up to the mid axillary line just below the axilla, which is then extended up to the iliac crest through the mid axillary line bilaterally (**Figure 10.7**).

Reflection of the posterior flap

The posterior flap of the scalp is reflected back up to the occiput and anteriorly up to the frontal ridge.

The posterior flap is then reflected back making superficial strokes by the scalpel on the

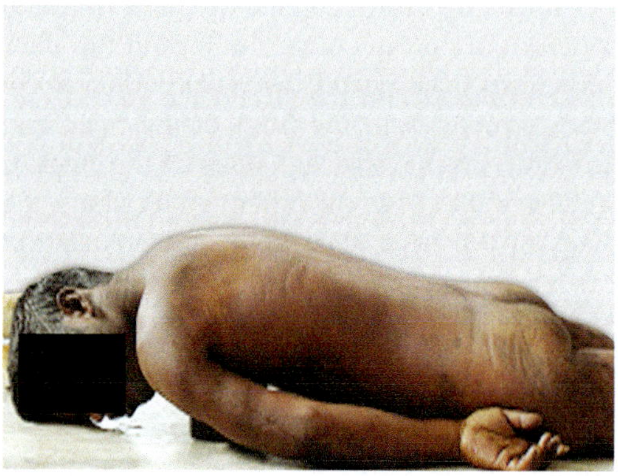

Figure 10.4 Positioning the body (incision on the back)

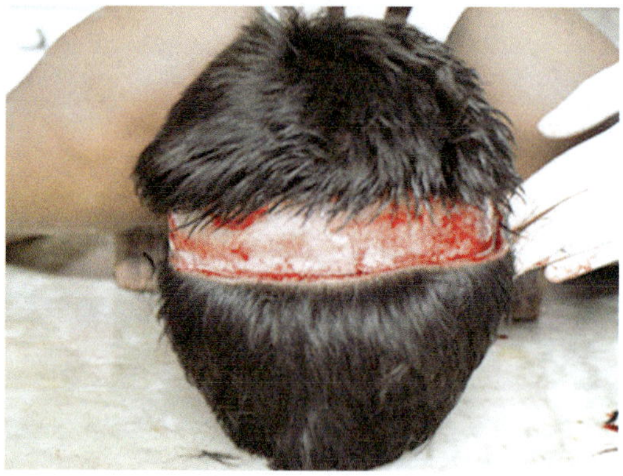

Figure 10.5 Scalp incision

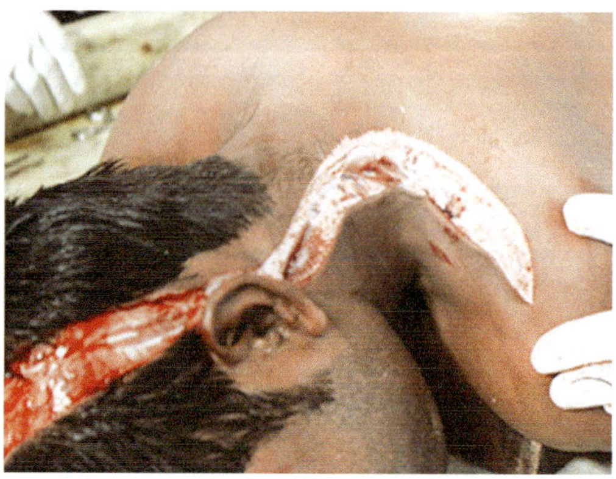

Figure 10.6 Extension of scalp incision on back

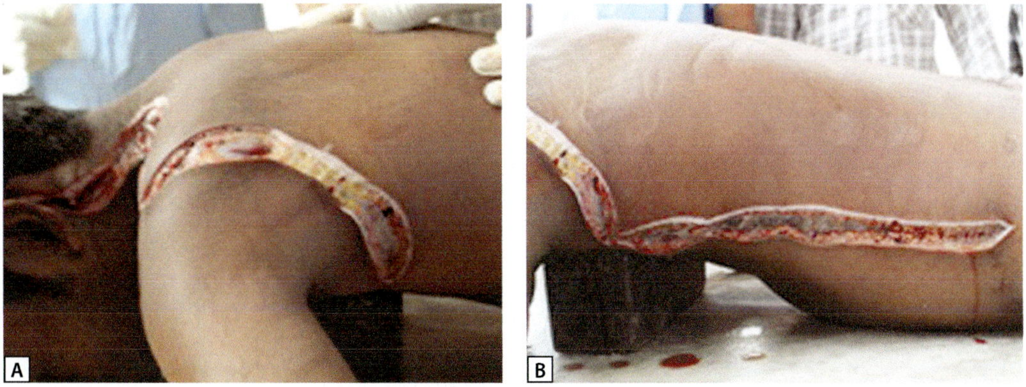

Figures 10.7A and B Extension of 4th incision on mid-axillary line

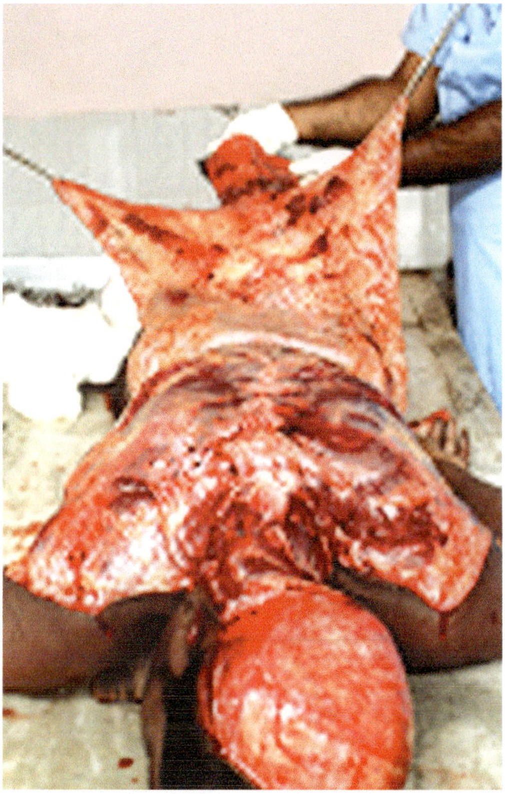

Figure 10.8 Reflection of the posterior flap

superficial tissues and continued through the neck, then the chest and back of the abdomen up to the superior border of sacrum. In this way, the whole flap of the skin is reflected up to the superior border of the sacrum exposing the whole of the back of the head, neck, chest and abdomen as a whole (**Figure 10.8**).

Exposure of the Anterior Aspect

Positioning the body

After completion of the examination of the posterior aspect, the flap of the skin is reflected back and the body is turned back to the supine position with a wooden block under the shoulder to keep the neck in extended position.

Incision in the front

i. A curved incision is made from the acromion process through the medial border of the shoulder joint to the mid axillary line bilaterally as was made posteriorly (**Figure 10.9A**).
ii. Another incision is made from the mid axillary line on the iliac crest bilaterally over the inguinal ligament, to meet at the symphysis pubis (**Figure 10.9B**).
iii. The skin with the superficial tissue is reflected up superiorly. Care should be taken not to injure the rectus sheath. The flap is reflected up, up to the root of the neck and then to the inferior margin of the mandible bilaterally taking care not to injure the neck structures (**Figure 10.10**).
iv. This way, the whole of front of the neck chest and abdomen is exposed.

Opening of the abdominal cavity

To open the abdominal cavity, a paramedial incision is made on the rectus near the symphysis pubis, which is extended upward by keeping the index and the middle fingers as guard up to the xiphoid process using a scissors or enterotome (**Figure 10.11**).

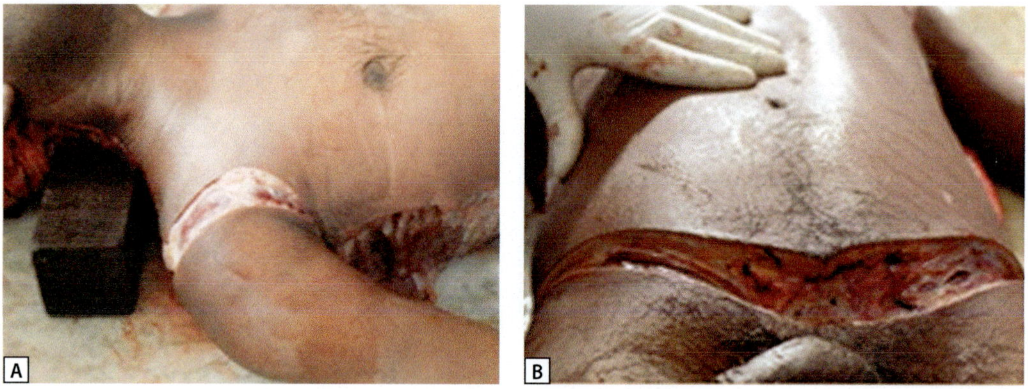

Figures 10.9A and B Incision in the front

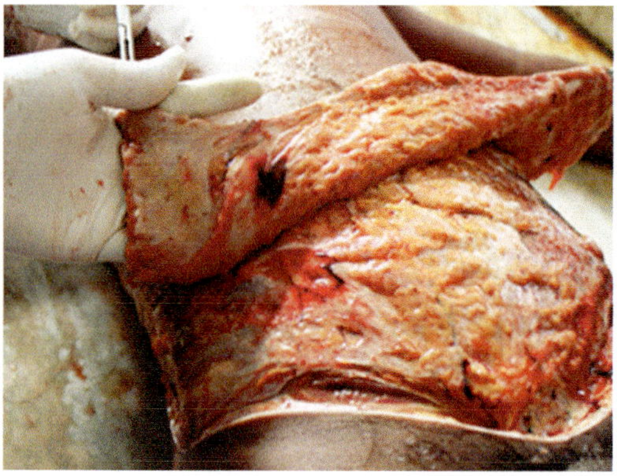

Figure 10.10 Reflexion of anterior flap of abdomen and chest

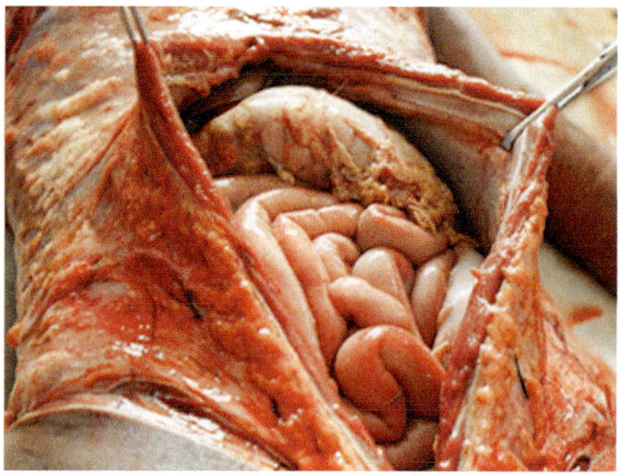

Figure 10.11 Opening of abdominal cavity

Opening of the thorax

The sternum is removed by cutting at the costochondral junction and then separating the sternoclavicular joint. Now, after separating the diaphragm, the whole of the thorax and abdomen can be examined later on (**Figure 10.12**).

In case of suspected pneumothorax, a syringe is filled with water and the needle is introduced into the thoracic cavity and piston is removed before opening the thorax; if collection of air is there, bubbles of air can be seen in the water in the syringe.

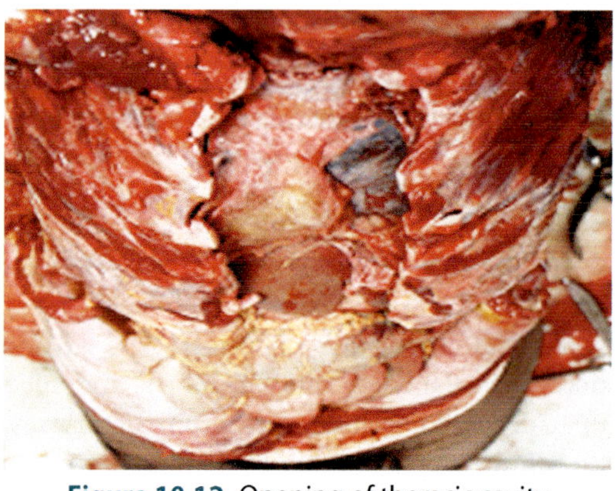

Figure 10.12 Opening of thoracic cavity

Opening the cranium

After removal of the scalp, examine the cranium for any fractures any other injuries. For opening the cranium, the vault of the skull is removed by using an autopsy saw and chisels (**Figure 10.13**).

Closing of the Incisions (Figure 10.14)

The sternum is replaced back to its position. The abdomen is closed by stitching the rectus.

Now the flap of the skin is replaced back. The incision on the inguinal ligament is stitched first then the bilateral mid axillary incisions up to the axilla. Then the stitches are continued in the front on the curved incision in the medial border of the shoulder and then on the incisions on both sides of the neck up to the mastoid process. The scalp is then stitched and the body is turned back to stitch the curved incision on the medial margin of the shoulder in the back.

Summary of the Cosmetic Autopsy Incision

i. Whole of the circumference of the neck, thorax and abdomen is visualized; so, better detection of the wounds, particularly in cases of death related to torture, burn,

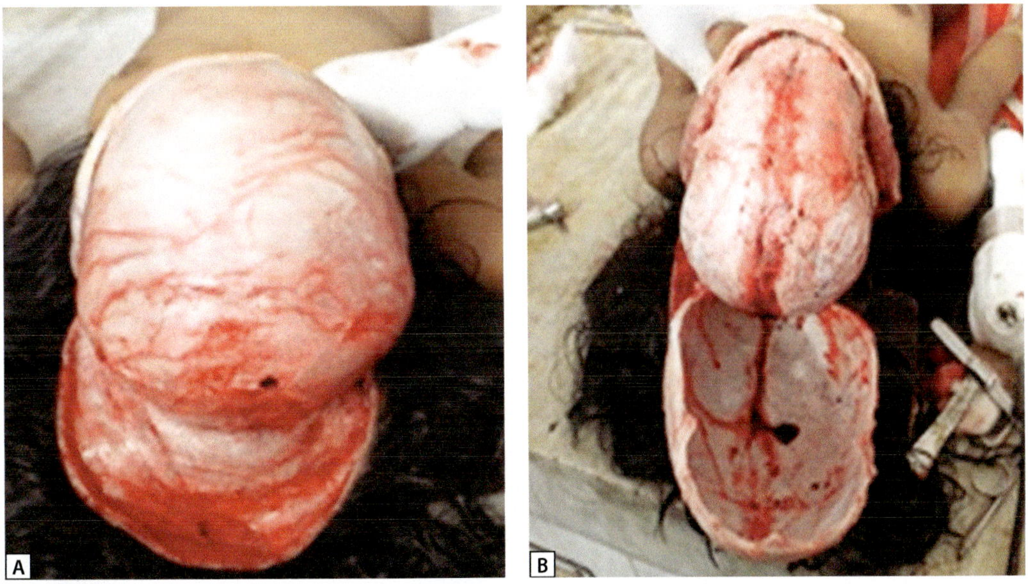

Figures 10.13A and B Opening of cranium

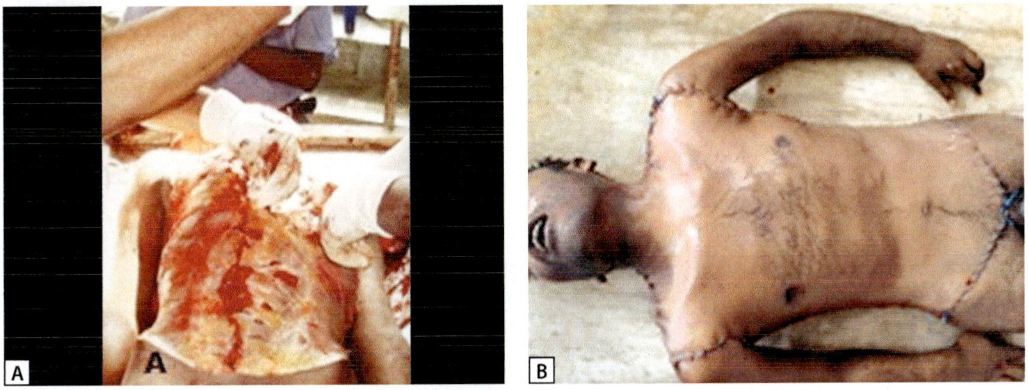

Figures 10.14A and B Closing the incisions

road traffic accidents and any other cases, where there is history of injury just before death of the person (**Figure 10.15**).

ii. No or minimal seepage from the cavities.
iii. Stitches can be kept hidden in the front of the neck, so, better acceptance for the relatives of the deceased (**Figure 10.16**).
iv. No separate incision is required for opening the spinal canal from the back.
v. The only disadvantage is that, it is more time consuming, requires 30 minutes more time in comparison to the "I" shaped incision.

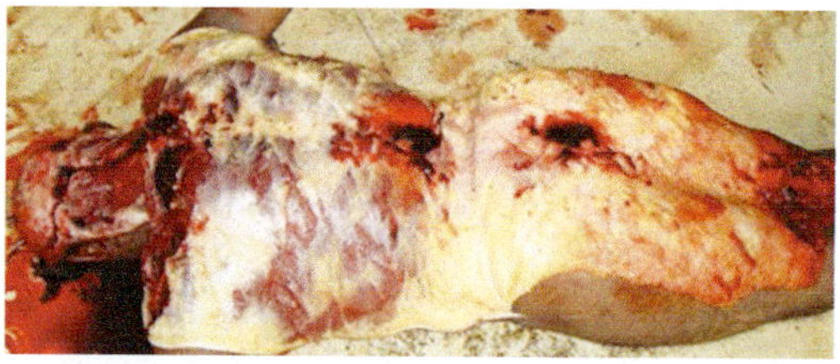

Figure 10.15 Deeply settled bruises on back of chest/abdomen seen after removal of the flap

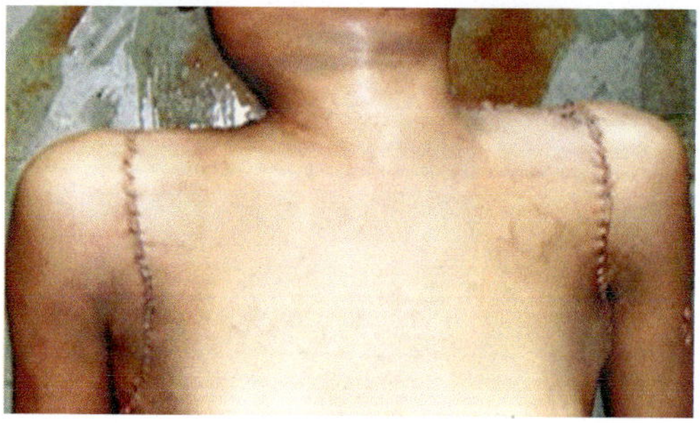

Figure 10.16 After stitches of 4th incision

For examination of the visceral organs, basically four techniques are used:[1,3,4,11]

Virchow's Technique: This is the most widely used method. Originally, it was accomplished in the order of opening the cranial cavity first, followed by the exposing the spinal cord from back, then the thoracic organs and then the cervical and the abdominal cavity. The organs are removed one by one.

Rokitansky's Technique: This is the method combined by in situ dissection combined with removal of the organs as organ blocks.

Ghon's Technique: The visceral organs are removed as organ blocks (en block removal).

Letuli's Technique: In this technique, all the organs including the cervical, thoracic and abdominal and the cervical organs are removed as a single block (en masse removal).

VISCERA EXAMINATION TECHNIQUE[1,3-6,10,11]

Dissection of Different Organs

Brain (Figure 10.17)

After removal of the cranial vault, the dura is exposed; examine it for any extradural hemorrhage, any injury or congestions. A nick is made in the dura, one cm lateral to the sagittal sinus, which is then extended both way to separate the sagittal sinus which is then pulled out and

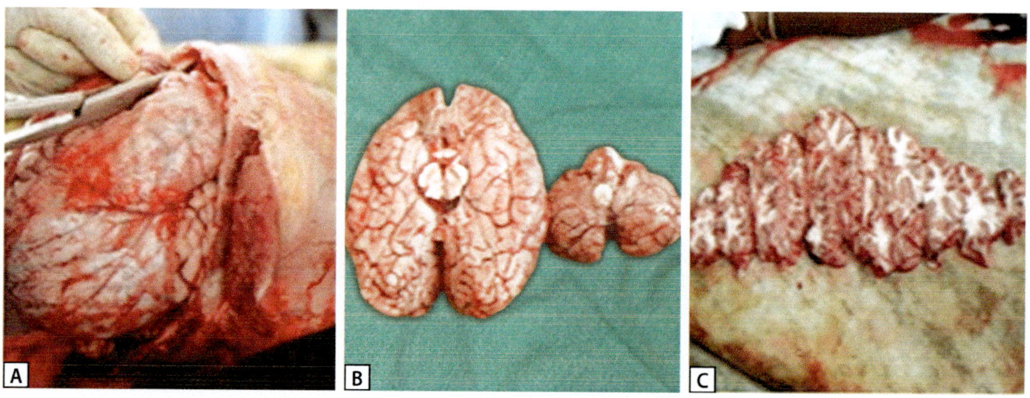

A B C

Figures 10.17A to C Dissection of brain

examined for any injury or abnormalities. One transverse incision is made on the dura from the sagittal margin to the temporal aspect, which will expose the subarachnoid space; look for any hemorrhage or any pathological findings.

Sometimes it becomes difficult to differentiate the subdural hemorrhage from subarachnoid hemorrhage. In such a situation, wash the surface with water and if goes off, then it is the subdural hemorrhage, otherwise, the subarachnoid hemorrhage.

The brain is then lifted by introducing one hand below the frontal lobes to expose the cranial nerves roots and cut them. Tentorium cerebellum is dissected near the bony margins to expose the cerebellum. Cut the remaining nerve roots and then the medulla as distal as possible; the brain can now be taken out of the cranial cavity. Examine the base of the skull, after stripping of the remaining dura, for any fractures.

The brain is then dissected by making multiple slices, about 1 cm thick, using the brain knife. For this, the cerebral hemispheres, the mid brain and the cerebellum are separated and all the ventricles are examined. Both cerebrums and also the cerebellum are sliced and examined. The mid-brain and the medulla should be sliced in transverse plane and any injury, hemorrhage or any other pathological changes are noted.

Spinal Cord

To expose the spinal cord, a midline incision is to be made from the back from the just below the occiput throughout the entire length of the spinal cord to expose the vertebrae (except in case or the fourth incision). The muscles are removed and the vertebral column is then removed by cutting the transverse processes to expose the spinal cord which can be removed by cutting the nerve roots.

Lungs

Both lungs should be separated at the hilum and examined for any congestion, its consistency, consolidation, edema, emphysema, atelectasis, any injury or other pathological changes. Petechial hemorrhage on the surface of the lung is very common in cases of death due to asphyxia except in cases of drowning. The trachea and the bronchi are to be opened and examined for any collection, pathological condition or any foreign material; presence of mud or sand particles in cases of drowning and shoot particles in cases of burn in the bronchi or beyond signifies its antemortem nature.

Heart and Great Vessels

The pericardium should be examined for any injury, congestions, adhesions or petechial hemorrhage; cavity should be examined for any collection and if present, the amount should be noted. The heart is separated by dissecting the great vessels.

For examination of the chambers, the most convenient method is dissection along the flow of the blood.

For this, an incision is made through the right border of the heart from one vena cava to come out through the other; a separate incision is made to the right auricle. Incision is then extended to the right ventricle through the inferior border of the heart up to the apex and then 1 cm lateral to the intraventricular septum upward to come out through the pulmonary trunk. The left atrium is opened by cutting between the pulmonary veins. The incision is then extended into the left ventricle through the left border up to the apex and then upward 1 cm left of intraventricular septum to come out through the aorta. Both sides of the heart should be examined for any thrombus or any other pathology particularly the in valves and the papillary muscles.

To examine the coronary arteries, transverse incisions are made on the arteries and look for any obliteration, thrombus, etc.

After removal of the organs, the thoracic cavity is examined for any injury or pathological condition. The ribs are cleared of the intercostals muscles and examined for any fracture.

Gastrointestinal Tract

The stomach should be removed tying at the two ends and is to be separated from the rest between double ligatures. Cavity is exposed by cutting at the greater curvature. Examine the mucosal surfaces for any congestion, hemorrhage, erosions, ulcerations or any other pathology and at the same time examine the content for type of food, state of digestion and for presence or absence of any suspicious materials or smell.

The intestines should be separated by cutting at the mesenteric margin and examined.

Liver: To be separated by cutting the ligaments and examined its surface for its appearance, color, congestion, injury or any other pathological findings. Liver is then examined by serial sectioning; gallbladder is to be examined for any calculi and also note whether distended or not.

Spleen: To be examined for its size and shape and for any injury or pathology.

Kidney, Ureters and Bladder: Both the kidneys are to be separated by removing the fatty tissue and peritoneal covering. Both the kidneys are dissected longitudinally in its convex border up to the hilum and then examined for any pathology, calculus, hemorrhages, etc. Ureters are explored up to their entry in to the bladder by slitting them open.

Urinary bladder is examined for any signs of inflammation, collections or calculus.

Prostate can be examined by pulling the urinary bladder upward and then dissecting at the urethra. It is then examined for any enlargement, or evidence or any malignancy if history suggested.

Genitalia

Male: Both the testis are examined and then dissected by longitudinal incision including epididymis and examined for any disease or injury.

Penis is examined for any injury, diseases or any congenital abnormalities.

Female Genitalia: Uterus is removed along with the ovaries and fallopian tubes by releasing them from the surrounding tissues; uterus is then released along with the cervix so as to facilitate the examination of the cervix. All these are then examined for the size, shape, consistency and the weight. Uterus is cut longitudinally and the cavity is examined for any pathology, collection, fetus or product of conception or any foreign body.

After removal of the organs, the abdominal cavity is examined for any injury or pathology, particularly in the peravertibral tissues, including the abdominal aorta and inferior vena cava and also the para-aortic lymph nodes.

After completion of the autopsy, all the incisions are stitched; body is washed and then handed over to the escorting police along with the articles preserved.

FETAL AND PERINATAL AUTOPSY

Refer to Annexure 14.

SAMPLES TO BE PRESERVED

While handling the medicolegal autopsy cases, certain standard guidelines are necessary to be maintaining to assist in the selection of appropriate specimens of the body fluids and tissue for postmortem biochemical and toxicological analysis.

Collection of proper autopsy specimen is an essential step in the process of toxicology case work.[13] Wrong collection of these specimens may greatly alter or negate chemical and toxicological analysis.

In case of suspected poisoning following is the list of samples of visceras preserved routinely are shown in **Table 10.2**.

However, it may not be possible to give the opinion regarding certain poisons or drugs without biological fluid analysis. Following biological fluid or sample (**Table 10.3**) may require to be preserved under curtain condition.

Other Body Fluids

In cases where blood and urine are not available, other available body fluids like pericardial[14] and

Table 10.2 Routine visceras to be preserved in a case poisoning

Viscera	Amount/quantities to be preserved
Stomach	Whole of it and its content
Intestine	Proximal 30 cm of intestine and its content, and in children whole of small intestine
Liver	Portion of liver, i.e. 500 g in adult, whole in children where weight may be less than 500 g, along with gallbladder
Kidneys	Half of each or one kidney

Table 10.3 Biological samples to be preserved in a case of poisoning or drug intoxication

Biological fluid or sample	Amount to be preserved	Preservatives to be used
Blood	10–20 mL	100 mg of sodium fluoride/10 mL
Urine	50–100 mL	100 mg of sodium fluoride or thymol/10 mL
CSF (by cisternal puncture)	30 mL screw capped plastic or glass container	100 mg of sodium fluoride/10 mL
Bile for drug estimation	20 mL	—
Vitreous humor (alcohols, diabetes and insulin related deaths)	10 mL collected from both eyes	Sodium fluoride (10 mg/mL)

synovial[15] fluids can be used for toxicological analysis.

Bone and Muscles

If bones[16] are available, the whole long bone (at least one) should to be collected and preserved for analysis. It is to be dried in room temperature and sealed in plastic bag. Bone marrow samples may be useful in drug identification (both qualitative and quantitative) in cases where all soft tissue has decomposed and missing. The skeletal muscle is also useful for toxicological analysis. A 100 grams of muscle tissue, i.e. the quadriceps muscle routinely can be preserved in SS (Saturated Solution) of common salt in a plastic or glass container.

Hair and Nail

Both hair and nails are useful samples for detection of chronic heavy metals poisoning or drug intoxication. Samples should be collected for analysis if poisonings are suspected, particularly to distinguish between episodic or continuous exposure or for those poisons which may have already been eliminated from the body by the time of death.

Hair can be plucked from the scalp with its whole root, shaft and tip. About 500 ng (about 20–30 number) of hair should be picked up and laid aligned by rolling into a clean plastic sheet with an indication of the scalp ends on the label. The entire nail from a toe or fingers should be preserved in a dried room temperature, sealed and labeled.

Maggots

In decomposed body, if maggots are present, 20 grams of maggots[17,18] can be collected in a plastic or glass container and preserved in SS of common salt or rectified spirit depending upon the poison. If drugs or intoxicants are detected, they could only have originated from tissues upon which the larvae were feeding. However, it is difficult to correlate the relation between the level of intoxicants in the larvae and the human. From this analysis, we can only have the qualitative information about intoxicant, etc.

Tablets, Powders and Syringes

These are especially useful in deaths in medical professional or drug addicts, who may use some medical substances that are difficult to detect once they have entered the body.

Hard plastic or glass containers are recommended for preservation for these items. The samples are best sent in their original state without adding any preservative in a refrigerated storage within few hours.

If it is not possible to send in time in an ideal state, due to lack of adept autopsy readiness, i.e. the cold storage facilities, quick transport arrangements, legal formalities and quick forensic laboratory services, etc. then the samples has to be put in ideal preservatives till they reach the laboratory. They should be preserved at 4°C temperature until they are analyzed. For long-term storage it has to be kept in freezer (-10°C) until analyzed and disposed off.

Preservatives used for Common Visceras

For preservation of viscera the commonly used preservatives are mentioned in **Table 10.4**.

Additional Samples to be Preserved Depending Upon the Circumstances

i. **Injected Poisons (or Snake Bite):** Skin along with subcutaneous tissue (portion of the vein in IV injection) around the injection (or bite) site within the radius of 2.5 cm and another similar sample from the opposite site as control, both in separate container.

ii. **Spillage on Surface:** Skin and subcutaneous tissue from affected site at least 2.5 × 2.5 sq cm size and control tissue from other site.

iii. **Inhaled Poisons:** One lung in polyethylene container for anesthetics.

iv. **Cerebral Poisons:** Half of the brain.

v. **Spinal Poison:** Spinal cord, half of brain.

vi. **Heavy Metal Poisons:** Portion of long bone, plucked hairs, nails and sample of muscles.

Apart from these, following samples are also required to be preserved depending upon the case:

i. **Insect Eggs, Maggots, Pupa:** In formalin or rectified spirit for identification, and along with 500 g of muscle in a container for entomological study for determination of time since death.

ii. **Stained Cloth:** Along with unstained portion, to be air dried.

iii. **Sample of Soils:** In exhumed cases, from above, below and all sides of the body or the coffin where the body was buried, along with control sample collected separately from some distance.

All the container of the samples should be sealed and labeled mentioning the nature of sample, preservative used along with other reference and sent to the chemical analyzer for analysis along with the sample of preservative used.

Table 10.4 Different preservatives used for viscera

Preservatives	Viscera
Rectified spirit	For all cases of poisoning except poisoning by carbolic acid, alcohol, phosphorous, paraldehyde, acetic acid, chloroform, chloral hydrate, ether, kerosine, where saturated solution of sodium chloride is used
Saturated solution of sodium chloride	For all cases of poisoning except poisoning by mineral acids or alkalis, aconite and other vegetable poisons and in case of poisoning by sodium chloride where rectified spirit is to be used

Custodial Death

In cases of death in police custody or death in prison, as per the direction of the National Human Rights Commission, video recording is to be done during the autopsy.

After completion of the autopsy, the recorded cassette is to be packed, sealed and sent to the inquesting authority that, in turn, is to send the same to the National Human Rights Commission. The name and all the references are to mentioned in the cassette before sealing. Details discussed in Chapter 27 (**Human Rights, Torture**).

REFERENCES

1. Pekka S, Barnard K. Knight's Forensic Pathology, 3rd ed. London: Arnold; 2004. p. 1.
2. Mukherjee JB. Forensic Medicine and Toxicology, 2nd ed. Calcutta: Arnold Publisher;1994. p. 7.
3. Krishan V. Textbook of Forensic Medicine and Toxicology—Principle and Practice, 5th ed. Elsevier: New Delhi; 2011. pp. 15-34.
4. Pillay VV. Textbook of Forensic Medicine and Toxicology, 16th ed. Hyderabad: Paras Medical Publisher; 2011. pp. 133-61.
5. Parikh CK. Medicolegal Postmortem in India. Bombay: Medical Publications; 1985.
6. Mathiharan K, Patnaik AK (Eds). Modi's Medical Jurisprudence and Toxicology, 23rd ed. New Delhi: LexisNexis; 2006. pp. 357-408.
7. Mahanta P. The medico-legal autopsy its religious and social attitudes. J Indian Acad Forensic Med. 2010;32(2):183-7.
8. Patowary AJ. The fourth incision—a cosmetic autopsy incision technique. Am J For Med Pathol. 2010;31(1):37-41.
9. Patowary AJ. The fourth incision—a few modifications in autopsy incisions. J Indian Acad Forensic Med. 2010;32(3):234-8.
10. Sheaff MT, Hopster DJ. Post Mortem Technique Handbook, 2nd ed. London: Springer; 2005.
11. Ludwig J. Handbook of Autopsy Practice, 3rd ed. New Jersey: Humana Press; 2002.
12. Rutty GN. Essentials of Autopsy Practices. London: Springer; 2006.
13. McCurdy WC. Postmortem specimen collection. Forensic Sci Int. 1987;35:61-5.
14. Moriya F, Hashimoto Y. Pericardial fluid as an alternative specimen to blood for postmortem toxicological analysis. Leg Med. 1999;1(2):86-94.
15. Oshima T, Kondo T, Sato Y, Takayasu T. Postmortem alcohol analysis of the synovial fluid and its availability in medicolegal practices. Forensic Sci Int. 1997;10(90):131-8.
16. Noguchi TT, Nakamma GR, Griesemer EC. Drug analysis of skeletonizing remains. J Forensic Sci. 1978;23:490-2.
17. Pouuder JD. Forensic entomotoxicology. J Forensic Sci. 1991;31:469-72.
18. Geoff ML, Ford WD. Entomotoxicology—A new area for forensic investigation. Am J For Med Pathol. 1994;15(1):51-7.

CHAPTER 11

Mechanical Injury

Putul Mahanta

LEARNING PLAN

- Learn different terminologies of medicolegal importance
- Understand the biophysics and mechanism of cell injury
- Know different types of injuries and their pathophysiologies
- Learn how features of injuries help in estimation of its age and the kind of weapons involved

SOME TERMS OF MEDICOLEGAL IMPORTANCE

Injury

The term injury is from the Latin word *injuria* (in-not, jus-the law). It is frequently used synonymously with the wound, but can have a broader use, including harm to tissues by heat, cold, chemicals, electricity, etc., in addition to physical violence. An injury is any damage to any part of the body due to the application of mechanical force.

Indian Penal Code defines an injury in **section 44** as "any harm whatever illegally caused to any person, in body, mind, reputation or property". Mechanical injuries are inflicted by means of physical violence.

Wound

In **medical point** of view wound is the break of the continuity of the tissues, created by external mechanical force. **Legally**, it can be defined as the breach of the full thickness of the skin, which excludes abrasions, bruises, internal injuries and fractures.

Trauma

It can be defined as bodily harm with or without the structural changes, ensuing from interaction with physicochemical agents, imparting energy to the tissues. It may cause morphologically apparent damage such as:

i. Wound.
ii. Physiological imbalances, e.g. reflex cardiac arrest by neuronic stimulation.
iii. Secondary effects like thrombosis, infection and obstruction of tubular organs.

Trauma is an insult to the state of well-being and may be physical or mental.[1]

Lesion

It is derived has come from the Latin word *laesio* (a hurt).

The word earlier meant injury, now more widely employed to include "any area of injury, disease or local degeneration in a tissue causing a change in its function or structure".

BIOPHYSICS OF INJURY

Energy to cause injury may be applied to tissues in different form. **Mechanical force** may induce impact, angulations, compression, traction, torsion, shearing and acceleration or deceleration as in RTA, etc.

Different body tissues have different dimensions of **elasticity** (the tendency of a body to return to its original shape after it has been stretched or compressed), **plasticity** (the property of being physically malleable) and **viscosity** (resistance of a liquid to shear forces).

Therefore, different body tissues have dissimilar **elastic limits** and are dangerous to different stresses.

Skin has a greater elastic limit than underlying fat and blood vessels, making subcutaneous bruising more common than skin laceration, e.g. torsion often causes spiral fracture of tibia but leaves soft tissues undamaged, compression often causes rupture of gas-filled lung or intestine, but muscle and skin are undamaged. The injury occurs when energy applied exceeds the elastic limits (or tolerance) of the tissues. Whether or not injury occurs following the application of energy, in whatever form, depends on **physical** and **biological factors** as mentioned follows:[2]

Physical Factors Affecting Injury

The physical factors affecting the injury are:[2]

- Degree of force or kinetic energy applied
- The area over which force is applied
- Duration of applied force
- Direction of force application

Degree of Force or Kinetic Energy Applied: Energy depends on the **mass** of the object causing injury and square of its velocity. The relation between force, mass and speed are as follows:

i. Force = Mass × Acceleration
ii. Kinetic Energy = 1/2 Mass × Velocity^2
iii. Crash energy = (mph)^2 × 0.034 (stopping distance in feet).

The Area over which Force is Applied: Same force spread over a larger area is less likely to injure at the site of impact. Edge or tip of knife allows a greater concentration of force applied to the site of impact. Edge of a board is more damaging than its flat surface. The heal of stiletto is more damaging than its sole and soft object deforms and flattens.

Duration of Applied Force: Longer duration of applied force allows tissues at the site of impact to deform and break up the applied energy, e.g. fall onto soft surface increases duration and area of impact, seat belt stretching retards the rate of transfer of kinetic energy to the body and spreads the area of impact over the trunk.

Direction of Force Application: If the direction of hitting object is glancing or with exiting bullet the release of kinetic energy (KE) is not complete. Therefore, some of its injuring potential is lost and completed when the hitting object come to on rest in the body.

Biological Factors Affecting Injury

The biological factors that affect wounding are:

- **Movement of the Involved Part**: While the involved part is fixed, it draws all applied energy, whereas the moving parts transform into kinetic energy to motion.
- **Anticipation and Coordination:** Rolling with a fall is the example of anticipation and coordination, viz. catching of a cricket ball.
- **Biomechanical Properties of Tissue**: Different tissues have different bio-mechanical properties like strengths and weaknesses. They are as follows:[2]
    - Skin is more elastic and resistant than its underlying tissues.
    - Blood vessels are more resistant to comp-ression than stretching.
    - Bone more resistant to bending than to torsion, hollow.

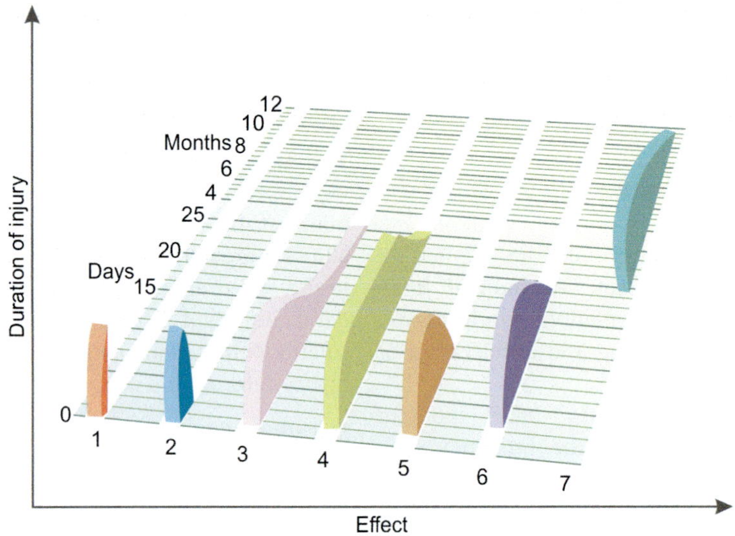

Figure 11.1 Schematic diagram demonstrating responses of tissue following an injury, 1. Clotting; 2. Vascular response; 3. Inflammation; 4. Scar formation; 5. Epithelial healing; 6. Contraction; 7. Scar remodeling

- Fluid-filled organs sensitive to compression.
- Brain more resistant to direct impact than rotational impact.
- Bone and joint may transmit force to a weak point.

PRINCIPLES OF CELL INJURY[3]

A number of general principles are relevant to most forms of cell injury. They are:

i. The cellular response to injurious stimuli depends on the type of injury, its duration and its severity.
ii. The consequences of an injurious stimulus depend on the type, status, adaptability and genetic makeup of injured cells.
iii. Four intracellular systems are particularly vulnerable: (a) Cell membrane integrity; (b) ATP generation; (c) Protein synthesis and (d) The integrity of genetic apparatus.
iv. The structural and biochemical components of a cell are so integrally connected that regardless of the initial locus of injury, multiple secondary effects rapidly occur.
v. Cellular function is lost far before cell death occurs, and the morphological changes of cell injury lag far behind both. Different responses of tissue following an injury are shown in **Figure 11.1**.

TYPES OF INJURY

Medical Classification

Energy may be applied to tissues in various forms, which may result injuries of different kinds as follows:

Mechanical Injuries

a. Due to **blunt force** impact: A moving object (KE) striking the body as in a blow or the moving body striking a fixed object or surface, as in case of fall, may cause abrasions, bruises, lacerations, fractures and dislocations of a bone, tooth or joint.
b. Due to **sharp edged** weapons: Knife tip or edge, broken glass, jagged metal when concentrated over a small area, requires little force to cut the tissues and may cause incised wound, chop wounds, stab wounds.
c. Due to **firearms:** High velocity, small mass projectile fired from gun causes firearm injuries, which is a punctured wound.

Thermal Injuries

Due to Application of Heat

Due to general effects of exposure to heat. Hot atmosphere may not cause any visible injury, but they may cause:

i. Heat hyperpyrexia (heat stroke or sun stroke).
ii. Heat exhaustion or heat collapse.
iii. Heat cramps or miner's cramps.

Due to Local Application of Heat

i. Burn (due to application of dry heat).
ii. Scald (due to application of moist heat).

Due to Application of Cold

i. Exposure to cold that may cause hypothermia.
ii. Local effects of exposure to cold: frostbite, trench foot and immersion foot.

Chemical Injuries

Chemical injury is as a result of chemical reaction with tissue releasing energy, as is the case with corrosive **acids** and **alkalis**.

Miscellaneous Injuries

a. **Electrical energy** causes electrocution: Flow of current may cause localized burn, if resistance is high.
b. **Blasting injuries**, which is a combination of mechanical and thermal injuries.
c. **Radiation injury**: Particles such as radioactive substances or radiation like X-rays, which is a form of electromagnetic radiation.
d. **Lightning injuries** (a combination of electrical, mechanical and thermal injuries).

Legal Classification

Legally, injury can be divided as simple and grievous injury.

Medicolegal Classification

It can be suicidal, homicidal and accidental. Fabricated and defense wounds has also tremendous medicolegal value.

ABRASION

The term abrasion is from Latin *ab-* from and *radere-* "to scrape"
Synonym: Scratch, graze
It is the simplest form of mechanical injury on a portion of the body surface involving epidermis or papillary dermis, or body lining epithelium caused by rubbing due to blunt force impact. Abrasion always occurs at the site of impact.

Mechanism of Abrasion

There is superficial crushing of epidermis or papillary dermis caused by **direct impact**. It is the process of scuffing, scratching, wearing down, marring or rubbing away. Abrasion injuries most commonly occur when exposed skin comes into moving contact with a rough surface, causing a grinding or rubbing away of the upper layers of the epidermis. It is more often seen in road traffic fatalities. Many abrasions have both a vertical and tangential component.

Abrasions are **clinically trivial**. Although they are painful, bleeding is slight and leads to crust or scab formation. The mechanism of production of abrasion is shown in **Figure 11.2**. It heals without scarring (by re-epithelialization). Abrasions are often associated with bruising and laceration.

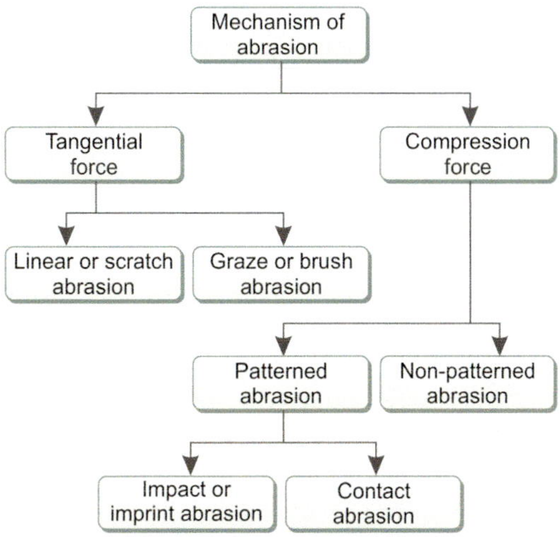

Figure 11.2 Mechanism of abrasion

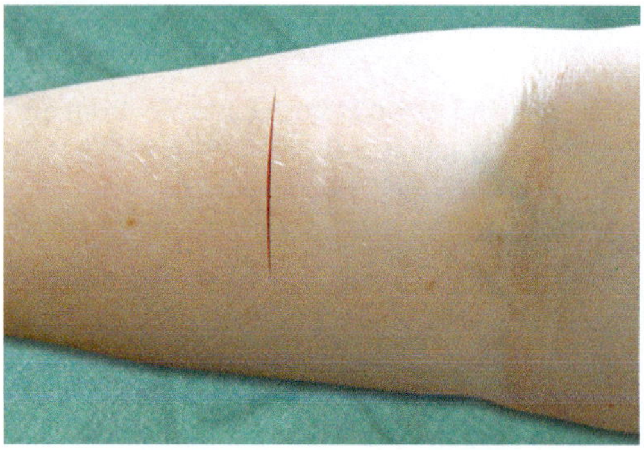

Figure 11.3 Linear abrasion

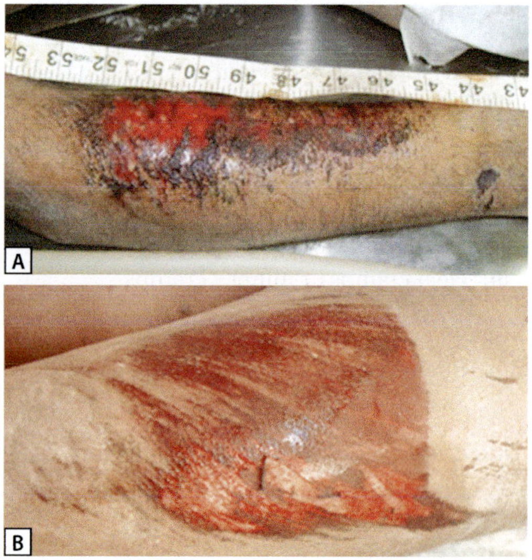

Figures 11.4A and B Scraping of epidermis in grazed abrasion

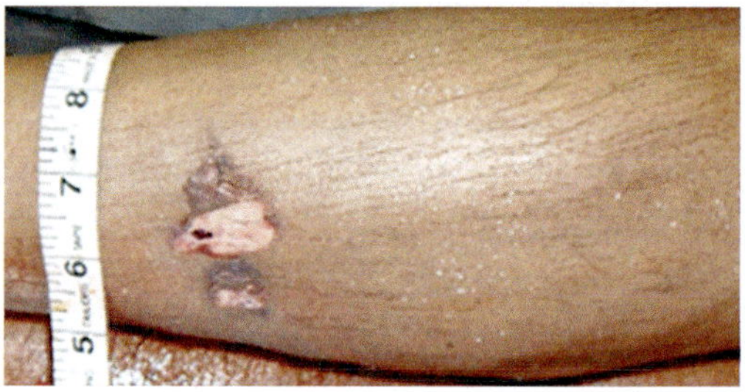

Figure 11.5 Abrasion showing tag

Types of Abrasion

On the basis of their features and manner of production, there are four types of abrasion.

Scratch or Linear Abrasion

These types of abrasions are caused due to:

i. Tangential or horizontal friction by the pointed end of weapons like needle, pin, thorn, etc.
ii. Or by the perpendicular friction with some linear object like nail or linear projection of vehicle.

There is loss or scraping of epidermis or papillary dermis due to this **tangential friction** or **impact** on sharp point. The abrasion is wider at the starting point and shows heaping of epithelium (accumulation) at the end (**Figure 11.3**). The direction of force is from the wider side to the narrower side of the scratch.

Graze or Brush Abrasion

It is also called sliding abrasion, gliding abrasion or scrape abrasion (**Figure 11.4**). This is due to a glancing (tangential) or horizontal impact by a moving objects to stationary body or the moving body against a rough wider stationary surface.

Scraping of **epidermis** is due to friction against a rough surface. Stratum corneum and superficial epidermal cells are removed, causing exudation of fluid. Deeper loss of epidermis may expose capillary loops in papillary dermis and cause bleeding. The graze abrasions are wider at the starting point and they get narrower at the end with heaping of epithelium at the end.

Direction of impact can often be assessed: starting edge has bevelled descent; a series of parallel furrows indicate direction of sliding motion; finishing edge has tags of heaped epidermis (**Figures 11.4** and **11.5**).

In road traffic accident (RTA), body is thrown across the rough road surface (gravel rash), falls or assault with a rough surfaced instrument, etc., resulting graze abrasion. When the friction force is extensive, grazed area resembles burn injury. Such graze abrasions are called as **brush burn** (**Figure 11.6**).

In graze abrasion, the abrasion shows uneven, longitudinal, parallel lines (grooves or furrows) with epithelium heaped up at the ends (**Figure 11.7**).

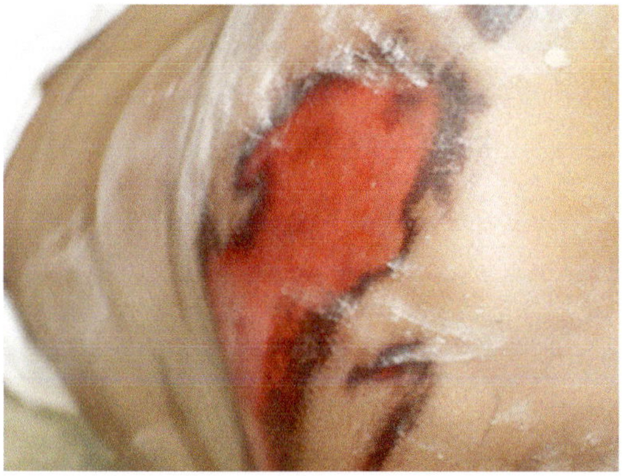

Figure 11.6 Brush burn

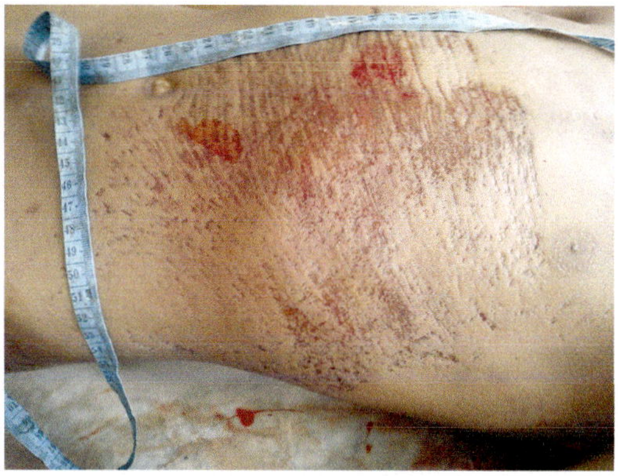

Figure 11.7 Abrasion over front of chest

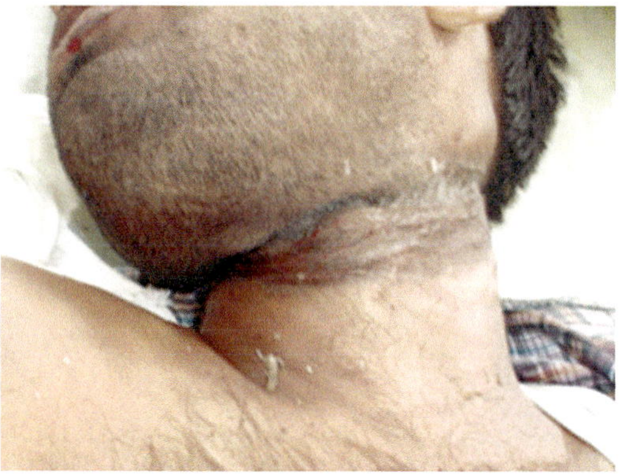

Figure 11.8 Pressure abrasions around neck

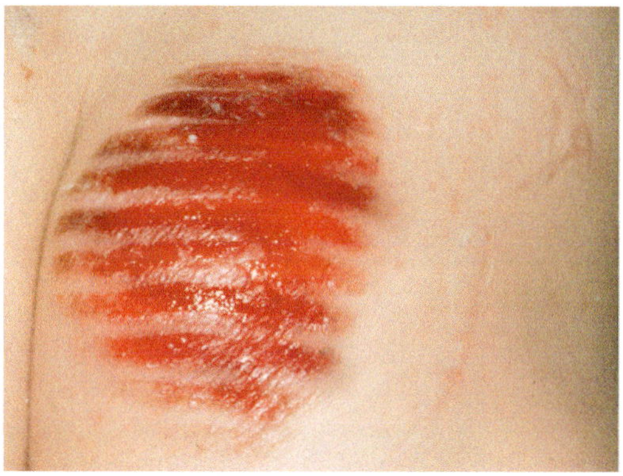

Figure 11.9 Imprint abrasion

Pressure Abrasion

It is also known as crushing abrasion. In some books, authors have also mentioned it to be imprint abrasion.

These are caused by direct vertical impact, which causes crushing of epidermis. The causative object may stamp its shape or surface pattern on the skin. Examples: Rope weaves in hanging (**Figure 11.8**) or ligature in strangulation, fabric weave of seat belt, clothes. In pressure abrasion, due to crushing, skin on getting dried up resembles parchment and appears brown to black.

Imprint Abrasion

It is also known as **impact** or **patterned abrasion** or **contact abrasion.** These abrasions (**Figure 11.9**) are produced when force is applied perpendicular to the skin. Direct vertical impact causes crushing of epidermis. When object strikes the skin, it leaves its impression over the skin.

Skin gets depressed or compressed as per the pattern of the object and reproduces the pattern of object. Whip marks on beating with whip; tyre tread mark or radiator grill mark over skin in RTA; **bite mark** (double crescent of spaced linear impressions) and **fingernail impressions** (crescentic) on neck in throttling (as shown in **Figure 11.10**), wrists, thighs and vulva in rape.

Healing of an Abrasion

An abrasion is healed by contraction of the injury and replacement of its lost tissues. Initially, it will be covered by red scab (**Figure 11.11**) composed of blood and lymph.

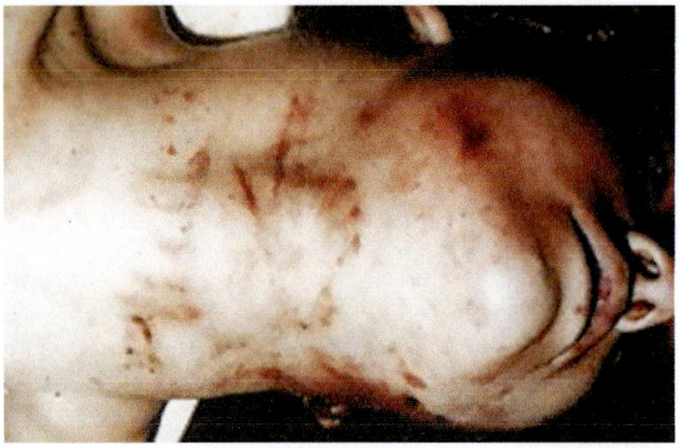

Figure 11.10 Manual strangulation (throttling) with imprint abrasions and bruises

Table 11.1 Age of abrasion

Age	Features
Fresh	Reddish, no scab
12–24 hours	Dark red scab
1–3 days	Reddish brown scab
3–5 days	Dark brown scab
5–7 days	Blackish scab shrinks and falling begins from margin
7–10 days	Scab falls off, leaving hypo pigmented area

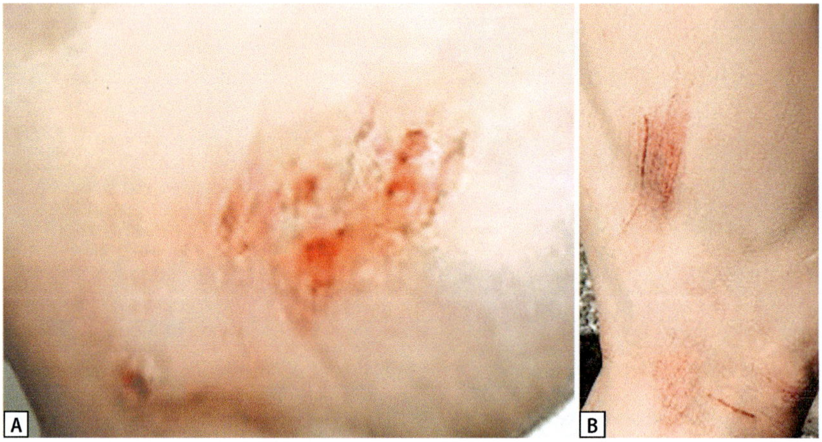

Figures 11.11A and B Dark red scabs

Microscopically, there is cellular infiltration seen at about 4-6 hours, and about 12 hours, three layers are identified consisting of surface zone of fibrin.

Age of Abrasion

The features from which age of abrasion is determined are mentioned in **Table 11.1**.

Bite Marks[2]

The marks may be abrasions, bruises or lacerations, or a combination of all these injuries. Clarity depends on contour of part bitten and the force applied. Animal bite is **deeply arched** or **'U-shaped'**. Human bite is near circular or shallow and oval shaped. Details discussed in the chapter of **Forensic Odontology** (**Chapter 7**).

Medicolegal Importance

1. It has significant forensic important and is the most informative of all injures.
2. Always reflect site of impact, frequently indicate causative object or surface and often indicate direction of impact.
3. Age of abrasions can be assessed.
4. Postmortem drying of abraded surface causes a golden yellow or reddish, leathery and **parchment-like** appearance.
5. Depth and breadth often useful for comparison with assailant and dragging of victim away from scene of crime may be helpful in crime investigation.
6. Presence of foreign materials (sand particle) may connect the criminal with the crime.

7. Abrasion near the breasts, neck, thighs, abdomen and vulva of a female indicates sexual violence, etc.
8. If seen in any site in children may be child abuse.
9. Self-inflicted or fabricated abrasion is usually over the accessible part.

CONTUSION

From middle English bruisen, from old English brysan-to crush.
Synonym: Bruise and Ecchymosis.
Contusion or bruise is the "escape of blood from ruptured small vessels (vein, capillaries, and arterioles) into the surrounding tissues" due to blunt force impact. The resulting discoloration is seen through the overlaying intact skin. The site, shape, size and severity of bruising are variable.

The term '**hemorrhage**' or '**bleeding**' means the escape of blood, from any part of the vascular system. It can either be external, from a skin wound, or internal, into a body cavity. Bruising is hemorrhage into the adjacent tissues. It may be seen in skin, muscle or any internal organ. Very small bruises, ranging in size from a pinpoint to a pinhead, may be described as petechiae, petechial or, alternatively, punctate hemorrhages. Hemorrhage or bleeding is the process which produces a bruise in tissues, but the term hemorrhage also encompasses bleeding which may not be associated with bruising, e.g. a bleeding nose or a bleeding stomach ulcer. **Petechiae** are the small, approximately **1–2** mm red or purple spot on the body, as a result of tiny hemorrhages of blood vessels in the skin.

Mechanism of Contusion

i. It is due to blunt force impact when a moving object strikes the stationary body; a moving body strikes a fixed target, i.e. fall.
ii. Usually the more elastic overlying skin is undamaged, but causing crushing or tearing of subcutaneous tissue or deep dermis. The extravasations of blood are due to rupture of blood vessel, which finally get collected surrounding tissues (**Figure 11.12**). The said collection may be associated with pain and swelling. Skin abrasion or laceration may also be present. It is less often associated with incised or stab wounds, which allow outward escape of blood from cut vessels. However, bruising may be external and internal.

In external or superficial bruising it rapidly comes out at the site of impact. Bleeding in the

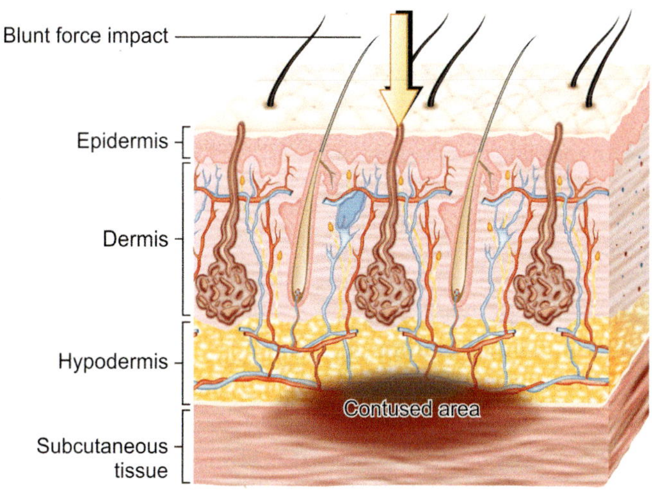

Figure 11.12 Mechanism of contusion formation

subcutaneous tissue may be seen through the semi-translucent skin.

However, **internal** or deep bruising is not visible through overlying fat and skin. They can be seen at the surface of the organ. Deeper bruise in muscle or internal organ, e.g. neck in strangulation, blows to chest or abdomen is not visible through overlying skin. The site of contusion not inevitably reflect site of impact. Hemorrhage into the adjacent tissues may continue for some time after impact under circulatory pressure. Extravagated blood passes over along the natural or traumatic planes of least resistance, influenced by force of gravity and movement of the body. For example:

1. Blow on head—bruise seen on cheek
2. Fractured jaw—bruising seen on neck
3. Fractured hip—bruise seen on thigh

Delayed Appearance

The deep seated bruise usually takes upto 24 hours to appear over the surface. Therefore, follow-up of the victim after 24 hours may bring out the unseen bruises. Ultraviolet light may disclose an otherwise unrecognizable bruise. Hemolysis of RBCs with time releases of breakdown pigments, which may spread outwards and stain the tissues over a wider area then the original intact red blood cells of the fresh bruise. Pigments may spread closer to the overlying translucent skin, thus becoming visible on the surface a few days after injury.

Degree of Force Enforced

i. As the skin has heavier limit of elasticity in comparison to underlying tissues like, fat and blood vessels hence, subcutaneous bruise is more common than skin laceration.
ii. It is not possible to measure the degree of force applied from the size of a bruise. However, heavy impact is generally causes a larger bruise.

The following factors regulating the severity of bruising:

i. **Body Site**: Apparent bony prominence (i.e. chin, cheeks), lax, vascular tissue (like, eyelid, orbit) and fatty tissues (buttocks) will bruise easily. Similarly, it is very rare to bruise the more resilient muscle of anterior abdominal wall although severe underlying visceral injury is present. Dense, tightly attached tissue, e.g. palms and soles, seldom bruises. Dense fibrous tissue physically limits collection of blood.
ii. **Age**: Infants have loose, delicate, fatty tissues, which bruise easily. Because of degenerative changes of blood vessels and connective tissues elderly people develop easy bruising.
iii. **Obesity** and **Sex**: Obese people bruise better than lean due to a greater proportion of subcutaneous fat. Females in general bruise better due to having a greater proportion of subcutaneous fat than men.
iv. **Presence of Disease**: There is spontaneous bruise in hemophilia, leukemia and platelet disorders. It is also seen in some infectious condition like meningitis, liver disorder, alcoholism, scurvy, poor nutrition and medications.
v. **Color of Skin**: It is more apparent in fair skin. Black skin may mask bruising. UV light may confirm the same.

Age of Contusion

Color changes begin at the periphery and progress towards center if the contusion is large. Smaller bruises may change color uniformly. Pigments, including bilirubin and hemosiderin are released from hemoglobin within degenerating red blood cells. A little bruise in a healthy individual may disappear in a week whereas a **love bite** mark may take 2 to 3 days to go away.

The **time course** is **variable**, which depends on adequacy of lymphatic as well as venous drainage, size and depth of bruise, anatomical site, age of the person and general health. Accurate timing of a bruise is not possible. Differentiating fresh from old is easier and often important in cases of repeated assault,

Table 11.2 Age of contusion

Age	Features	Caused by
Immediately	Dark red	Color of capillary blood
1–3 days	Bluish	Deoxyhemoglobin
Subsequent color changes are variable in timing and result from hemolysis by enzymes and cellular products.		
4 days	Bluish black to brown	Hemosiderin pigments
5–6 days or more	Green	Hematoidin pigments
7–12 days or more	Yellow	Bilirubin pigments
14–15 days (range 1–4 weeks)	Complete disappears	-

child abuse, etc. The features from which age of contusion is determined are mentioned in **Table 11.2**.

Why Color Change is Not Seen in Subconjunctival Hemorrhage?

The subconjunctival hemorrhages is the collections of blood under the conjunctiva (bruise), which do not show the normal color changes as the oxygen is present in the conjunctiva. The supply of O_2 comes either through eyelids or through the process of diffusion from the atmosphere through the cornea.

Differentiation from Postmortem Lividity

It is the settling of blood into the bottommost blood vessels under the force of gravity after the circulation ends. This results in a normal pinkish discoloration of the skin in the dependent parts of the body (**Figure 11.13**).

Blood vessels of the compressed part and the area will remain pale. Postmortem lividity sometimes may be confused with contusion. Distribution, pallor, oozing of blood from cut ends, engorged vessels, and washable blood stains can well differentiate a postmortem bruise. Incision over a true bruise reveals escape of blood into the tissues, which cannot be rinsed away (**Figure 11.14**).

However, release of blood cells and blood pigments into the adjacent tissues due to putrefactive breakdown may really be difficult to distinguish from bruising.

Postmortem Bruise

The possibilities of postmortem bruising is there, but it needs heavy force to give rise a small bruise. Only passive oozing from ruptured vessels after death is there. It occurs commonly in those areas of postmortem lividity, where blood is under tremendous physical pressure. It may also appear over bony prominences where tissues are crushed against the underlying bone, e.g. back of the head.

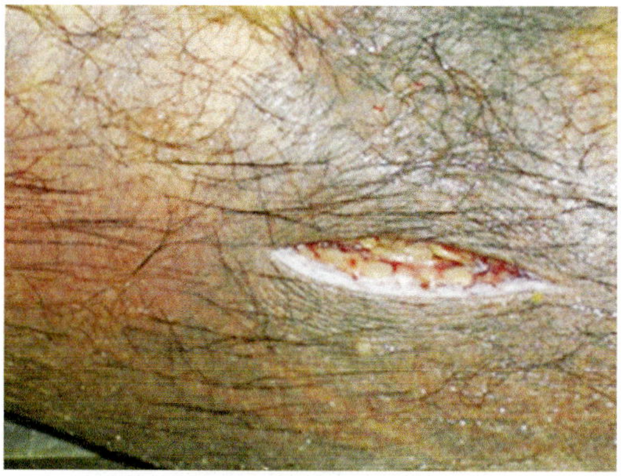

Figure 11.13 Postmortem incisions over hypostasis area

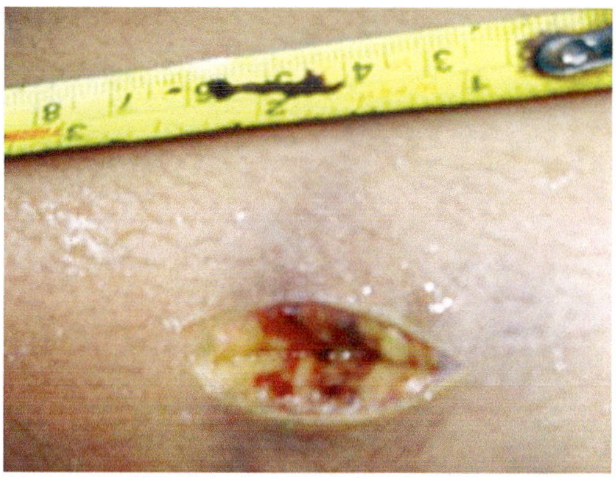

Figure 11.14 Postmortem incisions over contused area

Types of Bruising

Patterned Intradermal Bruise

These types of patterned intradermal bruises are produced due to hard, patterned blunt object with ridges or grooves. The part of the skin over ridges will be compressed and vessels remain intact. In the same way the skin is forced into the grooves resulting ruptures of the small dermal vessels. Here, bruise is situated in the sub-epidermal layer of skin resulting accumulation of a small amount of blood, near the epidermis which may demonstrate the obvious pattern of the causal surface (**Figure 11.15**) of the object/weapon.

Examples of patterned intradermal bruises are shoe thread marks, tyre marks (**Figure 11.16**), clothing, gun muzzle marks (**Figure 11.17**), etc. These may often be helpful to trace the outline of the object involved for later comparison.

Subcutaneous Bruise

This is the common type and is located in the subcutaneous tissues. Finger pad bruises are the example.

Finger pad bruises are round/oval, may be slightly larger than the finger tips which is due to outward spread of blood, and it is due to grip by fingertips in forceful restraint (**Figure 11.18**). In case of child abuse (limbs and face), rape (over the thighs), manual strangulation (neck), etc. they are common.

Tram-line or Rail-track Bruises

Produced due to a rod shaped weapon or stick. Vessels are centrally compressed and are not damaged commonly unless it is crushed onto bone. Rupture of vessels along edges of rod is because of traction. The bruise is limited to

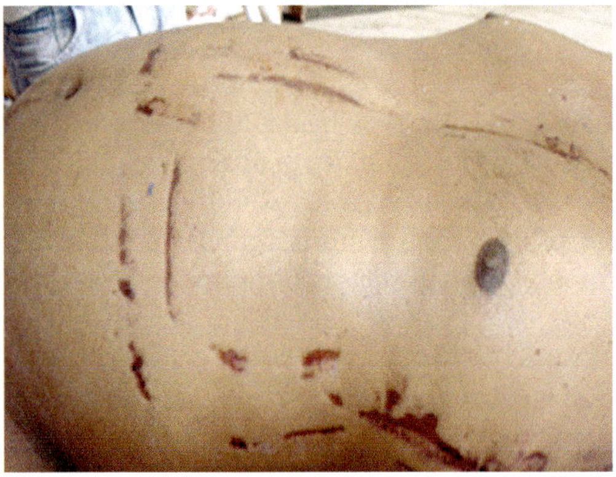

Figure 11.15 Patterned intradermal bruise

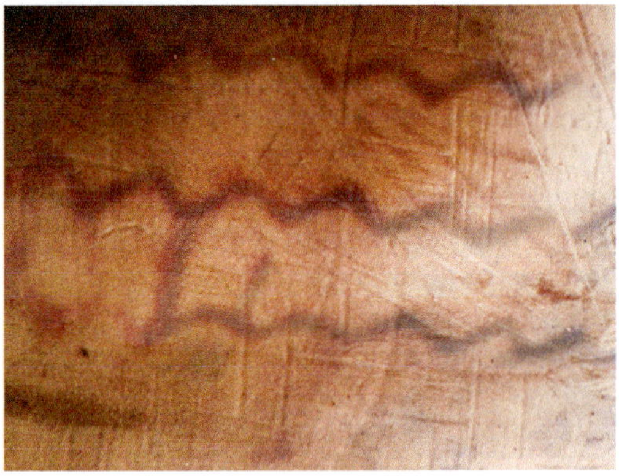

Figure 11.16 Tyre marks
(*Courtesy:* Dr Mrinal Halloi, GMCH, Assam)

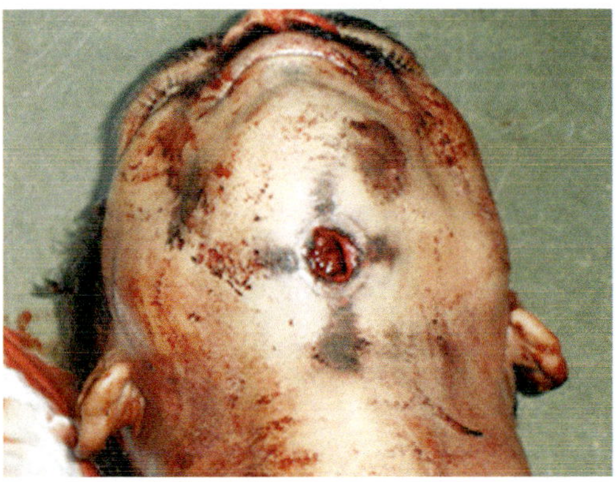

Figure 11.17 Muzzle marks of a gun

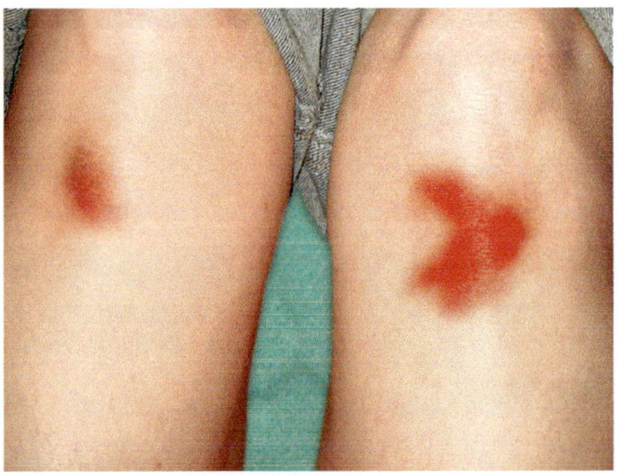

Figure 11.18 Finger pad bruises over legs

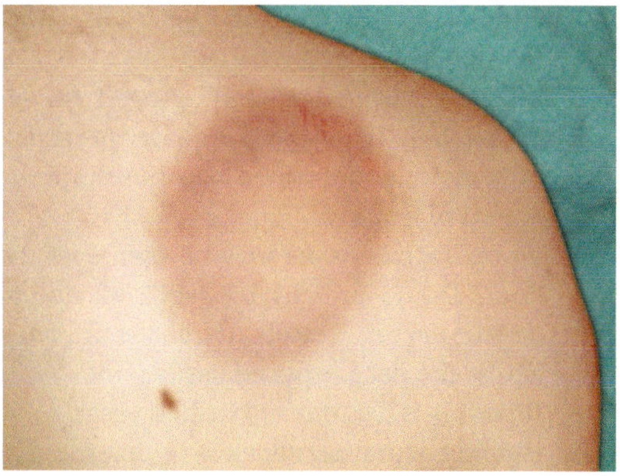

Figure 11.19 Doughnut bruise over back of chest

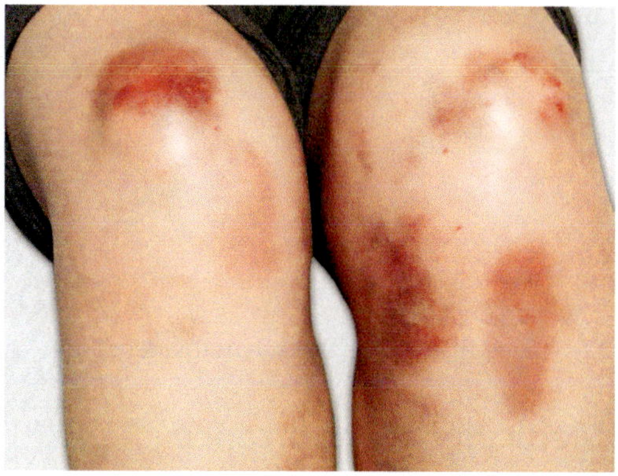

Figure 11.20 Counter pressure bruises over bony prominences

the convexity of the body surface of the object. Therefore, two parallel linear bruises, so-called 'tram-line' or 'rail-track' bruises are seen as a result of a hitting with a long object, which has a circular cross-section, such as stick.

Doughnut Bruise

They are due to a spherical object like cricket ball as shown in **Figure 11.19**. It gives a rough impression about the causative object.

Counter Pressure Bruise

These types of bruises are seen over bony prominences, viz. over shoulder blades, sacrum and back due to forceful restraint against hard surface. It is more common in muscles than skin (**Figure 11.20**).

Kicking or Shoe Foot Bruise

The shoe foot bruise may be produced by stamping, jumping leaving behind the pattern of the sole of a shoe. While peeking kick produces a scuffed abrasion, direct blow, i.e., the swinging kick may result in bruising besides laceration or imprint abrasion. Face, neck, loin, groin, back and chest are the common sites.

Love Bite or Hickey Bruise

As shown in **Figure 11.21**, it is not a true bite mark as it lacks the teeth marks of the individual.

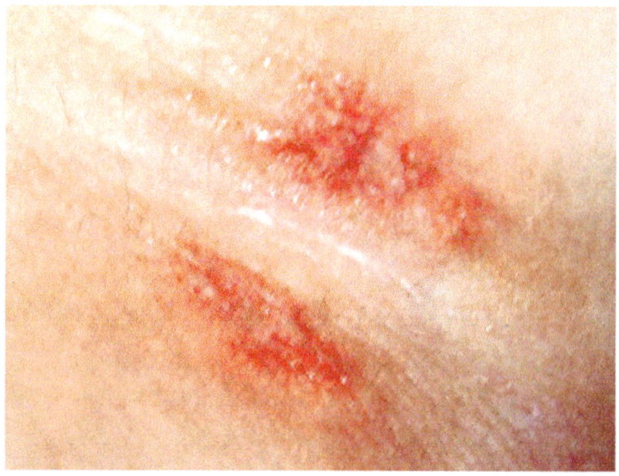

Figure 11.21 Love bite or hickey

Suction bruises are usually produced due to firm application of the lips against the skin, forming an air-tight seal, oral suction causing petechial bruises from rupture of numerous small vessels. Commonly found on teenagers and seen on neck, breasts and inner part of thigh in sexual assault. The same type of appearance may also be seen in the dental arches of a **true bite**.

Black Eye or Peri-orbital Hematoma (Figure 11.22)

There are many causes of peri-orbital hematoma. They are: Fist blow to the orbit, fractured skull, intracranial hemorrhage and blood tracking from forehead bruises. Blunt trauma to the face may cause abrasion, bruising, etc. over bony prominences.

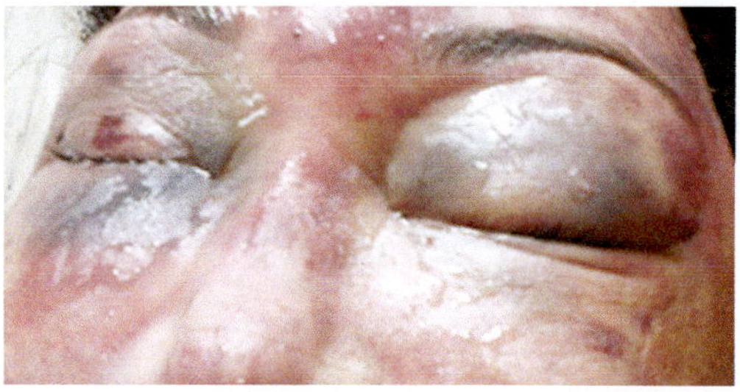

Figure 11.22 Black eyes (bilateral)

Medicolegal Importance

1. Cardiac resuscitation may cause sternal and cardiac bruising.
2. The age of the bruise can be determined. Different aged bruises hints repeated assaults as in child abuse, wife or husband battering and in alcoholics.
3. Injection sites may be accompanied with bruising.
4. Butterfly bruises may be present due to pinching of skin to test conscious level.
5. Character and manner of bruise can be identified. Usually, it is accidental or homicidal; rarely self-inflicted due to its painful and unimpressive nature.
6. Shape and size of the bruises are variable and is poor indicator of causative object.

Expanding upon a bruise dims its outline. A small hard object may cause bruise, immediately prior to death, may retain the pattern of the object.

LACERATION

From Latin *lacerare*—to tear.
It is a type of mechanical injury where there is full thickness tearing of skin or tissue due to stretching and crushing by blunt force impact. This is a three-dimensional injury which has length, breadth and depth.

Characteristics Features

1. **Shape**: Irregular, in a very few occasions, it may take the shape of the causing weapon.
2. **Size**: Less likely to match with the causative object.
3. **Dimensions**: Length and breadth are more than the depth of the injury.
4. **Margins**: Irregular and ragged edges associated with bruising or abrasion, bulging fat and crushed hair bulbs are the common features.
5. **Floor**: Tags of tissue may be seen over the floor. Tissue bridges in depth of wound (intact nerves, vessels, tendons) are seen across the deep exposed tissue.
6. **Bleeding** is less due to crushed vessels.
7. **Healing**: Duration depends upon extend of damage and associated infection. It leaves permanent scars due to damage to skin.

Mechanism: When the skin or other body structures are subjected to blunt forces, either by moving object or by fall induce laceration. The tissue due to pinning, crushing and stretching beyond the limits of elasticity causes in splitting and tearing.

Types of Laceration

Split Laceration

Here skin gets split due to compression against the underlying bone. Evidently, edges of the split laceration looks like clean cut on casual review thus it is also called **incised-looking** laceration.

Close inspection by magnifying lens reveal contused edges and presence of bridging of tissues. This type of laceration is commonly present over the bony prominences, where tissue is pinned, crushed and stretched against underlying bone, e.g. scalp, eyebrow, cheek, lower jaw, shin, dorsal aspect of hand, etc (**Figure 11.23**).

In incised-looking split laceration where there is confusion, hair root examination can prove the nature of injury, where the hair root will be crushed as shown in **Figure 11.24**.

Stretch Laceration

Due to overstretching of fixed skin tissues, it get lacerated with a flapping of the skin because of heavy frictional impact by a hard and rough blunt object. The flapping gives the direction

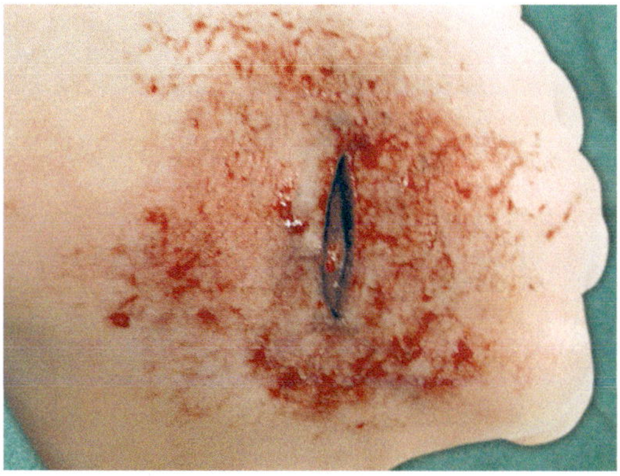

Figure 11.23 Split laceration

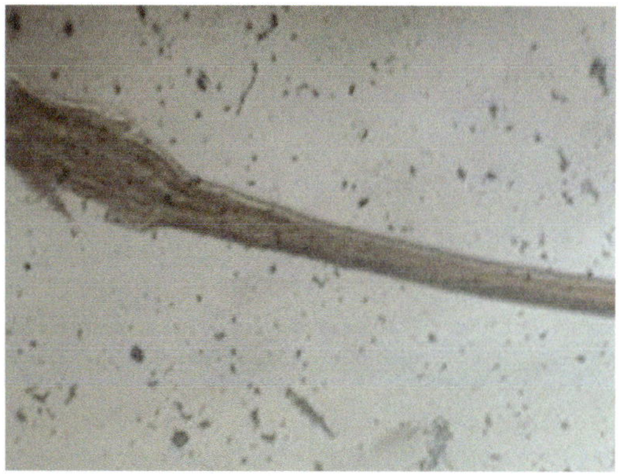

Figure 11.24 Crushed hair root due to blunt force impact

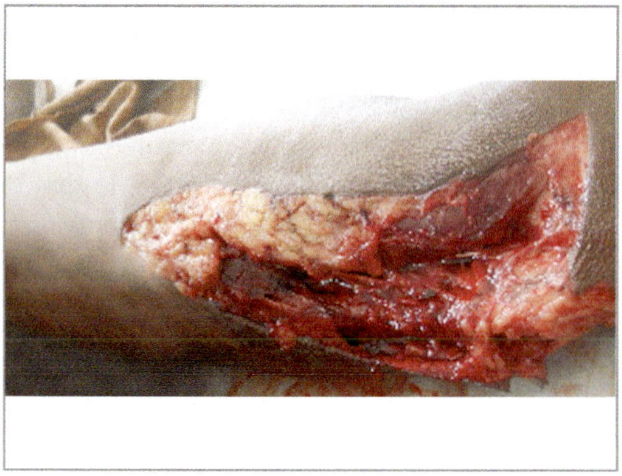

Figure 11.25 Avulsion laceration

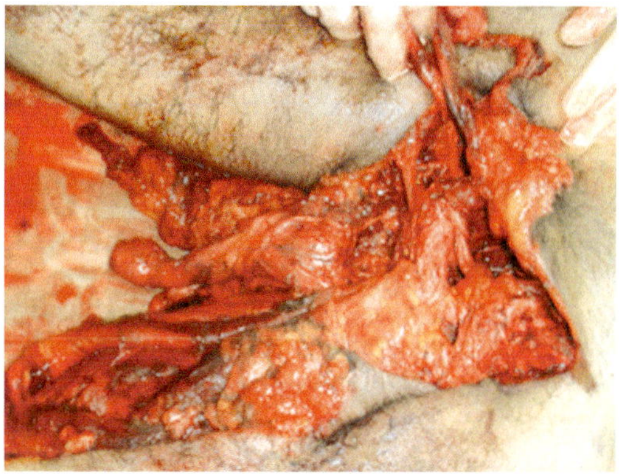

Figure 11.26 Crush laceration of pelvis

of force. It is usually seen when two ends of the fractured bones stretches the tissues beyond their limits. A blunt and projecting object if pulls the tissues obliquely against its elasticity, causes stretching and tearing of the involved tissues.

Avulsion Laceration

It is also known as flying or grinding laceration. Rolling or grinding movement of a car wheel may strip and split tissues involved (**Figure 11.25**). The involved parts are avulsed due to the weight of the grinding compression, having a pocket, which usually contains fat and blood.

There may be gross damage of tissues in avulsion, called **crush lacerations** which are commonly caused by run over cases by vehicles, as shown in **Figures 11.26** and **11.27**. Tissue bridging is a feature at the depth of wound.

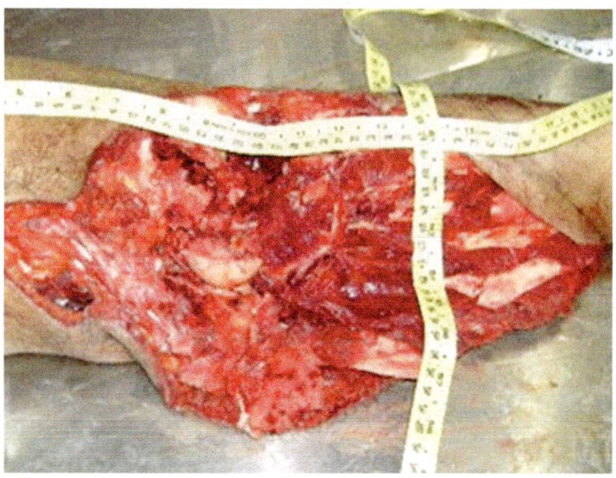

Figure 11.27 Crush laceration of leg

Tear Laceration

It is a common form of laceration. Here it is due to tearing of skin and subcutaneous tissues, which are being struck by an irregular hard object and

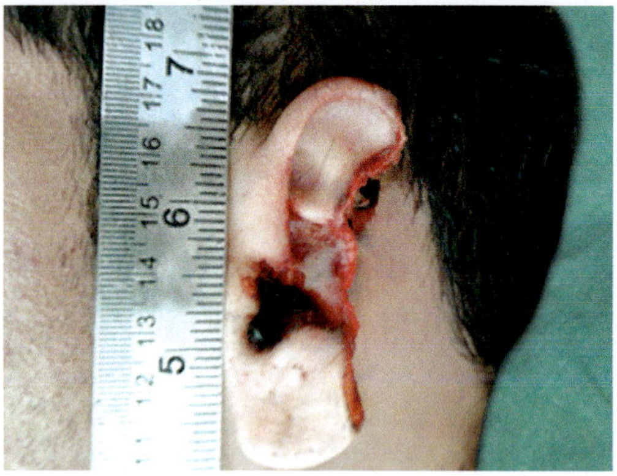

Figure 11.28 Tear laceration of left ear
(*Courtesy:* Dr Mrinal Haloi, GMCH Guwahati, Assan, India)

Table 11.3 Shape of laceration in relation to causative object

Shape of laceration	Object anticipation
Crescentic or circular	Round-headed object with an edge, viz. hammer head
Y-shaped	Linear round object such as metallic rod
Inside lips (trauma against teeth)	Blow to mouth
Flaying laceration	Rolling or stretching of skin over limb as in RTA (road traffic accident)
Stellate	Rolling or stretching of skin over limb in RTA mainly by object with a blunt round end

features, are similar to stretch laceration. It is deeper at start than its ending. The acting force from object splits the skin or tissues producing tear laceration, as shown in **Figure 11.28.**

Cut Laceration

This type of lacerations is produced by heavy to moderately heavy weapons with slight sharp edge as stated in some textbooks and is seen with chop wounds, when inflicted with a rusted uneven edge of heavy weapon. Here the margins may be abraded or contused.

Medicolegal Importance

1. Age estimation is difficult and unpredictable as they do not show uniform healing pattern.
2. It provides little specific information about the causal object. Shape and size of a laceration is not related to causal object and depth. Though shapes are variable, in certain situation it may be helpful, as mentioned in **Table 11.3.**
3. Trace evidence in wound like foreign body may be present. Grease, mud, etc, may be seen in wounds of vehicular accident.
4. It is rarely self-inflicted, usually accidental and homicidal.
5. A tangential component may give one clean-cut edge, other ragged, undercut or flap-like.
6. Surgical importance of laceration is that it often causes little external blood loss except scalp due to crushing and retraction of vessels. Associated internal injury or bleeding may be present. Wound infection is frequent and it heals by scarring.

Clinical Importance

1. Infection is very common thus retarding the healing process.
2. Bleeding is less due to crushed and retraction of the vessels except scalp.
3. Associated with internal injuries.
4. Heals by secondary intention with formation of scar. The time required will depend upon the extent of damage and severity of laceration.

INCISED WOUNDS

Latin ***incidere*** "cut into". Surgical term incision with scalpel.
Synonym: Cuts, slashes, slice wound.
It is defined as clean cut of the full thickness of skin (or other tissue) under the pressure of a sharp-edged weapon like knife, dagger, razor, *katari*, etc. Incised wounds have three-dimensions.

An incised wound (**Figure 11.29**) is **longer than its depth** due to **swipe** action.

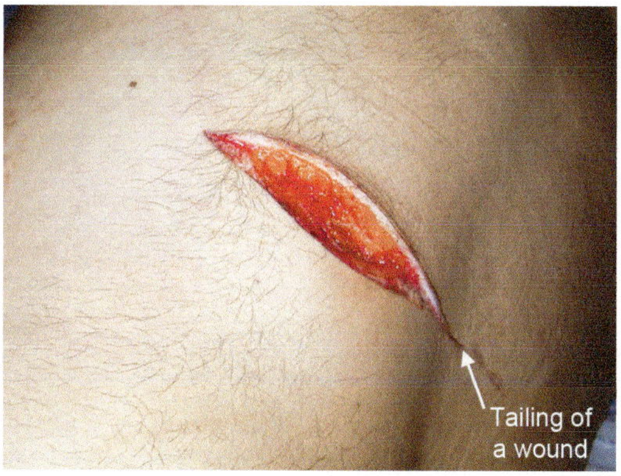

Figure 11.29 Elliptical shaped incised wound

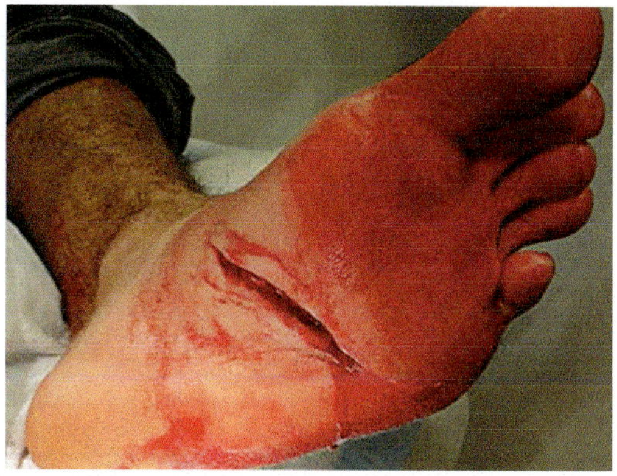

Figure 11.30 Incised wound over plantar aspect of foot

Instruments are sharp-edged, viz., knife, jagged metal and broken glass.

Characteristics Features

1. **Length** is more than its **breadth** and **depth** as shown in **Figures 11.30** and **11.31**. Length of the wound does not correspond with the length of the blade of the weapon when the incised wound is caused by drawing or sawing.
2. **Clean-cut edges** with everted margins, except the areas where the skin is wrinkled and loose.
3. Usually not associated with bruising or abrasion.
4. Underlying tissue is clean cut.
5. No tissue bridges.
6. Linear or **elliptical** shape, often gapes. They are deepest at the beginning, gradually becomes shallow, to finally end in a skin-deep scratch, known as '**tailing of a wound**'. With single-edged weapon, tailing is at one side and for double-edged weapon tailing is present at both the ends.
7. Jagged if inflicted through loose, folded skin as in scrotum.

Age of the Wound

Wound healing, or **cicatrization**, is an intricate process in which the skin (or another organ-

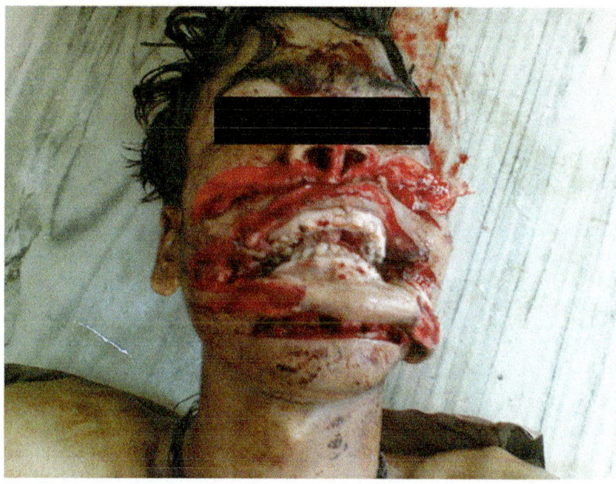

Figure 11.31 Incised wounds over face
(*Courtesy:* Dr Yogender Malik, BPS Govt. Medical College for Women)

tissue) repairs itself after injury.[4] In normal skin, the epidermis and dermis exists in steady-state equilibrium, forming a protective barrier against the external environment. Once the protective barrier is broken, the normal (physiologic) process of wound healing is immediately set in motion. The classic model of wound healing is divided into three or four sequential, yet overlapping,[5] phases: (1) Hemostasis, (2) Inflammatory, (3) Proliferative and (4) Remodeling.[6] Upon injury to the skin, a set of complex biochemical events takes place in a closely orchestrated cascade to repair the damage.[5] The chronologies of the healing process of a non-infected incised wound are given below (**Table 11.4**). If infected, the healing schedule shall be varied.

Table 11.4 Healing of incised wound

Time interval	Healing process
When fresh	Bleeding presents, fresh soft clot may be adherent to the margins, red, slightly edematous and tender
At 12 hours	Margins are red and swollen; blood clot dry up, leukocytic infiltration present
At 24 hours	Proliferation of connective tissues and vascular endothelium for revascularization
At 36 hours	Capillary network form with fibroblastic infiltration
At 48 hours	Capillary network completed, fibroblasts run across the new vessels
By 3–5 days	Vessels are thickened, many of obliterate; healing start by scar formation
By 6th day	Scab over the wound falls off or taken out easily, leaving a soft, tender, reddish scar which in course of weeks and months becomes less tender, whitish and firm

Table 11.5 Differences between laceration and incised wound

	Laceration	Incision
Edges	Irregular, abraded, crushed, contused and undermining of edges	Regular, not abraded, not contused, not crushed and no undermining of edges
Tailings	Irregular	Sharp pointed
Bleeding	Less due to crushed vessels	More due to cut vessels
Gaping	More	Less
Walls	Tissue strands present across wall	Tissue strands are absent across wall
Hair	Hair forced into wound, root of hair is crushed	Hair or its root may be cut clearly
If a bony base	May be fractured	Shows a clear cut

A laceration can be well differentiated from an incision by examining the edges, tailing ends, hair and its root, the floor and underlying bone, with the help of a hand lens (**Table 11.5**).

Medicolegal Importance

1. They reflect sharp edges, not the weapon type.
2. They give an idea about the site of impact and direction of force.
3. No trace evidence.
4. Age of the injury can be determined.
5. Profuse external hemorrhage and air embolism may be present.
6. Danger to life depends on site and depth.
7. Relative position of the assailant and victim can be determined.
8. Position and the characteristics of the wound usually indicate the mode of infliction.
9. Incised wounds may be as a result of **self-infliction**, **assault** or **accident** (rare).

Self-Inflicted or Suicidal Incised Wound

Self-inflicted injuries are produced by the person on his own body, in an attempt to bring false charge against somebody or in his defence. They are superficial and multiple and more or less parallel to each other and over the exposed and accessible parts of the body, opposite to the hand used. The common sites of election are wrists (**Figure 11.32**), neck (**Figure 11.33**), cubital fossae, chest, abdomen, groin, etc.

Suicidal Cut Throat (Figure 11.33)

The common features of suicidal cut throat are as follows:

i. Tentative cut incisions are present on left side of the neck if right handed and vice versa.
ii. One or more deep, sweeping cuts present and it is down from the left, across the mid-line.

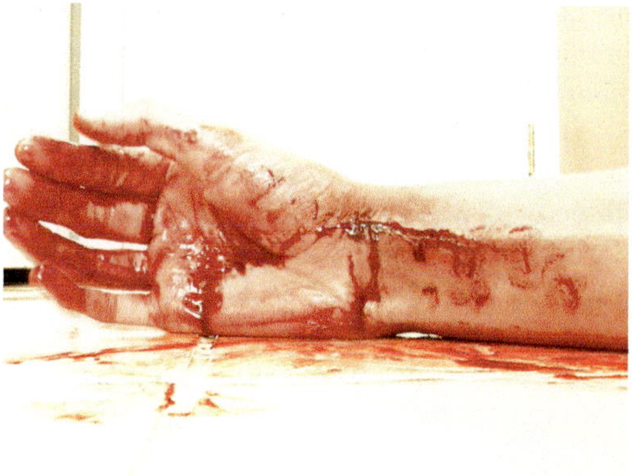

Figure 11.32 Suicidal tentative incisions over wrist

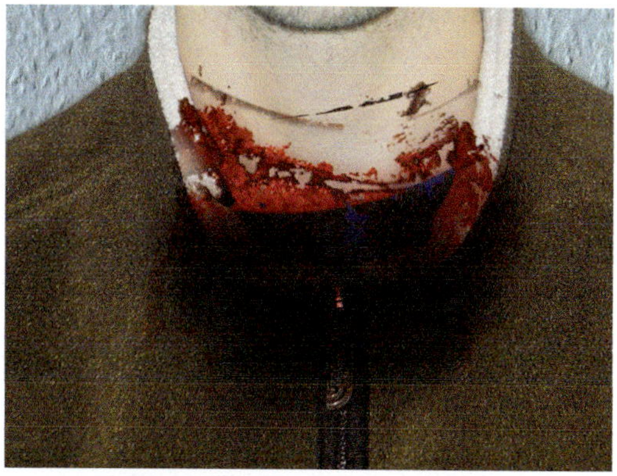

Figure 11.33 Suicidal cut throat

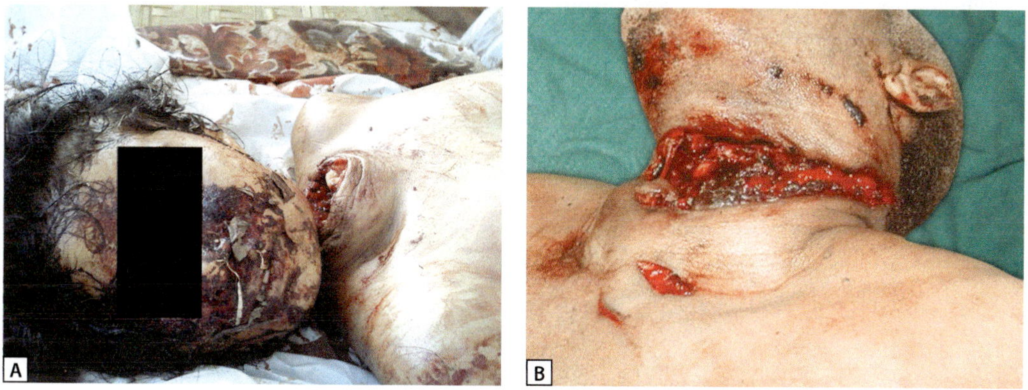

Figures 11.34A and B Homicidal cut throat

iii. The depth is shallow (beginning) to deep (central) to shallow (end).
iv. The incisions are usually through the level of thyrohyoid ligament.
v. Bleeding is venous, loss of consciousness is slow.
vi. Air embolism may occur.

Homicidal Cut Throat (Figure 11.34)

Compared to suicidal cuts, homicidal cut throat are:

1. Lack the deliberate choice of site. It may be aimed, but many miss.
2. The cuts lie both higher and lower across the neck.
3. There are no tentative cuts; all cuts are forceful and deeper.
4. Commonly no repetition in same track.
5. Slope of the track is backwards and downwards.
6. Associated with '**defense wound**' to hands and arms, etc.

Other Self-inflicted Injury

Fabricated Wound

i. Factious, forged or invented wounds are the injuries produced by a person deliberately, on his own body or on another person's body with his consent.
ii. Fabricated wound are usually seen over the inaccessible parts, viz. head, left arm, chest, abdomen and thighs.
iii. Fabricated wound are superficial and parallel.
iv. They are usually done in attempt to bring a false accusation on somebody else, in a way to prove or disprove the allegation.

v. To make a simple injury appear serious.
vi. By the assailant itself, to pretend self-defense.
vii. Fabricated wounds are usually incised wounds.
viii. Watchmen may pretend of forged injuries to defend themselves that they were on duty.
ix. Prisoners may bring charge of beating against officers.
x. Women to bring a charge of rape against her enemy.
xi. Clothes are not cut, if cuts they are not compatible with the nature of wounds.

Ordinarily to pretend incised wounds are used, though sometimes stab wounds or contusions or burns are produced. Lacerated wounds are rarely fabricated.

Parasuicidal Mutilation

Parasuicidal mutilations are usually seen over face, arms, trunk, etc. The people involve has low self-esteem.

Accidental Incisions

Accidental incisions are random pattern, usually single, often deep and forceful.

Defense Wounds

A defense wound is usually sustained when a victim places his hand often his palms (as shown in **Figures 11.35**), arm (lateral forearms) or other body part in harm's way to prevent or minimize the impact of a blow or slashing by a sharp weapon.

Though in most occasions, incised wounds are seen, abrasions, bruises, lacerations or punctured wounds were also seen in defense for self protection. Presence of wounds at these places, when identified as defense wounds, is very much helpful to ascertain the homicidal nature of the injuries or death.

Chop Wound

Definition

Chop wounds are type of incised wounds, which has clean cut edges, but an abraded margin due to inversion and friction against the sides of the wide blade on insertion with a fairly sharp moderately heavy weapons, like axe, chopper, *kukri*, *katari*, etc.

Features

i. These injuries are usually deeper and broader than the incised wounds (**Figure 11.36**).
ii. The dimensions of the wound correspond to cross-section of penetrating blade.
iii. While a heavy weapon, i.e. axe is applied, the heel end which is nearer to the assailant is deeper than the toe end (distal from the assailant). Hence, recognition of heal and toe ends are important to know the relative position of the assailant and the victim.

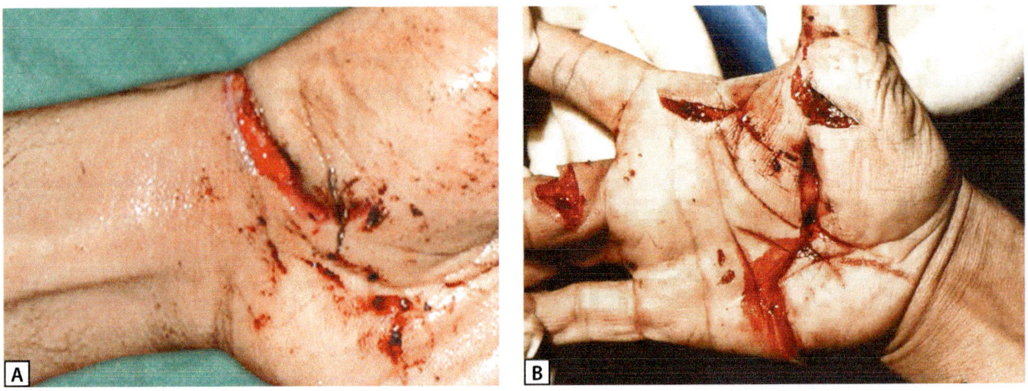

Figures 11.35A and B Defense wound on palmer aspect of hand

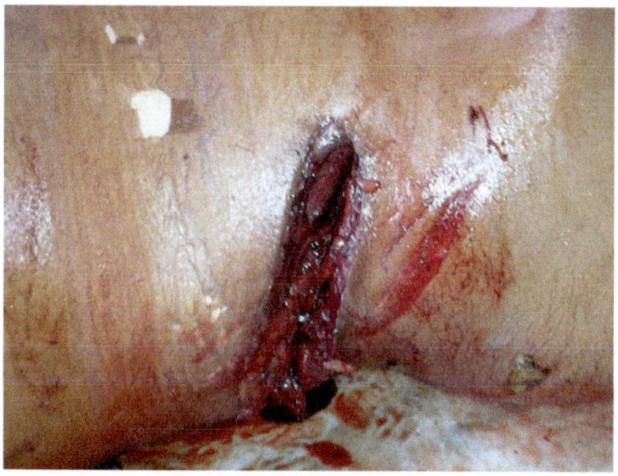

Figure 11.36 Chop wound

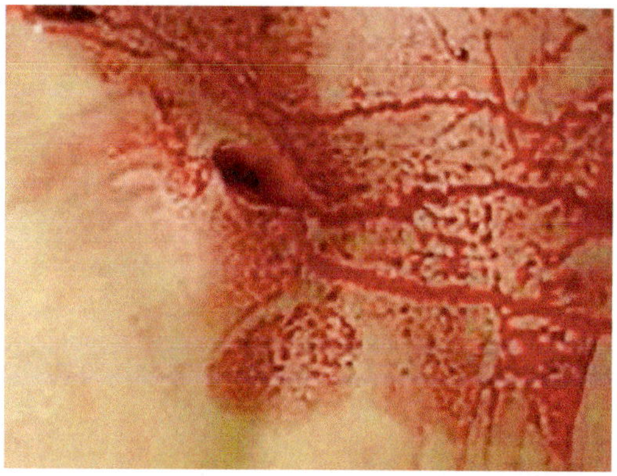

Figure 11.37 Stab wound to back of chest

Medicolegal Importance

i. Chop wounds are mostly homicidal in nature.
ii. It helps to ascertain the type of the weapon used.

STAB OR PUNCTURE WOUNDS

Synonyms: Penetrating wounds
Puncture wound is "a small hole made with a sharp pointed object" (**Figure 11.37**).
These injuries are caused by separation of the body tissues like (skin and soft tissues) under pressure of a sharp or blunt pointed object, the greatest dimension being its depth.

Classification

A. **Based on depth of penetration**

- Penetrating wound
- Perforating wound

B. **Based on the causative agents**

Stab or puncture wounds are caused by thrusting of three types of instrument causing three main types of injuries as follows (**Figure 11.38**).

a. Sharp/flat objects like knife and dagger that may cause **incised stab** wound.
b. Sharp and thin instruments like needle that may cause **needle puncture** wound.
c. Blunt, long and rigid objects like wooden stake, spike, screwdriver and cricket stump may cause **lacerated stab** wound.

All the three types of stab wound may be penetrating or perforating one as follows:

Penetrating Wounds

Penetrating wounds are the stab wounds that pass into, but not through any visceral organ. They are called penetrating wounds, when they enter a cavity of a body, i.e. wound terminating in the tissue or organ or cavity.

The penetrating wounds should be described in regards to the following points:[2]

A. Damage to the clothing (slashes, stabs through folds, blood flow and drip patterns, trace evidence) if any.
B. Site in relation to anatomical landmarks.
C. Shape of wound.
D. Alignment (horizontal, vertical, oblique).
E. Size: Length and breadth with margins.
F. Direction: In three planes.
G. Depth of wound.

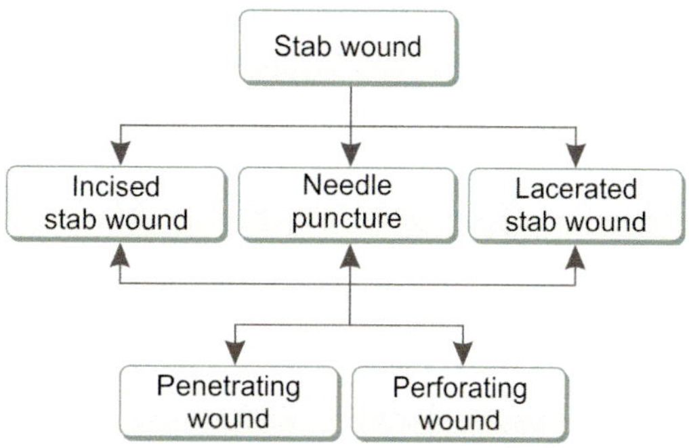

Figure 11.38 Classification of stab wound

Table 11.6 Description of penetrating wound

Description about	Information gathered
Shape of wound	Type of weapon, viz. Knife. Movement of knife in wound
Length and breadth with margins	Dimensions of the weapon and taper of blade
Direction in three planes	Direction of thrust
Depth of wound	Depth of thrust
Damage to tissues along track (external and internal hemorrhages, pneumothorax, air embolism)	Effect on victim, cause of death and amount of force used

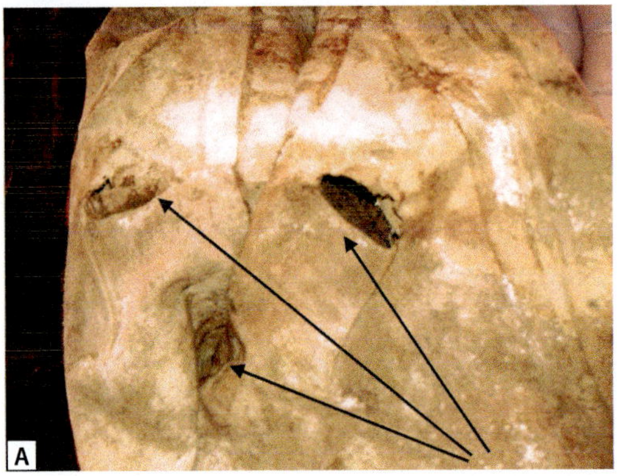

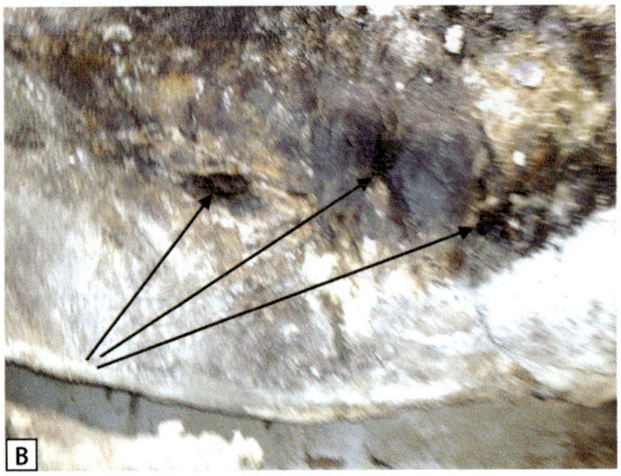

Figures 11.39A and B (A) Injury marks over cloth; and (B) Corresponding marks on the body

H. Damage of tissues along the track.
I. Effects like external and internal hemorrhage, pneumothorax and air embolism, if present should be noted.

Well-described penetrating wound may be helpful in providing a lot of useful information about the incident in question (**Table 11.6**).

Perforating or Transfixing Wound

These are the stab wounds derived from Latin word '*perforare*' (per—through and forare—to bore) and passes through and through an organ or whole thickness of any part of the body. When a weapon enters the body through the anterior abdominal wall giving rise to exit wound on posterior abdominal wall, then it becomes a perforating wound.

Features of Stab Wounds

i. Injury marks to clothing in the form of slashes, stabs, etc. may be present (**Figure 11.39**).
ii. Its depth exceeds its length on the body surface.
iii. Shape and size of wound often indicate the dimensions of the weapon.
iv. Stab wounds are commonly caused by a sharp/flat instrument like a knife (**stab wound**), a sharp and thin object like a needle (**needle puncture wound**) or rarely a blunt, long and rigid object like a wooden stake (**puncture**).
v. Stab wounds often appear trivial externally, but often cause more internal injuries and hemorrhage.
vi. **Stab wound length**: The length of a straight in and out stab wound is slightly shorter than the breadth of the blade due to stretching of the skin over the point of the knife on insertion and elastic recoiling of skin on withdrawal. Wound length and breadth of a stab wound must be measured to the edge taped together, because the wound is commonly shortened and widened into an oval shape because of skin elasticity, i.e., **Langer's lines** of **tension** and underlying muscle tone.

vii. Wound length is less than the breadth of the blade (reasons): (i) Stretching of skin over the point on insertion and subsequent recoiling on withdrawal and (ii) Tapered blade not fully inserted.

viii. Wound length is more than the breadth of the blade when: (i) Blade enters with an angle, i.e. the blade of the weapon does not pass straight in and out and (ii) On withdrawal, and the weapon **shakes**. Cutting edges extends the wound length.

ix. **Shape of Wound Indicates:**
   a. *Cross-section of the blade of the knife:* Double-edged blade leaves wound of slit shaped with two sharp ends, i.e. the tailing at both the ends, as shown in **Figure 11.40**. Single-edged knife may give similar wound due to clean splitting over blunt end, but when it is thin, single-edge blade it leave triangular slit with one sharp end and when it is thick, it leave slit with one sharp and one 'fishtail' end due to stretching and laceration over blunt edge.
   b. *Direction of insertion:* The upper edge is overhangs with beveling of lower edge. The direction of wound track through the tissues is measured at autopsy, with the body lying flat on its back. The position of internal organs is different during life, when standing, sitting and breathing. Therefore, it is difficult to ascertain at autopsy.

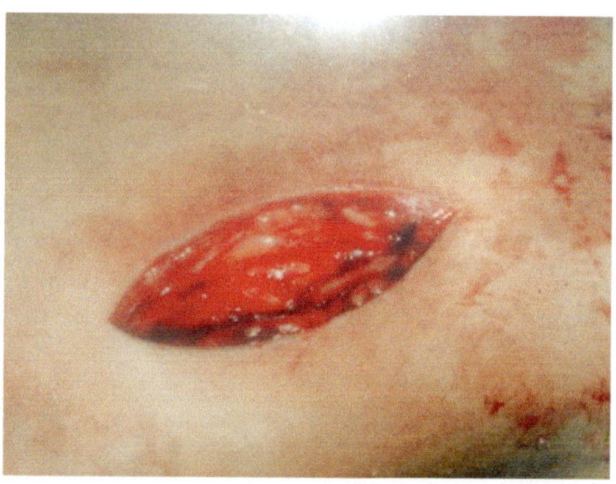

Figure 11.40 Eliptical shaped stab wound. Tailing at both end caused by double-edged blade

   c. *When the movement is little on withdrawal,* it leaves a notch; in a twisting movement, wound becomes crescentic.

x. **Wound Track Depth**: The depth of wound track is less than the length of instrument if not fully inserted. The depth of wound track is more than a length of the instrument if fully inserted and body surface compressed, e.g. abdomen, chest. A small penknife can perforate heart or abdominal aorta.

xi. **Degree of Force**: Depth of a wound is a poor indicator of force applied. With sharp pointed object slight pressure is required; whereas blunt tip requires greater force to penetrate the tissues. It depends on the sharpness off point, not of cutting edge.

xii. **Speed of Weapon's Approach** ($E=1/2\ mv^2$): A quick drive perforates the skin more easily than a slow and sustained speed. The damage of a bony is a useful index of depth and implied the force involve. The wearing garments and skin offers a considerable resistance. Hence, after being skin penetration, the blade slips easily through the underlying tissues, viz., muscle, internal organs and uncalcified cartilage, without any further force application.

xiii. **The Doctrine of Analogy is Stabbing a Melon**: Bone penetration requires appreciable force and that may even break the tip of a weapon. If the application is quick it requires less force to penetrate the skin than a slow and steady force. An imprint abrasion or bruising of the skin by the hilt of the knife may be produced due to the forcible introduction of the object.

xiv. **Effect of Counter-pressure of the Victim:** It may be exerted by falling or running onto the instrument. There are no needs to apply the rigid support to the knife if the tip is sharp and pointed.

Effects of Stabbing

1. The victim may not initially be aware about the injury.
2. There may be very little or no external bleeding.

3. Internal bleeding may be profuse and fatal or slow enough to take medical intervention.

Bleeding is the main effect. However, the time taken to incapacitate the victim and possible remedies to be accepted is very difficult to estimate during the incident.

The effect varies organ to organ as follows:

i. Stab wound to **heart** bleed profusely into the confined space of the pericardium with the development of cardiac tamponade if the pericardial injury is small. Stab to **left ventricle** may reseal partly, leading in slow blood loss or spontaneous healing if it is small whereas the thin-walled right ventricle is less likely to reseal including the great vessels.
ii. Stab to **lung** depends on the size of vessels cut to bleed. Bleeding is more if a large pulmonary veins and arteries are cut whereas peripheral stab bleeds less and may seal if lung collapses. Development of pneumothorax itself is fatal. Cutting of bronchus may obstruct airways.
iii. Stab to **abdomen** if penetrate great vessels, liver or spleen causes profuse bleeding into the abdominal cavity.
iv. Stab to **head** and face causes incursion of bone in the region of eye, nose and temple as the bones are thin here in these places.
v. Pulmonary **air embolism** from a partially stab jugular vein may be quickly fatal before much blood is lost. Exsanguinations are rapid if a carotid artery or jugular vein is stab or cut.

Puncture Wounds by Blunt Objects

Typical irregular, split, laceration like wounds are produced due to blunt force object where to penetrate the skin a greater thrust is needed. Inversion of skin on entry wound causes abraded margin. There may be bruising of the margins due to crushing and stretching of the tissues. Shape of puncture wound may indicate cross section of the object (**Figure 11.41**).

Associated Internal Injuries

Surface wounds may be informative of underlying damage, but are frequently the small markers of lethal underlying damages.

Concealed Punctured Wound

Concealed puncture wounds are caused over the concealed parts of the body, such as nostrils, fontanelle, fornix of the upper eyelids, inner canthus of eyes, axilla, vagina, rectum, nape of the neck, etc. These injuries are usually made by pins and needle-like objects and ordinarily difficult to locate.

Medicolegal Importance

1. The shape of the **stab wound** may indicate the class and type of the weapon, which may have caused the injury.
2. The depth of the wound will indicate the force of penetration.
3. Direction and dimensions of the **stab wound** indicate the relative positions of the assailant and the victim.
4. The age of the stab injury can be determined.
5. Position, number and direction of **stab wound** may indicate manner of its infliction.
6. Recovered broken fragment of weapon if found, will identify the weapon.

Type of weapon	Shape of injury
Hayfork	Elliptical
Ice pick	Round
Wooden stake	Cruciate
Poker	Stellate laceration
File	Triangular laceration
Scissors	Depends on degree of closure. 'Z'

Figure 11.41 Shape of puncture wound versus instruments

REFERENCES

1. Pillay VV. Mechanical injuries. In: Textbook of Forensic Medicine and Toxicology. 14th ed. Hyderabad: Paras Publishing; 2004. pp. 138-53.
2. Sadler DW. Department of Forensic Medicine, University of Dundee. [cited 2011 March 25]; Available from: URL:http://www.dundee.ac.uk/forensicmedicine/notes/woundsdws
3. Mitchell RN, Cotran RS. Cell injury, adaptation and death. In: Robbins Basic Pathology by Kumar V, Abbas AK, Aster J, 7th ed. New Delhi: Elsevier; 2003. p. 6.
4. Nguyen DT, Orgill DP, Murphy GF. Chapter 4: The pathophysiologic basis for wound healing and cutaneous regeneration. In: Biomaterials for Treating Skin Loss by Orgill DP, Blanco C. Woodhead Publishing (UK/Europe) and CRC Press (US), Cambridge/Boca Raton, 2009. pp. 25-57.
5. Stadelmann WK, Digenis AG, Tobin GR. Physiology and healing dynamics of chronic cutaneous wounds. Am J surg. 1998;176(2A Suppl):26S-38S.
6. Quinn JV. Tissue Adhesives in Wound Care. Hamilton, Ont. BC Decker, Inc. Electronic book.

CHAPTER 12

Firearm Injuries

Putul Mahanta, AJ Patowary

LEARNING PLAN

- Identification of the firearm and its structure
- Mechanism of firearm
- Identification of firearm injury
- How to find out the range/direction of fire
- Identification of weapon of offence

A **firearm** is a device, which propels a projectile by the force of the hot gases produced by combustion of explosive material in a closed chamber. **Firearm injuries** are generally caused by interpersonal violence, regardless of whether or not the victim was the intended target. Such injuries which are homicidal (common), suicidal and accidental, can be fatal.

TERMINOLOGIES

Ammunition is a term that came from the French "la munition", which covered all explosive material used for war, but which, in time, came to refer specifically to gunpowder, bullet, pellets, etc.

Forensic ballistics is the science dealing with the probe of firearms, ammunition and the troubles arising from their use.

Gun Ballistics (Figure 12.1): It is the work on projectiles from the time of shooting to the time of impact with the target. Gun ballistics is often broken down into the following four categories, which contain detailed information on each category.[1]

a. **Internal ballistics**, sometimes called interior ballistics, is the study of the processes originally accelerating the projectile, for example, the passage of a bullet through the barrel of a rifle.[2] It is also called proximal ballistics.
b. **Transition ballistics**, sometimes called intermediate ballistics, is the study of the projectile's behavior when it leaves the barrel and the pressure behind the projectile is equalized.[3]
c. **External ballistics**, sometimes called exterior ballistics, is the study of the passage

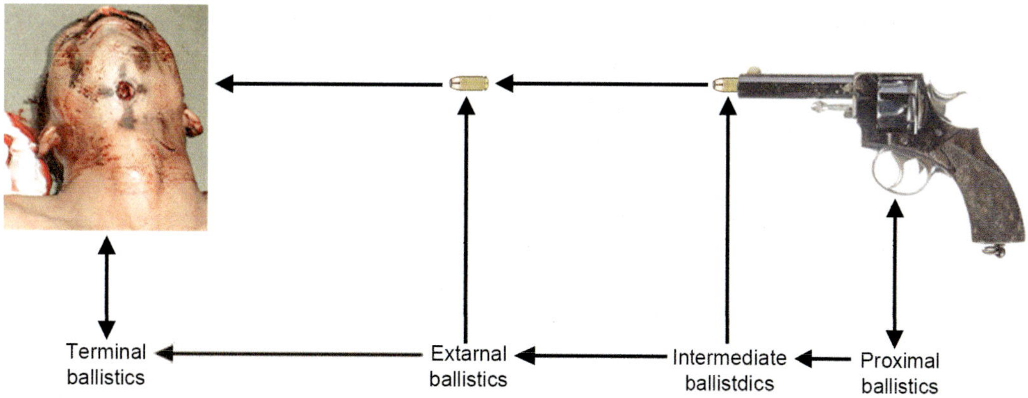

Figure 12.1 Gun ballistics

of the projectile through a medium, most commonly earth's atmosphere.[4]

d. **Terminal ballistics** is the study of the interaction of a projectile with its target, whether that be flesh (for a hunting bullet), steel (for an anti-tank round) or even furnace slag (for an industrial slag disruptor).[5]

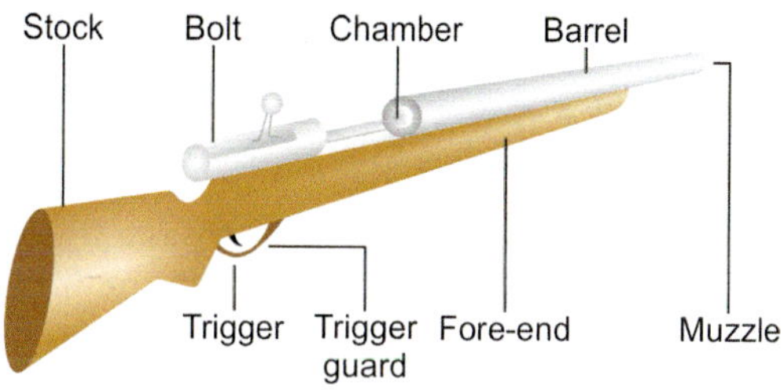

Figure 12.2 Different parts of firearm

GENERAL MAKE UP OF FIREARM

Every firearm weapon consists of three major parts:

- Stock or grip or butt
- Barrel
- Breech action

Stock or Grip or Butt

A **stock**, also known as a **buttstock** or **shoulder stock**, is a part of a rifle or other firearm, to which the barrel and firing mechanism are attached, that is held against one's shoulder when firing the gun. Stocks are also found on crossbows, though a crossbow stock is more properly referred to as a tiller.[6] The stock provides a means for the shooter to firmly support the device and easily aim it. The stock also transmits recoil into the shooter's body.[7] It can be held in hand in a case of pistol or revolver, or it can be supported on the shoulder, as mentioned, in a case of military rifle.

Barrel

It is a metal tube, through which the projectile travels, in the form of hollow cylinder of varying length according to type of gun. It is closed at the back end, called the **breech end**, and open in the front end, called the **muzzle end.** The inside of the barrel consists of three parts.

1. The **chamber**, at the breech or rear end of the barrel, which is wider than rest of the cylinder, to accommodate the cartridge or shot shell to be fired (**Figure 12.2**). The backside of chamber has a metal plate known as **breech plate** or **breech face** which has a central hole.
2. The front part of chamber is called taper, **lead** or **leed** in rifled arm and **chamber cone** in a smooth bore that connects the chamber to the bore.
3. The lead continues anteriorly as barrel. Lumen of the tube is called **bore**, which lies between the taper and the muzzle.

Breech Action

A breech action is connected to the barrel at the breech end to close the end of the barrel. It consists of (a) Bolt or block, (b) Trigger, (c) Hammer.

Bolt: The breech action consists of a receiver which contains a bolt or block that closes and locks a cartridge into the chamber. The bolt or the block can be opened to insert a new cartridge into the chamber. That part is called bolt which contains the firing pin, spring and trigger.

When the weapon is closed for firing, the barrel comes into position against a **flat block** of metal called **breech face**, which seals the breech end of the chamber. The block is pierced in its center to accommodate the **firing pin**, which is actuated by a spring and moves forward when hammer hits on its back on pressing the trigger.

Trigger: The lower part of firearm has a trigger used to initiate the firing process in the firing chamber of the weapon. This is carried out by inciting a striking device through a combination of spring and kinetic energy operating through a firing pin to strike and ignite the primer. When trigger is pulled, it causes hammer or striker to hit on the percussion cap of cartridge that causes ejection of bullet or pellet from muzzle end of barrel. The **trigger guard** is a metallic rim that surrounds trigger to prevent accidental firing.

Hammer or **Striker**: It is there in the posterior part of the chamber which hits the firing pin when trigger is pressed.

Mechanism

When the weapon is ready to be fired, the hammer is pulled back against a strong spring and is held back by the end of the sear, which rests in a notch known as the bent. When the trigger is pulled, the sear is freed from the bent and the hammer moves forward and advances the firing pin to the chamber from the central hole of breech plate. The moving firing pin then strikes the base of the cartridge, the percussion cap, as a result of which the primer is crushed in the anvil and sparks are produced, which in turn goes out through the vents and ignite the gun powder producing the hot gases responsible for propelling the projectile.

CLASSIFICATION OF FIREARMS

Modern firearms come in two chief forms:

- Smooth bore firearms
- Rifled firearms.

A smooth-bore firearm has a barrel that is altogether smooth on the inside, while a rifled firearm has spirally arranged grooves that help direct a bullet down the length of the barrel. Each type of weapon has particular uses and differing levels of power and accuracy.

Smooth Bored or Shotgun Firearms

A **shotgun**, also known as a **scattergun** or a **pepper gun,**[8] is a firearm that is usually designed to be fired from the shoulder, to fire a number of small spherical pellets called **shot**, or a solid projectile, i.e. **slug** (**Figure 12.3**).

Shotguns come in a wide variety of sizes, ranging from 5.5 mm (0.216535 inches) bore up to 5 cm (2 inch), and it includes breech loading, single-barrelled, double or combination gun, pump-action, bolt and lever action, semi-automatic and even fully automatic editions. The length of barrel varies from 52 to 72 cm.

A shotgun, in general, is a smooth bore firearm, which means that the inside of the barrel is not rifled. In the 19th century, these were commonly used on the battleground with breech loading rifled firearms, which were more accurate over longer ranges.

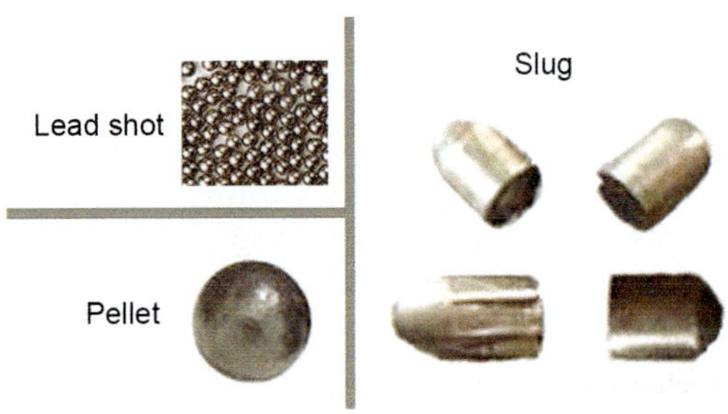

Figure 12.3 Lead shot, pellet and slug

The shot pellets from a shotgun disperse upon leaving the barrel, and the power of the burning charge is divided among the pellets, which means that the energy of any one ball of shot is averagely low.

Exceptions: Although shotguns are usually smooth bore weapons, which sometimes uses projectiles having rifling on its surface known as a slug. This heavy-duty projectile is used most often for very large game. Some modern-day muzzle-loaded hunting weapons also use as a smooth bore barrel. Advances in both weapon and projectile design, and more powerful gunpowder preparations, make these guns far more accurate than those of yesterday.

Types of Shotgun (Figure 12.4)

A. **Depending** on **length** of **barrel**:
   - Long barrel or shoulder rest
   - Short barrel or hand rest

B. **Depending** on **loading** of **ammunition** or **cartridge**:
   - Muzzle loading
   - Breech loading
   - Magazine loading

C. **Depending** on **number** of **barrel**:
   - Single barrel
   - Double barrel
   - Multi-barrel

D. **Depending** on **choking** of **barrel**:
   - Full choked
   - Three-quarter choked
   - Half choked
   - Quarter choked
   - Non-choked

E. **Depending** on **firing action**
   - Over-bolt action
   - Under-bolt action
   - Lever action
   - Pump action or auto loading model

Long Barrel (shoulder rest): All weapons of long non-rifled guns do not fire pellets, but group of missiles (shots, sometimes slugs in ghaffir and wads), the inner side of the barrel is smooth, not rifled. The barrel may be single, but most commonly is double-barrelled.

Sporting Gun: It is long non-rifled weapon, with single or double barrel. Sometimes one of the two barrels may be narrowed (**choked weapon**) toward the muzzle, this is to keep the charge of the shots in a compact group over a longer distance after firing, thus increasing the lethal range (**Figure 12.5**).

Ghaffir Guns: They are long non-rifled weapon, similar to sporting gun, but the cartridge is made of brass and the external wad is replaced by a corrugation of the end of the cartridge. It was used by ghaffirs. They are three types: Greener, Schneider and Remingoton.

Muzzle Loader: They are old-fashioned weapons not used nowadays owing to their near range, slow action and difficulty in loading. They were loaded from the muzzle end.

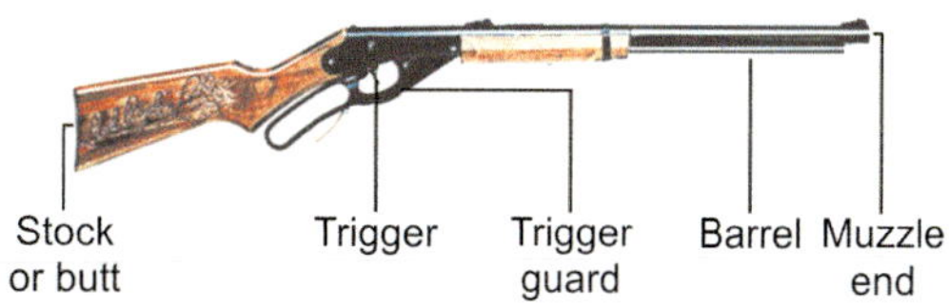

Figure 12.5 Different parts of sporting gun

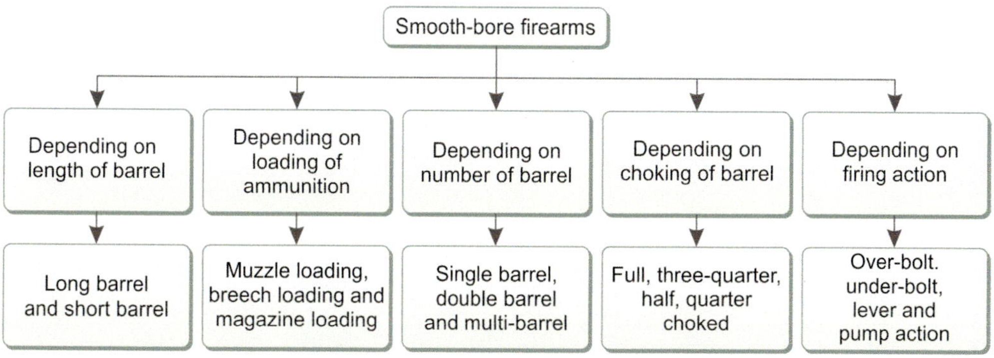

Figure 12.4 Types of smooth-bore firearm

Breech Loaders: They are used nowadays and can be classified into rifled as well as non-rifled weapons.

Magazine Loading: Magazine is a container on a repeating firearm that holds the receiver.

Uses of Shotgun

1. Typically shoot multiple missiles at short range; hunters often use them to bring down ducks, other birds and small games.
2. Police and military personnel also use smooth-bore guns as short-range weapon for controlling riot, etc.
3. Used for target shooting sports such as skeet, trap and sporting clays.

Bore or Caliber of Non-Rifled Weapon

In the US, the most commonly employed system is that of **gauge.** In this system, the bore denotes to the number of lead balls of equal size, each fitting the bore, which can be prepared from one pound (454 g) of pure lead. Hence, the 12 bore shotgun has a bore diameter such that 12 balls of lead, each fitting the bore, can be made from a pound of lead. Thus, the bigger the bore, the smaller the diameter of the barrel, e.g. the diameter of the barrel bore 4 is bigger than that of bore 10 (**Figure 12.10**).

It is to be noted that as the bore number increases, the inner diameter of barrel of shotgun decreases and the other way around. Each one has a fixed number that is written on the cartridge brass bases to the side of the percussion cap. The most common calibres are 12 and 16.

The bore diameter can also be stated in **inches**, e.g. modern 0.410 bore, where the bore diameter is stated in inches.

In the **meter system**, the bore diameter is stated in **millimeter**, e.g. 10 mm shotgun that has a bore diameter of 10 mm.

Choking

It is a design used in shotgun where the terminal few centimeters of the bore of muzzle is constricted so as to insure the shot pattern. In shotgun, choke basically measures the degree of constriction, which decreases the spread of the pellets thus reducing the diameter of the pellet pattern, expressed in thousands of an inch. Different degree of choke is shown in **Figure 12.6** and **Table 12.1**.

Shotguns may have **fixed** choke, which is one particular degree of choke, or **multi-**

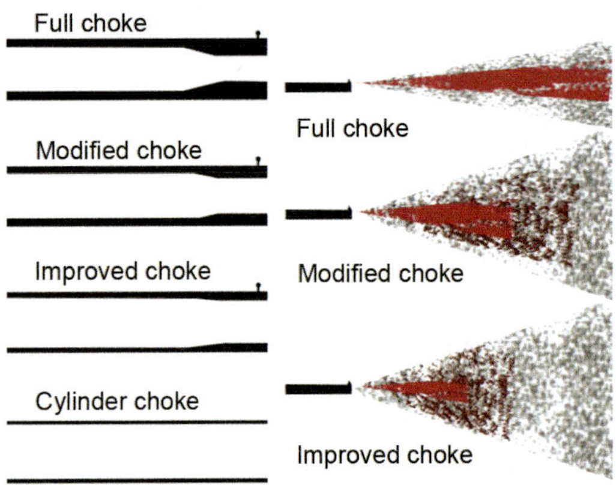

Figure 12.6 Choke of shotgun

Table 12.1 Various degree of choke

Degree of choking	Constriction of bore		Degree of constriction
	In mm	In inch	
Full choke	1.00	0.04	40/1000th of an inch
Three-quarter choke	0.75	0.03	30/1000th of an inch
Half choke	0.50	0.02	20/1000th of an inch
Quarter choke	0.25	0.01	10/1000th of an inch
True or improved cylinder	0	0	3–5/1000th of an inch

choke, which are interchangeable choke tubes screwing into the end of the muzzle, or possibly **poly-chokes**, which increase or decrease the degree of choke by turning a device attached to the muzzle end of the shotgun.

The degree of choke ranges from **true cylinder** which is the most open, to **full choke** which is the tightest. Other countries do use different measurements in some cases or different descriptions for a similar choke; for example, the American gun makers refer to the equivalent of UK half choke as modified but choke sizes commonly used by British gunsmiths are measured in thousands of an inch. **Non-choked shotgun** has the uniform size of barrel from muzzle end to breech end, hence this type of barrel is known as cylindrical type barrel or **cylinder bore**.

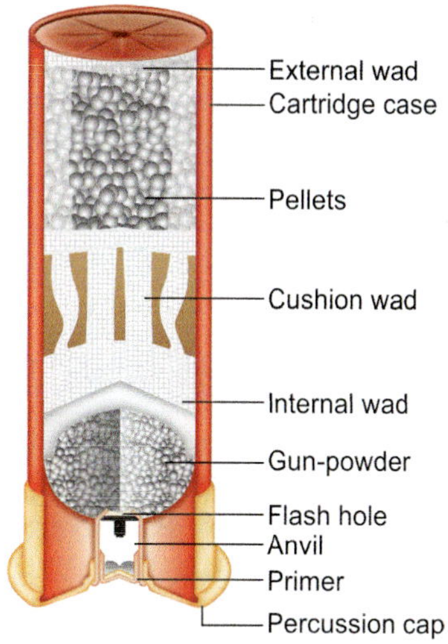

Figure 12.7 Shotgun cartridge

Cartridge of Shotgun

A cartridge is ammunition for firearms, which is loaded to the chamber. It is formed by a small copper percussion cap at the base, gun powder in the middle, internal wad then missile (shots or slug) and external wad on the top (or may be absent). A **shotgun shell** is a self-contained cartridge loaded mainly with lead shot or slug designed to be fired. The length of the cartridge varies from 5 to 7 cm.

A **shotgun cartridge (Figure 12.7) consists** of following: (i) Cartridge case, (ii) Primer or detonator, (iii) Propellant and (iv) Projectile.

i. **Cartridge Case**: It is cylindrical in shape made up of cardboard or plastic. It has two ends, one of which is closed and known as base. The base is made up of metal plate, usually of brass. The central part of it is known as percussion cap or primer cap. The primer cap contains detonator. The base may be grooved or rimmed. The other end is open and is covered by cardboard. The main function of the cartridge case is to hold the explosive agents together, to prevent backward leakage of gases and to provide waterproofed cover for gunpowder.
ii. **Primer or Detonator**: The percussion cap contains paste of substances known as primer, which when crushed produces sparks. It is basically to ignite the gun powder. It contains mercury fulminate or lead azide, which is a highly inflammable substance, potassium chlorate that act as an oxygen donor and powdered glass for friction for spark formation to ignite gun powder (through flash hole).
iii. **Propellant**: It is also known as gunpowder, which is placed next to detonator in the cartridge. Ignition of primer is needed for combustion of gunpowder. On firing, pulling the trigger pushes the firing pin inside the chamber to the base of the percussion cap; so, a spark is formed that ignites gun powder producing huge amount of gases inside the cartridge (trapped) pushing the missile to the target. Three types of gunpowder are: (i) Black powder, (ii) Smokeless powder and (iii) Semi-smokeless powder.

Black Powder: It is a mixture of 75% potassium nitrate, 15% charcoal (carbon) and 10% sulfur. It is of granular form and designated as FG, FFG, FFFG, etc. depending on the size of the grains. The more is the number of 'F,' the finer are the grains and the faster in burning. F stands for fine and G for grain, thus FG implies fine grain.

The powder grains are black, coarse or fine, without any particular shape. It burns with production of much heat, flame and smoke. Fine grains travel 60–90 cm or more. A single grain of black powder produces 200–250 cc of gas containing CO, CO_2, N_2 and H_2, etc. One gram of powder produces 3,000–4,500 cc of gas. The residues are alkaline in nature.

Smokeless Powders: Smokeless gun powder is composed of nitrocellulose and nitroglycerin. It takes different colors and forms (scales, granules, cordite, macaroni, etc.). It is of following types: (i) **Single Base**: Nitrocellulose (gun cotton), (ii) **Double Base**: Which is a combination of nitrocellulose and nitroglycerin and (iii) **Triple Base**: Consist of combination of nitrocellulose, nitroglycerin and nitroguanidine. They produce much less flame and smoke and are more completely burnt than black powder. They are most effective explosive that imparts higher velocity to the projectile.

A single grain release 800–900 cc of gas. One gram produces 12,000–13,000 cc of gas. The color varies from bright orange to bluish-black, and in shape from minute globules, flakes, square, rectangular, irregular disks, cylinders to longer threads.

Modern smokeless powder is composed of nitrocellulose. Other explosive ingredients like nitroglycerine and stabilizers such as diphenylamine (DPA), ethyl centralite (EC), methyl centralite (MC), hydroquinone or resorcinol and flash suppressors such as 2, 4-dinitroluene (2, 4-DNT) are also usually present.[9] The residue is neutral in nature. Smokeless powder is three times stronger than the black powder and is used nowadays in place of the black powder.

Semi-smokeless Powder: Semi-smokeless powder is a mixture of 80% of black and 20% of the smokeless type. The differences between black and smokeless powder are listed in **Table 12.2.**

Projectile: Smooth bore firearm has the projectile known as "**pellets or shot**" in addition to slugs and sabots (in some Ghaffir guns). The shots are small, multiple spherical balls, for the most part made of lead, but this has been partially replaced by bismuth, steel, tungsten-iron, tungsten-nickel-iron and even tungsten polymer loads.

Their size and number vary from one cartridge to another depending on the type of animal to be shot. Sometimes hand-made shots are used in sporting gun. In country-made firearms, the projectiles, in the form of glass pieces, metal pieces, stones, nails, etc. are used. Instead of shot, in some shotguns, slugs are used. Slugs are single projectile and larger than the pellets and are similar to bullets. It is of various types and used for game hunting and law enforcement application.

WAD

After the gunpowder comes the wadding. The main function of a wad is to provide a gas seal, since without a wad the gas would just blow through the shot rather than propelling it. The wad consists of three parts, the powder wad, the cushion and the shot cup. The wad is made of some soft material like felt, plastic, straw, paper, cardboard, etc.

The **powder wad** or **internal wad** acts as the gas seal and is placed firmly over the powder. It may be a paper or plastic part. The **cushion**

Table 12.2 Differences between black and smokeless powder

Differences	Black	Smokeless
Composition	Charcoal (carbon) 15%, sulfur 10% potassium nitrate 75%	Nitrocellulose, Nitroglycerin Nitroguanidine
Ignition of 1 g acquire	3,000–4,500 cc of gas	12,000–13,000 cc of gas
Nature of residue	Alkaline Carbonate-bicarbonate Sulfate-sulfates thiosulfate	Neutral Nitrate-nitrite

Table 12.3 Differences between external and internal wad		
Difference	**External wad**	**Internal wad**
Made of	Cardboard	Felt, plastic
Function	Keep shots in place	Separate powder and shots
Distance	1–3 m	Piston like action (3–10 m)

comes next, and it is designed to compress under pressure, to act as a shock absorber and minimize the deformation of the shot. It also serves to take up as much space as is needed between the powder wad and the shot. Cushions are almost universally made of plastic. The **shot cup or external wad** is the last part of the shell, and it serves to hold the shot together as it moves down the barrel. The external wad is a disk of cardboard covering the shots. The differences between external and internal wad are shown in **Table 12.3.**

Functions of the Wad

1. To seal gases developed on ignition of the powder, preventing them from escaping between the shots.
2. To act as a shock absorber and minimize the deformation of the shot.
3. To hold the shot together as it moves down the barrel.

Medicolegal Importance of Wad

- Diagnosis of firearm injury
- Differentiate between entry and exit wound from the presence of it
- Diagnosis of gunpowder (black or smokeless), thus may help in weapon identification
- Distance of firing estimation
- Determination of type of weapon (non-rifled weapon).

SMOOTH BORE FIREARM INJURY

The autopsy surgeon should be capable of answering the following while conducting the autopsy of a firearm death victim.

- Whether the weapon is rifled or smooth bored?
- The nature of projectile
- The nature of propellant
- The direction of firing
- The range of firing.

Multiple pellets are used in shotgun. The pellets after firing travels as a compact mass for certain distance. As the distance increases, the pellets start dispersing from each other. Further increase in distance of firing causes fall of some pellets on the ground because of gravitational force. However, some pellets still travel and strike the target causing multiple injuries. This section will describe the pattern of wounds seen at various ranges of fire, first described by Breitennecker in 1969.[10]

The following elements of the cartridge emerge on the discharge of a smooth bore weapon and all may contribute to the wound:

- Lead pellets
- Soot in the form of smoke and debris
- Unburnt and burnt propellant particles
- Flame and hot gases under pressure
- Carbon monoxide
- Wads either felt, cardboard or plastic
- Detonator constituents
- Fragments of the cartridge case.

Factors Altering Shotgun Wound: Factors altering shotgun wound are: Range of firing, size of the shot, nature of the explosive and type of the gun itself.

Range of Firing

The distance or range of firing by shotgun can be considered as follows:

- Contact and near contact range
- Close range
- Short range
- Intermediate range
- Long or distant range.

Injuries caused by shotguns are much bigger than those caused by handguns and vary from massive disruption of the skull and its contents when it strike the head during a contact discharge to the head, or to a widespread pattern of pellet holes when fired at a distance.

Entry Wound

Contact and Near Contact Range

In contact range, muzzle end is firmly held against the skin. Features of contact and near contact range of firing are:

i. The wound is **single**.
ii. **Shape of wound**, usually round or circular, equal to the size of bore (2–4 cm diameter). The wound is also often ragged caused by individual pellet and tearing caused by gases.
iii. **Muzzle marks** if the weapon is firmly held with the skin.
iv. **Burning** or **blackening** is minimal or absent altogether. If the muzzle is not pressed firmly or due to recoil of the gun, gas, soot and flame escape sideways and cause singeing and blackening of the surrounding skin.
v. The **margins** of the wound (skin) are charred by flame and abraded soiled with powder grains.
vi. **Smoke** or **soot soiling** in exposed parts of the wound and in the wound depths, particularly if clothing interposed between weapon and body.
vii. Because of blasting effect of gases within the wounds, the subcutaneous and deeper tissues sustain terrible disruption. The momentaneous vacuum bellow the skin may even cause expulsion of the soft tissues, i.e. fat through the wound.
viii. Some of the **unburnt powder** grains are driven into the wound track to some distance and found embedded in the wound and may cause bleeding in deeper tissue and contusion of the margins. **Wads** contained within the wound depths. **Cherry red** or **pink** tissues in wound track due to combination of carbon monoxide present in gases and hemoglobin, causing carboxyhemoglobin or carboxymyoglobin formation.

It is well known that gunshot wounding can produce fine droplets of blood spattered in a forward direction. Under certain circumstances of contact firing, because of blasting effect of muzzle and the negative pressure created inside the barrel, discharges like blood, hair, fragments of tissues and cloth fibers may be propelled backwards in the direction against the line of fire. The phenomenon of **back spatter** is most commonly seen in contact gunshot wounds of the head; its occurrence is not well recognized. Back spatter is a type of "blow-back" effect produced by discharge of a large volume of gas in a confined space (**Figure 12.8**).

Close or Contact Range Injuries to the Head

When fired into the head during a contact (hard or loose) or close-range shot up to about 15–30 cm or 6–12 inches, the pellets contained in the cartridge have not had time to spread, and they enter the body as a single mass. If the barrel of the shotgun is in tight contact with the head, a large volume of gas enters the cranium, so the effect will be massive destruction.

The explosive effect disrupts the cranium and its contents, so that pieces of skull and brain tissue are spread over a wide area. Determining the point of contact requires meticulous gathering of skull fragments and attempting to reconstruct the skull and head, in order to

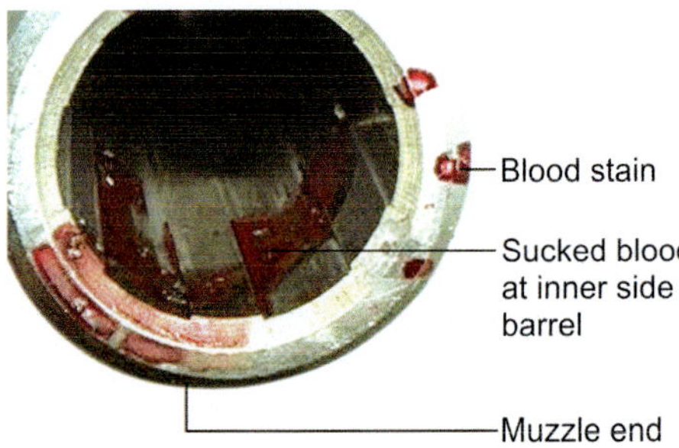

Figure 12.8 Back spatters on a gun barrel

find a hole, which will usually be heavily soot stained.[11,12]

The process of ejecting the mass of shot from the barrel results in production of '**secondary projectiles**', which include components of the cartridge such as wadding and metal fragments from the cartridge case, as well as flame, carbon deposits, soot, unburnt powder and gases. Contact wounds will not usually demonstrate features of these secondary projectiles externally unless there is loose contact where everything enters into the wound, whilst close range wounds usually demonstrate features of them all to a greater or lesser extent, depending upon how 'close' the weapon was actually discharged.

The severity of the effects depends, to some extent, on the gauge of the weapon. A 12 bore being more destructive than 20 bore due to relative differences in gas volume produced at discharge.

In forensic practice, most such contact or close-range shotgun wounds to the head are suicidal in nature. Favorite suicidal sites of selection are the roof of the mouth, the temple and under the chin. Where the entry point is the roof of mouth the escaping gas volume causes overstretching of the skin, and this causes splitting and tearing of the tissues around the mouth, nostrils and eyes.[12]

Close Range

Within a distance of **15** cm (about **6** inches), the pellets strike the target as a tightly packed mass and produce a single wound that is circular if strike is perpendicular to the skin or elliptical if strike is with an angle. The edges are inverted, may be clean or slightly ragged.

The skin surrounding the wound is blackened by smoke and burnt (singeing of hairs) by flame. The deposit of smoke is wider than gunpowder known as smudging, fouling or blackening. If the powder is smokeless, there may be grayish or white deposit on the skin round the wound. Unburnt particles of powder are embedded in the skin, producing tattooing, also known as stippling or powder peppering.

The deeper tissues show marked disruption. CO may be present in blood or tissues and looks cherry red. Wad will be in depth of wound and the pellets are found en mass.

Short Range

The short range comes within a distance of **15** cm to **one** meter (**6** inches to 3.28084 feet).

Within a distance of about **30 cm** (one foot), the pellets strike the target as a tightly knit mass and produce a single wound that is circular or oval, usually of 3–4 cm in diameter, depending upon the bore of the gun. The margins of the skin wound may be clean or slightly ragged. The skin surrounding the wound is blackened by smoke and burnt by flame along with the tattooing surrounding the wound. The deeper tissues show marked disruption along the track, and CO is present around the wound, hence the cherry red discoloration is found.

As the range of fire increases to approximately **30 cm** to **1.2 m**, the presence of secondary projectile damage is reduced.[13] Still the pellets strike the target as a single wound that has the edges which are rounded and scalloped. This appearance is known as "**rat-hole**" appearance because of resemblance to rodent teeth mark.

Extensive flame produced during shotgun discharge and hot combustion gases leaving the barrel at discharge rapidly cool and singeing or blackening of the wound edges is, therefore, not usually seen at distances beyond 30 cm. The tissues within and around the wound are not cherry red because they lacks CO at this range.

Similarly, hair singing is not usually seen beyond **30 cm**. In addition, soot marking tails off with increasing distance (20–40 cm), and the diameter of black staining reduces with increasing range of fire until it is absent (at about 50 cm). Powder tattooing similarly tails off with increasing range of fire and is not usually seen beyond 1 m.

Intermediate Range

The intermediate range is considered as distance of **1–4 m**.

As the column of pellets exiting the shotgun begins to spread due to the effect of air resistance, the wounds produced range from a large central hole, to one that has 'scalloped' edges. This is the result of some peripheral pellets being slightly separated from the main mass hitting the skin at the edges of the wound created by the central pellet mass. Up to approximately **1 m**, central wounds are still in the region of **2.5–4** cm in diameter, but then start to become scalloped.[13]

With increasing distance of fire, this scalloping will become more spectacular, till the central mass has diverged enough to give rise to a smaller central defect, but with a cuff of **satellite pellet** holes, and eventually, a widespread pattern of individual pellet holes with no discernable central hole.

The central mass of pellets tend to '**break down**' at about the **2 m** range, but this will depend upon the features of the arm involved, i.e. the gauge, barrel length, type of ammunition used, amount of choke, etc.

At a distance outside approximately **2 m**, there will be no soot staining or burning and no powder tattooing.

The shotgun cartridge '**wad**' initially travels with the central pellet mass, and in contact wounds, it will be found within the wound track. Beyond 1.5–1.8 m, the wad may not follow the pellet mass, and consequently strikes the body separately, giving rise to a separate area of abraded skin.[11]

Central defects are not normally seen by approximately **3 m** range. The **wad** will usually fall to the ground beyond approximately **2** m.[12,13]

In order to evaluate the estimated range of fire, detailed measurements are needed of the central hole, the area and pattern of satellite pellet holes, the presence or absence of soot, powder tattooing and wad abrasions. The presence of injuries or features associated with secondary projectiles is inversely related to the range of fire.

Distant Wounds

The distance range is more than **4 m**. Shotgun wounds made at a distance can be inferred by the widespread pattern of pellet wounds, i.e. small circular defects with abraded margins, and the complete lack of central wound or hole, soot staining and powder tattooing or other secondary projectile damage.

Knight in 1996[14] explains an old '**rule** of **thumb**' designed to estimate range of fire for distant shots as being **1/3rd** of the **spread** of **shot** in **cm's** = **range** of **fire** in **meters**. However, it should be noted that the only accurate method of determining range of fire for distant shots is by **test firing** the suspect weapon and ammunition and comparing patterns of shot produced with those seen on the victim.

Where the shot mass hits an intermediate object, such as a glazed door, etc. the pattern of shot dispersion will be increased substantially, the phenomenon known as **billiard ball ricocheting effect**; and so, great care should be taken when confirming shotgun pellet patterns if nothing is known about the circumstances of the wounding or evidence found at the scene.

The effective range for shotguns is approximately **50 m**, but the severity of wounds caused by these weapons rapidly diminishes with increasing range of fire, so that the mortality rate reduces to a few percent where the range is over 11 m, while closer range discharges (<5 m) give rise to a mortality rate of 85–90%.[13]

Exit Wound of Shotgun: Unlike exit wounds created by rifled weapons, shotguns do not generally give rise to exit wounds unless there is a contact wound to the head, for example (where the exit wound is actually a reflection of the explosive effect of the gases expanding in the enclosed cranial vault), or where there is a 'through-and-through' wound to a limb at close range. Head wounds demonstrate ragged and irregular exit defects due to fragmentation of cranial contents with everted edges.

Where the body is struck at increasing range, the shotgun pellets do not have enough energy to traverse the body, and particularly, they do not have the energy to pierce the skin at the exit site, and it is not uncommon to find pellets lodged just underneath the skin at the point of exit.

The Size of the Shot

The smaller the shot, the more smaller and irregular are the edges. The penetrating power of a large shot is greater than that of the smaller shot. At close range, the wounds produced by shot of various sizes are similar, but small shots usually lodge in the body.

The Nature of the Explosive

With smokeless powder, blackening and tattooing is less marked at all ranges than with black powder.

Type of the Gun Itself

The pattern of wound depends on the length of the barrel, the bore, absence or degree of the choke present. Shorter barrels usually produce greater deposits over larger areas.

Atypical missiles, such as pieces of stone, iron, beads of metal, seeds, etc. used in muzzle-loading guns, produce various irregular lacerated wounds, and the exit wounds are larger than the entrance wounds. The direction of the fire may be ascertained from the passage of individual shots through the clothes and tissues, from the grouping of shot marks and the direction of glancing shots.

Direction of Fire

While trying to determine from which direction a shotgun wound was inflicted, one may look cautiously at the wound margins to see if there is any undermining; the pattern of soot soiling and powder tattooing may also help to describe angles of fire. However, as range of fire increases, this will be more and more difficult, and the striking of intermediate targets, or attempts by the victim to protect vital organs against a shot may result in distorted wound and shot spread patterns making such reconstructions difficult.

Survivability

The ability of a victim to survive a shotgun wound depends upon the range of fire as well as the part of the body involved. Contact or close range injuries usually result in massive destruction, and clearly wounds involving the head or thorax result in instantaneous or rapid death.[15]

Balling or Welding of Shot

It results in the alteration of shot into a compact mass, and this can travel for few meters in this form. In such cases, a circular or oval entrance wound of about 5–10 mm diameter, surrounded by widespread, small, circular punctures; simulating the use of two different weapons.

This can occur due to faulty manufactured or old ammunitions, but this is rare. It can also be due to hand-loading of cartridges, if too much powder is used, if wads of incorrect kind are inserted, or sealing pressure on the wads is too high. The most likely cause is due to pouring of paraffin wax into the cartridge after removing the outer cardboard or by replacing some of the pellets by a large ball, which is held in place with wax.

Billiard Ball Ricochet Effect

In close range shots, while the shots are bunched, they strike one another upon impact on primary target, i.e. the skin or clothes, and spread out in a wide pattern as they pass through the body. This causes the shots to spread widely and may suggest a greater range of fire than actually occurred. Similar spread is seen if the shots strike any other intermediary object, e.g. door or window, before reaching the victim. The process is termed the billiard ball ricochet effect. The final shot spread as seen in X-ray gives a true picture of the range of fire, only when the range of fire is great enough that the shots are spread out, before striking the target. In decomposed and burned bodies where the skin pattern cannot be seen, the range of fire can be determined by X-rays.

Country-made Firearms

The injuries caused to the victim vary considerably depending upon the nature of missiles. Metal scraps may give rise to small incised or incised-looking wounds; punctured wounds may be produced by nails, and lacerations and contusions by stone pieces. The distance up to which the smoke, flame and carbon particles travel is about half of that from factory made firearm. The pellets commence to disperse at a distance of 30–45 cm. The muzzle velocity is low and the barrel can adapt a sub-caliber missile. As the characters of the firearms and components of the cartridge vary widely in country-made firearms, the data relevant to factory-made firearms to calculate the range of firing cannot be applied. For figuring the range of firing, the ideal method is to carry out test firing with the distrusted weapon.

RIFLED FIREARMS

Rifled firearms are the powerful weapons having **rifling** and fire bullets. In ammunition of rifled weapon, the cartridge is made out of a metal (brass) case with percussion cap in the base, gunpowder in the middle and a single missile, i.e. a bullet on the top.

Types of Rifled Firearms

A. **Depending on Length of Barrel**: (i) Short barrel or hand rest or hand guns, viz pistols and revolvers, (ii) Long barrel or shoulder rest gun, viz military rifle, AK-47, etc.
B. **Depending on Muzzle Velocity**: (i) Low velocity up to 1200 feet/s, (ii) Medium velocity up to 1200–2500 feet/s and (iii) High velocity, which are more than 3000 feet/s.
C. **Depending on the Firing Mechanism**: 1. Slide action, 2. Bolt action, 3. Lever action, 4. Semi-automatic and 5. Automatic.

The long barrel or shoulder rest gun designed to hit long distance. The short barrel rifles are called carbines.

Uses of Rifled Firearm

1. The concentrated firepower and accuracy of a rifle-fired projectile makes it an effective long-range weapon.
2. Hunters commonly use rifles for long-range shooting, often to bring down deer, bear or other big animals.
3. In tactical situations, rifling provides accuracy both to smaller weapons, such as handguns in close-range shooting, and to long-range combat or sniper weapons.

Rifling

Rifling is longitudinal **grooves** alternating with **ridges** (lands) running spirally along the inner side of the barrel (**Figure 12.9**). It has many functions as follows:

i. Rifling forces a **spinning** bullet (on its longitudinal axis) out from the muzzle. This spinning will **diminish the resistance** of **air and gravity** to the bullet that stabilize it during flight giving it a longer range and a more effective penetration and leave rifling marks on the bullet.
iii. Pattern of rifling is not uniform in every gun. It varies gun to gun; hence it is unique feature for that class of weapon. Therefore, it helps in identification of the weapon in question.

The marks sustained on the bullet during its flight through the barrel are of two types as follows:

Primary Markings: The marks produced by lands are known as primary rifling marking.

Secondary Markings: The secondary markings on bullets are caused due to certain individual characteristics of interior surface of barrel like minor projections or elevations or depressions.

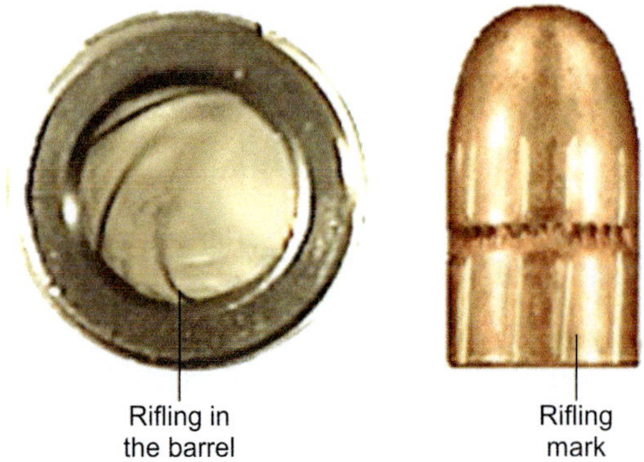

Figure 12.9 Rifling in the barrel and the marks left on the bullet[16]

The marks are specific for a particular gun, not common to all.

Bore

Rifled-bore weapon has grooves that help to guide a bullet down the length of the barrel. The caliber of a rifled firearm is the inner diameter of the barrel. It is measured as a distance between two opposite lands of the rifling (**Figure 12.10**). It is expressed in fractions of an inch or millimeter, viz 0.303 rifle (has caliber of 0.303 of an inch) or 9 mm pistol.

Rifle: A rifle (**Figure 12.11**) is a gun that has a long barrel. The bore of the rifle is rifled.

Short Barrel or Short Rifled or Hand Guns or Hand Rest

Pistols: A pistol is a hand-operated firearm having a chamber integrated with or permanently aligned with the bore. The cartridge is directly loaded into the chamber of the barrel or from magazine. It may be a single action or a semi-automatic.

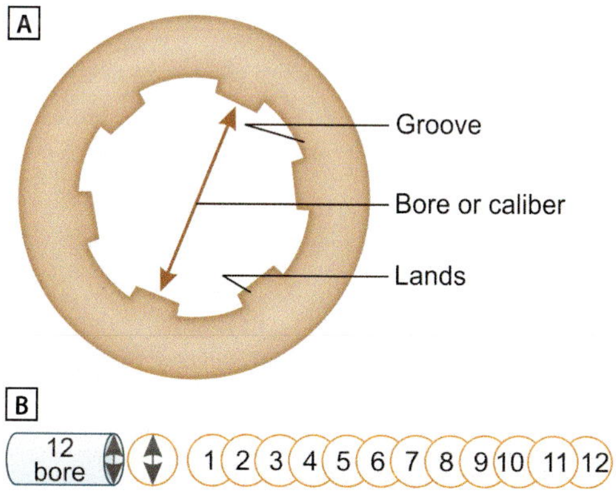

Figures 12.10A and B (A) Caliber or bore of rifled firearm, (B) Bore of Shotgun

Semi-automatic Pistol (**Figure 12.12**): Here magazine carries a number of cartridges, one on top of the other with spring like action. The cartridge is made of brass (copper and nickel) with a **groove** (for extractor hook ejection) at its base. The barrel has a sliding cover (sliding action) which moves backwards and forwards, it is pulled backwards before the firing to load the uppermost cartridge from the magazine into the breech. On firing, the power of the evolved gases will force the bullet out of the muzzle and will cause the sliding cover. It goes on firing every time the trigger is pressed, till the magazine is empty. Many a times, this type of weapon is mentioned as automatic pistol, but actually it a semi-automatic one.

Revolvers (**Figure 12.13**): A revolver is a hand-operated firearm with a revolving magazine that carries a number of individual cartridges that are loaded into revolving a chamber at the breech end of the barrel. It fires one shot at a time. Normally, it has five to nine chambers. The cartridge is made of brass with a rim at its base (**non-automatic**). The magazine revolves with each firing bringing a cartridge in alignment with the barrel.

Differentiating features between automatic pistol and revolver are shown in **Table 12.4**.

Cartridge of Rifled Firearm

It has the following parts: Cartridge case, detonator (primer), propellant (gunpowder) and projectile (bullet) as shown in **Figures 12.14** and **12.15**.

Cartridge Case: It is an elongated metal cylinder made up of copper and zinc. The base is flat which may have a rim except in an automatic or semi-automatic weapon, where the cartridge has an extractor groove near the base.

Table 12.4 Differentiating features of semi-automatic pistol and revolver

Differences	Automatic pistol	Revolver
Magazine	In handle spring loaded	Revolving cylinder
Cartridge base	Groove for extractor hook	Rim (well fitted cartridge) to fit in grooves of revolvers or pistols
Empty cartridge	Ejected automatically by extractor hook	Remains in the magazine

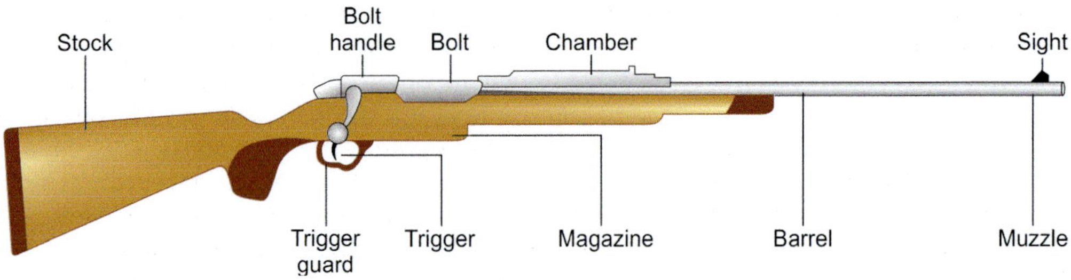

Figure 12.11 General features of a rifle

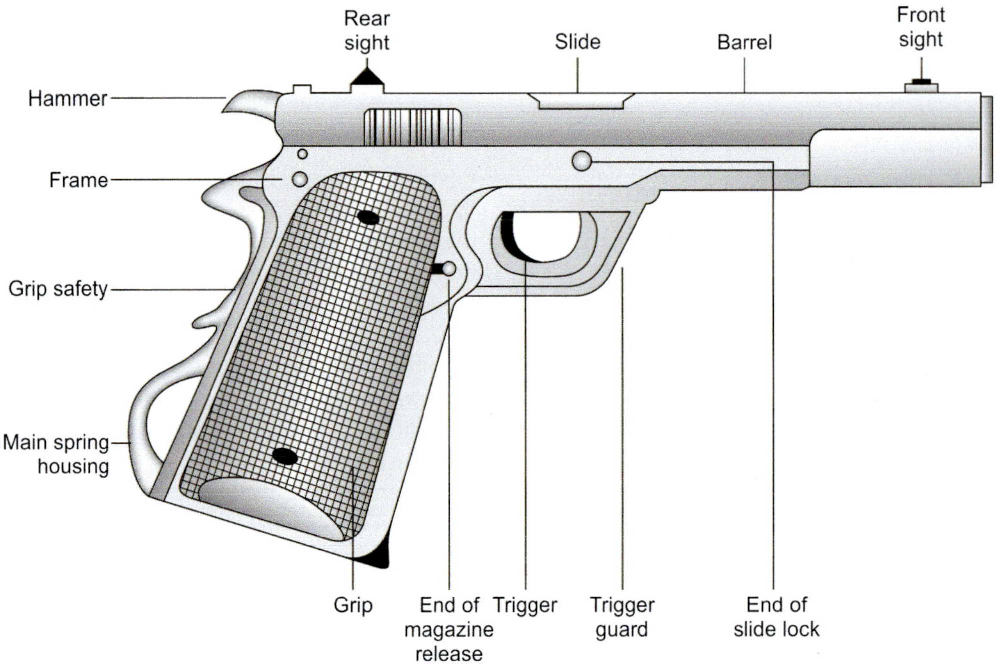

Figure 12.12 Semi-automatic pistol and its different parts

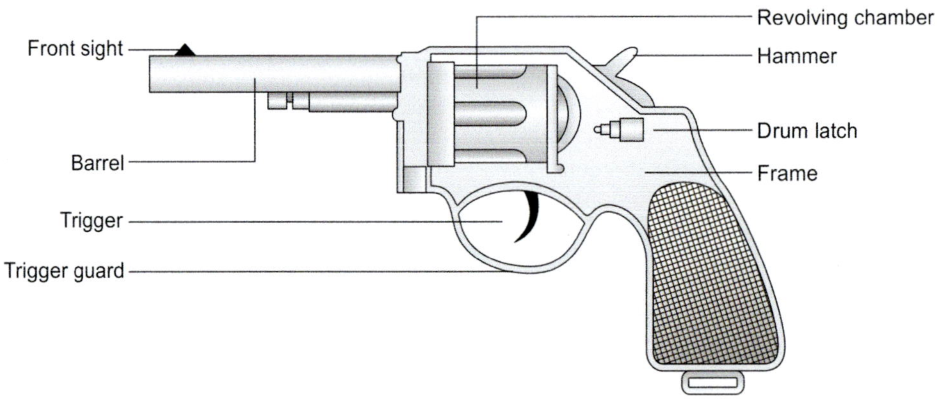

Figure 12.13 Revolver and its different parts

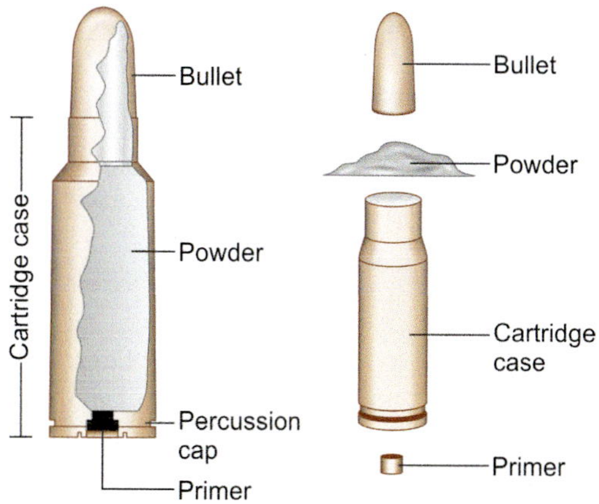

Figure 12.14 Different parts of cartridge of rifled firearm

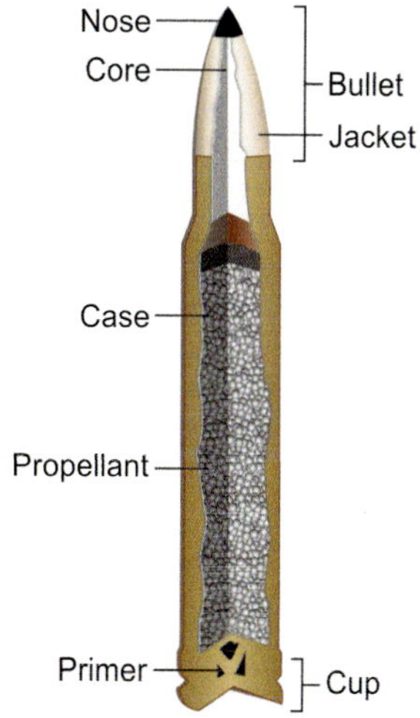

Figure 12.15 Longitudinal section of cartridge of a rifled firearm

Table 12.5 Different shaped bullet

Tip shapes	Ogive shapes	Heel shapes
• Full metal jacket • Soft point • Hollow-point nose (has a depression in the nose and is projected to amplify or 'mushroom' upon impact)	• Spitzer • Round nose • Flat nose • Semi-wad cutter • Square-nose or wad-cutter (soft metal bullet and used mainly for target hitting)	• Flat base • Boat tail

Detonator: Also called as primer and is stored in primer cup or percussion cap. The percussion cap has an igniter fitted in a circular hole, usually in the center of the base ending in to the anvil, having a flash hole in the middle which communicate with the rest of the inside of the cartridge case containing the gunpowder. The top end of cartridge case has hard grips for the base of the bullet.

Propellant: It is the gunpowder which lies in between the primer cap and the bullet and same as for smooth bore firearm. Low-power rim-fire cartridge may not comprise propellant but only a primer mixture in an empty rim. Intrinsically, those cartridges cannot produce tattooing.

Projectile

In rifled firearm, the projectile is a **bullet** that has base, body and nose. It is made of soft metal and in general is cylindrical. The nose may be round or ogive. The base may be flat or boat tailed (**Figure 12.16**). Classical bullet has rounded nose that has cognized as the round-nose soft bullet and is commonly used in rifles and revolvers. In revolver and pistol, the bullet is also short. The metal is lead with varying amounts of antimony added to provide hardness.

Some bullets have, near its base, a peripheral groove called 'cannelure', into which the end of the cartridge case is craped. The bullet in absence of cannelure is fitted in position by indentation on the circumference of the cartridge case. The caliber of a bullet is its cross-sectional diameter. In rifle, the bullet is elongated with pointed end. The different variants of bullet on the basis of shapes of nose and base (heel) are shown in **Figure 12.17 and Table 12.5.**

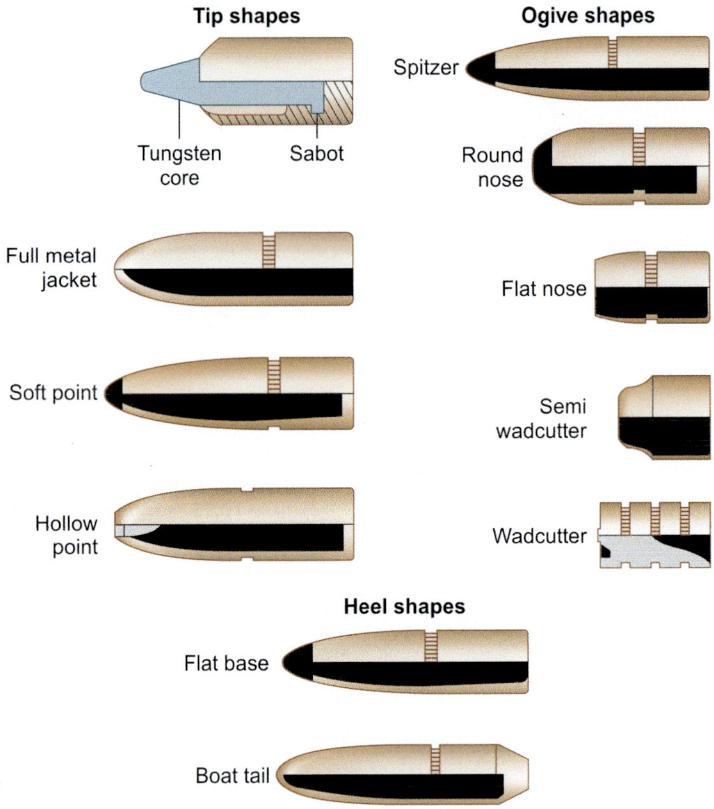

Figure 12.16 Different shaped bullet

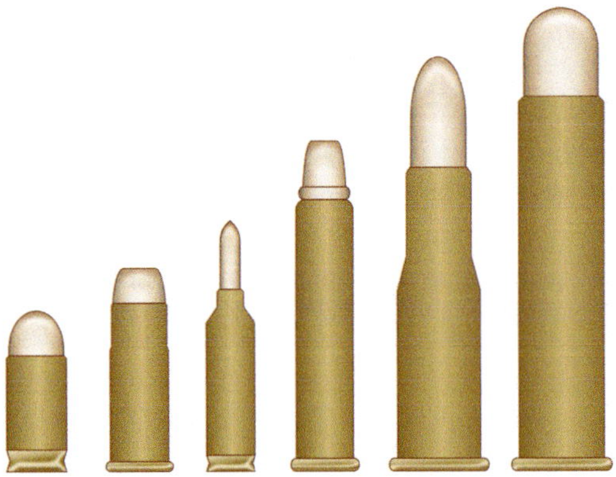

Figure 12.17 Cartridge showing different types of bullet nose

Jacketed Bullets

It has a cover and two type of cover are available:

i. **Full Metal Jacket**: Here the bullet has a soft core made of lead encased in a case of harder metal, viz gilding metal, cupronickel or, less ordinarily, a steel alloy. This case can cover round the entire bullet, or often just the front and sides with the rear left as exposed lead.

The bullet which is completely covered by the jacket is termed a **total metal jacket** round. The jacket allows for higher muzzle velocities than bare lead, without depositing significant amounts of metal in the bore. It also prevents damage to bores from steel or armour-piercing core materials. The appearance of FMJ bullet is extremely distinctive when equated to hollow-point or soft point bullets.

Historically, the first successful full metal jacket rifle bullets were invented by Lt **Col Eduard Rubin** of the Swiss Army in 1882.[17,18] Full metal jacket bullets were first used as standard ammunition in 1886, for the **French Mle** 1886 Lebel rifle.

ii. **Semi-jacketed Bullet**: The case is relatively thin, but tough jacket that cover the base and cylindrical part of body, leaving behind the nose partially or fully uncovered. This type is designed to expand like mushroom to cause more damage on target (**Figure 12.18**).

Mushroom Bullet: It is a semi-jacketed bullet that expands like mushroom when hit on target because of soft nose, which is not covered with jacket. They cause more severe and extensive damages.

Dumdum Bullet: This type of bullet was developed at Dumdum arsenal in India in 1890s by Captain Bertie Clay. Here the jacket does not cover the base, but covers the nose so as to form a hollow at its nose. The purpose is that when bullet strikes the body surface, it expands and produces large hole. There is a tendency for the core to blow off and leave the jacket in the rifling of the barrel blocking the loading of the next round. Hence, the design is discarded and replaced by the 'ball mark III' bullet, which has full jacket with a hole bored in the nose and filled with a short metal tube.

Explosive Bullet: Firebug bullets contain explosive at the front end. It is forbidden types of bullets; it may be dumdumized or devastator bullet. This bullet causes extensive damage to the victim and also danger for the treating doctors or surgeon. It may explode during surgery or during ultrasound or microwave diagnostic techniques, if it had failed to detonate in the body.

Frangible Bullet: Usually made up of compressed particles of metal (iron) and paint, that fragments on striking the object without causing any damage, but leaving the paint marks. It is used by US army and air force for training bullet for aerial gunners.

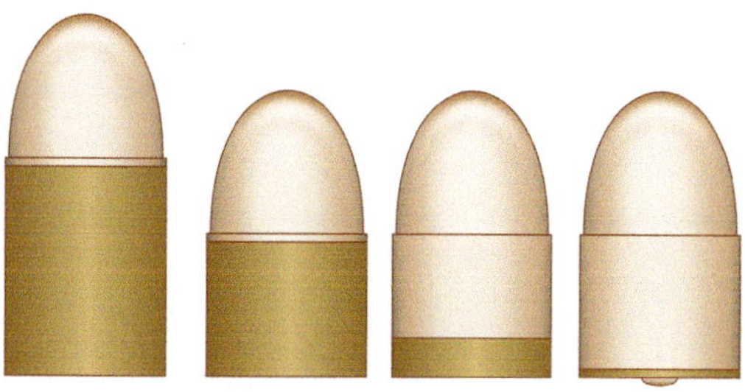

Figure 12.18 Semi-jacketed bullet

Plastic Bullet: It is made up of solid cylinder of polyvinyl chloride. It is commonly fired from a smooth-bore weapon and is effective up to 50–70 meters. Diameter is about 38 mm and is 10 cm long with 135 g of weight. They are used for riot control. Commonly it causes bruising and superficial circular laceration. Less commonly fracture skull, eye damage, fracture ribs, limb bones and contusions of liver, lung and spleen are reported.

Rubber Bullet: It is also known as 'baton round.' These are made up of rubber and commonly used by law enforcement agencies to control mob. Usually causes abrasion and bruises.

Tandem or 'Piggy-back' Bullet: This is a rare event but not unknown. A pair of bullets travels in tandem if the nose of one is in contact with the base of the other. It is observed when a bullet gets lodged inside the barrel and encounters a kick on its base by the nose of another bullet fired afterward. This impact results in carry-over of kinetic energy, i.e. the striking bullet loses kinetic energy whereas the lodged bullet gains kinetic energy. If the striking impulse is significant then the lodged bullet is unseated and becomes free to move in the forward direction along with the striking bullet, as a single projectile. These bullets moving unitedly inside the barrel come out from the muzzle in tandem. Usually, they tend to follow the same flight, but only for a short length because the two bullets unitedly form an unstable projectile. The bullets are thereafter separated and follow different flights.

If the tandem bullets hit the target ahead of separation, a single entry may be detected. If the bullets separate before they hit the target two entry wounds on the same or on different targets may be detected. The phenomenon of two separate regular entry holes by a single effective firing can be established if the recovered bullets are identified as tandem bullets. The identification of tandem bullets thus plays an important role in arriving at significant forensic conclusions. Examination of the base and the nose of the bullet is utmost essential for detection of this phenomenon.

An unusual case of a homicidal gunshot wound to the chest is reported in which two bullets were fired in union as tandem bullets from a handgun. At autopsy, two intact bullets were retrieved from the body of the victim, yet there was only one entrance wound and a single bullet track across the chest wall and thoracic organs. An examination of the weapon and ammunition supported the likelihood of tandem bullets and suggested the probable mechanism for this event. Very few similar cases have been documented.[19]

Souvenir Bullet: If the bullet lodged in tissue remains in the body and get covered by encapsulation of tissue then it is called souvenir bullet. Chronic lead poisoning may occur from such types of bullet.

Incendiary Bullets: Incendiary ammunition contains a compound that burns rapidly and causes fires. Incendiary projectiles, in particular, those intended for armor penetration, are more effective if they explode after penetrating a surface layer, so as to explode inside the target. Additionally, targets with onboard electronics or computers can be damaged by metal fragments when they explode on the surface. Ignition is often delayed by varying means until after impact.[20]

Armor-Piercing Bullet: It is a type of bullet designed to penetrate armor, a bullet that (almost) no armor or bulletproof vest can withstand. It is made up of a hard steel core surrounded by a lead sleeve, both carried in the usual type of jacket. On impact, the lead sleeve and jacket are arrested, while the piercing core continues to penetrate through the target.

Armor-piercing cartridges are also available as small arms ammunition, primarily for use as an anti-materiel round or to defeat body armor.

Devastator Bullets are modified by drilling out the bullet tip, and inserting a cylinder containing lead azide, which is explosive material.

Mechanism of Discharge of Projectile: Pulling the trigger on a loaded gun makes the release of the sprint action of the hammer and hammer hits firing pin, which in turn strike the cartridge base, detonating the primer. The latter event causes ignition of gunpowder in the cartridge. Gunpowder combustion brings on rapidly expanding gas, the pressure of which propels the bullet.

RIFLED FIREARMS OR SHOTGUN INJURIES

The injuries caused by rifled firearm are classed as either entrance or exit wounds. Atypical wounds, i.e. the grazing may also be present. The penetrating wound produced by the bullet over the body at the entrance is termed as **entry** wound and wound caused while leaving the body is termed as **exit** wound. The path travelled by the bullet between entry and exit wound is known as **track of injury**. The distance between the muzzle end and target is termed as **range of fire** (**Figure 12.19**).

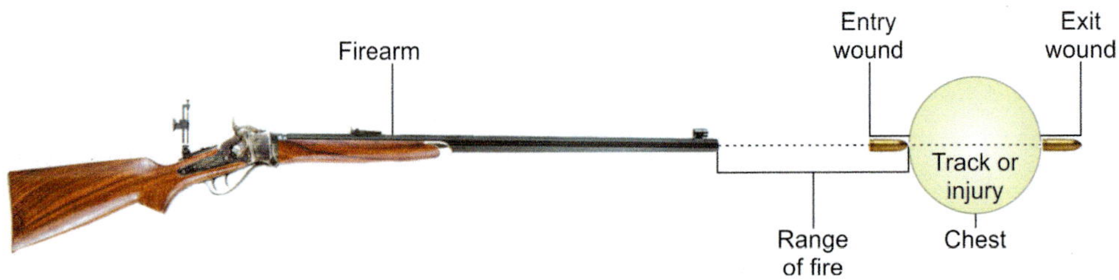

Figure 12.19 Range of firing, entry, track and exit wound

Table 12.6 Discharging components from muzzle end and effects	
Elements	**Effects on body**
Projectile (bullet)	Entry and exit wound
Smoke and soot	Smudging, blackening
Gunpowder particle	Tattooing
Gases	Blasting effect, cherry red discoloration
Flame	Scorching or singeing
Metal particle	Metal ring
Grease or dirt	Grease collar

Certain Features of Rifled Firearm Wound

1. The elements of the cartridge emerge on the discharge of a rifled firearm and all contribute to the wound are shown in **Table 12.6** and **Figure 12.20.**
2. The bullet on the body tries to penetrate the skin against its elasticity that result skin stretching. This attempt results in perforation of the skin with inverted margin. The bullet also causes abrasion. Due to elasticity of the skin, the margin of entry wound get retracted and appears small. Like that of entry wound the exit wound is not supported, hence causes eversion of the margins with larger sizes.
3. As the bullet penetrates the skin, friction between it and the epithelium results in the creation of an '**abrasion collar**'. This abrasion collar is caused by the bullet's scraping the margins of the skin on penetration and is characteristic of a gunshot wound of entrance. However, in some cases '**contusion collar**' instead of abrasion may also be present. Contusion collar is the bruise caused by the bullet trajectory to the human body. Abrasion collar and contusion collar also gives the direction of fire; the side in which it is more prominent is the direction from which the gun was fired and, if the abrasion collar/contusion collar is very uniform all around the margin of the wound, it means that the gun used was directly perpendicular to the site of entry. These two features are proof of an entrance wound. The abraded collar is reddish at first, but becomes reddish brown as it dries. Irregular and occasionally patterned abrasion collar is sometimes produced by coarse article of clothing scraping on the skin.
4. A black colored ring "**grease or dirt collar**", which is also known as '**bullet wipe soiling**' **or** '**soiling ring**', is seen as a narrow ring of skin, lining the defect. It is caused from the wiping of contents from the surface of the bullet as it passes through the skin, i.e. bullet lubrication, gun oil of interior of the barrel, lead from the surface of the bullet, barrel debris, etc. It is more marked in a distant firing though it can also be present

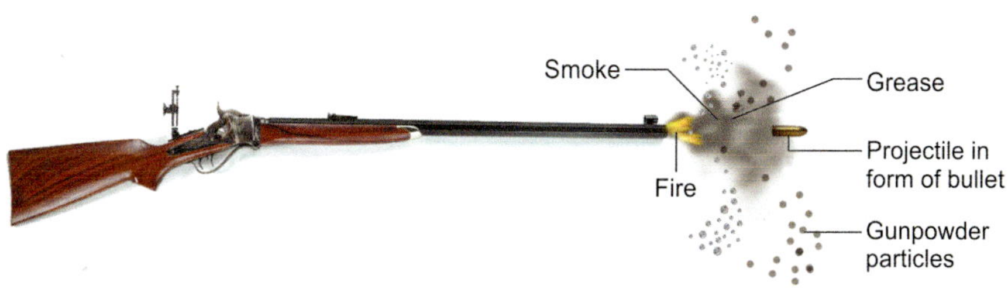

Figure 12.20 Discharging components from muzzle end

in near firing. Infrared photography distinctly points the presence of black ring round the bullet hole. **Dirt collar** is unlikely if the bullet is jacketed. By contrast, soot is dark in the center and fades towards the periphery.
The abrasion collar surrounds the dirt collar. When both grease and abrasion collar are present, then the grease collar is seen in the inner zone and the abrasion collar at the outer zone (**Figure 12.21**).

5. Singeing of the hairs may be present due to the escape of the flame through the muzzle end. The clothes may show evidence of burning. Evidence of burning is noted on microscopic examination in the edges of the contact and near-contact bullet wounds due to the flame of muzzle blast.
6. Tattooing begins when the muzzle to target distance exceeds one cm. The unburnt gunpowder and debris, causes punctate abrasions on target. It is also known as peppering or stippling. It is seen as small, discrete, black specks, and it does not wipe off.
7. The blackening or smudging is present due to deposition of smoke particles on the skin.
8. The carbon monoxide emerging from the gases combines with hemoglobin and leads to formation of carboxyhemoglobin and results cherry red coloration of the tissues.
9. A **metal ring** may also be present around the entry wound as a result of deposition of lead or other metal particles, which can be detected by neutron activation analysis or by X-ray.

Medicolegal Importance of Powder Marks

- Diagnosis of firearm injuries
- Differentiate between entry and exit wound
- Diagnosis of gunpowder, thus help in weapon identification
- Distance of firing estimation
- Direction of firing.

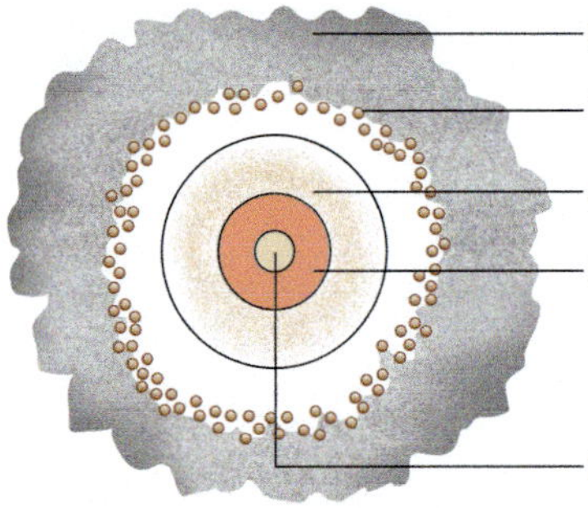

Figure 12.21 Effect of discharge of rifled firearm

In perpendicular firing, powder marks will be found in symmetrical distribution around the entry. In oblique firing, powder marks will be found in asymmetrical distribution around the entry, being more condensed at the nearest side of the assailant. In tangential firing, powder marks will be found only at the edge of the track, which is the near end to the assailant.

Entry Wound in Rifled Firearm

Entry wounds of gunshot are divided into four categories based on their **range of fire: Contact, close, intermediate and distant**. Entrance wounds over elastic tissue will contract around the tissue defect and have a diameter much less than the caliber of the bullet.

Contact Shot or Point Blank Shot

i. If the muzzle is pressed against the skin firmly (tight contact) when fired, the entire powder residue will be blasted into the tissues. Imprint abrasion of muzzle end may be present (**Figure 12.22**). If the seal between muzzle and skin is weak (loose contact), powder residue will be deposited on the cutaneous surface and the wound track.
ii. It is circular in size in areas of "loose" skin, viz abdomen and chest with blackened, singed skin margins.
iii. On head, where the scalp is tightly covering the skull, entry wounds can have several different appearances:

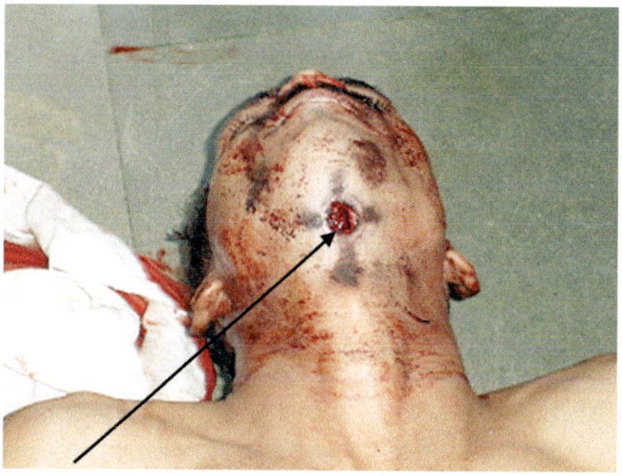

Figure 12.22 Entry wound of a bullet showing imprint abrasion of muzzle end

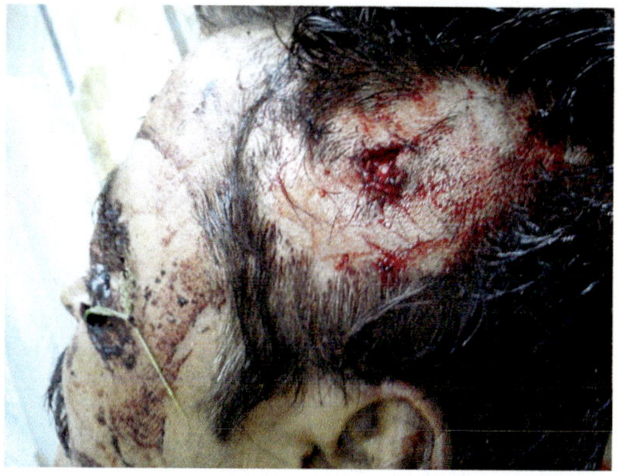

Figure 12.23 Stellate shaped entry wound in contact shot

(A) round wound with blackened, seared skin margins. (B) Stellate shaped wound, due to tearing of skin from explosive effect of gas dissecting between the scalp and skull (**Figure 12.23**). (C) Round wound with muzzle imprint, also due to gas expanding under the skin causing it to press back against the gun.

iv. '**Back spatter**' phenomenon may be present due to muzzle blast and negative pressure in the barrel that may suck blood, hair, fragments of tissue and cloth fibers inside.

Close Shot

i. Flame in revolver or pistol travel about 7.5 cm and in shoulder-rest gun, up to 15 cm.
ii. Circular entry wound (unless entering at an angle—then more tear-drop shaped).
iii. If the bullet enters perpendicularly, the wound will be circular and soot soiling, powder tattooing, stippling, etc. will be distributed circumferentially.
iv. Abrasion collar, grease collar may be present.
v. Inverted edges.
vi. **Stellate shaped** in higher velocity weapons, or hard contact over bony parts of the body, slit-like or irregular if bullet deformed or tumbling.
vii. Shallow angled wounds may '**graze the surface**'.

Intermediate Range Shot

i. As the range of fire increases, features of intermediate range wounds are seen. There is a gradual reduction in the amount of soot soiling seen around the wound, as well as a reduction in the amount of heat searing. Soot soiling is generally seen up to about 15 cm while powder tattooing can be found at up to 30–45 cm. These distances can be doubled for rifles.[14]
ii. Where small fragments of metal from the bullet or the barrel impact the skin surface, the term '**fouling**' is used. These fragments are not easy to remove (unlike soot, which can be wiped off), and where the victim survives an inflammatory reaction occurs to these foreign bodies.[15]
Unburnt explosive flakes may also be seen as small glistening and often colored particles, depending upon the manufacturer.
iii. As the range increases, the areas of skin **tattooed** increases up to the point till it start falling because of lack of energy (about **60–120** cm, depending upon the powder type).
iv. If the bullet enters the body at a very acute angle, it may travel just under the skin surface before coming to rest—when this occurs, there may be a series of interrupted surface bruises that follow the track. Intermediate range rifle wounds still result in massive internal damage.
v. Singeing and scorching absent.

Distant Shot

When the muzzle to skin distance is beyond the range of powder deposition, circular defects are seen with an abraded collar, but with no associated searing, soot deposition or powder tattooing.[21] Distant shots from rifles may result in a central defect with micro-tearing of the wound edges, and massive internal destruction. The important features of entrance wound at different ranges are summarized in **Table 12.7**.

Exit Wound

In general, exit wounds (**Table 12.24**) are larger than the entrance wounds. They are also more irregular in outline, and their edges are everted. They exhibit no abrasion collar, and they do not have any features of secondary muzzle product projectile impact, such as soot soiling or powder tattooing.[14,21]

The exit wound assist in ascertaining direction of firing, position of victim at the time of firing. The differences between entry and exit wound of a bullet are given in **Table 12.8**.

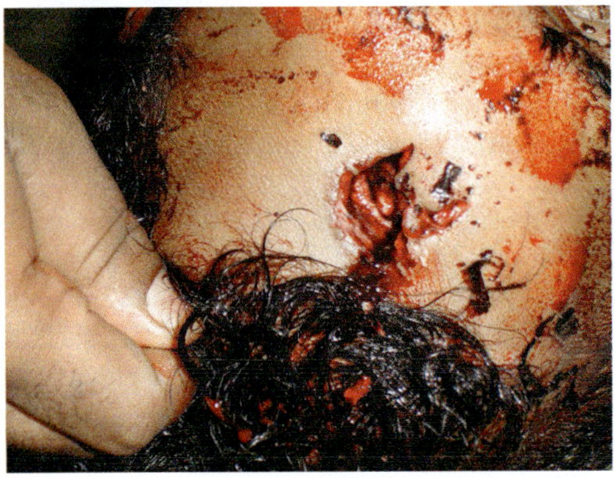

Figure 12.24 Exit wound of a bullet

Gunshot Wounds in Bone

Because the skull is formed of an inner and outer table, entrance and exit sites are ordinarily determined. When a bullet enters the skull, it produces a sharp-edged "punched-out" hole in the outer table, with a larger corresponding "beveled-out" hole on the inner table.

In flat bones like skull, the entry wounds are round with sharp margins (**Figure 12.25**) and show internal beveling (**Figure 12.26**). The inner table of the skull is more eroded than the outer table, producing a '**cone**' shape in the direction of the bullet path. Fragments of bone travel in the direction of the bullet path through the cranial vault.

Exit wounds may be more irregular and show external beveling, i.e. outer table of the skull is more eroded than the inner table, creating a cone shape facing outward (**Figure 12.27**). In the skull, gunshot wounds often produce multiple fractures due to rapidly increasing pressure as the bullet travels through the skull.

Table 12.7 Features of entrance wound at different ranges of fire

Features	Hard contact	Close range	Intermediate range	Distant range
Range	Contact with skin	< 7.5 cm	30–45 cm	>60 cm
Size	Larger than bullet	Bullet size	Smaller than bullet size	Smaller than bullet size
Shape	Variable	Circular	Circular	Circular
Muzzle imprint	Present	Absent	Absent	Absent
Edges	Everted	Inverted	Inverted	Inverted
Scorching	Present in deeper tissues	Present	Absent	Absent
Singeing	Present in deeper tissues	Present	Absent	Absent
Blackening	Present in deeper tissues	Present	Present up to 30 cm	Absent
Tattooing	Present in deeper tissues	Present	Present	Absent
Abrasion collar	May be absent	Present	Present	Present
Grease collar	May be absent	Present	Present	Present

Table 12.8 Differences between entry and exit wound

Features	Entry	Exit
Loss of substance	More	Less
Edges	Inverted except in contact firing, entry into a fatty area (skin stretched, but fat plug outward), putrefaction (due to the effect of gases)	Everted
Powder marks (burning-blackening, tattooing)	May be present depending upon the range of fire	Absent
Size	Smaller except contact firing, oblique firing shots (big central hole with smaller exit)	Larger
Regularity of the wound	More regular, circular except in very near firing	Irregular
Soiling ring	Present	Absent
Carboxy hemoglobin	May be present	Absent
Beveling of the flat bone	Internal beveling	External beveling
Microscopic examination around the wound	Embedded powder particles are seen, which is not seen by the naked eye Swelling and homogenization of dermal collagen fibers caused by the heat of the bullet along with the streaming of the nucleus	No embedded powder particles present No swelling and homogenization of dermal collagen fibers are found

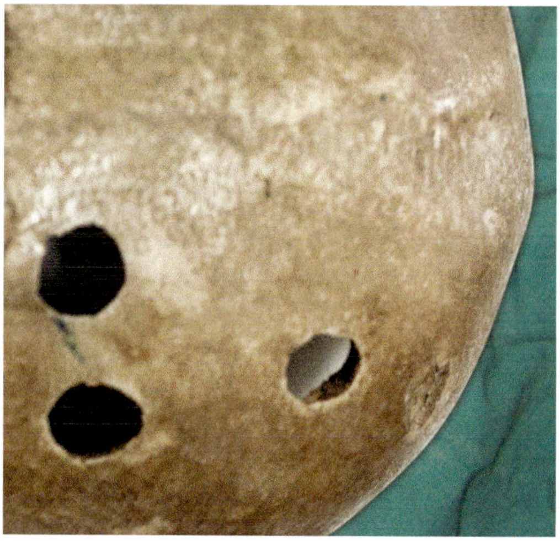

Figure 12.25 Bullet entry wound on skull showing outer table

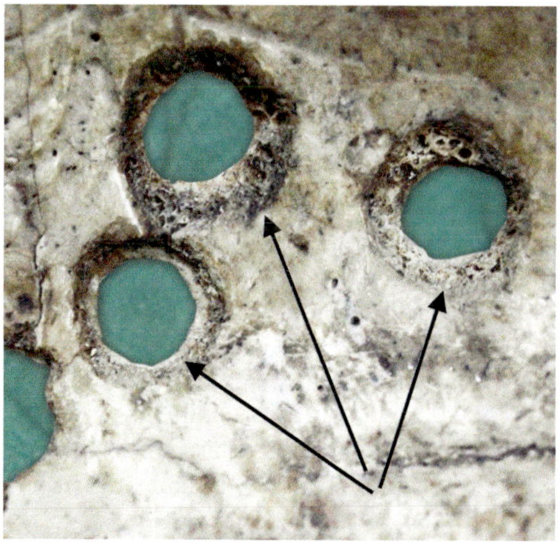

Figure 12.26 Bullet entry wound on skull with beveling in inner table

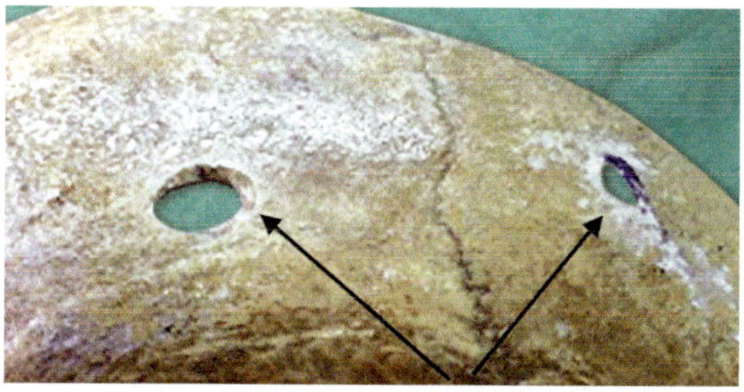

Figure 12.27 Bullet exit wound on skull with external beveling (outer table)

Unusual Effect of Rifled Firearm

i. **Single Entrance and Multiple Exits:** (a) when a bullet hits a bone in its course, it may break the bone into pieces which may act as separate missiles and may give rise single entry, but several exit wounds. (b) When bullet hits some intervening object and that moves along with the bullet acting as a separate missile (the phenomenon known as **secondary missile effect**). (c) The jacket of a bullet may separate from inner part upon impact on bone, producing two different exit wound.

ii. **Atypical Entry Wound**
   a. At close range, the entry wound may become atypically larger with everted margins. This is due to the presence of '**tail wobbles**' or '**tail wag**'. This is partly responsible for the great tissue damage and the large atypical entrance wound at short range.
   b. Gyroscopic effect of a bullet diminishes as it attains the end of its flight, when it begins to wobble and then to tumble. During wobble, yaw or tumble, the impact of the bullet may be sideways or even backwards with an atypical lateral movement, due to which an atypical lacerated wound is produced. The bullet traveling in an atypical fashion instead of traveling **nose-on** is named as '**yawning bullet**', and the bullet which rotates **end-on-end** during its movement is named a '**tumbling bullet**'. The quantity of tissue crush might be three times bigger when the bullet yaws to 90°.
   c. When silencers are used, the tattooing seen on the skin may be altered. Muzzle brakes and flash hiders may create peculiar blackening and tattooing patterns by allowing gases to pass in particular direction.
   d. **Ricochet Bullet**: It is one which before hitting the object, hits some interposing object first, and then after ricocheting and rebounding from that, strikes the object. This is rare, as most bullets on striking a hard coat break up or penetrate. Critical angle of the impact for ricochet for hard coats ranges from 10–30°. The bullet ricochets off at an angle smaller than the impact angle. The bullet may ricochet before or after hitting the body and may create a non-penetrating or a penetrating injury.
      The bullet may be deformed and flattened before hitting the skin. Thus it creates a big irregularly oval, triangular or cruciate entry wound with irregular abraded margins. As the bullet usually loses gyrating movements, abrasion collar may be absent. Burning, blackening and tattooing are also not seen as it usually a distant shot.
      Sometimes, a bullet may hit an object and then tumble and hit the body side on, producing an elongated wound of entry like a keyhole. On recovering the bullet, traces particles from which the bullet is deflected or has struck, e.g. soil, fibers, paints, etc. may be found. The nose of the bullet may be found facing the entrance wound due to deflection in the body. When the velocity is lost, the bullet only produces an abrasion or contusion.
   e. A bullet may hit the target producing a contusion and fall off to the ground. This is seen with relatively soft non-jacketed bullet fired from a firearm that has an eroded or worn barrel; and also when the ammunition used is of smaller size than the barrel of the gun.
   f. **Bullet Graze or Slap**: If a bullet hits the body surface at an acute angle, then it does not perforate the deeper tissues, rather a grazing wound is created. Commonly, it looks as reddish-brown, elongated, elliptical or triangular furrow or abrasion or laceration. The underlying dermis or the deeper tissue may or may not be involved, but the adjacent intact skin may be ecchymosed.

iii. **Bullet Striking the Skull without Entry Wound**: The bullets may graze or rub the top or sides of the cranium without producing any wound of entrance. The entry and exit wounds may be found on the scalp itself with about 2–3 cm diameter. It may be associated with an oval or elongated gutter-like depression (**gutter wound; key-hole defect**) of the intervening skull.

iv. **Single Firing, but Multiple Entry and Exit Wound**: A bullet may go through the arm and then the chest so that four wounds are ensued. A bullet going through the chest or abdomen and then thigh and lower leg, produces six wounds. This occurs when the person is running or sitting in an uncommon position. The bullet injuries through the irregular surfaces, such as the breast and buttocks, several re-entries and exits may occur. Examination of clothing and estimation of nitrites and nitrates and histological examination of the wound may be necessary. The features of re-entry wound that correspond to long-range wound may create confusion.

v. **Entry Wound Present, but Bullet not Recovered in the Body**: This is only possible when the bullet coming into the stomach is vomited out, coming into the windpipe and is coughed out, entering into the mouth and is spit out, entering the gastrointestinal tract is passed out with the feces, and when it is so deviated on coming in contact with some bone, that it passes out by the same wound as it entered.

vi. **Casualties with Blank Cartridges**: A blank is a type of cartridge for a firearm that contains primer, gunpowder and wadding, but no bullet or shot. When fired, the blank makes a flash and an explosive sound. Blanks are often used for simulation, training, and for signaling.

Deaths or injuries from blanks occur when blanks are fired by people who are unaware of their destructive capabilities. Actors in particular are at serious risk of injury from blank cartridges used on movie sets. Several famous actors, viz. Brandon Lee, Jon-Erik Hexum, etc., died in such mishaps.

vii. **Tear-gas Cartridge Gunshot Wounds**: Clarot, et al.[22] accounted a case of head injury caused by a tear-gas shell fired, in a case of suicide. The weapon was an 8 mm blank firing pistol loaded with a CS 8 mm cartridge. The discharge of blank firing guns or tear-gas cartridges produces a gas jet capable of causing pronounced close or contact range firings, often more so than other gunshot wounds, where the amplifying gases are able to follow the path of the penetrating projectile—unlike in the case of blank firing weapons.

viii. **Bullet Emboli**: Another surprise characteristic '**bullet emboli**', where a bullet or fragment affects an artery or great vessel and is carried into the bloodstream to lodge at another site distant from the wound track. However, this is more likely to occur in distant wounds from shotguns where the pellets are embolized.

ix. **Artefacts**: The external wounds may be altered by therapeutic procedures. Excision of wound margins and closure of wound by sutures may make it hard to identify correctly an entrance or exit wound. The marks of sutures may look as gunpowder tattooing. During hospitalization, victim may sustain '**Pseudo-gunshot wounds**', the trocar marks and drainage incision in chest and abdomen. A classical example of this is '**Kennedy phenomenon**' it is surgical alteration of the gunshot wounds on the neck of President John F Kennedy, which lead to difficulty in evaluation of that wound and the consequent controversy rose whether it was an entrance or an exit wound.

If there is any loose cartridge on garment and body is X-rayed with garments on, there may be misinterpretation. X-rays may also describe other metallic objects such as buttons, which resemble a bullet or stem of zipper giving the impression of a mushroom bullet and a dislodged crown from tooth may correspond a flattened bullet.

x. **Presence of Unexpected Bullet**: During the autopsy of firearm deaths, finding of unexpected bullets in the body is always a puzzle and may lead to a false conclusion.

Example of an old bullet: In case of a burned body, X-rays showed a bullet in the posterior wall of chest. This X-ray finding immediately raised suspicion of murder. However, when the bullet was located and removed, it was found to be well-enclosed by dense fibrous tissue.

Example of a new bullet: A man shot him in right temple and the bullet was found from the brain. There was, however, another bullet inside the stomach. The investigation showed a row of beer cans in his house's backyard, used as a target. Part of the beer in the cans that had bullet holes had been consumed. The man drank beer from each can and drank a bullet with the beer. Injuries such as punctured wounds and lacerations may resemble exit and entrance wound.

xi. **Concealed Firearm Wounds**: When the body is covered with blood, the blood clots may blur the wound. A wound in the mouth, nostril, ear or in the body orifices, e.g. rectum or vagina may not be detected, if due care is not taken.

xii. **Effect of Bullet in Fluid Filled Viscera**: When a bullet travels through fluid filled viscera such as the stomach filled with fluid, urinary bladder filled with urine, blood filled heart or CSF filled cerebral ventricles, etc., there produces a violent turbulence in the fluid as result of the bullet passing through it. As a result of this turbulence, extensive lacerations are seen in these organs.

Position of the Assailant

i. The distance of firing can be estimated from external and internal wads and degree of penetration of the bullets and shots dispersion, distribution of powder marks around the entry, but this method only tells that firing was perpendicular or oblique or tangential, etc.

ii. By joining the exit and entry wound with an imaginary line and extending that line by a distance equal to the estimated range, the end of the line indicates the position of the assailant. In this case, we must be sure during autopsy that the bullet passed in a straight line and is not deviated inside the body.

iii. In case, the missile stays inside the body, an imaginary line in the line of the tract will give the direction of fire, but must be sure that no deviation of the bullet occurred.

iv. When there is a deviation of the bullet, the straight line in the pathway of the bullet before deviation.

v. The position of the assailant may be ascertained by the presence of empty cartridges found on the ground at the scene of the crime in case of automatic weapons or foot print or eye witness.

Factors Affecting the Appearance of the Entry

i. **Type of the Weapon**: Whether it fires shots (central hole with or without dispersion) or bullets (single hole).

The length of the barrel also has an effect on the area of skin exhibiting soot soiling; a snub nosed revolver, for example, will spread soot over a larger area than from a pistol with a longer barrel.[15] The use of silencers on handguns reduces the area of soot soiling and powder tattooing and cause difficulties in determining range of fire.

However, powder particles leaving the muzzle are able to impact upon the skin surface, giving rise to powder tattooing at a distance of about 10 mm from the average handgun muzzle.

ii. **Distance of Firing**: In very near firing (less than 15 cm) the entry is lacerated with everted edges. In non-rifled weapon in near firing (less than one meter), the shots entering together as one mass make one central hole with no dispersion, but distant firing causes dispersion of the shots.

iii. **Direction of Firing**: Perpendicular firing causes a circular entry, oblique firing causes oval entry, and tangential firing causes a track over the surface (**Figure 12.28**).

iv. **Site of the Entry**: When the entry is in an area with a corrugated skin, e.g. axilla, it will be irregular in shape.

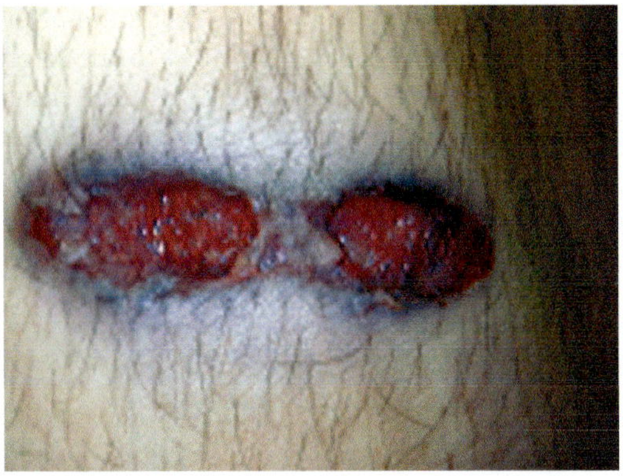

Figure 12.28 Tangential passage of a bullet

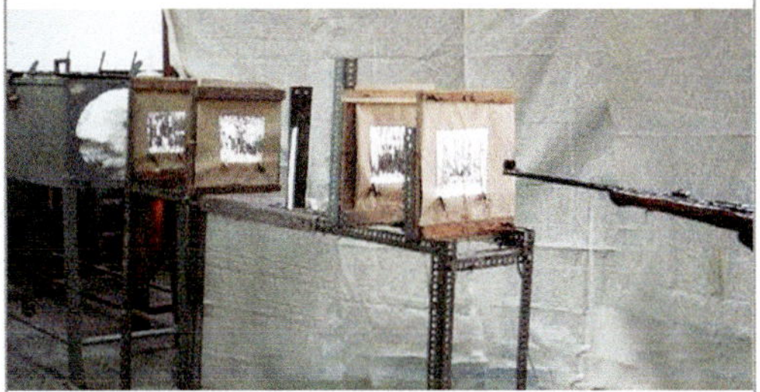

Figure 12.29 Test firing

v. **Type of Powder**: Dense black ring around the entry in case of black powder, and a faint grayish around the entry in case of smokeless powder.

IDENTIFICATION OF THE WEAPON

Weapon

(A) Its number: Each weapon has a specific number written on it. (B) Type and bore of the weapon (compared with the missiles extracted from the body or empty cases found in the scene of crime). (C) Fingerprints or blood stains. (D) Chemical analysis: Swab from barrel to detect the nature of powder and the time passed since firing.

Test Firing: The suspected weapon is loaded and fired into boxes packed with wool (**Figure 12.29**). The bullet that is recovered is known as the **test bullet** and the bullet recovered from the scene of crime or the body of the victim is known as the **crime bullet**. The test bullet and the crime bullets are then compared for the secondary markings under the **comparison microscope**. Similarly, the recovered cartridge case after the test firing as well as the one from the scene of crime are compared for the impression of the firing pin, etc.

The Missile

The bullet is examined for its type and caliber (compare with the suspected weapon) and for rifling marks.

Rifling Marks: The number, direction (clockwise, anticlockwise), breadth and depth of primary rifling marks are examined by comparison microscope. Identical marks means that suspected weapon may be responsible for the crime. Secondary rifling marks, microscopic scratches on the surface of the bullet due to irregularities and rust on the inside of the barrel, are also individual to each weapon. The bullet should not be held with metal instruments while recovering to avoid artefacts (preferably should hold with rubber tipped forceps or cover with cotton or gauze before holding).

The Wads: It gives an idea about the type (non-rifled) and caliber of the weapon.

Gunshot Wound Imaging

When bullets enter the body and fragment, especially after striking a bone, they can be seen on X-rays as '**scattered radiopaque**' fragments. However, when a semi-jacketed high-velocity bullet round fragments, it is seen on X-ray as a '**snow storm**' of fragments. Fully jacketed bullets usually do not fragment, and so, do not show these radiological features.

Imaging of gunshot wound victims may also detect a surprise characteristic, i.e. the '**bullet emboli**'.

i. **Dermal Nitrate Test/Paraffin Test**: For detection of the nitrates/nitrite from the gun in the fired hand, but due to high false positivity, it is omitted nowadays.

ii. **Neutron Activation Analysis (NAA)**: For detection of gunshot residue in fired hand or in the cloth or in entry wound.
iii. **Flameless Atomic Absorption Spectrometry** (FAAS).
iv. **Scanning Electron Microscopy-energy Dispersive X-ray Spectrometry** (SEM EDX): For detection of the metal particles like barium, antimony and lead in entry wounds.

Patterns of Gunshot Injuries

Evaluating whether an injury is self-inflicted is helped by knowledge of epidemiological data. The most common site for suicidal gunshot wound is the head (74%), usually the right temple (39%), followed by chest and abdomen. Men are more likely than women to shoot themselves in the head.

Karger, et al.[23] evaluated records of 624 consecutive gunshot autopsies in Germany and carried out binary logistic regression analysis in order to identify characteristics of suicidal and homicidal gunshot wounds. They said that females comprised more of the homicide victims than suicide victims (26.3% vz 10.6%).

Suicidal gunshots were fired from contact or near-contact range in 89% (7.5% of homicides), and the typical entrance wound sites were the temple (36%), mouth (20%), forehead (11%) and left chest (15%). However, uncommon sites did occur, including the back of the head, eye, ear and nape of neck.

They also analyzed the wound track in order to identify characteristics of suicide or homicide, and noted that in suicidal wounds to the right temple, the majority of tracks were oriented front-to-back and upwards (or parallel), while homicidal wound tracks were oriented back-to-front or downwards. Suicidal gunshots to the left chest were oriented right-to-left or parallel, while homicidal shots were frequently left-to-right. Shots were oriented upwards and downwards in both groups.

In a study conducted by AJ Patowary[24] in Assam, India, also confirmed that most common site of injury in homicidal firearm injury were in the chest (29.95%) followed by the head (18.27%).

It can hence be concluded that an analysis of wound patterns can give clues to the likely manner of death, but atypical patterns occur frequently, and a proper crime investigation and multidisciplinary approach is, therefore, crucial in all firearm deaths.

ROLE OF PHYSICIAN IN FIREARM INJURIES

Do's

i. Make good notes of the original appearances of the injuries before any surgical cleaning or operative interference.
ii. Remove any missiles, foreign bodies such as wads, bullets or shots and any skin from the margin of a firearm wound as well as the tract of the wound during treatment and preserve carefully for the police.
iii. Swab the skin around the wounds for powder residues.
iv. Draw the site, size and appearance of the wound.
v. Photograph of each injury (distant and close-up) with an appropriate scale in view.
vi. Look at radiographs before beginning the surgery to identify types of the projectile and their location.
vii. Look under the breasts, scrotum, axillae, groin and perineum for hidden inlet, exit or re-entry wound.
viii. Differentiate between firearm injuries and puncture wound by the presence of different characters of firearm injuries.

Don'ts

i. Push probes through loose tissue because this can result in art factual tracks with incorrect directionality.
ii. Handle the projectiles with metal instruments because forceps and clamps can distort rifling marks on lead projectiles and metal jackets.
iii. Forget to search for components of a shotgun charge that are not visible on a radiograph such as a plastic sleeve and fiber wadding.

REFERENCES

1. US Marine Corps. FM 6-40 Tactics, techniques, and procedures for field artillery manual cannon gunnery. Washington: Department of the army; 1996.
2. Interior ballistics. [cited 2012 March 22]; Available from: URL:http://www.ballistics.org/docs/InteriorBallistics.pdf
3. Ballistics Fields—Launch Dynamics—International Ballistics Society. Transitional Ballistic. [cited 2012 March 22]; Available from: URL:http://www.ballistics.org/docs/Ballistic%20Fields%20-%20Launch%20Dynamics.pdf
4. Ballistic Fields—Exterior ballistics. [cited 2012 march 22]; Available from: URL:http://www.ballistics.org/docs/Ballistic%20Fields%20-%20Exterior%20Ballistics.pdf
5. Ballistic Fields—Terminal ballistics. [cited 2012 march 22]; Available from: URL:http://www.ballistics.org/docs/Ballistic%20Fields%20-%20Terminal%20Ballistics.pdf
6. Tiller/Define Tiller at Dictionary.com. Online Etymology Dictionary. [cited 2012 March 23]; Available from: URL:http://www.dictionary.reference.com/browse/Tiller
7. Rifle Recoil—Chuckhawks.com: Gun and Shooting online. [cited 2012 March 23]; Available from: URL:http://www.chuckhawks.com/recoil_table.htm
8. Scattergun/Define Scattergun at Dictionary.com. [Cited 2012 March 23]; Available from: URL:http://dictionary.reference.com/browse/scattergun
9. Muller D, Levy A, Vinokurow A, Revreby M, Shelef R, Wolf E, et al. A novel method for the analysis of discharged smokeless powder residues. J Forensic Sci. 2007;52:75-8.
10. Breitennecker R. Shotgun wound patterns. Am J Clinical Path. 1969;52(3):258-69.
11. Dana SE, Di Maio VJM. Gunshot trauma. In: Payne-James JJ, Busuttil A, Smock W (Eds), Forensic Medicine: Clinical and Pathological Aspects. Greenwich Medical Media 2003.
12. Di Maio VJM. Gunshot Wound: Practical Aspects of Firearms, Ballistics, and Forensic Techniques, 2nd ed. CRC Press: 1999.
13. Cassidy M. Smooth-bore firearm injuries. In: Mason JK, Purdue BN (Eds), The Pathology of Trauma, 3rd ed. Arnold Publishers; 2000.
14. Knight B. Forensic Pathology. 2nd ed. Arnold Publishers; 1996.
15. Spitz WU (Ed). Spitz and Fisher's Medico legal Investigation of Death. Guidelines for the application of pathology to crime investigation. 3rd ed. Charles C Thomas Publishers; 1993.
16. Branson A. The Assassination of Robert Kennedy. Part 5-Sirhan Sirhan. Sott focus 2008 Jun [cited 2012 march 31]; Available from: URL:http://www.sott.net/articles/show/159511-The-Assassination-of-Robert-Kennedy
17. Bobinson H. The model 1911 Schmidt Rubin: the other Switzer. Guns Magazine. Find Articles.com. [cited 2012 march 31]; Available from: URL:http://www.findarticles.com/p/articles/mi_m0BQY/is_11_54/ai_n28573712/
18. Wood JB. The Gun Digest Book of Firearms Assembly/Disassembly. Centerfire Rifles. Volume 4. Krause Publications; 2003. pp. 631-5.
19. Bentley AJ, Busuttil A, Clifton B, Sibbald P. Homicidal tandem bullet wound of the chest. Am J Forensic Med Pathol. 1997;18(1):56-9.
20. Bullets for Beginners—GlobalSecurity.org. [cited 2012 March 31]; Available from: URL:http://www.globalsecurity.org/.../systems/munitions/bullets.htm
21. Besant-Matthews PE. Examination and interpretation of rifled firearm injuries. In: Mason JK, Purdue BN, The Pathology of Trauma. 3rd ed. Arnold Publishers; 2000.
22. Clarot F, Vaz E, Papin F, Clin B, Vicomte C, Proust B. Lethal head injury due to tear-gas cartridge gunshots. Forensic Sci Int 2003;137(1):45-51.
23. Karger B, Billeb E, Koops E, Brinkmann B. Autopsy features relevant for discrimination between suicidal and homicidal gunshot injuries. Int J Legal Med. 2002;116:273-8.
24. Patowary AJ. Study of pattern of injuries in homicidal firearm injury cases. J Ind Acad Forensic Med. 2005:27(2):92-5.

CHAPTER 13

Regional Injuries

Manjula Bai KH, Putul Mahanta

LEARNING PLAN

- Know about anatomical review of head
- Learn the pattern of injuries to the head, abdomen, limbs, etc.
- Know the different types of fracture of skull and intracranial hemorrhage

Regional injuries consist of injuries sustained to various regions of the body. The effects of injuries vary depending on the exact area of the body that is injured. A stab wound to a limb is unlikely to have fatal consequences, whereas a similar injury to the chest may well be fatal. The effects of a blow to the chest may be minimal, but the consequences of exactly the same blow to the head may be catastrophic.

BRIEF ANATOMICAL REVIEW OF HEAD

The head is vulnerable to injury, often with severe consequences. It is particularly susceptible to acceleration/deceleration and rotational forces because it is dense, freely mobile and relatively unstable. Injuries to the head are particularly dangerous because of the brain's vital role in sustaining the life of the individual. "Head injury" and "brain injury" are not identical, but cannot be easily separated. Head injury may not be associated with neurological deficits.

The brain is protected within the strong, bony cranial cage, but it is not well restrained within this compartment and injuries to the brain result from differences between the motion of the skull and the brain. Once the impact of a force crosses the protective threshold, life is invariably in danger. The external injury to the head and the face may or may not be representative of the internal injury and the extent of the danger of the impact. There are three main components of the head: the scalp, the skull and the brain.

Scalp

The scalp consists of five layers of tissue arranged from outside to inside in the following order: 1. Skin, 2. Dense connective tissue, 3. Galea aponeurotica, 4. Loose connective tissue and 5. Periosteum (pericranium).

Skull

The skull can be divided into two main parts as follows:

a. The **calvaria (brain box)**: The upper part of the cranium which encloses the brain. The calvaria or brain case is composed of eight bones: Paired parietal and temporal bones and unpaired frontal, occipital, sphenoid and ethmoid bone.
   The skull is not a homogeneous body, but is composed of panels of bone that differ in thickness and elasticity from individual to individual, and in the same individual in the different portions of the skull. The thickness of the calvaria ranges in the adult from 3 to 6 mm. It is thinner in the squamous portion of the temporal bone and much thicker in the midfrontal, midoccipital, parietosphenoid and parieto-petrous buttresses.
b. The **facial skeleton** that constitutes the rest of the skull and mandible.

Brain

The brain is a very important but delicate organ, protected by the following coverings from outside to inward as shown in **Figure 13.1**.

1. Bony covering of the cranium.
2. Three membranous coverings (meninges): Outer dura mater, middle arachnoid mater and inner pia mater.

Among the meninges, the dura mater is the thickest and toughest covering of the brain. It is the outer-most covering. It encloses the cranial venous sinuses and has a distinct blood supply and nerve supply.

The cerebrospinal fluid, which fills the space between the arachnoid and the pia mater (subarachnoid space), acts as a water cushion.

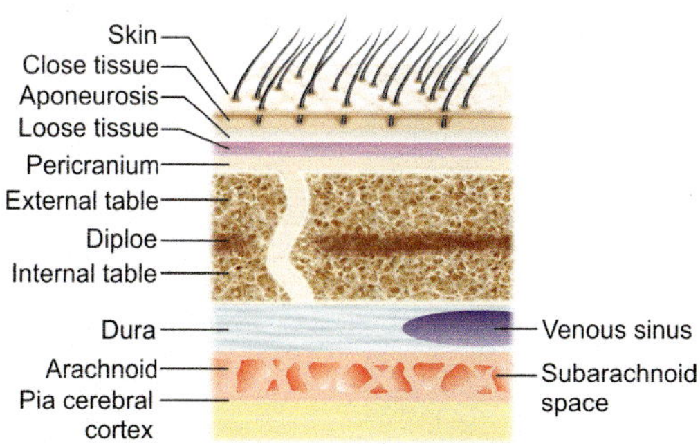

Figure 13.1 Anatomy (cut section) of the scalp, skull and meninges

Parts of the Brain

The brain consists of:

1. Cerebrum—two large cerebral hemispheres
2. Cerebellum—two small cerebellar hemispheres
3. Midbrain
4. Pons
5. Medulla oblongata

(3–5: Together form brainstem)

The cerebrum is the largest part of the brain and is made of two cerebral hemispheres, which are incompletely separated from each other by the median longitudinal fissure. The two hemispheres are connected to each other across the median plane by the corpus callosum. Each hemisphere contains a cavity, called the lateral ventricle. A thin layer of gray matter, called cerebral cortex, covers the surface of each hemisphere. The cortex is folded in a complex manner, so that there are a number of raised areas (gyri) that are separated by depressions (sulci). Each cerebral hemisphere is divided into four lobes—frontal, parietal, temporal and occipital. Their positions roughly correspond to the corresponding bones.

HEAD INJURY

External Injuries on the Head and the Face

Head and face may suffer blunt-force injury as other parts of the body. But it must be remembered that fatal blunt-force injuries inflicted with intention to kill a person will be on the head.

The scalp is vascular, hair bearing skin. At its base is a thick fibrous membrane called the galea aponeurotica. Lying between the galea and the skull is a very thin sheet of connective tissue that is penetrated by blood vessels (emissary veins) emerging through the skull, and beneath this connective tissue is the periosteum of the outer table of the skull.

The vascularity of the scalp, possibly the connection with the intracranial blood vessels, results in profuse bleeding if it is injured. Bleeding will also, very commonly, continue after death if the head is in a dependent position.

Specific Features and Peculiarities of Blunt Force Injuries on the Head and the Face

i. The scalp is easily injured by blunt trauma, as it can be crushed between the weapon and the underlying skull, which acts like an anvil. **Bruises** of the scalp are associated with prominent edema because this normal tissue response cannot spread and dissipate as easily as in other areas of the body. The easiest way to detect scalp injuries is by palpation, but shaving is essential for proper documentation and photography. On the scalp, a bruise is better palpated than seen due to the general bluish color of the scalp due to hair roots.

ii. **Lacerations** of the scalp will, if inspected carefully, reveal a band of **abrasion** adjacent to the laceration, and examination of the depths of the wound will reveal the bridging fibers that will confirm the true origin of these injuries. This is important because the relative thinness of the scalp and its immobility mean that blunt trauma can result in sharply defined injuries that may, at first sight, appear to be incised injuries.

iii. Tangential forces or glancing blows, either from an instrument or from a rotating wheel as in a road traffic accident, may tear large flaps of tissue, exposing the underlying skull. If hair becomes entangled in rotating machinery, portions of the scalp may be **avulsed**.

iv. Fist blow or a similar blow on the face may cause **abrasion, bruise** and if with a ring on a finger, may also cause **laceration.** Laceration with fist blow is common if the impact is on the molar prominence, on the eyebrows, on the forehead and in the inner aspect of the lips due to impact of the lips with the teeth behind. With fist blow, there may be **fracture** of the nasal bone with bleeding from the nose. Similarly, there may be **dislocation** of the teeth.

v. If on the eye, then there may be damage to the eyeball, dislocation of lens, displacement of the retinal vessels.

vi. **Blow** over the forehead and the eyebrows may cause black eye due to settling and accumulation of blood in the loose tissue of the eyelids. In addition to these, there may be subconjunctival hemorrhage.

vii. A fist blow on the ear may cause rupture or tear of the pinna and bleeding from the ear.

viii. A **forceful fist** blow on the temple may cause cerebral apoplexy and instantaneous death.

ix. Blow with a hard blunt weapon, other than fist, e.g. with a wooden or iron rod, will cause more severe and dangerous injuries, including fracture of the bone and internal injury. Externally, if a long rod-like weapon is used over the forehead, scalp, eyebrow or malar prominence, then an **incised looking split laceration** will be produced. Split laceration may also occur on the chin (**Figure 13.2**).

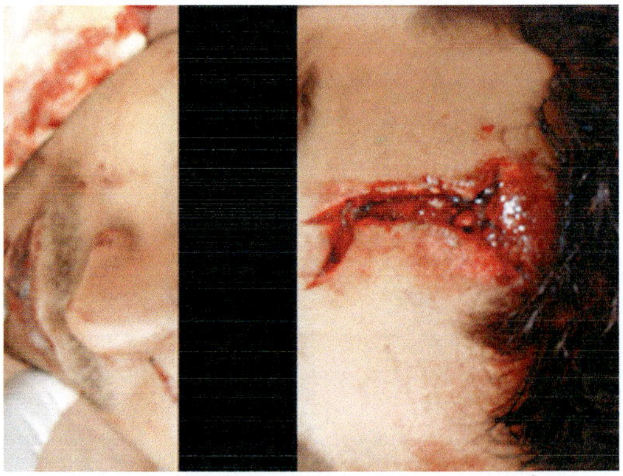

Figure 13.2 Incised looking split laceration

x. In case of **smothering**, there may be bruises, abrasions with occasional nail scratches present around the mouth and the nose with similar injuries on the inner aspects of the lips with occasional dislocation of teeth, fracture of the nasal bone and bleeding from the nose. In these cases, Petechial hemorrhage may be present in the conjunctiva, over the eyelids and the forehead.

xi. **Cut injury** over the face and the head is common only in homicidal circumstances. Stab wounds are comparatively uncommon on head and face.

xii. **Concealed punctured wounds** may be caused at the inner canthus of the eyes, over the nape of the neck and over the fontanelle in case of infants, all of which are homicidal in nature.

xiii. **Suicidal gunshot wounds** may be present on the palate inside the mouth cavity, over the temples, on the forehead, on the eyes and below the chin. All these suicidal wounds are likely to be contact wounds.

xiv. **In case of burn injuries**, except the part of the head covered by the hair, there may be any degree burn injuries. The scalp hair show singeing and give the smell of the fuel in suicidal and some homicidal cases.

xv. In case of **ingestion of corrosive agents**, there may be corrosion and stain on the angles of the mouth, over the lips, with evidence of trickling of the corrosive agents in front of the chin. Inside the mouth cavity, there will be signs of irritation, desquamation, hemorrhagic points, discoloration, depending on the type and concentration of the agent. In case of sulfuric acid, there is carbonization of the corroded area and white brittle appearance of the teeth. In case of corrosive alkalies, in addition to corrosion, there will be bleached, sodden and translucent appearance of the mucous membrane of the mouth and the tongue.

xvi. In case of **vitriolage**, or acid attacks, evidence of spilling of the agent will be there on the face. Pouring of acid or alkalies on the eyes may cause total damage of the eyes with loss of the eyesight.

Periorbital Hematoma

In case of hard blunt impact, the loose tissue of the scalp may show extravasations, which may be diffused or may form extensive, frank hematoma at times. In case of impact over the forehead or the front of the head, there may not be much accumulation of blood at the site of impact, but the extravasated blood may settle down into the tissue of the eyelid causing **black eye (Figure 13.3)**. Subcutaneous extravasations in the loose tissue of the scalp may be present all around the head or may be localized sporadically at and around the sites of impact. Other synonyms include Raccoon eyes or Panda eyes.

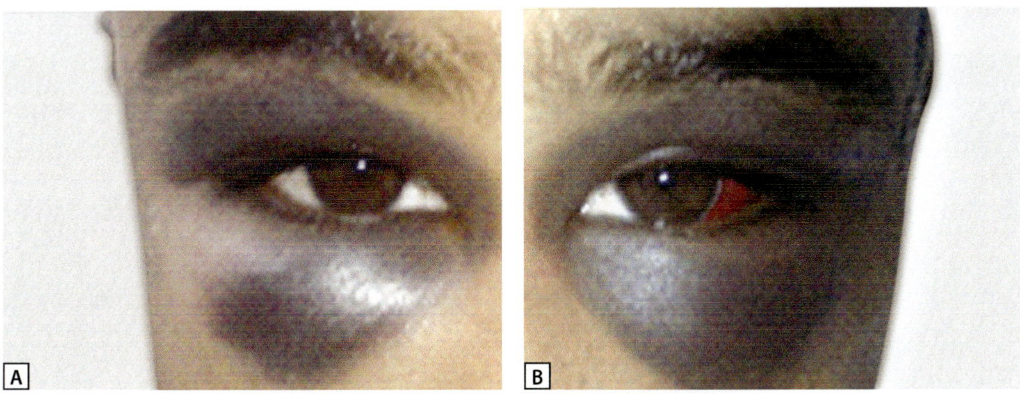

Figures 13.3A and B Black eyes
(*Courtesy:* Dr Ajay Kumar S, JNMC, Belgaum, Karnataka, India)

INJURY TO THE BONES OF THE HEAD

Fractures of Skull

Fracture of skull depends on the amount of force applied and whether the force applied is generalized (falls) or localized (stones, hammer, etc.), position of head when it was struck; area affected and thickness of the bone. Fracture of the skull bones may be simple or compound. However, irrespective of whether closed or open, the fractures of the skull bones may be of the following types:

Fissured or Linear Fracture

A fissure fracture (**Figure 13.4**) when involves only one table of skull is called as **crack** fracture. Crack fracture affects usually the inner table as it is comparatively brittle. Fissured fractures are caused due to impact with hard, tough and flat surface. This type of fracture is often the result of a fall on the ground or after being knocked down on the ground by a vehicle.

In the young child, the linear fracture may pass into a suture line and may cause diastasis fracture.

Comminuted Fracture

When a part of the skull bone cracks into pieces, it is termed comminuted fracture. This occurs often in radiating fashion, with the center being at the site of the impact and fissures radiating from that point in more than one direction, along the direction of radiation of the force of impact (**Figure 13.5**). Non-displaced comminuted fracture resembles a spider web or mosaic pattern.

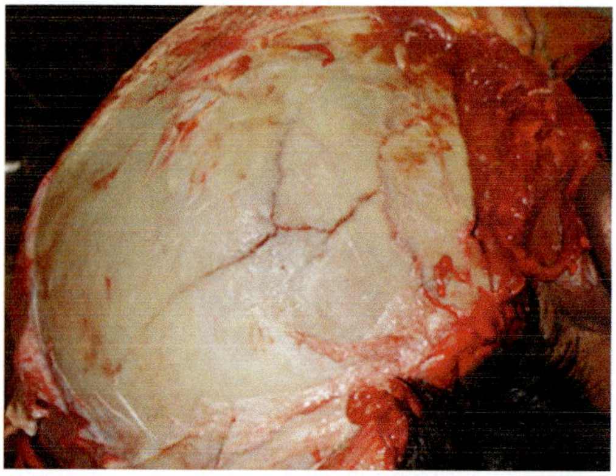

Figure 13.4 Fissured fracture

Depressed Fractures

Depressed fractures will force fragments of skull inwards and, due to the bi-layer construction of the skull, the inner table fragmentation will be much greater than the fracturing of the outer table. Fragments of bone can be driven into the underlying meninges, blood vessels and brain tissues (**Figure 13.6**).

Depressed Comminuted Fracture

This occurs due to forceful localized impact causing multiple linear fractures radiating from the site of impact with depression of the site of impact where the bone breaks into pieces.

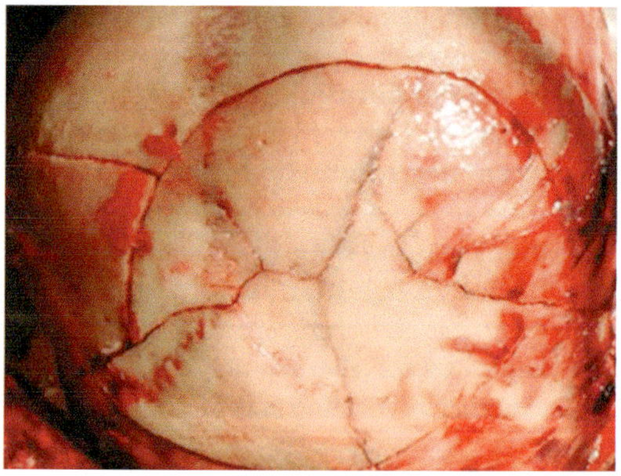

Figure 13.5 Comminuted fracture

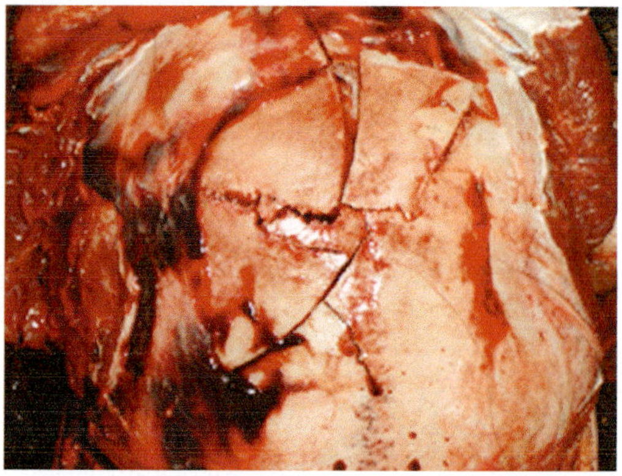

Figure 13.6 Depressed fractures

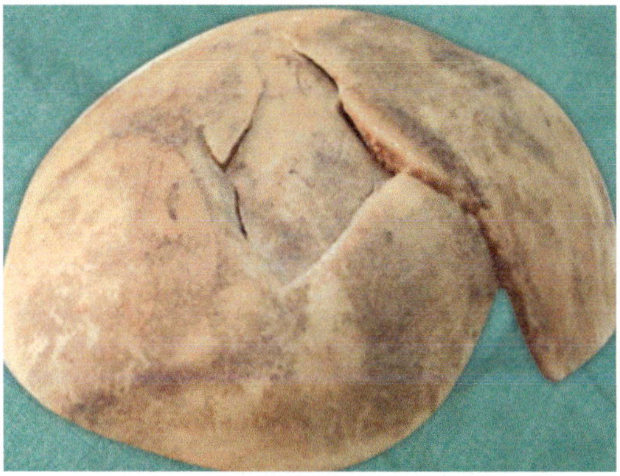

Figure 13.7 Fracture a la Signaturea or signature fracture

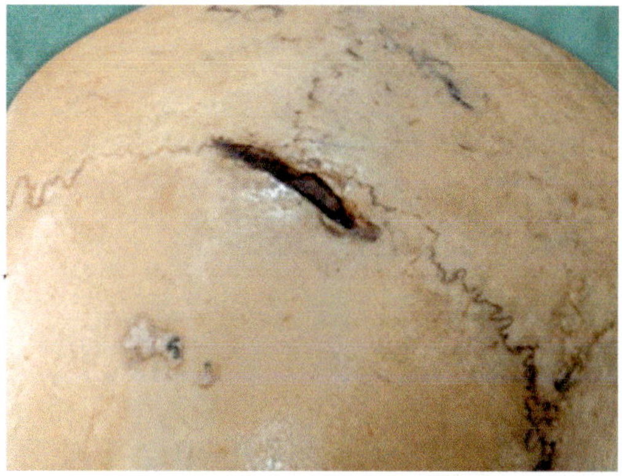

Figure 13.8 Perforating fracture

Depressed comminuted fractures are also called '**Fracture a la Signaturea** or **signature fracture**', because, like the signature, the weapon which has caused the fracture may leave its impression on the fracture, from which the shape and size of the striking part of the weapon can be known (**Figure 13.7**).

Thus, the depression may be circular, if the striking surface is circular; it will be elongated if the object of impact is an elongated one. This type of fracture may occur in case of primary impact by a vehicle. In such a case, from the size and shape of the fracture, part of the vehicle striking the head can be known.

In homicidal cases, if a hammer has been used, then that also can be guessed from the size and shape of the depressed fracture. Comminuted fracture or depressed comminuted fractures are also called as **radiating** fracture.

Pond or Indented Fracture

This type of fracture is seen in case of **infant skull**, where the bones are not yet fully calcified and hence are soft and yield on application of force. Thus, at the site of impact of the force there is a depression, but there is no cracking anywhere or there will be very small or minor cracking.

Penetrating Fracture

In this type of fracture, the skull is perforated by a sharp pointed object that involves both the outer and inner table. When a pointed knife blade, nail, etc. is passed into to skull, this type of fracture is commonly produced (**Figure 13.8**).

Bullet Fracture

In case of punctured wound of the head due to bullet, there will be punched in hole on the skull at the site of entrance of the bullet with beveling at the inner table, and at the site of the exit, there will be a punched out hole with beveling on the outer table of the skull.

In **Figure 13.9** bullet wound on the skull is shown: (**A**) Bullet entry wound on the skull on outer table, (**B**) Entry wound on the skull on inner table with presence beveling and (**C**) Exit wound on the skull on outer table with external beveling.

Gutter Fracture

Tangential impact by the sharp edge of a sword or a high-velocity bullet over some part of the skull bone may cause the superficial layer of the bone at the site of impact to be slashed out due to the glancing impact. Usually, the outer table of the skull is affected, and there is no effect on the inner table with any cracking of the bone.

Ring Fracture

This occurs due to indirect impact on the base of the skull, when a person falls from a height on his feet or buttock. The force travels along

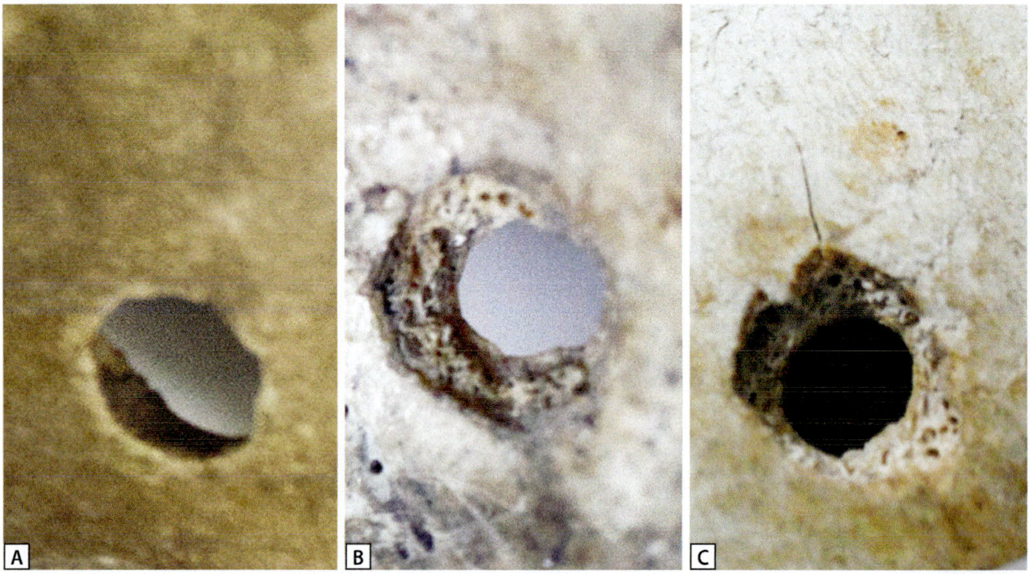

Figures 13.9A to C Bullet wound on the skull

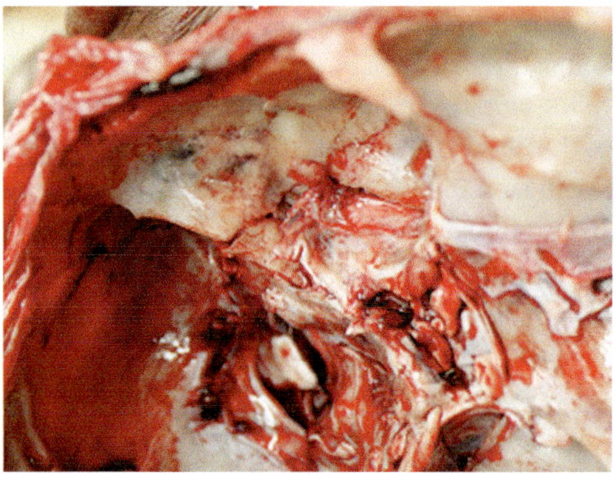

Figure 13.10 Ring fracture
(*Courtesy:* Dr Raktim Pratim Tamuli, TMC, Assam)

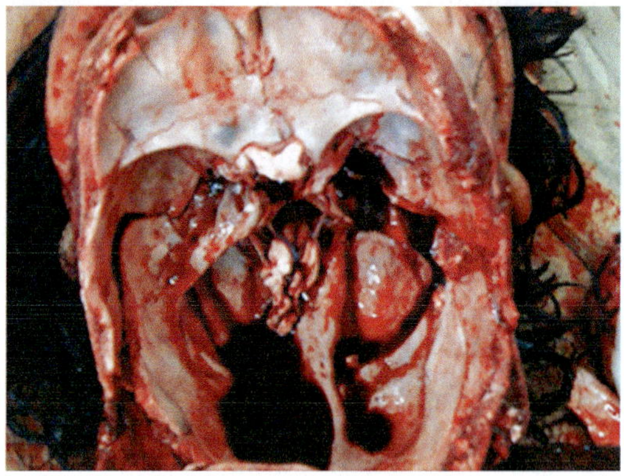

Figure 13.11 Hinge fracture
(*Courtesy:* Dr Raktim Pratim Tamuli, TMC, Assam)

the vertebral column and strikes the atlas and thence the part of the occipital bone around the foramen magnum. This may cause separation of the base of the skull from the rest. The separation starts about 2–4 cm (**Figure 13.10**) away from the foramen magnum and then travels by the side of the ear bones and base of the eye bones.

Sometimes the separated part of the base is pushed inside the cranial cavity. Ring fracture may be caused due to a shearing force resulting from an impact on the frontal or occipital bones. This is a type of basilar fracture.

Hinge Fracture

Hinge fracture of skull is a basilar fracture of skull involving middle cranial fossa and pituitary fossa dividing the base of the skull into anterior and posterior segments (**Figure 13.11**). It is associated with blows to the chin as sustained by boxers or motorcyclists who fall on the road surface striking the chin.

Cut Fracture

Sharp cutting heavy or moderately heavy weapon causes straight linear cut when, except the line of contact with the edge of weapon, there may not be any lack of continuity of the bony substance anywhere. If the edge is not very sharp and if the weapon is quite heavy, then there may be any of the conventional types of the fractures present along the direction of passage of the force (**Figure 13.12**).

Suture Fracture or Sutural Separation

When the impact is over a wider area of the head, there may be separation of the bones at the sutures shown in **Figures 13.13A and B**. In case of elderly subjects where partial calcification of the sutures have occurred, there may be fracture in the line of the sutural obliteration, if similar impact is applied on the head over an wider area.

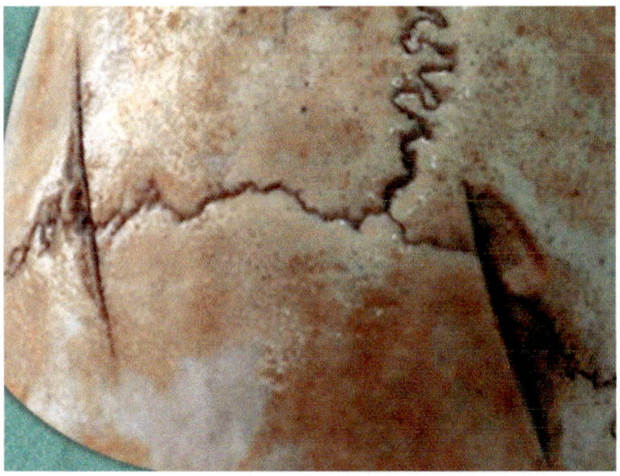

Figure 13.12 Cut fracture

Crush Fracture

In case of crushing of the head by heavy substance, the skull bones are crushed into numerous small pieces with total distortion of the structure of the head and the face. Such crush fracture of the skull bone is seen when the head is run over by the wheel of a heavy vehicle.

Heat Fracture

Heat fracture occurs when the head is exposed to intense heat. There occurs either dryness or desiccation of skull, resulting in outward curving of outer table with cracking or increased intracranial tension resulting in bursting of whole thickness of skull or sutural fracture or separation.

Contrecoup Fracture

When the impact is over the occipital region, then the force will be directed anteriorly. In course of its path, the force causes vibration. Wherever the force passes through a thin and weak bone in its path; it may cause fracture of that bone.

Thus, in a case of reasonably heavy impact on the occipital bone, there may not be any fracture at the site of impact due to toughness of the occipital bone, but the force, when passes anteriorly causes fracture of the thin orbital plates of the frontal bone. However, the mechanism of contrecoup injury to brain

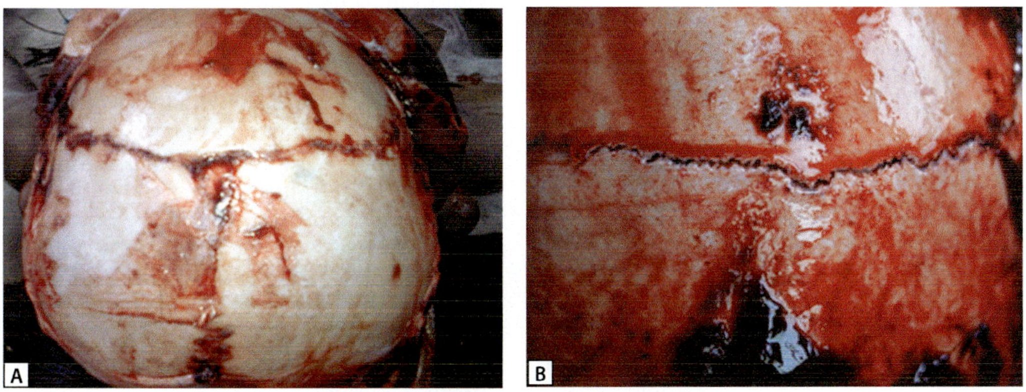

Figure 13.13A and B Suture fractures

is totally different. The coup and contrecoup injury is shown diagrammatically in **Figure 13.14** where the site of impact, coup injury and contrecoup injury at a place diagonally opposite is produced because of shearing action due to rotation of head.

In regards to mechanism of coup and contrecoup injuries, the criterion to be fulfilled is that the head is to move freely on the vertebral column during the moment of impact.

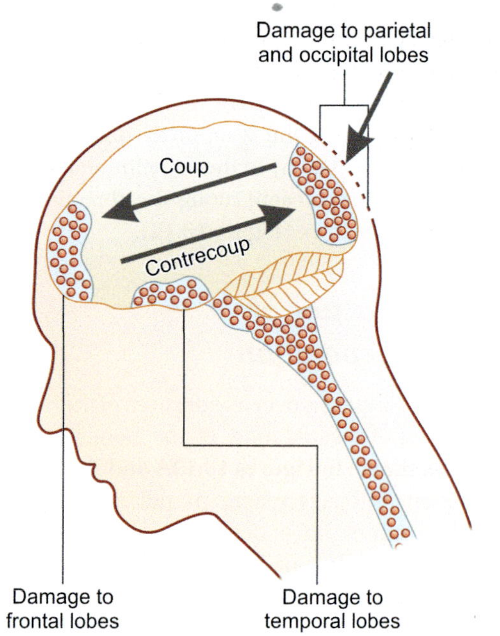

Figure 13.14 Coup and contrecoup injury of the brain

Mechanism of Fracture of Skull (Figure 13.15)

At the Base of the Skull

Fracture of base of skull (basilar fractures) may be caused:

i. **Due to direct violence like**:
   a. Upward blow over mandibular region of the face or chin.
   b. Penetrating injury through orbit.
   c. Penetrating injury through nose.
   d. Penetrating injury through mouth.
ii. **Due to indirect force like**:
   a. Fall from height on feet or buttock.
   b. Severe blow over vault.

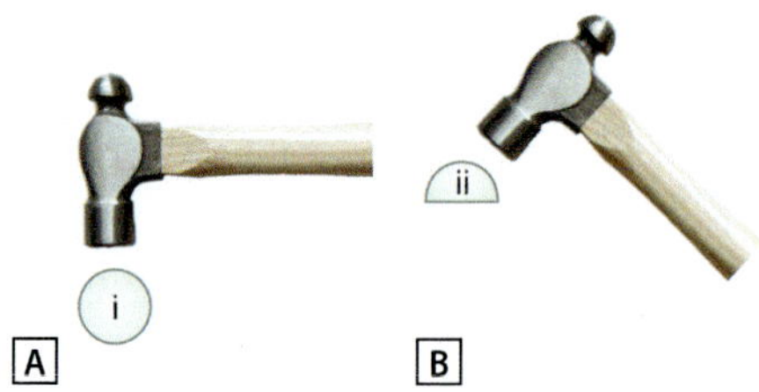

Figures 13.15A and B Mechanism of fracture of skull, (i) Shape of fracture circular (similar) being struck by the circular surface of hammer (A); (ii) Semicircular shape of fracture when struck by the when struck by the margin of hammer head (B)

Fracture may be:

1. **Longitudinal**: When base of skull is divided into right and left halves results from blunt force applied from front and back of the head or due to anteroposterior or postero-anterior compression.
2. **Transverse**: When base of skull is divided into anterior and posterior halves results from side to side compression.
3. **Ring fracture**: Also known as foramen fracture. This type of fracture occurs due to fall from height on the vault of skull, on feet, or on buttock; heavy blow on chin or nape of neck; violent twisting of head on vertebral column.

Fracture on the Anterior Fossa

Fracture at the anterior fossa of the base of the skull occurs mostly due to an impact in the front of the head. Fissured fracture of the orbital plates of the frontal bone may occur due to impact over the occipital bone posteriorly. If the anterior fossa fracture extends up to the sinuses, then there is a chance that this will lead to infection inside the cranial cavity. In some cases, fracture of the anterior fossa may be the extension, of fracture of the middle fossa.

Complications: Bleeding will be seen through nose (epistaxis) or mouth. CSF and brain tissue may escape through nose (rhinorrhea) due to tear of meninges and nasal mucosa. Leptomeningitis, frontal brain abscess due to passing of infection through nose. There may be cranial pneumatoceles due to involvement of paranasal sinuses. It may also be associated with subconjunctival hemorrhage and periorbital hemorrhage.

Fracture of the Middle Fossa

A linear fracture may extend across the middle fossa including the pituitary fossa. Such fracture commonly occurs due to heavy side-by-side compression middle fossa. Fracture may extend to the anterior fossa. Bleeding will be seen in the ear.

Complications: Bleeding (hemotympanum) and even CSF escape through ear (otorrhea) due to involvement of petrous part of temporal bone. Bleeding through mouth and Eustachian tube due to involvement of basi-occiput or sphenoid may occurs. Blood may enter into bronchial tree due to involvement of sella turcica.

Hinge Fracture: When the fracture line from the site of impact on the side or top of the head run down the temporoparietal bone and turn in and run across the base of the skull, often in the middle fossa to reach or pass through the pituitary sella. This fracture line may divide the floor of the skull into two halves the so-called hinge fracture. This is commonly seen in traffic accidents.

Fracture of the Posterior Fossa

These types of fracture occur due to direct impact over the posterior part of the skull.

Complications: Extensive extravasations behind mastoid process (Battle's Sign) and nape of neck. Cerebellar contusion and herniation of cerebellar tonsils when fracture line extends up to foramen magnum may occur.

Brain Injury

Injuries that have resulted in skull fractures or intracranial hemorrhage are clear macroscopic markers that significant force has been applied to the head and therefore to the brain. Sometimes, however, these markers are absent but, as a result of acceleration or deceleration, the brain has been significantly traumatized. Whatever the exact cause of the trauma may be, the effects on the brain as a whole are the same and **cerebral edema** usually develops, probably due to transudation of fluid into the extracellular space.

As edema develops, the brain swells and, the intracranial pressure rises and the brain is squeezed out of the spaces in the meninges and the skull. The cerebrum is forced downwards through the tentorium cerebelli and the cerebellum and brainstem are forced downwards through the foramen magnum (brain herniation). These movements produce secondary areas of injury in the unci of the cerebrum and the cerebellar tonsils. The weight of the edematous brain is increased and the surface of the brain is markedly flattened, often with hemorrhage and necrosis of the unci and the cerebellar tonsils.

Direct injuries to the brain from depressed or comminuted skull fractures result in areas of **bruising** and **laceration to the cortex**, often associated with larger sites of hemorrhage. Penetrating injuries from gunshots or from stab wounds will cause injuries deep into the white matter, and the tissue adjacent to the wound tracks will often be associated with contusion.

There is also another group of head injuries that do not result in either penetration or intracranial hemorrhage. The brain is injured in these cases by rotation or by acceleration/deceleration, which causes shearing between the different layers or components of the brain as each move in a different way or at a different speed. This shearing causes contusions and lacerations deep within the substance of the brain, but particularly in the region of the corpus callosum. Shearing is also associated with the so-called 'gliding lesions' that occur beneath the cortex and in the cerebral peduncles and brainstem. The shearing effects are also identifiable at a microscopic level, where the damage to the axons can be identified by the use of special staining techniques. These changes have been termed diffuse axonal injury.

Types of Traumatic Brain Lesions (Table 13.1)

Cerebral Concussion

Old term for cerebral concussion is **Commotio Cerebri**. It is sudden transient loss of consciousness from few seconds to few minutes. It is caused by a temporary (at times irreversible) derangement of neuronal activity without demonstrable organic change leading to unconsciousness or impaired consciousness due to direct violence to the head. This is also called "**stunning**". But there may be total cessation of the physiological functions and may be irreversible leading to immediate death. This is considered to be the result of sub-microscopic type of damage of reticular formation, diffuse neuronal injury and diffuse disruption of the nerve fibers in the white matter.

Rotational injuries to the head with distortion of brainstem or shearing strain are required for causation of concussion. There is good chance of recovery if vital centers are not affected and when consciousness is regained features of cerebral irritation due to cerebral edema may persist. It is characterized by contracted pupils, alteration of blood pressure and respiration and followed by post-traumatic and retrograde amnesia and confusional state.

There may not be any visible change in the brain or only scattered petechial hemorrhage may be detected. The 'cause' of the condition is the individual himself alone, which should not be linked with any circumstance of assault or accident. It cannot be denied that the condition may be a feigned one after an accident or assault to claim compensation. But that should not give an impression that the condition does not exist or that it is always negligible or trivial. In occasions, death occurred in circumstances, which appeared as post-accidental concussion.

The most constant post-concussional features are headache, dizziness and nervousness. There may be other features depending on the extent of internal pathology. Cerebral concussion is more commonly complained of in impacts received on the brain due to sudden deceleration of the moving head than in an impact received by a static head.

Table 13.1 Traumatic brain lesions
• Cerebral concussion
• Cerebral contusion
• Cerebral laceration
• Cerebral edema
• Cerebral hemorrhage
• Diffuse neuronal injury (axonal injury)
• Cerebral compression
• Cerebral irritation

Cerebral Contusion

These are foci of hemorrhagic necrosis on brain surface, wedge shaped in cross section with base in gray matter and tapering into white matter. Pia-arachnoid is intact and blood frequently spreads under it. May result from both coup and contrecoup lesion. Common sites are frontal and temporal lobes or, at times, the tonsillar region of cerebellum or medulla, even midbrain. These usually result from distortion of skull or rotational movement of brain in relation to skull. It may be associated with fracture of skull and is known as "fracture contusion". On organization the site looks yellow due to disintegration of blood pigments. This may result in brain abscess due to infection. Contusions are most severe in orbitofrontal cortex and temporal lobes. These may manifest clinically as focal deficits, progressive neurologic deterioration and late post-traumatic seizures.

There is also another group of injuries that are associated with head injuries, particularly the injuries that do not result in either penetration or intracranial hemorrhage. The brain is injured in these cases by rotation or by acceleration/deceleration, which causes shearing between the different layers or components of the brain as each move in a different way or at a different speed. This shearing causes contusions and lacerations deep within the substance of the brain, but particularly in the region of the corpus callosum. Shearing is also associated with the 'gliding lesions' of the cortex, cerebral peduncles and brainstem.

Cerebral Laceration

Cerebral laceration results from fractured skull as well as due to rotational and shear strain without fracture of skull, but usually associated with severe contusion. Common sites for such lacerations are frontal or temporal lobes and areas in contact with projections. Consciousness is lost if injury is severe or brainstem circulation is interrupted due to sudden displacement of cranial contents. Increased intracranial tension, either due to edema of injured tissue or bleeding from injured vessels, may lead to death. Healing of superficial surface lacerations may cause secondary epilepsy. Traumatic **porencephalic cysts** are glial cysts filled with CSF, resulting from healed deep lacerations.

Cerebral Edema

Sometimes, as a result of acceleration or deceleration, the brain has been significantly traumatized; and **cerebral edema** develops. The mechanism of cerebral edema is complex and appears to be due to transudation of fluid into the extracellular or perivascular space of brain. Generalized edema is usually associated with diffuse neuronal injury; however, focal edema is associated with cerebral contusions or lacerations. It usually results from increased permeability of cerebral vessels and increased intravascular pressure. Cerebral edema causes flattening of the cerebral convulsions, obliteration of sulci, herniation of cerebellar tonsils and compression of ventricles into slits. These movements produce secondary areas of injury in the unci of the cerebrum and the cerebellar tonsils. Rapidly developing diffused edema or localized edema of brainstem is fatal.

The shearing effects are also identifiable at a microscopic level, where the damage to the axons can be identified by the use of special staining techniques. These changes have been termed diffuse axonal injury.

Cerebral Hemorrhage

It is the accumulation of blood in the substance of brain. This may be either in the form of infiltration in the brain tissue or forming acute hematoma and results due to trauma or diseased condition. When cerebral hemorrhages are associated with gross contusion or laceration of brain as a result of trauma, then it is called primary or traumatic cerebral hemorrhage. These may be caused by shearing forces or penetrating injury that mechanically stretch and tear deep small-caliber arterioles, leading to petechial hemorrhages usually in frontal and temporal lobes. They are most prominent in white matter. Secondary or pathological cerebral hemorrhage result due to diseased conditions like hypertension and degenerative changes of vessels and is not due to trauma.

Diffuse Neuronal Injury (Axonal Injury)

This is a type of diffused neuronal damage due to widespread intracellular disturbances and damages to the synoptic junction between the neurons by interference of vascular mechanism. Concussion of brain is a mild form of diffuse axonal injury (DAI). It is almost universal to all patterns of traumatic brain injury. Mild DAI, with coma lasting for 6–24 hours, involves mainly subcortical part of parasagittal areas, resolves with mild or no permanent disabilities. Moderate to severe DAI, with coma lasting more than 24 hours, involves corpus callosum, cerebral peduncle and brainstem and has poor prognosis, with persistent vegetative state or death.

Though the macroscopic injury may not be detected, histological examination shows microscopic hemorrhage in the brain tissue. Depending upon the degree of injury, unconsciousness continues for six hours to more than 24 hours. If unconsciousness does not occur immediately and appears late, it can be presumed that the cause of unconsciousness is due to causes other than cerebral concussion; may be due to cerebral compression of any other cause and may not be traumatic. APP (beta apoprotein precursor) may be identified in the axons of the damaged nerves by immunohistological techniques. At later stages, retraction balls may be identified by silver staining techniques.

Cerebral Compression

Generalized swelling, hemorrhages in the layers of the meninges or space occupying lesions of brain causes cerebral compression. Brain being almost incompressible, effect falls on the CSF content in the ventricles and subarachnoid space. There occurs gradual decrease in the supply of blood to the brain due to increase in the intracranial tension. Unconsciousness is usually gradual as compared to cerebral concussion where unconsciousness is immediate. Cerebral irritation follows. Sectioning of brain reveals compression of the ventricles, sometimes into thin slits.

Cerebral Irritation

It is the resultant effect of head injury associated with superficial laceration of brain and cerebral edema. It may also due to large extradural or subdural hemorrhage. Symptoms appear from few hours to days. The patient may be aggressive, agitated or combative. The patient becomes comatose and unconsciousness gradually increases. Face is flushed, a pupil on the side of involvement becomes dilated and non-reacting to light, gradually there occurs, bilateral dilatation or may be constricted or even unequal and fixed. Pulse becomes slow and full bound, later on becomes weak, quick and feeble prior to death. Respiration becomes slow labored and stertorous, reflexes may be lost and unilateral paralysis of limb muscles many result. Patient usually dies of brainstem compression. If the patient recovers following surgery, may suffer from headache, loss of memory, epilepsy or hemiparesis. Presence of extradural hemorrhage, flattening or herniation or edema of brain, associated with fracture of skull is the usual postmortem findings.

INTRACRANIAL HEMORRHAGES

An **intracranial hemorrhage** is a bleeding within the skull. Hemorrhage inside the skull cavity may occur at different levels and at different sites. Intracranial hemorrhage may be traumatic or non-traumatic (pathological). When traumatic in origin, there may be accompanying fracture of the skull bone. **Extra-axial hemorrhage** occurs within the skull but outside of the brain tissue, and includes epidural, subdural and subarachnoid hematomas. **Intra-axial hemorrhage** is bleeding within the brain itself, or cerebral/intracerebral hemorrhage; and includes intraparenchymal hemorrhage, or bleeding within the brain tissue, and intraventricular hemorrhage, bleeding within the brain's ventricles. According to the levels, intracranial hemorrhages may be of the following types:

a. Extradural or epidural
b. Subdural
c. Subarachnoid
d. Intracerebral
e. Ventricular.

Extradural Hemorrhage (Figure 13.16)

It is also known as epidural hematoma or subperiosteal hemorrhage. The vessels involved in the trauma are **middle meningeal artery** (most common due to the peculiar site of involvement, i.e. temporoparietal site), **anterior ethmoidal artery** (frontal lobes), **transverse** or **sigmoid sinuses** (occipital lobes) and **superior sagittal sinus** (vertex area). Hence, extradural hemorrhage (EDH) is mostly arterial bleed and usually due to trauma. EDH is least common, but most fatal traumatic hemorrhage.

The accumulation of blood occurs most commonly in the temporal or temporoparietal region (**Figure 13.17**), with fracture of petrous part of the temporal bone. The fracture may be so small that there is a chance that it may not be detected during postmortem examination or by X-ray examination. The blood, which accumulates causes compression on the brain substance and exerts pressure effects.

The blood is not encapsulated and may not be absorbed for a long period and found adherent to the inner table of the skull (**Figure 13.17**). Thus, chronic cases of EDH are seen. **Chronic** EDH is more common on the posterior fossa. In most circumstances, EDH is traumatic in nature, may also follow surgery, bone eroding process though rare and occasionally due to blood dyscrasias in children.

Mechanism

In most cases, EDH occurs along with fracture of skull bone, and this fracture results in injury to the meningeal artery or its branches.

It is suggested that volume of 35 mL is needed for clinical signs to appear and a volume of 100 mL EDH is considered as fatal.[1]

Fate of EDH

In non-fatal cases, the hemorrhage may shrink due to escape of blood into scalp through the fracture site or may be reabsorbed or may be encapsulated to give rise chronic epidural hemorrhage.

Medicolegal Importance

EDH is usually associated with **lucid interval**. These are not contrecoup injury. It may be confused with heat hematoma and alcohol intoxication.

Subdural Hemorrhage

It is accumulation of blood in the subdural space, i.e. between dura mater and arachnoid mater **(Figures 13.18A to C)**.

Causes of Subdural Hemorrhage (SDH)

The causes are mentioned in **Table 13.2**. The most common site is lateral aspect of cerebral hemisphere and rarely the posterior cranial fossa, around the brainstem and cerebellum. Due to movement of brain relative to skull,

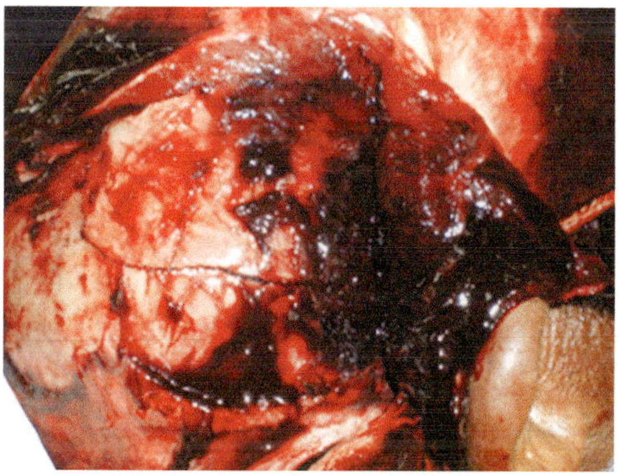

Figure 13.16 Extradural hemorrhage

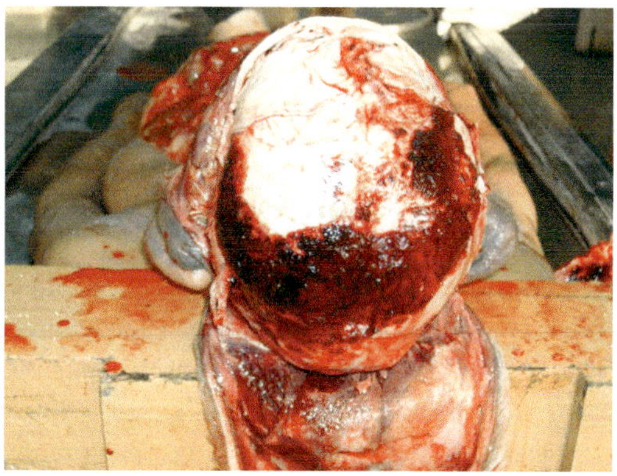

Figure 13.17 EDH over occipitoparietal areas

Table 13.2 Causes of subdural hemorrhage

Traumatic causes	i. Laceration or rupture of the superior cerebral veins ii. Rupture of the dural venous sinuses iii. Rupture of dura mater along with middle meningeal artery iv. Associated cerebral injury
Pathological causes	i. Tear of old adhesions of dura mater with brain ii. Diseases like: Blood dyscrasias, aneurysms, carcinoma, etc. iii. Hypertensive bleed within superficial part of brain due to rupture in subdural space

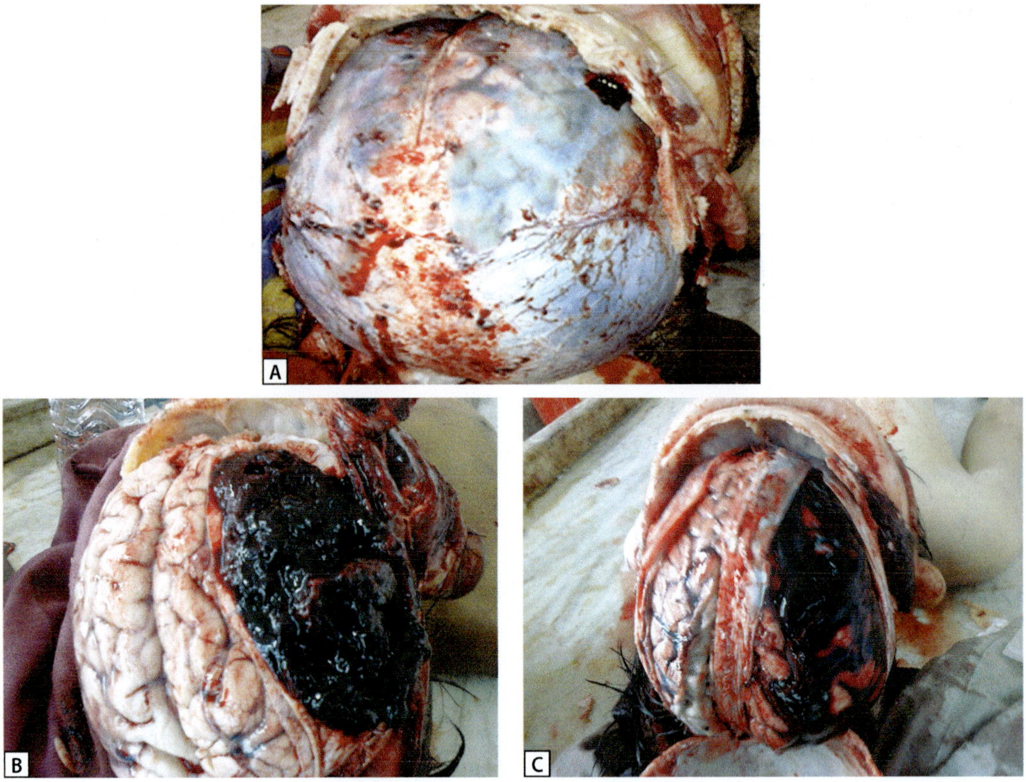

Figures 13.18A to C Acute subdural hemorrhages
(*Courtesy:* Dr Mrinal Haloi, GMC, Guwahati)

there occurs rupture (via shearing mechanism) of bridging veins; rarely, bleeding source may be cortical artery or oozing brain laceration. SDH are not usually associated with skull fractures. SDH was once considered most common intracranial birth injury. Bleeding is most commonly venous as against EDH where it is arterial. SDH may reach more than 100 mL before becoming symptomatic. It is usually associated with acceleration-deceleration injury like in falls, assault, vehicular accident or may be spontaneous.

Classification

Subdural hemorrhages are classified into three types:[2]

i. **Acute:** Patient presents within first 3 days of injury.
ii. **Subacute:** Patient presents between 3 days and 3 weeks.
iii. **Chronic:** Patient presents from 3 weeks to several months.

Primary or Acute SDH

Trauma is a common cause as it causes laceration or rupture of the superior cerebral veins; rupture of the superior longitudinal sinus leading to accumulation of the blood usually occurs at the dorsolateral aspects of the upper surface of either or both hemispheres.

Mechanism

It occurs because of change in the velocity of the head, either acceleration or deceleration with rotational component. It is common lesion than EDH and 35-100 mL is required to cause neurological signs.[3]

In the primary type, the blood over the dorsolateral aspects of the upper surface of the hemisphere may spread both anteriorly and posteriorly. The accumulated blood exerts pressure, as a result of which there is **widening of the sulci on the same side** and **flattening of the gyrus of the opposite side**. Pressure for a long duration may cause softening of the brain surface, particularly over the frontal area. Evacuation of the primary EDH gives good prognosis.

Subacute SDH

Here, blood accumulates in the layers due to hemolysis or mixing up with CSF. Surgically, it is usually evident after 3 days, whereas radiologically, it is seen after 7 days.

Chronic SDH

It is commonly associated with old people or with chronic alcoholics. In these individual, there is usually atrophy of brain, which results in increase in subdural space. This increase in subdural space permits more free movement of the brain within the skull. Hence, there is a higher risk of rupturing of bridging veins. Risk factors for chronic SDH include elderly with cerebral atrophy, chronic alcoholism, epilepsy, bleeding disorders, arachnoid cysts, cardiovascular disease (hypertension, arteriosclerosis).

On a non-contrast CT scan, acute SDH appear hyperdense whereas chronic SDH appear hypodense. SDH from natural causes is often bilateral, while traumatic variety is usually unilateral.[4]

Secondary SDH

Here the primary site of the hemorrhage is in the brain substance and the extravasated blood accumulates in the subdural space that result secondary SDH and occurs due to injury, i.e. laceration, etc. of the brain substance.

Secondary SDH may cause accumulation of blood on the medial aspects of the occipital lobe or in the midbrain or above the pons.

In the general conception, SDH is more common a phenomenon in young adults. When due to trauma, it involves victims of almost all ages and in many cases almost the whole of the surface of the brain. Even the base may have accumulation of the blood.

Fate of SDH

Small SDHs often spontaneously resorb; larger SDHs liquefy in about a week and form encapsulating vascular membranes (thicker outer membrane by about 7 days, and thinner inner membrane after 2–3 weeks). In due course of time, SDH may be organized and encapsulated. The macroscopic feature varies with age. Recent lesions up to weeks are red brown with a gelatinous membrane covering the surface. The contents are thick with central fluid part. Hematoma older up to months is firm with tough membrane. The central content may be liquid or firm.

Pachymeningitis hemorrhagica interna is other name for chronic SDH. After few days or weeks or even month, SDH may get organized and encapsulated to form a cyst and at times may get fibrosed and calcified. Prognosis of exploration of the secondary SDH is generally grave.

Medicolegal Importance

The SDH is very mobile and be gravitate to lower side and thus do not depends on the site of impact. Lucid interval is present. The clinical features may be mistaken for schizophrenia, pre-senile or senile dementia.

Subarachnoid Hemorrhage

Subarachnoid hemorrhage may be traumatic or natural in origin and occurs in the subarachnoid space, i.e. between arachnoid and pia mater surrounding the brain, as shown in **Figure 13.19** and is considered as most common traumatic intracranial hemorrhage.

It may be unilateral or bilateral or basal and may be localized or diffuse. The basal subarachnoid hemorrhage commonly proves fatal. As it becomes older, yellowish discoloration of leptomeninges are seen. The causes are given below:

a. **Traumatic Causes:** When traumatic, it may be primary or secondary. In primary subarachnoid hemorrhage, the vessels of the circle of Willis, anterior cerebral

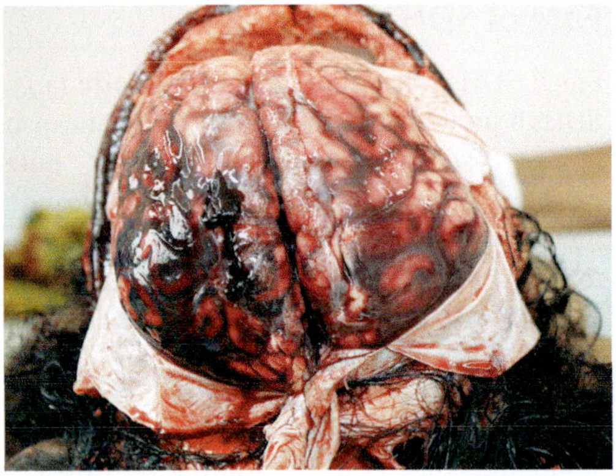

Figure 13.19 Subarachnoid hemorrhage

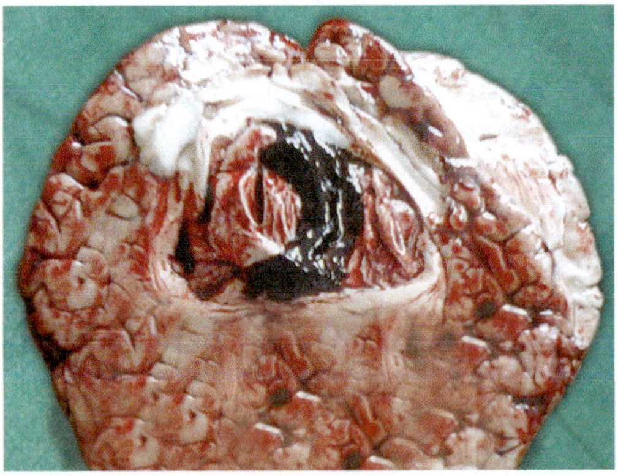

Figure 13.20 Intraventricular hemorrhage

artery and less commonly the posterior cerebral artery are involved. Young and elderly adults are the usual victims, and it is assumed that even in traumatic subarachnoid hemorrhage, trauma may actually be a minor factor in causing the hemorrhage. More important is the condition of the vessels. Secondary subarachnoid hemorrhage occurs due to contusion and laceration of the cerebrum, the blood defusing to the under surface of the arachnoid mater.

b. **Natural Causes:** Natural subarachnoid hemorrhage is primarily due to: Degenerative changes of the vessels in elderly persons; due to rupture of congenital aneurysm in the young, which usually occurs in small amount, mostly near the base of the brain; bleeding disorders and rupture of an intracerebral hemorrhage of non-traumatic origin into the subarachnoid space.

Intracerebral Hemorrhage

It is the accumulation of blood in the substance of brain. This may be either in the form of infiltration in the brain tissue or forming acute hematoma, and results due to trauma or diseased condition.

Traumatic intracerebral hemorrhage results due to trauma like:

a. Laceration of brain
b. Blunt trauma with or without fracture.

Non-traumatic or **pathological intracerebral hemorrhage** may be due to:

a. Malignant brain tumor, metastatic rupture of deep perforating vessels in elderly alcoholics
b. Diseases like hypertension, degenerative changes of vessels, septicemia, fat embolism, toxemia, Wernicke encephalopathy, etc.
c. Blood dyscrasias, anti-coagulant drugs, rupture of berry aneurysm, etc.

Intraventricular Hemorrhages

An **intraventricular** hemorrhage (IVH) is a bleeding into the brain's ventricular system (**Figure 13.20**), where the cerebrospinal fluid is produced and circulates through towards the subarachnoid space. It can result from physical trauma or hemorrhaging in stroke. Intraventricular blood is indicator of severe head trauma.

The IVH is always secondary, mostly to intracerebral hemorrhage or sometimes to subarachnoid hemorrhage. IVH is always fatal.

Causes

i. Traumatic.
ii. Non-traumatic (pathological) causes:
   a. Retrograde flow of subarachnoid hemorrhage into the ventricles.
   b. Rupture of arteriovenous malformation in the wall of ventricle.

c. Rupture of Berry's aneurysm of posterior communicating artery and bleeding into anterior portion of temporal horn of lateral ventricle
d. Rupture of Berry's aneurysm of basilar artery through the floor of third ventricle
e. Hemorrhagic stroke.

Medicolegal Importance

a. IVH is usually arterial in origin
b. If the IVH is the sole finding, it is the result of head striking a firm object as in a fall or fall-like injury
c. Brown or yellowish discoloration of the ependyma, choroid plexus and leptomeninges are due to deposition of hemosiderin and hematoidin and suggest the presence of old hemorrhage.

Other Injuries of the Brain

In case of blunt force impact, there may be fracture of the skull which, if is a depressed one, will in addition to the hemorrhages cause contusion or laceration of the meninges of the affected part. There may even be depression of the area injured (**Figure 13.21**).

When a static head is struck, there is usually similar lesion over the part of the brain of the area. But when the head being in motion, strikes a static or relatively static object, then, there will be coup lesion at the site of the impact and a contrecoup lesion at a site diagonally opposite to the site of the impact or the coup injury.

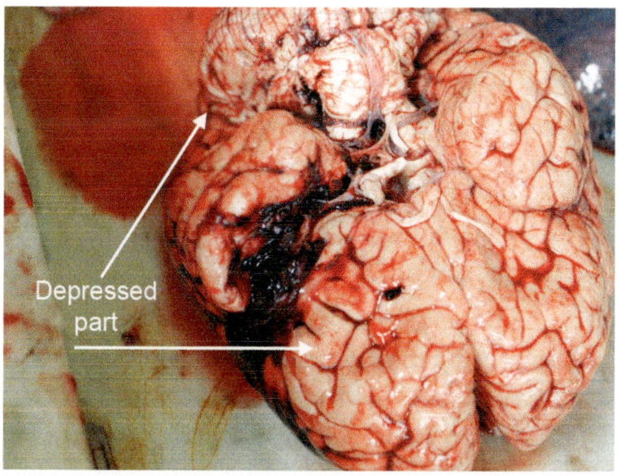

Figure 13.21 Mild subarachnoid hemorrhages with depressed part on one side

However, a lesion is not common over the occipital lobe in the coup-contrecoup phenomenon. Because, when there will be a coup lesion on the frontal lobe surface, then instead of contrecoup lesion on the diagonally opposite area of the occipital lobe, contrecoup lesion will be over the temporal lobe, possibly due to the uneven bony base at the middle and the posterior fossa. When the force does not strike the head perpendicularly over the mid part of the forehead or the occiput, there may be slight rotational movement of the skull cage and the contrecoup lesion may be due to the shearing effect causing lesions on the upper, middle or the lower surface of the temporal lobe. The contrecoup lesions may be on the vessels causing hemorrhages or may be on the surface of the brain causing contusion.

In case of use of a sharp cutting, heavy weapon, there will be incised wound on the brain matter with corresponding cut of the covering meninges. In these cases, there will be hemorrhages outside and in the layers of the meninges, but only a little bleeding will be there in the substance of the brain.

In case of a stab wound in the brain with a sharp cutting pointed weapon, there will be a narrow stab in the brain substance.

When a bullet enters the cranial cavity, there will be gross laceration of the meninges and the brain matter at the wound of entrance and exit, with a straight lacerated blind track. If the bullet strikes the bone on the opposite side of the entry, then it may take another course (backward) inside the brain or may pass out by making an exit wound.

In case of gross burn injury, there may be production of heat hematoma along with heat fracture of the skull bone.

Complications of the Intracranial Injuries

1. Meningitis is more likely if there is a communication between the inside of the cranium and the frontal air sinuses.

2. Subdural abscess.
3. Cerebral abscess.
4. Delayed meningitis.
5. Cerebral softening due to occlusion of the injured vessel.
6. Dissecting aneurysm, due to injury to the vessel, particularly to the carotid artery and its branches.
7. Arteriovenous communication between the terminal portion of the carotid artery and the cavernous vein due to fracture of the base of the brain.
8. Post-traumatic amnesia and neurosis.
9. Post-traumatic epilepsy.
10. Post-traumatic encephalopathy in boxer
11. Post-traumatic tumors like meningioma, malignant glioma and acoustic neurofibroma.
12. **Disability**:
    a. **Physical disability**: Paralysis, sensory disturbance, visual defects, headache, ataxia, epilepsy, etc.
    b. **Psychic disability** like lack of self-confidence.
    c. **Circumstantial disability**: When the person is not considered fit to continue in his job though he may actually be fit.

Post-traumatic Amnesia: After cerebral concussion, after a temporary period of stunning or suspended animation, the patient usually recovers fully within few minutes depending upon the degree of injury and, in the state of lucid interval, may relate the circumstance clearly but when becomes fully conscious can remember nothing about the moment of injury.

Retrograde Amnesia: Retrograde amnesia is mostly due to injury to frontal lobe. In this, there is loss of memory regarding moment of incident and recent events occurred some times before the incident or following the incident.

Post-traumatic Automatism: While in the state of amnesia the patient may unconsciously speak rationally or perform some criminal or violent acts, which he cannot remember afterwards and has medicolegal importance.

Post-traumatic Encephalopathy in Boxers: It is the disability which develops in a boxer after a long period. There is deficient memory, judgment and emotional balance, with lack of intelligence. There is loss of cortical cells and the cells of corpus striatum, and there is secondary overgrowth of neuroglia. Parkinsonism like state may develop.

Age of the Intracranial Injuries

Reasonably accurate relationship may be established between the infliction of the injuries and the time lapsed. This time interval in case of a SDH is related with the presence of the clotted state of the blood (3 weeks) or its liquid state (3 months).

1. At the beginning, there is presence of intact leukocytes (24 hours).
2. Fibroblastic infiltration occurs within the 2nd day and formation of cellular layer around the clot within 4th day, which gradually thickens.
3. Phagocytic activity starts by 5th day and break of the clot by the mid of the 2nd week.
4. Further thickening of the wall of the capsule occurs by the end of the 2nd week.
5. Further breakdown of the cells and completion of the healing may take some months or even a year or two.

HEAD INJURY AND LEGAL RESPONSIBILITY

This is a pertinent question raised, occasionally for the victims of the head injury. In fact, post-traumatic psychosis, mental defect, personality disorder, all may be considered to affect adversely the power of understanding of the sufferer. Obviously questions arise, how much civil responsibilities can these persons shoulder and how much should they be responsible criminally for their acts. Without bringing much controversy in the discussion, it can be safely said that, in some circumstances, the person may be wholly absolved from any responsibility, in some other circumstances the doctrine of diminished responsibility may be rightly considered and in the rest, he may be held fully responsible. It all depends on the nature of brain damage, extent of incapability and the circumstance in question.

Lucid Interval in Head Injury Cases

A person, who, due to sustaining intracranial injury, is unconscious and non-responsive to stimuli, may regain consciousness and behave normally for some time, only to be unconscious again after some period. This period when he behaves normally is termed lucid interval in head injury patients.

Punch Drunk

During the events of boxing, there may be minute hemorrhages in brain. The boxer may behave like a drunken person with cloudy consciousness, unsteady gait and blunting of faculties. It is essential to differentiate between drunkenness and cerebral concussion (**Table 13.3**). There are chronic changes in boxer's brain, which are both anatomical and microscopic lesions.

It is a chronic traumatic encephalopathy, also known as **dementia pugilistica**. Grossly affected brain may show some cortical atrophy and slight hydrocephalus, thinning of corpus callosum, diffuse axonal injury, hypothalamic anomalies, degeneration of substantia nigra, diffuse plaques and scarring of cerebellar folia. Throughout the brain substance, there may be scars and patches of gliosis. These persons also suffer from development of an Alzheimer's like condition, with neuro-fibrillatory tangles throughout cerebral cortex and brainstem though no senile plaques are present.

Vertebrobasilar Artery Injury

It has been recognized that blows to the side of the neck can give rise to fatal subarachnoid bleeding because of tearing or dissection of intrathecal course of vertebral artery allowing blood to track along the upper part of the vessel and enter the cranial cavity, where the artery penetrates the dural membrane of the foramen magnum.

Basilar artery and internal carotid artery can also give rise to the syndrome. The injury is manifested as skin bruising and bleeding into the deep neck muscles.

Mechanism of Vertebral Artery Trauma: The vertebral artery is injured due to: (i) Overstretching of atlanto-occipital membrane and (ii) Impact on muscles overlying the transverse process of upper cervical vertebrae. The damage to the vertebral artery occurs at the following places:

1. In the canal within the first cervical vertebrae.
2. Just below the axis, in the space between transverse process of Axis and Atlas.
3. As it emerges from the exit of the canal in the Atlas.

Table 13.3 Differences between drunkenness and cerebral concussion

Trial	Drunkenness	Cerebral concussion
History of	Consumption of alcohol	Head injury
Behavior	Non-cooperative	Calm and quite
Pupils	Dilated except in comatose case	Contracted; pin point in pontine hemorrhage
Pulse	Rapid	Slow and feeble
Respiration	Sighing	Shallow
Skin	Congested flush and warm	Pale and cold
Body temperature	Raised except in comatose	Raised in pontine hemorrhage
Examination of blood and urine	Evidence of alcohol	No alcohol

4. Within the subarachnoid space in the foramen magnum.

The most vulnerable points for trauma are: (i) At the penetration of dura, (ii) At exit from Atlas and transverse process and (iii) In osseous canal in Atlas. The demonstration of intracranial bleeding from the vertebrobasilar system is difficult since while removing the skull and brain at autopsy, the damage to vessels occurs, causing artefactual bleeding.

INJURY TO NECK

The neck can be, and often is, the site of many different types of injury. Its importance in forensic medicine is due to two features:

a. The presence of a large number of vital structures like: Throat and larynx, major blood vessels, major nerve trunks, the spine and the spinal cord.
b. The fact that it is of a size that can be grasped and easily held.

Ligature marks with intermittent abrasions on the skin of the neck is typical in hanging and strangulation. In case of strangulation with a ligature, in addition to the typical ligature mark with abrasions, there may be bruises on the skin (**Figure 13.22**). In case of strangulation by some hard materials like a rod, there will be extensive injuries over the surface of the neck, which may include abrasions, contusions and lacerations. These injuries may be of any dimension and may be placed at any level or site of the neck, but are most commonly present in front. In case of throttling, there will be abrasions and bruises representing the nail scratches and fingertip pressures, the sites and numbers of which will vary according to different influencing factors.

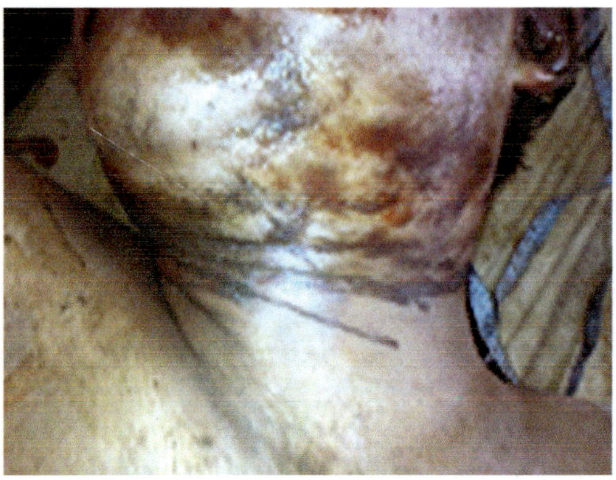

Figure 13.22 Ligature strangulation

In the subcutaneous tissue, the effect of ligature material compressing the neck is reflected by drying, whitening and glistening of the tissue, as is seen in case of hanging, but in a case of strangulation by ligature, instead of drying and glistening, the subcutaneous tissue may appear contused.

In case of strangulation by any other method, there should be gross damage to the soft tissue of the neck, which is most marked in case of throttling and strangulation by any hard blunt substance.

In violent asphyxial deaths, there may be laceration of the carotid sheath (strangulation by ligature) and transverse tear of the intima of the carotid artery (hanging). Among other injuries (related to violent asphyxia) in neck, there may be fracture of the hyoid bone (hanging and throttling, in victims above the age of 40 years), fracture of thyroid cartilage (strangulation), fracture of tracheal rings (hanging and strangulation) and fracture and dislocation of the 2nd and 3rd cervical vertebrae including bruise and laceration of the spinal cord with the covering meninges (judicial hanging). In violent asphyxial deaths injury to the sternomastoid muscles and contusion of the posterior wall of the esophagus may appear as important findings.

Apart from the injuries due to the violent asphyxiation, there may be sharp cut or stab injuries related to suicidal and homicidal deaths. Chop wounds on any side of the neck are almost always homicidal (**Figure 13.23**).

Decapitation cuts at the level of the neck may be homicidal cut throat or may be entirely postmortem in nature, where, after killing the victim by some other means, the body is decapitated. Decapitation (**Figure 13.24**) should compulsorily suggest homicidal nature of the death except when this occurs due to certain machineries or over a railway track or traffic accidents, when this may be accidental also.

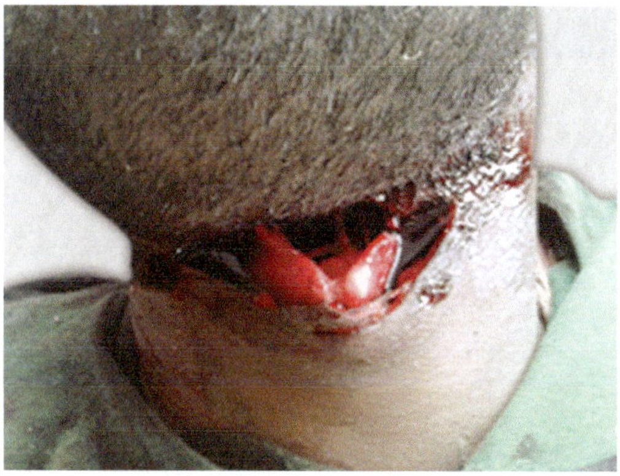

Figure 13.23 Homicidal cut throat
(*Courtesy:* Dr Mrinal Haloi, GMCH)

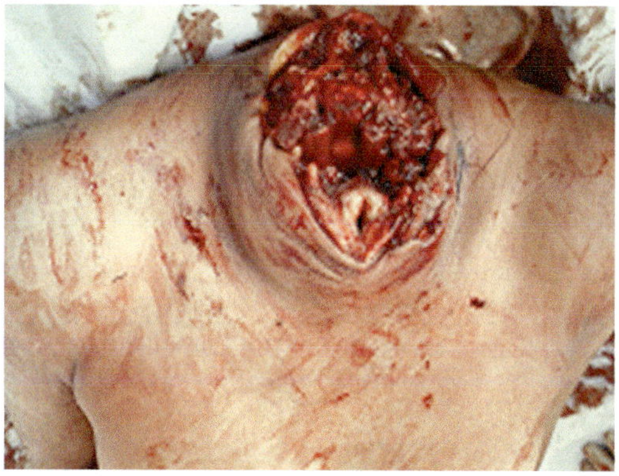

Figure 13.24 Antemortem separations of head (Homicidal)
(*Courtesy*: Dr Manoj Kr. Baishya, GMCH)

In the neck, incised or cut injuries may be either suicidal or homicidal in nature. From the features, it can be differentiated between homicidal and suicidal one (**Table 13.4**). Whereas incised wounds involving the front can be suicidal or homicidal, those on the back and many of the others, placed on either or both sides, go in favor of being homicidal in nature.

Stab injuries over the neck are mostly homicidal in nature. Chop wounds are homicidal irrespective of the site and level. These are also, usually more than one in number. Firearm wounds at the upper part of the neck, i.e. below the chin and the mandible go strongly in favor of being suicidal in nature, particularly if these are contact wounds. Any other type of firearm wound at any other site goes in favor of being homicidal in nature.

Causes of Death in Cut Throat Injury

a. When vagus nerve is cut it is neurogenic shock.
b. When carotid artery or jugular vein is cut it is hemorrhagic shock or venous air embolism.
c. When trachea or larynx is cut then it is due to edema of the glottis or aspiration pneumonia, etc.
d. Wound infection in late cases of death.

INJURIES ON THE CHEST

The chest can be subject to all kinds of injury and is particularly susceptible to both blunt and penetrating injuries. According to the different circumstances and weapon used, the nature of the injuries on the chest varies.

Chest injuries are: (a) Closed wounds like abrasion, contusion, etc., and (b) Penetrating or open wounds like stab or puncture wound.

In vehicular accidents, injuries are generally extensive. If it is a case of run over, there may be crushing of the chest with presence of tyre marks. In case of simple knock down, there will be primary impact injuries or extensive secondary injuries in the form of extensive grazed abrasion, bruise or laceration. There will be corresponding gross internal injuries in the form of subcutaneous hematomas, fracture of bones of thoracic cage like, clavicles, ribs and sternum at one or more than one place. There may be varying degree injuries to the intra-thoracic structures with or without rib fracture. These may be in the form of contusion or laceration and may involve pleurae, lungs and mediastinal structures, including the heart.

The heart may get separated at the base or ventricles may be ruptured, but the auricles may be spared. In traffic accident deaths involving the intrathoracic structures, there is invariably huge accumulation of liquid and clotted blood.

Table 13.4 Suicidal and homicidal cut throat injuries

Traits	Suicidal cut throat	Homicidal cut throat
Location	Placed high up, mostly situated on the upper part of left lateral side and partly on the right side of front of neck (right handed person)	Placed low down, mostly on either side of front of neck
Direction	Above downwards and from left to right (in right handed person)	Usually above downwards
Disposition of sloping	Oblique	Horizontal or downward sloping
Severity of wound	Main cut is less severe and superficial	Main cut is severe and deep
Hesitation cuts	Present on the initial part of the wound	Absent
Tailing of wound	Present on the last or terminal part of the wound	May or may not present at one or both the ends, depending upon the position of the victim and assailant
Signs of struggle and resistance	Absent	Present
Presence of defiance cut	Absent	Present
Associated injuries	Self-inflicted wounds over the accessible part of the body	Other homicidal wounds may be on other parts of the body /non-accessible parts
Types of weapon used	Light sharp cutting weapon	Usually heavy sharp cutting weapon
Presence of weapon	May be held in cadaveric spasm	Not so
Vessels involved	Usually jugular vein or carotid artery is cut at the site of commencement of the wound	Muscles, vessels of both sides are cut
Hemorrhage	Fair amount of blood tickles down over the front of the body	Blood usually tickles down on the sides of the neck
Cut marks on clothing	Absent	May show cut marks on clothing at corresponding level
Receipt of the dead body	Usually found with the face downwards	Usually in supine position
Foreign bodies in the clenched hand of the victim	Not detected	Foreign hair, fibers of fabrics, button of shirt, neck chain, etc, may be detected
Circumstantial evidences	Room may be bolted from inside, body found near or in front of the mirror	Place of incidence is open and accessible to others. Evidence of struggle and resistance is present
Suicidal note	May be detected	Absent

In late death cases, pneumothorax, pyothorax or hemothorax may be the cause.

Accidental blunt force injury on the chest may occur in fall from a height or getting pressed under a machine, in between buffers of two bogies of a train, or in other traumatic asphyxial circumstances. Crush injuries may be caused when the chest is compressed under the wheel of a vehicle or in between two rollers of a machine. The type of injuries and the depth of involvement will depend on the force of the impact and the type of the causative agent. The injuries may thus be anything from external abrasion to gross internal injuries.

Homicidal blunt force injuries are comparatively superficial with abrasions, contusions and occasional lacerations on the chest wall. With comparatively heavy force impact, there may be fracture of the sternum, clavicles and ribs, with corresponding internal injuries. In case of blunt force injuries of the internal organs of the chest, it may often be difficult to assess its extent from outside.

Incised wounds over the chest wall, if reasonably deep and chop wound are present, goes much in support of being homicidal in nature. Chop wounds are exclusively homicidal except in those rare circumstances where these may be accidental in nature. Self-inflicted incised wounds on the chest wall may be fabricated ones and bear the characteristic features of self-inflicted incised wounds as seen elsewhere. Deeper incised wounds on unapproachable parts of the chest wall are not suicidal in nature. It is not a necessity that incised wounds on the chest wall will be superficial in nature. Often their depth may be extended up to the chest cavity, particularly in case of chop wounds. Accidental incised wounds may result from fall on sharp edge of a cutting weapon or object or during operation of sharp cutting machinery. When a chop wound enters the chest cavity, the injuries to the internal organs will have similarity with penetrating wounds.

Penetrating wounds of the thorax are very much significant in many ways. Penetrating wound of the chest may give deceiving information about the length of the blade of the weapon and the direction of the penetration. When from the front, the length of the blade of the weapon may wrongly appear more than what it actually is and the direction of the wound may wrongly appear more upwards, when the lung is injured, due to backward and upward movement of the injured and collapsed lung, due to their posterior and upper attachment. The position is reversed when the stab is from the back and penetrates the lung. The depth or for that purpose the length of the blade of the weapon will appear shorter and the direction of the penetration will appear more upwards, than what it is.

Fatal suicidal stab wounds on the chest are typically located over the pericardial area of the anterior chest wall. With one centrally placed deep penetrating wound, there may be cluster of superficial tentative stab wounds.

Occasionally, accidental stab wounds may be sustained on the thorax due to either fall over the pointed projecting part of a weapon or object or accidental penetration of the chest wall by some pointing substance or weapon.

Stab wounds over the auricles, aorta or the superior vena cava shall be immediately fatal, whereas the same on the ventricles may not be immediately fatal, and may give sufficient time to undertake operative treatment. Stab wounds on the ventricles, particularly on the left ventricle may not be fatal if that does not reach the cavity of the ventricle. Death may not be quick even if the weapon has entered the ventricular cavity, if the direction of the wound is oblique in relation to the wall of the ventricle because in such a case the oblique opening of the ventricle will close during each contraction of the heart so that there will be minimum loss of blood. Similarly, hemorrhage will be minimal, if the weapon remains in situ with the blade occupying the space made by the penetration of the weapon.

In course of searching for the bullet or pellets or splinters of a bomb, difficulty may arise, particularly if these are lodged inside the lungs or the vertebral bones. Hence, it is very helpful if the body is X-rayed.

ABDOMINAL INJURIES

According to the different circumstances and weapon used, the nature of the injuries on the abdomen varies.

In vehicular accidents, the injuries are generally extensive. If it is a case of run over, there may be crushing of the abdomen against vertebral column with or without tyre marks. This is because of laxity of abdominal wall. In case of simply knocked down, there will be primary impact injuries on back side of the abdomen, or extensive secondary injuries in the form of extensive grazed abrasion, bruise or laceration, especially on back. There may be varying degree injuries to the intra-abdominal structures. These may be in the form of contusion or laceration and may involve liver, kidneys, spleen and stomach and intestine. The kidneys, spleen may get separated at the hilum, may be ruptured. Lacerations, avulsion or perforation of mesentery or gas-filled intestine and also injury to the vertebral column, particularly lumbar vertebra, can occur.

Because of rupture of liver, spleen, pancreas, cecum, urinary bladder, there is invariably huge accumulation of liquid and clotted blood in the peritoneal cavity. In late death cases, hemoperitonitis may be the cause.

Accidental blunt force injury of the abdomen may occur in getting pressed under a machine. Crush injuries may be caused when compressed under the wheel of a vehicle or in between two rollers of a machine. The type of injuries and the depth of involvement will depend on the force of the impact and the type of the causative agent. The injuries may thus be anything from external abrasion to gross internal injuries.

In case of blunt force injuries of the internal organs of the abdomen, it may often be difficult to assess its extent from outside.

Incised wounds over the abdominal wall, if reasonably deep and if they are chops, go much in support of being homicidal in nature. Chop wounds are exclusively homicidal except in those rare circumstances where these may be accidental in nature. Self-inflicted incised wounds on the abdominal wall may be fabricated ones and bear the characteristic features of self-inflicted incised wounds as seen elsewhere.

Often the depth of incised wounds may be extended up to the abdominal cavity, particularly in case of chop wounds. Accidental incised wounds may result from fall on sharp edge of a cutting weapon or object or during operation of sharp cutting machinery. When a chop wound enters the cavity, the injuries to the internal organs will have similarity with penetrating wounds.

Penetrating wounds of the abdomen are very much significant in many ways. Penetrating wound of the abdomen may give deceiving information about the length of the blade of the weapon and the direction of the penetration. From the front, the length of the blade of the weapon may wrongly appear more than what it actually is. **Hilt mark** is suggestive of complete insertion of blade of the weapon.

Fatal suicidal stab wounds on the abdomen are typically with one centrally placed deep penetrating wound, there may be cluster of superficial tentative stab wounds.

Occasionally, accidental stab wounds may be sustained on the abdomen due to either fall over the pointed projecting part of a weapon or object or accidental penetration of the abdominal wall by some pointing substance or weapon.

Stab wounds over the stomach or intestines are usually fatal because of development of peritonitis due to leakage of GIT contents and death is due to peritonitis.

There may be respiratory embracement due to upward pushing of diaphragm due to accumulation of fluid, blood or air secondary to perforation of GIT and intra-abdominal hemorrhage. There may be hemo or pneumothorax secondary to rupture of diaphragm.

Intra-abdominal injury may also be caused through the vaginal route, like in termination of pregnancy by a pointed instrument. Diaphragm injuries like rupture are generally fatal. If the diaphragm is ruptured, herniation of the organs may result.

INJURIES ON LIMBS

Self-inflicted or fabricated wounds are most commonly inflicted on upper limbs and sometimes lower limbs and other places. The self-inflected wounds are commonly seen on anterior aspect of the wrist and or forearm.

Incised slash defence wounds are common on posteriomedial aspects of forearm, dorsum of hand, wrist palmar aspects of hand. Incised wounds on palmar aspect can also be due to holding the single or double edged weapon with an attempt to prevent its use on him.

Amputation of limbs may be caused due to chopping.

Abrasion, contusions are due to struggle or falling on the ground if it is over the palm and back of the elbow. Injection marks over deltoid, cubital fossa, wrist and dorsum of the hand (should be searched cautiously).

On buttocks, linear bruise may be seen. Contusions grazed abrasion may be seen in traffic accidents. Old and recent injuries in a passive sodomite as per old or recent sodomy act.

Sprains, strains, ruptures and tears to the tendons, ligaments and muscles; dislocation, bone fractures and breaks; muscle avulsion injuries which are the tearing of a structure from the origin, for example, tearing the Achilles tendon from the base of the ankle or tearing a muscle from the bone (origin or attachment) can also occur due to accident or assault or homicidal act.

INJURIES TO PRIVATE PARTS

Injuries to private parts may be seen in sexual assault or otherwise. Nail scratches, bruise and rupture of hymen, congestion of parts of female genitalia or secondary sexual organs are common in sexual violation.

Injury to vaginal wall may occur while procuring termination of pregnancy.

Incised wounds of penis may produce fatal hemorrhage. Removal of testicles or kick over the scrotum may prove fatal from shock to nervous system. Wounds of the spermatic cord may be dangerous from hemorrhage. Incised wounds over scrotum may take irregular shape due to looseness of the skin (lacerated looking incised wounds) and due to presence and contraction of the superficial dartos muscles.

INJURIES TO THE SPINAL CORD

The spine is a complex structure with interlocking but mobile components. It is designed to flex to a great extent but lateral movement and extension are much more limited. The spine is very commonly injured in major trauma such as road traffic accidents or falls from a height, and severe injury with discontinuity is easily identified. However, sometimes the spinal injuries are more subtle and it is only after careful dissection that damage to the upper cervical spine and, in particular, disruption of the atlanto-occipital joint will be revealed.

For the survivors of trauma, spinal injuries may have some of the most crucial long-term effects because the spinal cord is contained within the spinal canal and there is little, if any, room for movement of the canal before the cord is damaged. The sequelae of spinal damage will depend upon the exact site and the exact type of the injury.

The spinal cord injury may be due to concussion, compression (fracture dislocation) or wounds. That the wound has penetrated the meninges is shown by the escape of cerebrospinal fluid.

The cord and nerves may be injured by:

a. Puncture
b. Extravasations of blood and the formation of a clot and
c. Subsequent septic inflammation.

Division or complete compression of the cord at or above the level of the **fourth cervical** vertebra is immediately fatal (as happens in judicial hanging). When the injury is below the **fourth**, the diaphragm continues forcibly in action, but the lungs are imperfectly expanded, and life will not be maintained for more than a day or two. When the injury is in the **dorsal region**, there is paralysis of the legs and of the sphincters of the bladder and rectum, but power is retained in the arms and the upper intercostals muscles act, the extent of paralysis depending on the level of the lesion. In injuries to the lumbar region, the legs may be partly paralyzed, and the rectal and bladder sphincters may be involved.

Whiplash Injury

Whiplash is a term used to describe a neck injury caused by a sudden movement of the head forwards, backwards or sideways. It is due to violent hyperflexion followed by hyperextension (whiplash), leading to compression of spinal cord without fracture of vertebrae. These injuries are produced on the front seat occupant or driver of the moving vehicle. Whip-lash injuries are usually seen after rear-end car collisions. Most of the time the injuries are in the form of fracture dislocation of the cervical vertebrae due to violent hyperflexion followed by hyperextension (whip-lash) associated with or without head injuries and also fracture of femur, pelvic, wrist when the moving vehicle is brought to sudden halt. Earlier these injuries were also called **railroad spine**. The wide varieties of symptoms seen are grouped as **whiplash-associated disorders**. A whiplash injury from an automobile accident is called a **cervical acceleration-deceleration injury**.

Rabbit Punch

Rabbit punch is the compression fracture of spine portion of cervical vertebrae due to hyperextension of neck due to sudden knock from the back.

Railway spine or **traumatic neurasthenia or concussion of the cord** is due to compression fracture of the vertebral column and compression of the spinal cord like collision of railway boogies.

Jefferson Fracture

It is the compression fracture of anterior and posterior arch of the atlas with lateral displacement of the soft tissues on to the axis, resulting from vertical impact of the head with straightened neck.

Hangman's Fracture

It is the fracture of pedicles of axis resulting from anterior dislocation of 2nd and 3rd cervical vertebrae with or without fracture of odontoid process, usually results in judicial hanging or due to forceful hyperextension and rotation of neck in vehicular accident.

Pithing

Pushing a needle in the nape of the neck between 1st and 3rd cervical vertebra may injure the medulla and upper cervical cord (vital centers) causing instantaneous death.

REFERENCES

1. Lindenberg R. Mechanical injuries of brain and meninges. In: Spitz WU (Ed) Spitz and Fisher's Medicolegal Investigation of Death, 3rd ed. USA: Charles C Thomas Publisher; 1993. pp. 585-636.
2. Kamal R. Acute subdural hematomas. In: Mahapatra AK, Kamal R (Eds), A Textbook of Head Injury, 2nd ed. New Delhi: Modern publishers; 2001. pp. 128-35.
3. Saukko P, Knight B. Knight's Forensic Pathology: Head and Spinal Injuries, 3rd ed. Arnold, London; 2004. pp. 174-221.
4. Pillay VV. Textbook of Forensic Medicine and Toxicology: Regional Injuries. 14th ed. Paras Publishing: Hyderabad. 2004. pp. 173-90.
5. Shepherd R. Simpson's Forensic Medicine. 12th ed. London: Arnold. 2003. pp. 70-8.

CHAPTER 14

Road Traffic Injuries

Putul Mahanta, Madhab Ch Rajbongshi

LEARNING PLAN

- Brief review of road traffic accident (RTA)
- Know the mechanism of injury production
- Pattern of RTA injuries and its pathophysiology
- Understand about accident prevention

Man is, basically, an aggressive animal. Therefore, the history of trauma dates backs right down to the time of evolution of human kind. As early as 460 BC, Hippocrates was aware of the danger to life caused by injury to liver and spleen. The motorized transportation media like vehicle, rail, airplane, etc. with fast moving vehicular traffic, vast urbanization, rapid industrialization and changing social patterns have contributed very greatly to the increase in the incidence of trauma to the human body. The injuries include injuries on road traffic, railways, watercrafts and aviation mishaps.[1]

Road traffic accidents (RTAs) represent a major epidemic of non-communicable disease in the present century. According to WHO report on Road Traffic injury prevention, the total number of RTA related deaths and injuries worldwide would rise by 65% between 2000 and 2020 if efforts in prevention, with new initiatives, were not intensified. India accounts for as high as 6% of world's RTA, although it has only 1% of world's vehicle.[2]

DEFINITION

Accident is 'an unexpected, unplanned occurrence, which may involve injury'.[3] A WHO advisory group in 1956 defined accident as "an unpremeditated event resulting in recognizable damage". It can also be defined as "occurrence in a sequence of events, which usually produces unintended injury, death or property damage".

WHO defines **RTA** as "an event occurring on a street, road or highway, in which at least one motor vehicle in motion is involved by collision or losing control, and which causes physical injury or damage to property".[4] They are no longer considered accidental. They are part of the price we pay for technological progress.

BRIEF REVIEW OF ROAD TRAFFIC ACCIDENT

Accidents constitute a veritable epidemic throughout the world. They rank now fourth among the leading causes of death in the world and account for approximately 8% of all deaths in the world, 7.9% in the developing countries and 7.5% in the developed countries. They are also chief cause of death among persons aged 10–24 years. Between the ages of 5 and 14 years, death due to injuries ranks fifth among boys and seventh among girls in the developing countries. In the developed regions, 57% of male deaths and 43% of female deaths in this age group are due to injuries, mainly traffic accidents.[5]

Globally, an estimated 3 million people die yearly from unintentional injuries, including those resulting from motor vehicle accidents, etc. About 8,85,000 lives are lost yearly in the world by RTAs, of which two-thirds (500,000) mortality is in developing countries. Of the non-fatal accidents, 10% or more people suffer from permanent disabilities. Motor vehicle accidents account for around 23.8% of reported mortality in males and 23.2% in females. In many countries, motor vehicle accidents rank first among all fatal accidents.[5]

In addition, for every death, there are as many as 30–40 minor injuries and 10–15 serious injuries requiring long periods for expensive care, nursing and treatment.[6]

India has one of the highest road accident rates in the world, one out of every 42 vehicles in the country met with an accident in 1986. In the US and Europe, the average is one in every 100 vehicles.[7] The death toll is about eight for every 1000 vehicles as compared to one in industrialized countries.[8] In 1991, 60,000 people were killed in road accidents, compared to 24,600 in 1980. The number of people injured in RTA is doubled in the past 6 years, touching 1.75 lakh. Studies done by WHO show that RTAs account for 2.5% of the total deaths. But in the 5-44 years group, it is as high as 10% and is among the six leading causes of death.[7]

According to a study conducted by the National Transportation Planning and Research Center (NTPRC) of New Delhi and Trivandrum, every 4 minutes, a person is killed or injured in road accidents in India, which has a network of 1,500,000 roads. Drivers were found to be at fault in about 45% of the accidents, which showed an increase of 8.3% a year during 1960–1980. Road deaths increased at the rate of 18.5% on an average during the same period. The study revealed that pedestrians accounted for 10% of the accident and mechanical defects for 6%. The study pointed out that the number of accidents per lakh population varied from 5.39 in Assam to 63.72 in Maharashtra. In case of accident rate per 100 sq km area, Kerala had the highest figure with 16.85, followed by West Bengal with 15.98. Accident number per 1000 km of road length was the highest in Maharashtra 242 against 168.87 in Gujarat and 145.17 in Tamil Nadu.[9] According to 1976 Statistics, the number of persons killed per 10,000 motor vehicles in India was 64.9 as against 4.7, 13.5 and 12.5 in America, France and West Germany.[10]

MECHANISM OF INJURY PRODUCTION

The dynamics involved in any injury by mechanical force have been thoroughly studied by **De Haven H.**[11] The extent of an injury sustained in a road crash is directly proportional to the degree of acceleration or deceleration to which the occupant of the vehicle is subjected. The 'G' formula is used to calculate the mean force involved in a "real-life" accident:

$$G = \frac{V^2 \times 0.034}{D}$$

In which G is equal to the force exerted by gravity, V is the velocity of the vehicle in miles per hour, 0.034 is a mathematical conversion factor and D is the stopping distance in feet.[12]

For example, if a car traveling at a speed of 50 mph strikes a dirt bank head on and plows ahead 6 inches before full deceleration occurs, the mean force is 170 G's. Thus, an occupant of the car who weighed 150 lb, would theoretically be exposed to a force of 25,000 lb (gravity time's body weight) (**Figure 14.1**).

$$G = \frac{(\text{MPH})^2 \times 0.034^*}{\text{Stopping distance (f)}}$$

(* Mathematical conversion factor or contant)

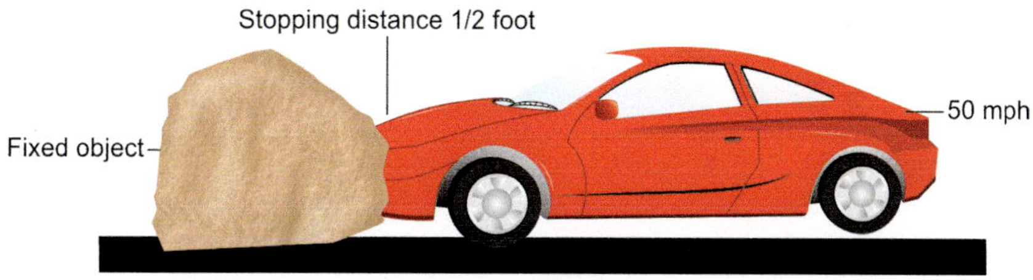

G = 170

Mean force absorbed by car (3600 lb) during decelaration—256 tons

Mean force absorbed by occupant (150 lb) during decelaration—12.7 tons

Figure 14.1 Mean force calculation in actual road accidents

He also stated that occupant is usually decelerated at a much slower rate than the vehicle and the stopping distance is much longer. Despite the massive forces to which the victims of road crashes are exposed, amazingly, many of them survive the accident.

PATTERN OF ROAD TRAFFIC INJURIES

The RTA victims may sustain variety of injuries. The victims may belong to three categories: (i) pedestrian, (ii) vehicle occupants and (iii) motor cyclist.

Injuries to the Pedestrians

Pedestrians, particularly the children and elderly people, are the most vulnerable road user. The dynamics of the crash depend on the following factors:

i. Relative heights of the impact site above the ground.
ii. Point of impact of vehicle in relation to the center of gravity of the pedestrian.
iii. The nature of road surface or ground, whether smooth or rough.

Impact below the center of gravity throws victim onto bonnet (or roof at greater speed). Victim acquires velocity of vehicle only to be thrown onto the road surface by violent braking. The **patterns** of injuries sustained by **pedestrians** can be **grouped** as follows:

i. Primary impact injuries
ii. Secondary impact injuries
iii. Secondary injuries.

This mechanism of pedestrian injury is called as **Waddle's Triad.**

Primary Impact Injuries

Indicating, which part of the body was struck first. These are caused when the pedestrian is hit by projecting objects of the vehicle, e.g. car bumper, mudguard, view mirror and handle of the door or, in case of Lorries, the load material projecting out. The site of primary impact would depend on the position as well as height of the pedestrian while being knocked down.

If a pedestrian is struck from behind, he may sustain a fracture dislocation of the thoracic spine or lumbar spine. An almost simultaneous impact on the buttocks may drive the femoral head through the acetabulum. Striae like superficial tears of the abdomen or inguino-femoral regions may be seen due to over-stretching of the skin.

If the pedestrian is facing the vehicle, he may sustain intra-abdominal injuries or injuries to the chest wall and thoracic contents. Sometimes, the pelvis may be fractured. Primary impact injuries are due to direct impact of vehicle against victim and may harbor trace evidence

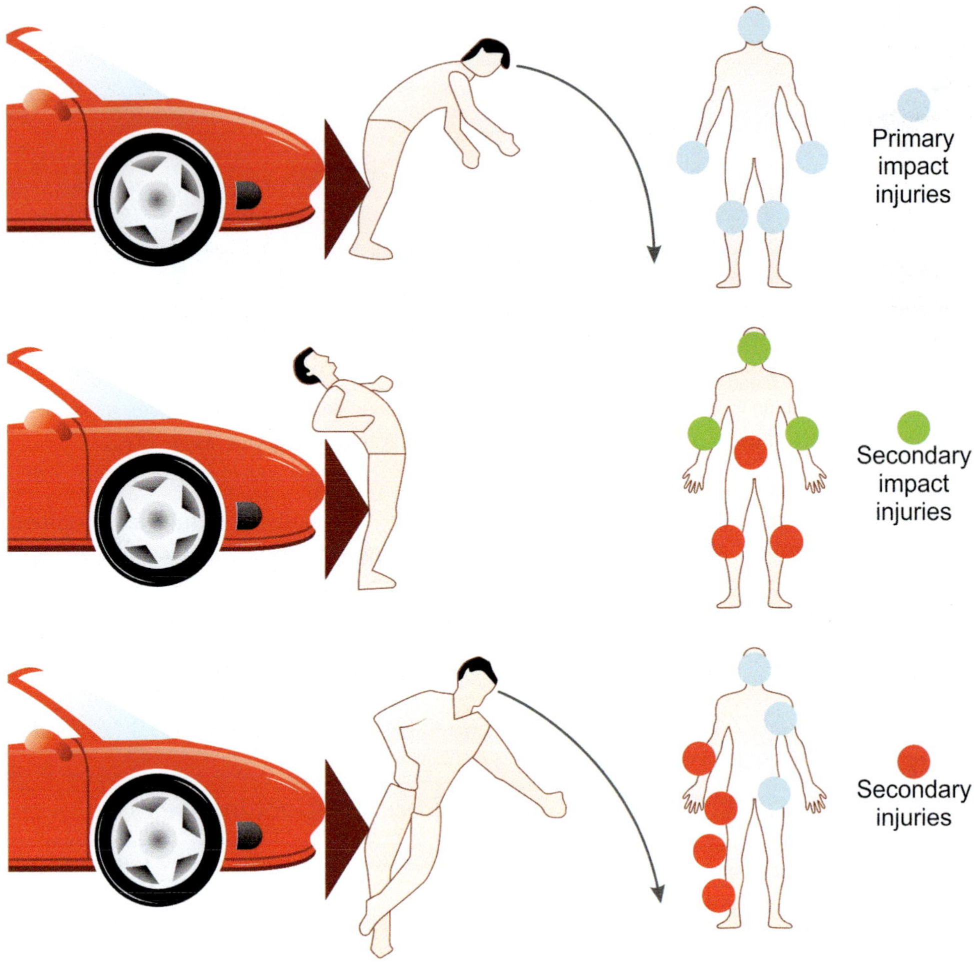

Figure 14.2 Dynamics of transportational of pedestrian injuries

(paint, metal) of evidential value in 'hit and run' collisions (**Figure 14.2**).

Secondary Impact Injuries

A secondary impact injury indicates whether further injuries were caused by the vehicle or not. These are due to a later (secondary) impact with the same vehicle such as being lifted onto the vehicle after primary impact or being run over.

If the point of impact is at or above the center of gravity, as is the case when children are concerned, the victim is directly thrown to the ground as a result of primary impact and may be run over by the same car, with consequent undercarriage injuries and stains from grease, oil, etc. The hot exhaust pipe may cause burns.

However, if the victim is an older child or an adult, the point of primary impact will be beneath the center of gravity, and it tends to lift the pedestrian up onto the bonnet or hood, or sometimes even on the road behind the vehicle, depending on the speed of the car. Secondary impact injuries may then occur from contact with the windshield and may result in severe head injuries and laceration. The body may then fall sideways and be run over by a passing vehicle.

Secondary Injuries

These are due to fall on ground or any other subject following an accident. These are due to being thrown to the ground or against some other object. They vary greatly in severity.

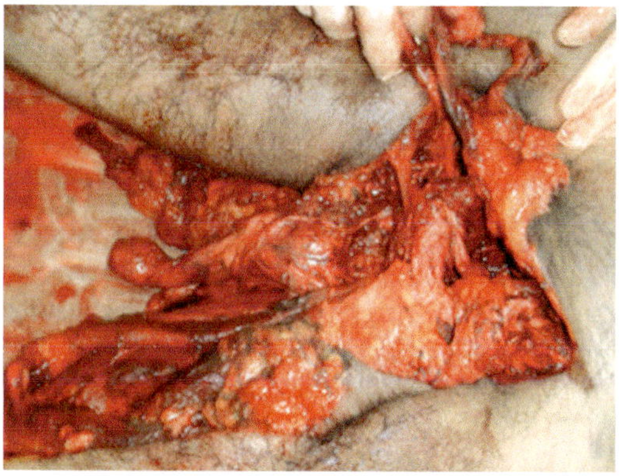

Figure 14.3 Flaying laceration

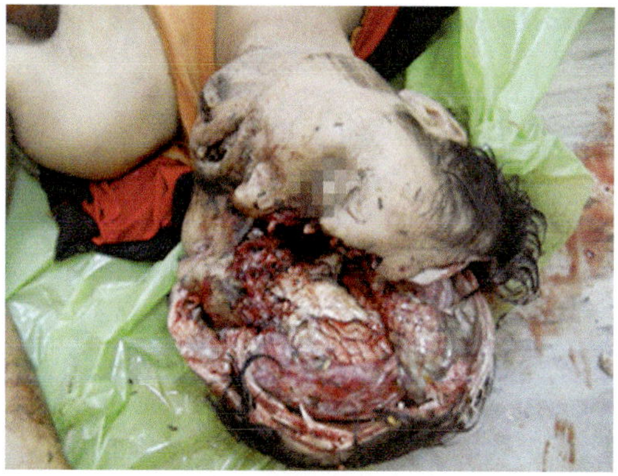

Figure 14.4 Run over by vehicle
(*Courtesy:* Dr Mrinal Haloi, GMC, Guwahati)

The distribution and nature of these injuries will be governed by the road surface, the speed of vehicle, the position of the victim and the amount of clothes on him.

Run Over Injury

Running over by a car may results in flaying lacerations if involve the limbs (**Figure 14.3**) and crushing of head if head is involved (**Figure 14.4**) or crushing of any part of the body.

Speed of impact cannot be estimated from the severity of injuries. It can only state whether injuries were mild, moderate or severe. **Skid marks** offer only objective evidence of vehicle speed as shown in **Table 14.1**.

About 50% of fatalities are hit at speeds less than 30 mph. 50% of those serious injured are hit at less than 21 mph.

Injuries to the Vehicle Occupants

In vehicular accidents cases, the occupants of vehicle sustain various types of injuries according to the position of the occupant. Vehicle occupants (**Figure 14.5**) move towards the point of impact. The occupants of a car are the following types:

1. Driver
2. Front seat passenger
3. Rear seat passenger

Table 14.1 Speed of impact versus fatalities

Speed of impact (mph)	Percentage of fatalities (%)
19–24	10
24–30	47
31–36	73

In vehicular accidents, a vehicle may sustain five main patterns of impact and they are:

- Front or head on impact
- Back impact
- Side impact
- Side swipe and
- Rollover and roof impact.

- **Head on** into a stationary object like a tree, another vehicle (speed and impact energy additive). The driver and front seat passenger may strike over the:
  i. Dashboard, windscreen and pillar's (impact mainly on skull and brain)
  ii. Steering wheel (impact on chest lacerating lung and heart).

  Parcel shelf (fractures of knees and pelvis) and pedals trap the ankles may occurs.

  Rear passenger may hit:
  i. Back seat or over into front
  ii. Deceleration causes whiplash (flexion and extension) neck, DAI (Diffuse Axonal Injury) and ruptured thoracic aorta.
- **Back or Rear impact** (speeds subtractive)
  i. Seats and head restraints support the torso (The body excluding the head and neck and limbs) and neck
  ii. Whiplash (extension and flexion) with no restraint
  iii. Risk of petrol fire.
- **Side impact (direct)**
  i. Risk of side intrusion
  ii. If left: Limb, spleen, left kidney and lung
  iii. If right: Limb, liver, right kidney and lung.

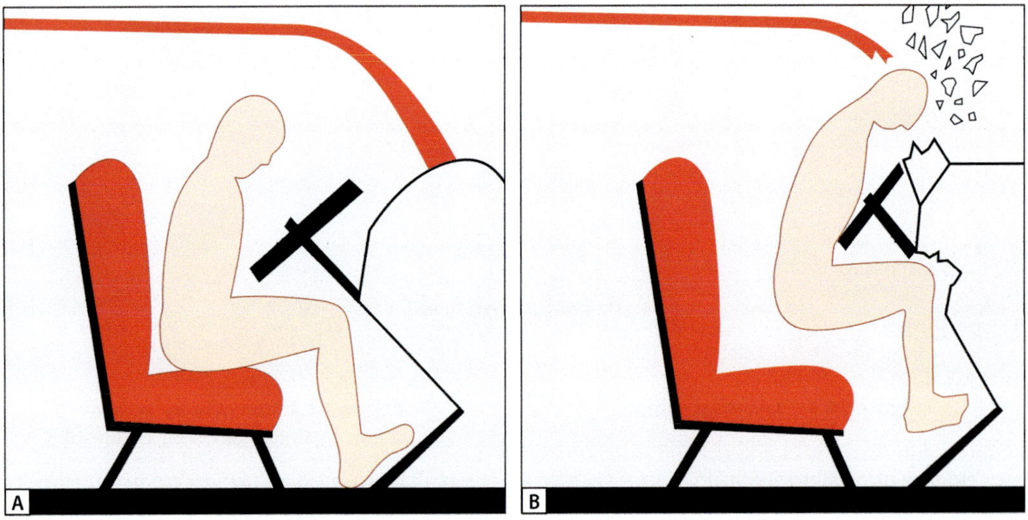

Figures 14.5A and B Movement of unrestrained front seat occupants in head on crashes, (A) Initial contact area; and (B) The final resting position

- **Side swipe (glancing):** Less risk of side intrusion.
- **Roll over:** Less damaging (rolling spreads the time of impact) unless occupant is ejected.

Whiplash Injury

This type of injury is due to sudden and violent acceleration or deceleration force applied to the occupant, usually, front seat passenger. When the vehicle comes to a sudden stop due to head-on obstruction, the head continues to move forward resulting acute hyperflexion. When the body comes to rest, then a reactionary hyperextension occurs as the head is pushed backwards. This double movement is known as whiplash. This may result in dislocation of the upper cervical vertebrae or, less commonly, a fracture-dislocation in the lower part of spine at the level of C_5 and C_6. Spinal cord may be contused or lacerated.

Seat Belt Injuries

Many injuries in accident are caused by the passenger's seat belt. Improper fastening of the seat belt or seat belt malfunction are common factors behind this kind of injuries. The type of seat belt injury a passenger receives depends on the seat belt design and how the seat belt was worn. It may be rarely more damaging than if a seatbelt is not worn.

A victim of a traffic accident who was wearing a seat-belt and who has superficial bruising or who complaints of pain may have visceral injuries.

The common seat belt injuries are:
- Bruising across chest and abdomen
- Neck injury and carotid artery rupture
- Fractured sternum, ribs and clavicles
- Lacerated mesentery, bowel
- Lumbar spinal injury.

Airbags Injury

Airbags drastically cut down both morbidity and mortality from vehicular crashes, but with the increased use of airbags, there has been a corresponding increase in the number of injuries descriable to these devices.

Injuries have been described resulting from all stages of airbag deployment, and all components of the system: from non-deployment, spontaneous deployment, the pyrotechnic used, expansion of the bag, contact with the bag and over-rapid deflation.[13,14,15]

Injuries ranged from the traumatic avulsion of a thumb to the development of a subdural hematoma with associated cerebral edema and respiratory arrest. Motor vehicle operators should be aware that although airbags can significantly reduce the severity of injuries sustained in frontal collisions, the module cover has the potential to inflict serious, even fatal injuries.[16]

SAFETY DEVICES

Seat Belts

A **seat belt (safety belt)** is a safety device designed to secure the occupant of a vehicle against harmful movement that may result during a collision or a sudden stop. It reduces the likelihood and severity of injury in a traffic accident by stopping the vehicle occupant from hitting hard against interior object of the vehicle, by keeping occupants positioned correctly for maximum benefit from the airbag, if the vehicle is so equipped, and by preventing occupants being ejected out of the vehicle. It is extremely effective in reducing mortality and morbidity in low- to medium-speed impacts as follows:

i. Diagonal strap restrains upper torso (prevents impact with steering wheel, upper dash board).
ii. Horizontal strap restrains lower torso and pelvis (prevents impact with lower dash, parcel shelf).
iii. Area of straps spreads deceleration force over a wider area than localized impact.
iv. Prevents ejection through windscreen or burst door.

Seat belts are the single most effective traffic safety device for preventing death and injury, according to the National Highway Traffic Safety Administration. Wearing a seat belt can reduce the risk of crash injuries by 50%.

Other Safety Features

i. Airbag (**Figure 14.6**) is a vehicle safety device.
ii. Crumple zones absorb impact energy and increase the duration of impact.

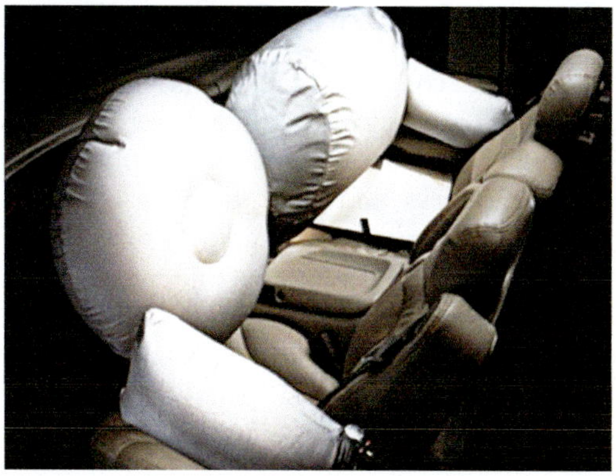

Figure 14.6 Airbags of a car

iii. Laminated windscreens deform without shattering and prevent ejection.
iv. Side impact bars.
v. Burst proof door locks to prevent ejection.
vi. Padded steering wheel and collapsible column.
vii. Breakable controls and mirrors, etc.
viii. ABS: Anti-lock braking system.

INJURIES OF MOTORCYCLISTS

Injuries sustained by motorcyclists are more dangerous than the car users. Accident and injuries sustained by motorcyclist may be due to:

i. Rash and negligent riding (high speeds)
ii. Instability of two wheelers
iii. Less or no protection
iv. Difficulties to see the road or object in front, etc.

Injuries associated with motorcycle accidents includes single vehicle accidents, collision with other motorcycle or standard vehicles and accidental striking of a pedestrian. If the impact is head on, more severe lesions can be expected, including rupture and separation of the heart from the aorta, crushing injury of the head and rupture of the abdominal viscera.[17] Primary impact injury may be to the leg only. Secondary impact injuries are on head, neck, chest and abdomen, etc. Helmet and leathers provide the only protection. Energy must be dissipated by sliding or rolling along the road.

Causes of Motorcycle Accident

The most common causes of motorcycle accidents are: alcohol and drugs, reckless driving, and environmental factors, e.g. pot holes, oil slicks and poor visibility. All types of injuries may be present. Besides other common injuries, abdominal injury also occur, which includes lacerations of the liver, spleen and kidney; rupture of the bowel and urinary bladder, and fracture of the pelvis.[18]

ACCIDENT PREVENTION

Thousands of accidents occur throughout the world every day. The failure of people, equipment, supplies or surroundings to behave or react as awaited causes most of the accident. Accident investigations determine how and why these failures happen. By employing the information gained through an investigation, a similar, or perhaps more disastrous accident may be prevented. It is important to carry on accident investigations with prevention in mind. There are currently no specific standards protocols for accident investigation.

RTA Reconstruction

This reconstruction is a scientific process of inquiring, analyzing and depicting conclusion about the causes and events during a vehicle collision. Reconstructionists are applied to conduct rigorous hit analysis and reconstruction to identify the collision causation and contributing factors in different types of accidents. This includes the role of driver, vehicle, road and the environment. The laws of physics and engineering principles such as conservation of linear momentum, work-energy methods and kinematics are the basis for this analysis and may arrive at use of software to compute useful quantities. The road accident reconstruction allows for rigorous analysis that an expert witness can be presented at trial. It is done in cases of fatalities. Results are also useful in arising recommendations for safety measures, including improving of safety aspects of motor vehicular designs. These reconstructions should be conducted by forensic medicine expert and forensic scientist, specialized units in law enforcement agencies.

Contributory Factors in Crashes

While this information is valuable in helping to identify ways of improving safety, care should be taken in its interpretation. The factors are largely subjective, reflecting the opinion of the reporting police officer and are not necessarily the result of extensive investigation. Some of the common factors associated with day-to-day traffic fatalities are:

i. Intoxication mainly alcohol, drugs, carbon monoxide, etc.
ii. Human factors: Reckless driving, high speeding, inattention, fatigue, inexperience, shoes, etc.
iii. Environmental factors: Fog, rain, ice, snow, leaves, sun, obstruction to vision, etc.
iv. Mechanical failure: Tyres, brakes, steering, etc.
v. Natural diseases: Ischemic heart disease, stroke, epilepsy, etc.

Apart from these, the following risk factors may also take active role in an RTA (**Figure 14.7**).

Preventive Measures

Seat belt, airbags and crash helmets are of very much important in preventing fatal injuries. An airbag is an occupant restraint system consisting of a flexible fabric envelope that prevents the vital part of the body like face, chest, etc. We can minimize or prevent the incidence of motor vehicular accident by following Haddon strategy.[19] In 1962, Haddon developed 10 strategies for injury prevention as mentioned in **Table 14.2.**[20]

Traffic Rules

Traffic rules and regulations of the roads are both the laws and the informal rules that may have been developed over time to help a neat and timely flow of traffic. With the replacement of ancient horse-driven carts with cars and trucks, the speed of the traffic increased,

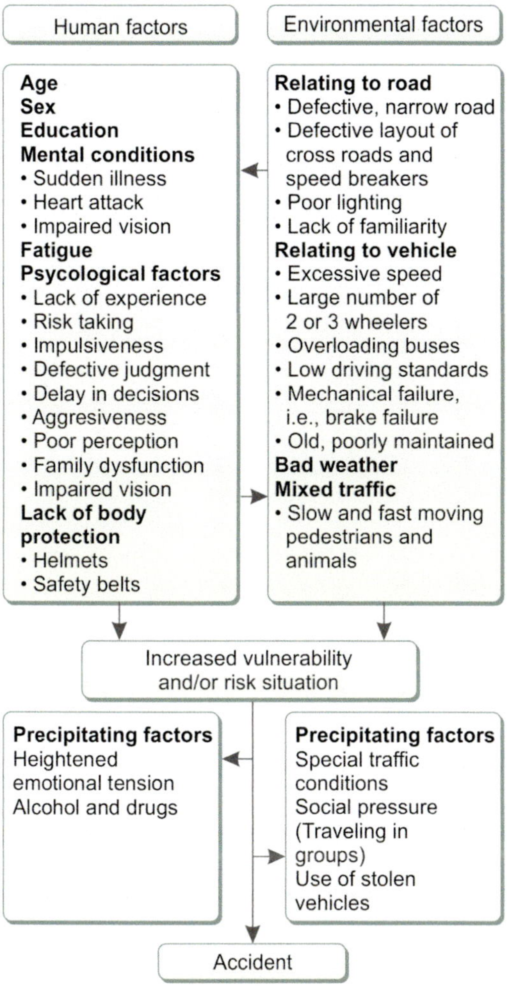

Figure 14.7 Various factors taking part in an accident

giving rise to the need for smooth roads and yet smoother traffic. So, to curb the need of the smoother traffic, some rules were devised. Almost all of the roadway traffic rules are built with devices meant to control traffic.

Table 14.2 Strategies for motor vehicle injury control; the Haddon counter measures

Strategy	Motor vehicle injuries
Prevent creation of the agent	Reduce the manufacturer of particularly dangerous motor vehicles
Reduce amount of agent	Improved vehicle engineering to prevent crashes; reduce the amount of argentous drivers, e.g. laws against driving under the influence of alcohol
Prevent release of agent	Reduce speed limits
Modify rate or spatial distribution of agent	Alternative transportation to limit the amount of vehicles in use
Separate the agent from the susceptible host in time and space	Remove pedestrians and bicyclists from vehicle traffic by the use of bike lanes, pedestrian over passes and sidewalks
Separate the agent from the susceptible host by interposition of a material barrier	Design improved vehicle safety mechanism, for example, seatbelts and air bags
Modify qualities of the agent	Design vehicle to reduce injuries, e.g. shatterproof windows, more absorbent front bumpers, better fire retardant materials and more foot room
Strengthen the susceptible host	Increase public awareness, e.g. pedestrian education and drinking-driving agents
Begin to counter the injury already done by the agent	Train medical staff and emergency medical services to respond speedily and appropriately to the crash and the injuries
Stabilize, repair and rehabilitate the injured host	Improve rehabilitation services

REFERENCES

1. Jhanjee A. A postmortem study of abdominal and pelvic trauma in central Delhi—A thesis for MD Forensic Medicine. Anil Aggrawal's Internet Journal of Forensic Medicine and Toxicology. 2000;1(2).
2. Epidemiology of RTA in India (Internet). Sir Ratan Tata Trust and Navajbai Ratan Tata Trust. [cited 2013 April 04]; Available from: URL:http//www.srtt.org/road_traffic_accidents.htm
3. Hogarth J. Glossary of health care terminology. WHO, 1978.
4. WHO. Economic Commission for Europe and the World Health Organization, Geneva; WHO; 1979.
5. WHO. The World Health Report 1995, Report of the director general WHO, 1995.

6. Ravindran Nair G. Swasth Hind 1982, 25(12):329.
7. India Today. May 15, 1987;143-8.
8. WHO. World Health Act. 1975.
9. Times of India. Times of India, 28th Oct, 1985.
10. Indian Express. Indian Express, 5th Sept, 1984.
11. De Haven H. Mechanical analysis of survival in fall. War Med. 1942;2:586.
12. Moore JO. Former director of Cornell automotive crush injury research programme: Personal communication.
13. Adams SL, Petri RW. Injury with spontaneous deployment of an automobile air bag. Acad Emerg Med. 1996;3:179-80.
14. Baruchin AM, Jakim I, Rosenberg L, et al. On burn injuries related to airbag deployment. Burns. 1999;25:49-52.
15. Smock WS, Nichols GR. Airbag module cover injuries. J Trauma. 1995;38:489-93.
16. Smock WS, Nicholas GR. Airbag module covers injuries. J Trauma-injury Infect Critical Care. 1995;38(4): 489-93.
17. Tedeschi CG, Eckert WG. Forensic Medicine; Vol. II. 1977. p. 853.
18. Parikh CK. Parikh's Textbook of Medical Jurisprudence, Forensic Medicine and Toxicology. 6th ed. 1999.
19. Mahanta P. A study of abdominal injuries in victims of road traffic incident in medico legal autopsy. 2001. pp. 190-1.
20. Haddon W Jr. A note concerning accident theory and research with special reference to motor vehicle accidents. Ann NY Acad Sci, 1963;107:635-46.

CHAPTER 15

Thermal Injuries

Adarsh Kumar, Putul Mahanta

LEARNING PLAN

- Learn about injuries due to heat and cold and their pathophysiology
- Understand the classification of burn
- Know the factors affecting prognosis of burn
- Learn about the electrical injuries and lightning
- Enumerate the postmortem changes

BRIEF REVIEW OF BURNS

Burn injuries have been a major cause of concern since prehistoric days to the present era of modern medicine.[1] The general belief that burns usually occur at the two extremes of age, indicating the accidental nature of infliction does not hold true as reported by Martin A Crore et al[2] and LPH Leenan et al[3] who described involvement of mean age of 30 and 28 years, respectively. Fire and burn injuries are second only to motor vehicle accidents as the leading cause of death in children of ages 1–4 years in the US. They are among the leading causes of injury and death in children of ages 1–18 years. Severe burns are considered the most catastrophic injury a person can survive, resulting in disfigurement, pain, emotional stress and tremendous economic costs.[4]

CLASSIFICATION OF THERMAL INJURIES

The skin constitutes about 15% of total body weight and is one of the largest organs of body. Physical agents (cold and hot) can cause both fatal and non-fatal injuries to it. These are the injuries produced by exposure of body to extremes of temperature and may be classified as (**Figure 15.1**):

Injuries Due to High Temperature (Heat)

1. **Generalized Effects of Heat**
   a. Heat Stroke
   b. Heat Hyperpyrexia
   c. Heat Cramps (Miner's cramps)
   d. Heat Exhaustion

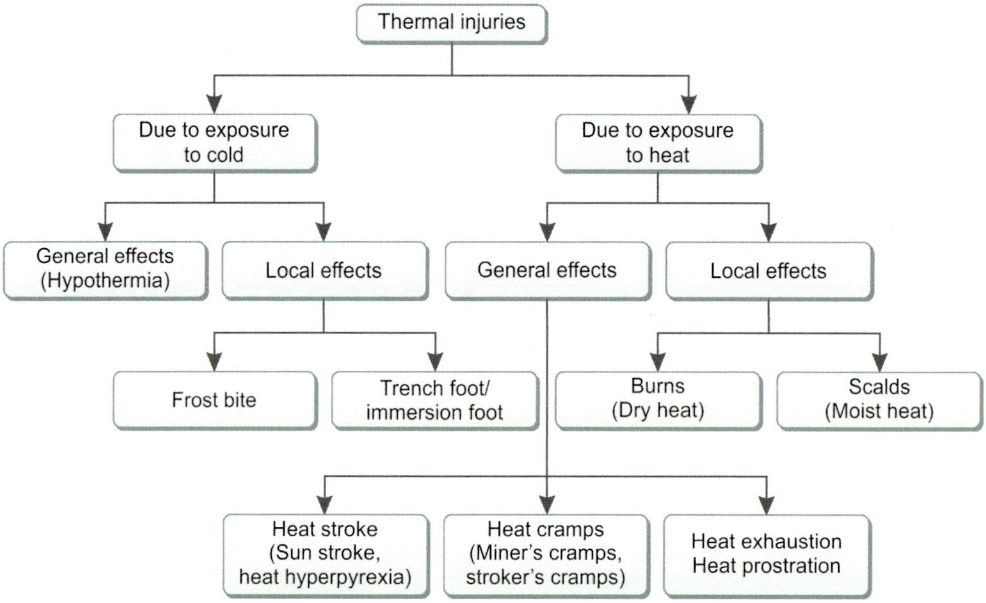

Figure 15.1 Classification of thermal injuries

2. **Localized Effects of Heat**
   a. Burns due to dry heat
   b. Scalds due to moist heat

Injuries Due to Low Temperature (Cold)

1. **Generalized Effects of Cold**
   Hypothermia
2. **Localized Effects of Cold**
   a. Chilblains (Pernio)
   b. Frost bite
   c. Trench foot or immersion foot

INJURIES DUE TO HIGH TEMPERATURE (HEAT)

Generalized Effects of Heat

They are produced when victim is exposed to abnormal hot environmental conditions, like that prevailing in our country. These conditions, although frequent, are not of much medicolegal significance as the attending circumstances are self-explanatory. The importance lies in the fact that such cases owing to their symptoms may be mistaken as meningitis. Another medicolegally important situation may arise in cases of death occurring in mine-workers, in which question of compensation arises. Of course, that has to be dealt as per Workmen's Compensation Act.

Heat Stroke

There occurs failure of thermoregulatory mechanism in body leading to sudden unconsciousness; hence, the name 'stroke'. It may further lead to fatality in a span of 5 minutes or delayed up to 3 days. It is seen typically when a person is exposed to direct sunlight during summer for considerably long period of time.

The onset is usually sudden with symptoms like headache, nausea, vomiting, feeling of exhaustion with lethargy, weakness in limbs and excessive desire for micturation. Face is flushed with dry, hot skin because of impaired sweating. Pupils get contracted, may be even pin-pointed, with sluggish light reaction. Body temperature may rise up to 43°C (109°F). Pulse becomes irregular, respiration is labored and person develops oliguria. The person becomes delirious and may have convulsion before being comatosed.

Heat Hyperpyrexia

Some authors equate hyperpyrexia with heat stroke, but both are different entities. Heat hyperpyrexia occurs because of malfunctioning of thermoregulatory center (not due to the failure), in which body temperature exceeds 41°C (106°F).

Other than environmental factors, hyperpyrexia may be associated with overdose of certain drugs like atropine, amphetamine and substances of abuse like cocaine. Several anesthetic agents like halothane and muscle relaxants like suxamethonium may also produce hyperpyrexia.

Heat Cramps

Synonyms: Miner's cramp, Fireman's cramp.

There occurs excessive loss of salt or water or both by way of perspiration. Painful spasms of voluntary muscles with flushing and dilation of pupil is seen. It is slow in onset and is non-fatal.

Heat Exhaustion

Synonyms: Heat collapse or heat prostration.

It is a condition of collapse, i.e. effect of heat over circulation without any rise in body temperature and usually seen following exposure to hot and humid atmosphere. Characteristic feature is prostration accompanied by evidence of peripheral vascular failure like hypotension, pallor and poor venous return. The patient recovers soon. Lethality is unusual, even if it occurs, it is due to sudden failure of heart.

All the above-mentioned conditions are frequently encountered in person working in mines, furnace, bakeries, laundries, etc., and marching soldiers. Alcoholism, hunger, lack of sleep, fatigue further predisposes a person to these generalized effects of heat.

Treatment

The victim should be removed immediately from the hot environment to a cooler place. Water should be given orally if possible. Hydrotherapy should be started at the earliest so as to bring down the body temperature. Intravenous fluids should be given with monitoring of electrolyte imbalance, chiefly sodium (hyponatremia).

Autopsy Findings

No specific findings are observed except that the body is dry and postmortem caloricity, which is appreciable in early period. Rigor mortis starts early as well as passes off early. Internal organs are congested and petechial hemorrhages may be found on lungs.

Medicolegal Importance: Deaths are usually accidental in manner.

Localized Effects of Heat

Various factors that determine the effects produced include:

- Intensity or degree of heat
- Period of contact or duration
- Material used for transmission of heat
- Nature of heat, i.e. dry or moist.

The more the intensity of heat, the greater is the damage caused. Minimum 45°C temperatures are required to produce any invisible damage. However, temperature of 60°C will produce the injury instantaneously. Duration of contact is directly related with visible damage. Hot metals or glass produces more damage in comparison to flame heat. The damage produced by dry heat (burns) and moist heat (scalds) vary greatly in appearance and are being discussed in detail.

Burns

Burns are injuries to tissues caused by heat, friction, electricity, radiation or chemicals. Burn fatalities are second to road-side accidents in numbers. Sections **324** and **326** IPC specifies any 'hurt' or 'grievous hurt', which is caused by 'fire or any heated substance' or 'corrosive' or 'explosive substance' is punishable more severely in comparison to unspecified means.

The usual circumstances under which a person sustains burn injuries are catching of fire by clothes worn by victim while doing household chores like cooking on a gas stove or kerosene oil stoves.

As per Criminal Law Amendment Act of 2013, there is addition of Section 326-A and 326-B, which deals with Vitriolage and related with burns. The same are being described as under:

Section 326A: Voluntarily causing grievous hurt by use of acid, etc.

Whoever causes permanent or partial damage to or deformity to or burns or maims or disfigures or disable any part or parts of the body of the person or causes grievous heart by throwing acid or by administering acid to that person or by using any other means with the intention of causing or with the knowledge that he is likely to cause injury or hurt shall be punished with imprisonment from 10 years to life and with fine. Provided that such fine shall be just and reasonable to meet the expenses of medical treatment of the victim and also any fine imposed shall be paid to the victim.

Section 326B: Voluntarily throwing or attempting to throw acid: Whoever throws or attempts to throw acid on any person or attempts to administer acid to any person or attempts to use by any other means with the intention of causing permanent or partial damage or deformity or burns or maiming or disfigurement or disability or grievous hurt to that person shall be punished with imprisonment from 5-7 years and fine

Classification of Burns

To know the extent of burn injuries, various scientists have classified them into various ways.

Wilson's Classification

It is most commonly used in medicolegal practice. According to this, various burn injuries can be categorized into three types, depending upon body layer involved.

a. **Epidermal:** There occurs reddening (erythema) and blister formation. These blisters contain serum rich in protein and chlorides and are surrounded by a zone of hyperemia (red line). These are painful and heal without formation of any scar.
b. **Dermo-epidermal:** When full thickness of skin is involved in burn injury including hair follicles, sweat and sebaceous glands. These are extremely painful due to involvement of sensory nerve endings and heal with formation of scar due to damage to all layers of skin.
c. **Deep:** When deeper tissues below skin are involved, viz. subcutaneous tissues, muscles and bones, etc. These are relatively less painful owing to destruction of nerve endings and heal with scar and contracture formation. Thus, they cause much disfigurement and loss of function of the part of body involved, chiefly when near a joint.

Dupuytren's Classification

According to depth of tissue involved, he classified burn injuries into six categories:

a. **First Degree:** When low degree heat is applied for very short duration, there occurs an erythema or redness over area of contact (**Figure 15.2**). It remains painful for a day or two and redness fades in few hours or a day. The covering superficial layer of epidermis may get devitalized and shedded off in few days.
b. **Second Degree:** The epidermis is affected completely. There occurs blister formation surrounded by a zone of hyperemia (**Figure 15.3**). The blisters contain serous fluid, which is rich in protein and chloride. These are very painful and if extensive; also produce hypovolemic shock. They usually heal in one week, without scar formation, may rupture and get infected.
c. **Third Degree:** The epidermis is completely destroyed with involvement of dermis. There occurs blister formation with red line. They ulcerate and may get infected and are extremely painful. They heal with formation of scar.
d. **Fourth Degree:** Whole thickness of the affected burn areas of skin is involved. These are not much painful owing to destruction of nerve ending. Usually these injuries followed by sloughing after some days.

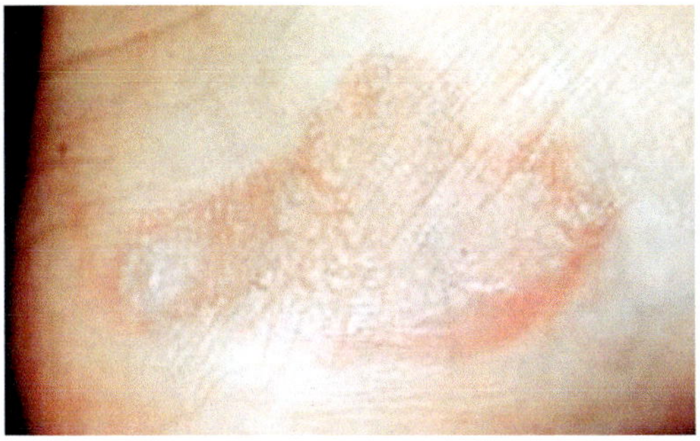

Figure 15.2 First degree burns

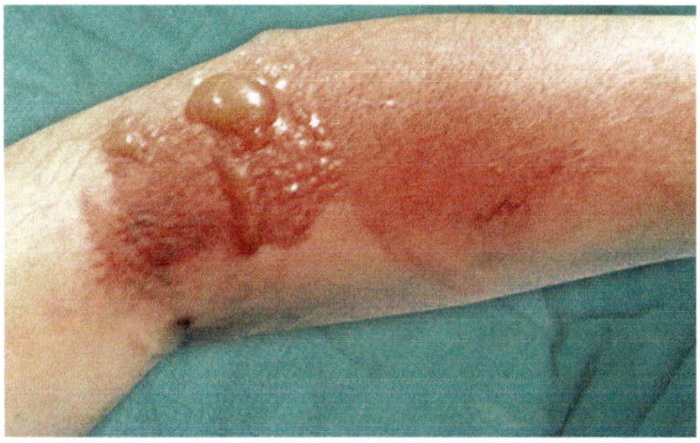

Figure 15.3 Second degree burns over forearm

e. **Fifth Degree:** Depth of lesion extends further and subcutaneous tissue is involved. These are less painful owing to total destruction of sensory nerve endings. These heal with deep scarring, produce contractures and when close to a joint, seriously hamper the movement at joint.

f. **Sixth Degree:** In this, muscles and bone are also involved. There occurs charring of the limb and heal with much difficulty with contracture formation (**Figure 15.4**).

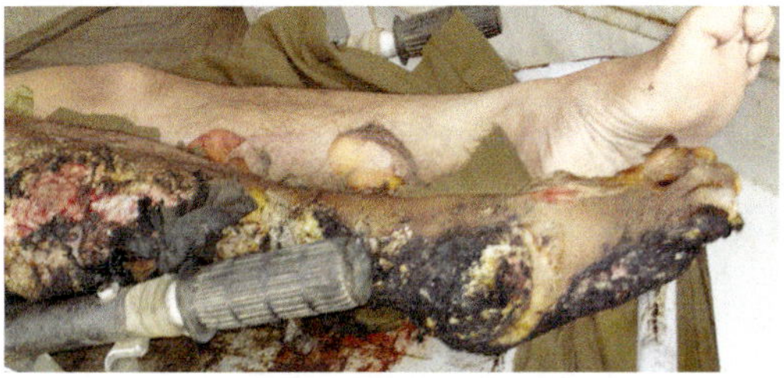

Figure 15.4 Sixth degree burns over right leg including thigh

Hebra's Classification

According to this, the burn injuries can be categorized into three groups by clubbing together the injuries classified by Dupuytren, i.e.

i. Epidermal: 1st and 2nd degree
ii. Dermo-epidermal: 3rd and 4th degree
iii. Deep: 5th and 6th degree

Factors Affecting Prognosis of Burns

Body Surface Area Involved

It is most important parameter that affects the prognosis in case of burn injury. To estimate the body surface area involved (**Figure 15.5**), "**Rule of Nines**", given by Alexander Wallace, is practiced clinically for calculating the amount of fluid, i.e. "ration" to be given to injured adult. However, it also helps in knowing the prognosis of injury.

For calculating approximate percentage of body surface area involved in children in practice "**Rule of Five**" is more simple. Lund and Browder's chart is otherwise used to calculate percentage of burns. According to rule of five, the body can be divided into following five parts each assigned as 20%. They are further subdivided into four quadrants/parts and assigned 5% for each (**Table 15.1**)

For calculating percentage in case of scattered burn injuries, '**Palm Rule**' has been found handy. According to it, the surface area of the palm of victim is approximately 1% of total body surface area (**Figure 15.6**).

Generally speaking, involvement of about one-third (33%) of total body surface area has grave prognosis and about 50% involvement of total body surface area is expected to be fatal in present Indian circumstances. However, with recent advances in modalities of treatment, prognosis is expected to improve. A recent Delhi High Court judgment for enforcing Government to construct separate burn wards in various hospitals with better treatment and patient care, one expects further improvement in near future.

Depth of Burn Injury

Deeper the burns, difficult are the healing processes, giving rise to more complications. Superficial burns will produce more pain, thereby causing neurogenic shock; whereas in

Head and neck	9%
Front of chest	9%
Back of chest	9%
Front of abdomen	9%
Back of abdomen	9%
Right upper limb	9%
Left upper limb	9%
Front of right lower limb	9%
Back of right lower limb	9%
Front of right lower limb	9%
Back of left lower limb	9%
Perineal area	1%
Total	100%

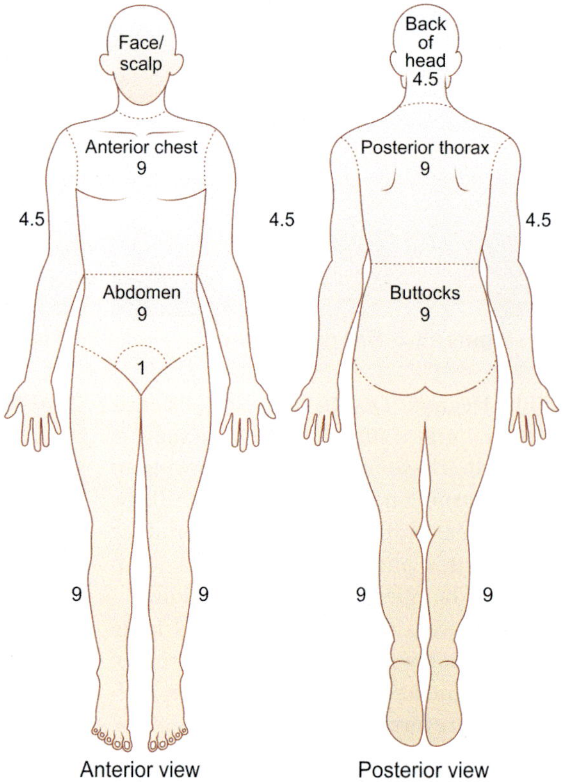

Figure 15.5 Rule of nine

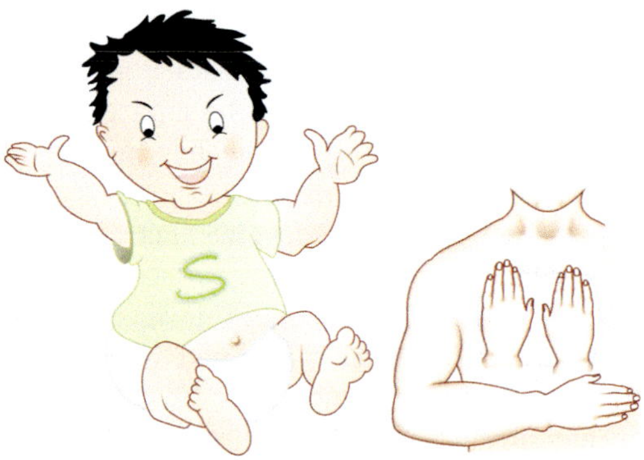

Figure 15.6 Rule of palm

Table 15.1 Rule of five

Body part	Five divisions	Subdivisions
Head and neck	20%	(5% × 4)
Abdomen	20%	(5% × 4)
Chest	20%	(5% × 4)
Upper Limb	20%	(5% × 4)
Lower Limb	20%	(5% × 4)

deep burns, although pain is less, hypovolemia is much severe. However, when we talk about the prognosis or fatality, body surface area involved is more important than depth of burn injury. To elaborate, one can say a deep wound over a small area has better prognosis than superficial burn over large area.

Calculation of Depth of Burn

First Degree: Epidermis

Second Degree: Dermis: (i) Superficial second degree (Superficial dermis), (ii) Deep second degree (Deep dermis).

Third Degree: Entire epidermis and dermis—full-thickness.

Superficial Dermal Burn: Characterized by tissue necrosis limited to upper third of dermis, zone of necrosis lifted off viable wound by edema and a small zone of injury as shown in **Figure 15.7**.

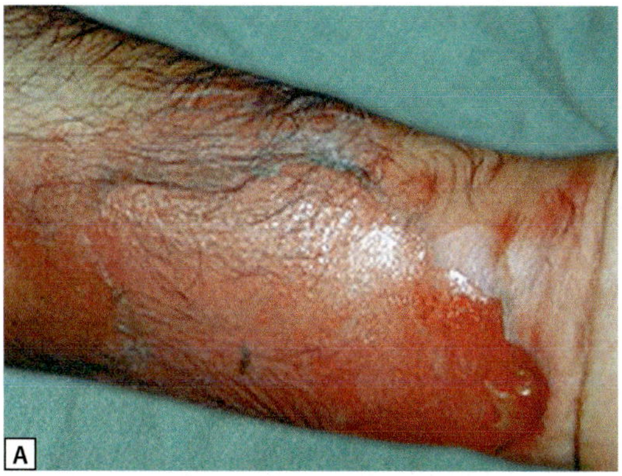

A

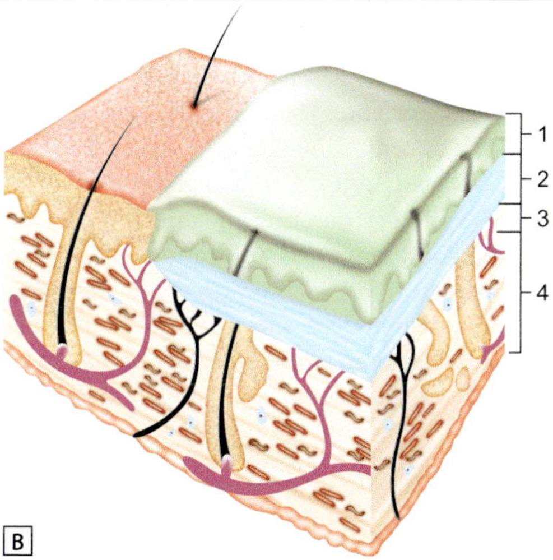

B

1. Zone of necrosis (Coagulation); 2. Edema layer; 3. Zone of injury (Stasis); 4. Normal tissue

Figures 15.7A and B Superficial dermal burns

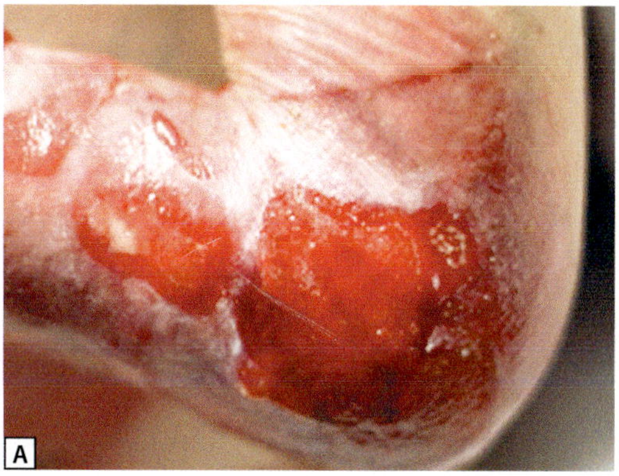

A

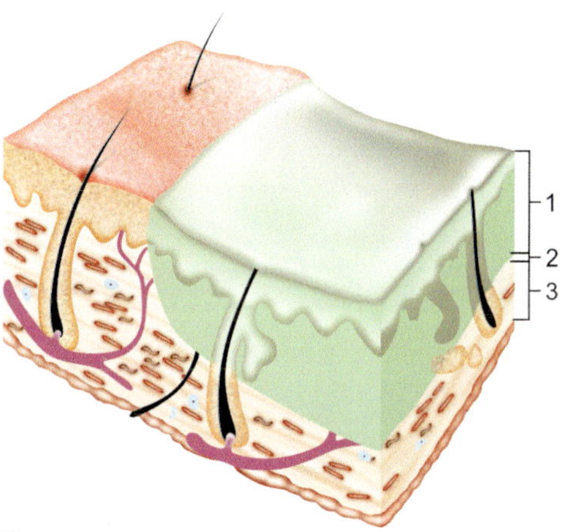

B

1. Zone of necrosis; 2. Edema layer; 3. Zone of injury (Stasis)

Figures 15.8A and B Deep dermal burns

Deep Dermal Burn: Characterized by zone of necrosis of majority of skin layers followed by a zone of edematous layer adherent to a zone of injury as shown in **Figure 15.8.**

Full Thickness Burns: Here there is total necrosis of epidermis and dermis with no remaining viable tissues of the skin (**Figure 15.9**).

Severity of Burn Injury

i. **Mild:** I°—When less than 10% of total body surface (TBS) area is involved.
ii. **Moderate:** II°—10-30% of TBS area; or III° < 10% TBS.
iii. **Severe:** TBS area 30-50%; or III°—10-20%; or with shock, airway burn, combined injury.
iv. **Major:** Total area > 50%; III° > 20%; or with severe complications.

Site of Burn Injury

Burns on neck, chest and abdomen have grave prognosis and over perineal region has worst prognosis.

Age of Victim

Victims in extreme age groups are vulnerable to lethal complications and succumb easily. In case of children, about 20% burns have been found to be fatal.

Sex of Victim

Males can cope up burn injuries better than females.

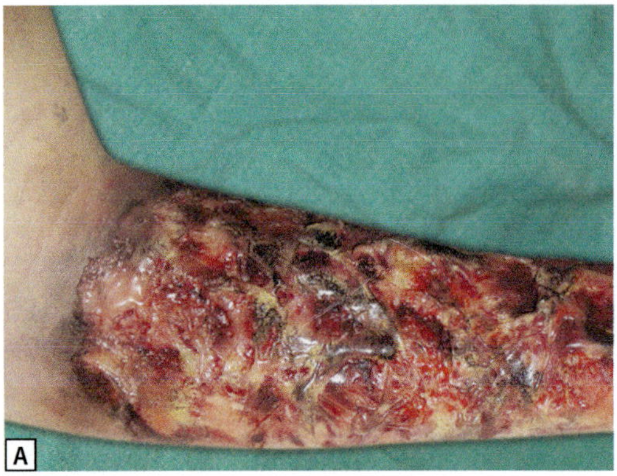

A

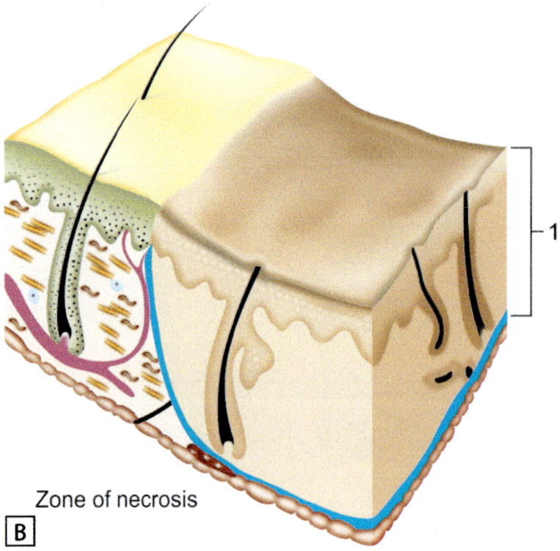

B

Figures 15.9A and B Full thickness burns

Intensity of Heat

More the intensity of heat, greater is the damage produced. A minimum temperature of 45°C is required to produce burn injury, though the time needed will be few hours. A temperature of about 60°C produces effect of burns in few minutes. A temperature of about 1000°C will completely incinerate the body in about an hour.

Duration of Exposure

Longer the duration of contact or exposure to heat, the graver will be the burns produced.

Cause of Death in Burn Injuries

Immediate Causes

a. **Neurogenic Shock:** Death may occur within few hours due to severe pain, especially in extensive superficial burn injuries.
b. **Suffocation:** Death may occur due to inhalation of smoke, CO, CO_2 and other irrespirable gases during conflagration. Cases are frequently encountered where practice of lighting 'Angithi/Sigri' during winter season inside the room is prevalent. It burns slowly and because of incomplete combustion of coal, CO and smoke are produced. Person while sleeping gradually inhales and surrenders to suffocation. Simultaneously, the cotton quilt, which a person wraps to cover himself, accidentally catches fire with slow burning angithi. It leads to production of huge amount of irrespirable gases and the person dies due to suffocation. Similarly, if a person tries to commit suicide by pouring kerosene oil over himself, smoke might enter the respiratory passage; thus person dies due to combination of suffocation and shock.
c. **Injuries:** The victim dies while attempting to escape from site of fire, by sustaining injuries from falling structure of building or hitting an object.

Early Causes

a. **Hypovolemic Shock:** Death occurs within 24–36 hours due to loss of fluid from burnt surface. More than half of fluid loss is fatal immediately.
b. **Pulmonary Edema:** Death occurs in a day or two due to pulmonary edema, glottic edema or laryngeal edema.
c. **Electrolyte Imbalance**, mainly hypokalemia, can also lead to death in early period after sustaining burn injuries.

Late or Delayed Causes

a. **Toxemia:** There occurs systemic absorption of various toxins in blood, which is produced at ulcerated areas after burns. Death due to shock as a result of toxemia usually occurs in 36–48 hours.
b. **Septicemia:** Signs of systemic infection usually appear by 48 hours after sustaining burn injuries. Most of deaths occurring after 48 hours are due to infection of serous membrane and internal organs like meningitis, pneumonitis, pericarditis, peritonitis, pleurisy and other complications.

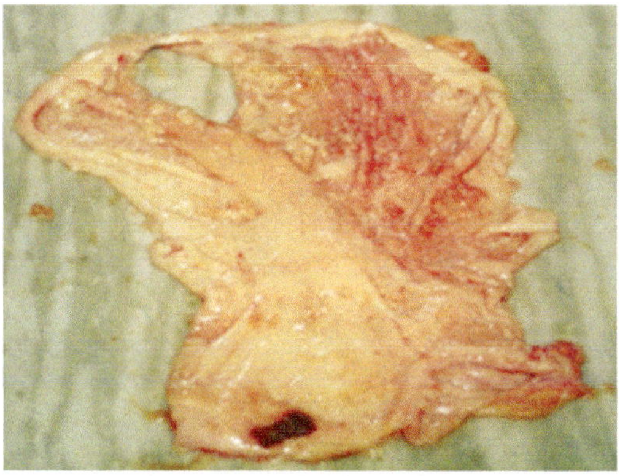

Figure 15.10 Stomach of a burnt victim showing Dupuytren's ulcer a late complication

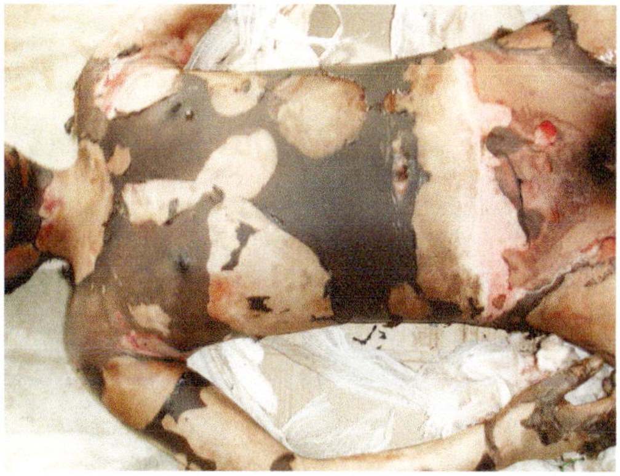

Figure 15.11 Extensive charring is seen all over the body (suggests Kerosene burn), erythema at places indicative of antemortem burns

c. **Renal Failure:** There occurs acute tubular necrosis, which leads to renal failure, and death occurs usually on 3rd/4th day.
d. **Gastrointestinal Ulceration:** Initially, there occurs ulcer formation in stomach due to prolonged confinement, which is called as Dupuytren's ulcer (**Figure 15.10**). Afterwards, ulcers may also be formed in duodenum, which is called as Curling's ulcer. These are late complications of burn injuries produced as a result of stress and local ischemia and person may succumb to death when there occurs uncontrollable bleeding from the site.
e. **Anemia and Hypoproteinemia:** The victim may die even after weeks, as he develops anemia and hypoproteinemia.

Postmortem Findings

a. **External:** The body must be carefully examined; as remnant of clothing (especially synthetic) may have got stuck on body parts where they are tightly placed. They should be removed carefully and examined for presence of any inflammable substance like Kerosene, petrol, etc. Even if no smell is perceivable, they should be preserved and sent to concern Forensic Science Laboratory so that they can be chemically identified.

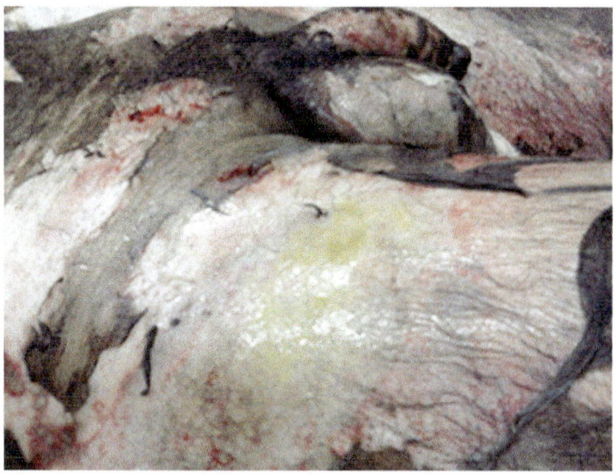

Figure 15.12 Erythema, slough at places (antemortem burns)

While preserving the clothing, extra precaution is to be taken by putting them into glass containers first and then sealing them before handing over to police official. The reason for it is that most inflammable materials are volatile substances and simply preserving them in a sealed box will defeat the purpose of preservation.

The body should be looked for the signs of vital reaction, like line of redness, tissue changes like sloughing, blister (**Figure 15.12**), etc.

b. **Internal Findings:** The nasal and oral cavities may show presence of carbon soot and are inflamed. Soot are often mixed with mucus and adhered on wall

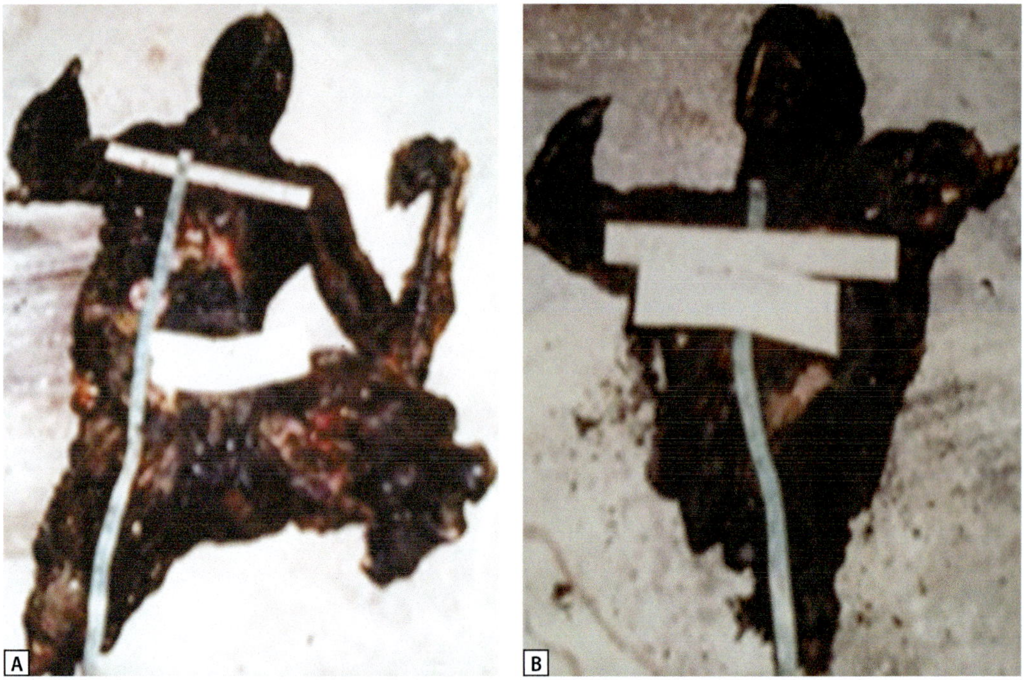

Figures 15.13A and B Partly incinerated bodies in pugilistic attitude with missing parts

of lumen of respiratory tract and below up to bronchioles. Mucosa over tongue and larynx may be edematous and show blistering.

i. Due to presence of excessive amount of CO_2 and CO, which produces asphyxiant effects, the tissues may assume bright red coloration owing to excessive amount of carboxyhemoglobin. The blood in the vessels is bright pink or red, thick and more fluid.
ii. All the organs are usually congested. Lungs may be deeply congested and edematous. In few cases, there may be blood-tinged discharge through nostrils, which occurs due to excessive secretion in lungs and rupture of capillaries. The mucosa of upper GIT is invariably reddened and may show ulcer formation (as described earlier; **Curling's** and **Dupuytren's** ulcer).

Pugilistic Attitude

Heat causes muscles of the limbs to stiffen and contract with arms becoming flexed and hands (fist) clenched, the appearance suggesting the boxer's attitude or fencing posture, as if the person was engaged in a fight at the time of death (**Figure 15.13**).

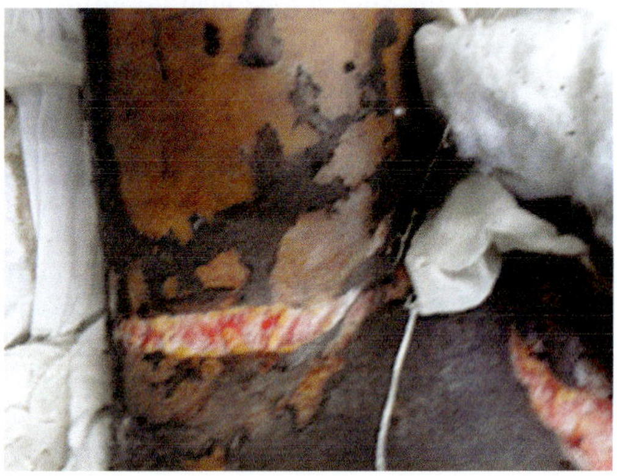

Figure 15.14 Heat rupture

Heat Ruptures

The contraction of the skin caused by the heat may tear the skin, producing ragged wounds resembling lacerations (**Figure 15.14**). When they are present on the scalp, they may be easily mistaken for antemortem injuries. Histopathological examination will reveal the fact.

Heat Hematoma

Due to intense heat, the capillary wall may get damaged and blood oozes out in the extradural space of skull and deposited as a firm, friable and cherry-red or chocolate-red colored clot and honeycomb in appearance, owing to vaporization of liquid part of blood consequent upon boiling of blood by intense, external heat. It is usually present over the side opposite to site of greatest damage, e.g. occipital and frontal regions. It is a postmortem phenomenon and, therefore, must be differentiated from antemortem extradural hemorrhage.

Most important findings are to be observed in the respiratory passage and blood, which will be extremely clinching towards the fact whether the victim was alive when the fire commenced. The tongue, fauces, larynx, trachea and bronchi are usually inflamed and contain soot often intimately mixed with mucous. If the deceased had inhaled very hot gases or fumes or, rarely, the flame itself, then the mucosa over the tongue and larynx may be edematous and exhibit blistering or shredding. Sometimes, some vomitus (presumably due to bouts of coughing) may also be present in the respiratory passages. Carbon-impregnated mucus may be swallowed and found in the esophagus and/or in the stomach.

Together with the soot, the inhaled smoke usually contains some carbon monoxide, which is therefore absorbed by the blood. The presence of carbon monoxide in the blood is often obvious from the bright pink appearance of the blood, the muscles and even the cut surfaces of the organs.

Medicolegal Aspects

The questions which usually arise in case of alleged death due to burns are:

i. Whether the death is due to burns or not?
ii. Manner of death, i.e. suicide, accident or homicide?
iii. Whether the victim was alive or dead at the time of burning?

It is ascertained by antemortem or postmortem nature of the burns. The points which help in differentiating are:

i. Presence of red line in the normal skin adjacent to burnt area.
ii. Presence of blisters, which contain serous fluid comprising of albumin and chloride. On puncturing, it shows red inflamed base surrounded by a zone of erythema or hyperemia.
iii. Presence of smoke in respiratory passage: It indicates the victim inhaled smoke and was alive when fire spread. The presence of soot over mouth and nostrils does not have any diagnostic value. The quality of soot inside respiratory passage depends upon type of fuel, combustibility of fuel, type of article burnt and of course the period of survival of victim.
iv. Laryngeal edema, which is caused by passage of hot gases into respiratory tract.
v. Raised carboxyhemoglobin level in the blood; exceeding 10%. Chain smokers may develop blood level up to 8–10%; therefore, it needs careful interpretation in such cases.
vi. Histological investigation reveals the same changes as occur in any other injury. Apart from these, dilated capillaries, tissue necrosis, hemorrhages, gas inside the vessels and cellular infiltrations are the significant findings which are seen as shown in **Figure 15.15**.

Few medicolegally important burn cases (Figures 15.16 to 15.20)

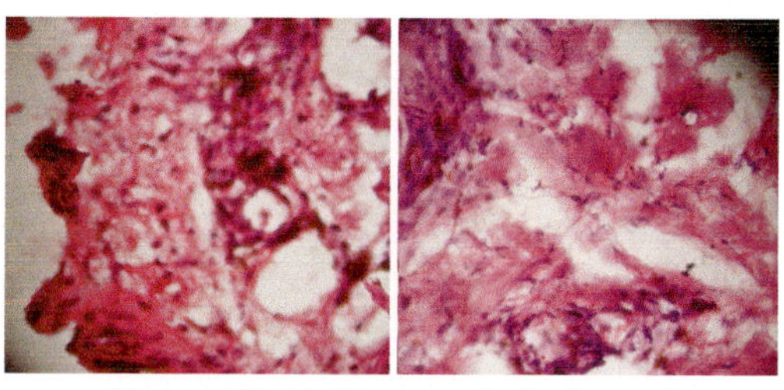

Figure 15.15 Microscopic findings of antemortem burn tissues (skin)

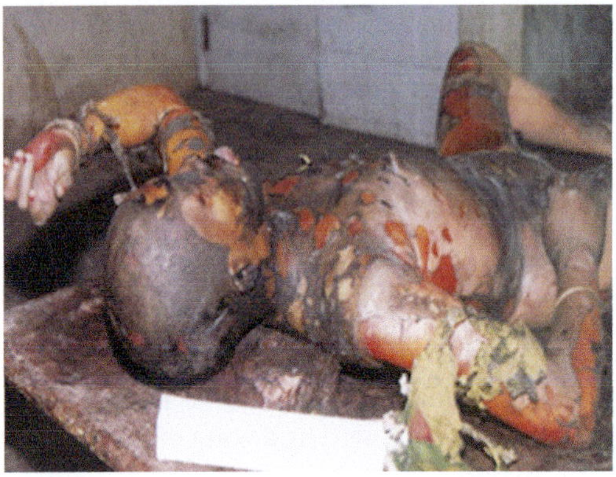

Figure 15.16 Burn injuries showing singed scalp hair, protrusion of tongue; blackening over upper part of chest, lower part of abdomen, and pelvis; erythema over scalp, left hand and right arm. Note the presence of remnants of clothing, i.e. yellow colored blouse over right arm, which needs be preserved and sent for chemical examination to know about nature of inflammable material used

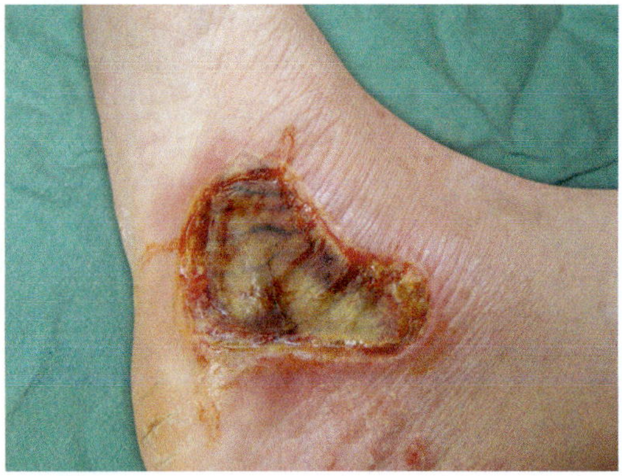

Figure 15.17 Deeply infected burns over leg with deposition of yellowish slough

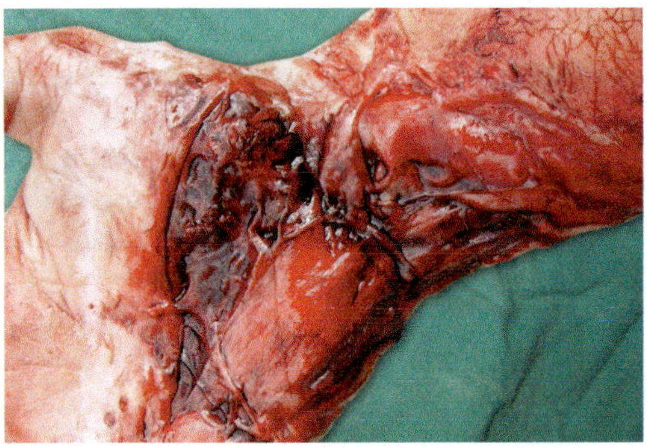

Figure 15.18 Granulation tissue formations over-hand following extensive burn injuries

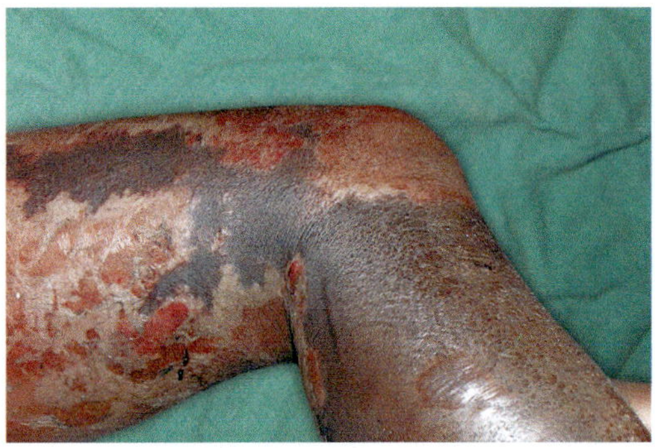

Figure 15.19 Healed areas of burn around the knee joint

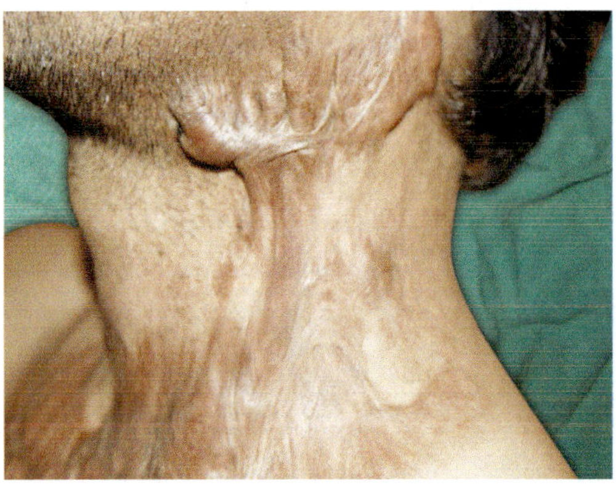

Figure 15.20 Keloid formations with contractures (sequelae of burns)

SCALD

A **scald** is a type of burn injury caused by application of hot liquids or gases, i.e. moist heat. Application of water of 50°C at vulnerable part will cause scald.[5,6]

Characteristics

i. It does not cause charring or singeing of body hairs (**Figure 15.21**).
ii. The size and shape of the scalds usually vary, but it has sharply demarcated margins, which correspond to the extent of fluid contact.

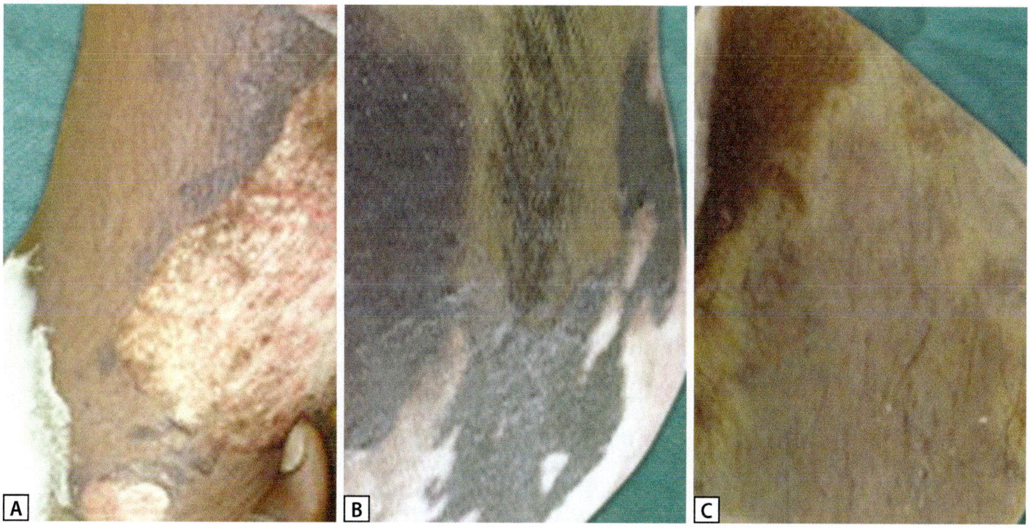

Figures 15.21A to C Antemortem scalds: No singeing of body hairs

iii. If the steam is inhaled, scalding may be inside the oral cavity, nasal mucosa, epiglottis and larynx.

Medicolegal Importance

i. Scalds are commonly accidental in nature that involves infants, toddlers and children.
ii. Suicide is very rare.
iii. It may be one of the ways of infanticide or battered baby syndrome.

INJURIES DUE TO LOW TEMPERATURE (COLD)

Generalized Effects of Cold

Hypothermia

In this condition, an individual's core body temperature falls below 35°C (95°F). Hypothermia involves the rapid loss of body heat, resulting in total body cooling.

Classification

i. Mild hypothermia begins when the core body temperature is 35°–32°C.
ii. Moderate hypothermia: Core body temperature is <32°–28°C.
iii. Severe hypothermia: Core body temperature is <28°C.

Causes

Extremely lean athletes are at risk because they have little insulating body fat. A combination of wind and moisture facilitates hypothermia, even if temperature is well above freezing.

Causes of Death

- Ventricular fibrillation
- Disseminated intravascular coagulation (DIC)
- Acid base imbalance
- Bronchospasm
- Pulmonary edema.

Postmortem Findings

i. Postmortem hypostasis is pinkish due to persistent oxyhemoglobin in the capillaries.
ii. Rarely skin is pale (white) and thus hypothermic deaths are also called as **white death.**[7]
iii. Skin may show erythematous patches or irregular red or violet patches on exposed part of the body. They are often present over extensor surfaces of large joints, such as the outer side of hips, the elbows and knees and at flank and face.[8]
iv. Viscera congested with fresh hemorrhage in the lungs.

v. Froth at nostril and trachea with evidence of bronchospasm.
vi. Ulceration with small hemorrhages of stomach mucosa.
vii. Kidneys show acute tubular necrosis.
viii. Urinary catecholamine levels and blood sugar is high, and there may be glycosuria.

Localized Effects of Cold

Chilblains (Pernio)

i. Chilblains are a painful abnormal reaction of the small blood vessels in the skin when exposed to cold temperatures with humidity. The condition is often confused with frostbite and trench foot.
ii. It usually occurs several hours after exposure to the cold temperate humid climates.
iii. The cold exposure damages capillary beds in the skin as it causes constriction of the small blood vessels, which in turn can cause redness, itching, blisters and inflammation.
iv. If rewarming of the skin happens too rapidly, there may be leakage of blood into the tissues, as the blood vessels do not respond quickly enough to this rewarming.
v. These conditions are not very common in countries where the cold is extreme, as the air is drier. The clothing used in these climates is protective. They are more likely to develop in those with poor circulation, but chilblains are still common in those with good circulation.

Frostbite

i. It is a medical condition where localized damage is caused to skin and other tissues due to freezing (<0°C). Frostbite is most likely to happen in body parts farthermost from the heart and those with large exposed areas.
ii. Symptoms include feeling of burning and pain, followed by progressive loss of sensation.
iii. The initial stages of frostbite are sometimes called "frost nip". Frost nip is less severe and involves only outer skin layers.
iv. These conditions usually involve the nose, ears, fingers and feet. Severe damage occurs when frostbitten tissue is thawed and refrozen. During outdoor activities in freezing temperatures, athletes need to be vigilant for early warning signs.

Trench Foot or Immersion Foot

i. Trench foot, also known as immersion foot, occurs when the feet are wet for long periods of time at a low temperature of 5°–6°C.
ii. It can be quite painful, but it can be prevented and treated.
iii. Symptoms of trench foot include a tingling or itching sensation, pain, swelling, cold and blotchy skin, numbness and a prickling or heavy feeling in the foot. The foot may be red, dry and painful after it becomes warm, and blisters may form, followed by skin and tissue dying and falling off. In severe cases, if untreated, trench foot can involve the toes, heels or the entire foot.

ELECTRICAL INJURIES

Electrical injuries, although relatively rare, are inevitably encountered by most of medicos working at emergency. The range of electrical injury is very broad, ranging from minimal injury to severe multiorgan involvement, with both occult and delayed complications, to death.

Electrical injuries have become a more common form of trauma with a unique pathophysiology and high morbidity and mortality. They encompass several types, viz. lightning injury,[9] high-voltage injury and low-voltage injury.[10-12] Clinical manifestations range from transient unpleasant sensations without apparent injury to massive tissue damage.[13] Some electrocutions are instantly fatal.

Severity of Tissue Damage

The severity of tissue damage is mostly depends on following:

i. Intensity of the current (Voltage applied and its duration)
ii. Type of current

iii. Pathways of the current through the body
iv. Resistance of tissues
v. Duration of exposure to the current

Body must form part of an electrical circuit so that current flows from an entry point to an exit point, if an electrical injury is to occur. The path taken from entry point to exit point depends on the relative resistance of possible exit points. Electrical injury takes shortest route between entry and best exit point.

Intensity of Current

The intensity of the current is measured in volts and amperes. Injury depends on quantity of electrical flow, such as

i. 30 mA applied to hand causes painful muscle spasm.
ii. 40 mA applied to hand causes unconsciousness.
iii. 50–80 mA for more than few seconds may often prove fatal.

High voltage can jump or arc through the air anywhere from an inch up to several feet, depending on the voltage. Thus, a person may be injured simply by coming too close to a high-voltage line. High voltage causes more severe injuries than low voltage and is more likely to cause internal damage.

Ohm's Law: Current varies directly with the voltage and inversely with the resistance.

$$\mathbf{V = I \times R}, \text{ and } \mathbf{I = V/R}$$

Voltage

Considerable voltage must be applied to dry skin to cause flow of 50 mA. Voltages of 240 or 100 volts (V) may be lethal if applied for long time. Very high voltage may be paradoxically safer as muscle contraction caused by shock may physically fling subject off the source. 240 V applied to hand may cause forearm muscle spasm, gripping the source and prolonging contact.

Type of Current

Electrical current is categorized as direct current (DC) and alternating current (AC). Direct current, such as current generated by batteries, flow in the same direction. Alternating current, such as current available through household wall sockets, changes direction 50–60 times per second. Alternating current is more dangerous than direct current. Direct current tends to cause a single muscle contraction often strong enough to force people away from the current's source. Alternating current causes a continuing muscle contraction, often preventing people from releasing their grip on the current's source. As a result, exposure may be prolonged.

Pathway of the Current

The path that electricity takes through the body tends to determine, which tissues are affected. Because alternating current continually reverses direction, the commonly used terms "entry" and "exit" are inappropriate with alternating current. The terms "source" and "ground" will be more precise. The most common source point for electricity is the hand and the second most common is the head. The most common ground point is the foot. A current that travels from arm-to-arm or from arm-to-leg may go through the heart and is much more dangerous than a current that travels between a leg and the ground. A current that travels through the head may affect the brain.

Resistance of Tissues

The skin is the major barrier to electrical current, having very high resistance. Burns occur when current flows because of the energy transfer to heat. Once inside the dermis, current flows more easily because of less resistance through electrolyte-rich cytoplasm and blood vessels. Resistance of dry skin is more than the wet skin.

Resistance of tissues is the ability to impede the flow of electricity. Most of the body's resistance is concentrated in the skin. The thicker the skin is, the greater its resistance. A thick, calloused palm or sole is more resistant to electrical current than an area of thin skin, such as inner arm. The skin's resistance also decreases when broken. If skin resistance is high, more of the damage is local, often causing only skin burns. If skin resistance is low, more of the damage affects the internal organs.

Thus, the damage is mostly internal if people who are wet or has broken skin come in contact with electrical current.

Duration of Exposure

As a rule, the longer the person is exposed to the current; the worse is the injury and damage.

Types of Electrical Injuries

Electrical injuries are of three types. They are:

i. Contact injury
ii. Spark burn or injury
iii. Flash burn injury

Contact Injury

Firm contact with conductor: When current is passed through the body, it heats up the tissue fluids to produce steam, which splits skin within epidermis or epidermo-dermal junction. When current ceases, the blister collapses to produce a raised white or gray ring with a depressed center. The mark may reproduce the shape of the conductor, e.g. linear wire or shaped metal object. A characteristic **entry point** or **entry wound** and **exit point** or **exit wound** is seen only with direct current.

Electrical Mark

The electrical mark is a type of localized thermal burn due to heat production when current flows through highly resistant skin. The entry wound seen, usually on hand, and exit or earthling point on leg (**Figures 15.22** and **15.23**).

There may be no skin mark, even in a case of fatality. If the skin is damp or the area of contact is wider (less resistance per unit area), then the heating effect is proportionately less, so marks on skin are unlikely.

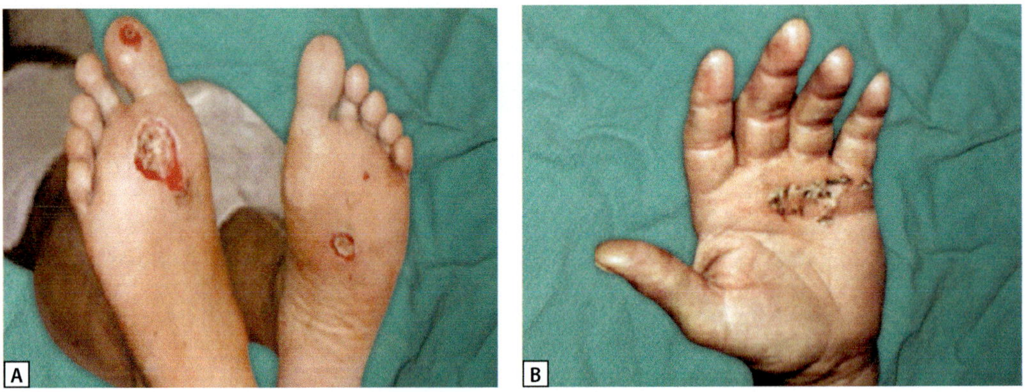

Figures 15.22A and B Exit wound on foot and entry wound on hand

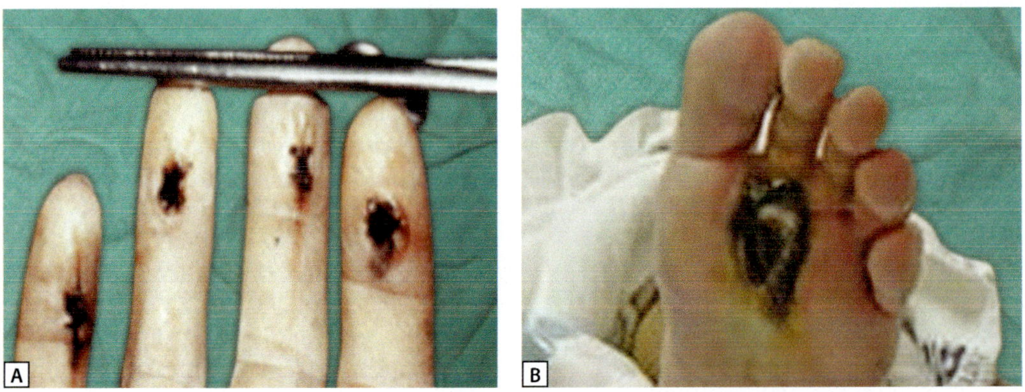

Figures 15.23A and B Entry wound on hand and exit wound on foot

Arteriolar spasm causes a surrounding areola of skin blanching around the central blister. The peripheral zone outside the blanched area may be hyperemic. The injury may thus appear as **blister** followed by areas of **redness** and **pallor** from center outwards. Smaller marks may appear as tiny white discs. Prolonged contact with domestic supply may cause severe burning with a wide area of epidermal peeling, hyperemia and deep charring and cooking of muscle.

Spark Burn

Spark burn or injury is due to lose contact with the electrical source. Current leaps the gap as a spark. 1000 V will leap few millimeters across dry air. 100 kV will leap up to 35 cm. Localized point of entry creates a very high temperature causing melting of epidermal keratin, which fuses into a slightly raised, hard brown or yellowish parchment like nodule on cooling (**spark burn injury**).

Flash Burn

It is caused due to contact with very high voltage, i.e. high tension wires and commonly seen with line-man working on the grid system. High voltage transmission cables may cause similar deep burns or multifocal spark lesions resembling **crocodile skin.**

Cause of Death in Electrocution

Electrocution may be fatal if current flows across a vital part of the body, e.g. hand to opposite foot:

- Across heart causes ventricular fibrillation (VF)
- Across chest causes respiratory muscle paralysis, i.e. respiratory failure
- Across head causes cardiac and respiratory center paralysis
- Burn, e.g. entry and exit on same hand may cause severe burn
- Secondary injuries sustained during the incident.

LIGHTNING

Clouds to ground lightning bolts are common physical process. This tremendous electrical discharge is caused by an imbalance between positive and negative charges. During a storm, colliding particles of rain, ice or snow increases this imbalance and often negatively charge the lower layers of storm clouds. Objects on the ground, like steeples, trees and the earth itself, become positively charged creating an imbalance that nature seeks to remedy by passing current between the two charges. Lightning is exceedingly hot; a hot flash can heat the air around it to temperatures five times hotter than the sun's surface. This heat causes surrounding air to quickly expand and vibrate, which produces the rolling thunder we hear a short time after seeing a lightning flash.

Lightning Injuries

Lightning is not only striking, but also dangerous. Around 2,000 people are killed globally by lightning every year. Hundreds more survive of lightning strikes, but suffer from a variety of life-changing ailments, including memory loss, dizziness, weakness, numbness, etc.

Although most injuries occur outdoors, a few people are injured indoors every year, including individuals who incur landline telephone-mediated strikes.[14,15] While use of cell phones, iPods and other portable electronic devices may change the pathway of lightning around a person, it does not increase the risk of injury except by distracting the individual from paying attention to warning signs, such as storm clouds and thunder.

The most important characteristic features of lightning injuries are multisystem involvement and widely variable severity.[16] Because persons struck by lightning have a better chance of survival than persons who experience cardiopulmonary arrest from other causes, resuscitation for persons struck by lightning must be instituted immediately.[17] Injuries range from tiny static electricity like exposures to cardiac arrest.[18-22] Internal burns are rare. Myoglobinemia is rarely encountered in lightning injuries, whereas cardiac and respiratory arrest, vascular spasm, neurologic damage and autonomic instability play a greater role.[23] Blunt force injuries from falling, being thrown by muscle contractions, or barotraumas from the explosive force of a nearby lightning strike may occur.[19]

Lightning strikes are primarily a neurologic injury that affects all three components of the nervous system: central, autonomic and peripheral.

Linear Lightning Burn Injury

These are the burns of size few cm to few inches and mainly found on part of the body where body offers less resistance (**Figure 15.24**).

Arborescent Marks

They are also known as fern leaf pattern or filigree burn or feathering or Lichtenberg figures. The mark has a feathered, arborescent or dendritic pattern and this injury is pathognomic of a lightning strike. The markings are seen on the shoulder and chest mainly, though the fern-like pattern of erythema can be found in the skin of other part of the body like foot (**Figure 15.25**).

Mechanism of Formation: Exact mechanism is not known. However, it can be due to deposition of copper on the skin. Some authors have mentioned that it might be caused due to staining of the tissues with hemoglobin from the lysed blood cells along with the pathways of the high voltage electricity—lightning and hydroelectric generators. These markings fade in due course of time over a period of 2 to 3 days.

Surface Burns

The burn areas are related to metallic ornaments worn or carried by the victims (**Figure 15.26**). Secondary burn injuries may be there because of ignition of wearing garments. Blisters, fissures or charring of deeper tissues and bones depends upon the degree of burn.

Complications

Although rare, serious lightning injuries are likely to cause primarily cardiac and neurologic injury.[24-26] Otologic injury and cutaneous burns have also been noted as frequent sequelae of this events.[25-30] Cataract formation resulting from lightning injury typically occurs within days to weeks of injury. This complication has been reported as late as 2 years afterward, but commonly occurs within the first week. The various complications of lightning strike are listed in **Table 15.2**.

Major complications are rare in mild and moderate lightning injuries, although musculoskeletal discomfort and subjective sensations of paresthesia, irritability and other non-specific neurologic sequelae may be present, depending on the location and intensity of the strike.

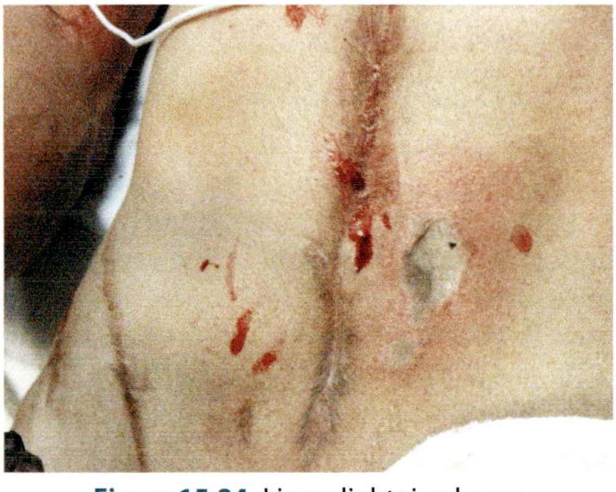

Figure 15.24 Linear lightning burns

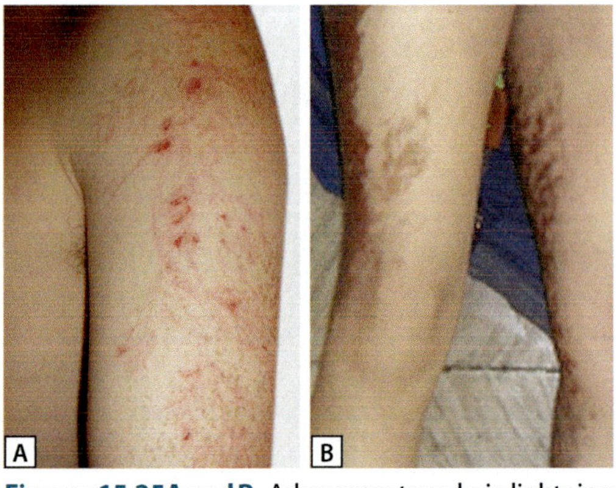

Figures 15.25A and B Arborescent marks in lightning

Table 15.2 Complications due to lightning strike

Cardiopulmonary complications
• Transient hypertension with ECG changes • Myocardial injury • Congestive heart failure • Dysrhythmia • Transient asystole • Atrial and ventricular fibrillation • Frequent premature ventricular contractions • Respiratory complications • Apnea • Hypoxemia
Neurologic complications: Damage to the central nervous system (CNS) is the second most debilitating group of lightning injuries[31]
• Immediate loss of consciousness • Seizures and convulsion • Amnesia and confusion • Dizziness • Sympathetic nervous system dysfunction • Retrograde amnesia • Hemiplegia, aphasia • Symptoms similar to post-concussion syndrome (e.g. headaches, nausea, confusion) • Neuromuscular pain • Chronic pain syndromes • Coma
Vascular complications
• Vasomotor instability • Arterial spasm and vasoconstriction • Vasodilatation • Intraventricular hemorrhage • Hematomas
Ophthalmic complications
• Cataracts • Macular holes • Corneal lesions and bleeding • Iritis and vitreous hemorrhage • Retinal detachment and optic nerve injury
Otologic complications[27]
• Ruptured tympanic membrane • Temporary hearing loss
Psychiatric complications
• Sleep disorders • Isolation or depression • Neuro-cognitive deficits including short-term memory loss, difficulty accessing or processing new information, attention deficit, personality change, distractibility or loss of ability to multitask

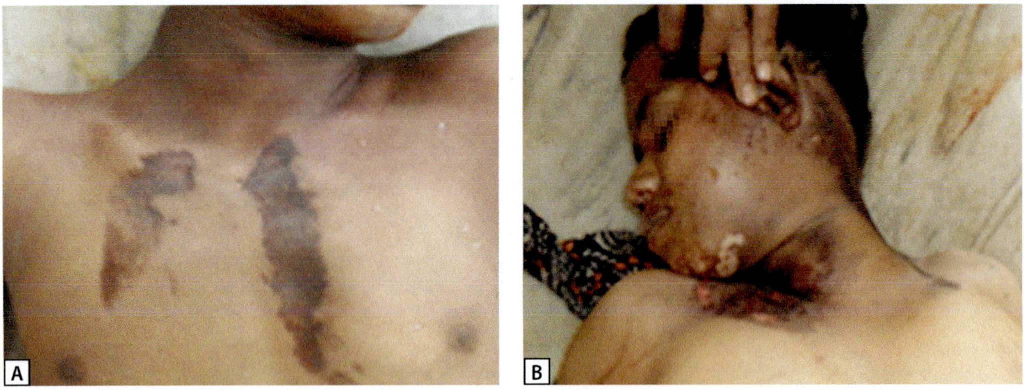

Figures 15.26A and B Surface burns due to lightning

There may be ear bleeding (**Figure 15.27**) because of rupture of tympanic membrane. The ruptured margins will be ragged, edematous with presence of oozing.

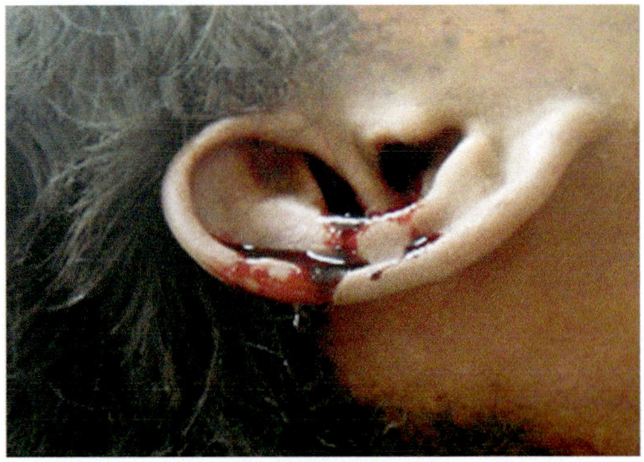

Figure 15.27 Ear bleeding due to ruptured tympanic membrane

Gastrointestinal (GI) complications of lightning injuries are similar to those following any major trauma.[32,33] Most common is gastric atony with gastric dilatation. Another complication seen in victims of lightning injury is GI bleeding, albeit a very rare complication. GI perforation is another rare complication of lightning injury.[33,34]

Though unusual with lightning strike, autopsy findings show hemorrhage and necrosis in the pancreas. In severe lightning injury, even with cardiopulmonary resuscitation (CPR) in the field, permanent neurologic deficit and hypoxic injury are common.

REFERENCES

1. Mahanta P. Fatal burn injuries in accidental vehicular crush: A medico legal study. J Indian Acad Forensic Med. 2010;32(1):66-9.
2. Crore MA, et al. Epidemiology of motor vehicular accident, JAMA. 1992;981:210.
3. Leenan LPH, et al. Internal fixation of open unstable pelvic fractures. J Trauma. 1993;35(2):220-5.
4. Herndon DN. Total Burn Care. London, WB Saunders. 1996.
5. Bull JP. Burns. Postgrad Med J. 1963;39:717-25.
6. Polson CJ, Gee DS, Knight B. The Essentials of Forensic Medicine, 4th ed. Pergamon Press, UK. 1985. pp. 271-350.
7. Dikshit PC. Thermal injuries. In: Textbook of Forensic Medicine and Toxicology, 1st ed. New Delhi: Peepee Publishers and distributors (P) Ltd; 2007. pp. 237-54.
8. Saukko P, Knight B. Knight's Forensic Pathology, 3rd ed. London: Arnold; 2004.
9. Blumenthal R, Jandrell IR, West NJ. Does a sixth mechanism exist to explain lightning injuries? Investigating a possible new injury mechanism to determine the cause of injuries related to close lightning flashes. Am J Forensic Med Pathol. Sep 26, 2011.
10. Browne BJ, Gaasch WR. Electrical injuries and lightning. Emerg Med Clin North Am. 1992;10(2):211-29.

11. Fontanarosa PB. Electrical shock and lightning strike. Ann Emerg Med. 1993;22(2):378-87.
12. Martinez JA, Nguyen T. Electrical injuries. South Med J. 2000;93(12):1165-8.
13. Dega S, Gnaneswar SG, Rao PR, Ramani P, Krishna DM. Electrical burn injuries: Some unusual clinical situations and management. Burns. 2007;33(5):653-65.
14. Andrews CJ, Cooper MA, Darveniza M. Lightning Injuries: Electrical, Medical and Legal Aaspects. 1992.
15. Andrews CJ, Darveniza M. Telephone-mediated lightning injury: An Australian survey. J Trauma. 1989;29(5):665-71.
16. Edlich RF, Farinholt HM, Winters KL, Britt LD, Long WB 3rd. Modern concepts of treatment and prevention of lightning injuries. J Long Term Eff Med Implants. 2005;15(2):185-96.
17. Lifschultz BD, Donoghue ER. Deaths caused by lightning. J Forensic Sci. 1993;38(2):353-8.
18. Cooper MA, Andrews CJ, Holle RL. Lightning Injury. Auerbach. Wilderness Emergencies. CV Mosby; 2006.
19. Cooper MA. Emergent care of lightning and electrical injuries. Semin Neurol. 1995;15(3):268-78.
20. Cooper MA, Holle R, Andrews C. Field J, (Eds). Electrical current and lightning injury. In: The Textbook of Emergency Cardiovascular Care and CPR. Lippincott, Williams and Wilkins. 2009. pp. 498-511.
21. Cooper MA, Johnson SA. Cardiopulmonary resuscitation and early management of the lightning strike victim. In: Ornato JP (Ed), Cardiopulmonary Resuscitation. Peabody, Mass: Humana Press; 2005.
22. Cooper MA. Lightning Injury Homepage. Lightning Injury. [cited 2012 12th Jan] Available from: URL:http://www.uic.edu/labs/lightninginjury
23. Cooper MA. Lightning injuries: prognostic signs for death. Ann Emerg Med. 1980;9(3):134-8.
24. Lichtenberg R, Dries D, Ward K, Marshall W, Scanlon P. Cardiovascular effects of lightning strikes. J Am Coll Cardiol. 1993;21(2):531-6.
25. Whitcomb D, Martinez JA, Daberkow D. Lightning injuries. South Med J. 2002;95(11):1331-4.
26. Fish RM. Electric injury, part III: cardiac monitoring indications, the pregnant patient, and lightning. J Emerg Med. 2000;18(2):181-7.
27. Offiah C, Heran M, Graeb D. Lightning strike: A rare cause of bilateral ossicular disruption. AJNR. 2007;28(5):974-5.
28. Miller SF. The long-term consequences of lightning injuries. Burns. 2003;29(1):97.
29. Norman ME, Albertson D, Younge BR. Ophthalmic manifestations of lightning strike. Surv Ophthalmol. 2001;46(1):19-24.
30. Janus TJ, Barrash J. Neurologic and neurobehavioral effects of electric and lightning injuries. J Burn Care Rehabil. 1996;17(5):409-15.
31. Cherington M. Neurologic manifestations of lightning strikes. Neurology. 2003;60(2):182-5.
32. Montalto M, Ancarani F, Manna R, Gasbarrini G. Globus pharyngis: Was it a stroke of lightning? Am J Gastroenterol. 2003;98(4):938-9.
33. Kilbas Z, Akin M, Gorgulu S, Mentes O, Ozturk E, Kozak O, et al. Lightning strike: An unusual etiology of gastric perforation. Am J Emerg Med. 2008;26(8):966.
34. Aslan S, Aydinli B, Ocak T, Akcay M. Lightning: An unusual etiology of gastrointestinal perforation. Burns. 2005;31(2):237-9.

CHAPTER 16

Medicolegal Aspects of Injuries

Anil Garg, Putul Mahanta

LEARNING PLAN

- Learn about the classification of offences
- Recognize different types of weapon
- Understand different legal issues of injuries
- Know about homicide and its classification
- Know the manner, modes and mechanism of death
- Understand to write injury certificate/report

INJURY

In Section 44 of Indian Penal Code (IPC), the word "**Injury**" denotes **any harm whatever illegally caused to any person, in body, mind, reputation or property**.

Note: In Sections of IPC, like 323, 324, 325, etc., offences related to human being, word **bodily injury** was used. It means other type of injuries like mind; reputation or properties are not included in these sections of IPC.

OFFENCE

Section 40 of IPC, the word "**offence**" denotes an act punishable by the Code. An Offence takes place in two ways, either by commission of an act or by omission of an act.

Classification of Offence

As per criminal procedure code, on the basis of bail, the offences can be:

Bailable Offences

It means an offence, which is shown as bailable in the first schedule, or which is made bailable by any other law in force for time being. It means that the person shall be offered to be released on suitable bail upon his arrest by the police or the court (informing about his right to be so released).

Non-bailable Offences

It means the person shall not be automatically entitled to be released on bail, but does not mean that the court may not order him to be released on a suitable bail with or without any conditions.

As per Section 2, Criminal Procedure Code, 1973, the offence/crime can be:

Cognizable Offence and Case

Cognizable offence or case means a police officer may arrest in accordance with the First Schedule or under and other law for the time being in force, without warrant.

Non-cognizable Offence and Case

Non-cognizable offence or "non-cognizable case" means in which a police officer has no authority to arrest, without warrant".

As per Section 320, Criminal Procedure Code, 1973, the offences are:

Compoundable Offences

These are those offences punishable under the sections of the Indian Penal Code, which can be compromised with the victim with or without the permission of trial court:

i. Compoundable offences, which may be compromised with the respective person (even without permission of court before which any prosecution for such offence is pending). For examples: 298, 323, 334 IPC, etc.
ii. Compoundable offences, which can be compromised with permission of court before which any prosecution for such offence is pending. For examples: 325, 335, 337, 338 IPC, etc.

Non-compoundable: 302, 304B, 307, 324, 326 IPC

Punishment: Section 53 IPC, describes the punishments to which offenders are liable under the provisions of this code are:

- Death
- Imprisonment for life
- Imprisonment, which is of two descriptions, namely: (i) **Simple** imprisonment; (ii) **Rigorous** imprisonment, that is, with hard labor
- Forfeiture of property
- Fine.

Warrant-Case: In Section 2 subsection (x), warrant-case means a case relating to an offence punishable with death, imprisonment of life and imprisonment for a term exceeding 2 years.

Summons-Case: In section 2 subsection (w), summon-case means a case relating to an offence, and not being a warrant-case.

TYPES OF WEAPON

Weapons can be classified as:

- Dangerous weapon
- Other weapons

Dangerous Weapon

Section 324 and 326 IPC described dangerous weapon as any instrument used for shooting, stabbing or cutting, or any instrument, which when used, is likely to cause death, etc.

Weapons are further classified as:

a. **Blunt weapon**
   - *Hard blunt weapon*: Stick, stone, fist, bat, hockey, etc.
   - *Soft blunt weapon*: Rope.
b. **Sharp weapon**
   - *Light sharp weapon with cutting edge*: knife, scalpel, razor, etc.
   - *Heavy sharp weapon with splitting edge*: Axe sober, hatchet, etc.
c. **Pointed weapon**
   i. *Blunt pointed/penetrating weapon*: By this weapon, the overlying skin is split and penetrated and there is also bruising of margins, e.g. scissors, screwdriver, poker, chisel, etc. Here the instrument is relatively dull in sharpness.
   ii. *Sharp pointed/penetrating weapon*: By this weapon, the overlying skin is cut and penetrated and there is no bruising of margins, e.g. double edged sharp dagger and knife, chisel, etc.

LEGAL ISSUES OF INJURIES

Assault

According to **Section 351** IPC, "Whoever makes any gesture, or any preparation intending or knowing it to be likely that such gesture or preparation will cause any person present to apprehend that he who makes that gesture or preparation is about to use criminal force to that person, is said to commit as assault."

Hurt

Section 319 IPC describes, "Whoever causes bodily pain, disease or infirmity to any person is said to cause hurt."

Grievous Hurt

Section 320 IPC describes that the following kinds of hurt only are designated as "grievous":

1. Emasculation (**Figure 16.1**).
2. Permanent privation of the sight of either eye.
3. Permanent privation of the hearing of either ear.
4. Privation of any member or joint.
5. Destruction or permanent impairing of the powers of any member or joint.
6. Permanent disfiguration of the head or face.
7. Fracture or dislocation of a bone or tooth.
8. Any hurt, which endangers life or which causes the sufferer to be during the space of 20 days in severe bodily pain or unable to follow his ordinary pursuits.

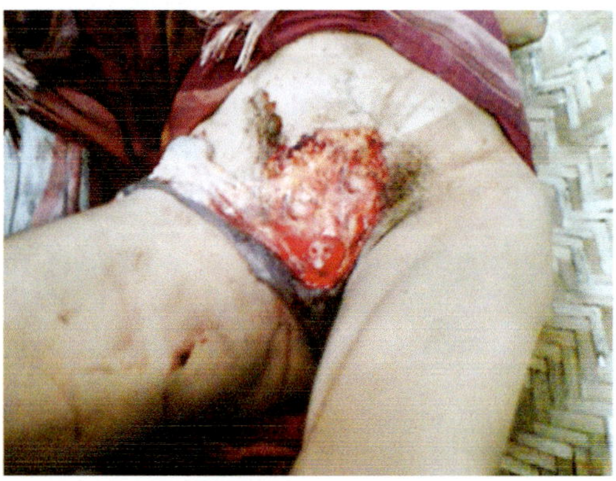

Figure 16.1 Excision of penis (Emasculation)

Voluntarily Causing Hurt

Section 321 IPC explains, "Whoever does any act with the intention of thereby causing hurt to any person, or with the knowledge that he is likely thereby to cause hurt to any person, and does thereby cause hurt to any person, is said voluntarily to cause hurt".

Voluntarily Causing Grievous Hurt

According to **Section 322 IPC**, "Whoever voluntarily causes hurt, if the hurt with the intend to cause or knows himself to be likely to cause is grievous hurt, and if the hurt which he causes is grievous hurt, is said voluntarily to cause grievous hurt".

Punishment for Voluntarily Causing Hurt

Section 323 IPC describes, "Whoever, except in the case provided for by Section 334, voluntarily causes hurt shall be punished with imprisonment of either description for a term, which may extend to one year, or with fine, which may extend to one thousand rupees, or with both."

Voluntarily Causing Hurt by Dangerous Weapons or Means

Section 324 IPC describes, "Whoever, except in the case provided for by Section 334, voluntarily causes hurt by means of any instrument for shooting, stabbing or cutting, or any instrument which, used as weapon of offence, is likely to cause death, or by means of fire or any heated substance, or by means of any poison or any corrosive substance, or by means of any explosive substance or by means of any substance, which it is deleterious to the human body to inhale, to swallow, or to receive into the blood, or by means of any animal, shall be punished with imprisonment of either description for a term which may extend to 3 years, or with fine, or with both."

This offence is cognizable, non-bailable, triable by any Magistrate and compoundable by the person to whom hurt is caused with the permission of the court.

Punishment for Voluntarily Causing Grievous Hurt

Section 325 IPC describes, "Whoever, except in the case provided for by section 335, voluntarily causes grievous hurt shall be punished with imprisonment of either description for a term which may extend to 7 years, and shall also be liable to fine.

This offence is cognizable, bailable, triable by any Magistrate and compoundable by the person to whom hurt is caused with the permission of the court".

Voluntarily Causing Grievous Hurt by Dangerous Weapons or Means

Section 326 IPC describes, "Whoever, except in the case provided for by section 335, voluntarily causes grievous hurt by means of any instrument for shooting, stabbing or cutting, or any instrument which, used as a weapon of offence, is likely to cause death, or by means of fire or any heated substance, or by means of any poison or any corrosive substance, or by means of any explosive substance, or by means of any substance which is deleterious to the human body to inhale, to swallow, or to receive into the blood, or by means of any animal, shall be punished with imprisonment for life, or with imprisonment of either description for a term which may extend to 10 years, and shall also be liable to fine. This offence is cognizable, bailable, triable by Magistrate of the first class and non-compoundable".

Voluntarily Causing Grievous Hurt by Use of Acids, etc.

Section 326A IPC describes, "Whoever causes permanent or partial damage or deformity to, or burns or maims or disfigures or disables, any part or parts of the body of a person or causes grievous hurt by throwing acid on or by administering acid to that person, or by using any other means with the intention of causing or with the knowledge that he is likely to cause such injury or hurt, shall be punished with imprisonment of either description for a term which shall not be less than 10 years but which may extend to imprisonment for life and with fine:

i. Provided that such fine shall be just and reasonable to meet the medical expenses of the treatment of the victim.
ii. Provided that any fine imposed under this section shall be given to the person on whom acid was thrown or to whom acid was administered. This offence is cognizable, non-bailable, and triable by session court"

Voluntarily Throwing or Attempting to Throw Acid

Section **326B** IPC describes, "Whoever throws or attempts to throw acid on any person or attempts to administer acid to any person, or attempts to use any other means, with the intention of causing permanent or partial damage or deformity or burns or maiming or disfigurement or disability or grievous hurt to that person, shall be punished with imprisonment of either description for a term which shall not be less than 5 years but which may extend to 7 years, and shall also be liable to fine.

Explanation 1 For the purposes of Section 326A and this section, "**acid**" includes any substance which has acidic or corrosive character or burning nature, that is capable of causing bodily injury leading to scars or disfigurement or temporary or permanent disability.

Explanation 2 For the purposes of Section 326A and this section, "**Permanent or partial damage**" or deformity shall not be required to be irreversible. This offence is cognizable, non-bailable, and triable by Session Court."

HOMICIDE

Definition: Homicide is killing of a human being by another human being.

Classification of Homicide (Figure 16.2)

Lawful Homicide

- Excusable homicide
- Justifiable homicide

Excusable Homicide: Here is no criminal intension and knowledge and caused unintentionally by an act done in good faith or in self-defense.

Justifiable Homicide: This is the homicide which is justified in the circumstances, which led to the killing of a person. This may occur (i) in the administration of justice, like execution of sentence of death, (ii) the maintenance of justice, e.g. in suppressing riots or executing arrest or killing in course of violent crime, e.g. a woman who kills a person who attempts to rape her.

Unlawful Homicide

- Culpable homicide not amounting to murder
- Murder

Punishment for culpable homicide (**Section 299 IPC**) not amounting to murder is described under **section 304 IPC**. Punishment for murder (**Section 300 IPC**) is described under Section **302 IPC**.

Culpable Homicide

Section 299 IPC describes, "Whoever causes death by:

1. Doing an act with the intention of causing death, or
2. With the intention of causing such bodily injury as is likely to cause death, or
3. With the knowledge that he is likely, by such act, to cause death, commits the offence of culpable homicide."

Illustrations

a. A lays sticks and turf over a pit, with the intention of thereby causing death, or with the knowledge that death is likely to be caused thereby. Z believing the ground to be firm, treads on it, falls in and is killed. A has committed the offence of culpable homicide.

b. A knows Z to be behind a bush. B does not know it. A, intending to cause, or knowing it to be likely to cause Z's death, induces B, who fires and kills Z. Here B may be guilty of no offence; but A has committed the offence of culpable homicide.

c. A, by shooting at a fowl with intent to kill and steal it, kills B who is behind a bush; A not knowing that he was there. Here, although A was doing an unlawful act, he was not guilty of culpable homicide, as he did not intend to kill B, or to cause death by doing an act that he knew was likely to cause death.

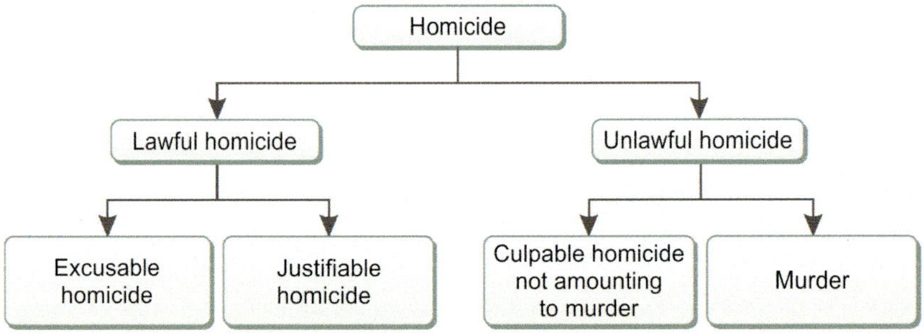

Figure 16.2 Classification of homicide

Explanation 1: A person, who causes bodily injury to another who is laboring under a disorder, disease or bodily infirmity, and thereby accelerates the death of that other, shall be deemed to have caused his death.

Explanation 2: Where death is caused by bodily injury, the person who causes such bodily injury shall be deemed to have caused the death, although by resorting to proper remedies and skilful treatment, the death might have been prevented.

Explanation 3: The causing of the death of child in the mother's womb is not homicide. But it may amount to culpable homicide to cause the death of a living child, if any part of that child has been brought forth, though the child may not have breathed or been completely born.

Murder

Section 300 IPC describes as, "Except in the cases hereinafter excepted, culpable homicide is murder,

Firstly: If the act by which the death is caused is done with the **intention** of causing death, or

Secondly: If it is done with the **intention** of causing such bodily injury as the offender knows to be likely to cause the death of the person to whom the harm is caused, or

Thirdly: If it is done with the intention of causing bodily injury to any person and the bodily injury intended to be inflicted is sufficient in the ordinary course of nature to cause death, or

Fourthly: If the person committing the act knows that it is so imminently dangerous that it must, in all probability, cause death or such bodily injury as is likely to cause death, and commits such act without any excuse for incurring the risk of causing death or such injury as previously mentioned.

Explanation 1:
When Culpable Homicide is Not Murder: Culpable homicide is not murder if the offender, while deprived of the power of self-control by grave and sudden provocation, causes the death of the person who gave the provocation or causes the death of any other person by mistake or accident.

The above exception is subject to the following provisons:

i. That the provocation is not sought or voluntarily provoked by the offender as an excuse for killing or doing harm to any person.
ii. That the provocation is not given by anything done in obedience to the law, or by a public servant in the lawful exercise of the powers of such public servant.
iii. That the provocation is not given by anything done in the lawful exercise of the right of private defense.

Explanation 2: Culpable homicide is not murder if the offender, in the exercise in good faith of the right of private defense of person or property, exceeds the power given to him by law and causes the death of the person against whom he is exercising such right of defense without premeditation, and without any intention of doing more harm than is necessary for the purpose of such defense.

Explanation 3: Culpable homicide is not murder if the offender, being a public servant or aiding a public servant acting for the advancement of public justice, exceeds the powers given to him by law, and causes death by doing an act which he, in good faith, believes to be lawful and necessary for the due discharge of his duty as such public servant and without ill-will towards the person whose death is caused.

Explanation 4: Culpable homicide is not murder if it is committed without premeditation in a sudden fight in the heat of passion upon a sudden quarrel and without the offender having taken undue advantage or acted in a cruel or unusual manner.

Explanation 5: Culpable homicide is not murder when the person whose death is caused, being above the age of 18 years, suffers death or takes the risk of death with his own consent.

Murder Distinguished from Culpable Homicide

"Culpable homicide" is genus, and "murder" is the specie. All "murder" are culpable homicide but not vice-versa; Narasingh Challan vs. State of Orissa, (1997) 2 Crimes 78 (Ori).

Punishment for Murder by Life Convict

Section 303 describes, "Whoever, being under sentence of imprisonment for life, commits murder, shall be punished with death. This offence is cognizable, non-bailable, non-compoundable and triable by Sessions Court".

Punishment for Culpable Homicide Not Amounting to Murder

Section 304 describes, "Whoever commits culpable homicide not amounting to murder shall be punished with imprisonment for life, or imprisonment of either description for a term, which may extend to 10 years, and shall also be liable to fine, if the act by which the death is caused is done with the intention of causing death, or of causing such bodily injury as is likely to cause death. Means any offence committed under section 299 (1) and (2) was punished vide this para. Also sometimes referred as 304 part (1).

Or

With imprisonment of either description for a term, which may extend to 10 years, or with fine, or with both, if the act is done with the knowledge that it is likely to cause death, but without any intention to cause death, or to cause such bodily injury as is likely to cause death. Means any offence committed under Section 299 (3) was punished vide this para. Also sometimes referred as 304 part (2).

SOME IMPORTANT IPC

Causing Death by Negligence

Section 304A describes, "Whoever causes the death of any person by doing any rash or negligent act not amounting to culpable homicide, shall be punished with imprisonment of either description for a term, which may extend to 2 years, or with fine, or with both".

Punishment is of imprisonment for 2 years, or fine, or both. Offence is cognizable, bailable, triable by Magistrate of the first class and non-compoundable, e.g. roadside accident due to rash and negligent driving.

Dowry Death

Section 304B IPC describes:

1. Where the death of a woman is caused by any burns or bodily injury or occurs otherwise than under normal circumstances within 7 years of her marriage, and it is shown that soon before her death she was subjected to cruelty or harassment by her husband or any relative of her husband for, or in connection with, any demand for dowry, such death shall be called "dowry death", and such husband or relative shall be deemed to have caused her death.
2. Whoever commits dowry death shall be punished with imprisonment for a term, which shall not be less than 7 years but which may extend to imprisonment for life. Punishment is of imprisonment not less than 7 years which may extend to imprisonment for life. Offence is cognizable, non-bailable, triable in Court of Sessions and non-compoundable."

Abetment of Suicide of Child or Insane Person

Section 305 IPC describes, "If any person under 18 years of age, any insane person, any delirious person, any idiot, or any person in a state of intoxication, commits suicide, whoever abets the commission of such suicide, shall be punished with death or imprisonment for life, or imprisonment for a term not exceeding 10 years, and shall also be liable to fine." Offence is cognizable, non-bailable, triable at Court of Sessions and non-compoundable.

Abetment of Suicide

Section 306 IPC describes, "If any person commits suicide, whoever abets the commission of such suicide, shall be punished with imprisonment of either description for a term which may extend to 10 years, and shall also be liable to fine." Offence is cognizable, non-bailable, triable at Court of Sessions and non-compoundable.

Attempt to Murder

Section 307 IPC describes it as, "Whoever does any act with such intention or knowledge, and under such circumstances that, if he by that act caused death, he would be guilty of murder, shall be punished with imprisonment of either description for a term which may extend to 10 years, and shall also be liable to fine; and if hurt is caused to any person by such act, the offender shall be liable either to imprisonment for life, or to such punishment as is hereinbefore mentioned.

Attempts by Life Convicts: When any person offending under this section is under sentence of imprisonment for life, he may, if hurt is caused, be punished with death."

Illustrations

i. A shoots at Z with intention to kill him under such circumstances that, if death ensued, A would be guilty of murder. A is liable to punishment under this section.
ii. A, intending to murder Z by poison, purchases poison and mixes the same with food, which remains in A's keeping; A has not yet committed the offence defined in this section. A place the food on Z's table or delivers it to Z's servant to place it on Z's table. A has committed the offence defined in this section.

Offence is cognizable, non-bailable, triable by Court of Sessions and non-compoundable.

Attempt to Commit Culpable Homicide

Section 308 IPC describes, "Whoever does any act with such intention or knowledge and under such circumstances that, if he by that act caused death, he would be guilty of culpable homicide not amount to murder, shall be punished with imprisonment of either description for a term which may extend to 3 years, or with fine, or with both, and if hurt is caused to any person by such act, shall be punished with imprisonment of either description for a term which may extend to 7 years, or with fine, or with both."

Illustration

A, on grave and sudden provocation, fires a pistol at Z. Under such circumstances that if he thereby caused death he would be guilty of culpable homicide not amounting to murder. A has committed the offence defined in this section. Offence is cognizable, non-bailable, triable at Court of Sessions and non-compoundable.

Attempt to Commit Suicide

Section 309 IPC describes, "Whoever attempts to commit suicide and does any act towards the commission of such offence shall be punished with simple imprisonment for term, which may extend to one year or with fine, or with both." Offence is cognizable, bailable, triable by any Magistrate and non-compoundable.

Voluntarily Causing Hurt on Provocation

Section 334 IPC describes, "Whoever voluntarily causes hurt on grave and sudden provocation, if he neither intends nor knows himself to be likely to cause hurt to any person other than the person who gave the provocation, shall be punished with imprisonment of either description for a term which may extend to one month, or with fine which may extend to five hundred rupees, or with both." Offence is non-cognizable, bailable, triable by any Magistrate and compoundable by the person to whom the hurt is caused.

Voluntarily Causing Grievous Hurt on Provocation

Section 335 IPC describes as, "Whoever voluntarily causes grievous hurt on grave and sudden provocation, if he neither intends nor knows himself to be likely to cause grievous hurt to any person other than the person who gave the provocation, shall be punished with imprisonment of either description for a term which may extend to four years or with fine which may extend to two thousand rupees, or with both." Offence is non-cognizable, bailable, triable by any Magistrate and compoundable by the person to whom the hurt is caused with the permission of court.

Act Endangering Life or Personal Safety of Others

Section 336 IPC describes, "Whoever does any act so rashly or negligently as to endanger human life or the personal safety of others, shall be punished with imprisonment of either description for term which may extend to 3 months, or with fine which may extend to two hundred and fifty rupees, or with both." Offence is cognizable, bailable, triable by any Magistrate and non-compoundable.

Causing Hurt by Act Endangering Life or Personal Safety of Others

Section 337 IPC describes, "Whoever causes hurt to any person by doing any act so rashly or negligently as to endanger human life, or the personal safety of others, shall be punished with imprisonment of either description for term which may extend to 6 months, or with fine which may extend to five hundred rupees, or with both." Offence is cognizable, bailable, triable by any Magistrate and compoundable by the person to whom hurt is caused with the permission of the court.

Illustration

Ram driving the car rashly and negligently hurts Krishan then he will be punished under this section.

Causing Grievous Hurt by Act Endangering Life or Personal Safety of Others

Section 338 IPC describes, "Whoever causes grievous hurt to any person by doing any act so rashly or negligently as to endanger human life, or the personal safety of others, shall be punished with imprisonment of either description for a term which may extend to 2 years, or with fine which may extend to one thousand rupees, or with both." Offence is cognizable, bailable, triable by any Magistrate and compoundable by the person to whom hurt is caused with the permission of the court.

Illustration

Ram driving the car rashly and negligently causes grievous hurt to Krishan then he will be punished under this section.

MANNER, MODE AND MECHANISM OF DEATH

Manner of Death

Manner means style or customary way of doing or accomplishing something. So manner of death means style or customary way of doing death. Manner of death is further classified as:

i. **Non-violent** or **Natural Death**: due to some disease, which is naturally going in human being.
ii. **Violent** or **Unnatural Death**: Depending upon how violence was used. The violent or unnatural death is further classified as:

a. **Homicide:** Death due to violence by another human being.
b. **Suicide:** Death due to violence by self on self.
c. **Accidental:** Death due to some accident likes motor vehicle accident, etc.

In India, as there is Police Inquest system, manner of death is to be ascertained by investigating officer dealing with the case. Doctor has no role in ascertainment of manner of death. But they may help to answer the queries raised by investigating officer for knowing manner of death, if asked. But in the USA, where Medical Examiner System is applicable, manner of death was ascertained by the medical officers.

Modes of Death

Modes of death means, the physiological condition/state present at the time of death of deceased or due to which death starts. Bichat described following modes of death:

- **Asphyxia**: Due to respiration system failure.
- **Syncope**: Due to heart or circulatory system failure.
- **Coma**: Due to brain functioning failure.

Mechanism of Death

Mechanism of death means physiological process or disturbances going on in the body leading to death of the deceased, e.g. toxemia, sepsis, metabolic acidosis and metabolic alkalosis.

INJURY CERTIFICATE/REPORT

Injury certificate/report is usually prepared by first attending medical officer who is the best judge for the victim with respect to injury reporting, as examined before any intervention. Injury reporting is usually done by emergency/causality medical officers (EMO or CMO) who is the first attending medical officer, in most of hospitals or by any other medical officer may be called upon to examine injured person.

Nowadays, in some states, like in Punjab and Haryana, injury certificate/report is being presented as computer typed report. Injury certificate/report can also be prepared as per **Annexure II** attached.

Data for Injury Certificate

Data should be noted in the injury certificate are as follows:

1. **Medicolegal Registration no**: This is unique number, which is related to the medicolegally examining doctor. This number tells that which doctor had done the MLR, in which hospital doctor has done the MLR and in which year MLR was done and what is the serial number of MLR in relation to particular doctor, e.g. Dr Anil Garg had done MLR at Gian Sagar Medical College, Patiala, then initial like AG (this may be two or more alphabet long to avoid confusion between two or more doctors having similar initial words working in same hospital). GSMCH for Gian Sagar Medical College and Hospital and year to be written as 12 or 2012. Next number of already issued injury certificate, e.g. AG/GSMCH/12/01. This tradition is followed in non-software based injury certificate. But nowadays in some hospitals, software-based injury certificates are issued where MLR registration number is issued uniquely by software and we can put this number in reference number.
2. **Name**: Then we have to note down the full name of the patient as per available document like Aadhaar number, etc.
3. **Age**: Exact age as per valid documents.
4. **Father's name/Husband's name**: Then full name of father or husband should be noted.
5. **Address**: Exact address of the patient should be noted as per available documents.
6. **Date** and **time of arrival**, **admission and examination**: It should be noted at appropriate columns.
7. **Consent**: This is the most important part of injury certification. It should be preferably

taken in patient handwriting in his/her language and then signed before starting medicolegal examination. Under section 53 CrPC, medicolegal examination of accused can be done on police request by not below sub-inspector by using reasonably necessary force. For the purposes of medicolegal examination, consent can be given by individual of sound mind of age 12 years or above, otherwise consent can be obtained from parents or guardian in charge of person below 12 years age, or unconscious patient or patient of unsound mind. Signature of patient or guardian should be taken at appropriate space provided on injury certificate. If patient or responsible person for consent is illiterate, the left thumb impression in male and right thumb impression in female should be taken in presence of third literate relative with his or her signature.

8. **Brought by**: The name of the friend or relative must be noted in the injury report along with father's name and complete address along with mobile or telephone number. If the case was brought by police official under section 53, 53A, 54 or 164A of CrPC, then the name and belt number of police official must be noted along with name of place of posting in Police Station. The application reference must be given in injury certificate.
9. **Place of incident**: In this point, exact place of incident of crime or assault should be noted.
10. **Name of concerned police station**: Depending upon the place of incidence mentioned above, the name of police station in whose jurisdiction incidence happened should be noted (it is for information and sending of injury report).
11. **Identification marks**: Two identification marks must be noted. Identification marks are, mole, scar, tattoo marks, birth marks, deformity, etc., identification marks should be described in respect of size, shape, vascularity, movement, location on the body and reference from two important surface markings. This should be described in layman language and not in medical language as applicable in injuries description. If no identification marks are found on the person of the patient/accused/victim undergoing medicolegal examination, his/her thumb impression must be taken.
12. **Place of examination**: Exact place of examination of the victim was noted like bed no, ward no.
13. **Brief history**: Alleged history regarding the incident was noted. Particularly alleged site of incident and person responsible for same may be noted.
14. **Examination part**: This is the most important part of injury certificate/report. The various entries in the injury certificate are mentioned in **Table 16.1**.

In the end, the injury certificate should be signed and stamped by the examining medical officer along with date and time of completion of examination.

Table 16.1 Description of an injury report

Column	Descriptions about the injury
01	Mention the serial number of injury
02	Here we mention the type of injury: like abrasion, bruise, laceration or incised wound, punctured lacerated wound
03	Here, size of wound in respect to length, breadth and depth should be noted and also special reference to color of abrasion, bruise with or without scab formation and edge or margins of lacerated and incised wound should be noted
04	In this column, location of wound is described and position of wound should be described from two nearest important bony landmarks
05	Here, nature of injuries was described as simple or grievous. If the injury is still kept pending or under observation from particular department. It should be mentioned in front of that particular injury
06	In this column, kind of weapon should be described in front of each injury as blunt or sharp or pointed or firearm, etc.
07	Here, the age of injury is described from color, margins and edges of wound
08	In this column, detail of department where injury is kept under observation may be mentioned

PROFORMA FOR INJURY CERTIFICATE

Medicolegal Registration No: ________ **Date:** ________

Reference: ________

Name: ________ **Age:** ________ month/years; Sex: M/F.

Son/daughter/wife of: ________ Resident of: ________

Date and time of arrival: ________

Date and time of admission: ________

Date and time of examination: ________

Consent for examination: ________

Brought/Identified by Mr/Mrs: ________ Constable No: ________

Police Station: ________

Place of incident: ________

Identification marks: 1. ________ 2. ________

Place of examination: ________

Brief history: ________

Injury Report

1	2	3	4	5	6	7	8
Sl. no	Type of injury, i.e. whether abrasion, laceration, incised, bruise, burn, etc.	Size of each injury in cm, i.e. length, breadth and depth, along with color of wound	On what part of the body inflicted	Nature of injuries Whether simple or grievous	By what kind of weapon inflicted or how caused blunt/ sharp force, fire	Age of Injury	Remarks (whether X-rayed, admitted under observation, where referred for further examination, or report or treatment or any other relevant information)

Station: ________ **(Signature and seal of the examining doctor)**

Date: ________

CHAPTER 17

Asphyxial Deaths

Sanjoy Das, Putul Mahanta

LEARNING PLAN

- Gordon's classification of death
- Know the classical signs of asphyxia
- Classify asphyxia
- Learn hanging and related issues
- Understand strangulation, suffocation and drowning

DEFINITION OF ASPHYXIA

Asphyxia literally means "pulselessness".

Asphyxia is a very broad term relating to the "inadequate aeration of blood". Thus, there is hypoxia (lack of oxygen) and hypercapnia (excess of carbon dioxide). The brain, being the most sensitive to lack of oxygen, is the earliest to suffer in all types of asphyxia.

Barcroft (1920) postulated that anoxia (absence of oxygen) in the blood is possible in three ways, namely anoxic, anemic and stagnant anoxia. **Peters** and **Slyke** (1931) added a fourth group and called it histotoxic anoxia.

GORDON'S CLASSIFICATION OF DEATH

Gordon (1944) clarified that lack of tissue oxygenation ultimately leads to cardiac failure and death. In this context, hypoxia is a more appropriate term as compared to anoxia.

1. **Anoxic Anoxia**
   Anoxic anoxia results from non-availability of oxygen to the lungs. This can occur when there is obstruction to the air passage, fixation of the chest, respiratory failure or lack of atmospheric oxygen.
2. **Anemic Anoxia**
   Anemic anoxia results because of reduced oxygen carrying capacity of the blood due to low or defective hemoglobin, as in severe anemia or carbon monoxide poisoning.
3. **Stagnant Anoxia**
   Stagnant anoxia results because of impaired circulation resulting in inadequate oxygenation of tissues as in cases of shock.
4. **Histotoxic Anoxia**
   Histotoxic anoxia results because of inability of tissues to utilize available oxygen. Histotoxic anoxia can be further classified as:

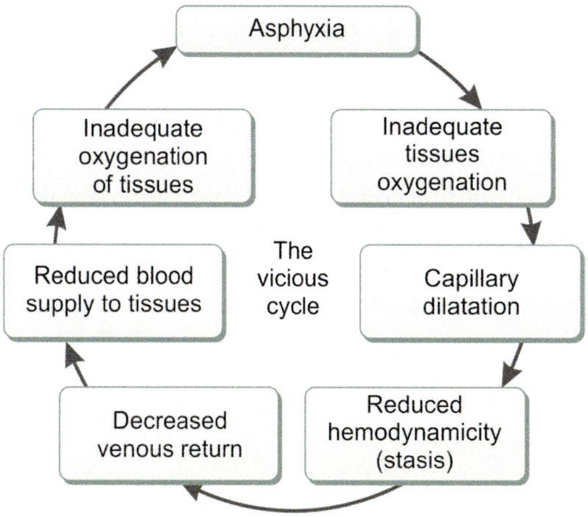

Figure 17.1 The vicious cycle of asphyxia

a. **Extracellular**: The enzyme activity of the cells is impaired, as seen in poisoning by hydrocyanic acid, where there is interference with the cytochrome oxidase enzyme system.
b. **Pericellular**: Decrease in permeability of cell membrane, as seen in cases of chloroform poisoning.
c. **Cellular**: Dumping of end products of cellular metabolism, resulting in prevention of further oxygen utilization, as seen in uremia, or there is inadequacy of foodstuff for metabolism.

Asphyxia Begets Asphyxia

Asphyxia after once setting in, causes further asphyxia, i.e. asphyxia begets asphyxia. Hence, a vicious cycle of it sets in. The vicious cycle of asphyxia is shown in **Figure 17.1**.

CLASSICAL SIGNS OF ASPHYXIA

The signs of asphyxia are neither very specific nor constant in all deaths. Many of these signs are modified, depending on the type of asphyxial death. Features are more pronounced when the obstruction or constriction, producing asphyxia, is more severe.

Cyanosis

"Cyanosis" is derived from the Greek word *saiaen* meaning dark blue. Thus, cyanosis is the blue color of the skin and mucous membranes. Due to lack of oxygen, there is rise in the level of reduced hemoglobin in the blood. When this level reaches a concentration above 5 g per 100 mL of capillary blood, bluish color becomes visible in areas with superficial capillary abundance like lips, nail beds, tongue, palate and tip of the nose. As the level of reduced hemoglobin rises, cyanosis becomes more pronounced.

After somatic death, tissue metabolism continues until molecular death supervenes. During this process, the arterial blood loses its oxygen and there is further increase in the concentration of reduced hemoglobin.

Moreover, after death, venous blood may mix with arterial blood due to cessation of circulation. Hence, cyanosis is actually significant only during or sometime after death. Sometimes, a pink color of postmortem lividity, in cold climate or in frozen bodies, may mask cyanosis that was present at the time of death. The appreciation of cyanosis may be altered due to racial differences, varying epidermal thickness and conditions like polycythemia.

Congestion

Capillary dilatation, consequent upon lack of oxygen, results in stasis of blood. This causes further decrease in oxygenation, resulting in diminished return of blood to the heart and further impairment of oxygenation. This causes more stasis of blood and a vicious cycle starts, producing congestion of visceral organs.

Presence of congestion along with right ventricular dilatation is a fair indication of asphyxia. However, care should be exercised in interpreting these findings and drawing inference from them as congestion may occur in many other forms of death.

Fluidity of Blood

Fluidity of blood is no more considered a sign of asphyxia. It has been established that fluidity of blood occurs due to fibrinolysin activity. The pronounced fluidity of blood in asphyxial deaths is probably due to the rapid fibrinolysis of blood in such cases.

Petechial Hemorrhages

These are small spots of capillary hemorrhage. Their significance and mechanism of production has remained a subject of controversy. The mechanism of production of petechiae is presumed to be related to hypoxic capillary dilatation and raised intracapillary pressure, usually above the site of obstruction. Their presence in the skin of face, eyelids and conjunctivae suggest that they occur above the site of obstruction, especially when neck veins are compressed.

Tardieu (1866) described pin-head size hemorrhages in the visceral pleura and pericardium and these were subsequently called "Tardieu's spots". These are petechial hemorrhages of varying shapes and sizes.

Pharyngeal Hemorrhage

It was thought that when pressure is applied upon the neck, large submucosal hemorrhages are produced behind the cricoid cartilage. It is now clear that congestion in the vessels and then subsequent rupture usually gives rise to such hemorrhages, even in cases where asphyxia does not occur.

CLASSIFICATION OF ASPHYXIA (FIGURE 17.2)

Non-mechanical

This includes all forms where there is depletion of oxygen, excess of irrespirable gases or impaired utilization and uptake of oxygen.

i. Carbon monoxide poisoning
ii. Carbon dioxide poisoning
iii. Poisoning by hydrocyanic acid

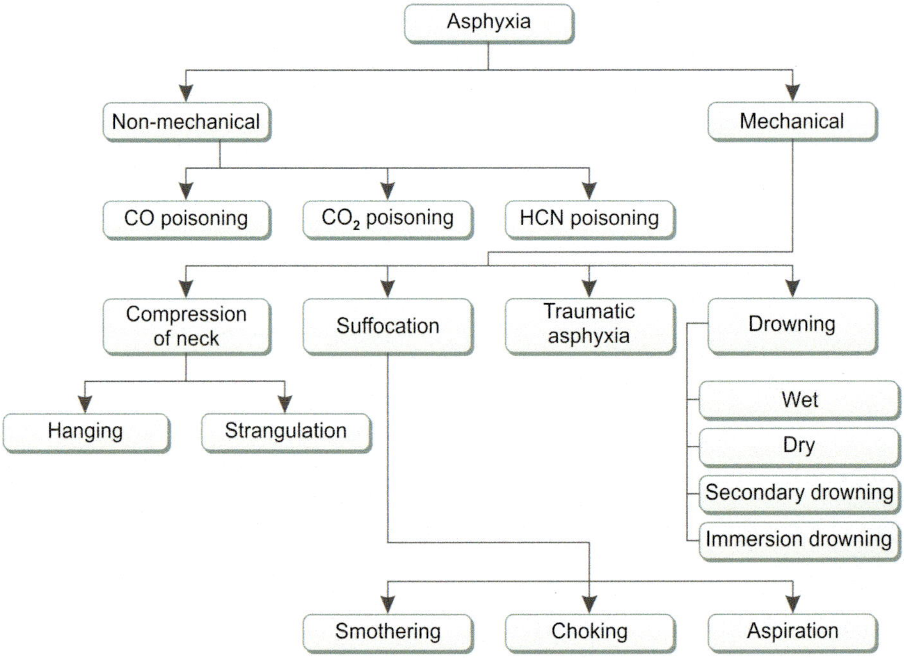

Figure 17.2 Classification of asphyxia

Mechanical

i. **Compression of neck**
   - Hanging
     - Complete
     - Partial or incomplete
   - Strangulation
     - Ligature
     - Manual

ii. **Suffocation** (obstruction of airway from outside or from within)
   - Smothering
   - Choking
   - Aspiration

iii. **Compression** and **fixation** of chest:
   - Traumatic asphyxia

iv. **Drowning**

HANGING

Definition

Hanging is a form of death where a body is suspended by a ligature round the neck and the force of constriction is the weight (or part of the weight) of the body.

When the point of suspension is high, the body is completely suspended with no part of the body touching the ground. This is termed as **complete hanging.** However, when some part of the body is resting on the ground, as in a kneeling, sitting, reclining and prone or any other posture due to a low point of suspension, it is termed incomplete or **partial hanging**.

Typical hanging is one where the knot is present in the occipital region. In this position, there is maximum constriction of the neck structures. If the knot is present anywhere other than the occipital region, it is known as **atypical hanging**.

The Ligature Material

The ligature used is usually one that is most readily available to the victim, as hanging is usually suicidal. The ligature material can be jute or nylon rope, wire, cloth, belt or even a sacred thread or any other material that the victim presumed to be strong enough (**Figure 17.3**).

The victim usually ties one end of the ligature to a high point, like a beam, ceiling fan or hook, and passes his neck through a noose on the lower end of the ligature material, while standing on a support such as a stool, chair or cot. The victim then jumps off or kicks off the support and the noose gets tightened around the neck. The noose can be a fixed or a slipping type with a granny or reef knot. Commonly, there is only one knot, but when there are two knots; one is not as tight as the other. However, in homicidal hanging, both the knots are tightly secured.

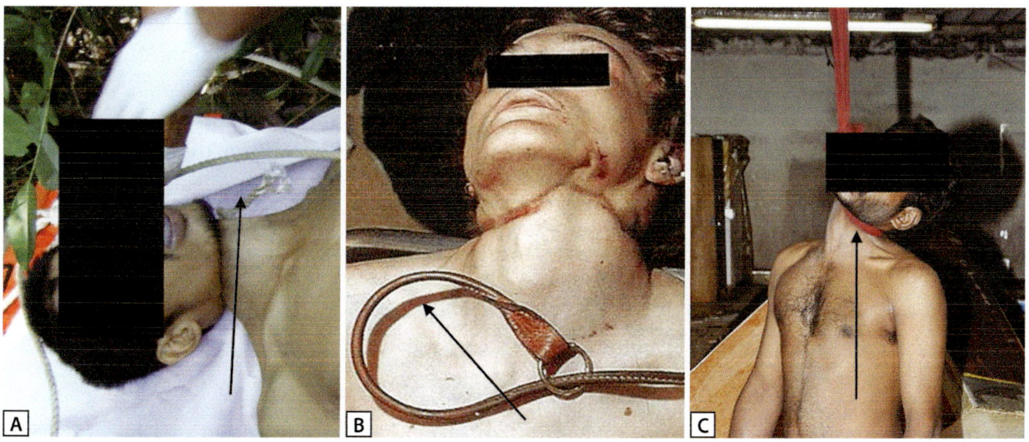

Figures 17.3A to C Different ligature materials, (A) Nylon rope; (B) Belt; (C) Cloth

Examination of Ligature Material

The type of the material, its length, thickness, strength and weave pattern is noted. The noose is cut away from the knot and the cut ends are tied. The thickness and the weave pattern will correspond to the ligature mark on the neck of the victim. The material should be strong enough to bear the weight of the body and the jerk at the end of the drop. Cloth ligatures like *saree*s, bed sheets and *dupatta* sometimes split longitudinally by the weight of the body, increasing the length of the ligature material so that the body comes to rest on the ground as in partial hanging, even from a high point of suspension.

Mechanism of Neck Constriction

Very little force is actually required to constrict the vessels of the neck. This is the reason why death occurs even in partial hangings, where the weight of the head only acts as the constricting force.

It has been shown by Hofmann and Brouardel that a tension of about 30 kg is sufficient to constrict the vertebral arteries, 15 kg to occlude the trachea, 5 kg for the carotid arteries and just 2 kg to close the jugular veins. Reuter (1901) and Polson (1985) reported even lower weights for closure of neck vessels and trachea.

Injury to the vagus nerve, spinal cord or base of the skull may also occur, depending upon the type of ligature, the force applied and the length of drop.

Sequence of Events in Hanging

Loss of Consciousness

Initially there is loss of power, ringing or hissing in the ears, flashes of light before the eyes, mental confusion and incoherence of thought. Unconsciousness supervenes rapidly. It is said that "once hanging, there is no return". This is due to the rapidity of loss of consciousness, coupled with the confusion and powerlessness. The victim cannot help himself even if there was a possibility of withdrawal.

Stage of Convulsion

The face is distorted, eyes suffused and livid, and there is violent effort to breathe. During this convulsive stage, the protruding tongue may be bitten by the teeth. Finally, the violent respiratory efforts cease, but the heart continues to beat for another 8–20 minutes.

Causes of Death in Hanging

1. **Asphyxia**: Asphyxia occurs due to occlusion of the air passages. The force of the ligature presses the root of the tongue against the posterior pharyngeal wall, thus blocking the airway. Asphyxia occurs in most cases, but pure asphyxia as a cause of death is uncommon.
2. **Venous Congestion (Apoplexy)**: The jugular veins are occluded with minimal tension of 2 kg, preventing venous return from the brain. Thus, there is venous congestion of the brain and cessation of cerebral circulation due to suboxia.
3. **Combined Asphyxia and Venous Congestion**: This is the commonest cause of death in hanging. In most cases of hanging, the air passages are not completely blocked, hence there is a combination of asphyxia and apoplexy.
4. **Cerebral Anoxia**: Pressure over large arteries of the neck impairs blood flow to the brain, which suffers from ischemia.
5. **Vagal Shock**: Pressure of the ligature over the carotid body or the vagus nerve may cause reflex cardiac inhibition and sudden stoppage of the heart.
6. **Fracture or Dislocation of the Cervical Vertebrae**: Whenever there is a long drop of 2 m or more, there is a sudden forceful jerk at the end of the drop, as in judicial hanging. This may result in fracture-dislocation of the upper cervical vertebrae, usually C_{2-3}, sometimes C_{3-4} and rarely C_{1-2}.

Fatal Period

In cases of fracture-dislocation of cervical vertebrae, death is instantaneous. Commonly death occurs in 5-15 minutes when occlusion of air passages is partial. The survival period is prolonged in cases of venous congestion alone.

Death may be delayed in some cases due to complications like pneumonia, encephalopathy, pulmonary edema or infections.

Postmortem Findings

General External Findings

The head is tilted to the side opposite to the knot. The face is usually pale and placid with eyes half closed (**Figure 17.4**).

But the face can also be suffused and swollen if the body was hanging for a prolonged period. The pupils are often dilated. The term "**Le facie sympathique**" has been attributed to rare cases where pressure over the cervical sympathetic will result in the eye of the same side to be open and its pupil dilated (**Figure 17.5**).

The tongue is usually protruded and bitten by the teeth and is swollen and livid (**Figure 17.6**). It may occasionally be drawn in. The protrusion of the tongue is due to the pressure of the ligature against the root of the tongue.

Dribbling of saliva from an angle of the mouth, usually from the angle opposite of the knot, over the chin and chest indicates that the person was alive at the time of hanging. This is the surest sign of antemortem hanging as dribbling of saliva is due to pressure of the ligature on the submandibular salivary glands is always an antemortem phenomenon. Sometimes, bloody froth may be present at the mouth and nostrils.

In the **Figure 17.7**, note the direction of dribbling saliva from angle of mouth. In this

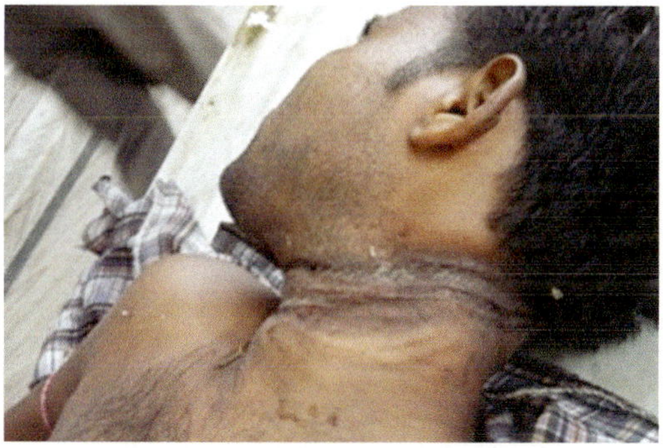

Figure 17.4 Head is tilted opposite to knot

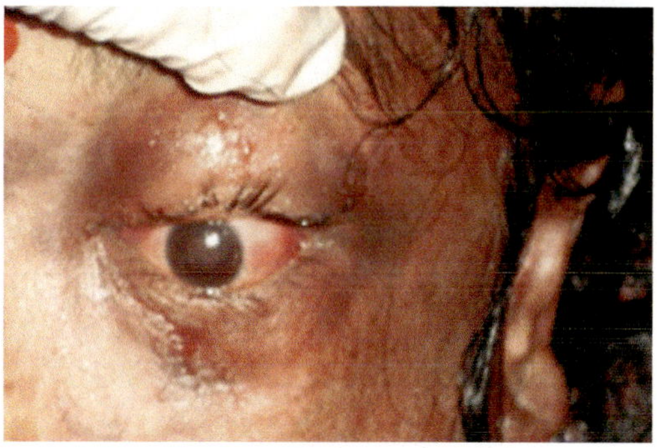

Figure 17.5 Dilated pupil with suffused and swollen face

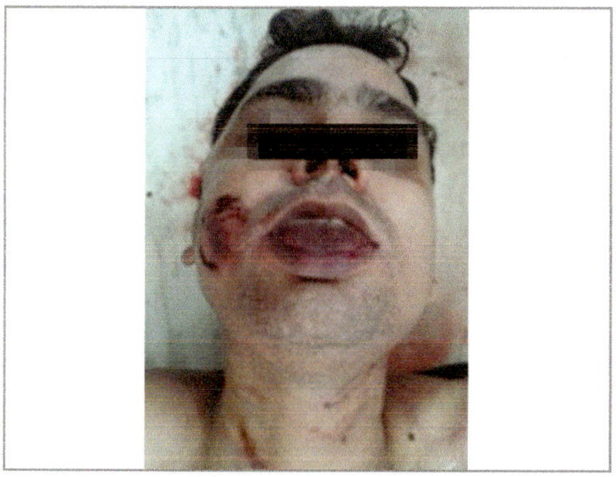

Figure 17.6 Protruded tongue bitten by the teeth
(*Courtesy:* Dr Mrinal Haloi, GMC, Guwahati)

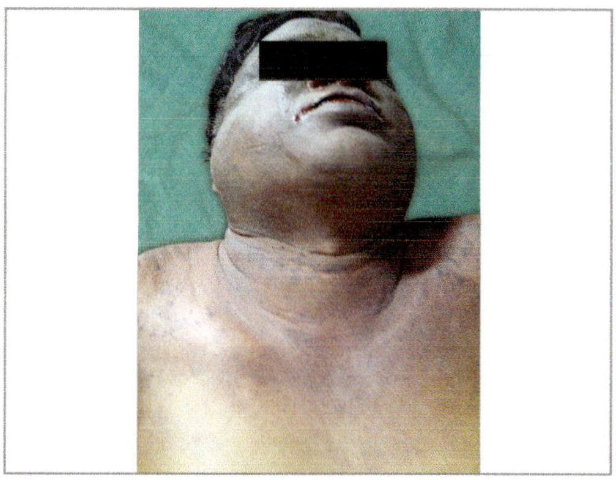

Figure 17.7 Ligature mark with dribbling of saliva from angle of mouth (In this case head was lying down from bed. Hence, the direction of saliva from angle of mouth towards head)

picture the dribbling of saliva is towards eyes and head as the person's head was lying down from bed to the floor at the time of committing suicide. The direction shows the position of head and knot. Also note the postmortem hypothesis, which is more pronounce over face and head.

Petechial hemorrhages may be found in the conjunctiva and above the ligature on the neck (**Figure 17.8**).

There will be **deep cyanosis** of the lips (**Figure 17.9**), fingertips and nail beds. This is more pronounced when the point of suspension was low or asphyxia was prolonged.

The hands are often clenched and sometimes there may be fibers of the ligature material between the fingers of the clenched hands.

The genitals may be turgid, resulting from hypostasis. This feature can be seen in both males and females, but cannot be attributed to the cause of death as it may occur in many other types of death. There may be emission of seminal fluid, which can be seen at the urethral meatus or inner side of the thighs (**Figure 17.10**). There may be escape of urine and feces due to relaxation of sphincters. Both these features are not of much value in the diagnosis of asphyxial death, as they may also occur in other forms of death.

There may be slight bleeding per vagina and per rectum, owing to the turgiscence and petechiae on the vaginal and rectal mucosa.

Postmortem staining, in a body that has been suspended for a long time after death, is typically described as of "**gloves and stockings**" type. It is observed in the forearms and hands as well as in the lower limbs.

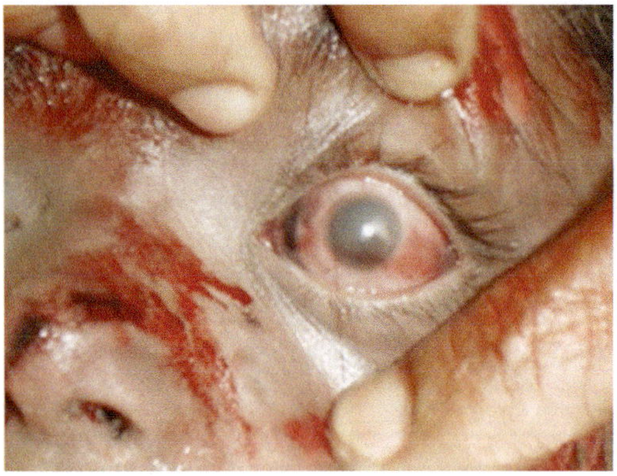

Figure 17.8 Subconjunctival hemorrhage

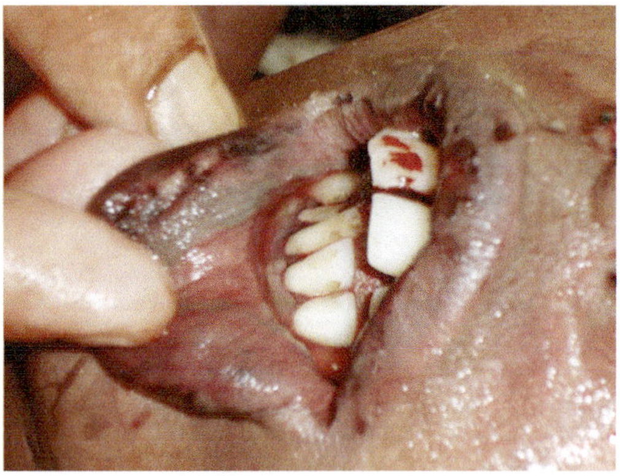

Figure 17.9 Deep cyanosis of the lips (with lip laceration)

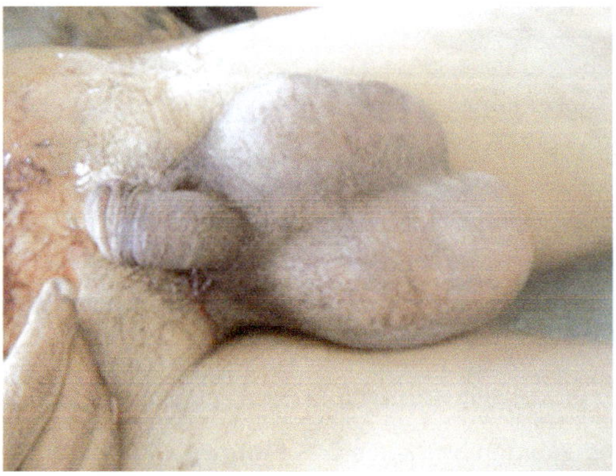

Figure 17.10 Emission of seminal fluid with turgid scrotum

Local External Findings

The neck may be stretched and elongated in case of prolonged suspension as shown in **Figure 17.11**. The main local finding is the mark produced by the ligature round the neck.

The **ligature mark** is a pressure abrasion. The prominence of this mark will depend upon the type of material used and the time for which the body was suspended after death. A strong but thin wire will produce a deep groove, while a soft ligature like a bed sheet will produce a shallow mark. If the body is brought down just after death, the ligature mark may be almost invisible. Presence of intervening material like a long beard in males, hair in females or thick neck scarves may make the ligature mark faint or absent over area of intervention.

Situation of the Mark

The ligature is typically described as being "**oblique, non-continuous** and **situated above** the level of **thyroid cartilage**" as shown in **Figure 17.12**. It travels obliquely upwards, following the lower border of the mandible towards the mastoids to become interrupted at the back, where there may be an irregular impression of the knot. The mark may be more circular and horizontal in case of partial hanging, where the neck and shoulders are at the same level.

Multiple ligature marks may be found when two or more loops are passed around the neck. In such cases, the initial loops may produce circular marks and the last loop will be oblique as shown in **Figure 17.13**.

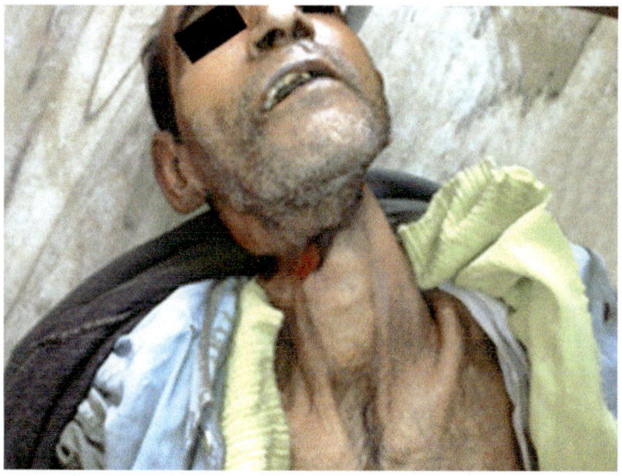

Figure 17.11 Stretched and elongated neck due to prolong suspension

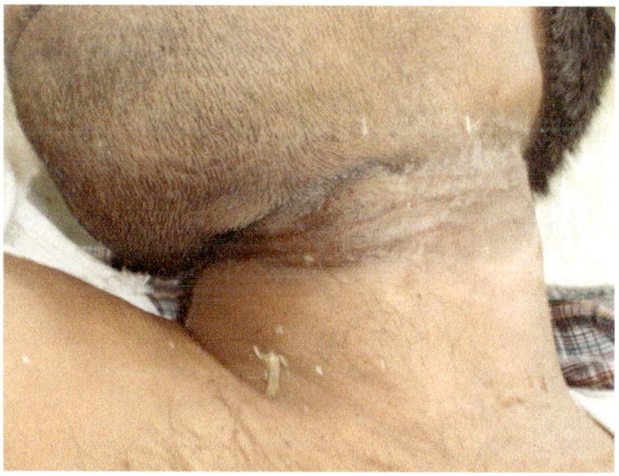

Figure 17.12 Oblique ligature marks around the neck

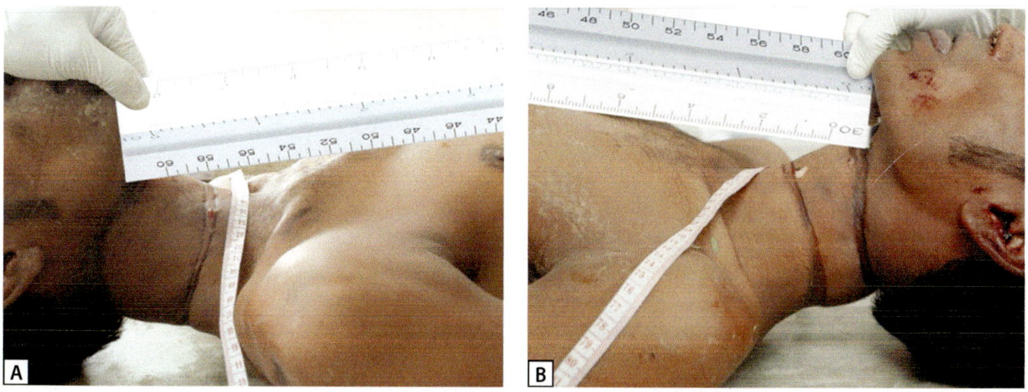

Figures 17.13A and B Multiple ligature marks: One transverse and one oblique
(*Courtesy:* Dr Raktim Pratim Tamuli, Gauhati Medical College, Guwahati)

The different oblique, non-continuous ligature marks found in a case of suicidal hanging are shown in **Figures 17.14A and B**.

General Internal Findings

These findings will, to a great extent, be influenced by the mode of death.

Tardieu's spots and marginal emphysema of the lungs may be seen, but these are more common in strangulation and suffocation. The lungs may be pale if the obstruction occurred at the end of inspiration or they may be edematous and exude dark fluid blood on cut section if the obstruction occurred at the end of expiration (**Figure 17.15**).

The right side of the heart, pulmonary artery and vena cava are full of dark fluid blood, while the left side of the heart is usually empty.

The abdominal organs are congested in most cases. The brain may be normal or even pale in cases of complete cerebral ischemia. However, it may be intensely congested in cases of pure venous congestion.

Local Internal Findings

Dissection of the neck is carried out after examining the cranial, thoracic and abdominal cavities. This prevents artefacts due to seepage of blood from the neck vessels and also offers a bloodless field of dissection. This was first observed by Schrader in 1940, who suggested that the brain be removed from the cranium and the heart be examined before examining the neck structures.

The preferred incision is a V-shaped one, with the limbs starting from the mastoid regions

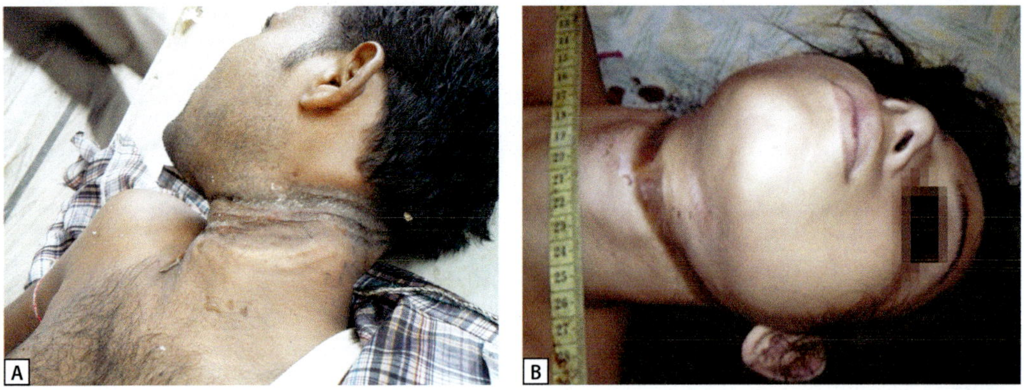

Figures 17.14A and B Oblique, non-continuous ligature marks around the neck

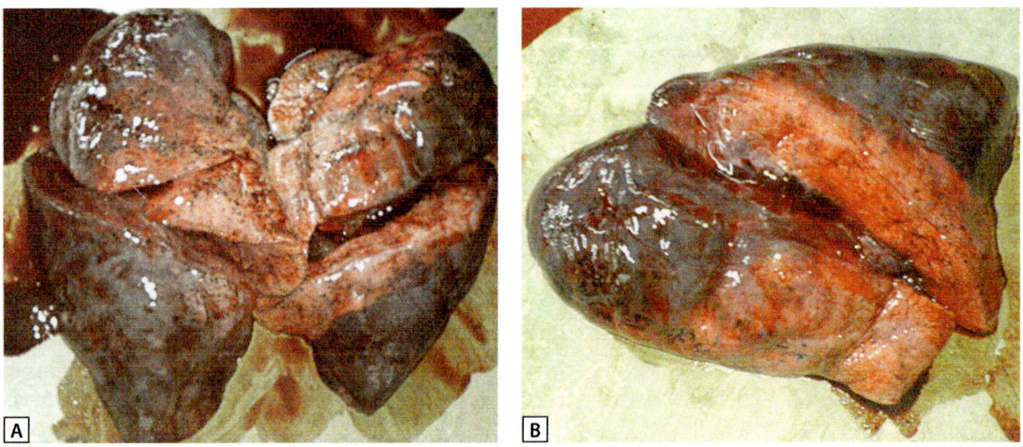

Figures 17.15A and B Congested lungs

and continuing to meet at the sternum. The skin is then carefully reflected, commencing from the apex of the 'V,' and a layer by layer dissection is done. Directly under the external mark, the subcutaneous tissue is condensed due to the pressure and looks dry, white and glistening. This is more marked if the body has been suspended for a long time. The epiglottis and tracheal mucosa is usually red and congested and rarely show tears.

In cases where there is a long drop, as in judicial hanging or when the victim jumps from a height, there may be much damage to the neck structures. The platysma and sternomastoid may be ruptured. The inner or middle coats of the carotid arteries may be ruptured and there may be extravasations of blood into the walls. There may be fracture and dislocation of the upper cervical vertebrae (commonly $C_{2\text{-}3}$, sometimes $C_{3\text{-}4}$ and rarely $C_{1\text{-}2}$) with tearing of the spinal cord. The cornu of the thyroid cartilage or the hyoid bone may be fractured, though rarely (**Figure 17.16**). All these features are observed only when there has been a substantial and violent jerk.

Microscopic and histological examination of skin and tissues may show tissue reaction, more prominently if death is prolonged.

Medicolegal Questions Related to Hanging

i. Whether the hanging was antemortem or postmortem?
ii. Whether the hanging was suicidal, homicidal or accidental?

Whether the Hanging was Antemortem or Postmortem?

Occasionally, a person may be killed and the body suspended to simulate suicidal hanging. It is important to know the actual cause of death in a suspended body. This can be assessed by examining the dead body and the scene of occurrence and critically evaluating the circumstances of the death.

Presence of a ligature mark alone does not indicate antemortem hanging, as this can also be a cadaveric phenomenon. Dribbling of saliva from the angle of the mouth is probably the most reliable sign of antemortem hanging. **Le facie sympathique** is also considered a sign of antemortem hanging. Other signs like rupture of the intima of the carotid arteries with extravasation of blood into its walls, epiglottis congestion, seminal emission and absence

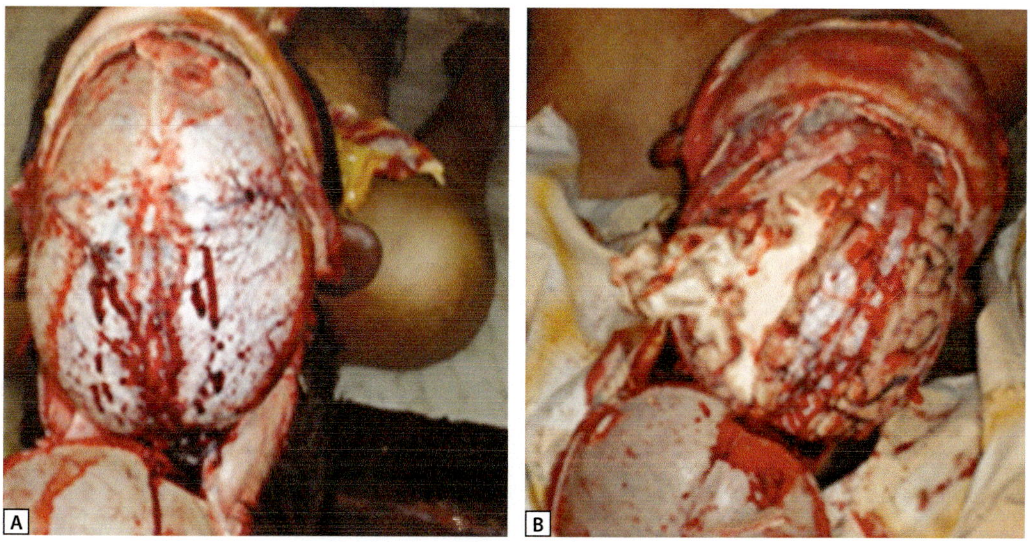

Figures 17.16A and B Congested brains

of any other fatal injury or poisoning are also important.

Examination of the scene of occurrence is important in assessing whether the hanging was ante or postmortem. Friction marks on the ligature material at the point of suspension and the direction of its fibers will indicate whether the body had been pulled up by someone else or it had dropped by its own weight. Similarly, a drag mark on the ground would indicate the possibility of a dead body being dragged by someone and then suspended.

Whether the Hanging was Suicidal, Homicidal or Accidental?

Hanging, as a rule, is usually suicidal, as it is presumed to be a painless means of committing suicide. Suicidal hanging has been observed even in blind persons and in extremes of ages. Circumstantial evidence plays an important role in deciding whether the hanging was suicidal, homicidal or accidental.

In suicidal hanging, the victim usually chooses an isolated place, but if it is a room, then the doors may be bolted from inside. Female victims in India usually take great care to dress themselves properly and securely prior to the attempt. Similarly, other articles may be found at the scene that would indicate preparedness by the victim for suicide. Approachability to a point of suspension and a suitable platform are points to be kept in mind. A suicide note may be recovered (**Figure 17.17**).

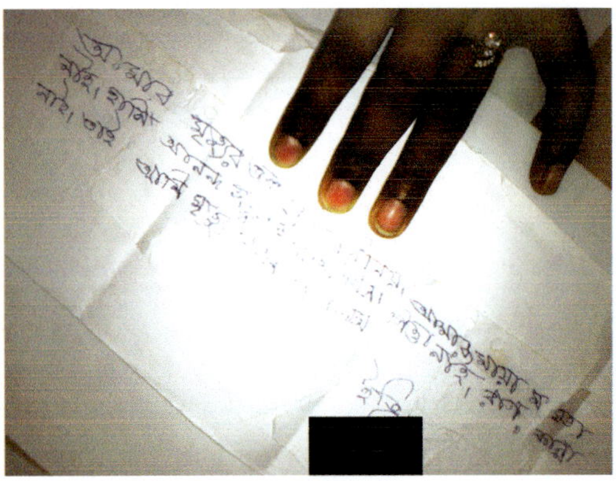

Figure 17.17 Suicidal notes in a case of suicidal hanging

Homicidal hanging is a rare phenomenon. Usually, more than one person is required to hang a conscious and healthy individual. However, if the victim is weak, intoxicated or a small child, then a single person may be enough. Footprints of multiple persons may be present at the scene. Signs of resistance by the victim like nail scratches, minor injuries, tearing of clothes, disturbed scene or drag marks will give rise to suspicion of homicidal hanging. Doors may be open or bolted from outside, it is also be possible that the victim may first be strangulated and then hanged.

Lynching

Lynching is a form of homicidal hanging by a mob. Lynching was practiced in the Southern American states where an angry mob used to snatch the accused person and hang him from a tree. This kind of homicidal hanging was resorted to when a black committed sexual assault on a white girl.

Accidental hanging may sometimes occur in children at play. A child may slip off a staircase and get hanged between its railings. Similar hangings may occur when a baby slips through the side rails of a cot. Children have been reported to have hanged to death while simulating judicial hanging at play.

Sexual Asphyxia

In some people sexual gratification is enhanced by producing mild asphyxia. Accidental death might occur during such sessions. The unfortunate victim, usually a male, may use various means to produce asphyxia, but the most common means is to pass a ligature around the neck and tie the free end to a higher point in such a way that lowering the head would produce mild asphyxiation. This is also known as **auto-erotic hanging.** The victim is usually naked with pornographic material found around him. The doors are closed from inside and curtains drawn. Some soft material, like handkerchief or towel may be present between the ligature and the neck.

STRANGULATION

Definition

Strangulation is a form of death where there is constriction of the neck, by a ligature or any other material, without suspension of the body.

Types of Strangulation

i. Ligature strangulation
ii. Manual strangulation by hands (throttling)
iii. Garroting (ligature strangulation by approaching the victim from behind)
iv. Mugging (compression of neck by elbow, foot or wrist)
v. Bansdola (compression of neck by means of sticks)
vi. Accidental strangulation.

Causes of Death in Strangulation

A combination of asphyxia and venous congestion is the usual cause of death in strangulation. Vagal shock may occur in cases of manual strangulation. In some cases, death may result from cerebral ischemia. Injury to the cervical vertebrae is rare.

Postmortem Findings

External Findings

Ligature mark is well defined, horizontal, situated below the thyroid cartilage and encircles the neck completely. **Multiple ligature marks**, each subsequent more prominent than the previous, is suggestive of homicidal strangulation (**Figure 17.18**).

Sometimes the ligature mark may be oblique and upwards if the victim had been dragged by the ligature. It may be faint or absent if a soft material has been used and released quickly after death. The transverse ligature marks with fingertip bruises and nail scratch abrasions (**Figure 17.19**) over the neck is homicidal.

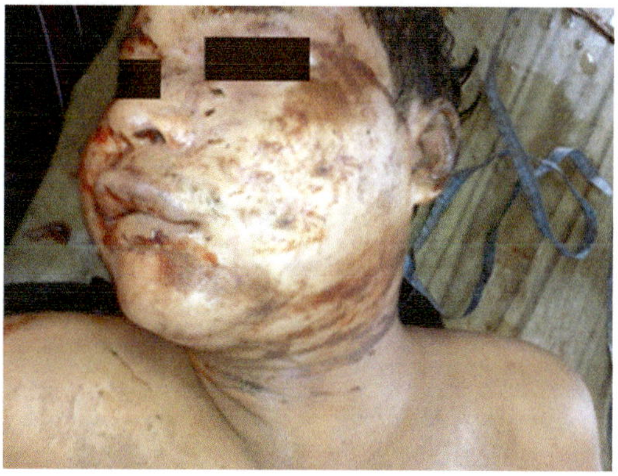

Figure 17.18 Multiple ligature marks with contusions and abrasions

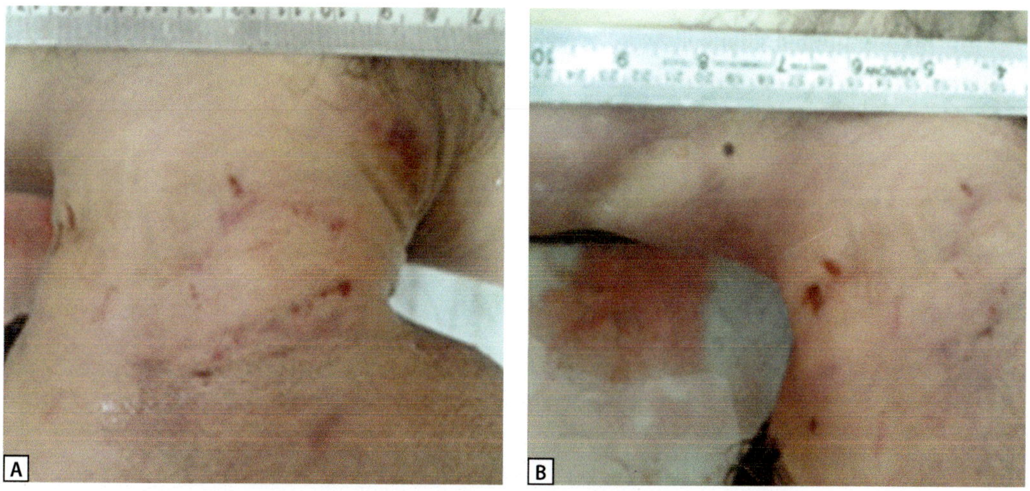

Figures 17.19A and B Faint ligature marks with fingertip bruises and nail scratch abrasions
(*Courtesy:* Dr Mrinal Haloi, Gauhati Medical College, Guwahati)

However, presence of fibers of the ligature material on the neck will indicate strangulation. A transparent adhesive tape may be used to lift these fibers off the neck for examination; Scratch abrasions may be seen under the ligature, indicating that the victim had struggled to remove the ligature. Fingernail scrapings of the victim may show skin fragments and blood (**Figure 17.20**).

In manual strangulation, multiple fingertip bruises may be present over the neck, usually along the windpipe, depending on whether one or both hands were used by the assailant. The various sized contusions of fingertip around the neck muscles (**Figure 17.21**) more towards the nape of the neck are homicidal.

There may be presence of crescentic nail abrasions over the neck. Distribution and number of fingertip bruises and nail abrasions in relation to the thumb with the fingers will not indicate whether one or both hands were used and also the handedness of the assailant.

If two sticks are used to compress the neck, as in **Bansdola**, there will be horizontal marks on the front and nape of the neck. Severe internal injuries are also common in such cases.

Internal Findings

The neck structures are examined after examination of the cranial and thoracic cavities. The subcutaneous tissue below the fingertip bruises and ligature mark will show extravasations of blood. There may be laceration of the carotid arteries and their internal coats with extravasation of blood into their walls. Fractures of the cornu of hyoid bones and superior cornu of thyroid cartilages may be observed (**Figure 17.22**). The fractures are usually common above the age of 40 years.

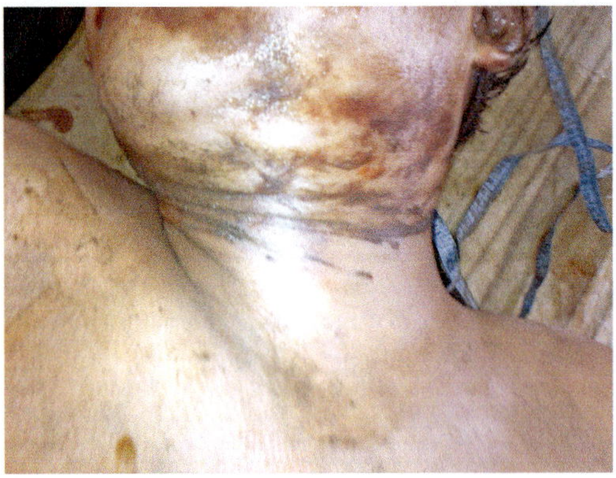

Figure 17.20 Faint transverse ligature marks with finger tip bruises and nail scratch abrasions

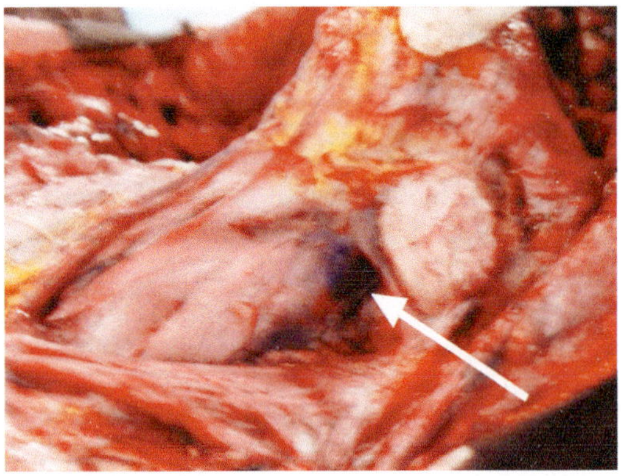

Figure 17.21 Contusion of muscles of the neck

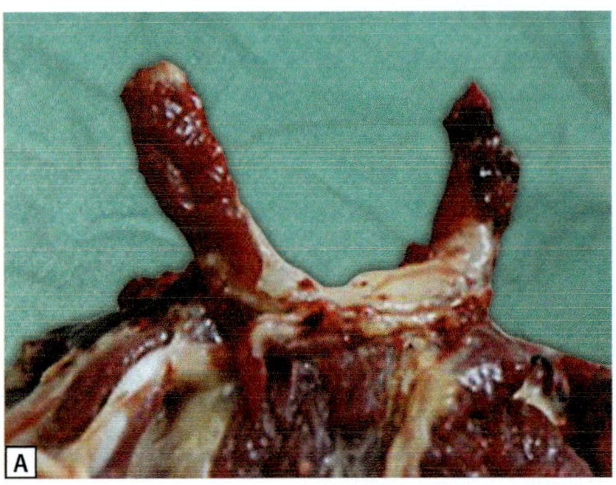

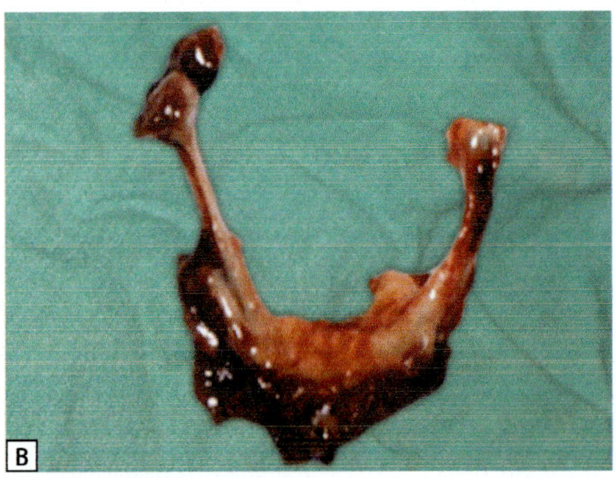

Figures 17.22A and B Fracture hyoid bone

The upper respiratory tract usually contains frothy blood and is congested. The lungs are congested with petechiae and exude dark fluid blood on cut section. The right side of the heart is full of dark fluid blood and the left side is empty. The brain and abdominal organs are congested.

Medicolegal Questions Related to Strangulation

i. Whether death was caused by strangulation?
ii. Whether strangulation was suicidal, homicidal or accidental?

Whether Death was due to Strangulation?

Injury to the neck structures as a result of violence and evidence of the use of a ligature material or other means will indicate death due to strangulation. Mere presence or absence of a ligature mark is not a conclusive proof of death due to strangulation, as skin folds and necktie, etc. may also look like ligature marks.

Whether Strangulation was Suicidal, Homicidal or Accidental?

Strangulation is commonly homicidal. Suicidal throttling is not possible as the victim cannot sustain pressure for duration sufficient to cause death by compression of the neck. However, a ligature tied around the neck and twisted to tightness by a stick below the mandible, may cause suicidal death by ligature strangulation.

In homicidal strangulation, the ligature is usually tied with one turn and one or multiple knots may be present. When there are multiple turns, each turn will be tighter than the previous one. There may be evidence of struggle, injuries, violence, intoxication or the hands and feet may be tied.

Accidental strangulation may occur sometimes as in cases of neck tie or dupatta getting caught in moving machine parts or between spokes of a moving wheel. Tightening of the umbilical cord around the neck of an infant may cause its death in utero or during childbirth.

SUFFOCATION

Definition

Suffocation is a form of death resulting from exclusion of atmospheric air from the lungs without constriction of the neck.

Suffocation can be caused by the following:

Smothering

Smothering occurs due to closure of the mouth and nostrils. Weak adults and children are sometimes smothered by using the palm, pillows or clothes (**Figure 17.23**) or hands (**Figure 17.24**). Smothering used to be a common means of committing infanticide in India.

Suffocation due to '**overlaying**' by the mother may kill an infant whose mouth and nostrils are blocked by the breasts of the mother during feeding. Suffocation can also occur due to plastic bags covering the head. It has been reported in substance abusers, who sniff or inhale toxic vapors. It is important to search the scene of occurrence for acetone, benzene, naphtha, toluene or other substances of abuse.

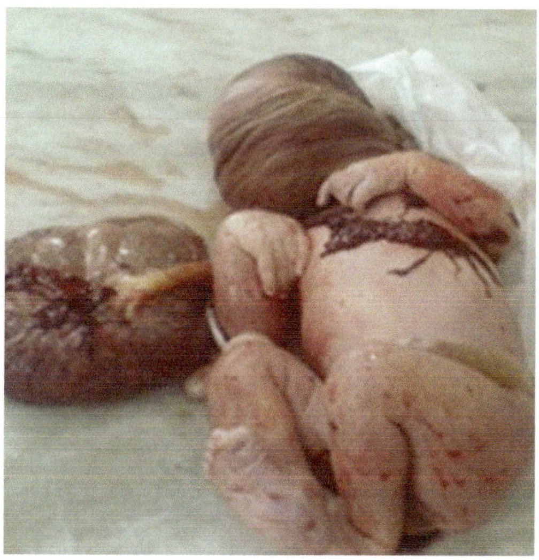

Figure 17.23 Smothering of newborn by using cloth

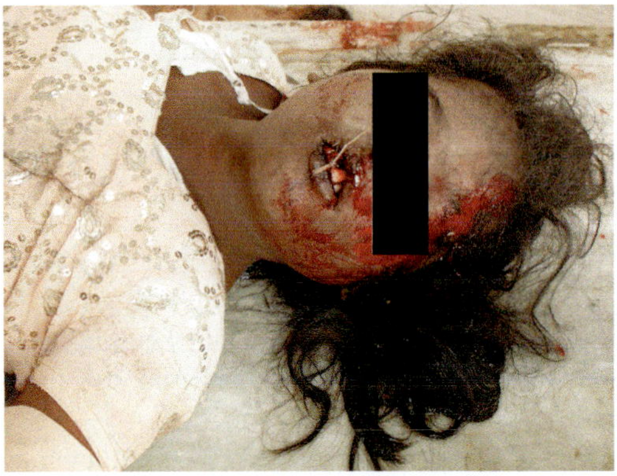

Figure 17.24 Smothering by using hand

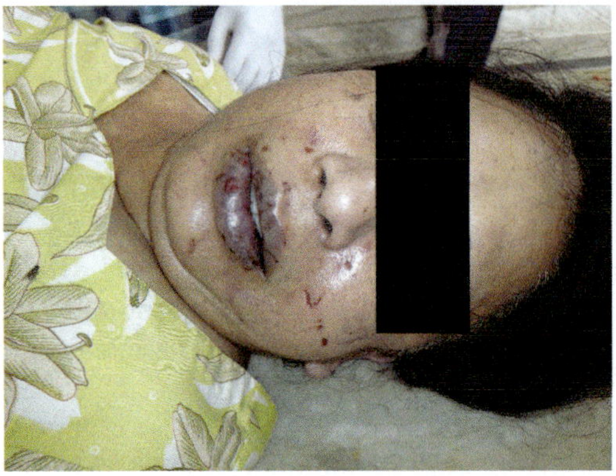

Figure 17.26 Multiple bruises and lacerations over the lips

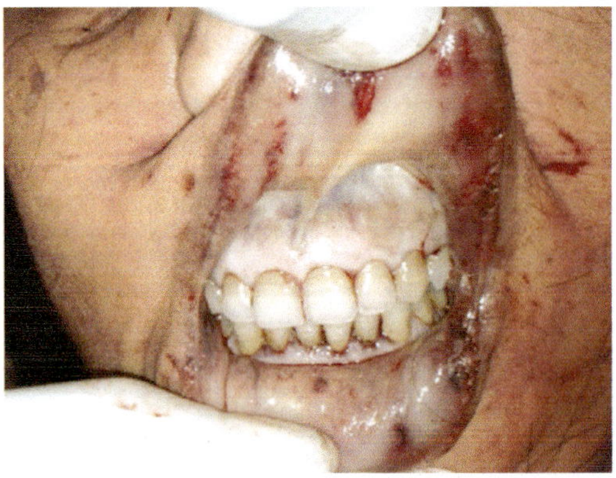

Figure 17.25 Multiple bruises, lacerations in the inner part of the lips

Smothering by using hand may leave multiple bruises and laceration around the mouth and inner part of lips as shown in **Figures 17.25** and **17.26**.

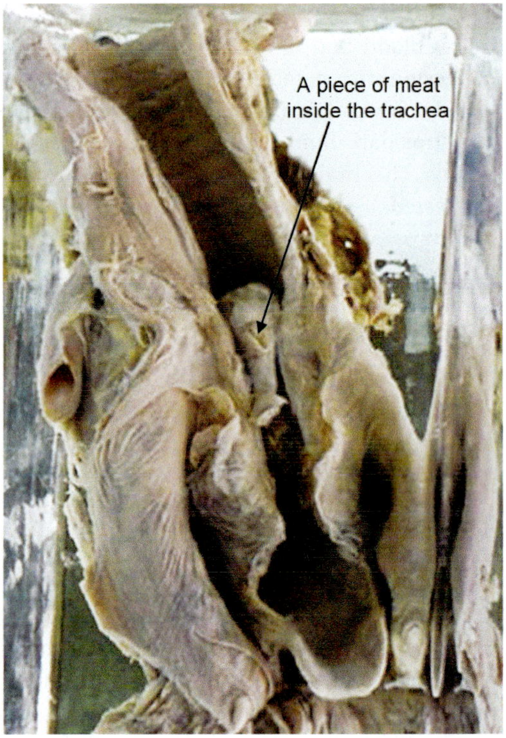

Figure 17.27 Choking due to obstruction of air passages from foreign bodies

Choking

Choking occurs due to obstruction of air passages from within. Foreign bodies (**Figure 17.27**) impaction, food or vomitus (**Figure 17.28**) particles, tumor, roundworms or bleeding caused as a result of complication of tracheotomy operation (**Figure 17.29**) can cause choking.

'**Café coronary**' is the term used to describe choking by a bolus of food, especially meat, in persons intoxicated with alcohol. The features include sudden breathlessness, restlessness and cyanosis and may appear like an attack of angina. Heimlich maneuver is employed to relieve choking in such cases.

Traumatic Asphyxia

This occurs due to fixation of the chest by pressure, thus restricting respiratory movements. Traumatic asphyxia may occur in victims

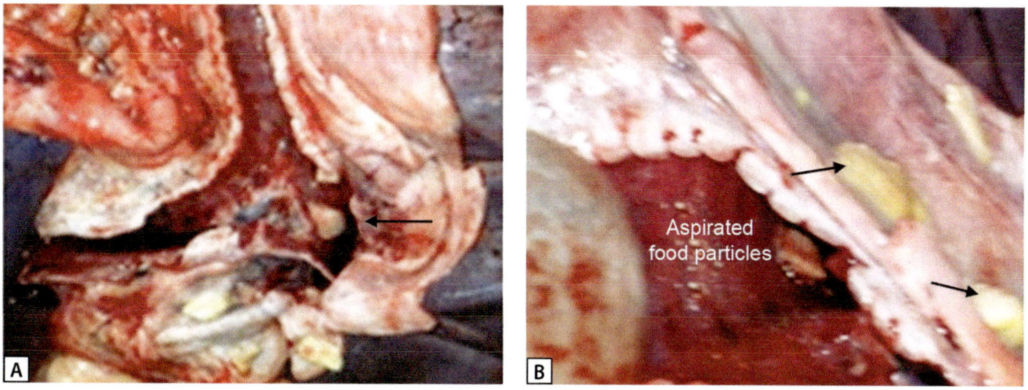

Figures 17.28A and B Food and vomitus particles in the air passage

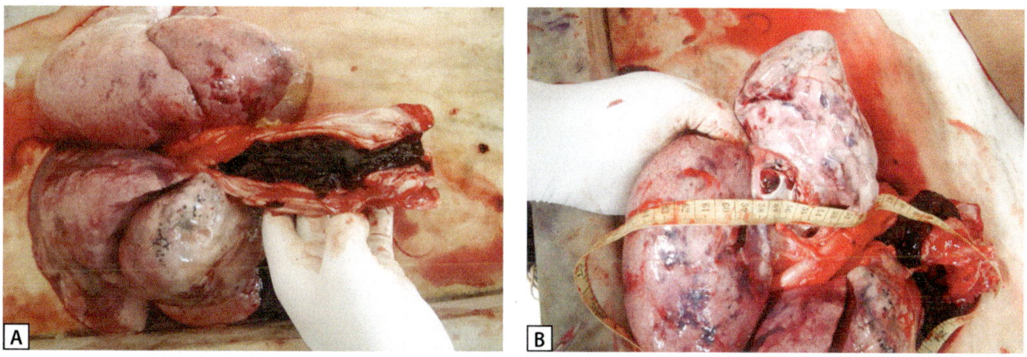

Figures 17.29A and B Choking due to obstruction of air passages from blood
(*Courtesy:* Dr Raktim Pratim Tamuli, TMC, Assam)

trapped under debris during earthquakes or in motor mechanics due to slippage of a jack and resting of the vehicle on the victim's chest. Asphyxial features are characteristically marked above the level of the pressure area.

In traumatic asphyxia, besides the signs of asphyxia there may be chest injuries (**Figure 17.30**) in the form of contusions and abrasion, etc.

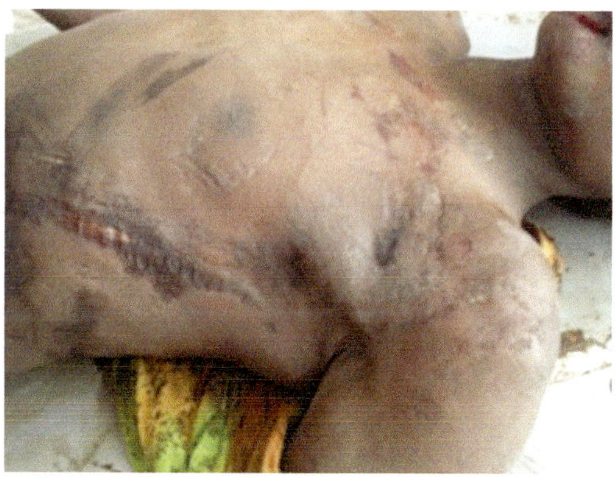

Figure 17.30 Chest injuries as a result of traumatic asphyxia

Inhalation of Irrespirable Gases

Smoke, carbon dioxide and carbon monoxide are the commonest offending agents.

Gagging

A soft material like cloth or paper is thrust into the throat of the victim, thus preventing air entry into the lungs. The postmortem findings consist of signs of asphyxia with abrasion of palate with edema of pharynx. Gag may be present inside the mouth.

Burking

Burke and Hare used a special technique to kill their victims for supplying dead bodies for anatomical dissections. The victim was thrown on the ground and the chest was compressed by kneeling over it, while the mouth and nostrils were closed simultaneously. Thus, this is a combination of smothering and traumatic asphyxia.

DROWNING

Definition

Drowning is a form of death in which atmospheric air is prevented from entering the respiratory passages due to submersion in a fluid medium.

Complete submersion is not necessary. Drowning can occur in very shallow water when only the mouth and nostrils are submerged. This is possible in intoxicated or epileptic individuals and infants.

Types of Drowning

1. **Wet Drowning (Primary Drowning)**: Inhaled fluid enters the lungs and fills up the air space. Wet drowning may occur in:
   a. **Fresh water**: In this case water from the lungs is absorbed into the bloodstream due to the osmotic gradient, resulting in hemodilution and hypervolemia. This will result in severe electrolyte disturbance, alveolar collapse, cardiac arrhythmia and death in a few minutes.
   b. **Sea water**: Body fluids are lost through the lungs, resulting in hypovolemia and hemoconcentration. There is pulmonary edema, electrolyte disturbances and bradycardia, resulting in death.
2. **Dry Drowning**: Fluid does not enter the lungs, but few drops of fluid entering the nasopharynx and larynx cause sustained laryngeal spasm.
3. **Secondary Drowning (Near Drowning, Post-immersion Syndrome)**: Death may occur due to delayed causes like aspirated foreign bodies, pneumonia, cerebral anoxia, electrolyte imbalance or metabolic acidosis.
4. **Immersion Syndrome (Hydrocution, Cold Water Drowning)**: Sudden fall into cold water or striking the abdomen or chest on the water surface, in inexperienced divers, may cause vagal stimulation, resulting in reflex cardiac inhibition and sudden death.

The Event of Drowning

A person who cannot swim will first sink to the bottom and then rises to the surface due to the buoyancy of air in the lungs. The breath is held instinctively. On rising to the surface, he inhales deeply and may take in some water; violent cough with forceful exhalation will result in inhalation of more water. He may sink to the bottom and rise to the surface repeatedly, drawing in more water each time, until his lungs are filled with water. He finally sinks to the bottom and becomes unconscious. There may be convulsions and memory panoramic views of past incidences preceding death. The hands are clenched in cadaveric spasm as the victim tries to grasp whatever is available within reach. Often, mud weeds and other aquatic material are held firmly in the clenched fists, thus providing proof of drowning.

In still water, the body remains at the bottom for about 24 hours. Rigor mortis develops and passes off. The body then floats to the surface due to the formation of gases of decomposition. As per '*Casper's dictum*', the rate of decomposition reduces to half for the duration of immersion in water and doubles once it is exposed to air. A body usually floats face downwards with the limbs and head submerged.

Causes of Death in Drowning

i. **Asphyxia**: This is the commonest cause. Death is due to cerebral anoxia.
ii. **Vagal Shock**: Occurs in people striking their abdomen and chest against the water surface. Very cold water can cause dyspnea in the thin and hypothermia in the obese.

iii. **Apoplexy**: Cerebral vessels may get ruptured due to excitement or struggle.
iv. **Concussion**: The head may strike against a solid surface or even the surface of water with great force
v. **Syncope**: May occur in flail individuals due to fall in cold water.
vi. **Exhaustion**: Attempts at trying to keep above the surface in non-swimmers may result in fatal exhaustion.
vii. **Injuries**: Injury may result from falling into shallow water and striking a hard surface. There may be fractures of the skull or cervical vertebrae.

Fatal Period

Even deep sea divers cannot hold their breath for more than 2 minutes. Asphyxia supervenes in about 2 minutes and the heart stops after few minutes. Resuscitation attempts fail after about 5 minutes of submersion. However, if vagal shock or syncope has occurred, resuscitation is possible even after 10–20 minutes.

The period of survival will depend on many factors. Individuals with more body fat will survive longer as fat increases the buoyancy as well as acts as an insulator in cold water. When the temperature of the water is below 10°C, survival is reduced to less than 3 hours, even in well-clothed persons with life jackets.

When death is delayed beyond 20 minutes and up to 4 days due to complications, it is termed as **post-immersion syndrome** or **near drowning.**

It is presumed that death occurs in 4–5 minutes in fresh water and 8–10 minutes in sea water. This has, however, been criticized by many workers.

Treatment

Resuscitation is almost impossible when the lungs are completely clogged with water. The commencement of resuscitation attempt should be immediate. The mouth and nostrils are wiped to remove mud, sand, weeds, etc. The victim should then be turned face downwards, with the head at a lower level than the feet. This helps to keep the mouth open and tongue drawn forwards, while allowing the water to flow out of the upper respiratory passages.

The victim is then quickly turned face upwards, the clothes removed, body dried with a towel and wrapped in warm blankets. Artificial respiration should be promptly resorted to if spontaneous respiration is absent. Sips of warm fluids may be given, once spontaneous respiration is established and the victim is conscious. Antibiotics and oxygen inhalation play a great role in preventing pneumonia.

Postmortem Appearance

External Findings

The body and clothes are wet, if examined early. Mud, sand and aquatic material may be found on the clothes, hair and face. The face is usually pale, eyes closed and conjunctiva congested.

Copious amount of fine, white, tenacious, lathery froth is present at the mouth and nostrils. The froth will reappear again and again, when it is wiped off or when pressure is applied over the chest. Occasionally the froth may be blood-tinged.

Aquatic material like grass, weeds, gravel, twigs or leaves may be found in the fists, clenched in cadaveric spasm. The fingertips may show abrasions, and there may be presence of mud and sand on the fingers.

Cutis anserina (goose skin appearance) is the puckered appearance of the skin when drowning has occurred in cold water. This is due to the contraction of the erector pili muscles from cold and subsequent rigor mortis. It is usually found over the anterior aspect of the body and the limbs. It can also be a postmortem phenomenon, before molecular death has occurred. Thus, cutis anserina is of little significance.

'Washerwoman's hands and feet' (Figures 17.31A and B) appearance is due to bleaching, soddening and wrinkling of the skin of hands and feet when the body was in water for a considerable time. This phenomenon will also

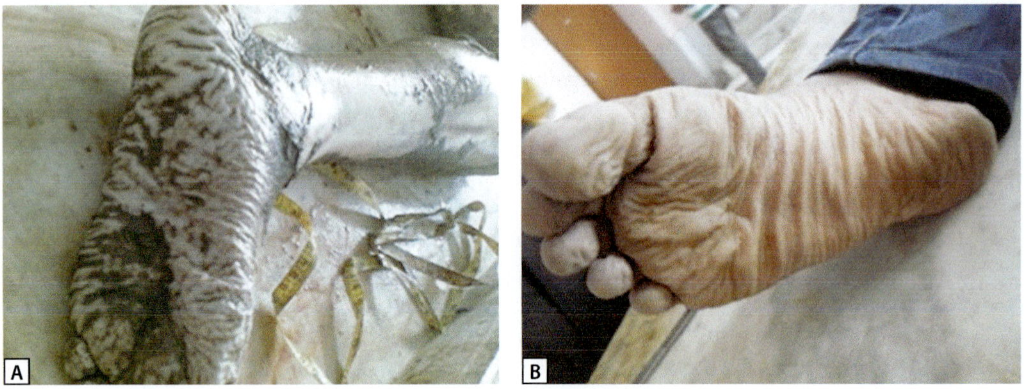

Figures 17.31A and B Washerwoman's feet

occur in a body thrown into water after death. Thus, this feature will only suggest that the body was lying in water for a prolonged period.

The scrotum and penis are usually contracted, especially in cold water. However, they may be swollen and turgid when the water is warm or when the body is removed from the water source.

Postmortem lividity is most marked in the head, neck, upper chest and limbs. This is due to the position in which the body floats. Rigor mortis occurs early in deaths due to exhaustion.

Internal Findings

The respiratory passages contain froth, watery fluid and aquatic debris. They may also contain regurgitated vomitus. Vomiting is caused by hypoxia of the brain and is drawn into the respiratory passages during forceful efforts to breathe.

On removal of the sternum, the lungs balloon out of the thoracic cavity. They are pale gray with reddish tints. The lungs are voluminous, edematous, doughy, pit on pressure and are indented by the ribs. Dark, frothy, blood-stained fluid exudes on cut section. There are patches of hemorrhages on the anterior aspect and margins of the lungs subpleurally. These are known as **Paltauf's hemorrhages**, caused due to rupture of alveoli during forceful expiration, thus indicating great struggle. Combination of all the above features is termed as '**emphysema aqueous**.' In unconscious victims, the lungs are simply filled with water, without froth in the respiratory passages. This is known as '**Edema aquosum**.'

The right heart and great veins are full of dark blood. This occurs due to obstruction of pulmonary circulation, caused by inhalation of water. Blood remains fluid because of dilution by inhaled water.

Water may be present in the stomach as a result of swallowing during struggle. This water may contain mud, sand, weeds and algae that match with those present in the source of drowning. However, it is possible that the victim drank water from the source, before entering it. It is also possible that water swallowed into the stomach may be forced out due to pressure of gases of decomposition. Sometimes, water may be found in the small intestine, and this is a reliable sign of antemortem drowning, as water from the stomach can reach the small intestine only by peristalsis, which is a vital process.

Hemorrhages in the middle ear and mastoid air cells have been reported and are presumed to be caused by barotrauma. However, such hemorrhages are also found in other types of death and are, thus, unreliable.

Histological Examination

Tissue from central and peripheral areas of each lobe of the lungs should be taken for histological examination along with tissue from kidneys, liver and cardiac muscles. Microscopic examination will reveal signs of acute oxygen deficiency. Histological findings in the lungs include alveolar dilatation, thinning of alveolar septa and compression of alveolar capillaries and areas of alveolar rupture.

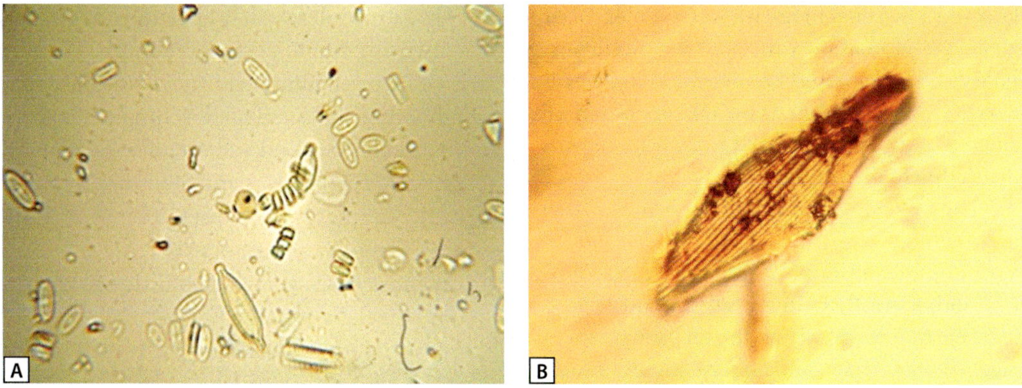

Figures 17.32A and B Some commonly found diatoms

Tests for Drowning

i. Gettler's test
ii. Diatom test

Gettler's Test

Alexander O Gettler (1921) studied the chloride content of blood from the right and left sides of the heart. Normally, it is about 600 mg per deciliter (dL) in both sides. He suggested that when the difference of chloride content in both sides is 25 mg per dL or more, it will indicate death due to drowning. He also found that the chloride content of blood from the left side of the heart is lower in fresh-water drowning and the reverse in sea-water drowning.

Diatom Test

Ravenstorf (1904) was the first to use the diatom test to diagnose death due to drowning.

Diatoms are unicellular algae with an outer coating of silica. This silica coat makes the diatoms resistant to heat, acids and putrefaction. They are found in all kinds of water bodies, where is enough sunlight to support photosynthesis. There are about 15,000 species of diatoms. They vary in size from 2 microns to 1 millimeter. They can be spindle-shaped, dumbbell-shaped, triangular, circular, etc. (**Figure 17.32**).

When a drowning person inhales water into the lungs, diatoms of size up to 60 microns can gain entry into the circulation via the ruptured alveoli. These diatoms can get deposited in distant organs like liver, brain or bone marrow. During postmortem examination, bone marrow is collected from a long bone (usually femur). This bone marrow is examined for the presence of diatoms after chemical digestion by acids, when all organic matter are digested.

The diatoms, being resistant to acids, remain intact and are seen by microscopic examination. Presence of diatoms in distant organs is considered as the surest sign of antemortem drowning, because diatoms can reach these organs only when the person is alive and the circulation is in progress. The diatoms are then compared with those found in the water sample collected from the source to confirm that the victim had drowned in that water body.

Medicolegal Questions in Case of Drowning

i. Whether death was caused due to drowning?
ii. Whether drowning was suicidal, homicidal or accidental?
iii. How long was the body in water?

Whether Death was Caused due to Drowning?

Sometimes a person may be killed by other means and the body be thrown into water. In a country like India, where there is an abundance of rivers, the poor inhabitants of river banks, at times, dispose of dead bodies into rivers after keeping a live coal in the mouth as an excuse for elaborate cremation rituals. These bodies may float downstream and be recovered many miles away. It cannot, therefore, be presumed that since a body was recovered from water, it was a death due to drowning.

The following points will confirm death due to drowning:

i. Copious amount of fine, white, tenacious, lathery froth at the mouth and nostrils.
ii. Froth present within the air passages.
iii. Water-logged and bulky lungs, exuding frothy, blood-tinged fluid on cut section.
iv. Presence of water containing mud, weeds, etc. in the stomach and small intestine.
v. Aquatic material held in cadaveric spasm between clenched fists.
vi. Positive diatom test.

Whether Drowning was Suicidal, Homicidal or Accidental?

Drowning is usually accidental, sometimes suicidal and rarely homicidal. Homicidal drowning is possible only in infants, small children and intoxicated persons.

Marks of violence may be found on the body of the victim due to accidental injury. The site, size and type of injury will give a fair idea as to whether they are accidental or homicidal. If the hands and feet are tied and weights are attached to the body in such a manner that it is not possible by the victim himself, then homicidal drowning should be suspected.

In most cases of accidental drowning, the victim is usually minimally clothed or wearing a swimsuit. A well-clothed body with shoes, wrist watch, etc. may give rise to suspicion of accidental drowning by falling into the water source. Bodies found in shallow water will exclude accidental drowning, except in intoxicated or epileptic individuals.

How long was the Body in Water?

A body will float to the surface of water due to formation of gases of decomposition. In flowing waters, the body will float to the surface some distance away from the site of drowning. This happens in about 24 hours in tropical waters.

CHAPTER 18

Anesthetic Procedures and Death

CB Jani, Putul Mahanta

LEARNING PLAN

- Learn about the classification of anesthetic deaths
- Identify the types of anesthesia used in surgical procedure
- Learn about death due to general anesthesia
- Know the medicolegal investigation of a case of "death on table"

BRIEF REVIEW

Since introduction of anesthetic agents in facilitating surgical procedures, it has been established as a boon. But, occasionally, it has turned out to be bane for treating doctors and even patient. Biomedical researchers have shown a reasonable concern in preventing and treating perioperative complications, whether surgical or anesthetic in nature or origin.

Incidences with reference to such complications (even death) vary with time and type of health care institutions. Lunn and Mushin[1] estimated the mortality directly related to anesthesia to be 1 in 166 in the year 1982. In subsequent years, it was reported to be 5-6 deaths/million anesthetic administrations.[2] Most current estimates of perioperative mortality range from 1 death in 53 anesthetics to 1 in 5,417 anesthetics.[3,4]

Such decline have been attributed to introduction of better monitoring devices, (i.e. multipara monitor-displaying indicators like pulse oxymetry, blood pressure, SpO_2, ECG and $EtCO_2$) of course coupled with better training of operative team members. However, to screen out "**exclusive anesthetic death**" among perioperative events may have many inherent limitations. For example, in case of death of a patient not having reasonable prognosis, hospital authorities (or even relatives of deceased!) may not opt for further investigation leaving no opportunity for recognizing anesthetic complication, if any. By and large, it shall be safe to conclude that such complications take place at larger scale than actually reported, at least in developing countries like India. Any scientific exchange of relevant aspects of such deaths pivot around reported experiences only.

CLASSIFICATION OF ANESTHETIC DEATHS

Gordon and Shaprio classified the anesthetic deaths into two broad groups:[5]

i. During the administration of anesthesia but not related to anesthesia.
ii. Death which are direct result of administration of anesthesia.

In first group, deaths are due to injury/disease which necessitated the surgical procedure, any other injury/disease diagnosed or even undiagnosed at the time of surgical procedures (undiagnosed one may be detected at autopsy only) and some complication of exclusive surgical nature. The second group includes deaths due to general, respiratory, cardiovascular or other systemic events.

In case of "**On-table**" complication/death, differentiation between these two groups is of prime significance. Usually, absences of objective evidence of features of group one shall raise suspicion of group two (exclusive anesthetic complication). Before further discussion, it is desirable to review pharmacology of commonly used substances used during procedures.

TYPES OF ANESTHESIA USED IN SURGICAL PROCEDURE[6]

Preanesthetic Medication

i. Pentazocine (fortwin)—opioid
ii. Butorphenol—opioid
iii. Tramadol—synthetic opioids
iv. Midazolam—benzodiazepine
v. Dynapar—NSAIDs.

Mechanism of Action

Anesthetic agent potentiates the action of inhibitory transmitter GABA to open Cl^- channels. Whatever may be the pathways, common adverse effects are either respiratory or cardiac in origin in the form of depression or dysfunction. The common agent and their side effects are shown in **Table 18.1**.

Table 18.1 Common agents and their effects

Type of anesthesia	Commonly used drugs	Side effects
General anesthesia	**For induction** Propofol: Used in form of oily liquid, superior than thiopentone sodium	Apnea lasting about 1 minute, fall of BP due to vasodilatation, bradycardia, pain during injection
	Thiopentone sodium (ultra short acting)	Intra-arterial injection produces pain, necrosis, gangrene; transient respiratory and cardiovascular depression
	For maintenance Halothane	Reduced cardiac activity, respiratory depression, abolishes pharyngeal and laryngeal reflexes, malignant hyperthermia in genetically determined cases
	Isoflurane	Increases heart rate, but not arrhythmogenic, respiratory depression
	Sevoflurane	Safe but degraded by sodalime and hence cannot be used in closed circuit
Short general anesthesia	Ketamine	Pharyngeal and laryngeal reflexes not abolishes, emergence delirium, hallucination and involuntary movement
	Propofol	Apnea lasting about 1 minute, bradycardia
	Midazolam	Non-irritating, shorter acting, used for intubation
Spinal anesthesia	Lignocaine heavy	Neurological side effects, respiratory arrest, coma
	Bupivacaine heavy	Prolonged QTc interval, cardiac depression
Epidural anesthesia	Plain lignocaine, bupivacaine plain	Larger amount required, less neurological complications
Local anesthesia	Plain lignocaine, bupivacaine plain	Shorter duration with immediate onset, larger amount required, motor functions not affected

Muscle Relaxant Used for Intubation[6]

Atracurium, vecuronium, pancuronium (almost obsolete) are long-acting agents. Succinyl choline is short-acting muscle relaxant used for intubation. Toxicity of muscle relaxants includes respiratory paralysis; fall in blood pressure, especially, in hypovolemic patient, cardiac arrhythmias and precipitation of asthma.

CAUSES OF DEATH DUE TO GENERAL ANESTHESIA

i. Overdose of anesthetic agent.
ii. Anesthesia to wrong patients.
iii. Wrong connection to gas machine, which may cause unexpected mixture of dangerous gases.
iv. Death due to hypoxia due to respiratory depression, hypoventilation, excessive muscle relaxation, laryngeal spasm due to inhalation of vomitus, etc.
v. Precipitation of myocardial ischemia because of use of IV pentothal which is depressing to heart.
vi. Wrong posture of the body leads to paralysis of a limb or its part.
vii. Faulty anesthetic equipment.
viii. Failure to diagnose the impending danger during monitoring of the vital signs.
ix. Unknown etiology.

Medicolegal Approach in a Case of "Death on Table"

Clinical Records

First and foremost task is to look for factor of "expectedness" of death in form of severity evaluation of pre-existing disease or injury. Mortality rate is directly proportionate to ASA (American Society of Anesthesiologists) rating. In case of complication with ASA rating I and II, there are more chances of some sort of surgical or anesthetic complication as the "expectedness" of death stands far less. However, this does not mean that in cases with ASA rating III and above, there is no contribution of surgical or anesthetic intervention. On the contrary, careful interpretation of findings is desirable to quantify contribution of disease or injury vis-a-vis iatrogenic complication. Pre-operative clinical records can give initial idea of what exactly went wrong. It can surely direct the investigator in right direction without prejudice to any of the factor, whether contributing or not. The different ASA rating and mortality rate are mentioned in **Table 18.2**.

Medicolegal postmortem examination in such deaths is almost mandatory in Indian states. It is always necessary to study the clinical records prior to conduction of autopsy.

Following, among other, questions may be looked for into clinical records:

i. Whether there was some pre-existing disease or injury which may lead to death?

Table 18.2 ASA rating and mortality rate

ASA rating	Severity of patient	Mortality rate
I	A normally healthy individual	0.1
II	Mild systemic disease	0.2
III	Severe systemic disease that is not incapacitating	1.3
IV	Incapacitating systemic disease that is constant threat to life	7.8
V	Moribund patient who is not expected to survive 24 hours with or without operation	9.4
E	Emergency operation	

ii. If yes, were they different from ones which necessitated procedure?
iii. Whether choice of anesthetic agent was suitable in terms of substance, dosages, rate and route of administration and combination?
iv. What was the "turning point" in operative events evident on monitoring gazette? What sort of pathophysiological event might have led to death?
v. Any other objective evidence of surgical or anesthetic complication.

Autopsy Examination

i. Like the routine medicolegal autopsy, complete and careful examination of external and internal surfaces is rule. All therapeutic marks, e.g. venesection, tracheotomy, intracardiac injections marks shall be noted.
ii. Remove the dressings and note the nature and amount of blood, pus or any other body fluid soaking the dressing. Weight them if heavily soaked.
iii. Describe the surgical wounds regarding their position, length of incision, number and type of sutures, whether intact or not.
iv. Underwater puncture of intercostal space: In water-filled chest, soft tissue flap emitting bubbles indicate pneumothorax. It can occur with excessive pressure to the airway, with normal pressure in patient with pre-existing lung disease, use of nitrous oxide, etc.
v. Dissection of internal organs as per conventional methods shall be done. Internal airway examination may reveal laryngeal edema, damage to trachea, aspiration of blood, gastric contents (more common in under-anesthetized patients) or any other foreign material. Airway management is a crucial task as majority of the substances depresses reflexes, and any shortcoming in that may immediately lead to fatal event. For example, if endotracheal tube reaches stomach instead of trachea, subsequent oxygenation can lead to cerebral hypoxia, as brain will be deprived of oxygen. In such case, some endotracheal injury may be evident along with marked distension of stomach with gas. Cerebral hypoxia is a histopathological diagnosis (and that is also not easy to be made quantifying different stages)[7] in which, at autopsy, only signs of asphyxia may be present in form of cyanosis and pulmonary edema. Pre-existing bronchial asthma, hypersensitivity reaction, fluid overload and aspiration of gastric contents may lead to bronchiolar spasm, leading to respiratory failure, obvious as pulmonary edema at autopsy.
vi. Dissection of heart shall be followed by special examination for air embolism. Air bubbles on puncturing left ventricle in water-filled pericardial cavity indicates air embolism. Pyrogallol test is also recommended by some authors.[7] Minimal invasive surgeries with use of distention media may encounter such event. Tubal ligation after creating pneumoperitoneum, uterine fibroid removal by endoscopy using distension media, (e.g. glycine) and similar procedures may witness air embolism due to entry of gas/air under pressure entering circulation from resection sites. Multi-para monitor will reflect abnormal changes in such case. In addition, coronary narrowing, myocardial infarction, myocardial hypertrophy or valvular heart disease shall also be looked for. Presence of such cardiac pathology shall be correlated to ASA rating as well as findings in clinical records.
vii. Other internal organs may show congestion without any obvious findings, but the surgical site shall also be looked for any undesired damage which has potential of developing hemorrhage and shock.

Preservation of Viscera and Other Materials for Analysis

It is advisable to preserve viscera for chemical analysis, even though quantitative drug analysis may not available at FSL, as it helps in excluding qualitative impurities of drugs and, of course, as a protocol for labeling an autopsy a negative one. Some recent analytical tests, i.e. **D-Dimer** for embolism, DIC, **serum trypsin**[8] for anaphylaxis are also valuable guide, if facility permits. In addition to viscera, injection site and/or any implant left in situ also may be subjected to analysis, if felt necessary.

As far as routine histopathological analysis is concerned, representation from almost all the organs shall be kept in mind.

In addition to conventionally preserved organs, i.e. brain, heart, lungs, liver, kidney, etc. Various workers have recommended other tissues as well for toxicological examination (**Table 18.3**).

Special investigations like immune histochemistry and enzyme histochemistry may be explored at advance tertiary care center and considering its cost effectiveness and availability, only suitable limited tests are advocated. The same applies to postmortem chemistry of blood and other body fluids of different nature, where time since death is additional factor for interpretation of results. A brief list of findings in different tissue is narrated herewith in **Table 18.4.**

Table 18.3 List of samples to be preserved at autopsy

Samples	How to preserve
Alveolar air	Should be collected with a needle and syringe under water by pulmonary puncture before chest is opened
Both lungs ligated at trachea (at least one full lung ligated at bronchus)	Placed in a nylon bag and sealed immediately
Brain (at least 100 grams)	Saturated solution of common salt
CSF (in a case of spinal anesthesia)	Sub-occipital puncture, or less recommended—aspiration from the brain's ventricle system after removal of the skull, or via lumbar puncture in normal sterile vial
Fat (2 grams from mesentry)	Saturated solution of common salt
Skeletal muscle (10 grams)	Saturated solution of common salt
Liver, kidneys (at least 100 grams)	Saturated solution of common salt
Blood (should be collected in syringe under oil before opening body cavity)	**For culture:** Blood to be injected in blood culture bottle with adequately nutritive media like brain-heart infusion (BHI) broth, etc. **For serology:** Serum from clotted blood (whole blood without anticoagulant)
Exudates (bacteriological examination)	Amie's transport media/ thioglychollate broth or any other proper transport media
Tissue samples (HPE)	Preserved in a 10% solution of formaldehyde in water
Skin (From injection site)	Saturated solution of common salt
Urine	After collection immediately refrigerated
Gases from heart, blood vessels	Before cutting open under water
Blood grouping and cross matching of blood	Clotted vial/oxalate

Table 18.4 Correlation between HP findings

Organ/tissue	Findings	Indications
Brain	Cerebral hypoxia (stage 1–4)[7]	Inadequate oxygenation
Heart	Myocardial infarction, coronary thrombosis, VHD, etc.	Pre-existing lesion
	Left ventricular hypertrophy	Malignant hyperthermia
Lungs	Edema, inflammatory infiltrate, etc.	Respiratory distress due to fluid overload or other reason
Liver	Necrosis	Halothane induced
Kidneys	Necrosis	Halothane induced
Supra-renals	Depletion of lipid contents in cortex	Hypovolemia
Skeletal muscles	Metabolic degeneration	Malignant hyperthermia

Precautions during Collection of Blood Samples

i. The site of collection of blood must be clean, dry and sterile.
ii. All the equipment used in collection must be clean, dry and sterile.
iii. The blood sample must be collected on the wall of the tube to avoid the hemolysis.
iv. Gentle mixing of the blood sample with the anticoagulant.
v. Avoid contamination of the blood samples with hair or dirties.
vi. The blood sample must be transferred directly to the laboratory under suitable conditions.

Interpretation and Opinion

In absence of availability of recent analytical tests, i.e. histochemistry, special stains, etc. interpretation of clinical records, conventional sources, i.e. postmortem findings and histopathological report forms the basis of opinion. If recent investigations are undertaken, they may be considered over and above the conventional sources.

The aim of the exercise shall be to quantify the anesthesia as principal factor or participating (even contributing!) factor.

If the autopsy findings positively suggest some specific complication, task becomes easy. For example, hemorrhage, internal airway obstruction, pneumothorax, air embolism, etc., if demonstrated, can form scientific basis in a positive way. Histopathological findings in such case may be generalized in nature. Usually, such deaths are ones where anesthesia is only participating factor.

Obscure findings at autopsy usually indicate anesthesia as principal factor and results of various analytical tests are not more than corroborative ones. The reason being, "exclusive anesthetic deaths" are more of physiological nature, leaving behind trace or minimal evidences. Common pathophysiological events in such deaths are respiratory failure, circulatory failure, electrolyte disturbances, cardiac arrhythmias (or even arrest!), malignant hyperthermia, anaphylaxis, vasovagal shock, hypoxic brain damage, etc.

REFERENCES

1. Lunn JN, Mushin W. Mortality Associated with Anaesthesia. London: Nuffield Provincial Hospital Trust, 1982.
2. Rosenbergh Henry. Mortality associated with anaesthesia. Expert Article Library [cited 2012 Jun 30]; Available from: URL:http://www.expertpages.com/news/mortality_ anesthesia.htm
3. Lagasse RS. Anesthesia safety: Model or myth? A review of the published literature and analysis of current original data. Anesthesiology. 2002;97(6):1609-17.
4. Arbous MS, Meursing AE, van Kleef JW, de Lange JJ, Spoormans HH, Touw P, et al. Impact of anesthesia management characteristics on severe morbidity and mortality. Anesthesiology. 2005;102(2):257-68.
5. Gordon I, Saphiro HA. Death associated with anaesthetic procedure. In: Forensic Medicine: A Guide to Principles. Churchill Livingstone. 1987.
6. Tripathi KD. Essentials of Medical Pharmacology. 5th ed. New Delhi: Jaypee Brothers Medical Publishers (P) Ltd; 2004.pp. 339-79.
7. Bernard Knight. Knight's Forensic Pathology, 3rd ed. CRC Press;2004.
8. Reddy KSN. The Essentials of Forensic Medicine and Toxicology. 29th ed. Hyderabad: K. Suguna Devi; 2010. pp. 338-41.

CHAPTER 19

Starvation Death

Putul Mahanta, Raktim Pratim Tamuli, Mrinal Haloi

LEARNING PLAN

- Learn types of starvation
- Know about factors influencing the fatal period
- Learn the clinical features and causes of starvation
- Understand the state of chronic starvation in a case of death
- Know about the postmortem findings
- Learn the medicolegal importance

DEFINITION

By definition, starvation is a process that may occur from the long and continuous deprivation of food needed to maintain the normal health. It can also be defined as an act of depriving the food or subjecting to famine.

Malnutrition is a state of poor nutrition, which can result from insufficient or excessive or unbalanced diet or from inability to absorb foods.

Cachexia is general lack of nutrition and wasting occurring in the course of a chronic debilitating disease. Emaciation means loss of body weight.

By depriving the body of nutrition, starvation slowly allows the body to consume its own reserves, including muscle, fat and organs, up to the point of complete system shutdown and death.

TYPES OF STARVATION

Starvation is usually of two types:

i. Acute starvation
ii. Chronic starvation.

Acute Starvation

This condition results from sudden and complete cessation of food and water.

Chronic Starvation

This condition results from gradual deficiency in the supply of food and water.

Fatal Period

If both water and food are completely withdrawn, death occurs in 10–12 days.[1,2] If food alone is withdrawn, death occurs in 6–8 weeks or even later. Death usually occurs when about 70–90% of body fat and 20% of the body proteins are lost. Newborns may survive for 7–10 days without food or water.[3]

Factors Influencing the Fatal Period

i. **Age**: The young adult suffer from deprivation worse than old, as the old person have a low requirement. Adults bear starvation better than the children do.
ii. **Sex**: Female withstands starvation for a longer period because of higher storage of fat in the body.
iii. **Nutritional Status of Body**: Fatty, healthy people bear it better than ill and thin.
iv. **Temperature**: Exposure to extreme of temperature hastens the death.
v. **Physical Exertion**: An active physical activity hurries death.

CLINICAL FEATURES

Acute Starvation

i. The person becomes hungry for the first 30–48 hours, followed by stomachache, which is relieved by pressure.
ii. Features after 4 to 5 days of starvation:
    a. General emaciation, absorption of the subcutaneous fat, eyes are sunken and glistening; mydriasis; hollowed cheeks with visible bony prominences.
    b. Dry and cracked lips, coated tongue with intolerable thirst.
    c. Thick and scanty saliva with weak and whispering voice.
    d. Dry, rough and inelastic skin, this may be wrinkled and pigmented.
    e. Thin abdominal concave and limbs, with loss of muscular power with progressive muscular weakness that may be severe in due course of time.
    f. Cardiovascular changes: Slow pulse at rest, paroxysmal tachycardia on exertion. The temperature is subnormal.
    g. Constipation is common, but diarrhea and dysentery may supervene towards the end of life.
    h. Scanty, turbid and highly concentrated urine, with evidence of acidosis.
    i. Constant weight loss is most marked.
    j. At the last stage, body is reduced to an extreme state of emaciation (**Figure 19.1**) characterized by prominent ribs, with concavities in the intercostal spaces and sunken supraclavicular fossae.
    k. Intellect remains clear throughout the period, though in some cases, delusions and hallucinations of sight and hearing occur.

Chronic Starvation

The changes following chronic starvation are constant and develop in a constant order as follows:

i. Loss of well-being, hunger and the hunger-pains
ii. Mental and physical lethargy and easy fatigability
iii. Progressive loss of weight, which is rapid in the first 6 months
iv. Increasing cachexia, the body weight is reduced by about 40% of the normal
v. Pigmentation and development of anemia
vi. Hypothermia, peripheral vascular stasis in the cold and hypotension

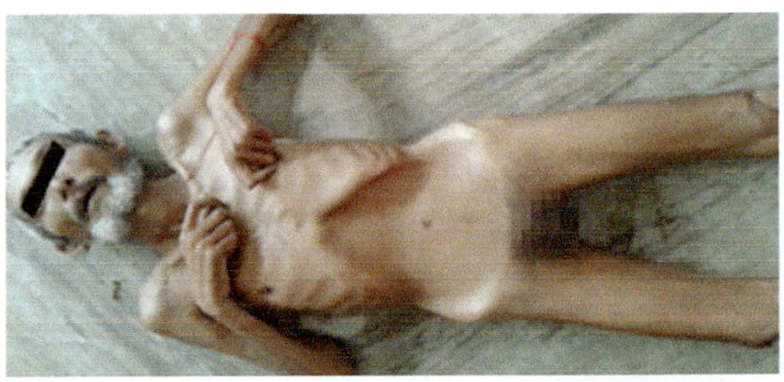

Figure 19.1 Emaciated body due to starvation
(*Courtesy:* Dr Mrinal Haloi, GMC, Guwahati)

vii. Extreme lethargy and loss of self-respect
viii. Edema, first in the feet then other parts of the lower limbs
ix. Reduced resistance to infection causes diarrhea, dysentery, tuberculosis, etc.
x. Lowered blood sugar, proteins, chlorides and cholesterol. NPN and urea are raised
xi. In females, irregular menstruation can occur.

Starvation Biochemistry: When food ingestion ceases, the body enters into a state of starvation. Initially, the body's glycogen stores are used up in about 24 hours. The level of insulin in the blood found low and the level of glucagon is very high. At this stage the main means of energy production is lipolysis. Gluconeogenesis converts glycerol into glucose. Two systems of energy enter into the gluconeogenesis: proteolysis provides alanine and lactate produced from pyruvate, while acetyl CoA produces dissolved nutrients (Ketone bodies), which can be detected in urine and are used by the brain as a source of energy. In terms of insulin resistance, starvation conditions make more glucose available to the brain.

CAUSES OF STARVATION

The main cause of starvation is an imbalance between energy intake and energy spending. This imbalance can arise from some medical conditions and/or circumstantial situations, as shown in **Table 19.1**.

Causes of Death

- Exhaustion
- Circulatory failure due to brown atrophy of the heart or recurrent infection
- Dehydration
- Hypothermia
- Electrolyte imbalance, etc.

POSTMORTEM FINDINGS

External Examination

i. Body is emaciated, characterized by prominent ribs, with concavities in the intercostal spaces and sunken supraclavicular fossae.
ii. Rigor mortis sets in and disappears early.
iii. Pale face, inelastic and pigmented skin, absorption of the subcutaneous fat, sunken eyes; mydriasis; hollowed cheeks with visible bony prominences.
iv. Dry and cracked lips, coated tongue.
v. Dry, rough with inelastic skin, this may be wrinkled and pigmented.
vi. Atrophied and darker muscles due to increase in lipochrome.
vii. Thin abdominal concave and limbs.
viii. Edemas are seen around the ankles and inside the thighs. In wet type, there is edema of the face, trunk and limbs with ascites and pleural effusions.
ix. Dry hair, lustreless with brittle nails.

Table 19.1 Causes of starvation

Medical conditions	Circumstantial causes
• Anorexia nervosa	• Famine: for any reason, such as political strife and war
• Bulimia nervosa	• Fasting without careful medical supervision
• Celiac Disease	• Poverty
• Coma	• Being trapped in pits, mines or landslides
• Major depressive disorder	• Neglect on the part of the parents or guardians
• Diabetes mellitus	• Wilful handling of food
• Digestive disease	• Wilful refusal to take food
• Constant vomiting	

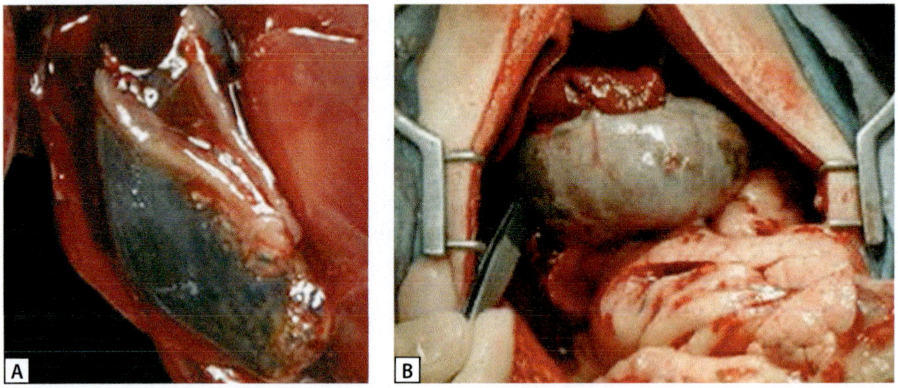

Figures 19.2A and B Distended gallbladders

x. Children's skeleton shows spinal curvature, rickets and dental defects. Osteomyelitic changes are seen in adult.

Xi. Body looks pale due to reduced blood volume and marked anemia.

Internal Examination

i. Fat is nearly absent in the subcutaneous tissues and also in the omentum, mesentery and in the internal organs, but the fat around the female breast and the orbit is persistent till last moment.

ii. Subepicardial fat becomes replaced by a watery gelatinous material.

iii. Stress fractures may occur.

iv. All organs and tissues are pale and shows changes of premature senility.

v. General reduction in size and weight of all the organs except the brain, which is sometimes pale and soft.

vi. Heart is smaller due to brown atrophy with empty chambers.

vii. Lungs are pale, collapsed and exude very little blood on cut section. There may be edema and hypostatic basal congestion (rarely).

viii. Stomach and intestines show atrophied mucosa stained with bile.

ix. Intestinal walls appear like tissue paper with atrophied mucosa.

x. Bowel contains offensive watery fluid and gas.

xi. Superficial extensive non-specific ulceration of the bowel like in ulcerative colitis is seen.

xii. Atrophied liver with necrosis due to protein deficiency may be seen.

xiii. Distended gallbladder with bile (**Figure 19.2**).

xiv. Spleen is shrunken.

xv. Kidneys show atrophy of the nephron.

xvi. Urinary bladder found empty.

xvii. Bones may show features of demineralization.

MEDICOLEGAL IMPORTANCE

i. Exclusion of diseases that likely to cause loss of weight, e.g. malignant disease, diabetes mellitus, tuberculosis, pernicious anemia, etc. is needed to establish starvation.

ii. Marked loss of weight and absence of fat, in absence of a disease, the condition goes in favor of starvation.

iii. Loss of weight and acidosis with ketone bodies in urine are the criteria to advice forced feeding.

iv. A person may fast voluntarily for the purpose of **suicide** or for the purpose of exhibition. To have the attraction of public, fasting may be undertaken, e.g. fast on to death.

v. To commit **homicide** this may be used as a means. Victim is usually an infant, which is illegitimate, or aged or feeble-minded person.

vi. Accidental starvation may occur during famine; being trapped in pits or mines, landslides, shipwreck, etc.

vii. Signs of self neglect and emaciation may be the sign of drug addicts, where the desire for the drugs is more than that of food.

viii. Starvation may be either due to psychiatric illnesses, usually of a paranoid schizophrenic nature or due to senile dementia.

ix. Lunatics and hysterical women may deny food.

x. Right to life, as guaranteed under Article 21 of the Constitution of India, does not include the right to die. Hence, such arrest with forcible feeding of individuals going on hunger strike is lawful.

REFERENCES

1. Vij K. Starvation and neglect. In: Textbook of Forensic Medicine and Toxicology. 3rd ed. New Delhi: Reed Elsevier India Pvt. Limited; 2005. pp. 267-9.
2. Pillay VV. Starvation. In: Textbook of Forensic Medicine and Toxicology. 14th ed. Hyderabad: Paras Publishing; 2004. pp. 249-51.
3. Reddy NKS. Starvation. In: The essentials of Forensic Medicine and Toxicology. 31st ed. Hyderabad: K. Suguna Devi; 2012.p. 312.

CHAPTER 20

Impotence, Frigidity and Sterility

Putul Mahanta

LEARNING PLAN

- Learn the impotence, frigidity and related issues
- Know about sterility and sterilization
- Understand artificial insemination and its legal issues

MALE IMPOTENCE

Synonym: Erectile dysfunction

Definition: Male impotence can be defined as the inability of a man to achieve and maintain an erection sufficient for mutually satisfactory intercourse with his partner. It is very common, and it occurs for a variety of reasons and at different ages.

Types of Impotence

- Temporary causes
- Permanent or organic causes.

Causes of Impotence

i. In extreme of age, impotence is observed.
ii. Usually, any disease can cause impotence by altering the nervous, vascular or hormonal systems. There are many diseases that may change the smooth muscle of the penis and cause impotence. The lists of common diseases are mentioned in **Table 20.1**.

Premature Ejaculation

This condition is often confused with erectile dysfunction. It is a condition in which the entire process of arousal, erection, ejaculation and climax occur very rapidly, often in just a few minutes or even seconds, leaving the partner unsatisfied. Premature ejaculation may be accompanied with an erection problem, but is generally treated differently.

Examination of a Case of Impotency

- Informed consent
- Details of history of illness
- Details of history of medication

Table 20.1 Causes of impotence

Traits	Diseases
Vascular diseases	Includes nearly half of all cases in men >50 years of age. The vascular diseases involving those are: Atherosclerosis, peripheral vascular disease, hypertension, prolonged tobacco smoking
Injuries	To the pelvic blood vessels, nerves, etc.
Medications	Antidepressants, antipsychotics, antihypertensive, antiulcer (cimetidine), hormonal (Zoladex, Lupron, finasteride or dutasteride) drugs that lower cholesterol, alcohol abuse, mind-altering agents, viz. Marijuana and cocaine
Systemic diseases	Diabetes, scleroderma, renal failure, cirrhosis, hemochromatosis, cancer
Diseases of the CNS	Epilepsy, stroke, multiple sclerosis, Guillain-Barré syndrome, Alzheimer's disease, Parkinson's disease.
Respiratory diseases	Chronic obstructive pulmonary disease
Diseases of endocrine system	Hyperthyroidism, hypothyroidism, hypogonadism
Penile conditions	Peyronie's disease, priapism (painful, abnormally prolonged erections)
Psychological	Depression, Widower syndrome, performance anxiety, general anxiety
Nutritional disorder	Malnutrition, zinc deficiency, etc.
Blood diseases	Sickle cell anemia, Leukemias, etc.
Surgical procedures	Procedures on the brain and spinal cord, retroperitoneal or pelvic lymph node dissection, aortoiliac or aortobifemoral bypass, abdominal perineal resection, proctocolectomy, radical prostatectomy, transurethral resection of the prostate, cryosurgery of the prostate, cystectomy, etc.
Congenital disease or malformation	Klinefelter's syndrome, cryptorchidism, phimosis, epispadiasis, etc.

- Details of history of surgery
- General physical examination
- Systemic examination
- Local examination for: Injuries, malformations related to genital tract, condition of genital organs (like testes, epididymis, cord, penis), and length of penis (mons to tip of glans). Usually the axis of the erect penis averages 26° to the horizontal ranging from 16° to 36°
- Penile sonography, pudendal arteriography, cavernosography can be done to assess the arterial and venous system.

Medicolegal Importance

- Nullity of marriage
- Divorce
- An alleged accused of disputed paternity and rape may claim to be impotent
- Compensation may be asked for causing impotence.

POTENCY TEST

This test is a medical examination that admits the authorities to prove potency, which basically means that the accused is physically capable of committing sexual assault. There are three male potency tests, which are carried on to prove manfulness. These tests are generally conducted by an Uro-Andrologist though a Forensic Expert can also opine on it with their help.

The tests are:

1. A semen analysis to evaluate certain characteristics of a male's semen to know male fertility.
2. Penile Doppler ultrasound to know how much and how well blood flows into and out of the penis. This test can tell which direction the blood is flowing. For an erection, blood must flow into the penis, but not flow out. A condition known as Venous Leak Syndrome, where the veins do not "shut off" at the right time, so too

much blood flows out of the penis, and the erection is not firm. Also, erectile dysfunction can be caused by nerve damage, like from diabetes.

3. Visual erection examination of penis is carried out in both states, aroused and flaccid, to check for any sort of dysfunction or damage. Morning erection of the accused is also important to be tested.

FRIGIDITY

Definition: It is a psychological fault with the female having an abnormal antipathy to sexual intercourse.

The term frigidity continues to be used in everyday oral communication, commonly as a derogatory term for women who are unaffectionate or are seen as sexually non-responsive. The term is frequently used to explain lack of interest or rejection by a woman, who originally was of interest to the person making the insult.

Types

- Temporary
- Permanent or organic.

Causes of Frigidity

i. In extreme of age sexual desire is low. As the female is a relative agent, age, as such, has no effect.
ii. Dyspareunia.
iii. Vaginal stenosis.
iv. Psychological causes are the most common cause of frigidity. They are: Vaginismus, fear, anxiety, shyness, sexual aversion disorder or sexual arousal disorder, etc.
v. Malformations or congenital disorders like: Total vaginal occlusion, intersex state like Turner syndrome, etc.

Medicolegal Importance

i. Nullity of marriage.
ii. Divorce.

STERILITY

Definition: Sterility is the inability of either a male or female to procreate. Sterility is a state of being unable to produce offspring; in a woman, it is an inability to conceive; in a man, it is an inability to impregnate. The newer term infertility is used rather than sterility.

Types of Sterility or Infertility

There are two types of sterility:

Primary Infertility

When a couple have never had children, or have been unable to achieve pregnancy after one year of living together despite having unprotected sexual intercourse, then it called primary sterility or infertility.

Secondary Infertility

When couples have had children or achieved pregnancy previously, but are unable to conceive at this time, even after one year of having unprotected sexual intercourse. Then it called secondary infertility.

Secondary infertility occurs more commonly than primary infertility, especially in developing countries where sexually transmitted infections are common. In many countries, induced abortion contributes much to secondary infertility. Generally, it accounts for 60% of the total number of infertility cases.

Causes of Sterility

The causes of infertility are varied and complex. According to studies from around the world, both men and women are affected by infertility: about 40–60% of causes are linked to female factors, and 20–40% is related to male factors.[1]

Causes of Male Sterility

i. **Age**: In men, sperm motility is reduced as the age advances, but overall fertility is not affected as much. There are many case reports describing men having children even after the age of 90 years.

ii. Blockage of the sperm tube.
iii. Problems of sperm production and quality following some diseases like mumps, etc.
iv. **Sexual problems:** Psychological conditions, viz emotional, psychological or physical stress. Impotence and premature ejaculation, where the man ejaculates before the penis is inside the woman's vagina, are another common cause.
v. Neurological damage due to leprosy.
vi. Medications such as methyldopa (antihypertensive drug).
vii. Surgery involving the penis, scrotum, prostate or pelvis, which can cause nerve damage.
viii. Alcohol consumption.
ix. Chronic diseases like diabetes can reduce the ability to have, and maintain, an erection due to vascular changes.

Causes of Female Sterility

i. **Age:** Age is an important factor in both the sex. Fertility declines in many women as the age goes, especially over 35 years of age, when the quality of eggs remaining in the ovaries is lower than when the women were younger.
ii. Blockage of the fallopian tube.
iii. **Ovulation Disorders:** Disorder in hypothalamus-pituitary-ovarian system, etc.
iv. **Uterine Factors:** Congenital malformation, fibroids, adhesion of the uterus due to infection or abortion can affect the possibility of pregnancy, either by interfering with the transport of male sperm or with embryo implantation.
v. **Cervical factors:** In some cases, cervical canal is so narrow that it prevents the passage of sperm into the uterus. Hormone imbalances, mainly low estrogen, can cause inadequate cervical mucus, or make it so thick that it blocks sperm transport.
vi. **Vaginal Factors:** Rarely, conditions like a vaginal septum that inhibits sperm transportation, and even the congenital absence of the vagina, can be causes of sterility.
vii. Extreme spasm of the vaginal muscles (as in vaginismus) during intercourse can prevent penetration of the penis, and so result in infertility.

Medicolegal Importance

i. Disputed paternity
ii. Compensation cases
iii. Sterility can be taken as a plea for adopting a child.

STERILIZATION

Definition: Sterilization is a procedure to make a male or female infertile without affecting his or her potency.

Types

Sterilization can be of two types:

- Voluntary
- Compulsory

Voluntary Sterilization

This procedure is usually undertaken by marital couple for the purpose of birth control.

Compulsory Sterilization

This procedure is carried out in some countries, but not practiced in India.

Methods

There are two methods: Temporary and permanent.

Medicolegal Importance

i. Legitimacy of child
ii. Divorce
iii. Disputed paternity

iv. Doctor may be charged if the failed procedures of sterilization result in unwanted pregnancy.

ARTIFICIAL INSEMINATION

Definition: It is the artificial deposition of semen in the cervix, vagina or uterus of a woman in an attempt to impregnate the woman.

Types

Artificial insemination is two types:

i. **Artificial Insemination Homologous (AIH):** It is when the semen of a husband of the woman is used.
ii. **Artificial Insemination Donor (AID):** It is when the semen of a person other than husband of the woman is used. This practice is not accepted in many of the Middle-East countries.

Indications of Artificial Insemination

i. Husband is impotent and the impotence cannot be corrected
ii. Husband is sterile
iii. Suffering from hypospadias
iv. Hostile vaginal secretion of the wife
v. Rh incompatibility.

Legal Precautions of Artificial Insemination Donor (AID)

i. Husband and wife must agree, and their consent must be taken in writing.
ii. Race and characteristic of the donor should resemble that like of husband.
iii. The donor should be healthy, potent and below the age of 40 years.
iv. Donor's wife must agree.
v. The donor should be of same blood group as that of the husband. There should no Rh incompatibility between donor and recipient.
vi. Donor should not be related to the woman undergoing artificial insemination.
vii. Complete secrecy is essential in order to avoid problems in the future between the married couple. A witness must be present, when insemination is done.
viii. The birth certificate should reflect that the husband is the father of the child, even though there is no biological connection between the husband and the child.

The procedures of insemination should be done at the ovulation period and can be repeated consecutively for 3 months if necessary.

Medicolegal Importance

i. Adultery: Donor and the recipient are not held guilty of adultery.
ii. Legitimacy: As the husband is not the biological father of the child, so the child will be illegitimate. Hence, adoption is needed.
iii. Danger of litigation
iv. Nullity of marriage and divorce
v. Incest: The risk of incest is more.
vi. Posthumous child.

SURROGATE MOTHER

The first recognized surrogate mother arrangement was made in 1976. Between 1976 and 1988, roughly 600 children were born in the US to surrogate mothers. The issue of surrogate motherhood came to national attention during the 1980s, with the Baby M case. In 1984, a New Jersey couple, William Stern and Elizabeth Stern, contracted to pay Mary Beth Whitehead $10,000 to be artificially inseminated with William Stern's sperm and carry the resulting child to term. Whitehead decided to keep the child after it was born, refused to receive the $10,000 payment, and fled to Florida. In July 1985, the police arrested Whitehead and returned the child to the Sterns.

A surrogate mother is a woman who provides her uterus for the growth of baby for others. A woman who bears a child for another person, often for an amount, either through artificial insemination or by carrying until birth another woman's surgically implanted fertilized egg. That means one that acts as, serves as or is a mother substitute.

Monetary compensation may or may not be involved in surrogacy arrangements. If the surrogate receives compensation beyond the reimbursement of medical and other reasonable expenses, the arrangement is called commercial surrogacy; otherwise, it is often referred to as altruistic surrogacy.[2]

Surrogate motherhood is a practice in which a woman (the surrogate mother) bears a child for a couple unable to produce children, usually because the wife is infertile or unable to carry a pregnancy to term. The surrogate is impregnated either through artificial insemination (usually with the sperm of the husband) or through the implantation of an embryo produced by in vitro fertilization. The surrogate traditionally gives up all parental rights, though this has been subject to legal challenge. It is a relationship in which one woman bears and gives birth to a child for a person or a couple who then adopts or takes legal custody of the child; also called mothering by proxy.

A recent study examined the impact of surrogacy on mother vs. child relationships and children's psychological adjustment at age of 7 years. Researchers found no differences among negativity, maternal positivity or child adjustment.[3]

REFERENCES

1. Causes of infertility. Openlearn LabSpace. 12.2 Types of infertility- LabSpace - The Open University. [cited 2013 Feb 4th]; Available from: URL:http://www.labspace.open.ac.uk/mod/oucontent/view.php?id=451924...1.4
2. Milliez J. Surrogacy: FIGO Committee for the Ethical Aspects of Human Reproduction and Women's Health. Int J Gynecol Obstetrics. 2008;102(3):312-3.
3. Golombok S, Readings J, Blake L, Casey P, Marks A, Jadva V. Families created through surrogacy: mother-child relationships and children's psychological adjustment at age 7. Dev Psychol. 2011;47(6):1579-88.

CHAPTER 21

Pregnancy, Delivery, Legitimacy and Paternity

Putul Mahanta

LEARNING PLAN

- Know why a female is examined for signs of pregnancy or delivery
- Learn the diagnosis of pregnancy in living and dead women
- Medicolegal issues relating to delivery
- Know about legitimacy and paternity

PREGNANCY

It is a state that occurs in a female, during her childbearing age, when an ovum gets fertilized by the spermatozoa. It is a physiological state in the female where she conceives and carries developing a product of conception in her womb until birth of a child.

When a Female is examined for Signs of Pregnancy or Delivery?

i. **Divorce:** Woman may claim to be pregnant to receive more alimony.
ii. **Adultery:** When having illegal pregnancy, as alleged by the husband.
iii. **Rape**: In defamation cases, if pregnancy is alleged, a greater compensation is secured.
iv. **Attendance in the Court of Law**: Advanced pregnant state is debarred from attending a court. A certificate has to be issued to the effect. The doctor should certify that the women is in a stage of advanced pregnancy and that she can go into labor anytime or that she would encounter a grave risk if she were made to attend the court in that time.
v. **Capital Sentence**: When a condemned woman alleges pregnancy to delay execution. However, the pregnant women will be pardoned for 6 months after delivery.
vi. **Inheritance**: To stop the heritage of a family with a view to acquire the property, a lady may complain about her pregnant state.
vii. **Infanticide**: In some cases of infanticide, the infant is subjected to a crime after a few minutes or hours of its birth. In such cases, the infant's body and the alleged mother are to be examined to prove the fact of recent delivery.

viii. **Interchange of Infant**: The mother may be required for examination.

ix. **If Pregnancy has been Suspected** to be the motive behind the suicide or murder of an unmarried women or a widow, the dead body is subjected to examine in order to confirm pregnancy to help judiciary.

DIAGNOSIS OF PREGNANCY IN LIVING WOMEN

Diagnosis of pregnancy in living women is done on the basis of presence of signs and symptoms in that particular female. These clinical features are divided into three major groups as shown in **Table 21.1**.

The Presumptive Signs

i. **Amenorrhea** is one of the important presumptive signs of pregnancy, which can also occur in the absence of pregnancy in the following conditions:

a. Debilitating diseases like pulmonary TB, severe anemia, etc.
b. Emotional disturbances like severe depression, etc.
c. Endocrinal disorders like hypothyroidism, etc.
d. Fear of pregnancy, e.g. after illicit sexual exposure
e. Intense desire for pregnancy of an infertile parent like pseudocyesis
f. Lactational amenorrhea, which is a natural cause.

Rarely, menstruation can occur in pregnancy in the first few periods due to incomplete fusion of the decidua vera with the decidua capsularies.

ii. **Changes in breasts** are quite characteristic in primigravida, but are of less value in multiparous women. The changes are (**Figure 21.1**):

a. Increase in size and slight generalized tenderness.
b. Nipple becomes prominent and secondary areola appears.

Table 21.1 Clinical features of pregnancy in living women

A. Presumptive signs	
Symptoms	*Signs*
• Amenorrhea	• Montgomery's tubercles
• Morning sickness	• Prominent nipple
• Quickening	• Expression of a clear secretion
• Excessive salivation	• Striae over the breast
• Perverted appetite	• Pigmentation on the skin
• Irritable temperament	• Linea nigra
• Easy fatigue	• Jacquemier's sign
• Urinary disturbances	• Pulsation on the vagina
B. Probable signs	**C. Positive or sure signs**
• Enlargement of the abdomen	• Fetal parts and movements
• Hegar's sign	• Fetal heart sounds
• Goodell's sign	• Fetal skeleton in X-ray plate
• Braxton Hick's contraction	• Features detected in sonography
• Ballottement	
• Uterine souffle	
• Laboratory tests	

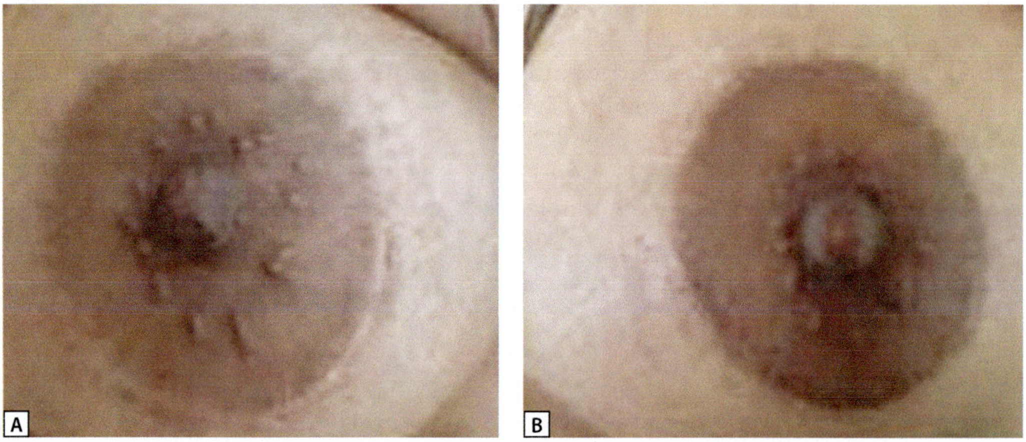

Figures 21.1A and B Hyperpigmentation of areola and nipple

c. Superficial venous engorgement over the breast.
d. Appearance of **Montgomery's Tubercles** (enlarged sebaceous glands).
e. Expression of a clear secretion from the breast usually starts at 12 weeks.
f. **Striae** over the breast, usually seen in the second trimester.

iii. **Morning Sickness** appears about the end of the first month and disappears 6 to 8 weeks. Nausea and vomiting are usually present in the morning, and passes off in a few hours.

iv. **Quickening**: From about 16th to 20th week, the pregnant woman feels slight fluttering movements in her abdomen, which gradually increases in intensity.

v. **Pigmentation of the Skin**: The vulva, abdomen and axilla become darker due to the deposition of pigment, and a dark line extends from the pubis to beyond the umbilicus, the so-called **linea nigra** (**Figure 21.2**).

vi. **Changes in the Vagina**: The mucous membrane of the vagina changes from pink to violet, deepening to blue as a result of venous obstruction, after the fourth week. This is known as **Jacquemier's sign** or **Chadwick's sign**. Pulsation may be felt in the vagina.

vii. **Urinary Disturbances**: During the early week of pregnancy, the enlarging uterus exerts pressure on the bladder and produces frequency of micturation. This gradually disappears after few months, as the uterus rises up into abdomen, and reappears a few weeks before term when head descends into the pelvis.

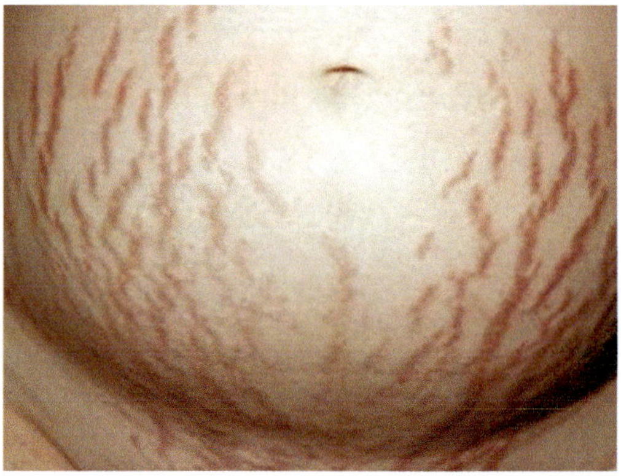

Figure 21.2 Abdominal wall showing linea nigra

viii. Easy **fatigability**.

ix. **Sympathetic Disturbances**: Salivation, perverted appetite and irritable temperament are the common complaints.

The Probable Signs

i. **Enlargement of the abdomen** (**Figure 21.3**)
   a. The uterus is just palpable per abdomen at 12 weeks.
   b. It is midway between the umbilicus and symphysis pubis at 16 weeks.

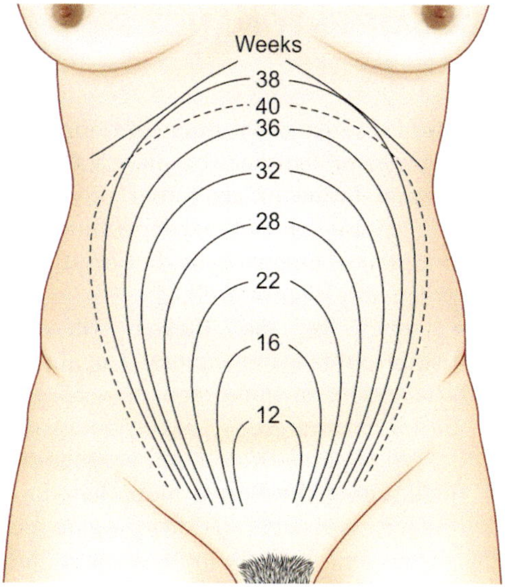

Figure 21.3 Fundal height of uterus

c. One finger below the umbilicus at 20 weeks.
d. At the umbilicus at 22 weeks.
e. One finger above the umbilicus at 25 weeks.
f. The portion between the umbilicus and xiphisternum is divided into three parts signifying uterine height corresponding to 28, 32 and 36 weeks of pregnancy.

At term, the fundal height comes down to the height at 32 weeks due to the enlargement of the head. The engagement of the abdomen can be due to other causes like ovarian cysts, tumors in the abdomino-pelvic cavity, ascites, uterine tumors and pseudocyesis, etc.

ii. **Uterus: Hegar's sign** is positive at about the six weeks. This is done bimanually. The left hand is kept per abdomen and the fingers of right hand are introduced per vaginally. The fingers of the two hands meet because of softening of the isthmus.
iii. **Cervix**: Softening of the lips of the cervix occurs from the second months from below upward. This is called **Goodell's sign**. Non-pregnant cervix is firm, feels like the tip of the nose, but the pregnant cervix feels soft like lips.
iv. **Intermittent Uterine Contractions**: These contractions occur throughout pregnancy and are painless. The frequency and duration are variable. Both frequency and duration increase as term approaches. These are known as **Braxton Hick's contraction.** In early pregnancy, they can only be detected by a careful bimanual examination. This is known as **palmar sign.**
v. **Ballottement**: This is the feeling obtained by the movement of the fetus in the amniotic cavity. Ballottement can be: (i) **Internal**—this is felt through vagina, give a tap to the fetus, it goes up and again strikes the hand after little while. (ii) **External**— this is felt per abdomen. Usually, this sign is present at 4th month of pregnancy and onwards.
vi. **Uterine Souffle**: It is a soft, blowing murmur heard on auscultation over the lateral aspect of the uterus, over the uterine arteries just towards the end of fourth month. It is synchronous with the mother's pulse. This sign is faulty because the same sound can be obtained over any vascular tumor like fibromyoma uteri, etc.
vii. **Laboratory Tests**: These are useful in detecting very early pregnancy. They are based on the reaction of test animals, to chorionic gonadotropins contained in the pregnant woman's blood or urine. **They are**: 1. Rapid rat test, 2. The Aschheim-Zondek test, 3. Friedman test, 4. Male frog test, 5. Galli Mainini test, 6. Hog Ben or female toad test, etc. However, these are obsoleted now days.
viii. **Immunological Tests**: The immunological test of pregnancy is done commonly. It is based on the fact that the pregnant woman urine contains a high level of chorionic gonadotropins. These tests utilize antibodies to react with another substance for the detection of hCG. It is very convenient and reliable and accuracy is 98%. Fallacy: It may be positive in case of hydatidiform mole, choriocarcinoma, pituitary tumors, etc.

Positive Signs or Sure Signs

i. **Fetal Parts and Movements:** Fetal movements are felt per abdomen after six months. Fetal parts can be identified by abdominal palpation by 36 weeks.
ii. **Fetal Heart Sounds (FHS.):** The fetal heart sounds can be heard by the ordinary fetoscope after 18–20 weeks. With **Doppler**, they can be heard over a full bladder as early as 8 weeks. Usual fetal heart rate is 120–160 per minute, and it does not synchronies with the maternal pulse rate. FHS is a definite sign of pregnancy which may not be heard in extremely obese patients or in patient with hydramnios.
iii. **X-ray Diagnosis:** It is useful after 16th week. Visualization of the fetal skeleton in an X-ray plate is a positive sign of pregnancy (**Figure 21.4**). Twins, congenital malformations of the uterus, hydatidiform mole, intrauterine death, tumors associated with pregnancy can also diagnosed by it. It also gives approximate maturity of the fetus in the late pregnancy.
iv. **Sonography:** It can alone give definite evidence of pregnancy. **Gestational ring** is seen by sixth week. Fetal heart beat can be made out by 12th week. It can detect intrauterine growth retardation and fetal malformation besides fetal maturity.

SIGNS OF PREGNANCY IN THE DEAD

i. **The Presence of Products of Conception:** Embryo or fetus or the placental tissues or membrane or any other products of conception in the uterus depending on the duration of pregnancy is the surest sign of pregnancy (**Figure 21.5**).
ii. **Changes in the Uterus:** Uterus is hypertrophied and increased in the size. The weight in non-pregnant is 50 g and of full-term uterus is 1 kg. At autopsy, the length of parous uterus is more than three inches long, the body is more than double the length of cervix. Its cavity is globular in parous and triangular in nullipara. Raised blood tinged areas at the placental site is found till 6 months after delivery.
iii. **Corpus Luteum:** The corpus luteum is formed in the ovary after the release of the ovum from the graffian follicle. A well-formed corpus luteum is found in one of the ovaries. It is not a reliable sign because it is also present in fibroids and other conditions causing over congestion. It can be present in delayed menstruation also.
iv. **Even in an Exhumed Body** which has been reduced to skeleton, fetal bones will be found in the remains and by DNA analysis of available tissues, paternity or maternity can be established.

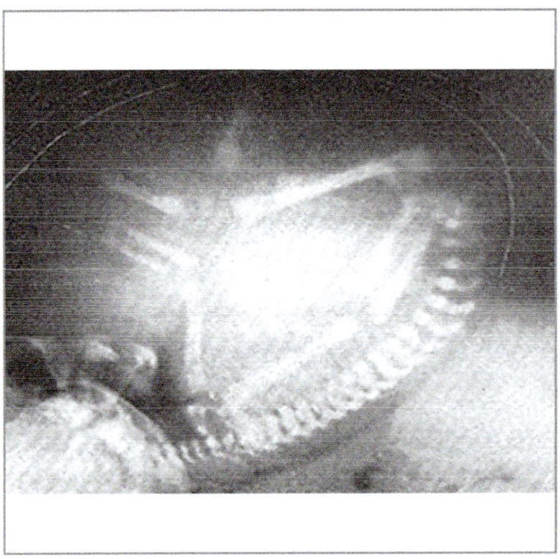

Figure 21.4 Fetal skeletons in an X-ray of abdomen

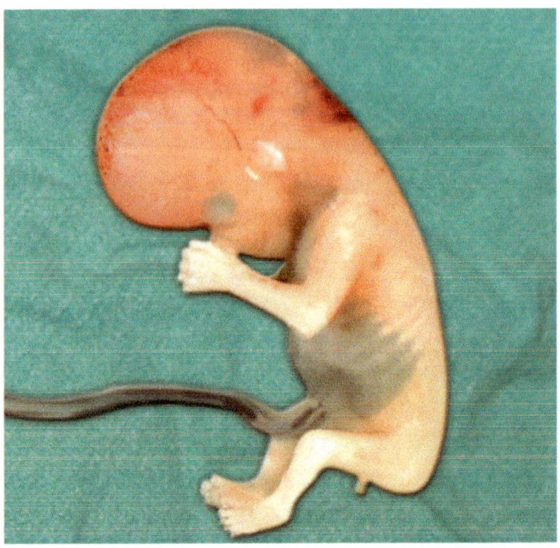

Figure 21.5 Product of conception

GESTATIONAL PERIOD

Average Duration of Pregnancy: The average duration is 280 days (from the first day of the last menstrual period, so that the actual period of gestation is about 270 days or less). The exact date of conception cannot be, however, be fixed. If the date of insemination is known, it may be possible to ascertain the date of approximate conception.

Maximum Period of Pregnancy: The maximum period accepted by English courts on medical evidence was 349 days. However, Indian law does not lay down any fixed limit of pregnancy.

Minimum Period of Pregnancy: Children born at or after 210 days of uterine life are viable, i.e. are born alive and able to survive. Children born after 180 days of uterine life may be viable and capable of continuing an independent life apart from their mothers. Infants born at still shorter periods have sometimes survived and grown up.

CERTAIN MEDICOLEGAL TERM

Posthumous Child

It is a child born after the death of its father, the mother being conceived by the said father before the death of her husband.

Super Fecundation

If the fertilization occurs of two ova of the same cycles either out of one or more than one act of coitus. The doubt usually arises whether the father of the infant is same or different. This could be proved by blood groups tests or DNA analysis after the birth of twins. Both ova do not always develop to maturity. One fetus may be aborted early and retained until the labor expels the other. The dead fetus may be flattened by pressure and may not be recognizable, and is referred to as **fetus compressus** or **fetus papyraceus**.

Superfetation

It is the fertilization of two ova of different cycle by two different acts of coitus. It is a possibility only within 3 months from the first conception when the ovary keeps on shedding ova. The age of one child will be more than the other.

Pseudocyesis (Spurious or Phantom Pregnancy)

Pseudocyesis is observed in patients nearing the menopause or in youngers who intensely desire children, and they suffer from some form of psychic or hormonal disorder. They may present with all the subjective symptoms of pregnancy associated with a considerable increase in the size of abdomen, which may be due to abnormal deposition of fat or to tympanites and occasionally due to ascites. Women may imagine fetal movement and pregnancy may go to full term and frank labor pains may occur, which ceases abruptly when the patients was told about the fact.

Suppositious Child

It is a child that is presented by a female and that female pretends that she has delivered the child, but in real sense, she is not the biological mother.

Birth in Helmeted (CAUL) Head

A caul (Latin: caput galeatum) is a piece of membrane that can cover a newborn's head and face immediately after birth. Death of the infant may occur due to suffocation.

DELIVERY

Delivery is a physiological process, which means the expulsion or extraction of the child at birth and at term. The term is not synonymous with labor, and delivery may even take place without labor as in case of Cesarean section.

The question of delivery arises in civil or criminal cases, where a medical man is called to prove or to disprove the allegation (**Table 21.2**). Before an examination, a written consent should be taken from the female to be examined, besides other formalities in a case of living.

Table 21.2 List of cases when a doctor is to examine a female for signs of delivery

Civil cases	Criminal cases
• Feigned delivery	• Abortions
• Disputed virginity	• Infanticide
• Divorce	• Concealment of the fact of birth
• Nullity of marriage	• Blackmailing
• Contested paternity	• Homicidal and suicidal cases
• Legitimacy	• Delivery following alleged rape
• Inheritance of property	• To delay execution of judicial death following delivery up to 6 months

Table 21.3 Color changes of Lochia

Duration of puerperium	Color of discharge	Nature of discharge
1–4 days	Lochia Rubra	Bright red discharge
By 5–9 days	Lochia Serosa	Serous and pale
By 9th days	Lochia Alba	Yellowish gray
By end of 15 days (usually by 2–3 weeks) all the signs will disappears		

Signs of Delivery

i. Signs of recent delivery—up to 2 weeks
ii. Signs of remote delivery—more than 2 weeks duration.

SIGNS OF RECENT DELIVERY IN THE LIVING

i. **General Indisposition**: More so in the first 48-72 hours. There may be mild reactionary fever in the first day. There may be after pains due to strong contractions of the uterus. Woman looks pale with sunken eyes, exhausted and ill looking with increased pulse rate.
ii. **Breast Changes**: Full, knotty, enlarged and engorged with milk. Dark secondary areola, well-developed nipple and Montgomery tubercles are seen. During the first 24 hours, colostrum can be expressed from the breast and subsequently milk expression occurs.
iii. The **Abdomen**: The abdominal walls are pendulous, wrinkled and show **stria gravidarum** especially in the flanks.
iv. The **Uterus**: Uterus is hard and contracted like a cricket ball after delivery. It is first below the umbilicus immediately after delivery and gradually decreases in size. Subsequently, it becomes a pelvic organ after 10-14 days.
v. The **Labia**: They are tender, swollen and bruised or lacerated.
vi. The **Vagina**: There may be bruises and lacerations caused at the time of delivery.

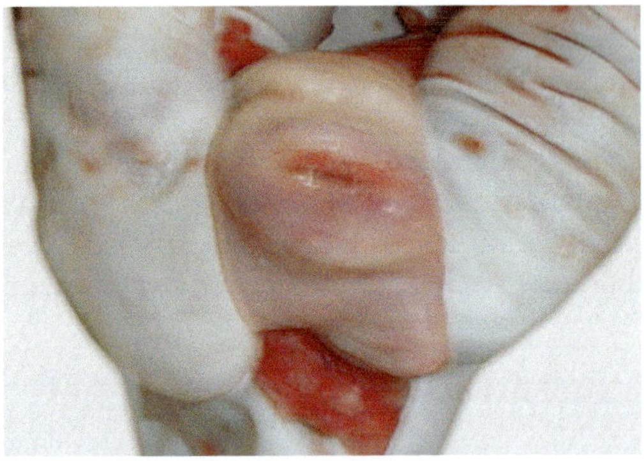

Figure 21.6 Parous cervix

Vagina is smooth, roomy, may show the presence of recent tears. Fourchette is invariably torn.
vii. The **Perineum**: The perineum sometimes may be lacerated.
viii. The **Cervix**: Immediately after delivery external os admits two fingers and after one week only one finger. Internal os closes within 24 hours of delivery. The cervix is soft, patulous and may show signs of injury (**Figure 21.6**). There may be tear or laceration at the angles.
ix. The **Lochia**: Lochia is the alkaline discharge from the uterus having a peculiar, sour, disagreeable odor that is composed of RBCs, WBCs, debris of deciduas, epithelial cells and bacteria. It lasts for two to three weeks after a delivery.
Lochia changes its color after delivery as time passes by as mentioned in **Table 21.3**.
x. **Intermittent Uterine Contraction**: They are usually present for the first 4-5 days.

xi. **Laboratory Test**: If the blood or urine gives a positive pregnancy test, it is strong corroborative evidence that the pregnancy has been recently terminated. Usually, blood and urine give positive result for up to 10 days after delivery.

SIGNS OF RECENT DELIVERY IN THE DEAD

In addition to the signs described above, the uterus is found to be enlarged, flabby, contains blood clots and the decidua is usually present. The area of placental attachment is seen. The uterus, immediately after delivery, weighs about 1 kg and 9–12 inches long. At the end of one week, it is 500 g in weight and 5–6 inches long. The **ovaries** and **fallopian tubes** are congested and a large corpus luteum is usually seen in one of the ovaries.

SIGNS OF REMOTE DELIVERY IN THE LIVING

i. **Abdominal Examination**: Striae and linea albicantes may be seen and the abdominal wall is relaxed.
ii. **Breasts**: Soft, pendulous, striae are present. In the lactating breast, nipples are prominent.
iii. **Vagina**: Roomy, relaxed, admits more than two fingers and rugae are absent. Posterior commissure and the fourchette are destroyed. Hymen is ruptured or absent and seen as nodules known as **carunculae myrtiformes**.
iv. **Cervix**: External os is transversely patulous and may have irregular margins.
v. **Uterus**: It is a pelvic organ but may be slightly enlarged. In lactating mothers, on the other hand, the uterus is smaller in size than normal.

SIGNS OF REMOTE DELIVERY IN THE DEAD

In addition to above signs, following features may be noted with the dead female.

i. Uterus is larger than nulliparous, more hypertrophied and bulkier than the multiparous uterus. The cavity is wider and more rounded or pear-shaped uterine cavity.
ii. The cervix is irregular; edges may show the signs of tears and lacerations caused during delivery. The external os is patulous, and irregular, admits tip of a finger and shows transverse slit-like opening and may have areas of healed scars (**Figures 21.7** and **21.8**).

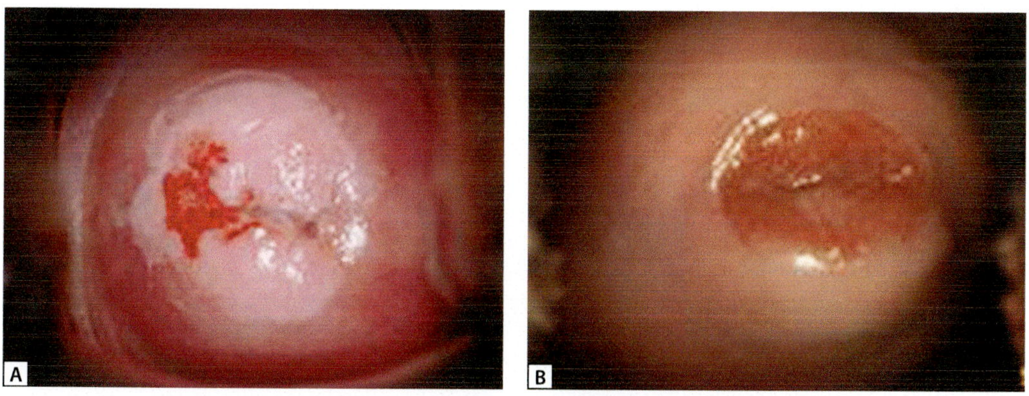

Figures 21.7A and B Parous cervixes with slit (Transverse) like external os

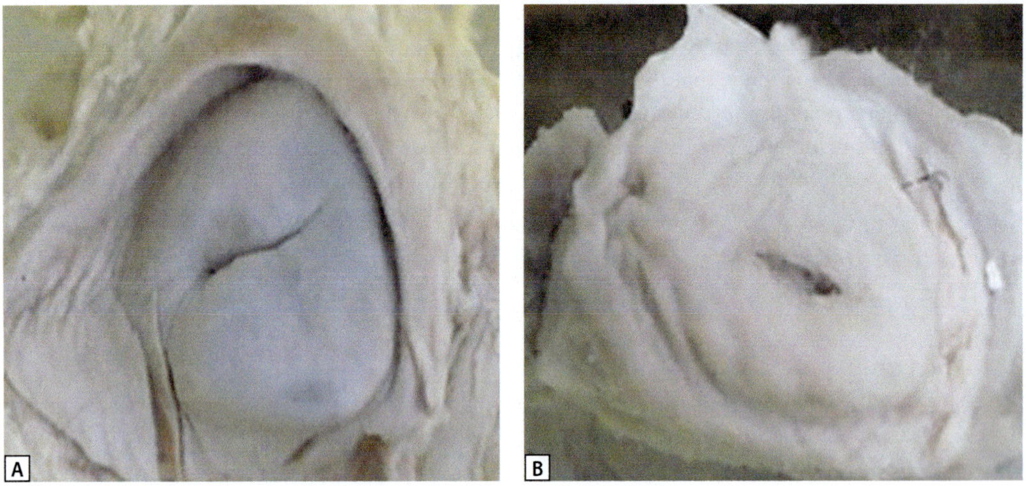

Figures 21.8A and B Parous cervixes with slit like external os (Wet specimen)

LEGITIMACY AND PATERNITY

Legitimacy is the legal state of a person born in lawful marriage. If a person is born during the continuance of a legal marriage, or within 280 days after the dissolution of the marriage by divorce or death of the husband, his birth is presumed to be legitimate.

Careful attention to the definitions of the words "legitimacy" and "paternity" is necessary because they are used loosely in the reported decisions. Some courts refer to a "presumption of paternity".[1]

The child becomes illegitimate, or bastard (slang), if it can be proved that the husband could not possibly be the father of the child by producing evidence that the alleged father is:

i. Below the age of puberty.
ii. Physically incapable to beget children.
iii. The blood groups of the child and the alleged father are not compatible.

When Question of Legitimacy Arises?

i. **Inheritance of property.**
ii. **Affiliation Cases**: A woman may allege a particular man to be the father of her child and file a case in the court for fixing the paternity. If the paternity is fixed on a certain person, he becomes responsible to support the child. Blood grouping and DNA analysis can prove the allegation.
iii. **Supposititious Children**: The woman feigns to be pregnant and delivers subsequently, or substitutes a male child for a female child, or substitutes a living child for a dead child, usually for the diversion of inherited property.
iv. **Paternity**: The question of paternity arises in contests over legitimacy, posthumous births or supposititious children.

Paternity can be determined from:

i. Parental likeness
ii. Atavism[2]
iii. Developmental defects
iv. Blood grouping
v. DNA analysis, etc.

REFERENCES

1. Contino v. Estate of Contino, 23 Fla. L. Weekly d1870, d1871 (Fla. 3d D.C.A. 1998).
2. TalkOrigins Archive. "29+ Evidences for Macroevolution: Part 2". Archived from the original on 29 October 2006. Retrieved 2006-11-08.

CHAPTER 22

Abortion and MTP Act

Putul Mahanta, Vijayanath V

LEARNING PLAN

- Understand the definition of abortion and its classification
- Know about medical termination of pregnancy (MTP) and MTP Act
- Know about criminal abortion, methods for induction
- Identify the evidences about abortion during life and death

DEFINITION OF ABORTION

It can be defined as an expulsion of the products of conception before the age of viability, i.e. 28 weeks of pregnancy. For international credence, the limit of viability is brought down to either 20 weeks or fetus weighing 500 g.

The terms abortion, **miscarriage** and **premature labor** are all synonymous from medicolegal point of view and signify premature expulsion of the fetus at any time of gestation before the full term. **Premature delivery** is delivery of fetus after 28th week of pregnancy, but before 40th week.

Abortion is a procedure to end a pregnancy. This procedures uses medicine or surgical intervention to remove the product of conceptus from the uterus **Figure 22.1**. Legally, the procedure is done by a licensed physician or someone acting under the supervision of a licensed physician.

INCIDENCE

Abortion, when induced in developed world in accordance with local law, is among the safest procedures in medicine.[1] However, unsafe abortions result in approximately 70,000 maternal deaths and five million disabilities per year globally.[2] An estimated 44 million abortions are performed globally each year, with slightly under half of those performed unsafely.[3] The incidence of abortion has stabilized in recent years,[3] having previously spent decades declining, as access to family planning education and contraceptive services increased.[4] Nearly 40% of the world's women have access to induced abortions within gestational limits.[5]

Study shows 10% of all pregnancies end in spontaneous abortions and 10% are induced illegally. 70% abortion occurs before the 16th weeks and, of these, about 75% occurs before the 8th week of pregnancy.[6]

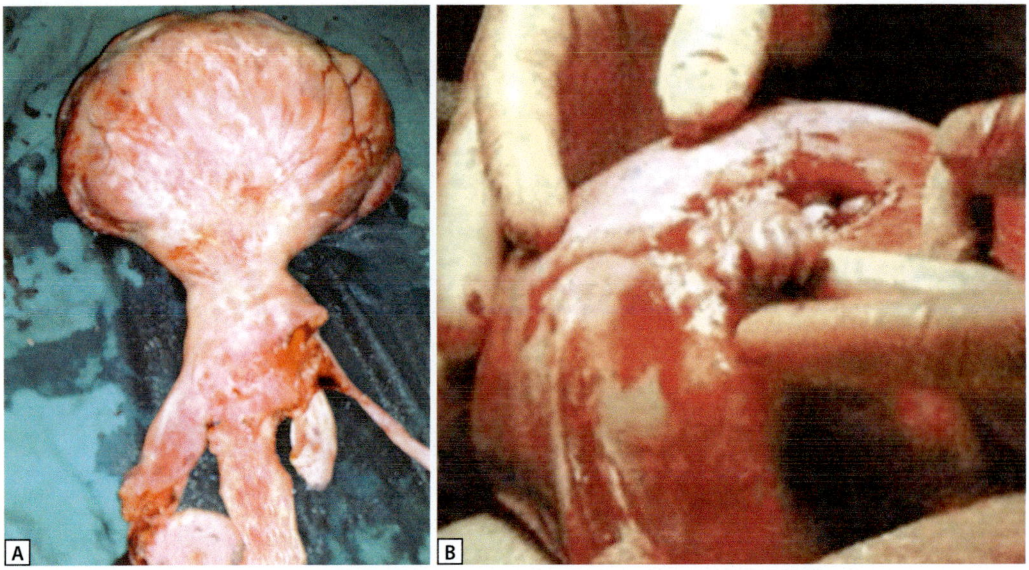

Figures 22.1A and B Gravid uterus containing product of conceptus

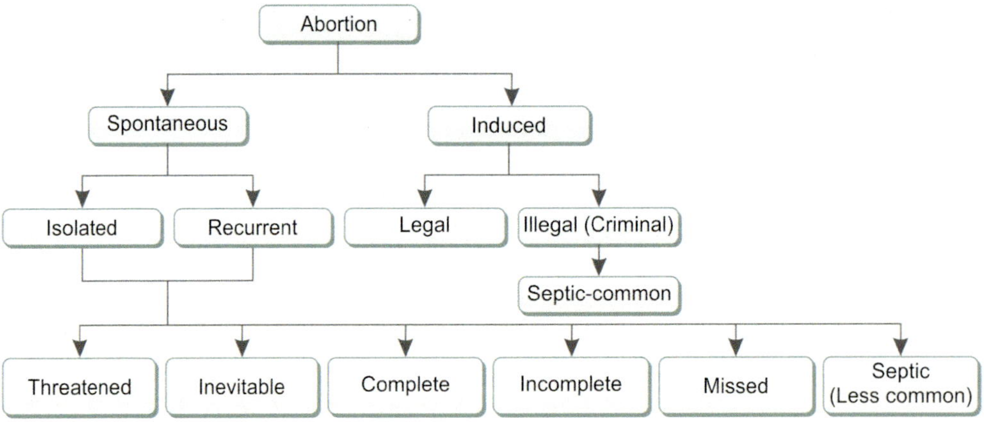

Figure 22.2 Classification of abortion

Medicolegal circumstances when an alleged victim is required for examination for the evidences of abortion:

a. A woman alleging abortion after a blow in an altercation.
b. A woman wishing to conceal abortion after being charged for it.
c. A woman complaining that a medical man produced abortion in her or gave her an abortifacient drug which resulted in abortion, etc.

CLASSIFICATION OF ABORTION

Abortion can be divided into the two major groups, viz spontaneous (Natural) and artificial or induced abortion as shown in **Figure 22.2**.

Spontaneous (Natural) Abortion

Natural abortion may be spontaneous or accidental in origin. The products are expelled days or weeks after the death of the embryo. Both

Table 22.1 Natural causes of abortion	
Maternal causes	
General causes	
Chromosomal abnormalities	Trisomy, triploidy, turner's syndrome, blighted ovum
Acute infections	Viral: Smallpox, rubella, infective hepatitis
	Bacterial: Streptococcal
	Parasitic like malaria, etc.
Chronic infections	Syphilis (mid trimester abortion), active pulmonary tuberculosis, toxoplasmosis, listeria monocytogens, etc.
Poisonings	Lead, copper or mercury poisoning, etc.
Chronic diseases	Hypertension, nephritis, diabetes, severe anemia, heart disease, toxemia of pregnancy, etc.
Psychological causes	Shock, sudden fright, etc.
Trauma	Physical trauma mainly to abdomen
Local causes	• Fibroids, cervical incompetence • Chronic pelvic inflammation, endometritis • Chronic retroversion • Excessive sexual intercourse during pregnancy causes hyperemia and abortion
Fetal causes	
• Death of fetus due to germ plasm defects • Hormonal imbalances • Hydatiform mole • Placental diseases, e.g. placenta previa and diseases of deciduas	

spontaneous and accidental natural abortion may be of maternal and fetal origin (**Table 22.1**).

The outcome of either a spontaneous or induced abortion are classified based on clinical presentation, as judged by the health care provider. It is important for the students to know the different categories:

Complete Abortion

It means that all parts of the fetus and placenta have been expelled through the vagina; nothing is left behind inside the uterus with closed cervix. No treatment is usually necessary. After a complete abortion which has been safely induced, the woman may feel light cramping pains in her abdomen, and bleeding from her vagina should be not more than the normal menstrual period normally.

Incomplete Abortion

An incomplete abortion is when part of the fetal tissue or placenta is still in the uterus and the cervix is open. In incomplete abortion without treatment, may increase risk of infection and this could be life-threatening for the woman.

Threatened Abortion

When a pregnancy is complicated by bleeding per vagina with closed cervix, this may signal a threatened abortion. There is a chance that the pregnancy may continue normally, provided the fetus is showing signs of life.

Inevitable Abortion

It is a clinical type of abortion where the changes have advanced to such a state, from where continuation of pregnancy is impossible. In this condition, the fetus is entirely inside the uterus, but it will end in the expulsion of the fetus. Often the woman has lower abdominal pain and a cervical change called effacement, when the cervix has pulled back and become thinner; then the cervix starts to dilate and open as like during a normal full-term labor. The contents of the uterus will often spontaneously come out, but if this does not happen soon, surgical intervention may be needed.

Missed Abortion

When the fetus is dead and retained entirely inside the uterus for more than four weeks, it is called a missed abortion.

Septic Abortion

Any abortion, associated with clinical evidences of infection of the uterus and its contents, is called septic abortion.

Artificial or Induced Abortion

This is a deliberate termination of pregnancy before the viability of the fetus and may be further grouped as: (A) Therapeutic or justifiable or legal and (B) Criminal abortions.

Therapeutic or Justifiable or Legal

An abortion is justifiable only if it is done in good faith to save the life of the woman, if it is materially endangered by the continuance of pregnancy. The World Medical Association in 1970 adopted a resolution on therapeutic abortion, known as '**Declaration of Oslo**'.

In India, it is performed either in accordance with the legal provisions of the **MTP Act 1971**, i.e. legal abortion or caused in good faith to save the life of the pregnant women.[7]

Precautions

a. Firstly an endeavor should be made to prolong the pregnancy as much as possible if there is no danger to the life of the mother.
b. Consent from woman is necessary before conducting the abortion. Consent of husband is not necessary.
c. The indication should be clearly mentioned.
d. It should be performed in a hospital or in the centers authorized by law.

Medical Termination of Pregnancy (MTP)

The **Medical Termination of Pregnancy Act passed in 1971** legalizes abortions on the following grounds:
- Therapeutic
- Eugenic
- Humanitarian
- Social.

Therapeutic grounds

These relate to conditions when the continuance of pregnancy involves risk to the life of the pregnant women or because of grave injury to her physical or mental health. The indications include the conditions such as:

i. Hypertension complicated by cardiac or renal failure
ii. Nephrotic syndrome
iii. Pulmonary hypertension
iv. Toxemia of pregnancy
v. Uterine hemorrhages, etc.

Eugenic grounds

These include the conditions in which the born child is likely to suffer from such physical or mental abnormalities that may lead the child to be handicapped. The conditions or diseases associated are:

i. Measles, small pox, chicken pox, viral hepatitis or other serious viral infections.
ii. Exposure to X-rays and other radiations.
iii. When the parents have some inheritable mental conditions or chromosomal abnormalities.

Humanitarian grounds

These include those cases where pregnancy has been caused by rape. Pregnancy, which has taken place due to such incidents, is presumed to constitute grave injury to woman's mental health.

Social grounds

These relate to the conditions: (i) When pregnancy in married women is the result of contraceptive failure and (ii) The environment of the pregnant woman during the pregnancy and after the birth of child would involve risk to her health.

Rules for Doing MTP

Qualification Required

i. Only a qualified registered medical practitioner possessing prescribed experience can terminate pregnancy; or
ii. A registered medical practitioner who has assisted in at least 25 cases of MTP in a recognized hospital; or
iii. A doctor with MD in obstetrics and gynecology or DGO qualification or has 6 months of experience in house-surgeonship in obstetrics and gynecology in a recognized hospital.

Place

i. Hospitals maintained or established by government.
ii. Non-governmental hospital may take up abortion if they obtain a license from Chief Medical Officer or Civil Surgeon of the District.

Consent

i. A female above 18 years of age with sound mind can give valid consent.
ii. The consent of the women is required before abortion: Written consent of the guardian is required if the woman is less than 18 years or a lunatic, consent of husband is not necessary.

Duration of Pregnancy

i. When the duration of pregnancy is below 12 weeks of gestation, one registered medical practitioner can do the MTP.
ii. Duration of pregnancy when above 12 weeks and below 20 weeks, then opinion of two registered medical practitioners are required to do the MTP.

Documentation and Record[8]

According to para 5 of MTP regulations, all approved centers are required to maintain an admission register in the format prescribed in form III. A fresh register should be started in each calendar year with new serial number generated by mentioning the year against the serial number. The admission register is a secret document. It should be maintained for at least 5 years from the last entry.

Methods for Induction of MTP

Medical Abortion

Medical abortion refers to the use of medication to terminate a pregnancy. The most widely used method worldwide, a woman is first given an oral dose of a progesterone antagonist, such as **mifepristone** (RU486) or the cytotoxic drug **methotrexate**. These drugs inhibit the action of progesterone in maintaining the pregnancy, and therefore, cause the embryo and placental sac to separate from the wall of the uterus. A prostaglandin analogue such as **misoprostol** is then given (vaginally, orally or sub-lingually) either at the time or up to 1–3 days later. The prostaglandin-like drug causes the contents of the uterus to be expelled. The combination of mifepristone and misoprostol for women in early pregnancy results in complete abortion in 93–98% of cases, with the remaining cases requiring consideration of a follow-up surgical procedure.[9]

The success rate is lower as the pregnancy advances. Although widely used overseas, mifepristone (RU 486) is so far only available in Australia under special circumstances in certain hospitals. These include KEMH (King Edward Memorial Hospital), where mifepristone is now being used for second trimester abortions. Some clinics are using methotrexate for medical terminations. Medical abortion with the prostaglandin analogue misoprostol alone has been used in Western Australia for some years, mainly for second trimester abortions. All evidence indicates that medical abortion is safe and acceptable to women. Women undergoing medical abortion need to be under close medical supervision and to have access to surgical treatment in case of an incomplete abortion or excessive bleeding.[9]

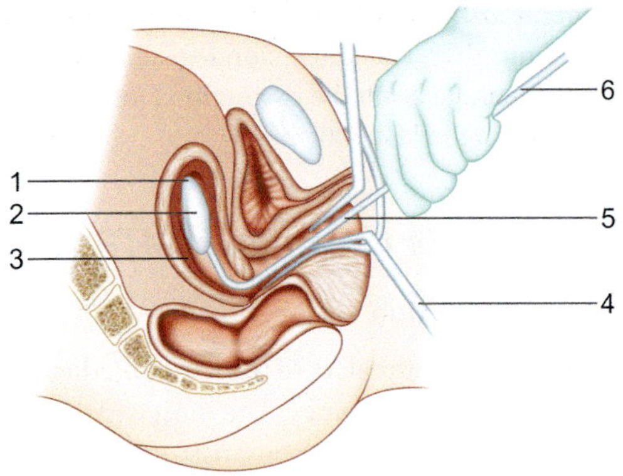

Figure 22.3 Vacuum-aspiration abortions: (1) Amniotic sac; (2) Embryo; (3) Uterine lining; (4) Speculum; (5) Vacurette (6) The vacurette is attached to a suction pump

Surgical Abortion

The common surgical methods are: Suction curettage (vacuum aspiration) or dilation and evacuation (**Figure 22.3**). In Western Australia, almost all early gestation terminations (up to 12 weeks) are carried out by vacuum aspiration or suction curettage (95% in 2005).[10]

The Royal College of Obstetricians and Gynecologists recommends that cervical preparation should be routine when the woman is under 18 or at a gestation of >10 weeks.[11]

Preparation of the cervix may include the administration of a prostaglandin or one of its analogues (such as misoprostol, gemeprost or mifepristone) or osmotic dilators (laminaria tents) placed in the cervix, where they absorb moisture and expand gradually to dilate the cervix.[12]

Criminal Abortions

Criminal abortion is one which is done not to save the life of the mother, but with some other intention, e.g. to injure the mother or to kill fetus. It is performed with the criminal intention to get rid of the products of conception. It is induced in the first trimester usually. Usually, a criminal abortion case comes to the notice of law if the woman dies to the ill effects of the abortion.

Motives for Criminal Abortion

Unmarried Girl and Widows: When the pregnancy is the cause of illicit sexual act, to avoid the shame they go for abortion, which is criminal.

Poverty: Poverty may be the cause of criminal abortion to avoid addition of a member to the family.

Female Feticide: Female feticide is the act of aborting a fetus because it is female. This is a major social problem in India. Fetal sex determination and sex selective abortion by medical professionals has today grown into a ₹ 1,000 crore industry. Social discrimination against women and a preference for males have been promoted.[13]

Legal Bearing

If the pregnant woman with consent gets criminal abortion done, both the abortionist and the woman are liable to punishment. If it is done without the woman's consent, only the abortionist is to be punished. **Abortionists** can be the **expert** or medically qualified, **semi-skilled** abortionist, such as midwives, nurses, chemists, etc. and lastly the **unskilled** abortionist.

Methods for Inducing Criminal Abortion

i. **Internal Use of Drugs**: Generally no drug, when administered orally, can lead to abortion unless given in very large dose, which are toxic to the mother herself.
   a. Drugs acting directly on the uterus: Ecbolics (prostaglandins, ergot, quinine, oxytocin, etc.) and emmenagogues, which promote the menstrual flow (savin, borax, apiol and estrogenic compounds).
   b. Drugs acting reflexly through the genitourinary tract like pennyroyal oil and oil of turpentine.
   c. Drugs acting through the gastro-intestinal tract: Emetics like tartar,

purgatives like croton oil, colocynth, castor oil, aloe, etc.

d. Drugs act as systemic poisons: **Vegetable poison** like unripe papaya seeds, unripe pineapple fruits, *madar* juice, *lal chitra*, seeds of Daucus carota. **Metallic poisons** like lead paste (consist of lead oxide and olive oil), copper, arsenic and mercury salts. Cantharides is used as an abortifacient.

ii. **Mechanical Violence**: This may be the general and local violence.

General (Violence) Methods

A. Acting **directly** on the uterus such as:
   - Pressing on the abdomen, e.g. blows, kicks, etc.
   - Tight fittings
   - Violent exercise like riding, cycling, jumping, skipping, etc.
   - Lifting heavy weights
   - Cupping
   - Alternate very hot and cold hip baths
   - Massage on the uterus through the abdominal wall, etc.

B. Acting **indirectly** on the uterus by promoting pelvic congestion or causing intrauterine hemorrhage.

Local Violence Methods

i. Rupturing of membranes of uterus by pointed tools like uterine sound, catheter, douche cannula, knitting needles, hair pins, etc. Drainage of liquor is followed by miscarriage.

ii. Introduction of laminaria tent: Laminaria tent is soaked in water and introduced into the cervical os. Afterward, membranes rupture and abortion may result.

iii. Abortion sticks: Commonly employed by *dai*s.

iv. Syringing: Employed usually by the doctor.

v. Passage of a low-voltage electric current through the lower abdomen. Its negative pole is applied to the cervix and positive pole to the sacrum or lumber vertebra. Passing of the electric current causes contraction of the uterus that expels the contents.

Legal Status of Criminal Abortion

i. **IPC 312**: For causing miscarriage (Para I -Punishment: Imprisonment for 3 years, or fine or both: Non-cognizable-Non-bailable: Triable by Magistrate of the first class: Non-compoundable. Para II- punishment: Imprisonment for 7 years and fine: Non-cognizable: Bailable: Triable by Magistrate of the first class: Non-compoundable).

ii. **IPC 313**: For causing miscarriage without women's consent (punishment: Imprisonment for life, or imprisonment for 10 years and fine: Cognizable-Non-bailable: Triable by Court of Sessions: Non-compoundable).

iii. **IPC 314**: Death caused by an act done with intent to cause miscarriage (Para I: Punishment: Imprisonment for 10 years and fine: Cognizable: Non-bailable: Triable by Court of Sessions: Non-compoundable. Para II: Punishment: Imprisonment for life or as above: Cognizable: Non-bailable: Triable by Court of Session: Non-compoundable).

iv. **IPC 315**: Act done with intent to prevent child being born alive or to cause it to die after birth (Punishment: Imprisonment for 10 years, or fine, or both Cognizable: Non-bailable: Triable by Court of Sessions: Non-compoundable).

v. **IPC 316**: Causing death of quick unborn child by act amounting to culpable homicide (Punishment: Imprisonment for 10 years and fine: Cognizable: Non-bailable: Triable by Court of Sessions: Non-compoundable).

Complication of MTP

The various complications of abortion, mainly of criminal abortions are mentioned in **Table 22.2.**

Table 22.2 Complications of criminal abortion	
Immediate cause	Hemorrhage (due to perforation of uterus, incomplete abortion, etc.), shock due to vagal inhibition, embolism (air, fat and amniotic fluid)
Delayed causes	Sepsis like peritonitis may occur early in the first three days in instrumental abortion or may be delayed by a week or more in non-instrumental cases, pyemia, generalized peritonitis, endometritis, tetanus, secondary hemorrhage, etc.
Remote causes	Pneumonia, pulmonary embolism, bacterial endocarditis, renal failure, jaundice, meningitis, empyema, systemic poisoning effects, etc.

Evidences of Abortion

Evidences during Life

There are signs of recent delivery with the women that depends on the type, procedure involved and duration of pregnancy. Common signs are:
- Blood-stained vaginal discharge
- Lax vagina
- Lacerations or signs of instrumentations in the vagina
- Presence of transverse slit cervical opening with patulous cervix (may or may not be torn)
- Bulky uterus
- Enlarged breasts.

Evidences after Death

Besides the signs of pregnancy, there may be presence of injuries caused by general violence, like:

i. Laceration, inflammation or corrosion of vagina.
ii. Cervical injuries.
iii. Uterus and appendages are to be preserved for chemical analysis as well as for histopathological examination to rule out any abortifacient and pathological disease.
iv. Site of attachment of placenta seen on opening the uterus.
iv. Fetus is examined for evidence of age.

Fabricated Abortion

It is false sort of abortion with malicious intention to accuse someone. The alleged female victim may allege a person that due to assault by the person, she has aborted and may produce menstrual pads, etc.

In these cases, the medicolegal expert must examine the uterine discharges carefully; the content may be nothing but the menstrual blood clots. Some woman may bring animal fetus or some products of it and may allege it to be the product of her conceptus. Precipitin test and DNA analysis will be helpful in this regard. Age of the fetus must be determined in every case. Histopathological examination can be helpful.

REFERENCES

1. Grimes DA, Benson J, Singh S, Romero M, Ganatra B, Okonofua FE, Shah IH. Unsafe abortion: The preventable pandemic. Lancet. 2006;368(9550):1908-19. doi: 10.1016/S0140-6736(06)69481-6. PMID 17126724.
2. Shah I, Ahman E. Unsafe abortion: global and regional incidence, trends, consequences, and challenges. J Obstetrics Gynaecol Canada.2009;31(12):1149-58. PMID 20085681.
3. Sedgh G, Singh S, Shah IH, Ahman E, Henshaw SK, Bankole A. Induced abortion: Incidence and trends worldwide from 1995 to 2008. Lancet. 2012;379(9816):625-32. doi: 10.1016/S0140-6736(11)61786-8. PMID 22264435.
4. Sedgh G, Henshaw SK, Singh S, Bankole A, Drescher J. Legal abortion worldwide: incidence and recent trends. Int FAM Plan Perspect. 2007;33(3):106-16. doi:10.1363/ifpp.33.106.07. PMID 17938093.

5. Culwell KR, Vekemans M, de Silva U, Hurwitz M. Critical gaps in universal access to reproductive health: Contraception and prevention of unsafe abortion. Int J Gynecol Obstet. 2010;110:S13-6. doi:10.1016/j.ijgo.2010.04.003. PMID 20451196.
6. Dutta DC. Haemorrhage in early pregnancy. In: Textbook of Obstetrics. 3rd ed. Calcutta: Dr. Mita Sen, MBBS. 1992. pp. 170-1.
7. Subrahmayam BV. Abortion and medical termination of pregnancy. In: Modi's Medical Jurisprudence and Toxicology, 22nd ed. Butterworths, New Delhi, India. 2001. pp. 581-603.
8. Sheier N. Medico legal aspects—medical methods for early abortion. Consortium on national consensus for medical abortion in India. [cited 2012 Oct 30]; Available from: URL:http//www.aiims.edu/aiims/events/gynaewebsite
9. De Costa CM. Medical abortion for Australian women: it's time. Med J Australia. 2005;183(7):378-80.
10. Straton J, Godman K, et al. Induced abortion in WA 1999-2005: Report of the WA abortion notification system. Perth, WA: Department of Health, 2006.
11. Royal College of Obstetricians and Gynecologists. The care of women requesting induced abortion. Evidence Based Clinical Guideline Number 7. London, UK, 2004.
12. The Royal Australian and New Zealand College of Obstetricians and Gynecologists. Termination of Pregnancy—A resource for health professionals. East Melbourne, Vic: The Royal Australian and New Zealand College of Obstetricians and Gynecologists, 2005.
13. UNICEF India. UNICEF. Female feticide in India. [cited 2012 Nov 12]; Available from: URL:en.wikipedia.org/wiki/Female_foeticide_in_India

CHAPTER 23

Infanticide

Putul Mahanta

LEARNING PLAN

- Know the motives for infanticide
- Learn the features of stillborn, deadborn and live birth baby
- Understand the viability of a child and the signs of maturity
- Know about the causes of infant death
- Learn about battered baby, shaken baby, Munchausen's and sudden infant death syndrome
- Know about female feticide, PCPNDT Act and related issues

DEFINITION

Though the legal definition and implications of infanticide vary from country to country, the medical concept is more or less ubiquitously accepted. **Infanticide** means unlawful destruction of an infant less than 1 year. In **Indian Law**, an infanticide is a murder and punished under section 302 IPC. In some of the Middle East Countries, like **Egypt** and **Libya**, it is defined as the homicidal killing of a newly born infant, during its first 15 days after birth, until the complete separation of the cord and healing of umbilicus. In **England** and **Germany**, there is a clear-cut distinction between homicide and infanticide and a charge of infanticide is less serious than a charge of murder, if committed by the mother due to stress-related factors under the effect of childbirth.

It must be proved that the child was born alive and that it died after its birth from criminal violence inflicted upon the child, in a trial for infanticide. The forensic medicine expert often examines the child's body and the alleged mother to prove the fact of recent delivery.

MOTIVE FOR INFANTICIDE

i. **Illegitimate Pregnancy**: An illegitimate child is one who is not born out of a lawful wedlock. The newborn baby is killed to avoid shame, disgrace from the society, mainly by unmarried girls and widows.
ii. **Inheritance**: To stop the heritage of a family with a view to acquire the property.
iii. Poor parents.

iv. In some families, female infants are seen with contempt.
v. Prostitutes do not want male children.

Feticide

Feticide is an act that causes the death of a fetus,[1] means killing of the fetus prior to death. In a legal context, "fetal homicide" or "child destruction" refers to the deliberate or incidental killing of a fetus due to a criminal human act, such as a blow to the abdomen of a pregnant woman. As a medical term, feticide is destruction of a fetus,[2] for example, as the first phase of a legally induced **abortion**.[3] Feticide does not refer to the death of a fetus from entirely natural causes, such as the **miscarriage** of a pregnancy.

Neonaticide

It is the killing of a newborn infant. The perpetrator is invariably the mother, and the cause of death is usually either asphyxia or abandonment.[4] In encyclopedia, **neonaticide** is defined as the killing of a newborn infant less than one month old. Although relatively uncommon, numerous cases of maternal neonaticide have been reported. As of 2007, only two cases of paternal neonaticide have appeared in the literature.[5]

Resnick coined the term neonaticide to describe the killing of a child of a less than 24 hours old. Although this tragedy is common amongst mothers, it is an exceptionally rare event among fathers.[5] **Filicide** is the killing of a child or a stepchild, aged between 0 and 18 years, by his or her parents.[6] Filicide is a broad term and includes neonaticide, infanticide and feticide.

MEDICOLEGAL QUERIES

A forensic medicine expert is often asked to answer the following queries while doing an autopsy in relation to infant death:

A. Is the infant born is stillborn or dead born?
B. Has the infant attained age of viability or not?
C. Was the child born alive?
D. If the child was born alive, how long did the child survive?
E. What was the cause of death?

Is the Infant Born is a Stillborn or Dead born?

Stillborn

Definition

A stillborn child (**Figure 23.1**) is one born after 28 weeks of pregnancy and which did not, at any time after being completely expelled, breathe or show any sign of life.

The child was alive in utero, but dies during the process of birth. Stillbirths occur more frequently among illegitimate and immature male children in primiparae. The incidence is about 5%.

Causes of Stillbirth

The causes are prematurity, anoxia of various types, birth trauma, especially intracranial hemorrhage due to excessive moulding, placental abnormalities, toxemias of pregnancy, erythroblastosis fetalis, etc.

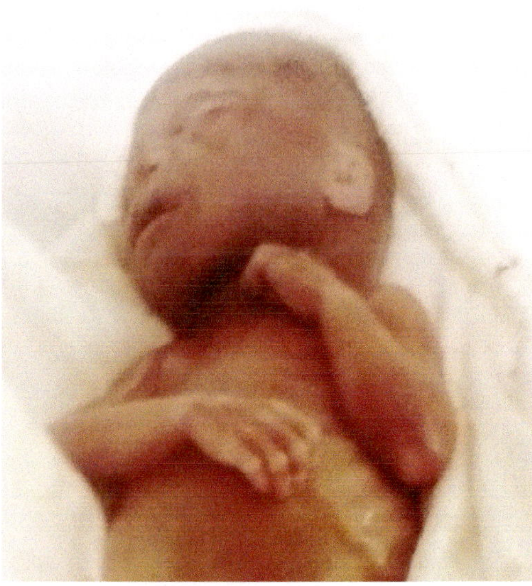

Figure 23.1 Stillborn baby

Postmortem Findings

As the child is born in sterile condition, putrefaction begins on the surface and extends inward whereas in case of newborn child which lived for some time, the bacteria inside the body may cause putrefaction to start in the abdomen. Signs of prolonged labor, i.e. edema and bleeding into the scalp, a caput succedaneum, and severe moulding of the head indicates stillbirth or death from natural causes shortly after birth.

Dead Born

Definition

A dead born child (**Figure 23.2**) is one who has died in utero and may show either sign of rigor mortis at delivery or signs of maceration or mummification.

Postmortem Findings

Maceration: It is an aseptic autolytic process. It is seen when the child remains in uterus for 3–4 days after death surrounded with liquor amnii but without air. Signs of maceration are not seen if the child is born within 24 hours after death. If air enters in the liquor amnii after death of the fetus, putrefaction occurs instead or maceration. The earliest sign of maceration is skin slippage, which can be seen in 12 hours after the death of the child in utero. The body of a macerated child is soft, flattened and emits a disagreeable smell. Serous fluid is contained in large blebs. Skin color is red. Tissues are swollen and sutures of the cranial bones are separated.

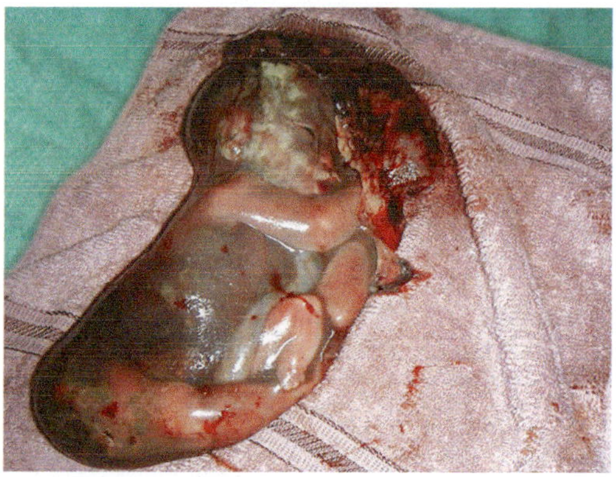

Figure 23.2 Dead born baby with signs of maceration

Abdominal X-ray examination may reveal an overriding of the fetal cranial bones, which is called **Spalding's sign**. In Spalding's sign, loss of alignment and overriding of the bones of the cranial vault occurs due to shrinkage of the cerebrum after death of the fetus. In the early stage, there is only loss of the alignment without overriding. The sign will develop earlier with a vertex presentation than with a breech. It may be detected within a few days of the death of the fetus, but often takes much longer time, sometimes even 2 to 3 weeks. The umbilical cord is red, smooth and thick. All the visceras lose their anatomical characters except the lungs and uterus.

Mummification occurs when the fetus dies from the deficient supply of blood, when liquor amnii is scanty and when no air enters the uterus. The fetus in such situation becomes dry and shriveled.

Has the Infant Attained Age of Viability or Not?

Definition

A **viable** child is one who is capable of an independent existence apart from its mother by virtue of a certain degree of development. Earliest viable are recorded is 174 days, i.e. 6 calendar months. Average viable age is 210 days, i.e. seven calendar months. Some factors which can help in assessing the viability include weight, crown-heel length and appearance of ossification centers. At 7 months, the average weight is 1.3 kg, and the crown heel length is 35 cm.

Signs of Maturity of a Fetus

i. Length: 47–50 cm.
ii. Weight: 2.5–3.5 kg.
iii. Hair: Thick hairs on head, about 4 cm long.
iv. Nail: Nails will be projected beyond the fingertip.
v. Eyes: Eyebrows and eyelashes are separated, membrane pupillaries has disappeared and eyelids are not adherent.
vi. The umbilicus is at midway between xiphisternum and symphysis pubis.

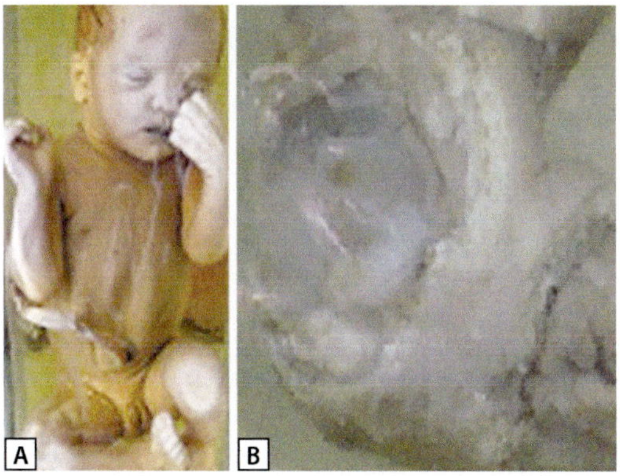

Figures 23.3A and B (A) Term male baby; (B) Center of ossification at lower end of femur (9 months)

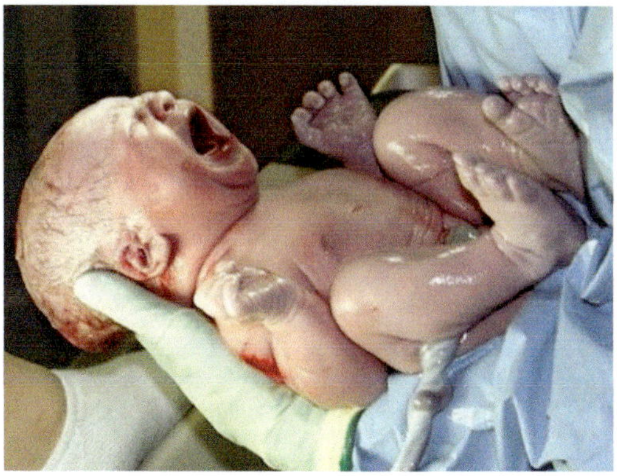

Figure 23.4 Live-born infant

vii. Testes are within the scrotal sac in case of a male child.
viii. The surest sign of maturity is the presence of a center for ossification at the lower end of femur, which appears as a circular red spot of 0.5 cm in diameter as shown in **Figure 23.3**. It appears in the 9th month of intrauterine life.

Was the Infant Born Alive?

A live-birth infant is said to be live born when, after complete extrusion from the mother, it displays some signs of vitality such as activities of heart, breathing, crying, etc. (**Figure 23.4**).

In Indian law, if any part of the child comes out of the uterus in a living condition, though the child might not have breathed, it constitutes a live birth. The death of such a child amounts to culpable homicide except in cases where it is done in good faith to save the life of the mother. It is essential to prove that the child was born alive and that the child was capable of an independent existence after it had been wholly or partially out of the womb of the mother.

Postmortem Findings

The following features of the dead fetus should be noted to establish the process of respiration on autopsy:

1. **The Shape of the Chest**: In a liveborn infant, because of the act of breathing, certain changes might have taken place. The shape of the chest appears flat before respiration, arched and rounded after breathing because of inflation of the lung due to the presence of air. The anteroposterior diameter in case of a live born infant will be increased.
2. **The Level of the Diaphragm**: Usually at the 4th to 5th rib position if respiration has not taken place and goes down to 6th rib position once the respiration takes place.
3. The findings of the lungs as mentioned in **Table 23.1** can be the vital determinates to prove the fact of live birth.

Some Other Useful Tests

i. **Static Test** or **Fodere's Test**: The lungs are ligated across their hila and separated. Approximate weight before breathing for both the lungs is 30–40 g and weight after breathing is 60–70 g. The weight of the lung increases on respiration because of the increase amount of blood circulating the lungs. A medicolegal role of this test has no significance, as the figures are in proportion to the size of the body of the infant and amount of respiration.
ii. **Hydrostatic** or **Floatation Test**: It is one of the important tests, but of limited value which should be done before giving an opinion. It can only be used as a suggestive note to live birth, but not conclusive.

Principle: Specific gravity of an unrespired lung is 1040–1050. It is heavier than a respired lung

Table 23.1 Deferences between respired and non-respired lungs

Appearances	Respired lungs	Non-respired lungs
Macroscopic size	Large, voluminous, filling the chest cavity and cover heart and thymus	Small, not filling the chest cavity and does not cover heart and thymus. They are placed by side of spine
Edges of lungs	The edges are rounded	Here it is sharp (**Figure 23.5**)
Color	Mosaic color because of air and blood	Uniform purple
Consistency	Crepitate and spongy	Liver like consistency (solid)
Surface	Not smooth	Smooth
Microscopic findings	Alveoli are extended, lined with flattened epithelium and increased vascularization	Small in size and collapsed, lined with low columnar epithelium and less vascularization
Flotation test	Floats	Sink

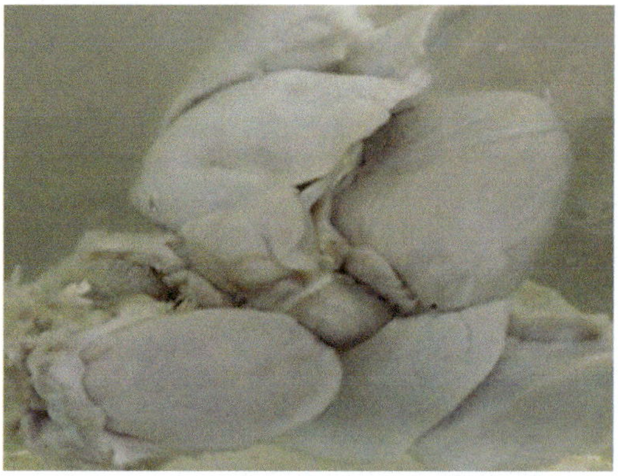

Figure 23.5 Thoracic visceras of stillborn baby

whose specific gravity is 940. The fetal lungs that have not breathed, therefore, sink in water and those that have breathed, float.

Method: A large bowl is filled with water. Rain water or distilled water should be used. Both the lungs along with trachea, heart and thymus should be removed and dipped into the bowl of water. It should be noted whether it floats or sinks. A ligature is tied around the bronchi, and lungs separated and again immersed individually. Then the lungs are cut into 12–15 pieces and each one tested. A piece of liver can serve as controls. If the liver floats, the test has no value, because it is clear that putrefaction has set in. If all the pieces of lung float, they are to be crushed under the weight and tested again.

Observation and Conclusion

1. For the whole structure consisting of the lungs, trachea and thymus to float, it must be fully inflated. It is a positive and conclusive proof of live birth.
2. If some pieces float while others sinks, it means feeble respiration has taken place.
3. If all cut pieces of lung float: Complete proof of inflating lungs. But if the pieces sink after pressure, no respiration has taken place.
4. If all cut pieces of lung sink: The child did not breathe, and it can be declared as stillbirth.

Fallacies of this Test

1. An inflated lung may be sinking in cases of thickened pleura, atelectasis of the lungs and congenital abnormalities of the lungs.
2. The unrespired lung may float because of putrefying gases or artificial inflation.
3. In cases of partial breathing such as might have taken place in the uterus or in the vagina, it may not show positive results because of the small quantity of air breathed.
4. It will show positive results in artificial inhalation.

   The test is unnecessary in the following conditions: When the age is below 180 days, i.e. 6 months of intrauterine life of the fetus, monster child (**Figure 23.6**), in a child with signs of intrauterine maceration and when milk is found in the stomach.
5. **Changes in the stomach and intestine: Breslau's test**: During the process of breathing, some amount of air goes into the stomach and duodenum. Presence of air in these organs is an evidence of live

Table 23.2 Changes seen with umbilical cord

Features	Time
Shrinkage of lumen of blood vessels	Just born
Dries up with blood clotting at the cut ends	After 2 hours
Drying of the portion of umbilical cord attached to the child	12–14 hours
Ring of inflammation at the base of the umbilical cord	36–48 hours
Falling of the umbilical cord because of sloughing	5–8 days
Healed wound or scar formation	8–12 days

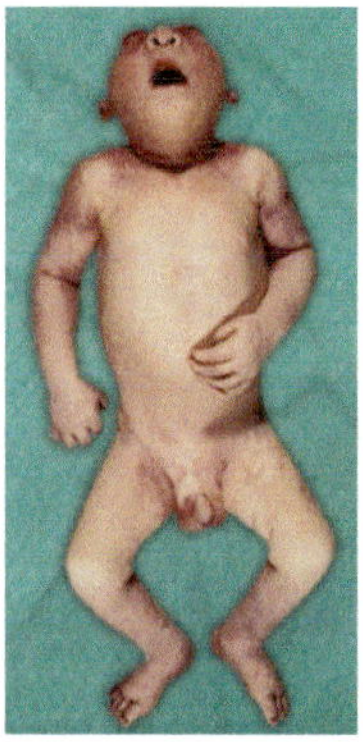

Figure 23.6 Anencephaly or monster baby

birth. The other possible contents to be found are blood, meconium and liquor amnii. Their presence indicates that the child had breathed and during the process of inspiration swallowed the contents. Presence of milk indicates that the child lived for a significant period. A microscopic and chemical examination is to be carried out of all such content.

6. **Changes in the kidney and bladder**: Uric acid crystals may be deposited in the pelvis of the kidney. Urine formation may or may not take place.
7. **Middle ear changes: Wredin's test**: It detects changes in the middle ear. This is the replacement of the gelatinous embryonic connective tissue by air in the event of respiration having taken place. There is the absence of a certain gelatinous matter from of the middle ear of the fetus, taken as evidence that a child has breathed and, therefore, had been born alive.

If the Infant was Born Alive, how long did the Infant Survive?

The assessment of the duration of life can be done by a careful examination of the following:

a. **Changes in the Skin**: The skin of the newborn infant is bright red with vernix caseosa covering the groin, axilla and folds of neck. It takes about two days for the removal of the vernix. The skin gets darker in the second or third day, finally turning into brick red and yellow. The normal color is assumed within a week's time. A macerated skin is an obvious conclusion that the child did not breathe.
b. **Changes in Caput Succedaneum**: During delivery, a swelling is formed on the scalp tissue, which contains blood or, more commonly, serum. The swelling disappears between one to three days after birth.
c. **Changes in the Umbilical Cord**: The changes are fairly reliable and prove to be a good guide for the medicolegal expert. The changes are shown in **Table 23.2**.
d. **Changes in the Circulation**: Fetal hemoglobin constitutes 80% at birth, 7–8% in 3 months and gradually falls by 6 months. Certain structures needed for fetus are not needed after the birth of the child, which is shown in **Table 23.3**.

What was the Cause of Death of the Infant?

The causes of death of an infant can be divided into three major categories, viz. natural, accidental and criminal cause, as shown in

Table 23.3 Changes in the circulation

Changes in the circulation and heart	Duration
Nucleated RBC	24 hours
Fetal hemoglobin present	Up to 6 months
Umbilical artery	
Contraction starts	After 10 hours of birth
Contraction completed	3rd day
Ductus arteriosus	
Contraction starts	Immediately
Contraction completed by	10 days
Foramen ovale: closure occurs by	2nd–3rd month or may remain open

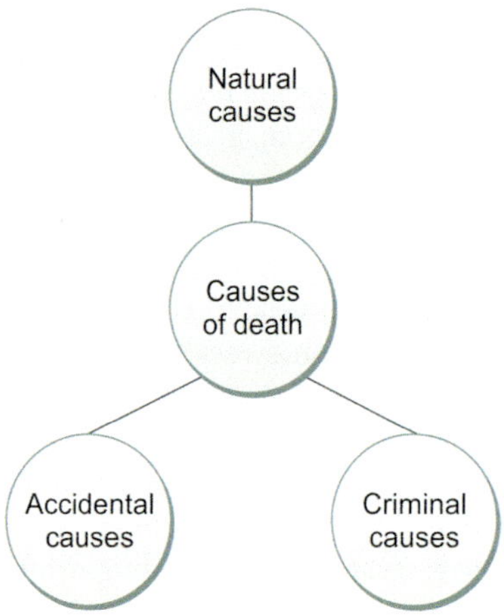

Figure 23.7 Causes of death of infant

Figure 23.7. The criminal causes may be the again divided into the act of **commission** and the act of **omission**.

Natural Causes

1. Immaturity: A premature child dies immediately after birth. But the question is whether the premature delivery has been natural or criminally induced so that the child should not live?
2. Congenital diseases: Syphilis, congenital lung, heart and brain diseases.
3. Congenital malformations of heart, blood vessels and in a case of monster.
4. Feebleness due to lack of general development of child, hemorrhage from the cord, stomach, rectum or genitalia.
5. Placental diseases: Placenta previa, abruptio placenta.
6. Neonatal infection, erythroblastosis fetalis, etc.

Accidental Causes

The accidental causes of death of a newborn could be during birth or after birth:

Death during Birth

1. **Prolonged Labor**: It results in injuries to the brain tissue with or without skull fractures. Rarely, the child may die due to exhaustion on account of prolonged and difficult labor.
2. **Cord Prolapse**: The mode of death is asphyxia, and in a postmortem examination of the child, the bronchial tubes will be seen to be filled with blood, meconium or liquor amnii.
3. Twisting of the cord round neck or knots of cord.
4. **Injuries** to the abdomen of a pregnant mother. Such injuries have usually blunted force impact, where the fetus is killed because of head injury or rupture of an important blood vessel. The differences between head injury in different circumstances are shown in **Table 23.4**.

Table 23.4 Differences between head injury in different circumstances

Trait	Precipitate labor	Difficult labor	Homicidal trauma
Type of mother	Multipara	Primipara	Any type
Site of fracture of skull	Parietal or frontal	Any site	Any site
Relation between fetal head and maternal passages	Fetal head is relatively smaller to room maternal passages	Fetal head is bigger than maternal passages	Fetal head may be bigger or smaller to the maternal passages
Caput succedaneum	Usually not present	Present	May be present
Moulding of skull bones	Usually not present	Present	May be present
Bruises	May be present over the presenting part		Anywhere on the body

5. **Death of the Mother**: The child can be saved if it can be delivered within 5-10 minutes of the mother's death.

Death of Child after Birth

1. **Suffocation**: If the child's head and face remain covered with the mother's blood or meconium or liquor amnii, the child will die of suffocation.
2. **Precipitate Labor**: This happens when sudden and rapid delivery takes place without the knowledge of the mother. It is only possible in multiparous women with large and spacious pelvis. The placenta is expelled out along with the child or the umbilical cord is torn. This child dies because of the improper place or expulsion from the uterus, e.g. a child falling into a lavatory pan, dies of suffocation or direct injury to the head or hemorrhage.

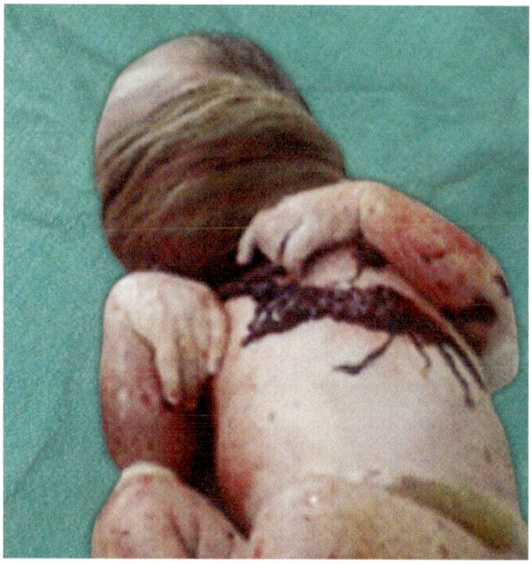

Figure 23.8 Face is covered with cloth to kill the newborn
(*Courtesy:* Dr Yogender Malik, BPS Govt. Medical College for Women)

Criminal Causes

The criminal causes of infant death may be the result of acts of omission or act of commission.

Act of Omission or Neglect: It is the improper assistance during labor or neglect on the part of the mother in regard to child's care such as:

1. Failure to provide proper assistance at the time of delivery.
2. Failure to cut and ligate the cord.
3. Failure to provide feed to the child.
4. Failure to remove the child from mother's discharge, resulting in suffocation.
5. Failure to protect from extremes of weather.

Act of the Commission: It is the use of mechanical force or poison to kill a child. The usual pro-cedures adopted to do such an act are:

1. **Suffocation**: It is done by pressing the face of the child against a pillow, any other cloth (**Figure 23.8**), cotton wool plugs or manually by fingers.

Table 23.5 Differences between accidental and homicidal strangulation by umbilical cord

Characters	Accidental strangulation by the umbilical cord	Homicidal strangulation by the umbilical cord
Cord twisting around the neck	Usually one	More than one
Cord's false knot	Present	Absent
Wharton's jelly	Normal	Displaced
Cord laceration	Absent	Present
Cord continuity	Attached to be placenta	May be cut
Constriction mark on neck	Mild	Deep
Length of cord	Longer than normal	Normal
Signs of respiration	Absent	Present

2. **Strangulation**: The materials used for strangulation are ropes, hands, garments or umbilical cord. The force applied is usually more than is actually required. The differences between accidental and homicidal strangulation by umbilical cord are shown in **Table 23.5**.
3. **Drowning**: This is rare. The more usual is first killing the child by some other mean and then throwing the body into a pool of water to conceal the crime.
4. **Burning**: Infanticide by burning is rare, but it may be used as a mode of disposal.
5. **Wounds**: The child may be killed by a stab incised wound, cut throat, etc.
   Fracture of head by blunt injuries.
6. **Poisoning**: It is also rare.

BATTERED BABY SYNDROME

Synonyms: Caffey's syndrome, non-accidental injury of childhood, child abuse syndrome and maltreatment syndrome in children.

Definition

A battered child is one who presents with injuries received as a result of non-accidental violence, inflicted by a parent or guardian.

Caffey (1946) first reported the unusual combination of recurrent subdural hematoma with fracture of long bones, but thought that the phenomenon could be due to metabolic abnormality. **Silverman** (1953) was the first to point out that both, subdural hematoma and bone fracture, were the result of severe recurrent trauma. Kempe, et al. (1962) coined the term "battered child syndrome", which is now frequently used.[7]

Features

i. The age of the child is usually under 3 years.
ii. More common in male.
iii. In addition to physical injury, there may be intentional deprivation of nutrition, care and affection.
iv. The classical features are obvious discrepancy between the nature of the injuries and the explanation offered by the parent and unexplainable delay between the injury and medical attention. Such children usually belong to broken families, lower socioeconomic group and may be illegitimate or unwanted.

Examination Findings

The battering child may show:

1. Fear and apprehension.
2. Bruises around the wrist, forearm, thighs and ankles, which form handles for adults to grip and swing the child.
3. Buttocks may show burns or whip marks.
4. Face and lips may be bruised. The frenulum of the tongue may be torn.
5. Circular bruises of 1–2 cm size, called 'six penny bruises', which occur due to the poking of adult fingers on the chest, abdomen and thighs.[8]
6. Signs of blunt trauma of different duration with inconsistent history of inflicting.

7. Crack fractures of the skull bones associated with intracranial hemorrhages.
8. Multiple rib fractures.
9. Fractures of bones mostly in the region of the metaphysis and epiphysis of growing bones. Periosteum elevations may be seen.

SHAKEN BABY SYNDROME

History

In 1946, the concept of "**shaken baby syndrome**" and the term "**whiplash shaken infant syndrome**" was introduced by **Dr John Caffey**, a paediatric radiologist.[9] The term described a set of symptoms found with little or no external evidence of head trauma, including retinal and intracranial hemorrhages with subdural or subarachnoid bleeding or both.[10] In 1971, **Dr Norman Guthkelch** proposed that whiplash injury caused subdural hemorrhage in infants by tearing the veins in the subdural space.[11]

Features

1. This syndrome involves vigorous manual shaking of an infant by the extremities or shoulders.
2. Diagnosed from a **triad of symptoms**: subdural hematoma, retinal hemorrhage and brain swelling.
3. The majority of cases there is no visible sign of external trauma.
4. Often fatal and can cause severe brain damage, resulting in lifelong disability.
5. Common age group younger than 1 year old, but may go up to 5–7 years.
6. SBS cannot be diagnosed by physical appearance alone, CT scans and MRI is very useful.

MUNCHAUSEN'S SYNDROME

Munchausen's syndrome is a term for psychiatric disorder known as factitious disorders, wherein those affected feign disease, illness or psychological trauma in order to draw attention or sympathy to themselves. It is also sometimes known as **hospital addiction syndrome** or **hospital hopper syndrome**. Nurses sometimes refer to them as **frequent flyers**, because they have returned to the hospital just like frequent flyers return to the airport. However, there is discussion to reclassify them as somatoform disorder in the DSM-5 (Diagnostic and Statistical Manual of Mental Disorders) as it is unclear whether or not people are conscious of drawing attention to themselves.[12]

Munchausen's Syndrome by Proxy

It is a type of child abuse commonly involving the mother. It consists of repeated pretensions of illness or the infliction of repeated minor injuries, with the object of gaining admission to hospital or obtaining medical care and attention. The child is brought to hospital with an induced sign and symptom of illness with a fictitious history. The child is frequently admitted to the hospital for medical attention for non-existent medical conditions.

Treatment

Medical professionals suspecting Munchausen's in a patient should first rule out the possibility that the patient does indeed have a disease state, but it is in an early stage and not yet clinically detectable. Providers need to acknowledge that there is uncertainty in treating suspected Munchausen patients, so that real diseases are not under-treated.[13] Then they should take a careful patient history, and seek medical records, to look for early deprivation, childhood abuse and mental illness. If a patient is at risk to himself or herself, inpatient psychiatric hospitalization should be initiated.[14]

SUDDEN INFANT DEATH SYNDROME

Synonyms: Cot death, Crib death, SIDS.

Definition

It is defined as the sudden death of an infant, which remains unexplained after a thorough case investigation, including performance of a complete autopsy, examination of the death scene and review of the clinical history.[15]

Risk Factors

- Incidence: 0.2–0.4% of live births
- Age: 2 weeks to 2 years, with maximum incidence between 3 and 7 months
- Sex: Male and female ratio—3:2
- Twins: Premature with low birth weight
- Crib deaths occur mainly at night or in the wee hours of the morning
- There is a prior history of running nose or coryza.

Etiology

1. Overlying of the infant by the drunken parents.
2. Prone sleeping position.[16]
3. Inadvertent smothering by soft cloth or pillow.
4. Sleep apnea, which causes hypoxia and respiratory depression.
5. Hypotonic babies, whose neck posture reduces the airway lumen.
6. Dust mite allergy.
7. Cow's milk allergy.
8. Calcium or selenium deficiency.
9. Viremia.
10. Hyperthermia or hypothermia.
11. Anaphylactic shock.

Autopsy Findings

Blood stained froth in the mouth; evidence of laryngitis may be present. Tracheobronchitis or congenital heart disease may be seen in some cases. Multiple petechial hemorrhages are seen sometimes in the heart, lung and thymus gland.

FEMALE FETICIDE

Female feticide is killing of female fetus. It is the act of aborting a fetus because it is female. This is a major social problem in India. Fetal sex determination and sex selective abortion by medical professionals has today grown into a ₹ 1,000 crore industry. Social discrimination against women and a preference for sons have been promoted.[17]

The practice of sex determination is widely prevalent in India and with increased availability of ultrasound machines; a corresponding decline in female birth rate was observed.[18]

In India, there is a constant decline in female births and problem is compounded by female feticide. There is continuous decline in the sex ratio from 972 females per 1000 males in 1901 to 927 females per 1000 males according to 2001 census, and these figures testifies the fact. Unfortunately, in many cases of feticide, qualified doctors are involved.[19,20]

The **Prenatal Diagnostic Techniques** (Regulations and Prevention of misuse) Act 1994 (PNDT Act 1994) was enacted for the check of female feticide. The Act was amended and is called as "The Preconception and Prenatal Diagnostic Techniques (Prohibition of sex selection) Act 2003 (PCPNDT Act 2003).

Objective of PC and PNDT Act 1996

1. Regulation for the purpose of detecting genetic or methods of chromosomal abnormalities or certain congenital malformations or sex-linked disorder.
2. Prevention of misuse of such technique for the purpose of prenatal sex determination leading to female feticide.

Thus, to fulfil the objectives not only genetic clinics or genetic laboratory, but also USG clinics or imaging centers, all have been brought under the purview of this Act. No person shall sell or buy any USG machine or imaging machine or scanner or any other equipment, capable of detecting the sex of fetus, to any other center or person not registered under this Act.

PCPNDT Act 2003[21]

Preconception and Prenatal Diagnostic Techniques Act 2003 (PCPNDT) prohibits sex selection before or after conception and the use of prenatal diagnostic techniques to determine the sex of the fetus.

Determination of sex can be as done by:

i. Amniocentesis
ii. Chorionic villous biopsy
iii. Ultrasound scans and imaging techniques.

Features of PCPNDT Act

i. The Act prohibits sex selection before or after conception.
ii. Regulates the use of prenatal diagnostic techniques.
iii. Gynecologist or RMP has to conduct prenatal diagnostic techniques at recognized place.
iv. Nursing home or RMP or hospital, where ultrasonography is used, have to display the board stating "hospital does not do sex determination test".
v. Prenatal diagnostic techniques can be conducted for purpose of determination of chronological or genetic or congenital abnormalities.
vi. Written consent of the pregnant woman is must to undergo PC and PND technique.
vii. Doctor contravening of the provisions of the Act shall be punished for 3 years imprisonment and fine of ₹ 10,000.
viii. Any person seeking help for sex selection shall also be held guilty and a provision of punishment for 3 years and fine of ₹ 50,000 is made under the Act.
ix. Doing sex determination test amounts to misconduct by Medical Council of India.[22]

Pre-requisite for Doing PCPNDT

PCPNDT should not be done unless any one or more conditions, mentioned below, are fulfilled:

i. History of two or more spontaneous abortions.
ii. Age of the pregnant women above 35 years.
iii. History of exposure to teratogenic drugs, radiation or infections.
iv. History of mental or physical deformities or genetic disease in family.

Indications

PCPNDT is carried out only to detect:

i. Hemoglobinopathies
ii. Ex-linked genetic diseases
iii. Chromosomal abnormalities
iv. Genetic or metabolic abnormalities
v. Congenital anomalies.

REFERENCES

1. Definitions of feticide. [cited 2012 Dec 17]; Available from: URL:http://www.dictionary.com
2. Borland's Medical Dictionary
3. The abortion (Amendment) (Wales) Regulation 2002 (Guidelines for doctors giving an abortion).
4. Di Maio VJM, Dana SF. Murder of infants and children. In: Handbook of Forensic Pathology. Lands Bioscience, USA; 1998. pp. 151-6.
5. Kaye NS. Families, Murder, and Insanity: A Psychiatric Review of Paternal Neonaticide.
6. Knight B, Singhal ML, Sahai VB. Infant deaths. In: HWV Cox's Medical Jurisprudence and Toxicology. 6th ed. Law Book Company; 1998. pp. 474-86.
7. Krahn LE, Bostwick JM, Stonnington CM. Looking toward DSM-V. Should factitious disorder become a subtype of somatoform disorder? Psychosomatics. 2008;49(4):277-82.
8. Bursztajn HJ, Feinbloom RI, Hamm RM, Brodsky A. Medical Choices, Medical Chances: How Patients, Families, and Physicians Can Cope With Uncertainty. New York: Delacorte, 1981; New York: Routledge, Chapman & Hall, 1990.
9. Johnson BR, Harrison JA. Suspected Munchausen syndrome and civil commitment. J Am Acad Psychiatry Law. 2000;28:74-6.
10. Willinger M, James LS, Catz C. Defining the sudden infant death syndrome (SIDS): Deliberations of an expert panel convened by the National Institute of Child Health and Human Development. PedPath. 1991;11:677-84.
12. Taylor BJ. A review of epidemiological studies of sudden infant death syndrome in Southern New Zealand. J Paed Child Health. 1991;27:344-8.

13. Karakus M, Ince H, Ince N, Arican N, Sozen S. Filicide cases in Turkey, 1995-2000. Croat Med J. 2003;44:592-5.
14. Mushin AS. Ocular damage in the battered-baby syndrome. BMJ. 1971;3:402-4.
15. [cited 2012 Dec 17]; Available from: URL:http://www.pediatrics.aappublications.org/cgi/content/abstract/54/4/396
16. David TJ. Shaken baby (shaken impact) syndrome: non-accidental head injury in infancy. J Royal Society Med. 1999;92(11):556-61.
17. Caffey J. On the theory and practice of shaking infants. Its potential residual effects of permanent brain damage and mental retardation. Am J Dis Child. 1972;124(2):161-9.
18. UNICEF India. UNICEF. Female foeticide in India. [cited 2012 Nov 12]; Available from: URL:http://www.en.wikipedia.org/wiki/Female_foeticide_in_India
19. Bardia A, Paul E, Kapoor SK, Anand K. Declining sex ratio: role of society, technology and government regulation in Faridabad district, Haryana. Natl Med J India. 2004;17:181-3.
20. Chaturvedi S, Chhabra P, Bhardwaj S, Smanla S, Kannan AT. Fetal sex-determination in Delhi—a population based investigation. Trop Doct. 2007;37:98-100.
21. Sharma BR. Female feticide in India: issue and concerns. J Indian Acad Forensic Med. 2008;30:157-60.
22. Pre-Conception and Pre-Natal Diagnostic Techniques Act, 2003.
23. Indian Medical Council (Professional conduct, etiquette and ethics) Regulations, 2002. Gazette of India dated 06/04/2002, part III, section 4.

CHAPTER 24

Virginity, Sexual Offences and Perversions

Putul Mahanta, Mukesh Yadav, AJ Patowary

LEARNING PLAN

- Know about the virginity and related issues
- Learn the classification of sexual offences
- Understand sexual harassment and punishments under Criminal Law Amendment Act, 2013
- Know about rape and related legal issues
- Learn the medical examination procedures of rape and sodomy victim and accused
- Know about incest and adultery
- Recognize unnatural sexual offences and sexual perversions

VIRGINITY

A **virgin** (*Virgo intacta*) is a female who has not experienced sexual intercourse. Originally, a virgin is a girl whose hymen is intact. **Defloration** means loss of virginity.

Signs of Virginity

A. Extragenital (Breast signs); B. Genital signs

Breast Signs

The breasts are firm, elastic, hemispherical and nonpendulous. There is a small under developed nipple with pink areola around it (**Figure 24.1**).

Masturbation, frequent sexual contact, and frequent handling make the breasts flabby and large.

Genital Signs

i. The labia majora are thick, firm, elastic and completely cover the labia minora

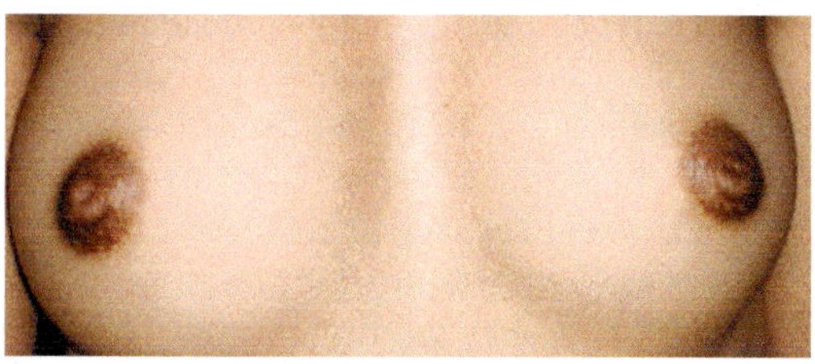

Figure 24.1 Virgin breasts

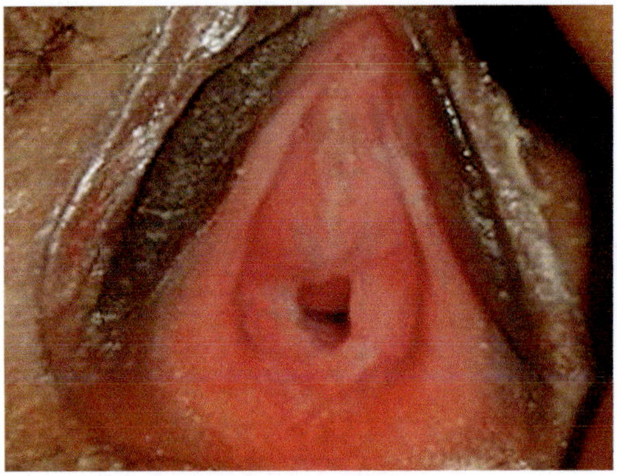

Figure 24.2 Intact hymen

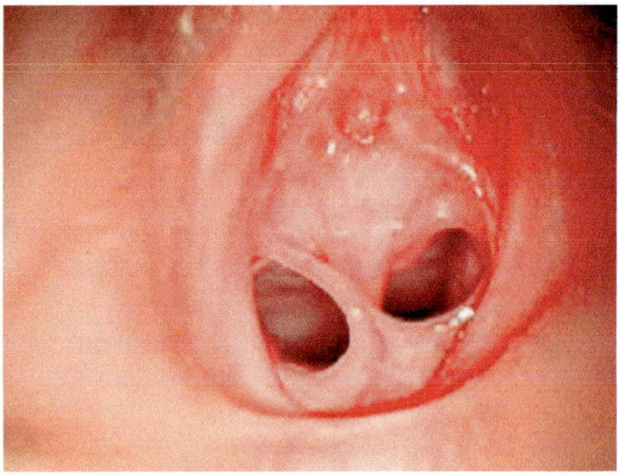

Figure 24.3 Septate hymen

including vaginal orifice. They are apposed together with each other.

ii. The labia minora are soft, small and pink in color in the form of a thin fold, which does not hang down, always lie behind the labia majora. In sexual habituation, they become dark, enlarged, and hang down from the labia majora.
iii. The clitoris is small with a narrow opening of the vestibule.
iv. Anterior commissure, posterior commissure and fourchette are intact and crescent shaped.
v. Hymen is intact **(Figure 24.2).**
vi. The vagina is narrow and tight with the presence of rugose.
vii. Vaginal orifice is small, which admits tip of little finger only.

HYMEN

What is Hymen?

Hymen is a thin fold of the mucous membrane in the opening of the vagina. It is lined on both sides with stratified squamous epithelium. Its shape is usually **semilunar** or **crescentic** and 1 mm thick. Embryologically, it is a remnant of the vaginal plates that develops between Mullerian duct and cloaca and has no useful function. The free margins are usually fimbriated having numerous notches. These may be mistaken for tears. The mucous membrane over the notches is intact.

What is the Hymen for?

Hymen has no purpose once birth has occurred. It is a remnant, covers to protect the reproductive parts when girl child was in the womb.

Types of Hymen

a. **Annular Hymen**: It has central opening.
b. **Septate Hymen**: A bridge of tissue divides the hymen into equal or unequal openings (**Figure 24.3**). Girls with a septate hymen may have trouble getting a tampon in or trouble getting a tampon out. The treatment for a septate hymen is a minor surgery to remove the extra band of tissue and create a normal sized vaginal opening.
c. **Crescentic** or **Semilunar**: This type of hymen has opening that is placed anteriorly.
d. **Cribriform** or **Microperforate Hymen**: Sometimes hymen is confused for imperforate, the hymenal opening appears to be absent, but has, under close examination, small openings. Cribriform hymen is a hymen with a number of small perforations.
e. **Fimbriated Hymen**: It has a central opening, but the margins are wavy or fimbriated and shows multiple notches (**Figure 24.4**).
f. **Infantile Hymen**: The infantile hymen has small and linear opening in the center.
g. **Imperforate Hymen**: The hymenal opening is absent. It requires minor surgery if it

has not corrected itself by puberty to allow menstrual fluids to escape.

h. **Congenital Absence of Hymen:** The frequency of congenital absence of the hymen has been found to be less than 0.03%.

The hymen is situated more deeply in very young girls. After coitus has taken place, the hymen becomes torn and takes a different shape. The tear is posteriorly or posterolaterally on one side or both sides. The normal hymenal opening admits one finger.

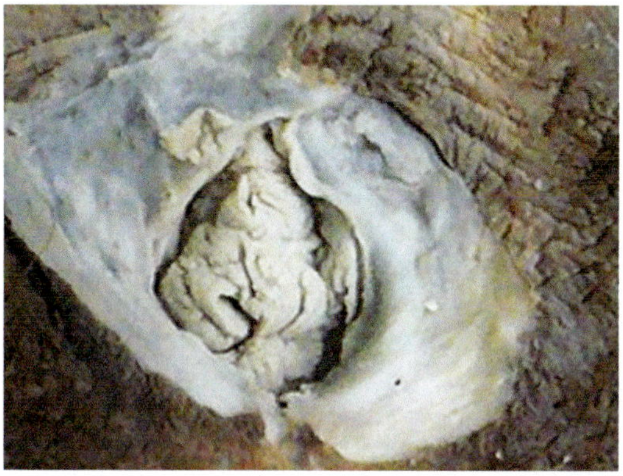

Figure 24.4 Wet specimen of fimbriated hymen

These are difficult cases where a definite finding of fact requires the experience of a medicolegal expert to prove the false virginity. It may be very loose, lax and tough, folded, so much so that it may not be even ruptured by a complete sexual intercourse. The differences between the virgin girl and deflorated women are shown in **Table 24.1**.

Rupture of Hymen

Generally, it is thought that a hymen ruptures the first time a girl has experienced sexual intercourse; however, due to the very active lifestyles we now lead, that is not inevitably the case. Some women are even born with a broken hymen. In **false virgins**, the hymen may remain intact even after sexual intercourse. The differences between true and false virgin are given in **Table 24.2**.

Table 24.1 Differences between virginity and defloration

Trait	Virgin	Defloration
Labia majora	Firm, thick, elastic, completely covers the labia minora	Loose, lax and the two folds are not apposed to each other
Labia minora	Small, pink color, thin folds, which cover the orifice of the vagina	Loose, thick, apart and hangs down, it is separate from the labia majora
Posterior commissure	Intact	Ruptured
Hymen	Intact, rigid and inelastic; the edges are distinct and regular with a narrow opening allowing little finger (**Figure 24.2**)	Torn or intact; in the later case it is loose, elastic, with a wide opening allowing passage of two or more fingers
Vagina	Narrow and tight with rugosities	Wider and laxed
Breast	Hemispherical, firm, non-pendulous, with small nipple and pinkish areola	Large, flabby and pendulous

Table 24.2 Differences between true and false virgin

Features	True virgin	False virgin
Definition	One who has never experienced sexual intercourse	One who has experienced sexual intercourse
Breast	Hemispherical, firm, non-pendulous, with small nipple and pinkish areola	Large, pendulous
Labia majora	Firm, thick, elastic, completely covers the labia minora	Loose, the two folds are not apposed to each other
Labia minora	Small, pink color, thin folds, which cover the orifice of the vagina	Enlarged, pigmented, separated, peep out
Clitoris	Small	Large
Hymen	Intact; rigid and inelastic; the edges are distinct and regular with a narrow opening allowing little finger (**Figure 24.2**)	Intact; loose and elastic; with a wide opening allowing passage of two or more fingers
Vagina	Narrow, apposed and tight with rugosities	Roomy, rugosity of mucosa partially lost

Hymen is ruptured by an act of sexual intercourse or may be due to other causes. When a ruptured following first act of coitus, the hymen is usually torn posteriorly at 6 o' clock position or may tear at posterolateral sites (5, 7, or 6 o' clock position) as bilateral tear. The tear extends from hymenal orifice to the vaginal wall. The tear is always complete and full. A sexually habituated female usually shows ruptured hymen with hymenal tags as irregular projections, known as carunculae hymenales. After vaginal delivery the hymen found completely absent only its remnants near the margin is present as an irregular thick area. This condition of the hymen is known as carunculae myrtiformis.

Causes of Rupture of Hymen Other than Sexual Intercourse

- Fall on a pointed object
- Masturbation
- Introduction of certain foreign bodies, e.g. solapith into vagina
- Instrumental medical examination
- Infections like diphtheria, scratching caused by thread worm infection
- Careless insertion of sanitary tampon, etc.

Medicolegal Importance of Virginity

The question of virginity comes up in civil cases like:

- Nullity of marriage
- Divorce
- Defamation .

In criminal case, it comes in relation to rape.

SEXUAL OFFENCES

In common parlance, **sexual offence** constitutes the most shocking crime against conscience and morality. The sufferings of a girl abducted, molested or raped far excel than that of the man committing it. It is the depraved passion and uncontrolled sex urges seeking gratification through force or fraud against the natural law of mating by mutual consent and as per accepted legal and social principles, that constitutes the root cause of almost every sexual offence. **Heterosexual** act between a male and a female with the help of their genitals meant for the purpose has been accepted all over the world for ages as a norm of normal sexual intercourse. When the sexual act transgresses the norms or rules of law, then it becomes illegal.

Classification of Sexual Offences (Figure 24.5)

Natural Offences

a. Rape
b. Incest
c. Adultery.

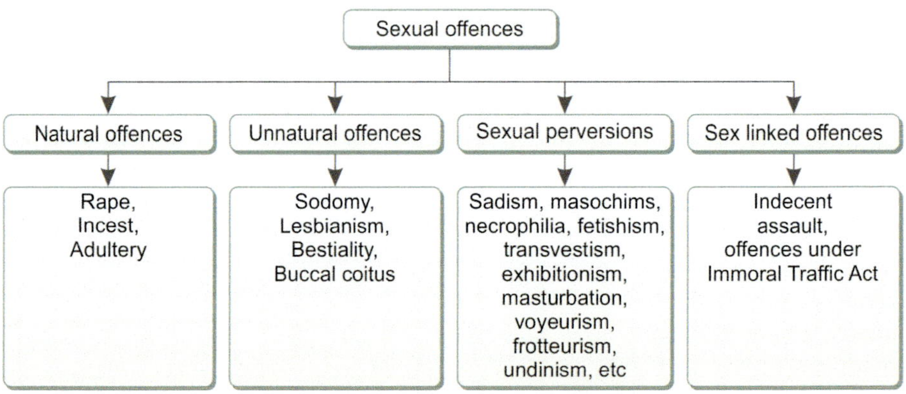

Figure 24.5 Classification of sexual offences

Unnatural Offences

a. Sodomy
b. Tribadism or lesbianism
c. Bestiality
d. Buccal coitus.

Sexual Perversions

a. Sadism (inflicting of humiliation or suffering)
b. Masochism (receiving of humiliation or suffering)
c. Necrophilia
d. Fetishism (use of non-living objects)
e. Transvestism (cross dressing)
f. Exhibitionism (exposure of the genitals)
g. Masturbation
h. Voyeurism (watching others engage in undressing or sexual activity, which is made a punishable offence after the Criminal Law Amendment, 2013)[1]
i. Frotteurism (touching and rubbing against a nonconsenting person)
j. Undinism, etc.

Sex-linked Offences

a. Indecent assault
b. Offences under Immoral Traffic Acts.

INDECENT ASSAULT (MOLESTATION), SEXUAL HARASSMENT AND PUNISHMENT

Indecent assault or molestation is an offence committed on a female with the intention or knowledge to outrage her modesty. Usually, the act involves the sexual parts of either or is sexually flavored. In such assaults, a man may try to kiss a woman, press her breast, touch or expose the genitalia or thighs, try to insert a finger in her vagina, etc. This is usually committed against children or adolescent girls and an adult. Unconsensual sexual act with a man by a female also comes under this term.

A medical practitioner can be accused of indecent assault if he examines a female patient by stripping her clothes without her consent and even with her consent in the absence of a female attendant.

Indecent Assault/Molestation (Section 354 IPC)

Whoever assaults or uses criminal force to any woman, intending to outrage or knowing it to be likely that he will thereby outrage her modesty, shall be punished with imprisonment of either description for a term, which shall not be less than one year but which may extend to 5 years, and shall also be liable to fine.

Such assaults are punishable under Section 354 IPC up to 2 years imprisonment and/or fine, but after amendment imprisonment may extend to 5 years (**Amended in 2013 by the Criminal Law Amendment Act, 2013**).[1]

After **Criminal Law Amendment, 2013**, new Sections 354A, B, C and D has been inserted after Section 354 IPC to cover 'sexual harassment,' 'voyeurism,' 'stalking,' etc.

Sexual Harassment (Section 354A, IPC)

1. **A man committing any of the following acts:**
   i. Physical contact and advances involving unwelcome and explicit sexual overtures; or
   ii. A demand or request for sexual favors; or
   iii. Showing pornography against the will of a woman; or
   iv. Making sexually colored remarks, shall be guilty of the offence of sexual harassment.
2. Any man who commits the offence specified in clause (i) or clause (ii) or clause (iii) of sub-section (1) shall be punished with rigorous imprisonment for a term which may **extend to 3 years** or **with fine** or **with both.**

3. Any man who commits the offence specified in clause (iv) of sub-section (1) shall be punishable with imprisonment of either description **for a term** that may **extend to one year** or **with fine** or **with both.**

Assault or Use of Criminal Force to Woman with Intent to Disrobe (Section 354B, IPC)

Any man who assaults or uses criminal force to any woman or abets such act with the intention of disrobing or compelling her to be naked, shall be punished with imprisonment of either description for a term which shall not be **less than 3 years but which may extend to 7 years and shall also be liable to fine.**

Voyeurism (354C, IPC)

Any man who watches, or captures the image of, a woman engaging in a private act in circumstances where she would usually have the expectation of not being observed either by the perpetrator or by any other person at the behest of the perpetrator or disseminate such image shall be punished on first conviction with imprisonment of either description for a term which shall **not be less** than **one year**, **but which may extend to 3 years**, and **shall also be liable to fine**, and **be punished on a second** or **subsequent conviction**, with imprisonment of **either description for a term which shall not be less than 3 years**, but **which may extend to 7 years**, and **shall also be liable to fine.**

Explanation 1: For the purposes of this section, "**private act**" includes an act of watching carried out in a place which, in the **circumstances**, would reasonably be expected **to provide privacy**, and where the victim's **genitals**, **posterior** or **breasts are exposed** or **covered only in underwear**; or the **victim is using a lavatory**; or **the victim is doing a sexual act that is not of a kind ordinarily done in public**.

Explanation 2: Where the victim consents to the capture of images or any act, but not to their dissemination to third persons and where such image or act is disseminated, **such dissemination shall be considered an offence under this section.**

Stalking (354D, IPC)

1. **Any man who:**
   i. Follows a woman and contacts or attempts to contact such woman to foster personal interaction repeatedly, despite a clear indication of disinterest by such woman, or
   ii. Monitors the use by a woman of the **internet**, **email** or **any other form of electronic communication**, commits the offence of stalking: **provided** that such conduct shall not amount to stalking if the man who pursued it proves that:
      i. It was pursued for the purpose of preventing or detecting crime and the man accused of stalking had been entrusted with the responsibility of prevention and detection of crime by the state; or
      ii. It was pursued under any law or to comply with any condition or requirement imposed by any person under any law; or
      iii. In the particular circumstances such conduct was reasonable and justified.
2. Whoever commits the offence of stalking shall be punished on first conviction with imprisonment of either description for a term which may **extend to 3 years**, and **shall also be liable to fine and be punished on a second or subsequent conviction, with imprisonment of either description for a term which may extend to 5 years, and shall also be liable to fine.**

Natural Offences

Heterosexual offences related to sex, in terms of sexual act conducted as per the rule of nature.

RAPE

According to the American Medical Association (1995), sexual violence, and rape in particular, is considered the most under-reported violent crime.[2] The rate of reporting, prosecution and convictions for rape varies considerably in different jurisdictions. The US Bureau of Justice Statistics (1999) estimated that 91% of US rape victims are female and 9% are male, with 99% of the offenders being male.[3] Rape is also recognized as an element of the crime of genocide when committed with the intent to destroy, in whole or in part, a targeted ethnic group.

Substitution of New Sections for Sections 375, 376, 376A, 376B, 376C and 376D

For Sections 375, 376, 376A, 376B, 376C and 376D of the Penal Code, the following sections shall be substituted, namely:

375 IPC

A person is said to commit "rape" if he:

a. Penetrates his penis, to any extent, into the vagina, mouth, urethra or anus of another person or makes the person to do so with him or any other person; or
b. Inserts, to any extent, any object or a part of the body, not being the penis, into the vagina, the urethra or anus of another person or makes the person to do so with him or any other person; or
c. Manipulates any part of the body of another person so as to cause penetration into the vagina, urethra, anus or any part of body of such person or makes the person to do so with him or any other person; or
d. Applies his mouth to the penis, vagina, anus, urethra of another person or makes such person to do so with him or any other person.

Under the circumstances falling under any of the following seven descriptions:

1. Against her will.
2. Without her consent.
3. With her consent, when such consent has been obtained by putting her or any person in whom she is interested, in fear of death or of hurt.
4. When her consent, when the man knows that he is not her husband and that her consent is given because she believes that he is another man to whom she is or believes herself to be lawfully married.
5. With her consent when, at the time of giving such consent, by reason of unsoundness of mind or intoxication or the administration by him personally or through another of any stupefying or unwholesome substance, she is unable to understand the nature and consequences of that action to which she gives consent.
6. With or without her consent, when she is **under 18 years of age**.
7. When she is unable to communicate consent.

Explanation 1: For the purposes of this section, "**vagina**" shall also include **labia majora**.

Explanation 2: Consent means an unequivocal voluntary agreement when the woman [person] by words, gestures or any form of verbal or non-verbal communication, communicates willingness to participate in the specific sexual act **provided** that, a woman [person] who does not physically resist to the act of penetration shall not by the reason only of that fact, be regarded as consenting to the sexual activity.

Exception 1: A medical procedure or intervention shall not constitute rape.

Exception 2: Sexual intercourse or sexual acts by a man with his own wife, the wife not being under 15 years of age, is not rape.

Punishment for Rape (Section 376 IPC and Other after Criminal Law Amendment, 2013)[1]

376 IPC

1. Whoever, except in the cases provided for by sub-section (2), commits rape shall be

punished with rigorous imprisonment of either description for a term which shall not be less than 7 years but which may extend to imprisonment for life, and shall also be liable to fine.

2. Whoever,
   a. Being a police officer, commits rape
      i. Within the limits of the police station to which such police officer is appointed; or
      ii. In the premises of any station house; or
      iii. On a woman in such police officer's custody or in the custody of a police officer subordinate to such police officer; or
   b. Being a public servant, commits rape on a woman [person] in such public servant's custody or in the custody of a public servant subordinate to such public servant; or
   c. Being a member of the armed forces deployed in the area by the Central or a State Government, commits rape in such area; or
   d. Being on the management or on the staff of a jail, remand home or other place of custody established by or under any law for the time being in force or of a women's or children's institution, commits rape on any inmate of such jail, remand home, place or institution; or
   e. Being on the management or on the staff of a hospital, commits rape on a woman in that hospital; or
   f. Being a relative, guardian or teacher of, or a person in a position of trust or authority towards, the person assaulted, commits rape on such woman; or
   g. Commits rape during communal or sectarian violence; or
   h. Commits rape on a woman knowing her to be pregnant; or
   i. Commits rape on a woman when such person is under 16 years of age; or
   j. Commits rape, on a woman incapable of giving consent; or
   k. Being in a position of control or dominance over a woman, commits rape on such woman; or
   l. Commits rape on a woman suffering from mental or physical disability; or
   m. While committing rape causes grievous bodily harm or maims or disfigures or endangers the life of a woman; or
   n. Commits rape repeatedly on same woman, shall be punished with rigorous imprisonment for a term which shall not be less than 10 years, but which may extend to imprisonment for life, and which shall mean imprisonment for the remainder of that person's natural life, and shall also be liable to fine.

Explanation: For the purposes of this sub-section,

a. "**Armed forces**" means the naval, military and air forces and includes any member of the Armed Forces constituted under any law for the time being in force, including the paramilitary forces and any auxiliary forces that are under the control of the Central Government or the State Government.
b. "**Hospital**" means the precincts of the hospital and includes the precincts of any institution for the reception and treatment of persons during convalescence or of persons requiring medical attention or rehabilitation.
c. "**Police officer**" shall have the same meaning as assigned to the expression "police" under the Police Act, 1861.
d. "**Women's or children's institution**" means an institution, whether called an orphanage or a home for neglected women or children or a widow's home or an institution called by any other name, which is established and maintained for the reception and care of women or children.

Punishment for Causing Death or Resulting in Persistent Vegetative State of the Victim

376A, IPC

Whoever, commits an offence punishable under sub-section (1) or sub-section (2) of section 376 and in the course of such commission inflicts an injury, which causes the death of the woman or causes the woman to be in a persistent vegetative state, shall be punished with rigorous imprisonment for a term which shall not be less than 20 years, but which may extend to imprisonment for life, which shall mean imprisonment for the remainder of that person's natural life or with death.

Rape by Husband upon his Wife during Separation [Punishment Increased from Minimum 2 Years to 7 Years]

376B, IPC

Whoever commits sexual intercourse [assault] with his own wife, who is living separately under a decree of separation or under any custom or usage, without her consent, shall be punished with imprisonment of either description, for a term which shall **not be less than 2 years but which may extend to 7 years, and shall also be liable to fine.**

Explanation: In this section, "sexual intercourse" shall mean any of the acts mentioned in clauses (a) to (d) of section 375.

Sexual Intercourse by a Person in Authority

376C, IPC

Whoever,

a. Being in a position of authority or in a fiduciary relationship; or
b. A public servant; or
c. Superintendent or manager of a jail, remand home or other place of custody established by or under any law for the time being in force, or a women's or children's institution; or
d. Being on the management of a hospital or being on the staff of a hospital and abuses such position or fiduciary relationship to induce or seduce any woman either in his custody or under his charge or present in the premises to have sexual intercourse with him, such sexual intercourse not amounting to the offence of rape, shall be punished with rigorous imprisonment of either description for a term which shall **not be less than 5 years but which may extend to 10 years, and shall also be liable to fine.**

Explanation 1: In this section, "**sexual intercourse**" shall mean any of the acts mentioned in clauses (a) to (d) of section 375.

Explanation 2: For the purposes of this section, Explanations 1 and 2 to section 375 shall also be applicable.

Explanation 3: "**Superintendent**", in relation to a jail, remand home or other place of custody or a women's or children's institution, includes a person holding any other office in such jail, remand home, place or institution by virtue of which such person can exercise any authority or control over its inmates.

Explanation 4: The expressions "**hospital**" and "**women's** or **children's institution**" shall respectively have the same meaning as in Explanation 1 to sub-section (2) of section 376.

376D, IPC

Where a woman [person] is raped [sexually assaulted] by one or more persons constituting a group or acting in furtherance of a common intention, each of those persons shall be deemed to have committed the offence of rape and shall be punished with rigorous imprisonment for a term which shall not be less than 20 years, but which may extend to life and which shall mean imprisonment for the remainder of that person's natural life and with fine, provided that such fine shall be just and reasonable to meet the medical expenses and rehabilitation of the victim; provide further that any fine imposed under this section shall be paid to the victim.

376E, IPC

Whoever has been previously convicted of an offence punishable under section 376 or Section 376A or Section 376C or Section 376D and is subsequently convicted of an offence punishable under any of the said sections shall be **punished with imprisonment for life, which shall mean imprisonment for the remainder of that person's natural life** or **with death.**

The **valid consent** must be free and voluntary, and given while she is of sound mind and not intoxicated by drugs or alcohol. The consent should be obtained prior to the act. A prostitute cannot be forced to have sexual intercourse against her will. Valid consent is also lacking if the victim lacks an actual capacity to give consent, as in the case of a victim who is a child, or who has a mental impairment or a developmental disability. Consent can always be withdrawn at any time, so that any further sexual activity after the withdrawal of consent constitutes rape.

In times gone by and in many countries even today, marriage is said to constitute at least an implied consent to sexual intercourse. However, marriage in many countries today is no longer a defense to rape or assault. In some jurisdictions, a person cannot be found guilty of the rape of a spouse, either on the basis of "implied consent" or because of a statutory requirement that the intercourse must have been "unlawful" (The British Virgin Islands under the Criminal Code, 1997). However, in many of those jurisdictions, it is still possible to bring prosecutions for what is effectively rape by characterizing it as an assault.[4]

In India, a husband cannot be guilty of committing rape on his spouse, if she is above 16 years, simply because, in marriage the wife consents to the husband for exercising the marital right of intercourse during the continuation of legal marriage.

Types of Rape

Rape can be categorized in different ways: for example, by reference to the situation in which it occurs, by the identity or characteristics of the victim, and/or by the identity or characteristics of the perpetrator.

Different types of rape include, but are not limited to: date rape, marital rape or spouse rape, gang rape, incestual rape, child sexual abuse, prison rape, war rape and statutory rape.[5]

Date Rape

Also called **acquaintance rape**, is a non-domestic rape committed by someone who knows the victim.[6] This constitutes the vast majority of rapes reported. It can occur between two people who know each other, usually in social situations, between people who are dating as a couple and have had consensual sex in the past, between two people who are starting to date, between people who are just friends and between acquaintances. They include rapes of coworkers, schoolmates, friends, and other acquaintances.

Spouse Rape

Also known as **marital rape**, wife rape, husband rape, partner rape or intimate partner rape (IPSA), is rape between a married or de facto couple. Research reveals that victims of marital/partner rape suffer longer-lasting trauma than victims of stranger rape.[7]

Gang Rape

Gang rape when number of assailants two or more than two; while in mass rape cases, number of assailants may be any in number but number of victims exceeds two or more.

One study showed that offenders and victims in gang rape incidents were younger with a higher possibility of being unemployed. Gang rapes involved more alcohol and drug use, night attacks and severe rape outcomes and less victim resistance and fewer weapons than individual rapes.[8] Another study found that group rape were more violent and had greater resistance from the victim than individual rape and that victims of group rape were more likely to seek crisis and police services, to contemplate suicide and seek therapy than those involved in individual assaults. The two groups were about the same in the amount of drug use and drinking during the assault.[9] Gang rape has now been categorized under the Criminal Law (Amendment) Act, 1983.

Incestual Rape

Incestual rape has been shown to be one of the most extreme forms of childhood trauma, a trauma that often does serious and long-term psychological damage, especially in the case of parental incest.[10]

Child sexual abuse is a form of child abuse in which an adult or older adolescent uses a child for sexual stimulation.[11,12] Different forms include asking a child to engage in sexual activities regardless of the outcome, exposure of the genitals, displaying pornography, sexual contact, physical contact with the child's genitals (except certain non-sexual contexts such as a medical examination), viewing of the child's genitalia for the purpose of sexual gratification or using children to produce child pornography.

Depending on the age and size of the child, and the degree of force used, child sexual abuse may cause internal lacerations and bleeding. In severe cases, damage to internal organs may occur, which, in some cases, may cause death.[13] Herman-Giddens et al. found six certain and six probable cases of death due to child sexual abuse in North Carolina between 1985 and 1994. The victims ranged in age from 2 months to 10 years. Causes of death included trauma to the genitalia or rectum and sexual mutilation.[14]

Protection of Children from Sexual Offences Act, 2012

The Act has been enacted and comes into effect in India in 2012. Under this Act, a child means any person under the age of 18 years. The salient features of the Act are as follows:

1. **Penetrative Sexual Assault** (**Section 3**): If a person penetrates his penis, any object or part of his body to any extent into the vagina, mouth, urethra or anus of the child or makes the child to do so with him or any other person or applies his mouth to the penis, vagina, anus, urethra of the child or makes the child to do so to him or any other person will constitute a Penetrating Sexual Assault on the child. The punishment for such act is imprisonment for a period not less than 7 years which may extend to imprisonment for life, and fine (**Section 4**).
2. **Aggravated Penetrative Sexual Assault** (**Section 5**): If such acts are done by a person such as a member of security forces, police officer, public servant, etc. The punishment for such act is imprisonment for a period not less than 10 years which may extend to imprisonment for life, and fine (**Section 6**).
3. **Sexual Assault** (**Section 7**): Whoever, with sexual intent touches the vagina, penis, anus or breast of the child or makes the child to touch the vagina, penis, anus or breast of such person or any other person, or does any other act with sexual intent, which involves physical contact without penetration is said to commit sexual assault. The punishment is imprisonment for a period not less than 3 years which may extend to 5 years, and fine (**Section 8**).
4. **Aggravated Sexual Assault** (**Section 9**): If such acts, are done by person, such as a member of security forces, police officer, public servant, etc. The punishment for such act is imprisonment for a period not less than 5 years which may extend to 7 years, and fine (**Section 10**).
5. **Sexual Harassment of the Child** (**Section 11**): Whoever uses any word, gesture or exhibits any body part of the body or makes the child do so with him any other person or shows any pornographic objects to the child will constitute sexual harassment of the child. The punishment for such act is imprisonment for a term which may extend to 3 years and fine (**Section 12**).

6. **Use of Child for Pornographic Purposes (Section 13):** Imprisonment for a term not less than 5 years, which may extend to 10 years or 11 life sentence depending upon the nature of the crime and fine (Section 14 (1) to (5)).
7. **Storage of Pornographic Material Involving Child (Section 15):** Any person, who stores, for commercial purposes any pornographic material in any form involving a child shall be punished with imprisonment of either description which may extend to 3 years or with fine or with both.

Apart from these, there are provisions for the abatement to commit an offence and attempt to commit an offence are also laid down. There is also provision for punishment for non-reporting the offence as well as the false reporting of the offence in this Act, thought the punishment for false reporting is kept comparatively less to encourage reporting.

The Act also has the guideline for the reporting, recording the statement, investigation as well as trial of such an offence.

Statutory Rape

It is a term used to describe sexual activities where one victim is below the age required to legally consent to the behavior. Although it usually refers to adults engaging in sex with minors under the age of consent, it is a generic term, and very few jurisdictions use the actual term "statutory rape" in the language of statutes. Different jurisdictions use many different statutory terms for the crime, such as "rape", "rape of a child", "corruption of a minor", "carnal knowledge of a minor", "unlawful carnal knowledge", or simply "carnal knowledge". Statutory rape differs from forcible rape in that overt force or threat need not be present.

Sexual offence is cognizable offence; some vital aspect about rape are described below:

1. **What constitutes rape?**
   The slightest penetration of the penis within the vulva, with or without emission of semen or rupture of hymen constitutes rape. There need not be a complete penetration, but it is essential to prove in a case of rape that actual penetration has occurred. Rape can occur even in absence of body injuries or semen in a genital tract, but such negative evidence does not exclude rape. Doctors should mention all the negative findings, but should not give his opinion that rape has not been committed. The circumstantial evidences are important in such cases.
2. The Indian Evidence Act has also been amended to shift the **burden of proving consent** to sexual intercourse from the victim to the rapist in limited cases.
3. Under the law, rape can only be committed by a man; and a woman cannot rape a man, although she may be guilty of an indecent assault upon him.
4. **Age of the accused**
   In India, there is no age limit; court is to decide the potency. Even old man commits rape on young girl. In the UK, a person less than 14 years is not charged for rape.
5. **Age of the victim**
   No age is safe from rape, as children of one year or even less and old women of 85 years have been raped. Children are frequently raped than adults as they are incapable to resist the act and also due to false belief that venereal diseases are cured by sexual intercourse with a virgin. One of the most salient and well-documented criminological aspects of rape is the unusually young age distribution of its female victims. Risk for women of rape victimization peaks in the late teens and early twenties, then declines throughout the lifespan.
6. Medical proof of sexual intercourse does not mean that it is a legal proof of rape. Rape is a cognizable offence, but it is not a medical condition. Rape is a legal term and not a diagnosis to be made by the medical doctors treating the victim. The medical officers should make the statement that there is evidence of recent sexual

intercourse. False rape is called simulated rape.

7. No specific time limit for lodging complaint of rape.
8. **Drink**, **drug** and **rape**: Date rape drug refers to a drug that can be used to assist in the commission of a rape, such as date rape. Drugs used to facilitate rape may have sedative, hypnotic, dissociative or amnesiac effects and can be added to a food or drink without the victim's knowledge.

The act of adding such substances to drinks is known as "**drink spiking**". The reasons for drink spiking range from personal amusement or maliciousness to theft or (sexual) assault.[15] The term "date rape drug" originated in American journalism in the 1990s, amid widespread reports that previously unknown herbs and pharmaceuticals were making rapes easier and more frequent. Most Americans still use the term in that narrow sense, to refer to what they consider "exotic" drugs, but alcohol and many other common substances can incapacitate a person and have been used in rapes.

Drug-facilitated Sexual Assault (DFSA)

In a recent case[16] in Delhi, Sessions Judge observed that "before I end, I deem it necessary to place on record the fact that while dealing with the case in hand this Court has observed that recently there has been an increase in number of cases where women have been surreptitiously administered drugs and sexually exploited thereafter." Interestingly the pattern of crime in all such cases has been observed to be almost similar. Rape of people under the influence of alcohol or drugs is not new, and rape of people who have voluntarily consumed alcohol or drugs are common. It is also not new to slip something into somebody's drink to incapacitate them. Law enforcement agents are seeing a pattern of women being surreptitiously drugged for the purpose of rape, particularly through use of odorless, tasteless incapacitating drugs that produce anterograde amnesia.

It is a matter of common knowledge that a large number of drugs are freely available in the market, which are used to assist in execution of Drug Facilitated sexual assault (DFSA). These are called date rape drugs or also predator drugs. Because of the effects of these drugs, victims may be physically helpless, unable to refuse sex and unable to remember what happened. Gamma hydroxybutyric acid (GHB), ketamine and benzodiazepines (Flunitrazepam, Rohypnol or Roofies, Rope and Roaches) are the most common date rape drugs.

This issue relating to free availability and sale of these date rape drugs is a matter of national concern. It is a known fact that detection of these drugs is difficult issue and unless a victim of DFSA seeks medical care within 72 hours of the assault, it is less likely that the tests would successfully detect the presence of these drugs, since most of them metabolize and get eliminated from the body within that period, resulting into a negative report.

Whenever a victim makes allegations of rape after being drugged, samples are required to be collected for detection and it is necessary for the law enforcement agencies to inquire the victim on effects of the drug felt by her after its administration. This is required to be done for making it possible for the laboratories to conduct not only a broad drug screen but also a specific drug screening (knowing the drug's effects and which drug to test for), which unfortunately is not followed in many of the cases. It is also obligated upon the Law Enforcement Agencies in case of allegation by victims of rape of being surreptitiously administered some drug to get the drug testing done as part of the **Rape Kit** (collection of blood, urine, sputum and hair samples) which again is not done regularly.

In the aforementioned case, the Court further added that the issue does not end here and the entire concept of date rape drugs is fraught with legal problems. For victims, it is extremely important to know if they consented or not or were drugged deliberately or voluntarily. For prosecutors, there is a difficulty in proving the intent or lack of consent where the rape or assault happened without witnesses (particularly in a private home) and where both parties were consuming drugs or alcohol since neither was able to legally give consent. Independent proof of forced consumption of drugs or forced sexual activity is seldom available. It is thus equally necessary for those dealing with the issues on the judicial side to be informed, updated and sensitized with the issues involved.

Needless to say, an information/awareness campaign on a large scale is the need of the hour. An informed debate with regard to the sensitization of general public as well as the law enforcement, prosecution, hospital and the forensic agencies about the date rape drugs is necessitated. This is required to be done so that the guilty does not go Scott free and justice is done to the victim.[16]

In most parts of the World, whether or not a drug was used is irrelevant to the issue of whether a particular incident is rape or not. The legal definition of rape in countries such as the US also covers a lack of consent when the victim is unable to say "no" to intercourse, whether the effect is due to drugging or simply alcohol consumption (**Rape-criminal law**).

9. **Anesthesia and rape**

   There have been many cases of women alleging of sexual molestation while regaining consciousness after anesthesia, sedatives and other drugs while undergoing surgery. Unfortunately, some doctors, dentists and oral surgeons use these drugs to rape their patients. Hence, it is necessary that when these drugs are administered, nurses or other chaperones are present in the room so that a hallucination can clearly be distinguished from rape.[17]

   It is impossible to have complete sexual intercourse with a woman during her natural sleep without her knowledge. When a woman takes an aphrodisiac or alcohol or other drugs voluntarily to increase sexual feelings and become the victim of sexual intercourse, the question of consent depends on the extent to which she had become affected. She can refuse consent if she is conscious. In such cases thorough/detailed history is needed besides analysis of samples of urine, blood, etc.

10. **Victim blaming**

   "Victim blaming" is holding the victim of a crime to be in whole or in part responsible for the crime. In the context of rape, this concept refers to the Just World Theory and popular attitudes that certain victim behaviors (such as flirting or wearing sexually-provocative clothing) may encourage rape.[18] In extreme cases, victims are said to have "**asked for it**", simply by not behaving demurely. In most Western countries, the defense of provocation is not accepted as mitigation for rape.[19] A global survey of attitudes toward sexual violence by the Global Forum for Health research shows that victim-blaming concepts are at least partially accepted in many countries. In some countries, victim-blaming is more common, and women who have been raped are sometimes deemed to have behaved improperly. Often, these are countries where there is a significant social divide between the freedoms and status afforded to men and women.[20] However, this is not practiced in India.

Examination of a Rape Victim

Different Objectives

i. To look for physical evidence.
ii. Collect and preserve all the trace evidences.
iii. Treat the victim for injuries, venereal disease, pregnancy and psychological damages, etc.

Procedures

All the cases of sexual offences are examined in India as per the provision laid down in the Section 164 (A) CrPC.

164-A. Medical examination of the victim of rape:

1. Where, during the stage when an offence of committing rape or attempt to commit rape is under investigation, it is proposed to get the person of the woman with whom rape is alleged or attempted to have been committed or attempted, examined by a medical expert, such examination shall be conducted by a registered medical practitioner employed in a hospital run by the Government or a local authority and in the absence of such a practitioner, by any other registered medical practitioner, with the consent of such woman or of a person competent to give such consent on her behalf and such woman shall be sent to such registered medical practitioner within 24 hours from the time of receiving the information relating to the commission of such offence.
2. The registered medical practitioner, to whom such woman is sent, shall, without delay, examine her person and prepare a report of his examination giving the following particulars, namely:
   i. The name and address of the woman and of the person by whom she was brought;
   ii. The age of the woman;
   iii. The description of material taken from the person of the woman for DNA profiling;
   iv. Marks of injury, if any, on the person of the woman;
   v. General mental condition of the woman; and
   vi. Other material particulars in reasonable detail.
3. The report shall state precisely the reasons for each conclusion arrived at.
4. The report shall specifically record that the consent of the woman or of the person competent to give such consent on her behalf to such examination had been obtained.
5. The exact time of commencement and completion of the examination shall also be noted in the report.
6. The registered medical practitioner shall, without delay forward the report to the investigating officer who shall forward it to the Magistrate referred to in Section 173 as part of the document referred to in clause (*a*) of subsection (5) of that section.
7. Nothing in this section shall be construed as rendering lawful any examination without the consent of the woman or of any person competent to give such consent on her behalf.[21]

Step of Examination

1. **Paper Documents**: A requisition for examination from authorized police officer or magistrate.
   However, in its 4th May 2000 judgment in relation to case of the State of Karnataka versus Manjanna, the Supreme Court recognized that the rape victim's need for a medical examination constituted a "medicolegal emergency". Second, it was also the right of the victim of rape to approach medical services first before legally registering a complaint in a police station. The hospital was obliged to examine her right away; they could always subsequently initiate a police complaint on the request of the victim. As a result of this landmark judgment, the doctor or hospital is now required to examine a victim of rape, if she reports to the hospital directly, and voluntarily, without a police requisition.
2. **Consent**: She should never be examined without her written informed consent taken in presence of witness. If the girl is below 12 years of age, or in case of the mentally challenged one, a written consent should be asked from parents or legal guardian. If the girl is more than 18 years of age a written consent should be obtained.
3. Two identification marks of victim should be noted.
4. Name, age and address should be noted.
5. Exact date, time and place of examination should be mentioned.
6. Name of the accompanying constables and persons who brought the victim for

medical examination should be noted. It is usually the police constable or officer.

7. Statements of the victim and brief clinical history are recorded.
8. A **female attendant** must be present at the time of physical examination of a female.

Gauhati High Court in Assam in a PIL filed in the year 2009 issued directions in its order dated 19.08.2010:[22] that the DGP, Assam, and the Health Department of the Government of Assam and all other concerned to ensure that a female victim of sexual offence is examined only by lady Government Doctor, and if there is no lady doctor available, a private female practitioner at state expense can be employed or vaginal smear be collected by a trained female nurse and examined subsequently by a lady doctor.

9. History of menstrual cycle.
10. General behavior, her mental state, gait, etc.
11. Examination of clothes.
12. Examination for physical development.
13. Collection and preservation of material evidence.

Examination Proper

The victim is allowed to stand on a large white paper and asked to remove her cloths of her own and any foreign material that may be falling on the sheet of paper is to be collected.

1. **Clothes**: If the clothes are same as those worn at the time of incident of rape, they should be carefully examined for the presence of blood or seminal stains, etc. Evidence of struggle like tears, if present, should be recorded. The vulval pads or vaginal tampons, if present, should be examined and preserved.
2. **Signs of violence**: Especially on the forearms, wrist, face, breasts (nail scratch abrasion, bruises, bite marks, etc., as shown in **Figure 24.6** and **Figure 24.7**), chest, lower part of abdomen, inner aspects of thighs and back should be looked and recorded.
   In addition to these marks, the female may experience difficulty in walking and pain in micturation or defecation. The gait of the victim should be carefully observed.[23] The whole body should be examined for any stains under the UV light so that any seminal stain or some other stain if any can be visualized which may not be visible in naked eye.
3. **General physical examination**: General physical development should be noted and for this, the height, weight and the physical development as well as the secondary sexual characters are to be noted.
4. **The Genitals**: The victim should be kept in lithotomy or knee-chest position in good light.
   Points to be Noted
   a. If the pubic hairs are found matted due to the presence of semen, they

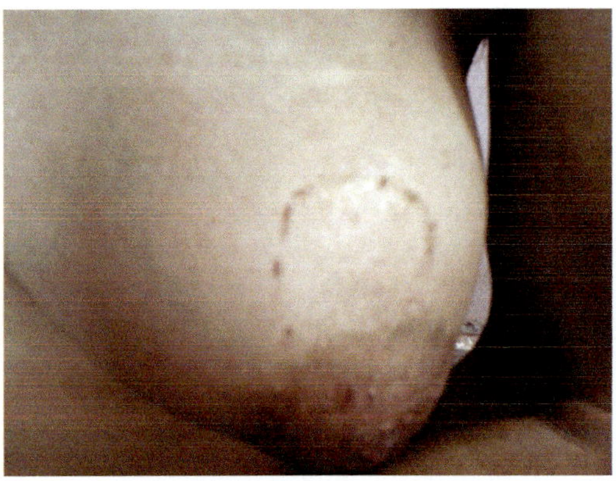

Figure 24.6 Bite mark on breast
(*Courtesy* Dr Mamata Devi Haloi)

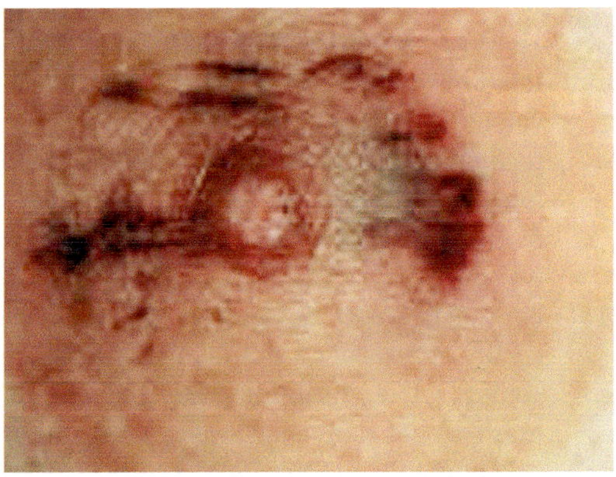

Figure 24.7 Bite mark on nipples

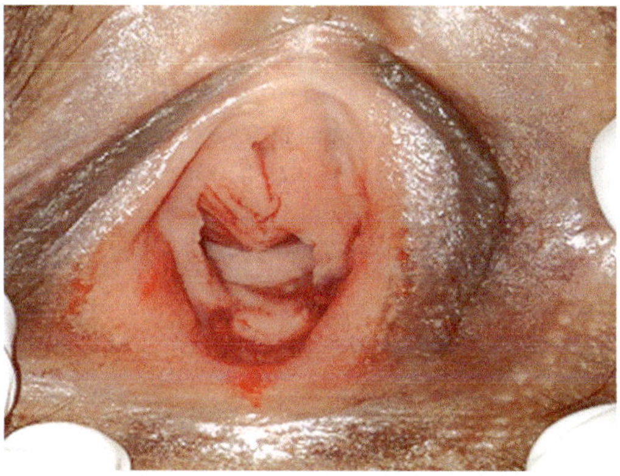

Figure 24.8 Recent hymenal tears (at 5 and 7 o' clock position)

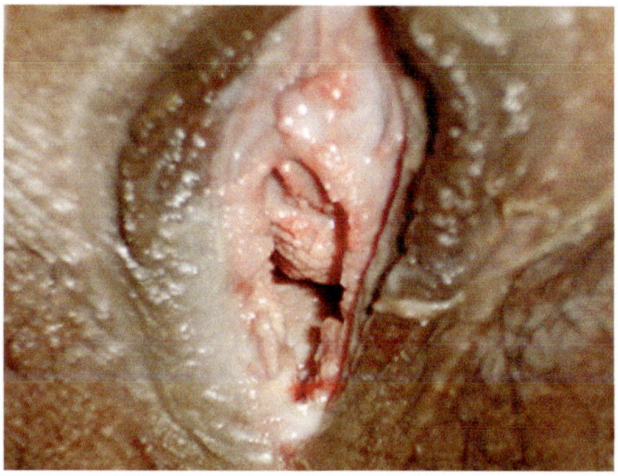

Figure 24.9 Old hymenal tear at 4 o'clock position with tear of posterior commissure

should be cut off and examined for the presence of human spermatozoa. Dried seminal stains, if found on the external genitals, should be scraped and preserved for subsequent examination. The dried scraped seminal stain is moistened with normal saline and slides prepared for microscopic examination.

b. Recently effused or dried blood, if found upon genitals, should not be forgotten, which may be bleeding due to menstruation, which is possible to be induced by sexual intercourse.
c. Bruising and laceration of the external genitals may be present with redness, tender swelling and inflammation.
d. The **hymen**, as a result of sexual intercourse especially in virgin is usually lacerated, having one or more radiating tears, more so in posterior part, the edges of which are red, swollen and painful and bleed on touch, if examined within 2 to 3 days after the act, which is known as **recent hymenal tear** (**Figure 24.8**).

   After 3 to 5 days, they heal and after 10 days become shrunken and look like small tags of tissues (**Figure 24.9**). Frequent sexual intercourse and parturition completely destroy the hymen, which is represented by several small tags of tissue, which are called carunculae hymenealis or myrtiformes. The fourchette and posterior commissure are not usually injured in cases of rape, but they may be torn, if the violence used is very great indeed.

   The hymen of small children is not usually ruptured, but may become red and congested along with the inflammation and bruising of the labia. If the violence used is appreciable; there is often laceration of fourchette and perineum.
e. The vaginal secretion from the posterior fornix should always be obtained by introducing a plain sterile cotton wool swab. The material obtained on the swab must immediately be transferred to a microscopic slide and spread out in the form of thin film and fixed in room temperature. After staining, the slide should then be examined for the presence of spermatozoa (**Figure 24.10**), which is a positive sign of recent sexual intercourse.

Detection of spermatozoa in slide, depends upon time since the rape. The presence of spermatozoa in the vagina after intercourse has been reported by **Pollak** (1943) from 30 minutes to 17 days, by **Morrison** (1972) up to 9 days in vagina and 12 days in the cervix. However, in the vagina of a dead woman, they persist for a longer period.[24]

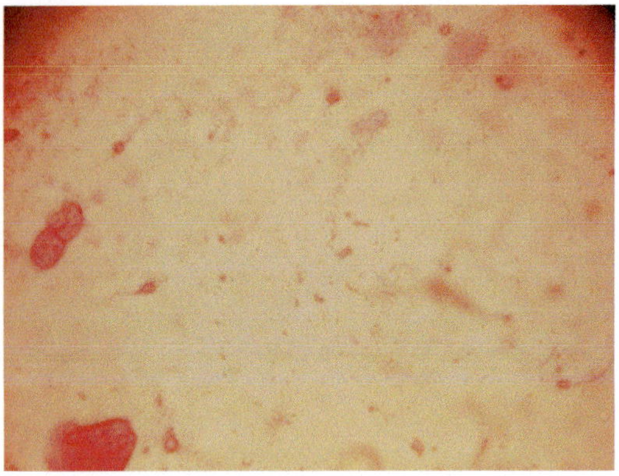

Figure 24.10 Spermatozoa in post-coital vaginal slide

Given normal sperm parameters in the area of motility, count, vitality and morphology, **how long can sperm survive in a woman**? That's a good question, but the answer is very difficult one and depends on a large number of variables including the individual longevity of sperm, the internal metabolic capacity of sperm, the environment of the vagina (body temperature, pH levels, relative acidity), the presence and the quality of cervical mucus, the ability of the sperm to get out of the vagina and into the womb, and the presence of sperm antagonists like immunity securing white blood cells.

Acid Phosphatase is an enzyme secreted by the prostate gland that is present in large amounts in seminal fluid. It, like prostatic specific antigen (**PSA**), is not unique to the prostate and can be found in other biological fluids including vaginal secretions. It is, therefore, considered a **presumptive** chemical test for the presence of semen and semen must be confirmed by other means (sperm detection or PSA detection using membrane test systems). Since seminal and vaginal acid Phosphatase cannot be discriminated, the only approach to differentiating semen in vaginal secretion is by quantitative analysis such as PSA or the microscopic inspection for sperm.

5. **Signs of venereal infection**: The existence of venereal disease in the female is not always a positive evidence of sexual connection. Any infection detected at post-rape screening may have been present previously. Therefore, it is absolutely necessary to examine the accused for the presence of either of these diseases as shown in **Table 24.3**.

Cytological Detection of Spermatozoa

The three most commonly used staining methods are: (i) Christmas tree, (ii) Hematoxylineosin, (iii) Alkaline fuchsin, and (iv) Gram's stains.

Alkaline fuchsin did not seem effective in detecting spermatozoa in vaginal samples. Compared with hematoxylineosin, Christmas tree stain appeared to be the most useful test in the first 72 hours. Two external factors were associated with decreased detection of spermatozoa: time since intercourse and sperm volume.

Specimens to Be Collected from Victim

Objectives

1. To confirm the allegations.
2. To establish a link between the victim with the scene; between the victims with the assailant.

Things are to Be Preserved

1. Avulsed scalp or pubic hairs.
2. Matted pubic hairs and any foreign hair recovered by combing the pubic hair.
3. 5 mL blood (plain) for grouping and 5 mL in EDTA for alcohol and drugs.
4. Urine for drug screening.
5. Nail scrapings.
6. Genital swabs. Three swabs should be taken: One from vulval margins, one from cervical margins and another from vagina (posterior fornix).
7. Saliva for secretor group.
8. Swabs from any soiled areas of skin.

Table 24.3 Sexually transmitted disease and its brief clinical features

Sexually transmitted disease	Clinical features
AIDS: Caused by the HIV virus that invades the immune system, resulting in "well carriers" to severe and fatal disorders. Spread by contact with infected blood, semen, vaginal fluids, needle sharing and maternal transfer mainly by unprotected vaginal and anal sex, unprotected oral sex, injection of tainted blood, needle-sharing, sharing objects and infected fluids, maternal blood to fetus	*HIV stage (1–14 years):* Flu-like symptoms may occur early or late; most look and feel well for years; infectious carrier; Skin and lung infections common in later years; HIV antibody test indicates infection; 25% of infants born to HIV mothers will be infected
Chlamydia: Caused by bacteria that commonly infects the genitals, anus and throat and is the most common STD. Spread through contact with infected semen and vaginal fluids; unprotected vaginal and anal sex, unprotected oral sex	Most women show no symptoms. Some may have slight vaginal discharge, pain on urination and during sex; frequent urination. Most men show discharge or itchy feeling in the penis; mild pain on urination; infection of anus or throat
Genital lice (crabs): Caused by the genital "crab louse", which transfers from the genital hair of one partner to the other, and lays eggs at the base of the hair. Spread by vaginal sex, protected or not; direct touch. skin-to-skin	Intense itching in the genital hair area. Itch in 5–10 days and produces small red bumps
Genital herpes (HSV): Caused by a herpes simplex virus with ulcerating blisters occurring on the genitals or anal area. Spread by unprotected vaginal sex, anal and oral sex; direct touch, skin-to-skin spread to the mouth	Many people feel fatigued, and have a fever. Painful blisters, itching, redden the skin, form into groups and ulcerate. Ulcers crust and may heal with scarring
Genital warts (HPV): Caused by human papillomavirus and occurs often on or in the genitals and anus. Genital warts are associated with cancer. Spread by unprotected vaginal and anal sex, unprotected oral sex	Soft, moist, pink growths on the penis, around anus, and on or in the female genitals. May become stalked like a cauliflower
Gonorrhea: Caused by bacteria that commonly infects the genitals, anus and throat. Spread by infected semen and vaginal fluids through unprotected oral, vaginal and anal sex *Incubation period:* 2–8 days	No symptoms or some vaginal discharge, pain on urination and frequency. Men usually notice thick yellow green discharge from the penis with pain, pain on urinating. If infected the rectum may have pain, bleeding and discharge. Sore throats if the throat is infected
Scabies: Caused by female mites which burrow under the skin to lay their eggs, causing skin irritation. Spread through close touch, skin-to-skin and shared personal items	Intense itching at night. Small red bumps and rashes develop 4–6 weeks after contact. Anywhere on the skin except head and neck.
Syphilis: Caused by the *Treponema pallidum* bacterium, develops a staged disease over years and is highly contagious, but cannot survive outside the body. Affects the skin and any organ. Incubation period: 2–8 weeks. Spread by contact with infected blood, semen, vaginal fluids or pus. It may spread from mother to unborn, direct touch, close body contact, unprotected oral, vaginal and anal sex, kissing, injecting blood (needle sharing)	*Stage 1:* Early stages show painless sores, swollen glands and skin rashes. Sores may be inside the vagina or anus and go unnoticed *Stage 2:* Rashes, new sores, flu-like symptoms, swollen glands, brain infection
Trichomoniasis: Caused by the single celled protozoan parasite *Trichomonas vaginalis*. Vagina most common site in women, and the urethra in men. Spread through unprotected vaginal sex	Itching, burning, irritation inside the penis; vaginal or vulval redness, unusual vaginal discharge, frequent painful urination; discomfort intercourse, abdominal pain

Evidence of Rape

- Marks of violence in both parties
- Marks of violence in genitals
- Presence of stains of semen or blood on clothes and body
- Presence of semen and spermatozoa in the vagina
- STD in both parties.

Rape Trauma Syndrome

It is a form of psychological trauma experienced by a rape victim that consist of disruptions to normal physical, emotional, cognitive, behavioral and interpersonal characteristics. The theory was first described by psychiatrist Ann Wolbert Burgess and sociologist Lynda Lytle Holmstrom in 1974.[25]

PROFORMA FOR EXAMINATION OF A SEXCRIME VICTIM

No. FM/SC: ______ Date: ______

Ref: ______ PSCaseNo: ______ U/S: ______

1. **Name:** ______ 2. **Sex:** ______
3. **Address:** ______
4. **Religion:** ______
5. **Marital Status:** ______ 6. **Age** (as told by the person): ______
7. **Occupation:** ______
8. **Accompanying** and **identifying Police**: No. ______ 9. **Name:** ______

   Signature: ______ **Date:** ______
10. **Male/Female attendant**:

    Name: ______

    Signature: ______ Date: ______
11. **Consent** for examination (Informed consent): ______ Date: ______
12. **Date of Examination:** ______ Place: ______ Time: ______
13. **Marks of Identification:** i. ______ ii. ______
14. **Case History:** From Police: ______ From Person: ______
15. **Physical Examination**:

    I. Height: ______ cm II. Weight: ______ kg

    III. Chest girth: ______ cm IV. Abdomen girth: ______ cm

    V. **Teeth:**

Right	8 (S) 7 6 5 4 3 2 1	1 2 3 4 5 6 7 (S) 8	Left
	8 (S) 7 6 5 4 3 2 1	1 2 3 4 5 6 7 (S) 8	

Temporary: ______ Permanent: ______ Total: ______

Space for teeth: ______

Contd..

Contd..

VI. **Hair**: A. Scalp:

B. Axillary:

C. Pubic:

VII. **Breast**:

16. **Menstrual History:** Menarche: Cycle: Last Menstrual Period:

17. Genital Examination:

A. Genital organs:

B. Vulva:

C. Hymen:

D. Vagina:

E. Cervix:

F. Uterus:

G. Evidence of venereal disease:

H. Vaginal swabs collected from:

18. Injury on the body:

19. Wearing garments: Evidence of struggle: Evidence of stain:

20. Mental condition at the time of examination:

21. Cooperation and behavior:

22. Intelligence and memory:

23. Gait:

24. **Report of radiological investigations:** Skiagram No.: Date:

25. Result of laboratory investigation:

26. **Opinion**: On the basis of physical examination and radiological investigations done on:.

I am/we are of the opinion that

Signature and seal of the examining doctor

The rape trauma syndrome (RTS) is divided into two phases, which can disrupt the physical, psychological, social or sexual aspects of a victim's life. The **acute or disruptive phase** can last from days to weeks and is characterized by general stress response symptoms. During the **second phase** the long-term process of reorganization, the victim has the recovery task of restoring order to her lifestyle and re-establishing a sense of control in the world. This phase is characterized by rape related symptoms and can last from months to years.

The early conceptualizations of the stress response patterns of rape victims are consistent with the diagnostic criteria of Post-Traumatic Stress Disorder (PTSD) of the DSM-IV within the major category of anxiety disorders. Burgess and Holmstrom present the only description in the literature of the manifestations of rape trauma in children and adolescents. In general, the RTS manifests itself similarly in children, adolescents and adults. The differences are consistent with the developmental stage of the young victim and the alternate affective and behavioral modes by which a youngster responds to stress. Thus, nausea, vomiting and bedwetting may occur along with the spectrum of life pattern disruption seen in adults. In addition to reacting to the threat to a life, feelings of embarrassment can be prominent, especially in adolescent victims. Many of the concerns of children and adolescents focused on how the event would affect them at school and the anticipated reactions of their peer group.

RTS describes a cluster of psychological and physical signs, symptoms and reactions common to most rape victims, during, immediately following and for months or years after a rape.[26] While most research into RTS has focused on female victims, males who are sexually abused (whether by male or female perpetrators) have also exhibited RTS symptoms.[27]

Medical Examination of the Accused

In case of accused, medical examination should aim to have the following points:

i. Injuries due to sexual act.
ii. Injuries (scratches, bite marks, etc.) due to resistance offered by the victim. They are often found if the female is healthy and spirited.
iii. Presence of blood and seminal stains on clothes and on body, especially on private parts.
iv. Presence of smegma is useful clue. It can refute the charge of false rape. Absence of smegma does not prove rape.
v. Capability of the accused to perform sexual act.
vi. Venereal disease.

Examination of the genitals: Penis is washed with normal saline and stained by Papanicolaou's stain. Presence of vaginal, cervical cells and Barr body suggest recent intercourse. Look for vaginal cells in glans. This is done by cleaning the organ with a filter paper and exposing the paper to Lugol's iodine. The paper becomes brown if vaginal epithelial cell present because of presence of glycogen.

Specimen to be Collected from Accused

i. Vaginal fluid stains, bloodstains, semen stains on the penis, on pubic hair, on the area around the male organ and thighs and on clothes. Smears from male organ, viz. coronal sulcus prepuce, penile shaft, urethral orifice; from pubic hair, from the surrounding skin should always be obtained to match the sample with that found of the clothes and body of the victim.
ii. Foreign hairs especially in the private parts and intermingled with pubic hairs. The doctor should collect them for further investigations.
iii. Fibers from the clothes of the victim. They are mostly on his clothes.
iv. Stains of cosmetics (lipstick, cream, powder, etc.) on the person and clothes.
v. The fingernail scrapings from the victim may contain vaginal fluid, skin, fibers, cosmetics, etc.

vi. Dust, dirt, flora or fauna from the scene, especially in outdoor cases.
vii. Clothes worn by the culprit at the time of occurrence must be taken into possession. They may carry stains, tears, hairs and fibers, flora and fauna and their fragments, dust and dirt from the scene.

Legal Procedure for Medical Examination

Section 53 CrPC: Examination of accused by medical practitioner at the request of police officer:

A. When a person is arrested on a charge of committing an offence of such a nature and alleged to have been committed under such circumstances that there are reasonable grounds for believing that an examination of this person will afford evidence as to the commission of an offence, it shall be lawful for a **registered medical practitioner**, acting at the **request of a police officer not below the rank of subinspector**, and for **any person acting in good faith in his aid** and **under his direction**, to make such an examination of **the person arrested** as is reasonably necessary in order to ascertain the facts which may afford such evidence and to **use such force as is reasonably necessary for that purpose.**
B. Whenever the person of a **female** is to be examined under this section, the examination shall be made only by, or under the supervision of, a female registered medical practitioner.

Explanation: In this section and in **Section 53A** and **54**

a. "**Examination**" shall include the examination of blood, blood stains, semen, swabs in case of sexual offences, sputum and sweat, hair samples and finger nail clippings by the use of modern and scientific techniques including DNA profiling and such other tests, which the registered medical practitioner thinks necessary in a particular case;
b. "**Registered medical practitioner**" means a medical practitioner who possess any medical qualification as defined in clause (h) of Section 2 of the Indian Medical Council Act, 1956 and whose name has been entered in a State Medical Register.

Section 53A, CrPC: Examination of person accused of rape by medical practitioner:

1. When a person is arrested on a charge of committing an offence of rape or an attempt to commit rape and there are reasonable grounds for believing that an examination of this person will afford evidence as to the commission of such offence, it shall be lawful for a registered medical practitioner employed in a hospital run by the Government or by a local authority, and in the absence of such a practitioner within the radius of 16th km from the place where the offence has been committed, by any other registered medical practitioner, acting at the request of a police officer not below the rank of a subinspector, and for any person acting in good faith in his aid and under his direction, to make such an examination of the arrested person and to use such force as is reasonably necessary for that purpose.
2. The **registered medical practitioner** conducting such examination shall, **without delay**, examine such person and prepare of his examination giving the **following particulars**, namely:
   i. The name and address of the accused and of the person by whom he was brought,
   ii. The age of the accused,
   iii. Marks of injury, if any, on the person of the accused,
   iv. The description of material taken from the person of the accused for DNA profiling, and
   v. Other material particulars in reasonable detail.
3. The report shall state precisely the reasons for each conclusion arrived at.
4. The exact time of commencement and completion of the examination shall also be noted in the report.

5. The registered medical practitioner shall, without delay, forward the report to the investigation officer, who shall forward it to the Magistrate referred to in section 173 as part of the documents referred to in clause (a) of sub-section (5) of that section [Inserted by the Code of Criminal Procedure (Amendment) Act, 2005, section 9].[21]

Section 54 CrPC: Examination of arrested person by medical practitioner at the request of the arrested person:

1. When a person who is arrested, whether on a charge or otherwise, alleges, at the time **when he is produced before a Magistrate** or **at any time during the period of his detention in custody** that the **examination of his body will afford evidence,** which will **disprove the commission by him of any offence** or which will **establish the commission by any other person of any offence against his body**, the **Magistrate** shall, **if requested** by the arrested person so to do **direct the examination** of the body of such person **by a registered medical practitioner** unless the Magistrate considers that the request is made for the purpose of vexation or delay or for defeating the ends of justice [Section 54 renumbered as sub-section thereof by the code of criminal procedure (Amendment) Act, 2005, Section 10].[21]
2. Where an examination is made under sub-section (1) **a copy of the report of such examination shall be furnished by the registered medical practitioner to the arrested person or the person nominated by such arrested person** [(Inserted by the code of criminal procedure (Amendment) Act, 2005, Section 10].[21]

INCEST

Incest is sexual intercourse between close relatives[28] that is illegal in some jurisdiction or is socially prohibited. This type of sexual activity and the nature of the relationship between people that constitutes a breach of law or social taboo vary with culture and jurisdiction. Some societies consider incest to include only those who live in the same household, or who belong to the same clan or lineage; other societies consider it to include "blood relatives"; other societies further include those related by adoption or marriage.[29]

It can also be defined as sexual intercourse by a man with a woman who is closely related to him by prohibited degrees of relationship, e.g. a daughter, granddaughter, sister, stepsister, aunt or mother. Instances between father and daughter and brothers and sisters are common. These cases usually have psychological features. Incest occurs (1) Between mental defectives; (2) Where alcohol removes the natural inhibitions; (3) Where close relatives have to live in intimacy; (4) Where brother and sister have been separated since childhood and (5) In some cerebral diseases.

Incest between adults and those under the age of majority or age of consent is considered a form of child sexual abuse[30,31] that has been shown to be one of the most extreme forms of childhood abuse, often resulting in serious and long-term psychological trauma, especially in the case of parental incest.[31] Prevalence is difficult to generalize, but research has estimated 10–15% of the general population as having at least one such sexual contact, with less than 2% involving intercourse or attempted intercourse.[32] Among women, research has yielded estimates as high as 20%.[31]

Father-daughter incest was for many years the most commonly reported and studied form of incest.[33] More recently, studies have suggested that sibling incest, particularly older brothers abusing younger siblings, is the most common form of incest. Some studies suggest that adolescent perpetrators of sibling abuse choose younger victims, abuse victims over a lengthier period, use violence more frequently and severely than adult perpetrators,[34] and that sibling abuse has a higher rate of penetrative acts than father or stepfather incest, with father and older brother incest resulting in greater reported distress than stepfather incest.[35]

Consensual adult incest is equally a crime in most countries, although it is seen by some as a victimless crime,[36] and thus it is rarely reported. Others argue that the increased mortality of babies from heterosexual incestuous couples is enough to criminalize the act.[37]

Most societies have prohibitions against incest. The incest taboo is and has been one of the most common of all cultural taboos, both in current nations and many past societies,[38] with legal penalties imposed in some jurisdictions. Most modern societies have legal or social restrictions on closely consanguineous marriages.[39] Incest is not a prosecutable offense in India by law.[40] Indian law does not recognize incest as a punishable crime, unless the child is a minor, in which case it is treated as child sexual abuse.[41,42]

ADULTERY

Adultery or **philandery** is a form of extramarital sex. It is sexual infidelity to one's spouse. It originally referred only to sex between a woman who was married and a person other than her spouse.[43] Extramarital sex that wilfully and maliciously interferes with marriage relations and "adultery is often cited as grounds for divorce".

Adultery is illegal in some countries. The interaction between laws on adultery with those on rape has and does pose particular problems in societies that are especially sensitive to sexual relations by a married woman and men. The difference between the offenses is that adultery is voluntary, while rape is not. In the traditional English common law, adultery was a felony. Although the legal definition of "adultery" differs in nearly every legal system, the common theme is sexual relations outside of marriage, in one form or another.

The law relating to the crime of adultery is present in **Section 497** of the Indian Penal Code. Simply the law declares it a crime for a man to have sexual intercourse with the wife of another man, without the consent of the husband; the consent may be explicit or implicit. The law also explicitly declares that the wife in such cases may not be prosecuted; the man is prosecutable and can be sentenced for up to 5 years (even if he himself was unmarried).

UNNATURAL SEXUAL OFFENCES

Offences related to sex, conducted against the rule of nature. This is the sexual intercourse against the order of nature with any man, or women, or animal. Any degree of penetration or any attempt at penetration is punishable. Proof of emission is not necessary.

Sodomy

Sodomy is the anal intercourse between two males, or between a male and female and one who practices sodomy is a "**sodomite**." It is also called **buggery**. It is called **gerontophilia** when the passive agent is an adult, and **paederasty**, when the passive agent is a young boy, who is known as **catamite**. A **pedophile** is an adult who repeatedly engages in sexual activities with children below the age of puberty. The only proof of sodomy is the presence of semen in the anus.

It is necessary that penetration, however little, should be proved strictly in order that the offence of sodomy is made punishable under section **377 IPC**. An attempt to commit this offence is punishable under Section **511**, IPC, with imprisonment for life or other imprisonment.

Opinion as to cause of the dilatation should be guarded and it should only be stated that it is consistent with entry of a penis. The consent of sodomy is of no value, as both partners are punishable.

Examination of Victim

1. Consent should be taken before examination.
2. History is taken as regards to sites of injuries and behavioral characteristics of assailant.
3. The victim is examined in the knee elbow position with proper lighting.
4. Presence of 3rd person is also needed.

Sign of a Habitual Sodomist

1. If the victim is a habitual sodomist, he lies easily in the knee elbow position, with prolapsed mucous membrane from anal canal.

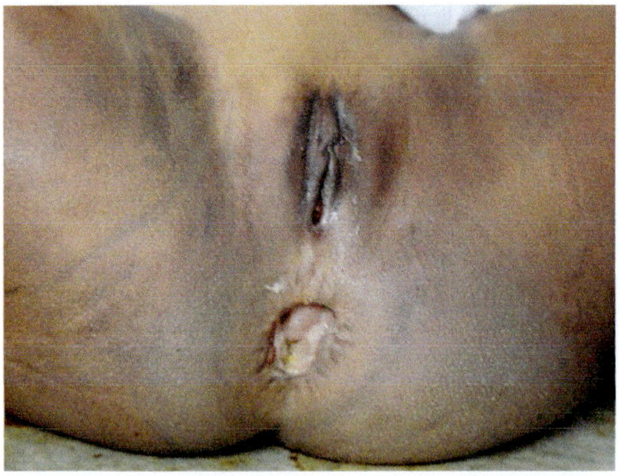

Figure 24.11 Dilated anus, lax sphincter, smooth rectal mucosa membrane and fissures

2. There may be old healed scars from previous stretching and splitting.
3. There may be feminine gait and manner of speaking.
4. Loss of usual mucosal folds, i.e. smooths mucous membrane.
5. Piles or fissures.
6. Evidence of any venereal diseases.
7. The anus dilated with keratinization of the mucosa as shown in **Figure 24.11**.

Signs in Unwilling Partner

1. The parts around the anus are usually tender due to bruising of the anal margins with splitting of the skin or tearing of the lining within the rectum and stretching of the anus itself.
2. Examination of the passive partner should include swabs for seminal fluid and lubricants. Foreign hair should be collected.

Examination of Assailant (Active Sodomy)

Assailant is examined for his age, mental condition and signs of resistance, bloodstains and venereal diseases. Victim's blood, hair or fecal stain may be found an assailant's clothes or private parts. Proforma for examination is enclosed (Annexure 5).

Tribadism or Lesbianism

Homosexuality means persistent emotional and physical attraction to members of same sex. Female homosexuality is known as tribalism or lesbianism. Sexual gratification of a woman is obtained by other women by simple lip kissing, generalized body contact, deep kissing, manipulation of breasts and genitalia, genital apposition, friction of external genital organs.

In some cases, enlarged clitoris is used as an organ of passion or some artificial penis or phallus may be used. Many lesbians are masculine in type, possibly because of endocrine disturbances. Such women are usually mentally defective or who suffer from nymphomania (excessive sexual desire) and hate opposite sex (men). Lesbians who are jealous of one another, when rejected may commit homicide, suicide or both.

Bestiality

It is the sexual intercourse by a human being with a lower animal. The animals involved include those that are kept on the farm or as pets in households. Vaginal intercourse is the most common. It is seen in person suffering from mental abnormalities. Cows, dogs and cats are common for female. Usually, the animal manipulates the genitalia with its mouth and the actual coitus is very rare.

Buccal Coitus

Buccal Coitus or Coitus per os (The sin of Gomorrah) falls within the provision, of and is punishable under section **377 IPC**.

Male organ is introduced into mouth, usually of a young child. Sudden accidental death from asphyxia may occur from aspiration of semen or impaction of penis in the lower part of pharynx. In such suspicious death, smears from trachea should be examined for sperms and acid Phosphatase. It is practiced mainly by prostitutes. Male prostitutes are called—**Eunuchs**, castrated eunuchs are called **Hijrahs** and eunuchs with intact genitalia are known as **Zenana**.

Section 377: Unnatural offences: Whoever voluntarily has carnal intercourse against the order of nature with any man, woman or animal, shall be punished with imprisonment for life, or with imprisonment of either description for term which may extend to 10 years, and shall also be liable to fine.

Explanation: Penetration is sufficient to constitute the carnal intercourse necessary to the offence described in this section.

IPC 377 criminalizes any penetrative sex that does not lead to reproduction, thereby criminalizing sexual expression by homosexuals, bisexuals and trans-sexuals.

Delhi High Court Ruling on Section 377 IPC

Delhi High Court allowing a petition and observed that "we declare that Section 377 IPC, insofar it criminalizes consensual sexual acts of adults in private, is violative of Articles 21, 14 and 15 of the Constitution. The provisions of Section 377 IPC will continue to govern non-consensual penile non-vaginal sex and penile non-vaginal sex involving minors. By 'adult' we mean everyone who is 18 years of age and above. A person below 18 would be presumed not to be able to consent to a sexual act. This clarification will hold till, of course, Parliament chooses to amend the law to effectuate the recommendation of the Law Commission of India in its 172nd Report, which we believe removes a great deal of confusion. Secondly, we clarify that our judgment will not result in the re-opening of criminal cases involving Section 377 IPC that have already attained finality. [Para 132, **Naz Foundation vs Government of NCT of Delhi and Others**, WP(C) No.7455/2001, Date of decision: 2nd July, 2009].[44] However, this was set aside Justice SJ Mukherjee and GS Singhvi of Honorable Supreme Court of India in the judgment dated 11th of December 2013 and hold that "we hold that Section 377 IPC does not suffer from the vice of unconstitutionality and the declaration made by the Division Bench of High Court is legally unsustainable". So, for now, the Section 377 IPC is a punishable offence, whether consensual or not and is liable for punishment as was mentioned before.

SEXUAL PERVERSIONS/ PARAPHILIAS

It comprises of acts aimed to obtain sexual gratification, without sexual intercourse and being taken up, usually, by psychopaths suffering from mental aberrations and conflicts due to socio-sexual maladjustments, inadequacies, psychosexual imbalances and abnormalities.

The nature of a paraphilia is generally specific and unchanging, and most of the paraphilias are far more common in men than in women. Paraphilias include fantasies, behaviors, and/or urges which:

- Involve nonhuman sexual objects, such as shoes or undergarments
- Require the suffering or humiliation of oneself or partner
- Involve children or other non-consenting partners.

A paraphiliac often has more than one paraphilia. Paraphilias often result in a variety of associated problems, such as guilt, depression, shame, isolation, and impairment in the capacity for normal social and sexual relationships. A paraphilia can, and often does, become highly idiosyncratic and ritualized. Few **common paraphilias** are narrated here as follows.

Sadism

The term is derived from the name of a French nobleman, the **Marquis de Sade**, infamous for his crimes and writings. Many of his stories were about sexuality, cruelty and torture.

In sadism, sexual gratification is obtained or increased from acts of physical cruelty or infliction of pain upon one's partner. To obtain sexual gratification, the sadist may bite, beat, whip, produce cuts, etc., or ill-treat or torture his sexual partner in many other cruel ways. This is practiced by both sex, but more common in male. It is also known as "Algolagnia" (Algos = pain, lagnia = lust).

The tendency towards sadistic behavior normally begins in adolescence or early adulthood. It may start with obsessive thoughts and sexual fantasies coupled with the desire to inflict physical or psychological torment or humiliation on another. It tends to be chronic in nature and usually increases in severity over time.

Sadistic behavior in men is thought to be the result of a distortion of the aggressive component of the male sexual instinct and sadistic acts are known to cause heightened levels of the male hormone, testosterone. Endorphins also play a part in the biology of sadism. The infliction of pain on others releases the same "feel good" chemicals that are released during any intense exercise session.

There is no known blanket cause for sadistic behavior. Treatment is highly individualized and must include psychotherapy as well as cognitive and behavioral therapies. Hormonal therapy may be successful in reducing levels of aggression.

Lust Murder

In extreme cases of sadism, murder serves as a stimulus for the sexual act and becomes the equivalent of coitus. This acts being accompanied by erection, ejaculation and orgasm. The murder may be the result of anger, jealousy, revenge, etc.

Sexual perversions are persistently indulging in sexual acts in which complete satisfaction is sought and obtained without sexual intercourse. The perverted behavior is really a repulsively abnormal and frequently cruel form of tension release that by its nature tends to operate under compulsion.

Masochism

This term is derived from the name of Leopold von Sacher-Masoch, an Austrian novelist. Being whipped by his wife used to be a stimulant for his literary work. It is opposite to sadism. Sexual gratification is obtained by the suffering of pain from being beaten, abused, tortured, humiliated, enslaved, degraded or dominated by their sexual partner.

It is more common in male. Sadism and masochism are rarely found in pure state. Combination of sadism and masochism is called **bondage**. This act of cruelty or pain may serve as a stimulant for or as a complete substitute for sexual intercourse.

Necrophilia (Phila - to defile or foul)

In this condition, there is a desire for sexual intercourse with dead bodies. It is said to have sado-masochistic foundation and that decomposition, foul smell and coldness act as a stimulus for sexual act. The corpse may be mutilated following intercourse. The offence is usually committed on a newly buried corpse or body waiting for burial. Murder for the purpose of necrophilia is very rare.

Fetishism

A fetish is an abnormal stimulus or object of sexual desire, e.g. part of women body or some articles belonging to her. Fetishism means the use of such objects for sexual gratification. The person experiences sexual excitement leading to orgasm from part of the body of a women or some article belonging to her that normally has no sexual influence on the mind, e.g. underclothing, brassiere, etc. which act as substitute for the female love object. It is almost exclusively seen in male.

It is harmless, but rarely it may drive the person to obtain his fetish object through violence, or other criminal act, e.g. object may be stolen, or women may be attacked either as part of robbery with violence, or because the fetish provides the trigger for rape or indecent assaults.

Transvestism

A transvestite (Trans = opposite; Vesta = clothing) is a person whose whole personality is dominated by the desire to be identified with the opposite sex. He wants to be thought of as a member of opposite sex. His dress, manner, occupational interests and associations are all designed to increase his feeling of being women. Sexuality with him is relatively unimportant. It is usually found in the males who obtain sexual pleasure by wearing female dress. There is no hormonal disturbance or genital abnormality.

Exhibitionism

It is a wilful and intentional exposure of the genitalia in a public place while in the presence of others, to obtain sexual pleasure. It may or may not be accompanied by masturbatory acts. It is mostly done by males, often to children or the persons of the opposite sex. The pervert adopts a childish method of attracting attention to himself, to experience sexual gratification at the time of the exhibition, without physical contact. Majority of them are psychopathic or suffer from compulsion neurosis. It is punishable offence in India. This is punishable under Section 294 IPC with imprisonment up to 3 months or fine.

Masturbation

Masturbation (onanism: ipsation) is the deliberate self-stimulation, which effects sexual arousal. Mild masturbatory exercises are common in both male and female. Techniques are mostly manual, by moving the penis against the bed or other object. Urethral and anal insertions or stimulations are rare. In females, a finger is gently and rhythmically moved over clitoris or labia minora or steady pressure is applied over these parts with several fingers or whole hand. The genitalia may be rubbed against a pillow, a bed or some other object. Sometimes, women may insert finger, etc. into the vagina. It is an offence only when practiced openly, e.g. in telephone booth, lavatories, etc.

Voyeurism or Scoptophilia

It is the counterpart of exhibitionism. The voyeur (so-called **Peeping Tom**) must see people undress in order to be sexually satisfied. There is a morbid desire to look at the sexual organs or other usually clothed parts of the body of one of the opposite sex or to watch sexual intercourse as a source of sexual satisfaction. The act of observation can also result in attempts at exhibitionism or masturbation. This perversion occurs in case of sever sociopathic personality disorder. It is rare in female. (Made punishable offence under Section 354-C, IPC, after Criminal Law Amendment, 2013).[1]

Frotteurism

Frotteurism is contact with another person in order to obtain sexual satisfaction. Sexual satisfaction is obtained by rubbing against persons in crowds. If they attempt intercourse, they have a premature ejaculation or they are impotent. It is an uncommon perversion and rarely occurs alone.

Undinism

In undinism, the sexual pleasure is often obtained by witnessing the act of urination by someone of the same or opposite sex. In some cases, pleasure is obtained by being urinated upon by the loved one or in urinating on him or her, but this is a rare.

SEMINAL FLUID

Seminal stains have to be detected in cases of rape or attempted rape, sexual murder of the female, sodomy and bestiality. Fertility of fluid has to be proved in disputed paternity.

The details about the seminal fluid, etc are discussed in **Chapter 27 (Forensic Serology).**

REFERENCES

1. The Criminal Law Amendment Act, 2013. (w.e.f. 02.04.2013).
2. American Medical Association. Sexual Assault in America 1995. AMA.
3. UCSC rape prevention education: Rape statistics. [cited 2011, January 04]; Available from: URL:http://healthcenter.ucsc.edu/shop/sexual_assault_prevention_education.shtml
4. Under the English common law, marriage has not been a defence to rape since 1991, see R v. R [1992] 1 A.C. 599.

5. UCSB's SexInfo. Soc.ucsb.edu. [cited 2010 Dec 31]; Available from: URL:http://www.soc.ucsb.edu/sexinfo/article/rape
6. Curtis DG. Perspectives on acquaintance rape. The American academy of experts in traumatic stress, Inc. 1997.
7. Finkelhor and Yllo (1985) and Bergen (1996).
8. Ullman SE. A Comparison of Gang and Individual rape Incidents. Violence and Victims 1999 [cited 2008, May 21]; 14(2):123–133. Available from: URL:http://www.ingentaconnect.com/content/springer/vav/1999/00000014/00000002/art00001
9. Gidycz CA, Koss MP. A comparison of group and individual sexual assault victims. Psychology of women quarterly 2006 July 28 [cited 2011 Jan 25]; 14(3):325–342. Available from: URL:http://www.blackwell-synergy.com/doi/abs/10.1111/j.1471-6402.1990.tb00023.x
10. Courtois CA. Healing the Incest Wound: Adult Survivors in Therapy. WW Norton and Company; 1988. p. 208.
11. "Child Sexual Abuse". Medline Plus. US National Library of Medicine. 2008.
12. Guidelines for psychological evaluations in child protection matters. Committee on Professional Practice and Standards, APA Board of Professional Affairs. The American Psychologist. 1999;54(8):586-93.
13. Anderson J, Mangels N, Langsam A. Child sexual abuse: a public health issue. The Justice Professional. 2004;17:107.
14. Herman-Giddens ME, Brown G, Verbiest S, et al. Under ascertainment of child abuse mortality in the United States. JAMA. 1999;282(5):463-7.
15. Drink-spiking—Introduction. National Health Service (England). [cited 2010 Mar 2]; Available from: URL:http://www.nhs.uk/Conditions/Drink-spiking/Pages/Introduction.aspx?url=Pages/what-is-it.aspx
16. Dr Kamini Lau, Addl. Sessions Judge. State vs. Harish @ Chirag, Sessions Case No. 25/2012, Date of judgment: 05.02.2013, date of punishment: 14.02.2013:110-112.
17. Balasubramaniam B, Park GR. Sexual hallucinations during and after sedation and anesthesia. Anesthesia. 2003;58:549-53.
18. Pauwels B. Blaming the victim of rape: The culpable control model perspective. Dissertation Abstracts International: Section B: The Sciences and Engineering. 2002;63(5-B).
19. Abrahms D, Viky G, Masser B, Gerd B. Perceptions of stranger and acquaintance rape: The role of benevolent and hostile sexism in victim blames and rape proclivity. Journal of Personality and Social-Psychology. 2003;84(1):111-25.
20. Attitudes to sexual violence 2005. [cited 2010 Dec 31]. Available from: URL:http//www.web.archive.org
21. The Criminal Law Amendment Act, 2005.
22. Dr. Lakshmi Kumari Goswami vs. The State of Assam & Ors., PIL No.75 of 2009, Gauhati High Court, Assam, date of judgment 19.08.2010, MemoNo.1742-1745/PIL Dated 25.08.2010.
23. Hicks DJ. Rape: Sexual Assault. In: Wynn RM (Ed). Obstetrics and Gynecology Annual, New York. Appleton-Century Croft, 1978; pp. 447-65.
24. GM Willot, Jr For Sc Soc 1975 Oct:270.
25. Burgess AW, Holmstrom LL. Rape trauma syndrome. Am J Psychiatry. 1974;131:981-6.
26. Sandoval, Johnathan. Handbook of Crisis Counseling, Intervention, and Prevention in the Schools.
27. Sarrel PM, Masters WH. Sexual molestation of men by women. Archives of Sexual Behavior. 1982;11:2.
28. "Incest" in Merriam-Webster's Dictionary.
29. Claude Lévi-Strauss. Elementary Structures of Kinship, Tr. by J. Bell and J. von Sturmer. Boston: Beacon Press. 1969 [1949].
30. Faller KC. Child Sexual Abuse: Intervention and Treatment Issues. DIANE Publishing; 1993. p. 64.
31. Shetty DH, Green AH. Child Sexual Abuse: A Handbook for Health Care and Legal Professionals. Psychology Press. 1988. p. 128.
32. Nemeroff CB, Craighead WE. The Corsini Encyclopedia of Psychology and Behavioral Science. New York: Wiley. 2001.
33. Herman J. Father-Daughter Incest. Cambridge, Massachusetts: Harvard University Press. 1988. p. 282.
34. O'Brien MJ. Taking sibling incest seriously. In: M Patton (Ed), Family Sexual Abuse: Frontline Research and Evaluation. Newbury Park, CA: Sage Publications. 1991. pp. 75-92

35. Cyr M, Wright J, McDuff P, Perron A. Intrafamilial sexual abuse: Brother-sister incest does not differ from father-daughter and stepfather-stepdaughter incest. Child Abuse and Neglect. 2002;26:957-73.
36. Wolf AP, Durham WH. Inbreeding, Incest, and the Incest Taboo: The State of Knowledge at the Turn of the Century. Stanford University Press. 2004. p. 169.
37. Khan R. "Ph. D". Unz Foundation junior fellow. Discover. Retrieved 5 March 2011.
38. Emile Durkheim. Incest: The Nature and Origin of the Taboo (tr.1963).
39. Kelly HA. Kinship, incest, and the dictates of law. Am J Juris.1969;14(1):69-78.
40. Hyderabad: Father-in-law held for incest. Criminal Records India. 26 October, 2010.
41. Incest in India. 12 August, 2009. [cited 2010 Dec 31]; Available from: URL:http://www.Ndtv.com
42. Incest and the conspiracy of silence. 30 April, 2009; [cited 2010 Dec 31]; Available from: URL:http://www.Indiatogether.org
43. Definition of Adultery. [cited 2010 Dec 31]; Available from: URL:http://www.Dictionary.com
44. Naz Foundation vs. Government of NCT of Delhi and Others, WP(C) No.7455/2001, Date of decision: 2nd July, 2009.

CHAPTER 25

Forensic Psychiatry

Vijayanath V, Deepanjali Medhi

LEARNING PLAN

- Learn the concept of forensic psychiatry
- Know about the classification of psychiatric disorders
- Identify the abnormal mental phenomena and disorders
- Understand the Mental Health Act
- Know about the judicial responsibility of insane offenders
- Learn the criminal and civil responsibility of insane offender

Forensic psychiatry is the branch of medicine that deals with disorders of the mind and its relation to law. It is as an auxiliary science of criminology. As per World Health Organization (WHO), **mental health** has been defined as "a state of balance between the individual and the surrounding world, a state of harmony between oneself and others, a coexistence between the realities of the self and other people and that of the environment". A Mental disorder is any psychiatric illness or disease whose manifestations is primarily characterized by behavioral or psychological impairment of function, measured in terms of deviations from the normative concept associated with distress or disease, not just an expected response to a particular event or limited to relations between a person and society.

Forensic psychiatry encompasses the interface between law and psychiatry in all aspects. Law is the sanctioning discipline and psychiatry is the therapeutic discipline. Forensic psychiatry is much neglected, ignored, misinterpreted and misunderstood discipline, however, among medical professionals. A forensic psychiatrist provides services, such as determination of competency to stand trial in a court of law to facilitate the adjudicative process. Forensic psychiatrists are also involved in the care of prisoners, both in jails and in mental health institutions. Forensic psychiatry team contains a variety of professionals, including Forensic Medicine expert, psychiatrist, psychologists, and nurses trained in forensic psychiatry as well as care workers. These teams have dual responsibilities—to promote both the welfare of their clients and to care for the safety of the public. The aim is not only to predict violence but also to prevent it by means of risk management.

Forensic psychiatrists often also do research work related to prisons, in which they go into prisons and assess and treat people suspected of having mental disorders. Most of the day-to-day work of these psychiatrists comprises care of very seriously mentally ill patients. Some also treat people with severe personality disorders and learning disabilities.

The patients who may require expert mental health professional's opinion in the judiciary are:

i. Who that harm themselves and others.
ii. Those who are incapable of looking after themselves and unable to handle welfare of their family and properties.
iii. Patients who are acting out to be dangerous due to psychiatric disorders.
iv. Spouse of mentally ill patients in cases of divorce, etc.
v. Patients who are having criminal and civil litigation as a consequences of mental illness.
vi. Mental patients who are going for some contract and want to make a will.
vii. Mental fitness certificate of the person is needed for adoption of child.

CLASSIFICATION OF MENTAL HEALTH DISORDERS[1]

There are two schools of classification of psychiatric disorders: one by WHO which is known as the "International Classification of Diseases ICD-10", of which chapter V (F) and sub chapters deals with psychiatric disorders, and the other is American system of classification, called as **Diagnostic Statistical Manual** (DSM). DSM classification is more useful for research purposes.

ICD-10 is more widely used for classification of psychiatric diseases. Here, the psychiatric diseases are classified into 10 broad groups as follows:

1. **Organic psychiatric disorders**—including Alzheimer's disease; dementia of vascular type and other dementias; organic amnestic syndrome; delirium other than alcohol or other substance induced; mental, personality and behavioral disorders due to brain disease or damage, etc.
2. **Psychoactive substance** induced mental and behavioral disorders—Following are some of the patterns of the drug-use disorders:
   a. Acute intoxication
   b. Withdrawal state
   c. Dependence syndrome
   d. Harmful use
   e. Withdrawal state with delirium
3. **Schizophrenia, schizotypal and delusional disorders**
4. **Mood (affective) disorders** are characterized by disturbances of mood and include:
   a. Mania (Manic episode),
   b. Depression (Depressive disorder),
   c. Bipolar mood disorder (manic-depressive psychosis),
   d. Persistent mood disorders (cyclothymia, dysthymia),
   e. Recurrent depressive disorder,
   f. Other types of mood disorders.
5. **Neurotic, stress related** and **somatoform disorders**
   a. Anxiety disorders (generalized anxiety disorder, phobic anxiety disorders, panic anxiety disorder),
   b. Obsessive-compulsive disorder,
   c. Dissociative (conversion) disorder,
   d. Somatoform disorders,
   e. Stress (acute stress reaction and post-traumatic stress disorder) and adjustment disorders.
6. **Behavioral syndromes** associated with physiological and physical disturbances:
   a. Eating disorders, e.g. anorexia nervosa, bulimia nervosa,
   b. Non-organic sleep disorders,
   c. Sexual dysfunction not caused by organic disorder or disease,
   d. Mental and behavioral disorders associated with puerperium,

e. Abuse of non-dependence producing substances.

7. **Personality disorders**
   a. Specific personality disorders, viz. Antisocial, borderline, paranoid personality disorder, etc.
   b. Habit and impulse disorder,
   c. Gender identity disorder,
   d. Disorders of sexual perversions (sexual deviations),
   e. Disorders associated with sexual development and orientation.
8. **Mental retardation**
9. **Disorders of psychological development include**
   a. Speech and language disorders
   b. Pervasive developmental disorders (autism).
10. **Behavioral and emotional disorders of childhood and adolescence**
    a. Attention deficit hyperactivity disorder (ADHD)
    b. Conduct disorders
    c. Tic disorders.

Some abnormal mental phenomena are defined below.

DISTURBANCES OF PERCEPTION

Hallucination

Hallucination is a false sensory perception occurring in the absence of any real external stimulation of the sensory modality involved.

Types of Hallucination

i. **Auditory hallucination**: It is hearing of sounds such as whirring noises and muffled whispers to organized sounds or voices talking or discussing about the patient. Auditory hallucinations are present in deafness also. Commonly, these are associated with psychosis, especially in schizophrenia and psychotic mood disorders. The command type of auditory hallucination is one where voices command or order the patient to follow the same, which usually is frightening or dangerous in nature. Examples: Commands to jump from the running train, to take the knife and stab oneself or sometimes even to kill others. In such situation, patient may feel compelled to carry out the orders and may indulge in criminal activities.

ii. **Gustatory hallucination**: A person feels tastes of sweet, sour, bitter, good or bad taste in the mouth, though there is no food in the mouth.

iii. **Olfactory hallucination**: These involve smell or odor. It is usually seen in depression, mostly as odors of decaying, rottening and dead things.

iv. **Tactile (Haptic) hallucination**: Primarily involves touch. Such hallucinations include that bugs are crawling over patients' body under the skin (formication). They are very commonly seen in alcohol withdrawal syndrome and chronic cocaine intoxication.

v. **Visual hallucination**: They can be formed images of animate objects, people or parts of people, especially head and faces. Religious images, fantastic creatures which may be similar to images in movies and on televisions and even animal's images, at times, may form visual hallucinations. These hallucinations are common in organic mental illnesses.

vi. **Synesthesia**: It is a type of hallucination where a stimulus is perceived by a sensory organ other than the one that should actually perceive it. Example: Visualizing music, hearing different colors, etc.

vii. **Lilliputian hallucinations**: Visual hallucinations of small animals and human beings are reported (person sees figures in reduced size like midges or dwarfs) in alcohol withdrawal delirium.

viii. **Hypnogogic** and **hypnopompic hallucinations** are predominantly visual hallucinations that occur during moments immediately before falling asleep and during transition from sleep to wakefulness, respectively.

Illusion[2]

It is a perceptual misinterpretation of a real external stimulus. They are perceptual distortions in estimation of size, shape and spatial relations and are commonly seen even in absence of psychiatric disorders, especially when someone is fatigued or excessively aroused. For example, when a person sees a dog and mistakes it for a lion or sees a string hanging to be a snake. Illusions are features of organic psychoses.

Types of Illusion

i. **Completion illusions** are seen in human with a tendency to complete a familiar and unfinished pattern. For example, to a person with an interest in reading, the word-'ook' might be misread as 'book' even though the faded letter was "L".
ii. **Affect illusions**: They can be understood in context with prevailing mood state. For example, a delirious person in a perplexed and bewildered state may perceive the innocent gestures of others as threatening.
iii. **Pareidolic illusions** are those where images are seen to form shapes; for example, seeing human faces in clouds. These illusions are the result of excessive fantasy thinking and a vivid visual imagery.

DISORDERS OF THOUGHT AND SPEECH

Derailment

It is a gradual or sudden deviation in the train of thought to a subsidiary thought without blocking.

Loosening of Association

It is a formal thought disturbance, where the ideas expressed have no logical connection or association with the next idea expressed and the speech therefore becomes irreverent.

Delusion

Delusion is a false belief that is firmly held despite objective and obvious contradictory proof or evidence and despite the fact that other members of the culture do not share the same belief.[3]

Delusion in a person is a symptom of mental disease. Delusions are found in schizophrenic psychoses, mood disorders, organic mental disorders and epilepsy.

Types of Delusion Depending on the Content

i. **Delusions of persecution**: The patient believes that their lives are being interfered from outside and feels that other people are trying to harm him. Persecutory delusions occur in schizophrenia, bipolar affective disorder, depression and organic psychosis.
ii. **Delusion of infidelity**: It is also known as pathological jealousy. It is a false belief that one's spouse is unfaithful.
iii. **Delusion of love (Erotomanic type)**: Here the patient will have a delusional conviction that another person, usually of higher status, is in love with him or her.
iv. **Delusion of guilt** and **unworthiness**: It is a belief that a person had committed sin and needs to be punished for same. It is common in patients with depression.
v. **Delusion of poverty**: The person wrongly believes that he is very poor, whereas **nihilistic** delusions are related to negative thinking and both are depressive delusions. In nihilistic delusion, patient believes that his body and everything related to it have ceased to exist, not even him.
vi. **Hypochondrial delusion**: It is an exaggerated concern about health, based not on real medical pathology but on unrealistic interpretations of physical signs or sensations as abnormal.
vii. **Delusion of influence** or **control**: Is a false belief that a person's will, thoughts,

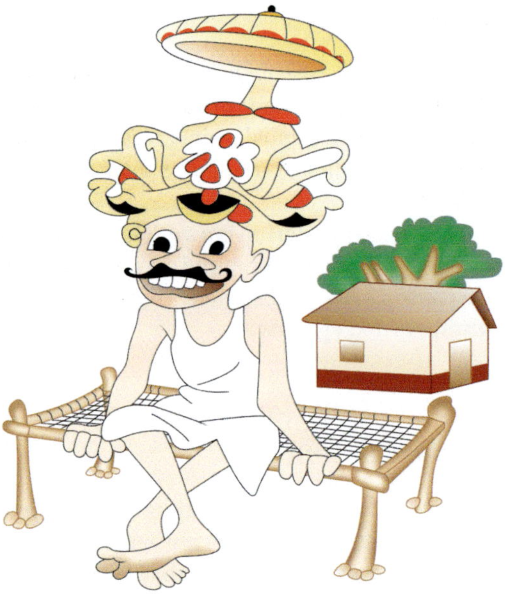

Figure 25.1 Delusion of grandeur

feelings and actions are being controlled by external sources.

viii. **Delusion of reference**: It is a false belief that behavior of other refers to oneself. Events, objects or other people have a particular and unusual significance for the patients, commonly of negative nature. For example, the patient may believe that people on television or radio are talking bad about them.

ix. **Delusion of self-accusation** or **self-reproach** is false believe of remorse and guilt about oneself.

x. **Delusion of grandeur**: The patient falsely believes that he is very rich, has lots of power and abilities. The diagrammatic representation is shown in **Figure 25.1**.

Echolalia

Psychopathological repeating of words or phrases of speech of one person by another; tends to be repetitive and persistent.

Circumstantiality

It is a kind of speech disturbance where there is digression of speech into unnecessary detail, distracting from central theme; however, the patient returns to the original theme at the end of the speech. This kind of speech may be seen in dementia and obsessive person.

Flight of Ideas

It is rapid succession of fragmentary thoughts or speech in which content changes abruptly to another topic, and speech may be very fast and, at times, also incoherent.

Word Salad

It is incoherent, essentially incomprehensible, mixture of words and phrases, commonly seen in far advanced cases of schizophrenia and organic brain syndrome.

Formal Thought Disorder

It is the disturbance in the form of thought rather than content of thought, may indicate presence of schizophrenia, e.g. thought broadcasting, thought insertion, thought withdrawal, thought reading, etc.

COMMONLY USED TERMS IN FORENSIC PSYCHIATRY PRACTICE

Abreaction

It is a psychological process by which repressed memory in unconscious mind, especially of a painful psychological experience or a conflict, is bought back to consciousness. In abreaction, the person not only recalls but also gets relieved of the repressed mental trauma, and it may be accompanied by appropriate emotional or affective responses. The concept is based on **Sigmund Freud**'s theory of psychoanalysis.

Affect

It is outward objective expression of the immediate, emotional experience attached to a thought, idea or an emotional stimulus, at a given time.

Euphoria

It is a state of feeling of emotional wellbeing. If it is seen in inappropriate setting, it may indicate mental disturbance.

Enuresis

It is a condition of urinary incontinence during sleep.

Aggression

It is forceful goal-directed action, which may be either verbal or physical.

Hypersomnia

Hypersomnia is excessive time spent in sleep.

Agitation

It is a state of severe anxiety associated with motor restlessness.

Ambivalence

It is a state of coexistence of two opposing impulses toward the same thing in the same person at the same time.

Aphasia

It is a disturbance in the comprehension or expression of language caused by lesions in the brain.

Compulsion

It is a pathological need to act on an impulse that, if resisted, produces anxiety. They are repetitive motor behavior in response to an obsession.

Coprolalia

Coprolalia is involuntary utterance of vulgar or obscene language.

Insight

It is conscious recognition of one's own condition. Insight refers to the conscious awareness and understanding of one's own psychodynamics and symptoms of maladaptive behavior, which is very much important in bringing effective changes in the personality and behavior of a person.

PSYCHIATRIC DISORDERS OF MEDICOLEGAL IMPORTANCE

Schizophrenia

Literally it means disintegration of mind. It is commonly known as 'split mind'. The exact reason of schizophrenia is not known, but it may be familial. There is a complete loss of reality contact in this condition. It is primarily a disorder of thinking (cognition) giving rise to symptoms of delusions, formal thought disorders and speech disturbances like loosening of association. There may be other disturbances of behavior, affect, perception (hallucinations) and personality deterioration.[3]

Eugen Bleuler classified it into four types:

i. Simple
ii. Hebephrenic
iii. Catatonic
iv. Paranoid

i. **Simple Schizophrenia:** It is the commonest type. It begins in early adolescence. It mainly affects the behavior of the person. There is all-round impairment of mental faculties. Person remains aloof, talks very little and is socially withdrawn. The motor activities are also quite less.
ii. **Hebephrenic:** It begins in early adolescence and young adults. In this type, the thought process is primarily deranged. Incoherence of thoughts, delusions and hallucinations are reported. The motor activities are also quite less. Often, conduct is impulsive and senseless. They also show inappropriate emotion (giggling) and inappropriate behavior like mirror gazing, making odd faces or gestures in front of the mirror, etc.

iii. **Catatonic:** In this type, the motor behavior of the person is primarily abnormal. There may be wild excitement and violent or may show very less motor activity (stuporous) or may exhibit abnormal motor behavior like catatonia. Sometimes in catatonic excitement, the person may be so violent that he may need to be restrained.
iv. **Paranoid**: Delusion is the primary thought disturbance in this type. The person may have delusion of persecution and believe that some persons are behind him and can kill him. He may have suspicion against his wife, parents, kids, friends and colleagues. It occurs more in males than in females. Other delusions like delusion of reference, grandeur, infidelity, love, control, thought broadcasting and thought withdrawal are also common. Usually, personality is well preserved, and these people are detected as suffering from mental illness after a long time. Auditory hallucinations are quite common. He may commit crime as he thinks people are after him.

Schizophrenia is a major mental illness and the patients have no insight about their illness. In India, schizophrenia is the commonest diagnosis made among criminal lunatics.

Schizophrenia and Offence

i. That schizophrenia disposes the patients to violence.
ii. Paranoid and catatonic excitement are the types most likely to be associated with violence.
iii. Violence is more common as a late accompaniment of the illness.
iv. Violence is more common in those patients who have recurrent exacerbations, rather than those who are continuously ill.
v. At the time of the offence the offender is generally psychotic and without insight.

Vivkkunen (1974) found that only one-third offended directly as a result of their delusions and hallucinations. The remaining two-thirds offended because of problems arising from stress produced within the family.

In **paranoid disorders** (**delusional disorders**), criminal acts may follow from delusional belief. Paranoids are more hostile than normal or other subgroups of schizophrenia. A well-recognized association is that of homicide associated with delusion of persecution.

Bipolar Mood Disorder

Mania

It is an elevated mood state characterized by elation, agitation, aggression, hyperactivity, hypersexuality and accelerated thinking and speaking.

Dementia

It is a mental disorder characterized by gradual impairment in intellectual functioning without clouding of consciousness. It is characterized by failing memory, difficulty in calculations, distractibility, alterations in mood and affect, impaired judgment and abstraction, reduced facility with language and disturbance of orientation.

It is a condition in which there is degeneration of mental faculties after they have been fully developed, unlike mental retardation.

Types of Dementia

1. **Pre-Senile:** Seen before 65 years of age
   a. Alzheimer's disease
   b. Pick's disease
   c. Jakob Creutzefeldt's disease
   d. Huntington's disease
   e. Vascular.
2. **Senile**: Starts usually after 65 years of age
3. **Secondary**: It can be because of:
   a. Epilepsy; head injury
   b. Syphilis
   c. Alcohol
   d. Cerebral tumors
   e. Myxedema
   f. Chronic neurological disorders
   g. Hypothyroidism
   h. Vitamin deficiencies.

Disorders of Consciousness and Other Higher Functions of Brain

Consciousness: It is a state of awareness of the self and the environment.

Confusion: It is a change in level of awareness in which a person is not able to think with his or her usual level of clarity.

Delirium: It is an acute reversible mental condition consisting of confusion that is impairment of consciousness, disorientation, impairment of recent memory, alteration of sleep-wake cycle, etc. It is also associated with emotional liability, hallucinations or illusions, and inappropriate, impulsive, irrational or violent behavior. It is usually seen in physical diseases (organic brain syndrome) as complication and in cases of substance withdrawal (alcohol, opioid, benzodiazepines, etc.).

Fugue: It is a kind of dissociative disorder characterized by a period of almost complete amnesia, during which a person actually flees from immediate life situation and begins a different life pattern, usually in a different place. Apart from the amnesia, other mental faculties and skills are usually unimpaired.

It is a state of altered awareness, with amnesia for the previous identity, with no memory of the fugue period when it is over.

Amnesia

It is partial or total inability to recall past experiences. Memory appears to be stored in several parts of the limbic system of the brain, and any condition that interferes with the function of this system can cause amnesia. Functional causes are psychological factors, such as post-traumatic stress disorder or may be due to, in psychoanalytic terms, defense mechanisms. Amnesia may also appear as a complication or squeal to brain disease or dysfunction due to head injury, encephalitis, etc.

Anterograde Amnesia: It is the loss of memory of the period following the brain injury. People may find themselves constantly forgetting a piece of information after a brain insult because the data have not transferred successfully from the short-term memory into permanent long-term memory as the brain insult happened at a particular point of time.

Retrograde Amnesia: It is the loss of pre-existing memories, beyond an ordinary degree of forgetfulness. This type of amnesia first targets the victim's most recent memories. The person may be able to memorize new things that occur after the onset of amnesia (unlike in anterograde amnesia), but is unable to recall some or all about his or her life events that happened before a brain injury.

Lucid Interval

It is a period of normalcy, during the course of an organic brain disorder. In this period, a patient is able to stand trial or testify for legal purposes and his testimony is accepted as evidence in the court of law as the person is in full capacity of mental functioning.

Somnambulism

Walking during sleep is known as somnambulism. Activities are confined to aimless wondering and purposeless repetitive behavior for a few minutes. This is kind of parasomnic sleep disorder involving the slow wave phase of sleep.

Narcolepsy

It is a pathological irresistible spells of daytime sleepiness or drowsiness lasting for 10 to 15 minutes, from which one can be aroused to a normal state of consciousness.

Obsessive–Compulsive Disorder

Obsession

It is a form of thought disorder. It is a persistent, intrusive and recurrent idea, thought or impulse that cannot be eliminated from consciousness by logic or reasoning. It is a disorder of possession of thought. They usually occur in neurotic people; however, these patients are well able to discharge the ordinary responsibilities of life.

The irrational idea or thought that is constantly entertained by the patient persists in spite of all efforts to remove it from persons mind.

Compulsion

When obsession converts into action, it becomes a compulsion. Normal persons also sometimes have obsessions, but they overcome them over a period of time. But once it becomes pathological, it may turn into obsessive-compulsive neurosis, e.g. a person goes to bed after securely bolting the door of his room, but he may once or twice check whether he has locked the door or not. A person with obsessive-compulsive disorder spends the whole night seeing whether the door is locked or not.

Mental Retardation

It is also known as mental sub-normality or oligophrenia. Mental retardation is incomplete or arrested mental development, which starts just after birth or early childhood and is characterized by limited intelligence. This group has been classified in the international classification of diseases by the WHO into four different categories:

Mild (IQ from 50 to 69)
Moderate (IQ from 35 to 49)
Severe (IQ from 20 to 34)
Profound IQ (less than 20).[4]

Some Old Terms for Mental Retardation

Idiot represents the lowest grade of mental deficiency. IQ is estimated to be less than 20. Such child usually has some body deformity like microcephaly, macrocephaly or hydrocephaly, curved bones, high-arched palate and irregular teeth. Usually, such a child is filthy in his habits and cannot manage their feeding and personal hygiene.

Imbecility covers child with IQ ranging from 20 to 50. Such children are unable to manage their routine daily affairs themselves, and these children may have poor memory and language.

Feeble mindedness (moron) is the children having IQ ranging from 50 to 75. These children may not have bodily deformities and capable of making their own living, even though they lack in initiation and ability for any work responsibility.

Impulse Control Disorders

Impulses are the sudden and irresistible force compelling a person to the conscious performance of some action without motive or forethought. A normal person may at times is capable of controlling the impulse, but a person with impulse control disorder may do things on impulse. Impulse related offenses are also seen in conditions of mental retardation, dementia, acute mania and epilepsy.

Types of Impulse Control Disorder

i. **Kleptomania**: It is pathological compulsion to steal objects or articles of little value.
ii. **Pyromania**: It is an irresistible desire to set fire to things.
iii. **Mutilomania**: An irresistible desire to mutilate animals.
iv. **Dipsomania**: An irresistible desire for alcoholic drinks at periodic intervals.
v. **Sexual impulses**: Compulsive urges to perform sexual intercourse, which may often be in a perverted way.
vi. Pathological gambling.
vii. Suicidal and homicidal impulses.
viii. Intermittent explosive (behavior) disorder.

Disorders of Anxiety

Anxiety is an unpleasant affective state and is defined as a fear for no adequate reason. It is also a psychological and physiological state characterized by somatic, emotional, cognitive, and behavioral components and displeasing feeling of fear and concern.

Phobia

Phobia is an irrational fear of an object, situation or activity leading to persistent avoidance of those. The fear is out of proportion to the demands of situation and unexplained. It is not under voluntary control.

Types of Phobia

i. **Acrophobia** is a morbid fear of height.
ii. **Agoraphobias** is fear of being away from home, in crowd or in situations from where easy exit is difficult, viz. Croweded bus, cinema hall, etc.
iii. **Nyctophobia** is a morbid fear of darkness.
iv. **Claustrophobia** is fear of staying in a closed or confined space.
v. **Mysophobia** is morbid fear of filth or contamination.
vi. **Xenophobia** is fear of strangers.

Feigned Mental Illness

Malingering

Malingering is feigning of disease to achieve some specific goal, for example, to avoid an unpleasant responsibility.

Insanity may be feigned by criminals to evade sentence of death or long-terms of imprisonment, by soldiers and policemen to leave the service and by businessmen to avoid contracts. The various differences between real and feigned insanity are shown in **Table 25.1**.

PSYCHOSIS AND NEUROSIS

These are the terms which have been used for many years to separate mental illness into two different categories, generally with the fact that gross reality testing and personality organization are in touch with reality or not, respectively.[3]

Psychosis

The term is very commonly used where there is loss of reality testing and impairment of some mental functioning. Psychosis is manifested by delusions, hallucinations, abnormal behavior and emotion. With gross impairment in reality testing, persons incorrectly evaluate the accuracy of their perceptions and thoughts and make incorrect inferences about external reality, even in the face of contrary have been proved beyond doubt. The most common of psychotic behavior is the presence of delusion, hallucination without insight into their pathological nature.

Neurosis

It implies a chronic or recurrent mental illness characterized mainly by anxiety. Neurosis is a mental disorder in which the predominant disturbance is a symptom or a group of symptoms which is distressing to the individual and is recognized by the person as unacceptable and alien and his reality testing is very much intact. The behavioral norms are very much in contact with reality.[5] The differences between psychosis and neurosis are shown in **Table 25.2**.

Table 25.1 Differences between real and feigned insanity

Trait	Real insanity	Feigned insanity
Onset	Gradual	Sudden
Motive	Absent, i.e. no crime	Present, i.e. crime
Predisposing factors	Positive family history, economic loss, grief, etc.	Absent
Signs and symptoms	Uniformly present	Present only when observed, not of any disease
Facial expression	Peculiar, vacant or fixed look	No peculiar changes
Insomnia	Present for several night	Cannot persist
Exertion	Can withstand exertion for several days	Cannot and breaks down
Habit, skin	Dirty, filthy, dry skin	Normal
Frequent examination	Does not mind	Resents for fear of detection

Table 25.2 Differences between psychosis and neurosis

	Psychosis	Neurosis
Contact with reality	Absent	Present
Insight	Not present	Present
Nature	May be genetic	Circumstantialities
Severity	Major	Minor
Treatment	Usually long-term	Usually short-term

Causes of Mental Illnesses[3]

The causes of mental illnesses can be:

i. Biological (organic, genetic)
ii. Psychological (stress, coping, personality)
iii. Social (poverty, unemployment, stigma, social changes).

Diagnosis of Mental Illness

i. Family history
ii. Personal history
iii. Physical examination
iv. Mental status examination
v. Psychometry (tools and scales).

MENTAL HEALTH ACT 1987

Before entering in depth about the forensic psychiatry, one has to know the law existing in the land. For the same, the Indian government has framed certain guidelines to safeguard the interest of the mentally ill people; the same has been put in the constitution by the title "**Mental Health Act 1987**". This is improved version of "**Indian Lunacy Act 1912**". The Act was amended keeping in mind about the treatment and care of mentally ill person and to make better provision with respect to their property and affairs.

The word **lunatic** has been derived from the Latin word "**luna**" which means "**moon**", as insanity was thought to be affected by the moon in ancient time. In the improvised version, different nomenclatures including the word 'lunatic' were removed as the older terminologies were very much stigmatizing and derogatory for the mentally ill patients.

Objectives of Mental Health Act

i. To regulate the admission to psychiatric hospital/psychiatric nursing homes
ii. To establish authorities (Both at Central and State levels) for licensing and monitoring the psychiatric hospitals.
iii. To supervise on working of these psychiatric hospitals, after their establishment.
iv. To protect the mentally ill people who are not able to look after themselves and sometime becoming dangerous to themselves or the society.
iv. To streamline the procedure about admission and discharge throughout the country.
v. To look for the maintenance charges of mentally ill person undergoing treatment in psychiatric hospitals.
vi. To provide the legal aid to mentally ill criminals at state expenses.
vii. To rename the offensive terminologies used in earlier act.

The Act has been categorized into 10 chapters consisting of 98 sections:

CHAPTER I (Preliminary):

It consists of definitions of certain terms like 'mentally ill person', 'mentally ill prisoner', 'cost of maintenance', 'inspecting officer', 'license', 'medical officer', 'psychiatrist' and 'psychiatric hospital/nursing home'.

The term 'mentally ill person' replaces the term 'lunatic' and means a person who is in need of treatment because of any mental disorder other than mental retardation. The term 'mental ill prisoner' replaces the term 'criminal lunatic' for whom detention in or removal to a psychiatric hospital or psychiatric nursing home, jail or any other place of safe custody may be required. The term 'psychiatric hospital' and 'psychiatric nursing home' replace the term 'asylum'. The differences between old and new terms are shown in **Table 25.3.**

Medical officer is a Gazetted officer who is appointed by the State Government.

Medical officer in-charge is the one who is in charge of the psychiatric nursing home or hospital.

Table 25.3 Differences in old and new terms

Old term	Present term
Lunatic	Mentally ill person
Criminal lunatic	Mentally ill prisoner
Asylum	Psychiatric hospital or psychiatric nursing home

Medical practitioner is the recognized medical practitioner under the provision of Act.

Mentally ill person is the one who is suffering from mental disorder, other than mental retardation.

Mentally ill prisoner is the one who is mentally ill and ordered by the court for detention in the psychiatric hospital or Jail.

Psychiatric hospital or nursing home is a hospital for the mentally ill persons, which is registered with proper competent legal authority.

Psychiatrist is a medical professional holding post-graduate or diploma or courses which have been mentioned in Medical Council of India.[6]

CHAPTER II (Mental Health Authorities):

A central authority for mental health services is envisaged, under the Central Government, with the following main functions:

i. In charge of regulation, development, direction and coordination with respect to mental health service under the Central Government.
ii. Supervision of psychiatric hospitals, nursing homes and other mental health service agencies under the Central Government.
iii. Advisor to the Central Government on all matters relating to mental health.

With above guidelines, a similar state authority for mental health services with similar functions is also envisaged for the various states.

CHAPTER III (Psychiatric Hospitals and Psychiatric Nursing Homes):

There is a provision for separate hospitals for:

i. Those under the age of 16 years.
ii. Those addicted to alcohol or other drugs which lead to behavioral changes.
iii. Mentally ill prisoner.
iv. Any other prescribed class or category.

The establishment or maintenance of psychiatric hospitals or psychiatric nursing homes is based on the following prerequisites:

i. **A valid license**, which is granted under the Act by the licensing authority under the following conditions:
   a. A receipt of an application for a license
   b. On enquiry, it is satisfied that such establishment or maintenance is necessary
   c. The applicant can provide the minimum facilities prescribed for admission, treatment and care of mentally ill persons
   d. The in-charge is a medical officer, who is a psychiatrist
   e. The license is neither transferable nor heritable.
ii. **The license can be revoked if the licensing authority is satisfied that**
   a. The psychiatric hospital/psychiatric nursing home are not being maintained by the licensees in accordance with the provisions of the Act.
   b. The maintenance is carried out in a manner detrimental to the moral, mental or physical well being of the inpatients.

In such a case, if any license is revoked, the inpatients can be transferred to any other specified psychiatric hospital/psychiatric nursing home. There is a provision for any aggrieved person to appeal against any order of the State Government.

There is a provision for an inspecting officer to inspect any psychiatric hospital/nursing home, record thereof, and to visit and interview patients in private receiving treatment and care therein. Any personal record of a patient so inspected is to be kept confidential. The inspecting officer may report the matter to licensing authority. In case, a mentally ill person's condition does not warrant admission, he can receive treatment as an outpatient.

CHAPTER IV (Admission and detention in psychiatric hospital or psychiatric nursing homes):

Admission (Figure 25.2)

1. **On a voluntary basis**
   a. A major mentally ill person (not minor) requests for admission as a voluntary admission.
   b. The guardian of a minor mentally ill person requests for admission of a minor as a voluntary patient.
2. **Under special circumstances**
   This clause provides admission of an unwilling patient on application by a relative or friend. This section stipulates the need for medical certificates from two medical officers (one should be from government medical officer) and maximum period of such admission would be 90 days only. At the same time, this section provides that mentally ill or his friend or relative may make an application to magistrate for discharge. Under such circumstances, the magistrate may conduct enquiries as necessary and then either pass a reception order or order the patient to be discharged.
   Illegal detention: Illegal detention is applicable to any unauthorized person who receives or detains a mentally ill person or an alleged mentally ill person in a psychiatry hospital for gain and also in case of detention in any place other than a psychiatric hospital. Illegal detention is punishable with imprisonment for a term which may extend up to two years or with fine or both.[6]
3. **Reception order on application.** This could be either on application by friends, relative or other people in the community. Further, the police, if it so feels, may pick up an alleged mentally ill person found wandering at large and produces him before a magistrate who may then issue a reception order. These procedures involve the magistrate being satisfied that the person is mentally ill and requires treatment. (A) This could be on the production of medical certificates. (B) The magistrate may have ordered for alleged mentally ill person be examined by medical officer and then pass the reception order under the following situations.
   i. Reception order on production of mentally ill person before magistrate.
   ii. As inpatient after inquisition.
   iii. As a mentally ill prisoner.

In addition to the above, magistrate can order detention of an alleged mentally ill person for short periods, pending report by the concerned medical officer (the period should not exceed more than 10 days in aggregate) or pending his removal to psychiatric hospital/ nursing home for a period not exceeding up to 30 days.

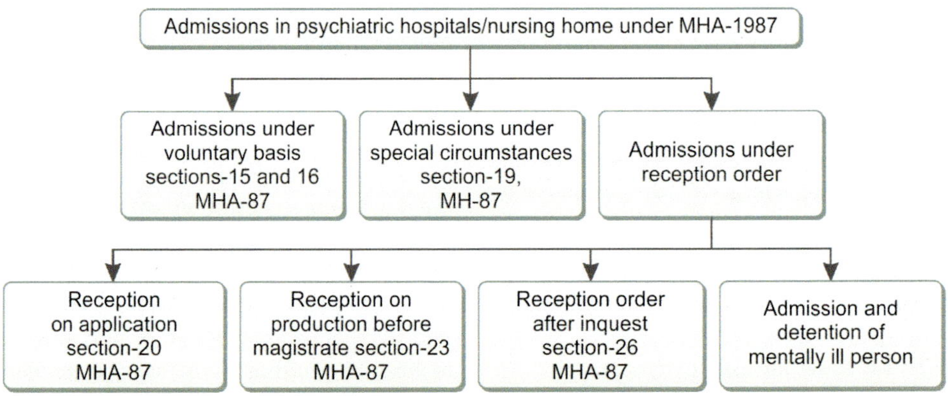

Figure 25.2 Admissions in psychiatric hospitals or nursing home under MHA-1987

CHAPTER V (Inspection, discharge, leave of absence and removal of mentally ill person):

The Central or State Government shall appoint, for every psychiatric hospital/nursing home, not less than five visitors, of whom at least one is a medical officer, preferably a psychiatrist and two social workers. The head of the medical services of the state shall be an ex-officio visitor for all psychiatric hospital/nursing homes in the state.

The assigned visitors are bound to inspect the psychiatric hospital/nursing home with the following guidelines:

i. Inspection at least once a month.
ii. At least three visitors should be present at the joint inspection.
iii. Shall write their remarks in the visitor's book regarding management and conditions of such psychiatric hospital/ nursing home and of the patients thereof.
iv. Shall not inspect any personal records of an inpatient which, in opinion of the medical officer in-charge, are confidential in nature.

The medical officer in-charge of psychiatric hospital/nursing home, where mentally ill prisoner is admitted, shall submit a special report regarding the mental and physical condition of such a person once in every six months. A leave of absence can be granted to any inpatient, on application by the petitioner/ applicant for admission or by a near relative on entering a bond with the medical officer in-charge along with or without sureties, except mentally ill prisoner. Such patients can be discharged without further formalities on the written instructions of two medical practitioners.

Discharge of mentally ill person from mental hospital

It is based on certain factors:

i. Recovery or cure,
ii. Request from the person who had brought petition,
iii. The order of an authority, on assuring proper care by the relatives,
iv. A judicial requisition confirmed to be sane.[7]

CHAPTER VI: Judicial inquisition regarding the alleged mentally ill person possessing property, custody of his person and management of his property.

CHAPTER VII: Liability to meet the cost of maintenance of mentally ill persons of detained in psychiatric hospitals or nursing homes.

CHAPTER VIII: Protection of human rights of mentally ill person.

Protection by human rights to mentally ill person

Mentally ill persons should be treated without violation of human rights, and they be subjected to any indignity or cruelty during treatment.[6]

CHAPTER IX: Penalties and procedures.

CHAPTER X (Miscellaneous):

i. Provisions as to bonds,
ii. Report of Medical Officer,
iii. Pension, etc. of mentally ill person payable by government,
iv. Protection of action taken in good faith.

Restraining of Mentally Ill

Restraint of insane may be, at times, necessary for combating violence and is legal in the following circumstances:

i. Immediate restraint,
ii. Reception directly into a mental hospital,
iii. Reception order on petition,
iv. Reception after Judicial inquisition,
v. Reception of criminally mentally ill.

Escape and Recapture of Mentally ill

Escaped mentally ill person from psychiatric hospital can be retaken or readmitted by any person of the society. The person can be a servant of the hospital, police officer or in-charge of hospital. This power of readmission is exercisable only for a period of one month from the date of his escape.[6]

JUDICIAL RESPONSIBILITY OF INSANE OFFENDERS

The issues of mentally ill offenders and their legal responsibilities are dealt in forensic psychiatry by the forensic psychiatrists who also play a very important role in identification, assessment and management of these offenders. Psychiatrists are often asked to give opinion, especially in relation to following two areas:[8]

1. Ability of the offender in decision making and action taking (competence to stand trial or to plead).
2. Criminal responsibility in relation to liability for criminal offences and the tort of negligence.

Thus, the laws related to mentally ill offenders are formulated according to the above two areas. Although, different countries of the world have their own system of jurisprudence, there are lots of similarities among laws of different countries in relation to mentally ill offenders, with borrowed ideas amongst themselves from common law jurisdiction. However, most of these ideas were borrowed originally from England and Wales.[9] Here the context will basically deal with the criminal liability of mentally ill offenders.

Criminal Liability of Mentally ill Offenders Arises in three Areas

i. Fitness to plead (fitness to stand trial),
ii. Mental state at the time of offence,
iii. Diminished criminal responsibility in certain situations.

CRIMINAL RESPONSIBILITY

The issue of influence of psychiatric disorders on criminal responsibility follows the principle that a person should not be regarded as punishable (culpable) unless he was able to control his own behavior and to choose whether to commit an unlawful act or not. Thus, based on this, in determining whether a person is guilty or not, it is necessary to consider his mental state at the time of the act.

Concept of The "Act"

In jurisprudence, "**Act**" means any event which is subject to the control of the human will. The emoluments of an act are:[10]

i. Its origin in some mental or bodily activity of the doer
ii. Its circumstances
iii. Its consequences.

Act of Omission or Illegal Omission (Section 32 IPC): Omission is covered within "act", if it is illegal. In Indian penal code, reference to the word "act" also extends to illegal omission. But it does not appear to be necessary that the omission should be intentional. An omission to act which is caused by "mental blackout" would be excused (cf. Bratty V. Attorney General for Northern Ireland, 1961).[10]

Mental State at the Time of Offence

Mentally ill offenders usually face trial in the same manner as other offenders, though consideration is given to their mental state in determining whether a person is guilty or not at the time of the act.[9] Before anyone can be convicted of a crime, the prosecution must prove that he carried out an unlawful act (actus reus) and an "intent" that he had a certain guilty state of mind necessary at that time to commit a crime (mens rea, i.e. guilty mind). When a person is charged with an offence, defense can be made that he is not culpable because he did not have a sufficient degree of mens rea.

This defense can be raised in three ways:

i. Not guilty by reason of insanity (section 84 IPC, **McNaghten rule**, 1843).
ii. Diminished responsibility (not guilty of murder, but guilty of culpable homicide not amounting to murder or manslaughter): There is lesser degree of criminal intent (mens rea).
iii. Inability to form "intent" because of automatism.

The degree of **mens rea** varies from crime to crime. For murder/culpable homicide, it is necessary to establish 'specific intent'. For manslaughter, it is sufficient to establish 'gross negligence'.

Various degrees and categories of mens rea exist and based on them, crimes can be classified and punishment framed against them. Lack of mens rea or "mental element" is, of course, a complete defense. Whilst there is no mental element requirement for all crimes (e.g. conviction of traffic offences based solely on street liability and does not require any degree of mens rea), most serious crimes require a mental element in the form of intention, recklessness, knowledge or belief and demand a consideration of what was the individual's purpose, awareness, foresight or realization at the time of committing the crime.[8]

Different Degrees of Mental Element or 'Mens Rea'[9]

i. **Intent:** The person perceives and intends that his act of omission will produce unlawful consequences.
ii. **Recklessness:** Recklessness is deliberate taking of an unjustifiable risk, e.g. D points a gun at P and pulls the trigger; if he does not know that the gun is loaded but realises that it may be, he is held reckless with respect to that circumstance, and whether he hopes it is unloaded or just does not care.[11]
iii. **Negligence:** "A man acts negligently when he brings about a consequence which a reasonable and prudent man would have foreseen and avoided".[11]
iv. **Blameless inadvertence:** "A man may reasonably fail to foresee a consequence of his act, as when a slight slap causes the death of an apparently healthy person or reasonably fail to consider the possibility of the existence of a circumstance for example, goods which are in fact stolen, are brought in the normal course of business from a trader of high repute".

Not Guilty by Reason of Insanity

Presence of mental disorder may give rise to a defense.[8] This may be raised by the defense (though it does not have the formal burden to prove it) or by the prosecution challenging a point made by the defense. For example, if the defense raises mental disorder as an explanation for lack of criminal intent, the prosecution may respond by arguing that the defense has, in fact, raised one of the defenses concerned with mental disorder. Defense of insanity was established by judicial answers to questions raised in McNaghten case in 1843 in England. This defense demands that the following matters should be established by the defense (This is one of those rare instances in which burden of proof lies on a balance of probabilities, on the defense).[8]

The defendant must have a **'disease of the mind'**.[8] This means that it is present if the defendant has a condition that has an internal cause, whereas there is no 'disease of mind' if there is an external cause. As an example, a person who has a brain tumor, has a 'disease the mind' as does a person with arteriosclerosis, schizophrenia (or other mental diseases), epilepsy, diabetes (provided the offender did not take insulin and caused offence in hyperglycemic state) or in sleep walking. On the contrary, a person with diabetes who commits the offence in hypoglycemic state after taking insulin (as an external cause) does not have 'disease of the mind'. So, there is difference between legal construct of 'disease of mind' (legal insanity) and medical approach (medical insanity). As per this definition of 'disease of the mind', many of the above conditions are identifiable with mental disorder which are actually not mental disorders. From this definition, it is difficult to ascertain whether a 'dissociative state' resulting from a 'psychological blow' amounts to 'insane automatism'. Supreme court of Canada recognized that psychological blow is an external cause giving rise not to insanity (a disease of the mind), but to automatism as a defense.

Lord Denning gave a different definition of disease of the mind: "Any mental disorder which has manifested itself in violence and is prone to recur is a disease of the mind, for which a person should be detained in hospital rather than given an unqualified acquittal".[12]

McNaghten Rule (Not Guilty by Reason of Insanity)

In 1843, Daniel Mc. Naghten, a wood turner from Glasgow, shot and killed Edward Drummond, private secretary to then Prime Minister of England, Sir Robert Peel. In the trial at the Old Bailey, a defense of insanity was presented on the grounds that McNaghten had been suffering from delusions of persecution and had believed that he was persecuted by spies and had gone to the police and other public figures for help. His delusional system gradually focused on against the Tory party and he decided to kill its leader, Sir Robert Peel, but mistakenly shot and killed Edward Drummond on 20th January, 1843. McNaghten was found not guilty on the grounds of insanity and was admitted in Bedlam hospital. Following McNaghten case, the Judges in England drew up rules which were not enacted in the law, but provided guidance in insanity pleads.[13]

The rule says: "To establish a defense on the ground of insanity, it must be clearly proved that at the time of committing the act, the party accused was laboring under such a defect of reason from disease of the mind as not to know the nature and quality of the act he was doing, or, if he did know it, that he did not know what he was doing was wrong or contrary to law".

The McNaghten rules have no statutory basis, but still accepted by court of law as having the same status as statutory law. If an offender is found 'not guilty by reason of insanity', the court may order his admission to a hospital for treatment rather than giving him acquittal in prison. These rules also says that every man is presumed to be sane if not proved otherwise, and insane person is also punishable, if he knows at the time of committing the crime that he was acting contrary to the law. Finally, it is the jury who decide whether the defendant was insane or not, based on different evidences and expert witness's (psychiatrist's) opinion.

INSANITY IN INDIAN PERSPECTIVE

In IPC, the insanity defense is described under section 84 (act of a person of unsound mind), which says, "Nothing is an offense which is done by a person who, at the time of doing it, by reason of unsoundness of mind, is incapable of knowing the nature of the act, or that he is doing what is either wrong or contrary to the law". This law also stresses that such incapacity must exist at the time of doing the act. Section 84 of IPC also considers epileptic insanity as a defense, which must exist at the time of commission of the act, e.g. murder. "Irresistible impulse" due to mental disease is covered by Section 84. Law presumes every person sane unless contrary is proved. Where any lunatic had "lucid interval", law presumes the offense to have been committed by the accused during lucid interval unless there is evidence to show that it was committed during the period of mental disorder. It is necessary for the accused to refute that presumption to establish his innocence.[10]

In IPC, burden of proof of insanity falls on the accused but burden upon him is not that heavy as it is on the prosecution but is the same as one which the party in civil proceedings has to discharge. The accused may discharge the burden by establishing a mere preponderance of probability by producing all the relevant evidence, oral, documentary or circumstantial before the court. When there is no motive (intention) for murder and mental condition of accused was not of normal person, protection under section 84 IPC can be extended to him. IPC is also concerned with 'legal' concept of insanity and not of medical view. In the background of medical opinion of accused suffering from paranoid schizophrenia, defense of insanity is available.[10]

In IPC, in order to constitute legal insanity, the 'unsoundness of mind' must be such as to make the offender incapable of knowing the nature of the act, or that he is doing an act contrary to law. It is the present state of mind at the time of neither offence, nor ante or past the offence, which only matters for the purpose of determining whether the accused was of unsound mind.[10]

Medical Insanity vs Legal Insanity

McNaghten rules follow a narrow concept of insanity as defect of cognitive abilities, i.e. loss of reasoning between right or wrong due to disease of the mind (legal insanity) and do not consider disturbances of emotions and will power (irresistibility/impulsivity), which are also affected in insanity. Thus, every type of insanity recognized by medicine may not form "legal insanity" unless the cognitive faculty of mind is impaired as a result of disease of mind (unsoundness of mind). Insanity is a defense because not knowing what he was doing or not knowing the moral nature of his act, the insane person is incapable of forming the intensions that are required for unlawful acts, e.g. killing. He does not have the mens rea (guilty mind) for any offence. As such, the word insanity has no technical meaning in law or in medicine. It comprises of a degree of mental disturbance so menacing and so disabling that the person may be considered legally immune of certain responsibilities arising out of unlawful acts done by him.[14]

On the contrary, medical insanity, which also considers problems of emotions and will power, may warrant the question of "diminished responsibility". For the above reason and growing concern against capital punishment, the defense of diminished responsibility for murder was introduced in England in 1957.

Diminished Responsibility

In English law, the defense of diminished responsibility is a defense only to the charge of murder, and if this defense is established, the offender is convicted for the crime of manslaughter only. The concept of diminished responsibility is based upon a broader definition of mental abnormality than the concept of insanity accepted in McNaghten rule. This is described in Homicide act, 1957, section 2 as follows: "Where a person kills or is party to a killing of another, he shall not be convicted of murder if he was suffering from such abnormality of mind (whether arising from a condition of arrested or retarded development of mind or any inherent causes or induced by disease or injury) as substantially impaired his mental responsibility for his acts and omissions in doing or being party to the killing." Original rationale of this partial defense was to avoid the capital punishment but its current use is quite wide, viz. a defendant can argue of irresistible impulses produced by mental disorder such as 'emotional immaturity', 'mental instability', 'psychopathic personality', 'reactive depressed state' and 'premenstrual tensions', and 'defense of diminished responsibility' can be pleaded for the charge of murder under such circumstances.[8]

Automatism

If a person has no control over an act, he cannot be held responsible for it. If such a state of automatism arises from a 'disease of the mind', it is referred as 'insane automatism' and then the appropriate defense is 'insanity' and McNaghten rules apply. In English law, insane automatism, accepted to occur in epilepsy, hyperglycemia in diabetes patient (insulin was not taken by him), hypoglycemia (but not caused by insulin), sleepwalking, etc. Other conditions of automatism have been described in sleep disorders and violence: confusion on sudden awakening (sleep drunkenness), night terrors and rapid eye movement sleep behavior disorder (Howard and d'Orban, 1987).[9]

Intoxication

According to **IPC 85** (Act of a person incapable of judgment by reason of intoxication caused against his will), nothing is an offense which is done by a person who, at the time of doing it is, by reason of intoxication, incapable of knowing the nature of act, or that he is doing what is either wrong or contrary to law; provided that the thing which intoxicated him was administered without his knowledge or against his will.[10]

Section 86 IPC (offence requiring a particular intent or knowledge committed by one who is intoxicated) again says that a person who does the act in a state of intoxication shall be liable to be dealt with as if he had the same knowledge as he would have had if he had not been intoxicated, unless the thing which intoxicated him was administered to him without his knowledge or against his will.[10]

Voluntary intoxication is not a defense if it affects person's state of mind to form the criminal-specific intent in relation to the crimes murder, theft, burglary, etc. Self-induced intoxication is not a defense to those crimes for which evidence of "basic intent" is only required (e.g. manslaughter, rape, indecent assault and common assault).[10]

Lastly, intoxication, whether voluntary or involuntary, appear as defense based only on the grades of criminal intent, which may be hampered to form to commit the crimes due to the influence of the substances on the brain.

Fitness to Stand Trial or Plead

The notion that a defendant should be mentally able to participate in the court proceedings has been observed, at least in some form, in England and other Western countries since the 14th century. This requires that the defendant should be able to stand trial of being guilty or not guilty.

The present-day application of this was largely defined in the landmark decision of American Supreme Court in Dusky vs. the United States, cited by Mossman et al.[15] The Supreme Court determined that key test of competency to stand trial is whether the defendant has sufficient present ability to consult with his lawyer with a reasonable degree of rational understanding and whether (he or she has) a rational as well as factual understanding of the proceedings against him.[15] Thus, if an accused of a crime is deemed to have mental illness and not fit to stand trial, the court can order for psychiatric opinion regarding his fitness to stand trial to defend himself. The issue may be raised by the defense, the prosecution or the judge. If the accused is found unfit to plead, court may issue an order to admit him in a hospital for psychiatric treatment till he is fit for trial.[16]

In determining fitness to plead, psychiatrist needs to determine how far the defendant can:

i. Understand the questions asked,
ii. Understand the nature of the charge,
iii. Understand the differences between pleading guilty and not guilty,
iv. Able to instruct his counsel,
v. Able to follow the evidence presented in the court,
vi. Able to challenge the selection of jurors.

A person suffering from severe mental illness may still be fit to stand trial. Determination of ability to stand trial can be done by using some structured instruments other than the clinical psychiatric assessment of mental status.

In 1965, Robey[17] published the first criteria for competency to stand trial checklist. There exists, at present, lots of other checklists, structured or semi structured interview schedules with their own strengths and weaknesses. Among them, the most commonly used one is Mac. Arthur Competence Assessment tool–Criminal Adjudication (Mac CAT CA).[18] However, these tools should be used in concert with a more comprehensive clinical examination, rather than using as a substitute.

Restoration of Competency to Plead Trial

All efforts need to be made to improve the mental condition of an insane offender so as to improve his competency to a sufficient level to stand trial, providing treatment for the different conditions—medical, substance abuse or other neuropsychiatric disorders affecting mental status. Deficits in competency due to some conditions like developmental disabilities (mental retardation), static traumatic brain injury and neurodegenerative disorders are difficult to resolve, but acute exacerbations of some psychiatric disorders like psychotic conditions can be treated very well. But, question arises whether a defendant can be forced to take medications to improve his competency or not. This issue was addressed by American Supreme Court in 2003 in the famous case Shell vs. The United States,[19] wherein the court specified several conditions for the involuntary administration of medications as follows:

i. Importance the restoration must be evaluated on a case by case basis
ii. The medication must have minimal side effects
iii. There are no other options of restoration
iv. The medication is appropriate for the treatment of the disorder that caused the incompetence in the first place.

Psychiatrists play an important role in determining criminal responsibility of mentally ill offenders, but it is not always an easy task for them to establish whether the person was suffering from unsoundness of mind at the time of committing the crime, as often he is brought for evaluation long after the act. Psychiatric evaluation and observation can comment on the present mental state of the individual but comment about mental state at the time of the offense is often difficult, as that maybe based only on reliable history of the illness which is also quite likely to be fabricated in most of the occasions.

CIVIL RESPONSIBILITIES OF INSANE

i. **Management of property**: If he is unable to take care of himself or manage his properties, the court will appoint a guardian or a manager after inquisition.
ii. **Contracts:** As per Indian Contract Act of 1872, if it is proved that at the time of signing a contract either of two parties was insane, then the contract becomes legally invalid.
iii. Child custody and adoption.
iv. Marriage.
v. Testamentary capacity or capacity to make a valid will.[14]

Marriage and Mental Health Problems

Marriage may be stressful for vulnerable people, which may lead to the development of mental health problems. Major mental health disorders may be effect of marital disharmony or vice-versa. Certain mental disorders may be one of the grounds for the divorce, which is accepted by law.[14]

According to Hindu Marriage Act[20] Section 5(ii) introduced by Act 68 of 1976, if at the time of marriage any party is incapable of giving a valid consent due to unsoundness of mind; or though capable of giving consent, has been suffering from mental disorder of such a kind or to such an extent as to be unfit for marriage and the procreation of children; or has been subject to recurrent attacks of insanity or epilepsy, the marriage shall be voidable and can be annulled by a decree of nullity under Section 12 of the Act.

Divorce can be granted under Section 13 of the Hindu Marriage Act on a petition filed by either spouse on the ground that the other party has been incurably of unsound mind or has been suffering continuously or intermittently from mental disorder of such kind and to such extent that the petitioner cannot reasonably be expected to live with the respondent.

The term mental disorder here means mental illness, arrested or incomplete development of mind, psychopathic disorder or disability of mind and includes schizophrenia. Psychopathic disorder here means persistent disorder or disability of mind (whether or not including subnormality of intelligence), which results in abnormally aggressive or seriously irresponsible conduct and whether or not requires or is susceptible to treatment.[20]

Testamentary Capacity[21]

Common Grounds for Invalid Testamentary Capacity

i. Inability in understanding the situation
ii. Difficulty in attention and information processing

iii. Language problems
iv. Memory disturbances
v. Impaired higher mental functions
vi. Paranoid delusions.

Most of the time, doctors are asked for an opinion whether a person has or did not have the mental capacity to make such a will. The above-mentioned points have to be kept in mind while assessing the testamentary capacity. The examination for such situation should be started only after the written request from the competent authority.

Responsibility in Disorders of Body Functions

i. **Somnambulism:** It is a condition in which a person walks during his sleep. It is also known as 'sleep walking.' It is the aimless wandering with incomplete arousal from sleep, along with acute anxiety. But person rarely injures himself. It is similar to automatism.
   Such person, if commit a crime, is not criminally responsible.[6]
ii. **Somnolence:** This condition is mid-way between sleep and wakefulness, also known as 'sleep drunkenness.' If such person is suddenly aroused from sleep, he may commit some crime due to confusion. He is not criminally responsible for his actions.[7]

Hypnotism: Hypnosis and Crime

It is also a sleep-like state, induced by suggestion. But it is very difficult to convince a person in hypnosis to commit some act, which he would not do in normal circumstances. It is a wrong impression that a person may commit murder under hypnosis.

Delirium: Disturbance of consciousness, where there is impaired orientation, recent memory, thinking with blunted other critical faculties of brain like perception. During the early stages, patient may become restless, with altered sleep-wake cycle, later he or she may completely lose self-control, may remain excited and may talk incoherent or irrelevant. It may be associated with delusions and hallucinations. Usually occurs due to physical exhaustion, loss of fluid and electrolytes, drug intoxication or as a complication of any organic medical condition. Such person is not criminally responsible for actions committed during his delirium.

REFERENCES

1. World Health Organization. The ICD-10 Classification of Mental and Behavioral Disorders; WHO; Geneva; 1992.
2. Casey P, Kelly B. Fish's Clinical Psychopathology: Signs and Symptoms in Psychiatry. 3rd ed. Gaskell; 2007.
3. Gelder MG, Andreasen NC, Lopez Ibor JJ Jr, Geddes JR. New Oxford Textbook of Psychiatry. 2nd (Indian) ed. Noida: Oxford University Press; 2011.
4. Sadock BJ, Sadock VA, Ruiz P (Eds). Kaplan and Sadock's Comprehensive Textbook of Psychiatry, 9th ed. Philadelphia; 2009.
5. Oyebode F. SIMS' Symptoms in the Mind: An Introduction to Descriptive Psychopathology, 4th ed. Birmingham; 2009.
6. Sharma RK. Insanity and forensic psychiatry. In: Concise Textbook of Forensic Medicine and Toxicology, 3rd ed. New Delhi; 2011.
7. Vyas JN, Ahuja N. Textbook of Postgraduate Psychiatry, 2nd ed. New Dehli; 1999.
8. Gunn M, Wheat K. New Oxford Textbook of Psychiatry, 2nd ed. Vol 2. Secion 11.1. pp. 1895-907.
9. Gelder M, Gath D, Mayou R, Cowen P. Forensic psychiatry. In: Oxford Textbook of Psychiatry, 3rd ed.1996;pp. 769-73.
10. Sarkar PC. Sarkar on Criminal Major Acts with Practice, Procedure and State Amendments, 6th ed. 1999. p. 14.
11. Ormerod DC. Smith and Hogan's Criminal Law, 11th ed. Butterworths, London; 2005.

12. Lord Denning. Bratty vs. Attorney General (1963) Appeal Cases 386.
13. McNaughten's Case (1843)10 Clarkson and Findley Law reports 200.
14. Nambi S. Legal Aspects of Psychiatry:Indian Perspective. Manashanti Publications; 2008.
15. Mossman D, Noffsinger SG, Ash P, et al. AAPL practice guideline for the forensic psychiatric evaluation of competence to stand trial. J Am Acad Psychiatry Law. 2007;35;S3-72.
16. Dawes SE, Palmer BW, Jeste DV. Adjudicative competence. Curr Opinion Psychiatry. 2008;21(5):490-4.
17. Robey A. Criteria for competency to stand trial; a checklist for psychiatrists. Am J Psychiatry. 1965;122; 616-23.
18. Otto RK, Poythress NG, Nicholson RA, et al. Psychometric properties of the Mac Arthur Competence Assessment Tool-Criminal Adjudication. Psychol Assess. 1998;10;435-43.
19. Heilbronn K, Kramer GM. Involuntary medication, trial competence, and clinical dilemmas; implications of Shell v. United States for psychological practice. Prof Psychol Res Pract. 2005;36;459-66.
20. Hindu marriage Act 1955. Commercial Law Publishers (India): Delhi, 2007.
21. Indian Succession Act 1925.

CHAPTER 26

Postmortem Artefacts

Putul Mahanta, Thejaswi HT

LEARNING PLAN

- Know the definition of postmortem artefact
- Identify different types of artefact
- Learn how an artefact creates interpretational problems

DEFINITION

Artefact can be defined as any alteration or introduction of a new feature(s) into the cadaver, which is physiologically and pathologically unrelated to its natural state and is likely to cause interpretation problems for the investigators unfamiliar with the phenomenon. It is imperative for the doctor to know the various types of artefacts, so that erroneous conclusions may be avoided, which otherwise lead to the inquest heading in the wrong direction and, rarely, may lead to miscarriage of justice.[1]

TYPES OF ARTEFACT

Postmortem artefacts can be grouped as follows:

- Agonal artefacts
- Artefacts related to changes after death
- Third-party artefacts
- Artefacts acquired during autopsy
- Artefacts of environment.

Agonal Artefacts

Aspiration of gastric contents is a common agonal artefact seen in natural deaths as a terminal event or due to handling of body or due to resuscitation. Without clinical corroboration of aspiration of gastric contents, the exact autopsy diagnosis of such aspiration is to be regarded with reservation. In a series of routine medicolegal autopsies, gastric contents were shown to be present in a quarter of all cases, irrespective of the cause of death.[2]

Artefact Related to Changes after Death[1]

Artefacts Related to Rigor Mortis

The development and pattern of appearance of rigor mortis are of some help in determination of time since death.[3] The partial breaking of the state of rigor due to the handling of the cadaver may lead to an erroneous determination of

Table 26.1 Hypostatic artefacts mistaken for injuries[7]

Area of lividity	Misinterpretation	Misdiagnosis
Neck and face	Internal neck bruising and ocular petechiae	Strangulation
Prinsloo-Gordon hemorrhages	Pharyngeal bruising	Strangulation
Scalp	Scalp bruising	Blunt trauma to head
Vulva	Vulvar bruising	Sexual assault
Spinal meninges	Antemortem epidural hemorrhage	Neck or back trauma

time since death. The same can be expected if the body is preserved in cold storage, which decreases the pace of postmortem changes.

At times, in infants and children, there may be marked dilation of the anal orifice during the postmortem. We know that immediately after death and before the development of rigor mortis, the whole body goes into the state of primary relaxation. In children, the anal sphincter loses tone and dilates, and in some cases, may be fixed by rigor mortis and may continue to persist even after the same has faded. Thus, anal dilation alone is not a marker for penetrative anal abuse of children prior to death.[4] This is particularly important because of the recent wave of child abuse cases being highlighted in the media, and overzealous misinterpretation of this phenomenon is a real threat.

Rigor affecting the heart may simulate concentric hypertrophy of the heart, and in all such cases, it should be confirmed by Fulton's technique of heart dissection.[5]

Artefacts Related to Postmortem Lividity

Certain poisons may change the color of the postmortem lividity, i.e. bluish-purple to cherry-red color in CO poisoning, bright-red color in HCN poisoning, etc. Thus, abnormal discoloration of it should raise these suspicions. If the bodies are kept in cold or in refrigerated condition, they turn pink.

Postmortem ecchymoses, otherwise called 'vibices', are tiny spots, at a time round to oval bluish-black hemorrhages, limited to livor mortis region. It is result of subcutaneous capillaries and smaller venules due to increased intravascular pressure from pooling of blood. This feature can again be mistaken for bruises.[6]

Big areas of hemorrhage that occur in the tissues behind the esophagus at the level of the larynx, caused due to leakage from the venous plexuses, can be mistaken for being due to strangulation. Simultaneously, pooling of blood in the posterior aspects of the viscera, including lungs can appear like visceral contusion. **Table 26.1** summarizes the artefacts involving postmortem lividity.

Artefacts of Brain

i. Convolutions of the brain are flattened as a whole due to edematous changes of the brain which are common findings, but partial flattening of the cerebral convolutions is due to contact with the cranium, especially the occipital lobe, is a postmortem artefact. Thus, measuring the weight of the brain in important in all postmortem cases in order to objectively confirm the presence of edema.
ii. In raised intracranial pressure, there is grooving of the unci, but the same can be present in normal cases as an artefact.
iii. Rough removal of the brain may cause artificial damage to the ponto-medullary region or to the midbrain-pons junction.

Artefacts of Liver

The surface of the liver may be stained with bile. However, the undersurface of the liver in contact with transverse colon may also show greenish coloration due to decomposition.

Artefact of Postmortem Hemorrhage

i. A postmortem injury may cause hemorrhage.

ii. The postmortem bleeding may collect in the body cavities due to wounds in respective system and may produce artefact.
iii. Postmortem blunt trauma may cause laceration of blood vessels and displace red cells into the adjacent tissue spaces that resemble bruise.
iv. Due to distension and leakage from the venous plexuses, there may be bleeding in the tissues behind the esophagus on the anterior surface of the cervical vertebrae that may mislead sometimes.
v. Sometimes in hanging cases, there may be postmortem bleeding from the anus if deceased had hemorrhoids and the suspension duration is long. A gravitational force due to the upright position of the body facilitates postmortem per-rectal bleeding from the ulcerated hemorrhoids.[8,9]

Artefacts of Hair

The growth of hair stops immediately after death, though it may grow after death in some cases. The reason of postmortem pseudo growth of the beard is shrinkage of skin and subcutaneous tissue. The growth in the hair may also be misled by rigor mortis development in the erector pili muscle.

Artefacts of Decomposition

i. Bloated face misleads to obesity.
ii. Bloody and fluidly discharge from the mouth and nostrils may be misinterpreted as antemortem hemorrhage due to trauma.[10]
iii. Localized areas of lividity may be difficult to differentiate from antemortem bruises.[11]
iv. Blood may be accumulated in the occipital areas of scalp due to gravity that may appear as a confluent bruising.
v. Displacement and accumulation of blood in the tissues of the neck in drowning may simulate antemortem hemorrhage due to strangulation.
vi. The darker blood due to decomposition appear congestion, may be mistaken as signs of asphyxia.
vii. The gaseous distention due to decomposition may give false feeling of antemortem obesity.
viii. A deep groove, feigning ligature mark, may be seen around the neck in decomposed bodies if the deceased was wearing tight shirt or dupatta/cloth around the neck.
ix. Presence of air in right side of the heart due to decomposition may mislead air embolism. But in decomposition, it is not present in adequate quantity. It can be confirmed by pyrogallol test.[12]
x. Postmortem blebs due to putrefaction may be mistaken for burn blebs.
xi. Regurgitated gastric juices may cause tanning of skin of the face and neck, which may simulate antemortem burns.
xiii. Focal autolysis in pancreas may be misguided for pancreatitis. It is because of the action of its enzymes. Inflammatory reaction and fat necrosis are not found in such cases.[13]

Third-party Artefact

Artefacts of Emergency Intervention

i. The needle prick (injection) marks over the body mainly in the cardiac region seen. It may be associated with contusion over the precordial region. Postmortem bruises may also be seen over the injection site.
ii. A ring-like bruise may be seen due to defibrillator applied to the chest.
iii. Fractures of the ribs and sternum in a commonly encountered resuscitation artefact. The location of these rib fractures is mainly in the medioclavicular line, thus close to the sternal joint, whereas sternal fractures are located horizontally in the lower two thirds. The sternum fractures are seen through the middle of the body and manubrium.[14] Liver may be lacerated due to direct manipulation of the right hypochondriac region and also by a push and pull effect on the liver ligaments and the diaphragm.[14]

iv. Air embolism may be induced because of energetic resuscitation with a thoracotomy and internal cardiac massage, etc.
v. Emphysema, occasionally with sub-pleural blebs, air in the mediastinum or tension pneumothorax are seen while artificial respirator is used for resuscitation. There may be rupture of esophagus and lung due to the administration of oxygen by tube.
vi. Introduction of IV cannula into the neck vein may cause hematoma and diffuse bleeding into the tissues alongside the larynx. This may create bruises of the neck tissues that may be mistaken for homicidal strangulation.
vii. Introduction of a laryngoscope may induce injuries around the mouth, palate and larynx. There may be gastric dilation on esophageal intubation.
viii. Tracheal intubation is one of the most common interventions in the treatment of life-threatening situations. Because securing of the patient's airway deserves fast intervention, unintentional injuries cannot always be avoided. Even the assistance for intubation, namely traction and hyperextension of the neck, may lead to injury of the cervical soft tissue.[15]
ix. Placing of a subclavian or internal jugular central venous catheter may induce pneumothorax. Similarly, hemothorax, pneumothorax and pulmonary artery tear may be caused by pulmonary artery wedge catheter.
x. A faint and broad ligature mark may be associated with a cervical neck collar used for the purpose of stabilization neck in some cervical injuries.
xi. Imprint abrasions may be seen over both the leg and hand, produced by postmortem ligature to facilitate transportation.
xii. Introduction of a chest tube may look like stab wound. Chest tube may be found in a pre-existing stab would or gunshot wound altering the original scenario.

Artefacts Induced in Firearm Wounds

Kennedy Phenomenon: Whenever firearm cases are presented to autopsy surgeons, differentiating entry wound from exit is one of the key purposes of the postmortem examination. It would not be difficult in fatal firearm cases as the body will be directly sent to mortuary, preserving the characteristics of the firearm wounds. But if the same are altered during surgical intervention prior to death, artefacts can be induced, resulting in individual features of entry and exit wounds being permanently altered. This is called 'Kennedy Phenomenon', as surgical intervention, which was immediately carried out on John F Kennedy, made differentiating entry from exit wound difficult, further fuelling the controversy surrounding his assassination.[16]

Rayalaseema Phenomenon: Likewise, artefacts can be deliberately introduced in the firearm cases to misguide the investigators. Maoists deliberately altered the firearm entry wounds by mutilating it with bayonets or daggers. Likewise, a bullet can be implanted in the stab wound. Since such cases were reported from Rayalaseema region of Andhra Pradesh, it is called Rayalaseema phenomenon.[17]

Artefacts of Animal and Insect Bites

i. Rodents bite-marks are frequently encountered in forensic practice as shown in **Figure 26.1**.
The morphological appearances of these postmortem injuries are summarized in **Table 26.2**.
ii. The bites by dogs, cat and other animal leave different types of injuries that may resemble stab wounds.
iii. Bite marks by ants can cause many irregular, serpiginous, scalloped areas of superficial skin loss, and small punctate and scratch-type lesions may be often observed on the body. Usually, ant injuries are orange-pink to yellow in color and diffusely scattered over the skin surface. These injuries consist of small and rather shallow gnawed holes that can be easily misinterpreted as antemortem abrasions or resulting from strong acids. No bleeding is associated with such skin lesions, but sometimes

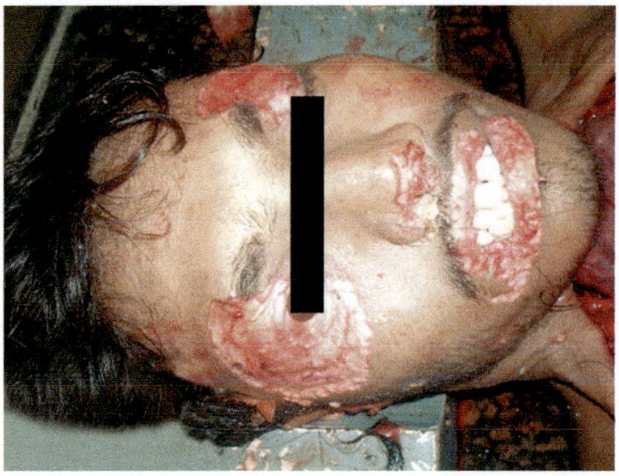

Figure 26.1 Rodent bite-marks
(*Courtesy:* Dr Anand P Rayamane, Global Institute of Medical Sciences, Bengaluru)

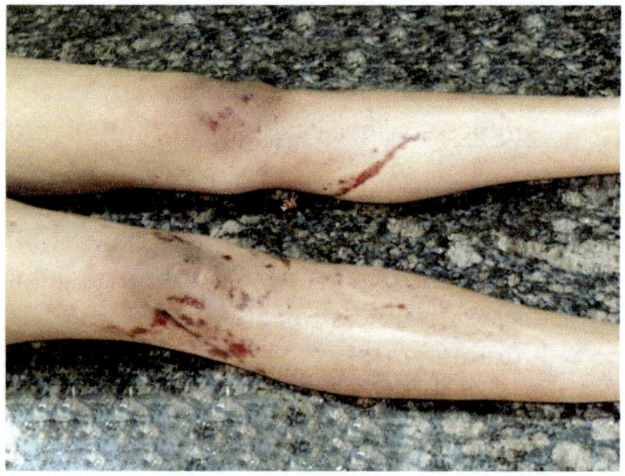

Figure 26.2 Ant bite marks on the lower limb
(*Courtesy:* Dr Anand P Rayamane, Global Institute of Medical Sciences, Bengaluru)

Table 26.2 Morphological aspects of postmortem injuries due to rodent activity[18]

Appearance of injuries
• Circular • Crater-like hollow defect
Injury margins
• Irregular edges: finely scalloped and serrated • Circumscribed 1–2 mm intervals within the wound edges • Protruding indentations up to 5 mm • Focal distinct parallel cutaneous lacerations
Preferred localization
• Exposed and unprotected parts of the body (face, hands) • Moist parts of the body (eyelids, nose, mouth)
Characteristics
• Hold on gnawing on a certain spot

considerable hemorrhage can take place, especially where removal of superficial layers of skin occurs in congested parts of the body (**Figure 26.2** in Case report 1). On histopathological examination, signs of vital reaction are not found.[19]

Artefacts Induced at the Time of Handling of the Cadaver

Due to rough handling of cadaver at the time of transportation, postmortem injuries may be produced to the cervical spine in the form of 'undertaker's fracture', which is the subluxation of the lower cervical spine due to tearing of the intervertebral disk at about C6–C7.[1] Also, bony prominences may be contused or abraded due to poor handling.

Tear of the wearing apparels during transport may appear to be due to antemortem struggle.

Artefact of Embalming

The procedures of embalming may change the pattern of pre-existing injuries and also create some injuries that look like of stab wound.

Embalming destroys detection of certain poisons, and postmortem toxicological detection of poisons, especially alkaloids and organic poisons, will be difficult. Similarly, it becomes extremely difficult to analyze the viscera for the heavy metal poisoning.[20]

Artefact of Exhumation

The excavators may cause fracture, laceration or stab wound, etc. at the time of excavation. The fungal and bacterial growth may produce artificial bruises. Contamination with the adjacent soil may change the chemical analysis result, arsenic being most common.

Artefacts in Toxicological Analysis

A false result is expected when there is incorrect procedure at any levels involving collection of the biological samples, storage and proper usage of the preservatives and labeling. If the tests are not carried out within reasonable duration, they may lead to wrong outcome.

Artefact acquired during Autopsy

i. During neck dissection, air may enter the neck veins which may lead to air embolism. Likewise, pulling of dura in sagittal line may cause entry of air to the blood vessels.
ii. Partial sawing and forceful pull of the skull cap or use of semi-sharp instrument may cause fractures of skull, which may pose problem in differentiation between antemortem from postmortem fractures.
iii. On rough and tight grasping and extracting of neck structures, there is possibility of fractures of thyroid cartilage, mainly in old person.

Artefact of Environment

Freezing of Cadaver

The normal color of hypostasis changes to pink if the cadaver is kept in extreme cold environment like refrigerator. This may create confusion in differentiation between postmortem hypostasis and bruises.

Artefacts Due to Burns

i. Heat ruptures of the cadaver body part may resemble that of lacerated or incised wounds.
ii. Heat hematoma may assume the appearance of extradural hemorrhage.
iii. Pseudo areas of strangulation mark may be observed around the neck due to unburnt tighten cloth.

MEDICOLEGAL IMPORTANCE

Ignorance of artefacts leads to:

- Wrong interpretation of cause of death.
- Wrong interpretation of manner of death.
- Wrong interpretation about time since death.
- Wrong interpretation about criminal intervention.

Ultimately leading to miscarriage of justice!

Case Report No: 1

A 26-year-old lady was found hanging in the morning, at about 08:00 hours, in her room with her pajamas and legs being blood stained. Since her pajamas were blood stained, it raised a serious suspicion of rape and murder. She was last seen alive the previous night. However, the room was secured from inside and the access to it was through a solitary door which had to be the broken before gaining entry to the room. During postmortem examination, other than characteristic presence of ligature mark, there were presence of multiple reddish colored, irregular, serpiginous, scalloped areas of superficial skin loss, and small punctate and scratch-type lesions around the lower limbs and the lining of her undergarments (**Figures 26.2 and 26.3**). Some red ants were still crawling over the body. Thus, it was concluded that the bleeding was the result of postmortem ant bites. It was limited to the lining of the undergarment lining because of the presence of firm elastic bands lining it, which limited the entry of ants further into perineal area. Since the body was in the state of suspension for 6–8 hours, the resultant pooling of blood aggravated the postmortem blood loss.

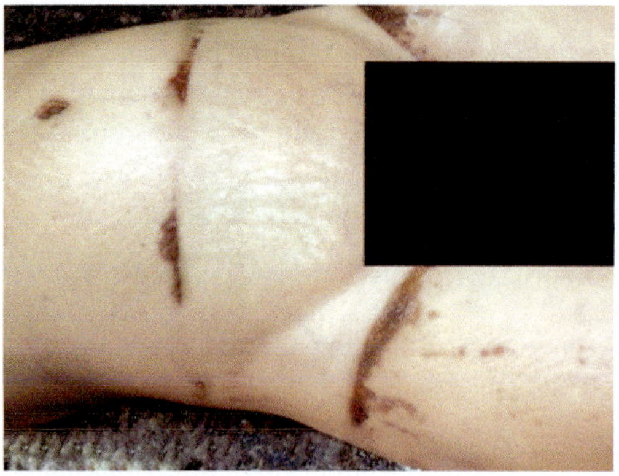

Figure 26.3 Ant bite marks along the lining of her undergarments
(*Courtesy:* Dr Anand P Rayamane, Global Institute of Medical Sciences, Bengaluru)

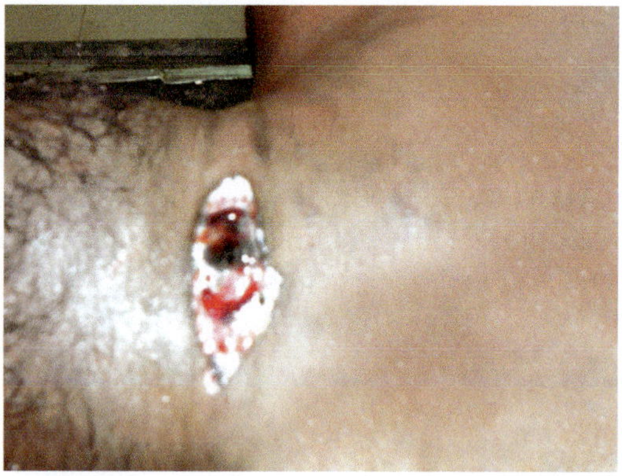

Figure 26.4 Postmortem predation by aquatic animals mimicking strangulation/stab injury
(*Courtesy:* Dr Anand P Rayamane, Global Institute of Medical Sciences, Bengaluru)

Case Report No: 2

One young male who, along with his friends, had gone to the lake for picnic, accidentally slipped and drowned. The body was retrieved about half a day later. However, when it was recovered, the relatives of the deceased observed the presence of injuries in the front of the neck (**Figure 26.4**) and back of the right hand, which raised serious suspicions of murder. During medicolegal autopsy, the neck was properly exposed by placing a plank below the shoulder, which showed the presence of lacerated wound measuring 4.5 cm × 1 cm × variable depth of 0.3–0.5 cm. On further examination of the wound with a hand lens, the edges were found to be soft, not swollen and containing multiple serrations with hollow defects. When layered dissection of neck was carried out, none of the vessels and airway was injured and there were no presence of vital reactions. Similarly, after drying of the body, multiple wounds around the front of the leg with irregular margins and pale-yellow-colored surface of the wounds without any features of vital reaction was observed (**Figure 26.5**).

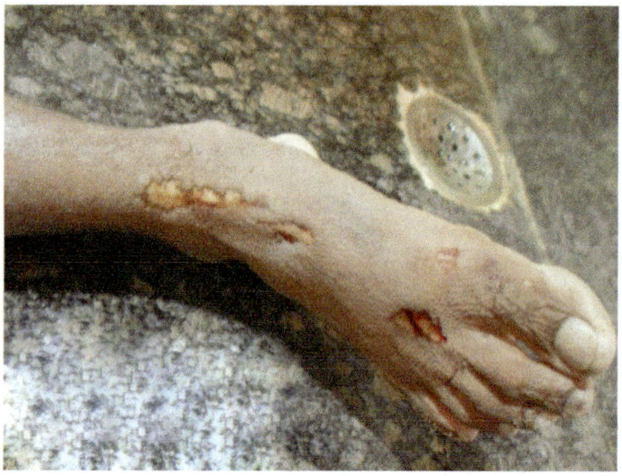

Figure 26.5 Postmortem predation by aquatic animals
(*Courtesy:* Dr Anand P Rayamane, Global Institute of Medical Sciences, Bengaluru)

Visceral examination showed the presence of large amount of frothy fluid in the trachea and main bronchi. The lungs were markedly overinflated with costal impression on their anterior and lateral surfaces and showed sub-pleural hemorrhages. Furthermore, the weight of the lungs was elevated (720 g for the left and 790 g for the right). No other pathological finding was found to explain the death at the macroscopic examination, and the cause of death was given as asphyxia due to antemortem drowning.

REFERENCES

1. Saukko P, Knight BH. Knight's Forensic Pathology. 3rd ed. London: Hodder Arnold; 2004.
2. Knight BH. The significance of the postmortem discovery of gastric contents in the air passages. Forensic Sci. 1975;6(3):229-34.
3. Anders S, Kunz M, Gehl A, Sehner S, Raupach T, Beck-Bornholdt HP. Estimation of the time since death-reconsidering the re-establishment of rigor mortis. Int J Legal Med. 2013;127(1):127-30.
4. McCann J, Reay D, Siebert J, Stephens BG, Wirtz S. Postmortem perianal findings in children. Am J Forensic Med Pathol. 1996;17(4):289-98.
5. Sheaff MT, Sheaff MT. Postmortem Technique Handbook. London: Springer; 2005. p.155.
6. Tsokos M. Forensic Pathology Reviews, Vol. 3. New Jersey: Humana Press; 2005. pp. 183-237.
7. Pollanen MS. Forensic pathology and the miscarriage of justice. Forensic Sci Med Pathol. 2012;8:285-9.
8. Kanchan T, Menezes RG, Manipady S. Haemorrhoids leading to post-mortem bleeding artefact. J Clin Forensic Med. 2006;13(5):277-9.
9. Bhardwaj DN, Sharma SK, Gupta S. Haemorrhoids leading to post-mortem artefact: A case report. Med Sci Law. 2005;45(3):265-6.
10. Rutty GN. Essentials of Autopsy Practice, Vol. 1. Springer, London; 2001.
11. Burke MP, Olumbe AK, Opeskin K. Postmortem extravasations of blood potentially simulating antemortem bruising. Am J Forensic Med Pathol. 1998;19(1):46-9.
12. Brenda LW. Handbook of Autopsy Practice, 4th ed. New Jersy: Humana Press: 2009. p. 281.
13. Tomita Y, Nihira M, Ohno Y, Sato S. Ultra structural changes during in situ early postmortem autolysis in kidney, pancreas, liver, heart and skeletal muscle of rats. Leg Med (Tokyo). 2004;6(1):25-31.
14. Tsokos M (Ed). Forensic Pathology Reviews, Vol. 1. In: Mario D. Injuries Resulting From Resuscitation Procedures. New Jersey: Humana Press; 2004. pp. 293-303.
15. Jaeger K, Ruschulte H, Osthaus A, Scheinichen D, Heine J. Tracheal injury as a sequence of multiple attempts of endotracheal intubation in the course of a preclinical cardiopulmonary resuscitation. Resuscitation. 2000;43(2):147-50.
16. Karmakar RN. Forensic Medicine and Toxicology. Kolkata: Academic Publisher; 2006. p. 158.
17. Sharma RK. Concise Textbook of Forensic Medicine & Toxicology. 3rd ed. New Delhi: Global Education Consultants. 2011. p. 88.
18. Tsokos M, Matschke J, Gehl A, Koops E, Püschel K. Skin and soft tissue artefacts due to postmortem damage caused by rodents. Forensic Sci Int. 1999;104(1):47-57.
19. Campobasso CP, Marchetti D, Introna F, Colonna MF. Postmortem artefacts made by ants and the effect of ant activity on decompositional rates. Am J Forensic Med Pathol. 2009;30(1):84-7.
20. Vij K. Textbook of Forensic Medicine and Toxicology: Principles and Practice, 4th ed. New Delhi: Elsevier; 2009.

CHAPTER 27

Forensic Serology

Akash Deep Aggarwal, Putul Mahanta, Monika Garg

LEARNING PLAN

- Identify blood stain and sources
- Characterization of unknown blood
- Blood spatter analysis for crime reconstruction
- Paternity testing
- Semen identification in rape cases
- Other body fluids like saliva, etc.

Dr Edmond Locard (1877-1966), the father of modern Forensic Sciences, studied medicine and then law in France. He formulated the basic principle of forensic science: "Every contact leaves a trace", the Locard's exchange principle.

The various types of **forensic evidence** include physical, biological, drug and other physical evidence, including firearms and fired ammunition, fingerprints, tool marks, tire tracks and footwear impressions, hair, fibers, glass, paint and other trace evidence. The term "**trace evidence**" is generally thought as any type of evidence occurring in sizes so small that it can be transferred or exchanged between two surfaces without being noticed. The instrumentation may be required to detect the presence of trace evidence. The identification and comparison of these materials can often associate a suspect to a crime scene or with another individual. **Forensic serology** is the detection, identification and typing of body tissues, either in native form or as stains or residues left at a crime scene. It is the application of the study of blood, semen, saliva and other body fluids, to legal matters.

Biological Evidence consists of body fluids or other bodily tissues, the examination of which may identify the donor, e.g. blood, semen, saliva, sweat, urine, bone, hair and skin. Biological traces evidence is a branch of forensic biology, which deals with trace evidence of biological origins.

BLOOD

Serological evidence consisting of blood and other body fluids is commonly encountered in offences related to the body. Blood, evidence is of value in such crimes as murder, rape, assault, abortion, robbery, burglary, hit-and-run accidents and law violations. It may aid an investigation by locating the crime scene, by identifying the weapon used, by proving or disproving a suspect's alibi and by eliminating suspects. DNA profiling can be performed on any biological substance. It can also be used for the identification of bodies when samples from parents and/or children of the missing person are available.

Blood is a fluid, normally red in color, containing plasma and blood cells. Plasma is composed of water along with glucose, hormones, vitamins, proteins, minerals, chemicals, etc. Blood cells include red blood cells (erythrocytes or RBCs), white blood cells (WBCs) and platelets as shown in **Table 27.1**.

Detection of blood is interfered by many factors, including contamination, putrefaction, heat, bacterial growth and chemical action.

Information to be Determined

1. Analysis must be performed on a stain **(Figure 27.1)** to determine that it is blood, since the appearance of blood varies greatly depending on the age, weather and other factors.
2. If the sample is blood, the species origin must then be determined. Usually, it is necessary to determine, if it is human blood.
3. If the blood is human, further classification will be achieved by isoenzyme and DNA analysis. Different individuals have different types due to the genes they received from their parents. Each type has a certain percentage of occurrences in the population. If one's blood type is different, the person is eliminated as the possible source. Most important is the determination of the blood group.
4. The sex of the person from whom the sample originated can be determined.
5. DNA profiling of blood stains is performed when necessary for individualization. Generally, DNA analysis will be limited to three or four samples per case, the victim's blood, suspect's blood and one or two questioned samples. This may also include paternity testing.
6. Additional information can be obtained from the size, shape and distribution of blood spatters at the scene. It may be determined how much blood has been shed; the age of a stain; part of origin of blood; occupation of the person; any disease condition and contents like alcohol, poisons, narcotics, etc. This information can be used to reconstruct the events that occurred during the commission of the crime.

Table 27.1 Serologically important components

Plasma (55%)	Hematocrit (45%)
• Water (93%)	• Erythrocytes 99%+
• Proteins (7%)	• Leukocytes
Fibrinogen	• Platelets
Albumins, globulins, etc.	
• Others: Electrolytes, gases, nutrients, lipids, hormones, waste, etc.	

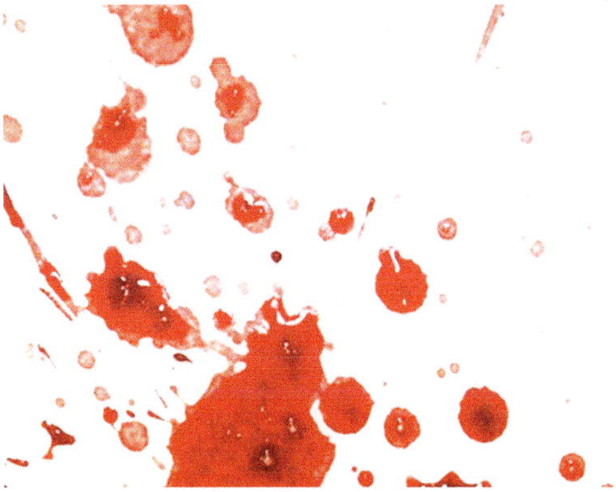

Figure 27.1 Blood stains on the floor

Location of a blood stain is usually visible and needs to be photographed and collected. Stains may be found at crime scene, on the accused, victim, weapons, vehicles or en-route in the form of stain, smear, streak, splash, spray, print, clot, pool, etc. Some techniques to make stains more visible include use of strong oblique light; colored lights; ultraviolet rays; infrared rays and luminol sprays.

Blood Spatter Stains

It is examined for:

- Position and movement during and after crime
- Place of impact
- Manner of impact
- Number of impact
- Pattern or types
- Direction and force of blow.

Pools are the best place for sample collection. Collection of a stain depends on its location and form. It may be scraped, cut, lifted, dislodged or collected as per form in a bottle or envelope. Chain of custody is maintained with proper packing, labeling, sealing and other formalities.

Classes of Blood Stains

i. Blood at the crime scene can be in the form of pools, drops, smears or crusts.
ii. Pools of blood obviously have more evidentiary value in obtaining a wet sample.
iii. Drops of blood tell the height and angle from which the blood fell. The blood spatter analysis says that blood which fell perpendicular to the floor from a distance of 0–2 feet would make a circular drop with slightly scratched borders.
iv. Drops of blood from a higher point would have more articulated plant structure fraying off the borders (a sunburst pattern).
v. A blood spot on the wall or floor leave the direction of force of the blow **(Figure 27.2).**
vi. The direction of the applied force is the direction towards the tail of the splatter or stain or spot. In particular, the largest area of the splatter is the point of origin **(wave cast-off pattern).**

Liquid samples may be collected in vials of sodium fluoride/oxalate/citrate vial without preservative, on a cotton gauze piece for dried blood. **Wet** stains may be collected on clean cotton gauze or filter paper, which may be moistened with saline. Adsorbent materials like clothes may be dried and preserved.

Dried blood stains **(Figure 27.3)** are collected from stained areas, with unstained areas as control, by cutting or combing or scraping, etc. These may be lifted with cotton gauze or filter paper moistened with saline or inert gums.

In forensic practice, wet blood has more value than dried blood because more tests can be run. For example, poisons, alcohol and drug content can be determined from wet blood only.

Evaluation of Blood

Presumptive/Catalytic Tests

Benzidine test (Adler test), phenolphthalein test (Kastle Meyer color test), Leuco-malachite green test, Ortho-toluidine test and luminol reagent test are for presumptive identification

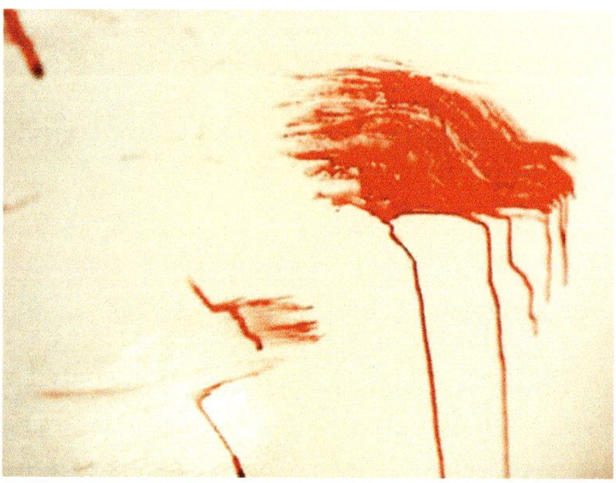

Figure 27.2 Blood stains on the wall showing the direction

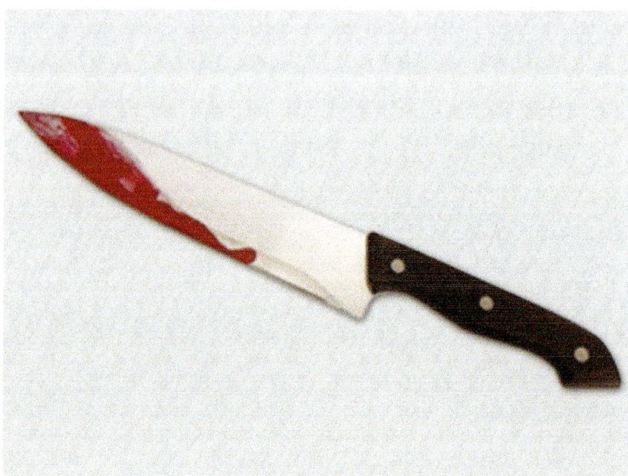

Figure 27.3 Dried blood stains over the knife

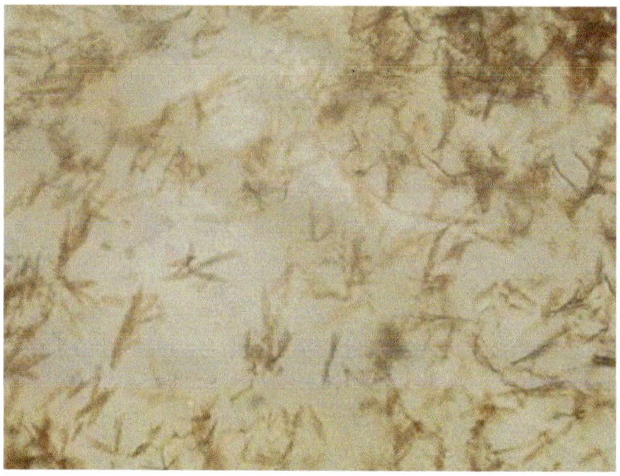

Figure 27.4 Takayama test showing crystals of hemochromogen

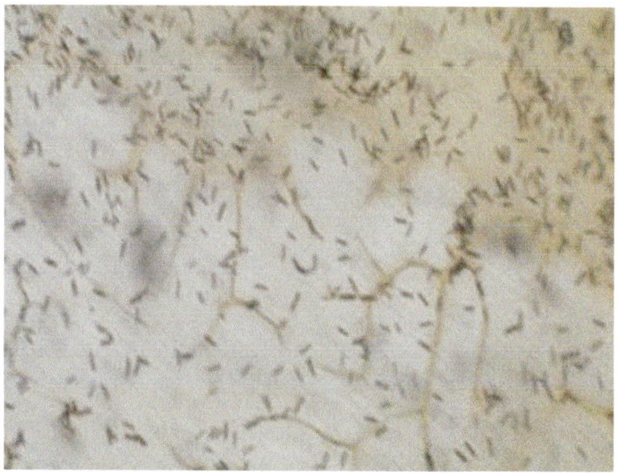

Figure 27.5 Teichmann test showing crystals of hematin hydrochloride

of blood, indicating that blood may be present. These tests are based on peroxidase like activity of heme group of hemoglobin. In these tests, the specimen is mixed with the reagent, followed by addition of hydrogen peroxide; positive color tests give blue, red, green/purple reaction, respectively. Commercially available Hemastix® strips can be used. False positive colored catalytic test reaction can be given by various chemical oxidants and catalysts; plant or animal tissues.

Confirmatory/Crystal Tests

Takayama Test: Take a drop of the suspected stain on a glass slide and add 2–3 drops of Takayama reagent. A cover slip is applied and slide is heated gently. Then it is observed under a microscope for the presence of characteristic crystals. The test gives good result, even with old stains. It is delicate and more reliable.

Features of the Crystals (Figure 27.4): These are the crystals of hemochromogen, which are salmon pink, needle shaped, feathery, arranged in rosettes if the stain is of human blood.

Teichmann Test: Take a drop of the suspected stain on a glass slide and 2-3 drops of glacial acetic acid and a crystal of sodium chloride is added. Then it is covered with a cover slip and gently heated and observed under microscope. The test may be negative if the stain is old, washed or treated by chemicals, the presence of too much salt, moisture in the acid and overheating conditions.

Features of the Crystals (Figure 27.5): These are the crystals of hematin hydrochloride, which are yellowish to red to brownish black, rhombic shaped crystals, arranged in clusters or in single if the stain is of human blood.

Individualization

This is possible using various components like enzyme types probabilistic graphical models (PGM), adenylate kinase (AK), glyoxalase (GLO), lactate dehydrogenase (LDH), blood groups (ABO, MN, Rh, Kell, Duffy, Lutheran, etc.); serum proteins (haptoglobin, globin, Gc, etc.); hemoglobin and DNA profiling.

Naked-Eye or Visual Examination

Visual examination of blood is imperative and determine the stain number, size, amount, age, direction (tip indicates direction of travel), relative movement, etc. **UV** and **IR examination** may reveal washed or invisible blood stains on various surfaces and even minute blood traces. On naked-eye examination, the non-coagulated blood is thick, viscid and bright red or bluish, depending on the source or region. Antemortem bleeding causes coagulation with separation of serum. The clot can be taken out

Table 27.2 Differences between ante- and postmortem bloodshed

	Antemortem bloodshed	Postmortem bloodshed
Hemorrhage	More	Less
Sprouting	Present	Absent
Clots	Firm and elastic color does not come out with washing	Usual absent. If present, it is small and loose. Color comes on easily for washing

en mass from the spot, but leaves an impression, due to the fibrinous network which results in the clot formation. The postmortem clot cannot be taken en mass and it leaves no impression on the spot. Roughly, three layers (Lines of Zahn) are detected in the mass: One by the platelets, second by the RBC and third by WBC. **Table 27.2** summarizes the differences between ante- and postmortem bloodshed.

Stains Resembling Blood

- Rust stain: Bleached by any oxide
- Vegetable stains: Bleached by any oxide
- Synthetic dye stains: Reacts with nitric acid
- Mineral stains: Reacts with nitric acid
- Other stains, viz grease, tar, which dissolves in chloroform.

Blood Stain and Sources

i. Hemoptysis: Bright red, frothy, alkaline in reaction.
ii. Hematemesis: Dark and acidic reaction.
iii. Menstrual: Vaginal epithelial or endometrial cells present and acidic in reaction.
iv. Per vaginal bleeding in abortion: Clots and products of conception may be seen.
v. The blood of insects: Crushed appendages or parts of insects may be seen.
vi. Bleeding from injury of the victim or accused: Venous/arterial—ante- or postmortem can be known. If it is from the nose, it may contain nasal mucosa or nasal hair.

Age of Blood Stain

i. When fresh: Red blood begins to dry after 3–5 minutes of exposure to air.
ii. Within 24 hours: Reddish brown in color.
iii. As time passes: Darker.
iv. Fresh blood dissolved easily in water, which depends on the quality.
v. Fluorescence decreases with age.
vi. Enzymatic activity: Antigens, Geno-products, Rh, etc. gradually diminishes with the passage of time.
vii. Adenylate kinase, phosphoglucomutase, the acid phosphate enzyme is late to diminish as age progresses.

Microscopic Examination

Microscopic examination is important for species of origin (shape of RBCs, Barr body, Davidson body), the body part of origin (arterial/venous, nose, mouth, vagina, anus, menstrual, hemoptysis, vomitus), diseases (leukemia, syphilis, infection, pus), etc.

The **human RBC** is biconcave, spherical and non-nucleated (**Figure 27.6**). The average diameter is 7.3 microns, the maximum breadth is 2.5 microns and the minimum is 1 micron.

The **non-mammalian RBCs** are nucleated and its sizes vary (**Figure 27.7**), whereas the RBCs of **mammalian of camel type** are oval and are non-nucleated as shown in **Figure 27.8.**

On treatment by reducing or oxidizing agents, the components, especially, hemoglobins have characteristic absorption spectra or band on **spectrophotometry** and **spectroscopy**. Even less than 0.1 mg of the blood sample is sufficient for doing this test. Using **electrophoretic** techniques, when subjected to an electric field, due to inherent polarity, body proteins move towards opposite polarity. **Chromatography** using acetic acid, methanol and water solvent systems has also been employed.

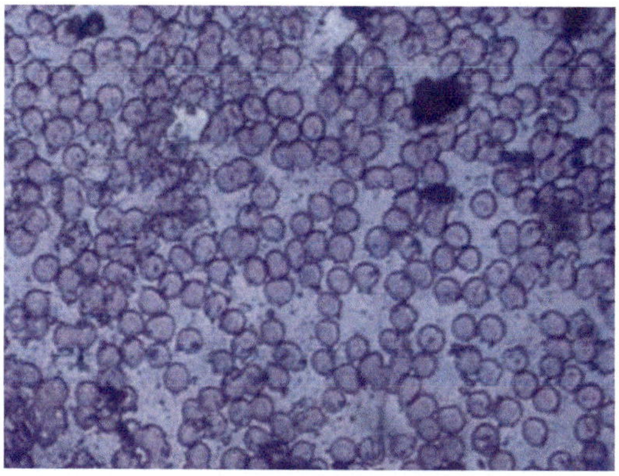

Figure 27.6 Human blood showing biconcave, spherical, non-nucleated RBCs

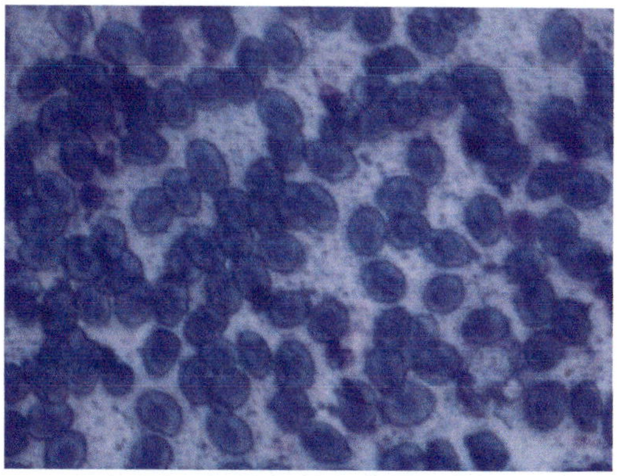

Figure 27.7 Non-mammalian blood showing nucleated RBCs

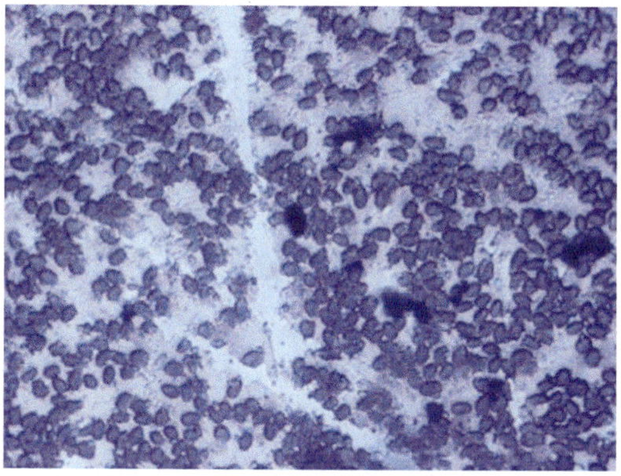

Figure 27.8 Mammalian blood of the camel type showing oval and non-nucleated RBCs

Sex Chromatin Test (**Nuclear Sexing**): Cells (more with female cells) usually show a collection of chromatin material (due to X chromosome) called **Barr bodies**. Barr and Bertram demonstrated it in 1949. It is the small Plano convex mass lying near the nuclear membrane (**Figure 27.9**). In the buccal smear, the percentage of nuclei having chromatin body ranges from 0–4 in males and 20–80 in females.

Similarly, **Davidson body**, which is a nuclear attachment of drumstick form, is also useful. It is found in up to 6% of cells in females and is absent or rarely found in males. Davidson bodies can be demonstrated in the peripheral smears with Leishman or Giemsa stains. Davidson demonstrated these neutrophilic drumsticks as dense chromatins head 1.5 μm in diameter and are attached to the nucleus by a threadlike connecting piece.

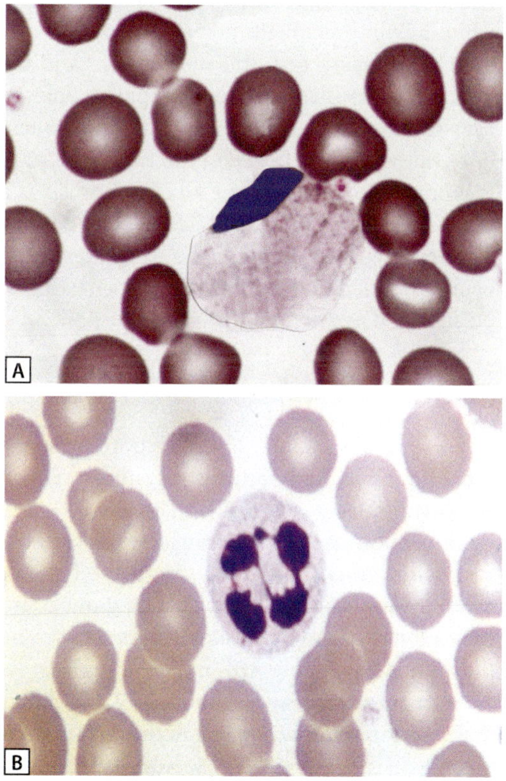

Figures 27.9A and B (A) Barr body; (B) Davidson body

Identification of the Davidson body in the neutrophils is very simple, cost effective and rapid method to determine the genetic sex of the individual. Presence of Barr bodies and Davidson bodies are the positive evidence of sex.

Species Origin

Origin determination tests are based on immunological principles that the immune system produces antibodies, which are specific proteins to counteract foreign proteins (antigens). These principles are used to produce **antihuman serum** in animals like rabbits. When the antihuman serum (antibodies) comes in contact with human blood (antigens), their results the precipitation reaction and the formation of large antigen-antibody complexes that will precipitate. **Ring precipitation test** involves layering of a dilute saline extract of blood stain on top of antihuman serum, forming a layer of interface, which on heating, leads to the formation of a white line, a precipitate between two layers. In the **Gel diffusion test**, the stain extract and the antihuman serum are placed in separate holes in agar-gel-coated plate, where a white precipitate line will be formed between the two if the stain is human blood. **Crossover electrophoresis** is a more sensitive technique which involves passing of electric current through the gel plate. While using these techniques, simultaneous testing of positive and negative controls must be done.

Blood Grouping

There are 30 major blood group systems, including the ABO and Rh systems, which are currently recognized. The study and identification of **agglutinogens** (antigens) and **agglutinins** (antibodies) form the basis of classification of blood into various groups and their identification by serological methods. The most important being ABO and Rh systems.

The presence of anti-A and anti-B antibodies in the serum differ according to the AB antigens present on the red cells. Those with A antigen on the red cells (group A) have anti-B in the serum. Those with the B antigen on the red cells (group B) have anti-A in the serum. Those with both A and B antigens on the red cells (group AB) do not have any anti-A or anti-B in the serum. Those without A or B antigens on the red cells (group O) have both anti-A and anti-B in the serum.

Forward Grouping (cell grouping) is determining whether or not the AB antigens are present on the red cells; we test them against potent and specific anti-A and anti-B. Using these two reagents, we can determine the ABO cell group. Anti-A, by definition, will react only with the group A antigen; similarly, anti-B will react only with the group B antigen. It is also necessary to carry out a **reverse grouping test** (serum grouping) by testing the serum against known group A and group B cells.

Three manual methods can be used when performing blood grouping: Glass **slide or tile** (white porcelain) method; **Tube method** (glass or plastic) and **microwell or microplate** method. Newer techniques are **column technique** (Sephadex gel) and **solid phase** tests.

In fluid, blood samples, the presence or absence of an antigen is ascertained by whether or not the red cells are agglutinated. In dried blood stains, the cells have ruptured and therefore, direct agglutination tests are no longer feasible. The antigens, in the ABO system, survive for many years and retain the capability of combining with specific antibodies. Three methods, which are routinely used for ABO blood grouping from dry stains, are described below:

Mixed Agglutination

In this test, the sample piece of stained cloth is cut into small pieces and the fibers are teased. Then they are added to tubes along with antisera of A, B, O types. After a period of absorption, unbound antibody is washed away, fibers are then suspended on indicator cell suspension of appropriate group, agglutination occurs between the absorbed antibody and the indicator cells so that, in the presence of a specific antigen. The fibers, when viewed with a microscope, are seen to be coated with a layer of red cells of the same specificity as the stain. Clumps of red cells seen adhering to the fibers is a positive reaction and the group can be known by the antisera, which clumped the blood to the cloth fibers.

Absorption-Inhibition

It is the classical method of detection of antigens in dried blood stains. In this technique, the sample and anti-sera are allowed to react with each other for a longer period. After a suitable period of absorption, the residual sera are tested with red cell suspensions of appropriate groups and the degree of agglutination is compared with that of controls tested in parallel from the unstained substrate.

Absorption-Elution

This test is similar to mixed agglutination test, but the clumps are noticed on the walls of the test tube rather than the sample cloth fibers. This technique can be used to find the blood group from body tissues also. After absorption and subsequent washing away of unbound serum, the combined antibody is eluted, usually by raising the temperature to about 56°C; then tested with indicator cells of the appropriate group. Agglutination indicates the presence of an antigen of the same specificity as that of the indicator cells. This method is more sensitive than mixed agglutination.

Secretors

The A and B antigens are found not only on red cells, but also in persons termed secretors, in a soluble form in the serum including saliva, semen and other body fluids. About 80% of individuals inherit the secretor (Se) gene that produces these soluble antigens. To determine if a person is a secretor, the principle of antibody neutralization, followed by agglutination inhibition is utilized, where the presence of agglutination means a negative test, and no agglutination is interpreted as a positive result.

Rh System

The **Rh system** has two genes (D and CE) that are inherited together to give a number of Rh haplotypes. Where a person inherits a D gene, their red cells are positive when tested with anti-D and that person is said to be RhD positive. Where a person does not inherit a D gene, their red cells are negative when tested with anti-D and that person are referred to as RhD negative.

DNA Typing

DNA testing can be used to further individualize the sample. Another genetic marker, human leukocyte antigen (HLA) can also be useful in paternity testing. However, DNA matching, when properly done, is the gold standard for assessing paternity which has been discussed in the **Chapter 8.**

Medicolegal Importance of Examination of Blood

Civil Importance

1. Identity of the individual.
2. Paternity or maternity issues.
3. Divorce and nullity of marriage cases (intersex and presence of some forbidden diseases).
4. For disputes arising out of affiliation case, the suppositious child (child of others).
5. Compensation cases related to workmen's welfare considerations (who are exposed to different toxic agents).
6. Civil negligence issues arising in hospital or medical practices (chemotherapeutics and blood transfusion).

Criminal Importance

1. Identification of the victim or offender of a crime.
2. Cause of death (e.g. detection of poison or some other pathology, responsible for the death).
3. Time of death (different chemical and biochemical tests of blood may be helpful).
4. Criminal abortion cases.
5. Sex offence.
6. Establish relationship between the offence, the offender, the offended (victim of the offence) and the offending agent.
7. Criminal negligence and other criminal charges.
8. Malingering cases.

SEMEN

Semen is a human body fluid present in human males. It is a viscid mucilaginous fluid with faint yellow color and characteristic odor called seminal odor. It is a suspension of spermatozoa in seminal plasma. Semen consists of spermatozoa (10%), seminal plasma (90%) and epithelial cell (<1%). Seminal plasma contains proteins, salts, organics (including flavins, which are the source of its UV fluorescence, and choline) and some cellular material. The components originate from several sources, including the seminal vesicles and the prostate gland. The prostate is the source of the enzyme acid phosphatase and the protein prostate specific antigen, or p30 protein.

Collection of Material

Dried or drying seminal fluid is collected with a wet throat swab. Fluid from vagina is collected by a pipette/throat swab. A portion of cloth containing the stain is cut out, dried and preserved. The pubic hairs should be plucked and placed in a small container. Stains on smooth surface should be gently scraped off with the portion of a knife into a glass container.

Vaginal/anal/penile swabs should be sent along with their smears on slides. Swabs should be taken on sterile gauze/cloth and their smears prepared on sterile slides. These should be dried in air at room temperature (37°C) and swabs dispatched in a sterile test tube and slides in clean wrappers.

Fluid from the vagina is collected by a pipette/throat swab. Stains on smooth surface should be gently scraped off with the portion of a knife into a glass container.

Physical Examination

It is the visual examination. To the naked eye, seminal stains generally appear translucent or opaque spots, at times with yellowish tint and darker border (map like outline), depending on the color and thickness of substrata, which, if absorbent, also acquire stiffness due to dried semen. On good substrata, seminal stains may appear to be fluorescent under ultraviolet light. Semen is very fluorescent by nature and the fluorescence can be observed in dark as well as light textiles when illuminated by an intense UV light.

Microscopic Examination

The best single confirmatory test for semen is the presence of spermatozoa themselves. Microscopic detection of spermatozoa (**Figure 27.10**) involves the direct examination of wet stains, whereas for dry stains, they can be dissolved in normal saline. Analysis of vaginal fluid or stain extract or swab extract or fresh semen, followed by staining of extract using Christmas tree stain or methylene blue or hematoxylin eosin stains may be done. Based on the principle that Y-chromosome is fluorescent to quinacrine, fluorescence microscopy can be done to detect both intact spermatozoa as well as the disconnected heads.

They undergo disintegration within a few months, but may be found up to 5 years. It length is 50 to 55 micron and consist of head, neck and tail. The head is oval and flattened when seen in front and pear shaped in profile.

Motility of sperms at room temperature: Motility of spermatozoa can be observed by putting a drop of mucus removed from vagina on a glass slide, which should be diluted with a drop of normal saline.

Motility persists for about 3 hours, 50% are motile by 8 hours and 10% for 24 hours. At body temperature, motility persists for several hours. In living persons, motile sperms are usually seen up to 6 hours after ejaculation into the vagina. Complete sperms are seen up to 24 hours and occasionally up to 2 to 3 days. Then they separate into heads and tails, which can be identified up to 120 hours. In the dead,

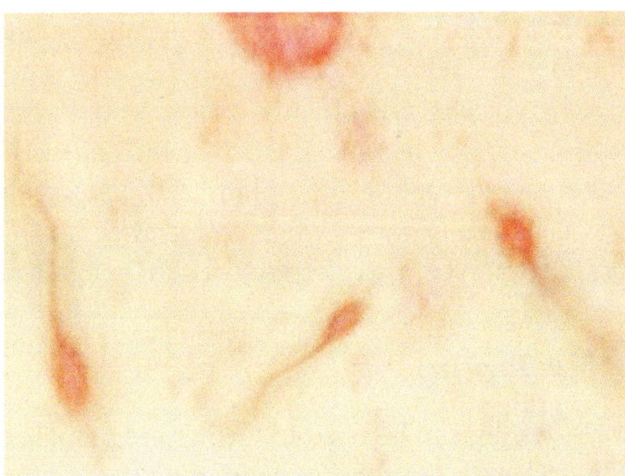

Figure 27.10 Showing human spermatozoa

sperms may be seen in the vagina up to 1 to 2 weeks. Sperms are destroyed by decomposition, but not by drainage or the action of the vaginal secretion. It may be found up to a fortnight in the uterine cavity.

Chemical Examination

The tests used to detect seminal stains are:

1. **Florence Test** to detect choline. A few drops of water solution of the stain is extracted and taken to a slide and a drop of florence reagent (solution of iodine in water containing potassium iodide) is poured and allowed to mix slowly under a cover slip. Dark brown crystals of choline periodide, generally needle shaped, forms within a few minutes. Non-specifics and false negative results are common.
2. **Barberio Test** to detect spermine. A few drops of Barberio's reagent, when added to spermatic fluid, produces crystals of spermine picrate (needle shaped, rhombic and of yellow color).
3. **Acid Phosphatase Test** (Brentamine Fast Blue Test). Human semen contains unusually high concentrations of acid phosphatase, which can therefore be the basis of a screening test. The stain extract is placed in a cavity on a porcelain tile and two drops each of citrate buffer and aqueous solution of disodium phenyl phosphate are added. After 10 minutes, the phenol is detected by the addition of 2 drops of phenol reagent and 2 drops of sodium carbonate. Blue color develops, which indicates the presence of acid phosphatase.
4. **LDH Isoenzyme Method**: Seminal stains are extracted with water and mixed with sucrose; then subjected to vertical polyacryl amide gel electrophoresis; isoenzyme bands are revealed by staining. This method gives a specific biochemical detection of spermatozoa in semen in the presence of vaginal fluid, blood, nasal secretion, saliva and urine. Seminal isoenzymes were found to be stable 11 four weeks after storage in tropical conditions. The method gave substantially more positive results than microscopic identification of spermatozoa when applied to a large number of relatively old stains on actual crime articles.
5. **Acid Phosphatase Isoenzyme Test**: Seminal stains are extracted with water and are used in polyacrylamide gel electrophoretic method followed by staining. The method is sufficiently specific and applicable to semen derived from normal, oligospermic, azoospermic and vasectomized individuals, with stains as old as 4 weeks.
6. **Creatine Phosphokinase:** Normal seminal fluids content: 385–14000 U of CPK/W. Diagnosis: >400V of CPK/mL. Advantage: Enzyme is stable and can be demonstrated in old status of 6 months. Serological typing of the semen is possible by precipitin method.
7. Ammonium molybdate test (Phosphorus)
8. **Prostate Specific Antigen (PSA):** PSA, also known as seminin, semenogelase, γ-seminoprotein and P-30 antigen is a glycoprotein produced almost exclusively by the prostate gland.
9. Enzyme-linked immunosorbent assay (ELISA), the SEMA® assay, for a seminal vesicle-specific antigen (SVSA).

Florence test, Barberio test and acid phosphatase tests are presumptive tests for semen; however, the first two are considered obsolete. The two most commonly used confirmatory tests for semen are microscopic examination and prostate specific antigen. One-step ABAcard® p30 Test and PSA Semiquant® Kit are immunochromatographic one-step tests for the detection of p30. Precipitin reaction with antihuman semen serum (or antihuman blood serum in case of secretors) and specific blood group antisera are used to determine whether a stain is human semen and blood group, respectively.

Vaginal swabs in rape cases are a mixture of fluids from the victim and attacker; and ABO types found in this fluid can be used much as blood typing to eliminate a suspect in a rape, but cannot accurately identify him. Secretor antigen matching of semen is similar to blood typing.

In living victims, sperms remain motile for 4–6 hours. Thereafter, first tails are lost, and then heads and tails undergo fragmentation. The survival of sperm heads and sperm remnants in various body orifices is highly variable. In general, these may remain in the vagina for up to a week, in the rectum for 2–3 days and in mouth for less than a day. In the vagina of a dead body, sperm may remain up to 2 weeks.

VAGINAL FLUIDS

Swabs from rape suspects' penis or any foreign object can be tested for glycogen containing epithelial cells. Periodic acid Schiff (PAS) reagent stains such cells bright magenta when viewed under microscope. This test may be falsely negative in the pre-menarche and post-menopausal.

SALIVA

Saliva is a mixture of many components as follows:

i. 99% water
ii. Mucin (protein helps in swallowing)
iii. Amylase (enzyme to help digest carbohydrates)
iv. Buccal cells (good source for DNA).

An adult produces about 1–1.5 liters of saliva per day. Saliva is not uncommon at crime scenes, especially those involving sexual assaults, murders, food, bites or on other objects.

Testing of saliva involves detecting presence of alpha amylase. The most common presumptive tests are starch-iodide test and Phadebas reagent color test.

Starch-Iodide test: A simple test for saliva involves mixing starch, iodine and a suspected saliva sample together. Starch and iodine are deep blue in color when mixed together. The amylase of saliva breaks down starch and the color fades, which takes about 15 minutes at 37°C.

It may reveal ABO antigens, and thus blood type in secretors, and may yield DNA for profiling.

SUGGESTED READING

1. Guidance manual on ABO and Rh blood grouping. Blood Reagent Laboratory, National Institute of Biologicals, Ministry of Health and Family Welfare, Government of India, Noida. 2013.
2. Newton DE. Forensic Chemistry. New York: Checkmark Books. 2007.
3. Lyle DP. Howdunit Forensics. Cincinnati: F+W Media. 2008.
4. Reddy NKS. Sexual offences. In: The Essentials of Forensic Medicine and Toxicology, 31st ed. Hyderabad: K. Suguna Devi; 2012. p. 407.

CHAPTER 28

Crime Scene Investigation

RK Gorea, Abdul Wahab Ali Abuderman, Putul Mahanta

LEARNING PLAN

- Learn about the crime scene
- Understand how to carry out crime scene investigation
- Know the "must for crime scene investigations"
- Learn about "do nots of crime scene investigations"

The crime scene is the place where the crime takes place and where the evidence of crime may be present. For the successful prosecution of the case, the best thing is to harvest this evidence of crime. This is possible only through the scientific investigation of the crime scene. Examination, collecting the relevant evidence, preserving this evidence for systematic analysis and documenting the whole process is crime scene investigation. This should be done as early and as systematic as possible by the experts to retrieve and preserve the evidence.

WHAT IS CRIME SCENE?

A **crime scene** is a place (**Figure 28.1**) where an offense took place and comprises the area from which most of the physical evidence is recalled by law enforcement officers, forensic scientists or in rare circumstances, forensic medicine specialists to collect the circumstantial evidences or to support in collection of trace evidences, etc.

Purpose

The aim of crime scene investigation is to find out the truth through physical evidences which

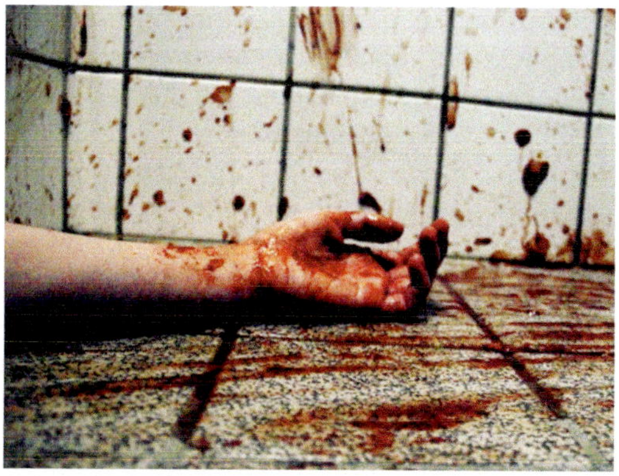

Figure 28.1 A crime scene

may be present at the crime scene. The essence of crime scene investigation is that evidence of crime should be used to prosecute the criminal, as eyewitnesses may turn hostile, but the physical evidence will never turn hostile unless scientific methods are not adhered to.

How It Should Be Done

Principle of crime scene investigation is that it should be done according to the established scientific principles, in a systematic manner and as soon as possible. On getting the information, usually nearest police officer, who is called the first responder, reaches the crime scene, and then the investigative police officer reaches the crime scene. Both these officers will have different responsibilities. Sometimes both these responsibilities may be performed by the same officer.

First Responders

Usually, first responders may not be the investigating officer, but any other police officials. In such circumstances, first responders have some duties. They should scan the entire area and identify the crime scene. The first responding officer has the duty to preserve the life of victims wherever possible. They should take care of the safety of witnesses, other people and property. They have the duty to protect the crime scene so that evidence of the crime is not tampered with or contaminated knowingly or unknowingly. He has the responsibility to call for medical help and ambulances. He should inform the medical and other paramedical people the importance of protecting the evidences and should note the names of the people entering the crime scene.

If the crime scene is in open space, it is important to evaluate and prioritize the collection of evidence which is likely to degrade or be lost due to environmental conditions. He should contact the person who has informed the police. He should remain alert and keep his eyes and ear open. He should inform the superior persons. He should document everything, which he has observed or done.

Investigating Police Officer

He should brief the investigating officer upon his arrival and hand over the charge to him, including all the documentation. This is the only opportunity when investigating officer can know the initial situation of the crime scene, and this opportunity should be fully utilized. The initial responding officer can help him in maintaining law and order situation, but should act now under his guidance.

Usually investigating officer should do a crime scene walk and draw a plan for further investigation and determine what is needed more in terms of experts and equipment, keeping in view the assessment of the case. Crime scene may be single or multiple. He needs to identify safe areas for keeping the evidences and apparatus for crime scene investigation.

EXAMINATION OF THE CRIME SCENE

After assessing the crime scene, the area should be cordoned off with the available means, e.g. twigs, vehicles, cones or tape. Additional police help may be needed and may be called to protect the crime scene. While determining the boundaries of the crime scene, it must be remembered that it is difficult to expand the boundaries of the crime scene but very easy to reduce the boundaries.

Always maintain a record of the persons entering the crime scene area. A common approach path should be marked and all the evidence on it must be collected before it is allowed to be used as a common approach path. There should be a systematic search pattern. Initial photography should be done before moving anything. Forensic photographer should do the initial photographic documentation.

Identification of Evidence

Evidences may be in the form of persons, e.g. witnesses of crime, or may be in the physical form at the crime scene, e.g. objects used for crime like a knife (**Figure 28.2**) or gun used to

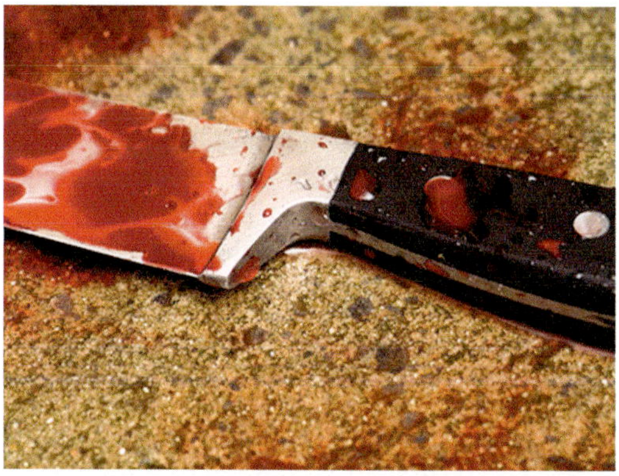

Figure 28.2 Blood stained knife at a crime scene

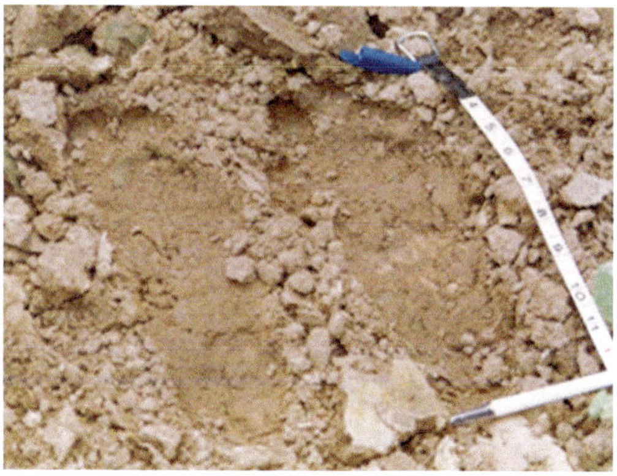

Figure 28.3 Footprints in mud

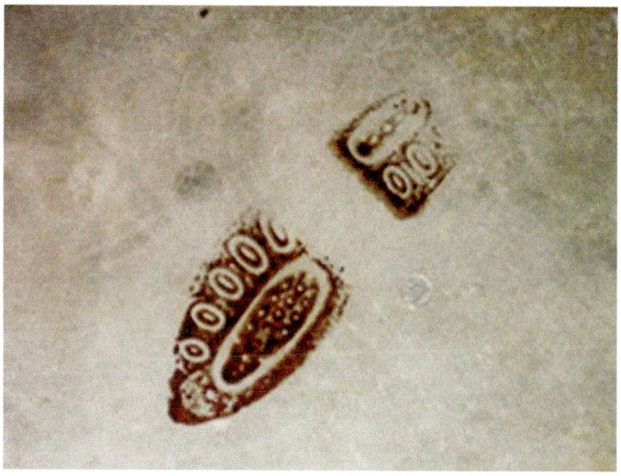

Figure 28.4 Shoe print at the crime scene

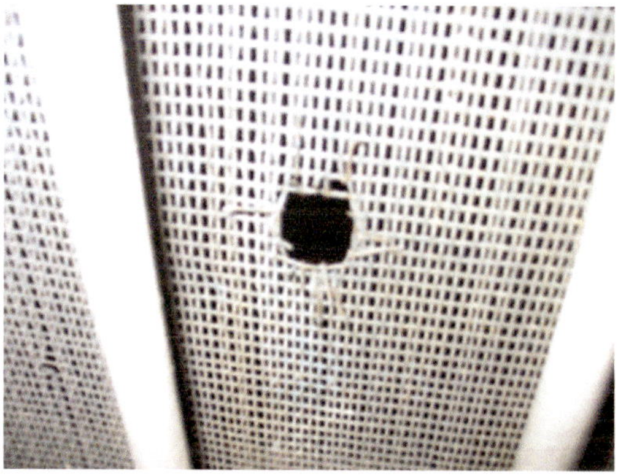

Figure 28.5 Bullet entries in an iron net in a window from outside (Photograph from inside)

kill a person or the impressions left at the crime scene, e.g. fingerprints, foot prints (**Figure 28.3**) or shoe prints (**Figure 28.4**). Sometimes, there may be trace evidences like fallen hair, blood stains, seminal stains or other stains at the crime scene. Physical evidences play a crucial role in the successful prosecution of the cases (**Figure 28.5**).

Collection of the Evidence

Collection of the evidence is an important step of scene process. Biological evidences deteriorate quickly as compared to other evidences; so, these evidences should be collected on priority. Keeping in view the environmental conditions, all those evidences should be collected early, which are likely to be affected by environmental conditions. Determine the sequence of collection of evidence keeping with the environmental conditions and portability of the evidences.

Use of personal protective equipment should be encouraged to prevent cross contamination of the evidences. Do not forget to take control samples and elimination samples. Evidence collection kits should be used wherever possible.

Preserving the Evidence

Once evidences have been collected, it is essential to preserve them so that these evidences are not degraded or decayed. It is also important that evidences reach safely to the labs and do not contaminate the environment or harm the public at large or persons carrying these evidences to the laboratories. Select the proper packaging material and containers depending upon the evidence so that the evidence will not get damaged. In biological samples, use the proper preservatives and preserve them at the right temperatures. Drying the stains also help in preserving. Seminal stained swabs should also be dried before these are packed as this will prevent growth of fungus on these swabs. Clothes should also be dried in shade if these are having wet stains. Evidences should be stored securely before these are transported to the proper agency.

Sending Evidence to the Proper Agency

It is always useful and helpful if the investigating officer knows where to send each sample he has collected, and this helps in saving time and this is particularly useful for biological samples as such samples degrade very quickly. Proper labelling of the samples and containers should be done. Evidence should be properly sealed and sample seal should always be sent for comparison. It is important to know the guidelines of the laboratory where the samples are being sent. If some forms are required to be filled, these must be properly filled and attested.

Maintaining Chain of Evidence

It is very important to maintain the chain of handing over the evidence till it is finally examined and reported. It should be well documented. This chain should not be broken and should be well documented.

Documentation of the Whole Process

This is as crucial as other parts of crime scene investigation. This should be recorded with the minute possible details. If there will any flaws in it, these flaws are likely to be exploited by the defense attorneys. The documentation can be in the form of notes, drawings, sketches, photographs and videos. Measurements and scales are important part of the documentation. Photograph the area with a scale in it. Wide angle camera is very useful. While photographing, proper lighting arrangements should be there. Alternative light source is important if the natural light is not sufficient. One of the conditions which can be well documented by photography is bloodstain pattern.

Every document should be properly labeled with case number and date. Documentations is record of crime scene investigation, which can be easily accessed, presented and cross examined and will showcase the accuracies and faults of the investigation in a truthful manner.

Final Survey of Crime Scene

A final survey of the crime scene should be done so that nothing is left to be done which is desired to be done. Debriefing should be done to all the responders so that everybody knows what has been done and nothing that needs attention has been ignored. Photographers, forensic scientists and technicians, doctors if involved, and all the investigators should review the proceedings together along with initial responders. Take care of dangerous material at the crime scene before leaving the scene.

Review the documents to see that these are accurate and complete.

Precautions

Crime scene investigation should be done as early as possible so that evidence is not contaminated, altered or destroyed wilfully or by natural decay. Early identification of the victim is essential as this will be the central point of most of the evidences. Name of all the persons entering the crime scene must be recorded, and their fingerprints and shoeprints must be taken to rule out artefacts in the crime scene.

MUST FOR CRIME SCENE INVESTIGATIONS

1. Protect the crime scene till the arrival of the crime scene investigators.
2. The outdoor crime scene should be given priority over indoor crime scenes.

3. It should be done without any loss of time.
4. Photograph the crime scene.
5. Document the crime scene.
6. Chain of evidence should be maintained.
7. Crime scene investigators must be trained and they should periodically update their knowledge and skills for the recent advances.
8. Crime scene investigators must have all the equipment needed for investigation.
9. In certain hazardous situations, persons especially trained to handle those situations should be used, e.g. radiological, chemical and biological hazards.
10. The approach should be objective.
11. Must have relevant crime scene investigation equipment, which will vary from crime scene to crime scene.
12. Plan according to environmental conditions.
13. Limit persons entering a crime scene as this will minimize the contamination of the scene.
14. Show compassion to victims, his family and friends.
15. Compile all the written material together into a case file.

DO NOT'S OF CRIME SCENE INVESTIGATIONS

1. Do not allow contamination of the crime scene.
2. Do not allow suspects to roam freely as he may alter or destroy the evidences and may be a threat to witnesses and others.
3. Do not ignore the minor details and trace evidence.
4. Do not ignore statements of witnesses, victims and suspects.
5. Do not ignore physical threats, e.g. gas leaks.
6. Do not ignore to record dying declaration if needed.
7. Do not spit, smoke and eat at the crime scene.
8. Do not touch or remove anything unless utmost necessary for the safety of people.

If necessary, obtain the search warrants required to meet the law of the land. Take consent of the people wherever required, preferably written. Be sure that crime scene investigation is complete in all respects before leaving the crime scene and crime scene is safe for the public.

Through social media, public should be made aware of importance of crime scene investigation and protection of the evidence at the crime scene before the arrival of the police. The public should prevent onlookers from entering the crime scene and should help the investigating police officers to reduce the crime in the society.

Investigation of death is very important and medical persons should be involved in such situations so as not to miss important clues, which can be appreciated by medical persons only. It is important that medical persons are part of the crime scene investigation in such cases. Inclusion of medical persons in crime scene investigation will serve a dual purpose. It will help in preserving the life of the victims wherever possible as well as safeguarding and collecting the biological evidence in a relevant manner.

Collection of material for DNA profiling is especially important is such cases. Suitable material should be collected, preserved and sent to labs for DNA profiling. FTA cards are useful for preserving most of the liquid biological fluids for DNA profiling.

If we will investigate the crime scene properly, it will create a sound basis upon which lies the process of sound and successful prosecution of the criminal. In the process of investigation, we should not forget that we are scientific persons and we should not under do or overdo the process, and we should stick to the scientific principles and should always overcome sentiments which tend to favor the quick conclusions of our mind which may not be always correct.

There should be a zeal to solve the crime and crime scene, officials should have proper training and equipment. The integrity of the crime scene official is a must. The crime scene investigation will be valuable evidence based tool to successfully prosecute the case. Precise and truthful crime scene investigation will be like justice done at the crime scene.

A Case Report

Things are not always what they seem to be at first sight. Many times, homicide cases go undetected because of the lack of suspicion and inadequate investigation in the field of criminal chain. Such a case was reported where a women burns victim was sent for autopsy in an unsuspected manner. The 35-years-old married women were found dead following burn injuries in her in laws' rented house, where she resided with her husband. Her husband claimed it to be a simple accidental burn following LPG leakage. A brief history of the incident produced a great amount of confusion to the autopsy surgeon. Hence, the investigating officer was advised to arrange for crime scene investigation (CSI), which was carried out immediately before the autopsy proper. Some very important substantial evidences were gathered from the CSI. The scene of occurrence of the incident confirmed along with the autopsy findings, to be a homicide case. And at autopsy, contused scalp and massive subdural hemorrhage, besides others, confirmed the diagnosis.

CHAPTER 29

Medicolegal Importance of People Living with HIV/AIDS

Putul Mahanta, KK Bairagi

LEARNING PLAN

- Learn the ways of HIV (Human Immunodeficiency Virus) transmission
- Know the rights and privileges for patient living with HIV/AIDS
- Declaring HIV status of positive individuals in death certificate
- Offences, penalties as under The Drugs and Cosmetic Act, 1940
- Learn about the approach to medicolegal autopsy of AIDS case
- Know about universal precautions

HISTORY

In 1981, the first case of AIDS was identified among gay men in the United States, acquiring the designation, GRID (Gay-Related Infectious Disease).

Scientists later found evidence that the disease existed in the world for some years prior, i.e. subsequent analysis of a blood sample of a Bantu man, who died of an unidentified illness in the Belgian Congo in 1959, made him the first confirmed case of an HIV infection.

AIDS awareness was soon brought to the public's consciousness, when popular film star, Rock Hudson, died of AIDS on October 2, 1985, shortly after making public his AIDS on July 25, 1985, thus becoming the first major public figure to announce that he had AIDS.

The first HIV infected case in India was reported in 1986. Since then, the numbers of individuals affected with HIV virus are increasing and it is estimated that in 2006, there were about 2.45 million Indians are living with HIV infection.

BRIEF REVIEW

An increase in HIV infection poses serious problems not only for medical services, but also to its legal system. Some of the more immediate medicolegal problems surrounding (HIV)/AIDS are: informed consent to the testing for HIV antibodies, the maintenance of confidentiality (privileged communication) and the question of whether healthcare workers may refuse to treat HIV/AIDS patients.[1]

The acquired immunodeficiency syndrome (AIDS) was first recognized in 1981 and is caused by the human immunodeficiency virus (HIV-1). HIV-2 causes a similar illness to HIV-1, but is less aggressive and restricted mainly to Western Africa.

In 2003, WHO estimated that there were over 40 million people living with HIV/AIDS, 5.3 million new infections and 3 million deaths. Many different cultural, social and behavioral aspects determine the regional characteristic of HIV disease.

India has a population of 1.2 billion, around half of whom are adults in sexually active age group. The first AIDS case in India was detected in 1986 and since then, HIV infection has been reported in all states and union territories. The spread of HIV in India has been uneven. Although much of India has a low rate of infection, certain places have been more affected than others. HIV epidemics are more severe in the Southern half of the country and the far North-East. The highest estimated adult HIV prevalence is found in Manipur (1.40%), followed by Andhra Pradesh (0.90%), Mizoram (0.81%), Nagaland (0.78%), Karnataka (0.63%) and Maharashtra (0.55%).[2]

Remember, HIV infection is a virus infection and AIDS is a stage and not a disease.

MODES OF TRANSMISSION

HIV is present in blood, semen and other body fluids such as breast milk and saliva. Exposure to the infected fluid leads to the rise of contracting infection, which is dependent on the integrity of the exposed site, the type and volume of body fluid and the viral load. HIV can enter either as free virus or within the cell. The major modes of spread are sexual, parental (blood or blood product recipients, injection drug users and those who experiencing an occupational injury) and vertical. The transmission rise after exposure is >90% for blood or blood products, 15–40% for vertical, 0.5–1.0% for injection drug use, 0.2–0.5% for genital mucous membrane and <0.1% for non-genital mucous membrane.

Worldwide, the major route of transmission (>70%) is heterosexual. About 5–10% of the HIV infections are in children and more than 90% of these are infected during pregnancy, birth or breastfeeding. There have been approximately 100 definite and 200 possible cases of HIV acquired occupationally in healthcare workers.[3]

RIGHTS AND PRIVILEGES FOR PATIENTS LIVING WITH HIV/AIDS UNDER INDIAN LEGAL SYSTEM

Individual Rights

- Informed consent
- Confidentiality and (right to) privacy
- Privileged communication
- Gender equality
- Right against discrimination
- Right of workers (right to employment)
- Personal liberty
- Right to marriage
- Right to information
- Right to free treatment.

Informed Consent

When an individual has any type of HIV testing performed, whether it is a test to diagnose HIV infection or simply to monitor the progress of the disease, he has a legal right of informed consent as per "**National HIV Testing Policy**". If it is done without informed consent, it is considered as a deficiency in service under the Consumer Protection Act. The consent should preferably be taken in written.

This means that no tests can be performed without the person's expressed consent, and before the testing, the person is to be informed of why it is necessary. Therefore, the patient will have the **right to refuse** the procedures, etc. If the tests are performed, the results have to be given, if requested as well. Hence,

- HIV test cannot be treated as any other diagnostic test
- Consent to another diagnostic test cannot be taken as implied consent to an HIV test
- Specific consent for HIV test is necessary
- An HIV test must be preceded by informed consent.

Informed consent in the context of HIV/AIDS implies conducting pre and post-test counseling. Failure to conduct pre and post-test counseling implies no consent.

Confidentiality and Privacy

A number of laws regarding HIV and AIDS have been put in place at the state, national and international levels to protect the confidentiality of HIV positive people. With very few exceptions, the revealing of an individual's HIV status is purely at their own discretion. There should not be any breach of confidentiality without a higher public interest being served.

The physician may apprize laboratory workers who are handling the blood of an HIV infected person, and the information is kept in the patient's medical records to inform the other doctors that are given access to those records, means the access is to be limited to service providers only. No one other than the service provider should know about the positive status of HIV/AIDS of the patient.

In many states, a physician also has the duty to tell a patient's sexual partner, if the physician thinks that the patient is withholding his/her HIV status and, as such, is a danger to the partner after due counseling. After counseling the client, the disclosure can be made to the sexual and needle sharing partner.

Sometimes, however a physician may reveal the information about the patient to protect a healthy person against a communicable disease to which he is about to be exposed. Hence, the notification can be given to the healthcare providers.

Court Case

Mr............................ X vs........... Hospital Z (1998) 8 SCC 296

Dr Tokigha Yepthomi

AIDS Patient: Apollo Hospital gave information to prospective wife—marriage called off—sued hospital for damages

Supreme Court: Case dismissed

Court Held: In the event of clash between two fundamental rights—Patient's right to privacy and the girl's right to lead a healthy life, the right which would advance public morality would alone be enforced by the court.

Case Law[4] on HIV Positive Patient's Disclosure to Interested Parties

Various questions related to HIV positive patient that came before the Supreme Court for consideration are as follows:

1. Whether a person suffering from HIV contracting marriage with a willing partner after disclosing the factum of disease to that partner will be committing an offence within the meaning of Section 269 and 270 IPC?
2. To clarify that there is no bar for the marriage, if the healthy spouse consents to marry in spite of being made aware of the fact that the other spouse is suffering from the said disease.

Questions Related to Practical Difficulties in Disclosure

1. What rights and obligations arise in such context as to the right to privacy or confidentiality?
2. Whether such persons are entitled to be married or not, or in the event such persons marry, they would commit an offence under law?
3. Whether such right is suspended during the period of illness?

In such a case[4] involving the disclosure of HIV status of patient to would be in-laws, the Supreme Court observed "in our view, this Court had rested its decision on the facts of the case that it was open to the hospital or the doctor concerned to reveal such information to persons related to the girl whom he intended to marry and she had a right to know about the HIV positive status of the appellant. If that was so, there was no need for this Court to go further and declare in general as to what rights and obligations arise in such context as to right to privacy or confidentiality or whether such persons are entitled to be married or not or in the event such persons marry they would commit an offence under law or whether such right is suspended during the period of illness".

Answer: SC (Supreme Court) observed that the appellant's right was not affected in any manner in revealing his HIV positive status to the relatives of his bride-to-be.[9]

Employment and Discrimination

There should not be any discrimination against HIV positive persons in society, including employment, services, particularly, the health. An HIV-positive person is not required to divulge their HIV status to their employer or co-workers.

HIV positive person cannot be denied employment or removed from his job unless:

- He is incapable of performing his job due to repeated ailments; or
- He poses a substantial risk to his fellow workers (MX V. ZY AIR 1997 Bom 406).

In a landmark judgment, the Supreme Court of India protected the freedom of employment and held that "government jobs or services cannot be denied to any person on the ground that he/she is infected with HIV virus".

The Constitution of India was granted the right to equality before the law **(Article 14)**. Indian Constitution has prohibition of discrimination on the grounds of religion, race, caste, sex or place of birth (**Article 15**).

If a person whose spoken or written words lead to hatred against people living with HIV/AIDS, it could invite punishments. An AIDS patient cannot be denied employment or sacked from the workplace.

Discrimination in Health Care

Discrimination may be in form of:

- Refusal to treat
- Physical isolation in wards
- Early discharge
- Delays in treatment
- Prejudicial comments and behavior.

Personal Liberty

Civil suit under the law of tort may be filled to claim compensation for violation of fundamental right to personal liberty.

The Constitution of India, under **Article 21**, has given the guarantee of the right to life and personal liberty. It is the fundamental right of HIV positive individuals to have access to adequate treatment provided by government.

Public Health Matters

- Protection of public health
- Prevention of disease
- Regulation of conduct
- Access to health care, etc.
- Establishment of infrastructure for services.

Considering the Public Health Matter

1. HIV infection is not a notifiable disease.
2. Spread of infection of diseases is an offence under **Section 269** and **270 IPC**.
   If a person **unlawfully** or **negligently** does an act to spread the infection of disease dangerous to life, he/she shall be punished with imprisonment of either description for a term, which may extend up to 6 months or with fine or with both under **Section 269 IPC**.
   If a person **wilfully** or **malignantly** does an act to spread the infection of disease dangerous to life, shall be punished with imprisonment of either description for a term, which may extend up to 2 years or with fine or with both under **Section 270 IPC**.
3. There is no provision of forceful HIV testing in India. An informed written consent is needed.
4. A doctor has an absolute duty to treat a patient to save the life of a patient (Paramanda Kataria vs Union of India, 1989). It is unethical on the doctor's part

to refuse treatment or any investigating procedures for an HIV infected person. A doctor may be held guilty of professional misconduct for this unethical behavior.[5]
5. A doctor in a public hospital is bound to treat a patient, including an HIV positive (**Article 14**).
6. The common law doctrine is applicable between the doctor and patients in relation to confidentiality (**Section 126 of the Evidence Act**).
7. The MTP Act does not indicate termination of pregnancy of an HIV positive mother.
8. If a person is infected by HIV because of any act done by a rash or negligence, it may constitute an offence under **Section 304, 336 IPC**.
9. The disposals of hospital wastages are included under **Biomedical Wastage Rules, 1998.** Under the Section 11 of the Act, the provision of an incinerator is must event for a 30 bedded hospital.
10. The **Prevention of Immoral Traffic** (PIT) Act makes a punishable offence for soliciting selling sex.
11. Oral and anal sex is considered as an offence under **Section 377 IPC**.
12. If infection results in a sexual partner and the HIV positive partner knew his HIV status before the sexual encounter occurred, he may face charges of grievous hurt under **Section 320 IPC**.
13. Divorce is granted if one partner suffers from venereal disease under the Hindu, Muslim, Christian and Parsi family laws. But it is not mentioned about the HIV infected spouse.

The civil rights of a citizen of India are protected by:
- Constitution
- Customary law
- Common law
- Statuary law and rules
- Regulations and legislation.

The Constitution of India Grants

1. The right to equality before law (**Article 14**).
2. Prohibition of discrimination on the grounds of religion, race, caste, sex or place of birth (**Article 15**).
3. Equality of opportunity in matters of public employment (**Article 16**).
4. Protection of certain rights regarding freedom of speech, etc. (**Article 19**).
5. Protection of life and personal liberty (**Article 21**) to all citizens of the country (including an individual with HIV and AIDS).

SOME LEGISLATIONS FOR CONTROL OF HIV

1. The Acquired Immunodeficiency Syndrome (AIDS) Prevention Bill No XX of 1989.
2. The Goa, Daman and Diu Public Health Act, 1985, Section 53 (i), (vii).
3. Indian Railway Act, 1989 (24 of 1989).
4. The Drugs and Cosmetic Act, 1940, amended in 1993.
5. The Delhi Artificial Insemination Act 1995.

DECLARING HIV STATUS OF POSITIVE INDIVIDUALS IN DEATH CERTIFICATE

There have been repeated queries about the disclosure of a person's HIV status by various authorities like insurance companies, the Court of Law and other Government Officers. The HIV status of an individual is secret information and cannot be publicly disclosed. However, concealing information for insurance claims, etc., can also, not be justified.

The HIV infection is usually not a direct cause of death and the death is usually due to some opportunistic infection, treatment failure and other causes. The death certificate issued by a hospital usually mentions "immediate cause of death" and "underlying disease". Hence, in the death certificate of a known case of HIV/AIDS, the doctor should mention "**Immunodeficiency**" in the "underlying cause". The same may be certified if asked by a Court of Law or an insurance company or any other Government organization (as per memorandum of NACO with the approval of the Secretary (DAC) and DG, NACO).

OFFENCES, PENALTIES AS LAID UNDER "THE DRUGS AND COSMETIC ACT, 1940"

Offence: Manufacturing for sale or selling whole human blood IP (Indian Pharmacopoeia) without a valid licence as required under clause (c) of Section 18.

Penalty: Imprisonment for a term which shall not be less than one year but may extend up to 3 years and with fine not less than 5,000 rupees, under Section 27 (b) (ii) of the act.

Offence: Manufacture for sale or selling whole human blood IP contaminated with HIV or hepatitis B virus or not sterile is an offence under the 16 (1) (a) of the Act.

Penalty: Imprisonment for a term which shall not be less than 5 years, but may extend up to a term of life and with fine which shall not be less than 5,000 rupees, under section 27 (a) of the Act.

The whole human blood IP contaminated with HIV or hepatitis B virus likely to cause death or is likely to cause such harm as should amount to grievous hurt under **Section 320 IPC**. Under **Section 304 IPC,** action can be taken against the blood bank for supplying infected blood to a person, resulting in death of the person due to HIV infection.

Offence: Manufacture of whole human blood IP for sale or selling which is not labeled in the prescribed manner is misbranded within the meaning of section 17 (b) of the Act.

Penalty: Imprisonment for a term which shall not be less than one year but may be extended to 2 years and with fine under section 27 (d) of the Act.

Offence: Manufacture of whole human blood IP for sale or selling, which is not in accordance with the conditions of a licence issued for such purposed.

Penalty: Imprisonment for a term which shall not be less than one year but which may extend to 2 years and with fine under section 27 (d) of the Act.

Notation to be used in Case Sheets

People living with HIV/AIDS (PLHIV) is preferred notation used for HIV infected cases. Case sheets should be endorsed with "PLHIV" and not with HIV positive.

AN APPROACH TO MEDICOLEGAL AUTOPSY OF HIV INFECTED CASE

In an HIV infected dead case, certain confusions arise in the mind of autopsy surgeon. They are:

1. Whether the HIV infected dead case is infective or not? Till how long the corpse remains potentially contagious?
2. What are the precautions to be taken doing the autopsy?

Explanations 1: The dead body of an HIV infected person is certainly infective. The blood and body fluids of an HIV infected case remain infective for a considerable time and the period is disputable.

Viable human immunodeficiency virus (HIV) could be isolated from blood at autopsy up to 21 hours after patient's death and viable HIV was isolated up to 14 days from spleen specimen.[6] However, HIV antibodies had been detected from postmortem vitreous humor specimens up to 34 hours.[7] For detection of HIV antibodies, serum is considered as more reliable specimen.[8]

HIV infection can be transmitted from dead body to the doctor or staff handling autopsy even up to 3 weeks at room temperature. The route of transmission remains a blood borne, i.e. through cut surfaces.

Further, cultures of blood and effusions from the refrigerated bodies have reportedly shown viable virus at nearly 17 days postmortem. Such information conveys that there was no well-defined safe period at which the virus ceases to be an infective risk.[9]

Explanations 2: The entire staff member dealing the infected body should take the precautionary measures. The staff needs to follow not only the several barrier precautionary methods, but also the instruments or mortuary table or equipment need to be disinfected in a prescribed manner after completion of examination, etc. All the autopsies need to be carried out with total universal precautions in order to curtail the infective risk.

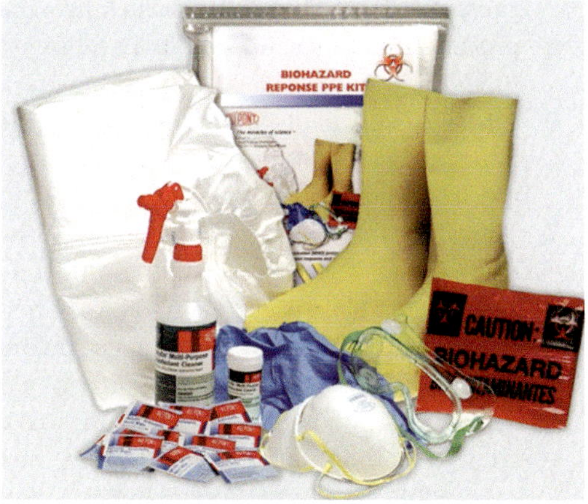

Figure 29.1 AIDS/HIV safety kit

UNIVERSAL PRECAUTIONS

1. The human immunodeficiency virus has been isolated from blood, body fluids and tissues. Hence, all the persons doing autopsies coming contact with blood, body fluids and tissues should follow universal precautions to prevent themselves from contacting the infections. Entry to the work complex should be restricted only to the trained hospital staffs. No unauthorized person should be admitted to the autopsy room to minimize the exposure.
2. The autopsy surgeon should be properly clothed with the "**AIDS/HIV suit**" before removing the body from the bag to the table and handling the case. The staffs transporting the infected body to mortuary should also wear the protective clothing or AIDS/HIV safety Kit (disposable) available in the market (**Figure 29.1**). The AIDS suit should consist at least the items mentioned in **Table 29.1**.
3. During autopsy, production of aerosol of biological material during sawing bone, etc. may pose a problem, hence a vacuum dust exhaust and filter should present by side of the table. After use, the same should be disinfected with 2% aqueous glutaraldehyde solution for 4 hours.
4. Biological samples required for further analysis should be collected in leakproof containers.
5. The body should be rolled in a plastic sheet on completion of postmortem examination and should be sealed with waterproof tape. After this, the packed body to be placed in a plastic bag for carrying for the last

Table 29.1 AIDS/HIV safety kit (Disposable)

Contents	No
Disposable head cap	1
Disposable face masks with bacterial filter and goggles	1
Proto gown/plastic apron (fluid proof) disposable surgical gown with full sleeves with elastic cuff	1
Disposable shoe covers with elastic top	2
Gloves: Disposable pre-sterilized latex gloves ISI mark (7½ and 8")	4
Disposable PVC drapes; Size: 150 cm × 140 cm	1
Disposable protective glasses, transparent glasses, zero power, adjustable holder	1
Disposable garbage bags: Black color; size: 50 cm × 30 cm	1

rites, etc. The relative should also follow the precautionary measures while handling of the body.

6. All the instruments including disposable items, etc., should be placed in puncture-proof container.
7. The reusable instruments should be placed in a 2% aqueous glutaraldehyde solution for 4 hours and then to be washed with clean water and autoclaved before further use or reusable instruments should be decontaminated by soaking in 0.5% chlorine solution for 10 minutes and then thoroughly washing and rinsing, and then either autoclaving for 20 minutes unwrapped at 15 lbs/in^2 pressure at 121°C or by soaking in 2% glutaraldehyde solution for 8–10 hours and then rinsing with boiled water and storing it dry.
8. Sodium hypochlorite solution is used to disinfect the mortuary room, including autopsy table, wall and floor, etc.
9. All the biological stuffs thus left should be disposed of as per the guidelines of **Bio-medical Wastage Rules, 1998.**
10. For handling of dead bodies certain recommendation are to be followed as mentioned in the following box:

Recommended procedures and precautions for dead bodies

- Hepatitis B vaccination is recommended for all staff who are likely to come into contact with dead bodies.
- Avoid direct contact with blood or body fluids from the body. Nursing and other personnel who handle dead bodies must wear protective clothing as mentioned above. They should cover all cuts and abrasions with waterproof bandages or dressings.
- Wound drainage and needle puncture holes should be disinfected with 0.5% Chlorine solution and dressed with impermeable material. Chlorine solution must be freshly prepared.
- Extreme caution should be exercised when removing intravenous catheters, other devices, etc., which are sharp. They should be disposed into puncture resistant containers.
- Rectal orifice should be plugged with swabs soaked in Chlorine solution while gentle suction is recommended for other body orifices, to minimize defacing of patient's general appearance.
- The body should be cleaned and dried.
- After identifying and attaching to the body the identity label, the body should preferably be placed in a robust plastic bag of not less than 150 mm thick, which should be zippered or closed tightly with tapes and bandage strips (Pins are not to be used) before being placed on mortuary trolley and transported to the mortuary.
- The outside of the plastic bag should be wiped with chlorine solution.
- Disposable items should be discarded into red plastic waste bag, which should be securely tied up and sent for disposal.
- Used linen or protective clothing should be autoclaved or soaked in chlorine solution for 30 minutes.
- Equipment should be decontaminated, cleaned and autoclaved as mentioned above.
- All surfaces should be disinfected with chlorine solution.
- After removing protective clothing and gloves, hands should be washed thoroughly.

In conclusion, it can be stated that no policy or laws can alone combat the spread up of the infection of HIV. The fear and prejudice that lies among the medical professional, needs to be tackled at the state and national level by creating a logical approach to stop the spread of infection.

REFERENCES

1. Van Wyk C. AIDS: Some medico-legal aspects. Med Law. 1991;10920:139-53.
2. NACO (2011) 'Annual Report' 2010-2011.
3. Hunter JAA. Human immunodeficiency virus infection and the human acquired immunodeficiency syndrome. In: Davidson's Principles and Practice of Medicine, 19th ed. London: Churchill Livingstone; 2002. p. 108.
4. Rajendra Babu S, Reddi JPV, Kumar JA. Mr. "X" vs. Hospital "Z" Appeal (Civil) 4641 of 1998, Date of Judgment: 10.12.2002.
5. Indian Medical Council (Professional conduct, etiquette and ethics) Regulations, 2002.
6. Karhunen PJ, Brummer-Korvenkontio H, Leinikki P, Nyberg M. Stability of human immunodeficiency virus (HIV) antibodies in postmortem samples. J Forensic Sci. 1994;39:129-35.
7. Klatt EC, Noguchi T. AIDS and infection control in forensic investigation. Am J Forensic Med Pathol. 1990;11:44-9.
8. Pepose JS, Pardo FS, Donegan E, Quinn TC. HTLV-III ELISA Testing of cadaveric sera to screen potential organ transplant donors. JAMA. 1986;256:864.
9. Krishan V. Acquired immunodeficiency syndrome: medical, social, ethical and legal implications. In: Textbook of Forensic Medicine and Toxicology: Principles and Practice, 5th ed. Haryana: Elsevier; 2011. p. 378.

CHAPTER 30

Human Rights, Custodial Torture and Deaths

Adarsh Kumar, PC Sarmah, Thejaswi HT

LEARNING PLAN

- Know about torture and different related issues
- Understand custodial death investigations: NHRC guidelines
- Know some of the statutory safeguards

"You can chain me, you can torture me, you can even destroy this body, but you will never imprison my mind" .... **Mahatma Gandhi**

> "Torture is wound in the soul so painful that sometimes you can almost touch it, but it is also so intangible that there is no way to heal it. Torture is anguish squeezing in your chest cold as ice, heavy as a stone paralyzing, as sleep and dark as the abyss. Torture is despair and fear and rage and hate. It is a desire to kill and destroy including yourself"
>
> **Adriana P Bartow**

The very name '**HUMAN RIGHTS**' signifies the basic power and privilege that naturally belongs to an individual just by the virtue of being human.[1] Human right is a form of natural rights, which are considered 'beyond the authority' of any ruler, government or international body to dismiss and 'not dependent' upon the laws, customs, or beliefs of any particular culture or government. These are indeed 'universal and inalienable,' which usually include, but not limited to right to life and liberty, freedom of thought and expression and equality before the law irrespective of nationality, race, religion, sex or any other discriminatory factors.[2,3] Even though the concept is not new, it came into wider use after World War II. This was natural as the world was coming to terms with the unprecedented unpardonable ghastly atrocities committed by Japan and Nazi Germany, which aptly can be described as crimes against humanity.[4] The first solid step was The Universal Declaration of Human Rights (1948) under the aegis of newly formed United Nations, which was perhaps the turning point in the history of humanity, as it recognized and defined human rights in its various contours on a global scale and has since been elaborated in subsequent international treaties, regional human rights declarations, national constitutions and laws. Its very preamble eloquently states that "recognition of the inherent dignity and of the equal and inalienable rights of all members of the human family is the foundation of freedom, justice and peace in the world...."[5] This was closely followed by The Geneva Convention, which extensively defined basic war-time rights of prisoners, civilians as well as military personnel, established protocols for protection for the wounded and protections for civilians in and around war zones.[6] Thus, this was the beginning of protracted and concerted efforts by the governments around the world to establish human rights as an inalienable aspect of modern governance.

Whenever a human rights issue comes up, the role of healthcare professionals takes the center stage. In the immediate aftermath of the World War II, many unethical shocking stories of human trials, mass exterminations, on the pretext of research, carried out by the Nazis were unearthed. What was more disturbing was that physicians were an intricate part of this and were even tried before the International Military Tribunal, in what is now known as Nuremberg Trials.[6] The World Medical Association took cognizance of the same and the Declaration of Helsinki was adapted in 1964, which is regarded as a foundation document of ethics on human research.[7]

Immediately after getting independence, when the constitution of India was drafted, human rights issue was well enshrined in it. The Article 21 of the constitution states, 'No person shall be deprived of his life or personal liberty except according to procedure established by law'.[8] Thus, it is a fundamental right of every citizen to enjoy basic human rights. Time and again the interpretation of this very article have been debated and the scope of its application has been constantly expanding. In the Supreme Court of India's judgment in the DK Basu Vs State of West Bengal Case, it was reiterated. It was clear that the precious right, which guarantees human rights to every citizen guaranteed by the constitution cannot be denied to convicts, under trials, detainees and other prisoners in custody, except according to the procedure established by law by placing such reasonable restrictions which are permitted by law.[9] Any form of torture or cruel, inhuman or degrading treatment would fall the breach of Article 21 of the Constitution, whether it occurs during an investigation, interrogation or otherwise. Thus, torture is considered a direct violation of the fundamental rights guaranteed by the constitution and also breach of Article 5 of the Universal Declaration of Human Right. The custodial torture by the law enforcement agencies is a serious issue as the government agencies and personnel with the sacred duty of upholding the laws of the land indulging in the gruesome abuse of their power is a serious aberration on the state. Before proceeding, let's understand different terminologies we come across while dealing with the issue.

SOME IMPORTANT TERMINOLOGIES

Custody

Literally, the word custody means the protective care or guardianship of someone or something.[10]

Arrest

Arrest means the taking, seizing or detaining of the person of another, either by touching or putting hands on him or by any act which indicates an intention to take him into custody, and subjects the person arrested to the actual control and will of the person making the arrest. In other words, it can be labeled as "to deprive a person of liberty by taking him into custody, especially under lawful authority, usually in response to a criminal charge".[11]

Police Custody

Police custody does not always means proper arrest, as it includes restriction on the movements of the person concerned.

Detention

Detention is the process when a state, government or citizen lawfully holds a person by removing their freedom of liberty at that time. This can be due to (pending) criminal charges being raised against the individual as part of a prosecution or to protect a person or property. Being detained does not always result in being taken to a particular area (generally called a detention center), either for interrogation or as punishment for a crime.[12]

Imprisonment/Incarceration

It is the detention of a person in prison, normally as punishment for a wrongdoing (custodial sentence). The purpose is to use it as a state tool for punishment and also as a means to deter general public against breaching the rule of law. During this period, prisoners are also rehabilitated.[13]

Deaths during Police Action

India is the largest democracy in the world, and time and again, we can see public demonstrations and political rallies, which are used as tools to register their grievances. Section 144 of the Criminal Procedure Code (CrPC) empowers a magistrate to prohibit an assembly of more than five people in an area. Many times, law enforcement officials are forced to use physical force in order to maintain law and order. While officers try to disperse unlawful assembly, they are used to using physical force. It might range from using non-lethal tactics like batons (lathis), water cannon, lachrymatory agents (tear gas) etc. to deadly tactics like use of firearms. Time and again, we come across fatalities, which create huge debate among the media, human rights associations and civil society regarding disproportionate use of force in order to accomplish the task. The most common causes of deaths include blunt trauma to the body by use of police batons. Constabularies also practice neck hold maneuvers as a means of subduing suspects resisting arrest or to control prisoners who are combative and unmanageable. There are two types of such maneuvers. The carotid sleeper and choke holds.[14]

a. **Carotid sleeper**: The carotid sleeper is designed to compress the common carotid arteries and produce transient cerebral ischemia. Another aspect involved is that it results in carotid sinus stimulation, which leads to bradycardia, at times, precipitating cardiac arrest. Once the person is weakened, complete recovery is expected.
b. **Choke holds**: The exercise is designed to occlude the airway by forearm compression of the front of the neck. This is similar to the earlier maneuvers, only that the pressure is directly applied to the airway. The fatal consequences of the neck holds can be due to pre-existing natural diseases, like underlying coronary artery disease, cardiac arrhythmias and atherosclerosis, which multiplies the risk. To further complicate the matter, subjects might be under the influence of alcohol, narcotic and psychotropic drugs, which increases the chances of arrhythmias.[15]

Thus, it is imperative that such deaths are transparently investigated not only to determine the cause of death, but also to instil public confidence in the institution.

TORTURE

Torture can be simply described as the act to inflict intense physical, psychological, emotional pain in order to punish, coerce or afford sadistic pleasures. According to 1984 United Nations Convention Against Torture, it is defined as "any act by which severe pain or suffering, whether physical or mental, is intentionally inflicted on a person for such purposes as obtaining from him or a third person information or a confession, punishing him for an act he or a third person has committed or is suspected of having committed, or intimidating or coercing him or a third person, or for any reason based on discrimination of any kind, when such pain or suffering is inflicted by or at the instigation of or with the consent or acquiescence of a public official or other person acting in an official capacity. It does not include pain or suffering arising only from, inherent in or incidental to, lawful sanctions".[16]

World Health Organization's working group, in the year 1986, came up with a new definition for torture as "The inter-human infliction of significant, avoidable pain and suffering by an organized group according to a declared or implied strategy and/or system of ideas and attitudes. It comprises any violent action that is unacceptable by general human standards and relates to the victims' feelings".[17] Organized violence includes "torture, cruel inhuman or degrading treatment or punishment" as in Article 5 of the United Nations Universal Declaration of Human Rights (1948). Imprisonment without trial, mock executions, hostage-taking or any other form of violent deprivation of liberty, also falls under the heading of organized violence.

Meanwhile, World Medical Association, in the year 1975, came up with the Declaration of Tokyo, which is a set of guiding principles for the practicing physicians around the world on the matters pertaining to torture, other inhuman or degrading treatment or punishment in relation to imprisonment and detention. It was unanimously agreed that doctors by getting involved with torture perpetrated by anyone by their act of commission or omission tantamount to breach of their basic ethical assurance undertaken in the Hippocratic Oath. The policy, without mincing words, directed the brethren to refuse to participate in, condone or give permission for torture, degradation or cruel treatment of prisoners or detainees.[18]

Laws against Torture

The UNDHR had a wider role to safeguard various aspects of human rights, in general, and torture. Specific International treaties were passed with the passage of time. The most important is United Nations Convention against Torture and other Cruel, Inhuman or Degrading Treatment or Punishment (United Nations Convention against Torture) in the year 1984. Some salient features of this are as follows:

i. Each State Party shall take effective legislative, administrative, judicial or other measures to prevent acts of torture in any territory under its jurisdiction.
ii. No exceptional circumstances whatsoever, whether a state of war or a threat or war, internal political instability or any other public emergency, may be invoked as a justification of torture.
iii. An order from a superior officer or a public authority may not be invoked as a justification of torture.
iv. No state party shall expel, return ("refouler") or extradite a person to another state where there are substantial grounds for believing that he would be in danger of being subjected to torture.

Interestingly, even though India has signed the treaty, it has not ratified the same till date.

History of Torture

Torture has been practiced throughout the recorded history. The Ancient Indians, Romans, Jews, Egyptians and many others cultures in history included torture as an integral part of their justice system. "Arthashastra", which is a 4th Century BC treatise by Kautilya on the art of ruling, proves the same. It recommends cutting off the right hand or nose for theft; cutting off the nose and ears for abetting in theft and adultery. There were also different forms of death penalty: death with torture for murder in a quarrel; death by impaling for theft of royal animals ....the list continues. Romans followed crucifixion, Jews practiced stoning. All these acts of torture were considered necessary (as to deter others) and good (as to punish the immoral) in order to uphold the law of the land. Also torture was deemed a legitimate means to obtain critical information about any alleged crime perpetrated by the suspects and extract confessions, etc.

Few methods of torture used to practice in ancient times worldwide are shown in **Figures 30.1** to **30.7**. (*Courtsey:* Personal visit of **Dr Adarsh Kumar** to Torture museum at Amsterdam, the Nederlands).

From the late 18th century, many European countries began to abolish torture. Napoleon Bonaparte openly discouraged use of torture to obtain information from the enemy, as he realized its ineffectiveness.

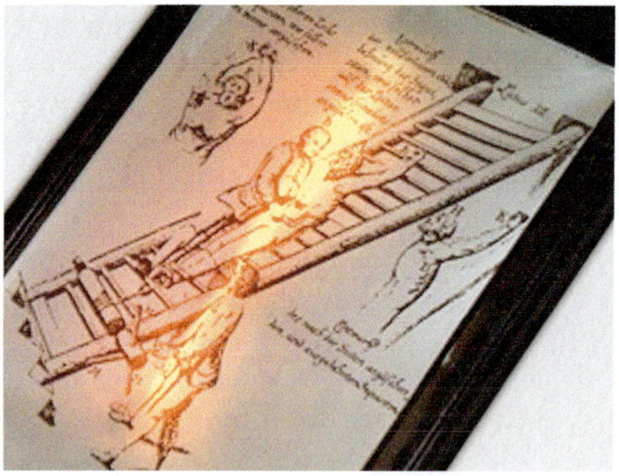

Figure 30.1 Torture methods practiced in Spain

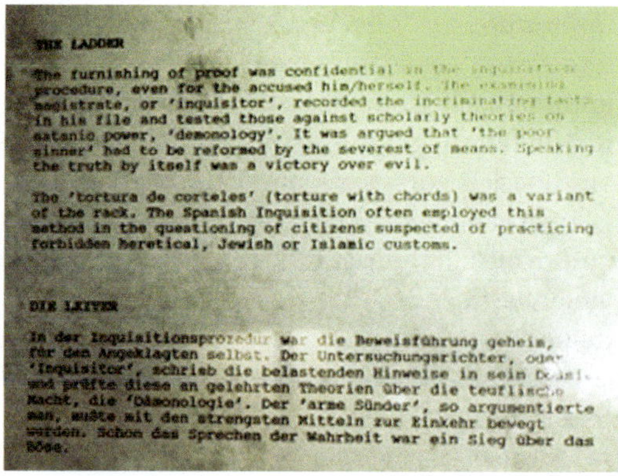

THE LADDER

The furnishing of proof was confidential in the [illegible] procedure, even for the accused him/herself. The examining magistrate, or 'inquisitor', recorded the incriminating facts in his file and tested those against scholarly theories on satanic power, 'demonology'. It was argued that 'the poor sinner' had to be reformed by the severest of means. Speaking the truth by itself was a victory over evil.

The 'tortura de corteles' (torture with chords) was a variant of the rack. The Spanish Inquisition often employed this method in the questioning of citizens suspected of practicing forbidden heretical, Jewish or Islamic customs.

DIE LEITER

In der Inquisitionsprozedur war die Beweisführung geheim, für den Angeklagten selbst. Der Untersuchungsrichter, oder 'Inquisitor', schrieb die belastenden Hinweise in sein [illegible] und prüfte diese an gelehrten Theorien über die teuflische Macht, die 'Dämonologie'. Der 'arme Sünder', so argumentierte man, mußte mit den strengsten Mitteln zur Einkehr bewegt werden. Schon das Sprechen der Wahrheit war ein Sieg über das Böse.

Figure 30.2 Torture methods practiced in Spain (written document)

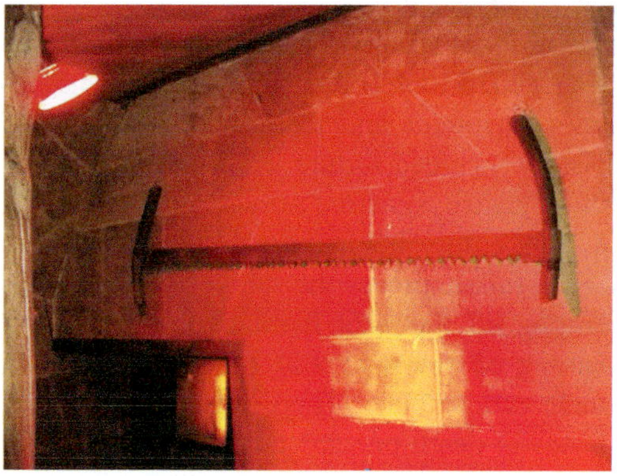

Figure 30.3 Torture methods practiced in Germany (The Saw)

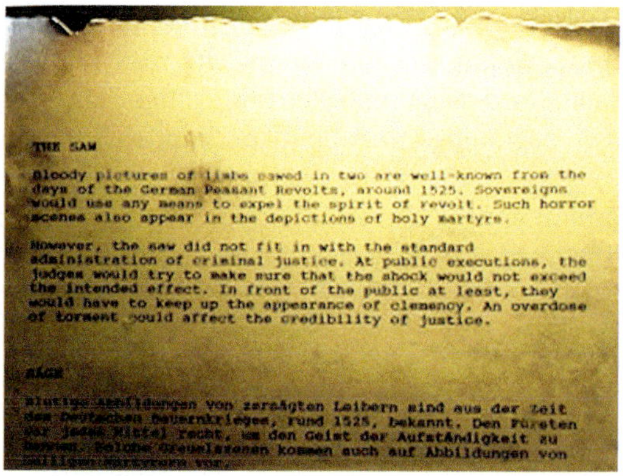

THE SAW

Bloody pictures of limbs sawed in two are well-known from the days of the German Peasant Revolts, around 1525. Sovereigns would use any means to expel the spirit of revolt. Such horror scenes also appear in the depictions of holy martyrs.

However, the saw did not fit in with the standard administration of criminal justice. At public executions, the judges would try to make sure that the shock would not exceed the intended effect. In front of the public at least, they would have to keep up the appearance of clemency. An overdose of torment would affect the credibility of justice.

SÄGE

Blutige Abbildungen von zersägten Leibern sind aus der Zeit des Deutschen Bauernkrieges, rund 1525, bekannt. Den Fürsten war jedes Mittel recht, um den Geist der Aufständigkeit zu [illegible]. Solche Greuelszenen kommen auch auf Abbildungen von heiligen Märtyrern vor.

Figure 30.4 Torture methods practiced in Germany (written document)

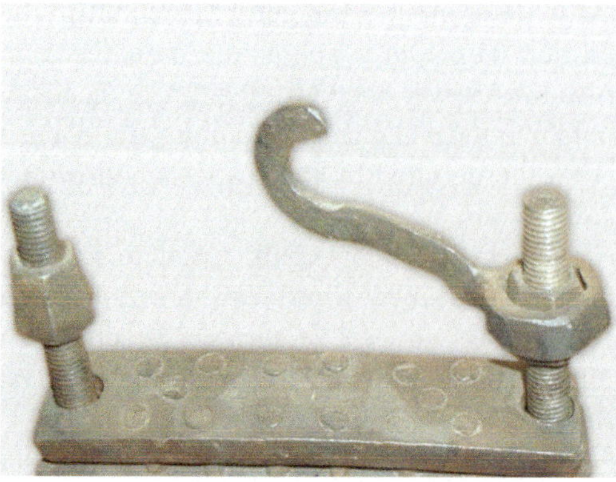

Figure 30.5 Cheapest method to extract confession practiced in Germany

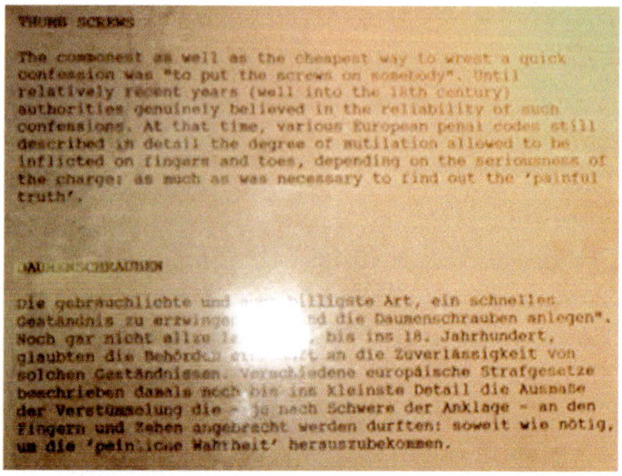

THUMB SCREWS

The commonest as well as the cheapest way to wrest a quick confession was "to put the screws on somebody". Until relatively recent years (well into the 18th century) authorities genuinely believed in the reliability of such confessions. At that time, various European penal codes still described in detail the degree of mutilation allowed to be inflicted on fingers and toes, depending on the seriousness of the charge: as much as was necessary to find out the 'painful truth'.

DAUMENSCHRAUBEN

Die gebräuchlichte und [illegible]billigste Art, ein schnelles Geständnis zu erzwingen, [illegible]nd die Daumenschrauben anlegen". Noch gar nicht allzu l[illegible], bis ins 18. Jahrhundert, glaubten die Behörden [illegible] an die Zuverlässigkeit von solchen Geständnissen. Verschiedene europäische Strafgesetze beschrieben damals noch bis ins Kleinste Detail die Ausmaße der Verstümmelung die – je nach Schwere der Anklage – an den Fingern und Zehen angebracht werden durften: soweit wie nötig, um die 'peinliche Wahrheit' herauszubekommen.

Figure 30.6 Torture methods practiced in Germany (written document)

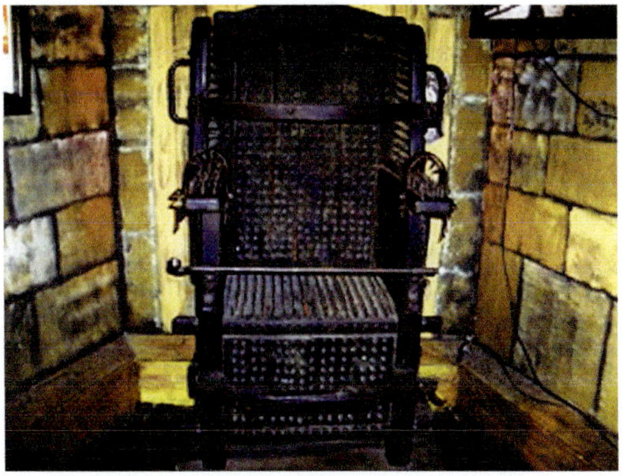

Figure 30.7 Torture Chair – probably most gruesome method

Purpose of Torture

Broadly, use of torture was justified for following reasons:

i. To solve crimes as a tool of interrogation
ii. To maintain social control
iii. To defend the ruling state from internal and external threats
iv. To force confessions
v. Ethnic cleansing
vi. Extortion.

Who are the Perpetrators?

State actors like police, prison staff, military officers, including their intelligence wing, and non-state actors like criminal syndicates, terrorists, militias and insurgents. At times, role of health professionals being passively involved cannot be ruled out.

Where it Occurs?

It occurs in the custody or control of the party not just limited to interrogation room, lockup or prison. It may be executed in unofficial 'secret' locations.

Types of Torture

Types of torture:

a. Physical torture
b. Sexual torture
c. Psychological torture
d. Pharmacological torture
e. Torture murder

Few torture methods along with its consequences are described below.

Physical Torture

The severity, extent and appearance of injuries depend on the various factors like the age of the person, sex, presence/absence of clothing, built and nourishment, presence of any pre-existing illness, type of the offending object, the force of impact, number and duration of the each session of beatings, time interval between the sessions of beatings and time interval between the torture and examination. Some of the torture maneuvers are mentioned below. These, by no means, are exhaustive but will help us gain understanding of the concept of torture investigation.

1. **Repeated Beatings**: Severe forms of blunt trauma, including beatings on the back and buttocks: It is common practice to repeatedly hit on the back of the person with sticks and lathis. On external examination, there may be presence of abrasions, contusions or lacerations. Often presence of fracture can be detected and confirmed only by radiological investigations. If the victim is alive, deep-seated contusions can be detected by MRI. However, if the victim is dead, special precautions have to be taken during autopsy, which is described later.
2. **Beatings on the Soles of the Feet (Phalanga)**: Also known as 'bastinado,' foot whipping is a process in which soles of the feet are repeatedly beaten with lathis/rods. Usually, the victim is immobilized before this act. The physical findings vary from case to case and change over time. These changes can be summarized as follows:
   Immediate Signs and Symptoms: Swelling of the foot associated with severe pain. At times, it is associated with the extravasations of blood and hematoma, leading to discoloration of foot. Fractures of tarsals, metatarsals and phalanxes

may be present and the same can be documented and confirmed by radiological investigations. Long-term complications include prolonged and continuous presence of intense pain. There will be loss of soft tissues in the heels. Because of the pain, walking is impaired. Speed and distance are dramatically reduced. Typically, the torture victim is only able to walk a limited distance, after which he will be overwhelmed by the excruciating pain which will be relieved by taking rest.

3. **Prolonged Handcuffing, Restraint and Shackling**: The true reason for subjecting the detainees to these procedures is to prevent them from escaping. But often, they have been used as a means of punishment, humiliation, coercion and to extort bribe. The Supreme Court of India in Prem Shankar Shukla vs. Delhi Administration (1980) case held that handcuffs are prima facie inhuman. The Court recognized the need to secure the prisoner from fleeing but asserted that this does not compulsorily require handcuffing and issued directives on use of handcuffs. Nonetheless, globally restraint and shackling are used on the detainees. The use of leg irons is widespread in Pakistan. The prolonged shackling and restraint was allegedly used by the US military in its Guantanamo Bay detention camp, a detainment and interrogation facility. In China, many euphemisms are given to shackling to morph the agonizing nature of the process.
4. **Positional Torture**: Many forms of positional torture are practiced around the world. Characteristically, the victim is tied in unnatural positions, which cause severe discomfort and pain. A small compact cell, dubbed as 'the refrigerator', is used to keep the victim immobile for hours or days. Depending on the type of position and the duration, injuries to soft tissues of the body may be produced, which are difficult to recognize even after radiological examination.
5. **Suspension for long Hours**: Suspension of the victim by a rope tied to the ceiling is a common form of torture that can result in immense discomfort and pain with little visible external injury. Different types include crossed suspension, butchery suspension, reverse butchery suspension, flexed forward suspension, Palestinian suspension, parrot perch suspension, etc. Depending upon the type and duration, characteristic brachial plexus injuries can lead to paralysis of the arm, involving segments of upper limbs. While conducting clinical examination of such victims, along with external examination, one has to look for any peripheral neurological deficits.
6. **Crushing Injuries**: At times, the victims are made to spread their hands on the floor only to be stamped repeatedly by the torturer with heavy leather boots, leading to fractures of the carpal, metacarpal and phalangeal bones. Another type of crushing, which was practiced in Punjab during 1980's, is called "Ghotna". The most common method is, with the victim seated or lying on the back and a Ghotna (a wooden pole used to pound spices and grains) is rolled up and down the front of the thighs with one or more individuals standing on it. Occasionally, with the victim prone, it is rolled over the hips till the calf, avoiding the bony areas. The direct effects are extensive bruising and inability to walk, and even years later, there is usually pain on walking longer distances. On examination, there may be scarring on the bony points, with noticeable tenderness on thigh muscles.
7. **Abnormal Stretching**: "Cheera", the Punjabi word for tearing, is the pet name given to this torture maneuver. The victim is seated on the floor, often with one torturer supporting him from behind and two others forcefully stretching the legs up to 180°, causing extensive hematomas in the groin region. Sometimes, the pelvic girdle is injured and, rarely, femur is fractured. At times, it is accompanied by repeated kicking of the external genitalia, adding further insult and injury. The victims usually develop long-term disability and can never walk or stand in normal way.

8. **Burning and Scalding**: Cigarette burns or burns with other instruments (branding) is also practiced around the world. If cigarette is deliberately stubbed out and held immobile on the skin, the scar is often characteristically circular, about 1 cm in diameter, with a hyper-pigmented periphery and an atrophic, hypopigmented "tissue paper" center (**Figure 30.8**). Acid burns may leave a trail, indicating the victim's posture. Scarring tends to be more elaborate, and in some cases, may lead to keloid formation. Heated metal objects often leave scars of distinctive shape of the offending object can be seen.
9. **Electric Shocks**: Electric shocks have been used commonly by torturers because they cause immense pain but seldom leave identifiable physical signs. Usually genitals and breasts are targeted and the victim is humiliated and serious bodily injury is threatened. Sometimes, an electrode is inserted in the anus, which may lead to uncontrolled urination and defecation, accompanied by terrible pain and hopelessness. Occasionally, electrodes can leave small burn injury. After sometime, it may lead to small hyperpigmented patch. On external examination, this can be inconclusive but have corroborative value.
10. **Prolonged Exposure to Hot or Cold Temperatures**: Sometimes, victims are subjected to prolonged exposure to either hot or cold temperatures. In hot climatic places like deserts, they may be tied under direct sunlight, needless to say without food or water, causing various effects like exhaustion and heat stroke. In cold places, they may be exposed to sub-zero temperatures without cloths, leading to variety of conditions like chilblains, frostbite, trench foot and, in extreme cases, hypothermic shock.

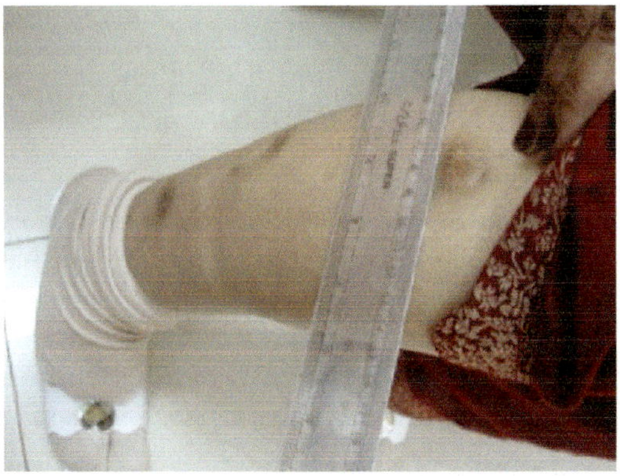

Figure 30.8 Typical appearance of cigarette burn

11. **Trauma to the Eyes**: Repeated punches to the face over the orbit can cause serious damage to the orbital complex. The spectrum of damage sustained may range from simple contusion around the periorbital region to serious injuries like retinal hemorrhage, dislocation or subluxation of ocular lens and detachment of retina. Sometimes, chilli powder or some other irritant may be smeared to the eyes. In China, police officials use 'tiger balm', a powerful analgesic ointment, causing serious damage to the eyes.
12. **Trauma to the Ears**: 'Telefono' is a slang that is used to describe hard slapping to the ear(s), usually leading to the rupture of the tympanic membrane. Sometime, it might lead to serious damage to the middle ear ossicles or even the inner ear.

Rape or Other Sexual Torture

It usually begins with forced nudity, making the victims helpless, enhancing the psychological horror of the impending torture. This is usually accompanied by verbal abuse, mock execution and threats which will only add to mental anguish. This is followed with forceful insertion of the penis into vagina, mouth or anus. Sometimes, the torturer will do this until he achieves sexual gratification. At times, it is just a symbolic ritual. There may be constant verbal threat of inflicting the victim with HIV and STDs and, in case of females, the threat of becoming pregnant adds to the anguish. In women, there may be mutilation of the breasts and genitalia, and in men, there may be hematoma in testicles due to repeated squeezing. Sometimes, a smooth lathi is lubricated with oil and smeared with chilli powder and then inserted into anus, causing unimaginable pain and suffering.

While examining such victims, a multidisciplinary team has to be constituted to look into various aspects of this atrocity.

Psychological Torture

These maneuvers, apart from causing physical pain, are intended to inflict greater psychological harm to the victim.

1. **Prolonged Sleep Deprivation**: Prolonged lack of sleep does have severe psychological consequences. Significant cognitive impairments, including deficits in memory, reasoning, learning and decision-making may happen. The UN Committee against torture has noted that sleep deprivation for prolonged duration constitutes torture.
2. **Sexual Humiliation**: Here victims may be forced to perform humiliating acts like prolonged nudity, human nude pyramid, performing sexual exercises with animals, forced sexual encounters between brother and sister, often exploiting cultural and religious sensitiveness leading to enormous shame, guilt and worthlessness.
3. **Mock Execution**: A mock/sham execution is a trick which is deliberately played by the torturer. Here the victim(s) might be blindfolded, transported to remote place, made to dig their graves, followed by holding a gun to their head and pulling the trigger, often shooting near, but not touching the victims. The psychological trauma during the act is very intense as the victim literally counts his/her last breath. This will continue in the immediate aftermath and the victim may feel that it is a planned rehearsal, and there is a real possibility of the execution in the future. This was practiced many times on the American hostages during the infamous Iran hostage crisis of 1979, where the Revolutionary Guards repeatedly subjected the hostages to a mock execution.
4. **Near Asphyxiation**: The most common way of inducing asphyxia to near-death is called 'submarino'. Here, the head is immersed in water for minutes at a time to the point of drowning, then brought out and immersed again. Sometimes the victim may be suspended head down and with the help of the rope and pulley, the same act is executed. To further cause psychological distress, the water bath might be contaminated with sewage and fecal matter. In another method, called 'dry-submarino', the head is inserted in a plastic bag and the bag is tightened in the neck, stopping the air supply to the nostrils creating near asphyxiation. Another infamous method, called "Waterboarding", has a history that dates back to the middle ages and recently practiced by the US in the aftermath of 9/11. Victims are strapped to a board or made to lie in a supine position with their heads lower than the rest of their bodies, their faces covered with cloth, and water is poured over their mouths to create the sensation of drowning.
5. **Forced Breach of Religious or Cultural Prohibitions or Taboos such as Dietary Codes**: Sometimes, orthodox Islamic victims may be forced to eat pork. Anything that will hurt the religious/cultural sentiments can be used including desecration of the holy books.
6. **Prolonged Solitary Confinement.**
7. **Sensory Bombardment**: The use of very powerful lights and loud music may lead to mental distress and disorientation.
8. **Use of Animals**: Sometimes victims might be threatened with impending attack by ferocious animals like dogs. In some parts of the world, snakes, spiders, scorpions, etc. are used to instil fear in the mind of victims.

Pharmacological Torture

Here psychotropic and/or other chemicals are used to induce pain and agony. Victim is forcibly injected with addictive drugs so much so that he becomes addicted to it only to be denied of the drug and forced to go through withdrawal symptoms. Unless they comply with the demands of torturer, drug will not be given to them. Strong acids/alkalis are used to cause burns.

Torture-Murder

It is a loosely defined term to describe a murder, where death has been preceded by the torture of the victim, involving "exceptional brutality or cruelty". Slow slicing (Lingchi) or 'death by a thousand cuts' was a form of torture and execution used in China from roughly AD 900 until it was banned in 1905. The punishment worked on three levels: as a form of public humiliation, as a slow and lingering death and as very strong public deterrent. The same was practiced in erstwhile Taliban ruled Afghanistan, where they imposed strict sharia law by their extreme interpretation of religious texts. For many crimes, the punishment was public execution, but not before gruesome inhuman torture.

Role of Medical Professionals in Tackling Torture Menace

There are many ways in which a physician can be complicit. He can be directly involved in overviewing the torture by monitoring the vital parameters of the victim. Sometimes, by using his medical knowledge, he can innovate gruesome yet relatively safe ways to torture. More commonly, they may help the torturers by declaring the victims physically fit for the torture. They can also help cover up the crime by issuing false certificate, purposefully ignoring vital signs of torture.

Ethics and Medical Profession

The fundamental idea behind medical ethics, as enumerated in Hippocratic oath, is the maxim 'Primum non nocere' (which translates to 'first do no harm'), and 'non-maleficence' is one of the principal law of medical ethics that all physicians are bound to. Thus, it is against the elementary part of medical ethics to, either by acts of omission or commission, get involved in torture. Health professions have unimpeachable role in fight against human-rights abuse. Simple documentation of suspected/confirmed torture can be a part of critical prevention and accountability measures. It is further obvious that without sound documentation of the injuries suspected to have been caused due to torture, any serious investigation at a later stage will be compromised.

Consequently, internationally accepted standard protocols for torture investigations and documentation of torture and ill-treatment were formulated. The most important of them are as follows:

1. **Model protocol for a legal investigation of extra-legal, arbitrary** and **summary executions** (**"Minnesota Protocol"**) by United Nations, in the year 1989, for dealing with the deaths due to torture/extra judicial killings.[19]
2. **Manual on effective investigation and documentation of torture and other cruel, inhuman** or **degrading treatment or punishment** (**"Istanbul Protocol"**) formulated by International Rehabilitation of Council for Torture victims in the year 1999. The UN General Assembly and UN Commission of Human Rights have given recognition to it as an important tool in fight against torture and degrading punishments.[20]

The main purposes of these protocols are to provide minimum standards for the effective documentation of torture, both in living and dead. This can be brought to the notice of various agencies that can constitute a thorough probe and perpetrators of the crime can be punished in accordance with the law. This is even more important, as the wrongdoers are usually law enforcement officials and will try hard to use every trick in the book to discredit the sanctity and validity of the medical document, thereby drastically reducing the strength of the case.

Republic of India, keeping with the letter and spirit of its commitment to the people of India and international community, passed the bench mark legislation: The **Protection of Human Rights Act, 1993 (amended in 2006)**. This act was passed for the formation of National Human Rights Commission (NHRC) and States Human Rights Commission for the better protections of human rights and all matters connected with it. Thus, NHRC, a premier autonomous institution, was created which defined the human rights as "rights relating to life, liberty, equality and dignity of individuals guaranteed by the constitution or embodied in the International covenants".

CUSTODIAL DEATH INVESTIGATIONS: NHRC GUIDELINES

1. According to 176 CrPC, magisterial inquest must be carried out on all the custodial deaths.
2. In the year 2005, it was further clarified that only in cases of suspected unnatural deaths, Judicial magistrate should investigate, and in others, executive magistrate shall conduct the inquest. This was essential because it was soon realized that majority of the custodial deaths were due to natural diseases like tuberculosis, old age and other disease conditions.
3. A model autopsy pro-forma was formulated, based on Minnesota protocol, and it was advised to conduct the postmortem examination according to it.
4. The postmortem examination should be conducted by the board of doctors and one of them preferably should be a Forensic Medicine expert.
5. Video-recording of the autopsy is mandatory. Further, in the year 2010, it was clarified that the responsibility of arranging the videography lies with the District Magistrate and not with the physicians/ hospital authorities.
6. While performing the autopsy, one must take special precautions and every attempt must be made to unearth deep-seated contusions. especially in the back of the body, including the gluteal region.
7. An incision should be made in both palms and soles to look for any deep seated collection of blood.

Note: Fourth incision, as advocated by Dr AJ Patowary, a new approach for evisceration which was primarily intended for aesthetic purpose, can also be used to detect deep seated muscular contusions.[21] Likewise, special incisions must be made to detect injuries to the soles and palms as mentioned above.

Some Statutory Safeguards

Indian Evidence Act, 1872

A confession to police officer cannot be proved as against a person accused of any offence (Section 25 Evidence Act) and confession caused by threats from a person in authority in order to avoid any evil of a temporal nature would be irrelevant in criminal proceedings as, inter-alia, provided in Section 24. Thus, even though custodial torture is not expressly prohibited by law in India, the evidence collected by illegal means, including torture, is not accepted in courts.

Code of Criminal Procedure, 1973

Sections 46 and 49 of the Code protect those under custody from torture, who are not accused of an offence punishable with death or imprisonment for life and also during escape.

Section 54 of the Code is a provision that, to a significant extent, corresponds to any infliction of custodial torture and violence. According to it, when an allegation of ill-treatment is made by a person in custody, the magistrate is then and there required to examine his body and shall place on record the result of his examination and reasons thereof.

Sections 167 and 309 of the Code have the object of bringing the accused persons before the court and so safeguard their rights and interests, as the detention is under their authorization.

Indian Police Act

Sections 7 and 29 of the Act provide for dismissal, penalty or suspension of police officers who are negligent in the discharge of their duties or unfit to perform the same. This can be seen in the light of the police officers violating various constitutional and statutory safeguards along with guidelines prescribed.

Alleged Victim of Custodial Torture: Photographic Documentation of Injuries

Figure 30.9 shows multiple pattern bruises.

Figure 30.10 shows traumatic swelling in one limb (dorsal aspect of left hand).

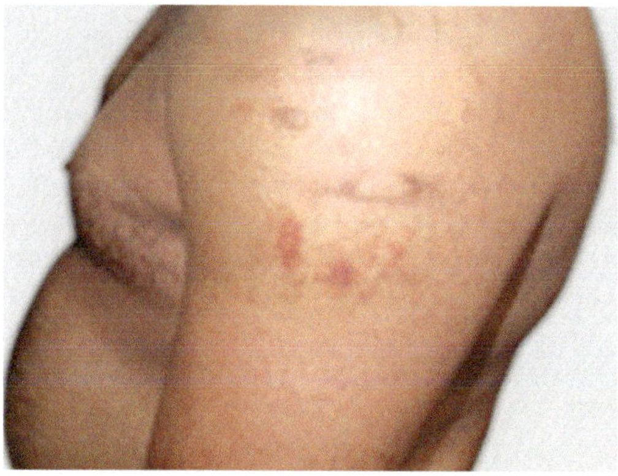

Figure 30.9 Injuries over the left arm

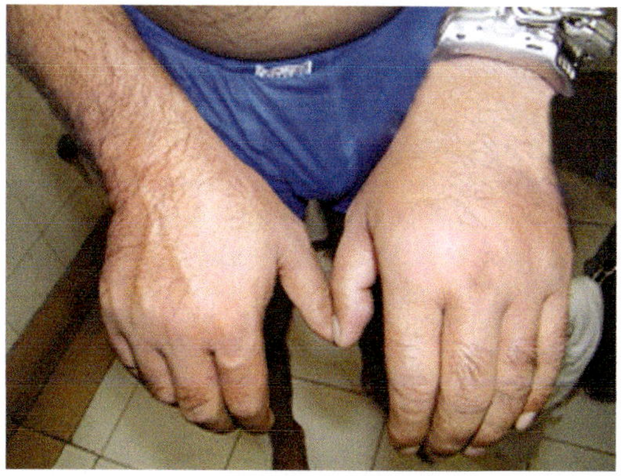

Figure 30.10 Traumatic swelling of dorsal aspect of left hand

REFERENCES

1 Gardner J. Simply in virtue of being human: the whos and whys of human rights. J Ethics Soc Philosophy. 2008;2(2):1-22.
2. Ralph M. Natural law and human rights. Am J Juris. 1991;36(1):1-14.
3. Alfredsson G, Eide A (Eds). The Universal Declaration of Human Rights. The Hague: Martinus Nijhoff Publishers; 1999.
4. Phillip A. International legal responses to the holocaust and genocide after Nuremburg. BC Third World LJ. 1988;8(47):47-63.
5. The Universal Declaration of Human Rights [Internet]. 2012, [Cited 2012 Dec 25]; Available from: URL:http://www.un.org/en/documents/udhr/
6. Lifton-Robert, Robert J. The Nazi Doctors: Medical Killing and the Psychology of Genocide. 1st ed. London: Macmillan; 1986.
7. Declaration of Helsinki: Bulletin of the World Health Organization. 2001;79(4):373-4.
8. Constitution of India [Internet]. 2012 [cited 2012 Dec 25]; Available from: URL:http://lawmin.nic.in/olwing/coi/coi-english/coi-indexenglish.htm
9. DK Basu vs. State of West Bengal. 1997 (1) SCC 416.
10. The free dictionary by Farlex [Internet]. 2012 [cited 2012 Dec 29]; Available from: URL:http://www.thefreedictionary.com/custody
11. Wikipedia contributors, "Arrest," Wikipedia, The Free Encyclopedia. [Internet] 2013 [cited 2013 Jan 12]; Available from: URL:http://en.wikipedia.org/w/index.php?title=Arrest&oldid=552824931
12. Wikipedia contributors, "Detention (imprisonment)," Wikipedia, The Free Encyclopedia. [Internet] 2013 [Cited 2013 Jan 12]; Available from: URL:http://en.wikipedia.org/w/index.php?title=Detention_(imprisonment)&oldid=549300667
13. Wikipedia contributors, "Imprisonment," Wikipedia, The Free Encyclopedia, [Internet] 2013 [Cited 2013 Jan 12]; Available from: URL:http://en.wikipedia.org/w/index.php?title=Imprisonment&oldid=544394264
14. Vanezuis P. Compressive neck injury II: Manual strangulation. In: Pathology of Neck Injury, 1st ed. London: Butterworths; 1989. p. 62-4.
15. Reay DT, Eisele JW. Death from law enforcement neck holds. Am J Forensic Med Pathol. 1982 Sep;3(3):253-8.
16. United Nations Treaty Collection [Internet]. 2013 [cited 2013 Jan 12]; Available from: URL: http://treaties.un.org/Pages/ViewDetails.aspx?src=TREATY&mtdsg_no=IV-9&chapter=4&lang=en
17. World Health Organization (WHO). The Health Hazards of Organized Violence. Report on a WHO Meeting. Veldhoven; 1986. p. 22–5.

18. WMA Declaration of Tokyo [Internet] 2013 [cited 2013 Jan 12]; Available from: URL:http://www.wma.net/en/30publications/10policies/c18/index.html
19. UN Manual [Internet]. 2013 [cited 2013 Jan 12]; Available from: URL:http://www1.umn.edu/humanrts/instree/executioninvestigation-91.html
20. Istanbul Protocol: Manual on the Effective Investigation and Documentation of Torture and Other Cruel, Inhuman or Degrading Treatment or Punishment. Geneva: United Nations Publications; 1999.
21. Patowary A. The fourth incision: a cosmetic autopsy incision technique. Am J Forensic Med Pathol. 2010;31(1):37-41.

CHAPTER 31

Techniques in Museum

Akash Deep Aggarwal, Putul Mahanta, Monika Garg

LEARNING PLAN

- Learn the functions of a well-organized museum
- Know the museum techniques
- Learn about the supplements in specimen preparation
- Understand the organization of specimens

FUNCTIONS OF A WELL-ORGANIZED MUSEUM

The making of a good museum involves meticulous planning at the time of autopsy, grossing and careful handling thereafter. "Medical museum is a library not comprised of books, but the things themselves on which books are written".

It should aim to:

i. A permanent exhibition of common conditions for undergraduate and postgraduate self-education (**Figure 31.1**).
ii. A collection of specimens illustrating rare conditions.
iii. A collection of specimens which can be used as the basis of a quiz, slide programs, medical exhibitions, examination viva-voce, lecture demonstrations, etc. (**Figure 31.2**).
iv. A permanent source of gross and histopathological material for teaching, research, etc.
v. A permanent source of photographic material, both gross and microscopic for exhibition, publications.

Even small museums, in addition to their teaching value, play a part in recording the history of medicine, since a common disease of today may well be the rarities of tomorrow. To fulfil such a purpose, it is essential that original shape and color of specimens is retained and that accurate records of patient's medical history and, if possible, relevant photographs and radiographs, are readily available (**Figure 31.3**).

It is important that a museum does not become a static, unchanging collection of plated specimens; efforts should be made to regularly update catalogue entries, incorporating clinical follow-up; any subsequent necropsy, etc. Similarly, old established specimens should be replaced by subsequent, more satisfactory material.

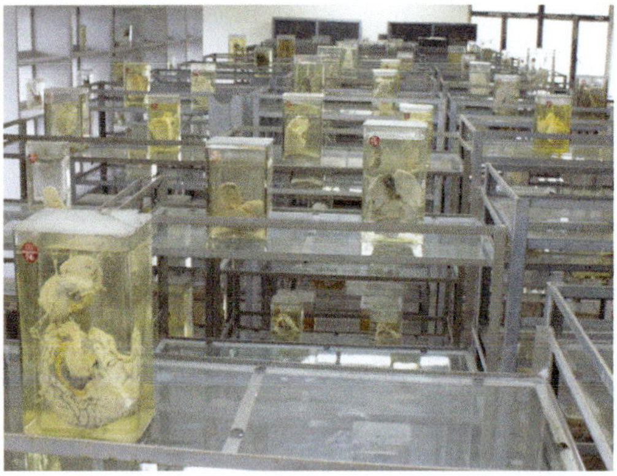

Figure 31.1 Museum showing different specimen

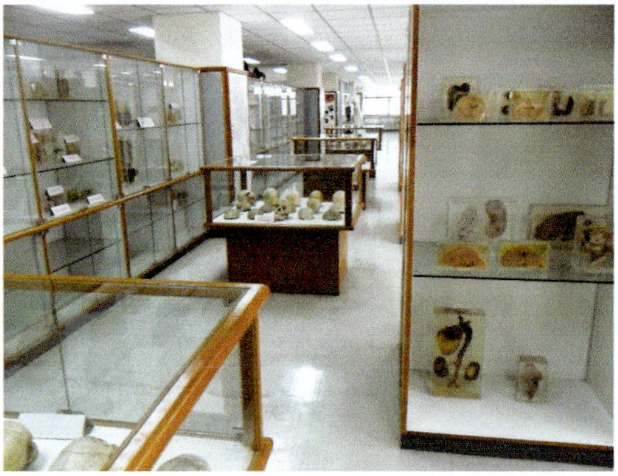

Figure 31.2 Museum showing arrangement of specimen

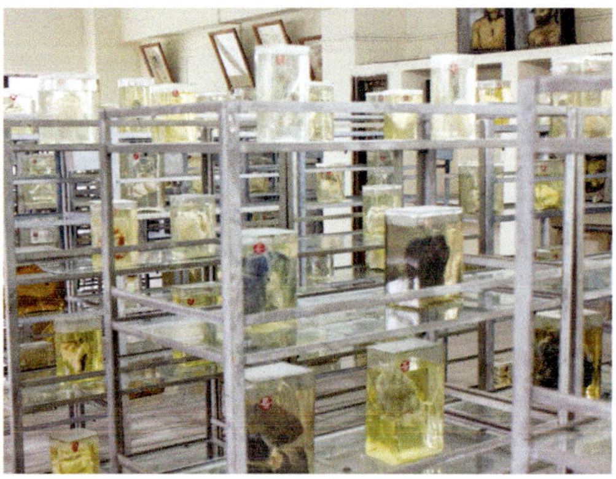

Figure 31.3 Different division of museum

BASIC MUSEUM TECHNIQUES

A specimen, dealt with to produce a permanent museum mount, undergoes the following procedure:

- Reception
- Preparation
- Fixation
- Restoration
- Preservation
- Mounting

Reception

Source of specimen for the museum are operating theaters, mortuaries or pathology grossing room. A proper record must be maintained for receiving the specimen in the reception book. It should include diagnosis, name of patient, deceased or donor, postmortem number, histological section number and institution name. On arrival each, specimen is given an excision number and this number is tied to the specimen. Liver specimens must always be stored separately.

Preparation

The best museum specimen is only possible if it arrives in a fresh unfixed condition, so that it can be dealt accordingly. Any gross trimming or dissection necessary should be carried out immediately. Cut surface of the specimen should be smooth and even; this is achieved by using a continuous stroke with a long-bladed sharp knife. The usual type of brain knife may be used, but a butcher's knife with a 14 inch blade is preferred because even large organs may be cut with one long stroke. Any blocks necessary for histological investigation are taken at this stage only. Specimen retains its natural color in unfixed stage, so it should be photographed in this stage. Each and every museum should have an attached preparation room equipped with necessary facilities, including preparation tables with running water (**Figure 31.4**).

Fixation, Restoration and Preservation

Most formalin-based fixatives turn the natural color of organs into a uniform gray-tan.

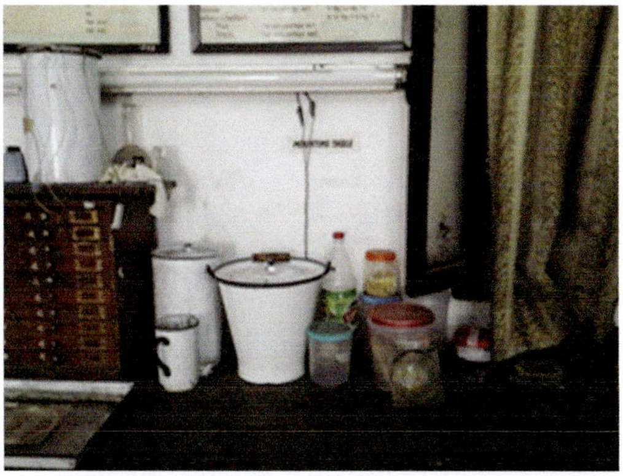

Figure 31.4 Specimen preparation table

Fortunately, there are several mixtures that had better preserve the original color of the organs. Modifications of the commonly used Kaiserling solution have been suggested by many authors.[1-8]

Kaiserling's Solution

1. **Kaiserling I** (fixing fluid): for 1-5 days, vary according to thickness of the specimen; best results are obtained by fixing in the dark.
   - 30 g potassium acetate
   - 15 g potassium nitrate
   - 200 mL formalin solution
   - 1000 mL water.
2. **Kaiserling II** (color restoring fluid): Transfer to 80% alcohol (1-6 hours), and then in 95% alcohol until the color fully returns (2-24 hours).
3. **Kaiserling III** (mountant fluid): They contain
   - 200 g potassium acetate
   - 400 mL glycerin
   - 2000 mL water.

Pulvertaft: Kaiserling Method

After K-I and K-II, for mounting the Kaiserling III fluid is used as:

- Glycerin: 300 mL
- Sodium acetate: 100 g
- Formalin: 5 mL
- Water: to make 1000 mL
- Sodium hydrosulfite: 0.4% is added immediately before sealing the jar.

Lundquist: Kaiserling Method

This method was developed to avoid the use of alcohol, which tends to stiffen and cause contraction of the specimens.

i. **Kaiserling I**: Suspend the specimen in 10-20 times its volume of fluid. Just after the fixation has been completed (avoid over fixation), wash thoroughly in running water and re-trim so that all cut surfaces are resurfaced.
   - 200 g potassium acetate
   - 45 g potassium nitrate
   - 80 g chloral hydrate
   - 444 mL formalin
   - 4000 mL tap water.

ii. **Kaiserling III**: Transfer to mounting solution for 12 hours. Replace the mounting solution for permanent mounting.
   - 10 g potassium acetate
   - 5 g chloral hydrate
   - 10 mL glycerin
   - 90 mL tap water.

Additional Points in the Fixing of Museum Specimens

i. The specimen should be placed in an adequately large container with 3–4 times its volume of fixative for a period of 3 days for a small specimen, and up to 14 days for large specimens, especially whole lung, liver and limbs.

ii. To ensure adequate fixation, specimen should always be injected with fixative if this is possible. Whole brain must be fixed in this manner by injection into the basilar artery, after first washing through with saline solution to remove the blood. After injection of the fixative, the basilar artery is tied off with a long length of linen thread; brain is then transferred to a bucket containing fixative and suspended by the thread from a glass or wooden rod laid over the top of the bucket so that the brain remains suspended in the center of the fixing fluid. Lungs, whole limbs and kidneys are more easily and speedily fixed by injection.

iii. The globe or orbital specimen is fixed in 10% formalin for 24–48 hours. After an overnight, wash in running water, eye is stored in 10% alcohol until cutting. To prevent eye collapse, some alcohol is injected into the vitreous.
iv. Specimen containing much blood should not be washed with water at any time, either before or after fixation. If excess blood has to be removed, the specimen should be washed with saline solution or formal saline.
v. Specimen should not rest on a flat surface of container. All container should be lined with fixed soaked or cotton wool.
vi. Cystic cavity, if unopened, are inflated with fixative; or if opened are packed with cotton wool soaked in fixative so as to maintain their natural shape.
vii. Bile stained or bile-containing specimens must be fixed and stored separately or they will stain other specimens.
viii. Specimen of skin or intestine should be pinned out on a lint-covered piece of cork to maintain the shape.
ix. Thymol crystals may be added to prevent mould.
x. Rejuvenator solution may be used to restore color (Pyridine 100 mL, sodium hydrosulfite 100 g, distilled water 4 liter).

Specimen Containers

1. **Glass Jars**: Thick-walled circular or rectangular glass jars epitomized the traditional organ museum. Glass is inert to fixatives and aggressive mounting fluids, such as oil of wintergreen. However, glass jars are heavy, cumbersome to transport, break easily and can cause injury. Glass jars with lids may be used for those specimens that are to remain in the museum (**Figure 31.5**).
2. **Polyethylene Terephthalate** (PET) **Bottles**: They are inert, translucent and thin; can easily be cut with scissors or a blade in order to adapt properly to the size of the jar. PET sheets can be easily cut and sutured to the specimen and does not visually hinder the display. Have good tensile strength and high degree of impact resistance.

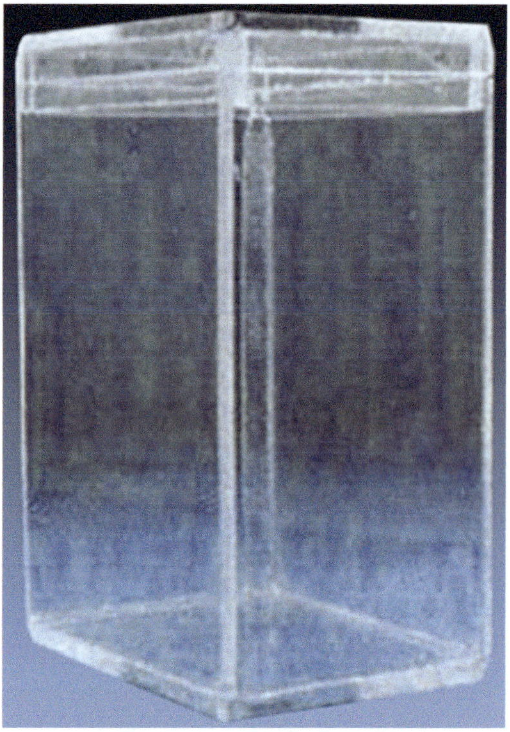

Figure 31.5 Museum glass jar

3. **Plastic Bags**: Although mounting museum specimens in plastic bags are convenient, portable and inexpensive, but specimens cannot be palpated and they may not display the abnormalities clearly as with other methods.
4. **Perspex** (Acrylic glass or Plexiglass) **Museum Jars**: It can be constructed of any size. They can be completely filled with mounting solution. A specimen can be attached to rigid supporting plates. They are light and strong. It can easily bend and can withstand heat up to 110–150°C. Surface is smooth and easily bonded using chloroform or ethylene dichloride. It is easily cut and polished. The thickness varies from 1.5, 3, 5, and 6 to 12 mm.

Construction of the Jar

Jar can be constructed by museum technician or can be obtained by manufacturing units.

The jar must be with an extra 3.75 cm in height, and 2.5 cm in width and depth of the specimen.

Mounting of the Specimen

To support the specimen in the jar, it is attached to the specimen plate which should have an extra 2 cm border at edges. The specimen is firmly held against the plate with the help of nylon thread. It is now placed in a container having K III. Any pieces of tissue floating from its surface should be removed or reattached.

To overcome this problem, immerse the specimen in 20% gelatin solution for half an hour and then suspend in refrigerator to set. All the air is expelled and allowed to stand form 24 hours. If the mounting solution is clear and no debris appears, it is ready to be sealed. It may be done by self-tapping screws, rubber stopper or polythene rod. Now the jar is thoroughly washed, dried and the accessories or reception number is written clearly (**Figure 31.6**).

Labeling of the Specimen

Since any label affixed to the outer surface of a container is exposed to the vicissitudes of handling, one must always attach a label directly to the specimen. These labels must be made of material capable of resisting the chemical action of the mounting fluid and must not unnecessarily obscure the specimen.

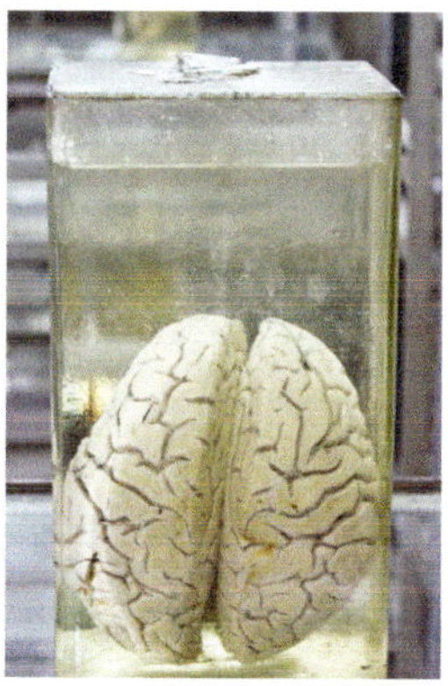

Figure 31.6 Museum glass jar showing specimen

SPECIAL MUSEUM TECHNIQUES

Gross Staining

There are number of stains used to demonstrate the presence of normal or abnormal constituents in gross specimens.

a. **Iron**: Slices of liver, pancreas, heart or other tissues are placed for several minutes in a 1–5% aqueous solution of potassium ferrocyanide and then are transferred to 2% hydrochloric acid. The specimens are then washed for 12 hours in running water. In the presence of abundant hemosiderin, the tissue will turn dark blue rapidly. Mount in 5% formalin saline.
b. **Fat**: When differential fat staining is desired, the freshly trimmed, fresh or formalin-fixed specimen is immersed in a saturated solution of Sudan III in 70% alcohol. The fat will stain bright red. Non-fatty structures are decolorized by placing the specimen in 95% alcohol. After the differentiation is complete, the tissue is washed and mounted in formalin solution.
c. **Calcium**: Immerse the specimen for 12 hours in 1:10000 solution of alizarin red S with just enough potassium hydroxide to render the solution basic. For differentiation, transfer the specimen to a solution of equal parts of alcohol and glycerin and expose the jar to sunlight. Alizarin dyes stain calcium pink. After several days, mount the specimen in Kaiserling solution that is made alkaline by adding a small amount (1:1000) of potassium hydroxide.
d. **Hematoxylin and Eosin Stains**: Tissues such as the intestinal mucosa can be stained with alcoholic eosin or hematoxylin.
e. **Myocardial Infarction**: Tetrazolium staining has emerged as the most popular method. The nitro blue tetrazolium (NBT) will not cross membranes and, therefore, can only be used with sliced tissue. The triphenyl tetrazolium chloride (TTC) will cross the cell membrane, and for that reason, it can be used to both stain slices as well as be included in the perfusate. At

the time of staining, the monobasic and dibasic sodium phosphate solutions are mixed to give a pH of 7.4 and then an equal amount of the 2% TTC solution is added. Then add few drops of N/10 NaOH solution to restore pH. On incubation at 37°C in this medium, the surviving tissue should turn a deep red (TTC) or a dark blue (NBT). Once the color has been established, fix the slice in 10% formalin for 20 minutes. The living tissue is colored and the infracted tissue is a pale tan color.

Bones

The same process of maceration is used to prepare the bones to preserve. After removing most of the adherent soft tissues as can be removed easily, the bones may be buried or put into tank of water and left for several months. Another method is by boiling in tap water or very dilute sodium hydroxide, and removing tissues at intervals. Another gross method for hard bones is autoclaving in N/10 sodium hydroxide for 5 minutes. Following removal of soft tissue, fat is removed by immersion in chloroform for 3–4 hours. Then dry and bleach in hydrogen peroxide.

Photography

It is useful to photograph the specimen, as they provide a permanent record and can be used in lectures, programs and possible publication. Photography is usually best carried out when the specimen is in its fresh state. If not possible, then it is done after treatment with K-II (80% alcohol).

Both macro and micro photographs must be a part of any museum. They should be preferable encased in perspex sheets with perspex cement avoiding air bubbles. Window mats may be used to prevent contact of photograph surface with glass or perspex sheets.

Other Techniques

These include:

a. **Paraffin embedding** using perfusion fixation with formalin alcohol solution, xylene and covering with melted paraffin.
b. **Plastination** method of Gunther von Hagen's using fixation in formalin, freeze substitution in acetone and forced impregnation of polymers, followed by curing and hardening.
c. **Injection, corrosion and clearing** technique for vessels, airways and hollow viscera using barium sulfate, resins, vinyl-acetate plastics, glycerin, contrast media and acids.
d. **Transparent specimens** of embryos, etc. (Dawson's or Spalteholz techniques), formalin fixation followed by maceration of soft tissues in 1% KOH and staining with Alcian Blue 8GX and Alizarin Red S.

Organization of Specimens

It is essential that the entire specimens are easily located and are accompanied by all the relevant information; with proper numbering, indexing and cataloguing. Museum must be well-lit, preferably with fluorescent lighting. Organized layout must incorporate display cabinets with semi-transparent displays, wall mounts, table stands and benches, etc. into various sections according to systems or chapters. Teaching displays can be in various forms like photographs, radiographs, mounted and un-mounted specimens (wet and dry), drawings, diagrams, models, charts, microscopic preparations, etc.

Arrangement: Specimen can be either classified by an anatomical system or by disease system, i.e. all tuberculosis specimens. All parasite diseases should be put together.

Numbering: Decided on anatomical division of the collection like: "**C**" for cardiovascular and "**R**" for respiratory, etc. followed by a number to indicate the main anatomical subcategories like C1 for heart, C2 for valve, C3 for arteries, C4 for vein, etc. This is then followed by a point and then the number indicating the disease process. C 1.1 for congenital heart disease, C 1.2 for inflammatory condition of heart. These numbers are then followed by the appropriate specimen especially C 1.11, C 1.12, C 1.13, e.g. for congenital heart disease.

The systematized nomenclature of pathology (SNOP) can be used in labelling with range of colors for a differential labelling system.
Red Label: Rare condition.
Yellow Label: Good examples in common condition.
Green Label: Less satisfactory example of common condition/less common condition.

Labels may be encased in Perspex sheets, fixed on cardboard sheet stands, stick-on labels on jars with cello tape covering, etc. Since any label affixed to the outer surface of a container is exposed to the vagaries of handling, we may attach a label directly to the specimen. These labels must be made of material capable of resisting the chemical action of the mounting fluid and must not unnecessarily obscure the specimen. Where specimens are used for exams, then numerical systems may be employed.

VIRTUAL MUSEUMS

Also known as an electronic museum, digital museum, hyper-museum or online museum; available either on local intranet or World Wide Web. These may include interactive environments using 3D models or virtual reality. Apart from photographs and videos, they can include power point presentations, eBooks, video slideshows, flipcharts, flashcards, glossaries, catalogues, etc.

These virtual collections are a searchable index of teaching material consisting of specimens representing the gamut of macroscopic and microscopic findings, along with descriptive case histories. These specimens offer students an opportunity to see for themselves real examples of cases, which they will otherwise see only in textbooks.

REFERENCES

1. Kaiserling C. Weitere Mittheilungen über die Herstellung möglichst naturgetreuer Sammlungspräparate. Archiv F Pathol Anat. 1897;147(3):389-417.
2. Whitney WF. Kaiserling's method for the preservation of specimens with their natural colors. J Boston Soc Med Sci. 1897;1(10):14.
3. Hall IW, Herxheimer G. Fixation—hardening: Preservation of macroscopical specimens. In: Methods of Morbid Histology and Clinical Pathology. London: William Green; 1905. p. 28.
4. Lundquist R, Robertson HE. Proposed modification of the Kaiserling method for preservation of specimens for display purposes. J Clin Lab Med. 1924;10:665-7.
5. Pulvertaft RJV. Museum techniques: a review. J Clin Pathol. 1950;3(1):1-23.
6. Culling CFA. Museum technique. In: Handbook of Histopathological Techniques: (including museum technique), 2nd ed. Washington: Butterworths; 1963. pp. 417-49.
7. Waters BL (Ed). Museum Techniques: Handbook of Autopsy Practice. 4th ed. Totowa, NJ: Humana Press; 2009. pp. 131–6.
8. Natarajan S, Boaz K, Ranjan J. Museum mounting techniques: Revisited econo-mode. Indian J Pathol Microbiol. 2012;55(2):260.

CHAPTER 32

Forensic Science Laboratory

Yogender Malik, Pooja Malik Puri, Pushpendra Malik

LEARNING PLAN

- Know the historical development of forensic science in India
- Common types of physical exhibits encountered in the field of forensic science laboratory (FSL)
- The organizational set up of FSL
- A brief account of some of the tools and techniques used in FSL

FORENSIC SCIENCE IN INDIA

The term "**Forensic Science**" is really an umbrella description relating to the practice of any science within a legal context.[1] But, nowadays, its scope has widened and regulatory authorities take its help for variety of reasons like pollution monitoring and control, to save endangered species, etc. Forensic Science is not new to our country. Some references related to code of law, fraud detection and prevention, secret and occult practices, etc. are found in the famous book "Arthashastra" by Kautilya, which was written about 2000 years ago.

The Chronological Order of Few Events Related to Forensic Science in India is as below[2] (Table 32.1)

Three central laboratories working under the aegis of Directorate of Forensic Science Services, Ministry of Home Affairs, and Government of India are:

CFSL, Hyderabad: Center of Excellence in Chemical Sciences

CFSL, Chandigarh: Center of Excellence in Biological Sciences

CFSL, Calcutta: Center of Excellence in Physical Sciences

The Central Forensic Science Laboratory, New Delhi, is under the direct control of Central Bureau of Investigation. In the year 2012, three new Central Forensic Science Laboratories (CFSL) have been established at Bhopal, Pune and Guwahati.[3]

FORENSIC SCIENCE LABORATORY

Forensic laboratories basically deal with the analysis of physical exhibits recovered from the

Table 32.1 Chronological order of few events related to forensic science in India

1849	The first Chemical examiner's laboratory was established at Chennai, then Madras Presidency, under the department of health followed by similar laboratories at Calcutta (1853), Agra (1864) and Bombay (1870)
1892	Anthropometric Bureau (adapting Bertillon's System) was established at Calcutta
1897	Indian Police officers, Khan Bahadur Aziz-ul Haq and Rai Bahadur Hem Chandra, evolved the Fingerprint Classification System and the first fingerprint bureau of world was established in Calcutta
1898	The first department of explosives was established in Nagpur
1904	The Government Handwriting Expert was appointed with his office in Bengal
1905	First Central Fingerprint Bureau (CFPB) was established at Shimla.
1906	The Government Handwriting Expert redesignated as Government Examiner of Questioned Documents (GEQD) with the office shifted to Shimla
1910	The Imperial Serologist to Govt. of India was appointed in Calcutta
1915	The footprint section was established under CID, Govt of Bengal
1917	Note forgery section was established under CID, Govt of Bengal
1922	Central Fingerprint Bureau was abolished
1930	Ballistic laboratory was established at Calcutta
1935	Forensic Science Laboratory was established at Lahore
1952	The first State Forensic Science Laboratory was first established in Calcutta Medical College by Govt. of West Bengal
1955	Central Fingerprint Bureau was restarted under Intelligence Bureau
1957	First Central Forensic Science Laboratory was established at Calcutta in Independent India
1961	Forensic Science Laboratory (Lahore) was shifted to Chandigarh and renamed as Central Forensic Science Laboratory in 1978
1965	The Central Forensic Science Laboratory was established at Hyderabad
1986	The administrative control of CFPB was shifted to National Crime Record Bureau, Delhi
1998	DNA Typing was started at Calcutta.

scene of crime, victims and the suspects. These are the most valuable evidences to prove the circumstances of crime.

In India, the Government operates the Forensic Science Laboratories in the various regions of the country, although few private laboratories have also developed in the due course of time. There is a state Forensic Science Laboratory (FSL) in every state with few exceptions.

Common Types of Physical Exhibits Encountered in FSL

Body Fluids: Mainly include blood, semen, vaginal secretion, saliva, menstrual exudates, urine, sweat and feces in liquid or dry form. These are recovered from the body of the victim, accused or from the scene of crime, weapon of offence, incriminating locations, etc. in cases of assault, murder or rape.

Body Tissues: Include various visceral organ samples that are collected at the time of autopsy along with the blood, urine and stomach contents for toxicological analysis. Toxicological analyses of poisoning cases constitute the major bulk of workload in Forensic Science laboratories. The test for quantitative as well as qualitative detection of a particular poison or its group is usually undertaken in the laboratory. Nowadays, so many varieties of poisons are being used for cattle poisoning or for procuring stupefaction or for some other criminal motive. Well-equipped Forensic Science Laboratories with modern scientific gadgets will not find toxicological analysis to be very difficult job.

Drugs: Include the controlled substances, plant materials, powders, tablets, capsules or other preparations and paraphernalia for identification. Some of the common examples include: morphine, codeine, diacetyl morphine (heroin), *charas*, *hashish*, *ganja*, etc.

Fibers: Fibers of vegetable, animal, synthetic or other origin recovered from the scene of crime; blood stained clothings of the victim or that of the assailant may show corroboration of the said fibers, which will be helpful in cases of recovery of fibers of garment from clothings worn by the accused.

Fingerprints: Fingerprints are unique and permanent and can be encountered in wide variety of crime like theft, murders and sexual assaults as the suspect must have touched some of the objects at the scene of the crime. The fingerprints on the scene of crime can be visible or latent. The prints have to be lifted from various surfaces for identification and comparison with the fingerprints taken from the suspect.

Explosive Materials: In the recent past, because of militant/terrorists upsurges, political upheaval, communal violence, subversion and sabotage by foreign infiltrators in different parts of India, various types of sophisticated firearms, implements and gadgets are being used indiscriminately, using explosives of great detonating, destructive and devastative properties because of their constituents like RDX, etc.

Bomb squad of Forensic Science laboratories, with help of Bomb-hut, if present, will have to handle and tackle such explosives, to take note of their fire/destruction power and to undertake other tests, etc., for future reference in courts of Law.

Firearms and Projectiles: A bullet recovered from a dead body or scene of crime has immense medicolegal significance, like that of a finger printing in the sense that the primary markings and secondary markings are specific for the particular firearm. By test firing, comparing these markings over the crime bullet under a comparison microscope will help to identify the alleged weapon of offence.

Glass: In hit and run cases, the broken fragments of glasses from the head lamp, wind-screen, etc. recovered from the scene of crime or in the body of the offending car that caused the accident, will have to be examined as to their refractive index, specific gravity, chemical composition, so as to be subjected to spectroscopic and UV light examination tests to ascertain the source of the glass, thus connecting the accident with the vehicle in question.

Hair Specimens: These are collected from the body of the victim or/and the accused or nearby locations in the scene of crime need be examined in the laboratory to identify its source, if human or animal part of the body it has come from, it is approximate. Age, sex, how it was separated from the body, any evidence of dying drug intake or disease, etc. Blood-stained hair sticking to mudguard/body, etc., of hit and run car, in cases of traffic accidents or pubic hairs of the victim or assailant found sticking in the genitals of the opposite sex in cases of sex assaults or presence of animal hairs around the genitals of the accused suggesting bestiality, etc., are the important medicolegal cases that are investigated in Forensic Science laboratories.

Tool Marks and Tyre Marks: The tool marks are the negative impressions produced on surfaces by the objects such as a pry bar or screw driver, may possess wear features that can provide unique characteristics for comparison with the impression. The tools marks like the fingerprints and footwear marks are unique and provide a link between crime scene and the criminal.

The tyre marks left at the scene of motor accident can be compared with the test mark caused by the tyre of the alleged car of offence. The tyre marks can also give a clue to the possible make of the vehicles.

Questioned Documents: They are the physical exhibits that may consist of handwritten, typed, photocopied or printed material that are examined for evidence of forgery. This may include the letters, suicide notes, forged wills, cheques, records, tickets, etc. Not only the forged documents but the counterfeit currency also forms important physical exhibit in these cases.

THE ORGANIZATIONAL SET UP OF FORENSIC SCIENCE LABORATORY

The organizational set up in a FSL varies in size as well as capabilities throughout the world. The forensic laboratory offers multidisciplinary services and is usually divided into divisions based on the types of physical exhibits examined. FSL, generally, has divisions as shown in **Table 32.2**. Out of these a medicolegalist is concerned mainly with toxicology, serology, biology, ballistics and explosive division.

A BRIEF ACCOUNT OF SOME OF THE TOOLS AND TECHNIQUES USED IN FSL

In forensic cases, the physical exhibits are often encountered in minute quantities or traces: like there may be a chip of the paint, small strand of hair, and smear of ink or a drop of blood. Similarly the exhibits submitted for the examination may be in their pure form or may be adulterated. Thus, the forensic examiners have no control over the quantity and the quality of the physical exhibit submitted for the analysis. So, techniques used

Table 32.2 Organizational set up of FSL

Division	Types of exhibit analyzed	Examples of related crimes
Biology	Blood, semen, saliva, other body fluids, bones, teeth, hair, fibbers, diatoms, maggots and insects, botanical evidences like: leaves, wood, seed, etc.	Murder, suicide, rape and drowning
Toxicology	Viscera for detection poisonous substances, drugs, intoxicating substances, fumigants, insecticides and pesticides	Suicide, murder and accident cases
Chemistry	Chemical analysis of poisons, alcohol, unknown drugs, arson and fire residues and petroleum products like adulterated petrol, lubricating oil, etc.	Adulteration, dowry death cases, accidents, arson and burning cases, etc.
Serology	Blood, semen, saliva, other body fluids	Rape, murder, assault, paternity disputes
DNA profiling	Blood, semen, saliva, other body fluids	Rape, murder, assault, paternity disputes
Voice analysis	Recorded tapes	Extortion, drug smuggling, wagering-gambling investigations, money-laundering, tax evasion, threats, terrorist activities, organized crime activities, etc.
Cyber/ Computer	Computers hard disc, mobile phones	Data acquisition and storage, stealthy access to systems, identity collection and theft, misdirection of communications
Physics	Paint chips, glass pieces, erased numbers on vehicles and other valuable gadgets, tool marks	Cheating, burglary, accident, murder, hit and run cases
Ballistics	Firearms, cartridge cases, bullets, pellets/wads, clothes, etc.	Murder, suicide, accidental firing, etc.
Explosive	Post-blast residues and explosive material	Explosive cases
Fingerprints	Fingerprints lifted from the scene of crime	Theft, burglary, murder, etc.
Questioned document	Hand writings, typewritten and printed matter which includes suicide notes, threat letters, cheques, wills and counterfeit currency	Cheating, forgery, suicide, scams and frauds, etc.
Lie detection (polygraphy unit)	Suspects, victims or witnesses	Theft, dacoity, rape, murder and other white collar crimes

in the forensic analysis should be rapid (give the results quickly), sensitive (require the very small quantity of sample) and specific (identify the sample positively).[4]

Photography

Photography is the primary tool used in forensic science. It is helpful in recording the scene of crime and related areas along with sketches. Photographs are the permanent visual record of the scene, which can be later used in court trials and hearings.

The photographs must be able to produce detailed recordings of all the available evidence at the scene, including overview photographs as well as accurate images of tire marks, fingerprints, footprints, blood spatters, bullet holes and other unique evidence at the scene. Apart from this, from a medicolegalist point of view, the photographs must also be able to demonstrate the location and the type of injuries sustained through accidents or assaults and photographs of dead bodies for the purpose of identification must be recorded.

Some special techniques such as microphotography, florescence, ultraviolet and infrared photography are being used in forensic photography and are extremely helpful in cases like old injuries, bite marks, detection of latent blood stains, metal traces, certain body fluids like semen and saliva, etc.[5]

Microscopy

A microscope is the instrument that is used to produce the highly magnified image of an object that cannot be otherwise seen with the unaided eye. As mentioned before, the forensic exhibits are often encountered in trace quantities, and it is often difficult to detect them. But the microscopic examination of exhibits can provide information about the type, probable source and also the composition of the exhibit under question. The microscopic examination is the simplest, quickest and least destructive method of the physical exhibit examination. The side by side microscopic comparison of the physical exhibits (mainly the bullets, cartridge case, fibers, tool marks, etc.) is usually most discriminating means of determining the source, i.e. whether the two exhibits originated from the same source or not.

The technique of forensic microscopy can be applied to almost any type of exhibit like: hair, fibers, glass, paint chips, bullets and cartridge cases, blood, semen, pollens, seeds, leaves, diatoms, teeth and bones, tool marks, fingerprints, gunshot residues, soil, etc.[6]

Chromatography

It is basically used to separate a mixture into its components based on their attraction to stationary liquid or solid. The most common type of chromatography used in Forensic Science is gas chromatography. The gas chromatography is a method for separating the components of a solution and measuring their relative quantities. It is a useful technique for chemicals that do not decompose at high temperatures and when a very small quantity of sample (micrograms) is available. In gas chromatography, a sample is rapidly heated and vaporized at the injection port. The sample is transported through the column by a mobile phase consisting of an inert gas usually helium, nitrogen or hydrogen.[7]

Sample components are separated based on their boiling points and relative affinity for the stationary phase, which is most often a viscous liquid (wax) within the column. The higher a component's affinity for the stationary phase, the slower it comes off the column. The components are then detected and represented as peaks on a chromatogram. The term gas-solid chromatography (GCS) and gas-liquid chromatography (GLS) refers to the nature of the stationary phase which is either a solid alone (GSC) or a liquid distributed on the surface of a solid (GLC).[8]

Electrophoresis

As the name indicates, electrophoresis is used to study the properties of charged particles and also as a separating technique. As an analytical tool, it is simple, rapid and highly sensitive.

Electrophoresis, which simply means to move particles through a liquid or gel by electromotive force, allows for proteins and nucleic acids to migrate in response to an electric field. Their rate of migration depends on the strength of the electric field, their net charge, the size and shape of the molecules, temperature of the medium in which the molecules are moving and the ionic strength of the buffer used.

Most electrophoresis is done in the presence of stationary matrices.[9] Polyacrylamide and agarose are commonly used. The pores of polyacrylamide gels are appropriate for separating proteins and small nucleic acids. Agarose gels are appropriate for separating DNA, RNA and large proteins.

Spectrophotometry and Colorimetry

Spectrophotometry and colorimetry are based on the absorption of light by a matter. The basic difference between the two is the type of light used. In spectrophotometry, monochromatic light is used, while in colorimetry, polychromatic light is used. Whenever a light falls on the colored solution, some portion of it is partly absorbed (I_0) and some passes through. The intensity of incident light (I) is decreased due to the absorption. The ratio I/I_0 are called transmittance T. Colorimetry and spectrophotometry in visible (VIS) or ultraviolet (UV) region are very useful method in forensic analysis. Any measurement is performed at a given wavelength. The Beer Lambert Law defines the basic relationship between the absorbance, the thickness of sample through which the light passes and the concentration.[10]

Neutron Activation Analysis

Neutron activation analysis (NAA) is a non-destructive, highly precise and accurate analytical technique capable of determining many elements (e.g. Al, Au, Ag, As, Ba, Ca, Cd, Co, Cs, Cu, Fe,, Hg, K, Mg, Mo, Na, Ni, Rb, Sc, Se, Sn, Sr, Ti, U, V, W, Zn, Zr,, Ce, Nd, Eu, Gd, Tb, Dy, Ho, Tm, Yb, etc.) in almost all types of forensic samples. It has very low detection limits.[11] It involves irradiating the unknown samples and reference materials with neutrons in the nuclear reactor to produce unstable radioactive nuclides. Many of these radionuclides emit gamma-rays with characteristic energies that can be measured utilizing specific detectors. The rate at which the gamma-rays are emitted from an element in the sample is directly proportional to its concentration. Samples, as small as 1 mg, can be quantitatively measured by NAA. Detection limits are in the parts per million to parts per billion range, depending on the element and sample type.

Narco Analysis

The term "Narco-analysis" has been derived from the Greek word "nark", which means the anesthesia. Narco-analysis is used as tool for criminal investigation in which the subject is induced with drugs like sodium pentothal to make him fall in a hypnotic state so as to make him reveal some information which may be reluctant to reveal while in conscious state. The drug depresses the central nervous system of the body. It is believed that in such a trance-like situation, the individual cannot speak anything but the truth. The statements given by the subject recorded on a video cassette. In India, the first narco-analysis was done in the FSL, Bangalore, in 2001, on an individual associated with offences committed by Veerappan, the famous Indian dacoit.[12]

Brain Mapping

Also called as Brain Fingerprinting, it is a technique in which certain words or pictures are presented before a subject onto a computer screen and then on the recognition of familiar stimuli, brain activity in the form of brain waves is recorded. It is a known fact that brain is central to all human activities. It plans, executes and records all the functions. So, if the subject has any information related to crime, it will be recorded in the brain. Brain fingerprinting is based on a specific measurable response known as P300, which is emitted by the brain of a subject who has relevant information stored in the brain. The concept was given by Dr Lawrence Farwell in 1992, and it utilizes a technology called as MERMER (Memory and Encoding Related Multifaceted Electroencephalographic Response).[13]

The technique can be applied only in situations where investigators have a sufficient amount of specific information about an event or activity. These technologies provide the 99.9% accurate result towards crime victims, falsely accused innocent suspects.[14]

Polygraph (Lie Detector)

It is a continuous graphic record of blood pressure, pulse, respiratory rate, heart rate, sweatiness of fingertips, i.e. electrodermal reaction changes or galvanic skin resistance and movements of arms and legs. Out of this, respiratory rate and galvanic skin resistance are more dependable. Examiner is called psychophysiologist. This instrument does not, as the nick name suggest, detect lies. This can only detect whether deceptive behavior is being displayed.

Mechanism: Fear produces sympathetic stimulation which produces rise in BP; slow-down of breathing and suppression and relative change in skin resistance.

Types: Keeler polygraph (in 1930, Leonard Keeler developed modern polygraph) and Stoelting deceptograph.

Uses:

i. Criminal investigations
ii. Before being hired for a job.

Attachments: For respiratory rate, two pneumographs (tubes) are applied on chest and abdomen.

Galvanometer which measures skin ability to conduct electricity is applied on two finger-tips.

Procedure: Uncomfortable experience of polygraph test is referred to as "going on the box". Only two people should be there in the room while examining. Examinee sits on chair facing the instrument and the examiner facing him.

Pre-test Interview

It takes about 1 hour. It is an interview between the examiner and the examinee. This is done with mutual consent of subjects and examiners satisfaction. Basic explanation of attachment is given to the subject. Test questions are formed in yes/no type.

Design Questions: These are specific to issue under investigation and are reviewed with examinee

i. Three categories of questions
ii. **Irrelevant questions**: These have no bearing with incidence of offence.
iii. **Relevant questions**: There are the questions which directly implicate him with commission of the offense or having knowledge about some aspect of offense.
iv. **Control question**: These are generalized in nature and relate to bad acts he might have committed sometimes early in life and should not have forgotten. Control questions are asked for proper understanding and interpretation of graphic curve imprinted with answered and mental reaction of subject to relevant question.

Sequence: Irrelevant question → relevant questions → irrelevant question → control question.

In Test

A total of 10–11 questions of yes/no type, which are clearly understood by the subject, are asked. There are only 3–4 questions relevant to the issue or crime. All other are control questions. A question is asked every 20–25 seconds and polygraph chart recorded in 3–4 minutes. The test is repeated 2–3 times to check possible errors.

Response Recording

Response is recorded on single paper and difficult adverse responses, intensity of responses and time and extent of exciting reaction are noted.

Subjects Unsuitable

Subjects with psychotic personality, over-reactive personality, drug addicts and persons who are deceptive by nature, restless and non-cooperative are unsuitable for this test. They require special preparation and need time to be fit for test.[15]

Gradwohl's borderline IQ or below mental age 11 cannot be vividly examined (Abraham and Weinstein, 1974).

How to Trick the Device?

The device can be tricked by consuming sedatives, applying antiperspirant on fingertips, putting tacks placed in shows and biting tongue, lip or cheek during examination.

Illustration

Gay Ridgway, "**The Green River Killer**", was given polygraph test which he deceived. He was let go and eventually killed 48 women before he was finally prosecuted.

Legal Value of NARCO Analysis, Brain Mapping and Polygraph Examination

The Supreme Court of India has questioned the value of brain mapping (detects suspect's familiarity with information by measuring brain activity triggered by exposure to words, sounds and images), narco-analysis (the intravenous administration of hypnotic medication which induces the subject to talk freely) and polygraph examination (lie-detector testing).[16]

DNA Profiling

Please refer to Chapter 8 for details.

REFERENCES

1. Wyatt J, Squires T, Norfolk G, James JP. Oxford Handbook of Forensic Medicine. New York: Oxford University Press; 2011. p. 496.
2. Nanda BB, Tiwari RK. Forensic Science in India: A Vision for Twenty First Century. New Delhi: Select Publishers; 2001. pp. 29-39.
3. [cited 2013 March 10]; Available from: URL:http://www.dfs.nic.in/dfss_jurisdication
4. Sharma BR. Forensic Science in Criminal Investigation and Trials, 4th ed. New Delhi: Universal Law Publishing Company; 2012. pp. 21-9.
5. Williams R, Williams G. Ultraviolet, Infrared, Florescence Photography. [cited 2013 March 18]. Available from: URL:http://www.forensictv.net/Downloads/digital_imaging_and_photography/uv_ir_and_fluorescence_photography_by_profs_robin_and_gigi_williams.pdf
6. Wheeler BP, Wilson LJ. Practical Forensic Microscopy: A Laboratory Manual, England. John Wiley and Sons Inc. 2008.
7. Fowlis IA. Gas Chromatography Analytical Chemistry by Open Learning, 2nd ed. Chichester, John Wiley and Sons Inc; 1995.
8. Gowenlock AH. Varley's Practical Clinical Biochemistry, 6th ed. CBS. 2002. p. 49.
9. Encyclopedia of Physical Science and Technology, 3rd ed. [cited 2013 March 10]. Available from: URL:http://dx.doi.org/10.1016/B0-12-227410-5/00218-0
10. [cited 2013 march 10]; Available from: URL:http://www.lfhk.cuni.cz/chemie/documents/dentistry/zs/zs06.do
11. [cited 2013 march 10]; Available from: URL:http://www.pub.iaea.org/MTCD/publications/PDF/te_1215_prn.pdf

12. Panda B. Narco-Analysis and its Evidentiary Value in India. [cited 2013 March 18]; Available from: URL:http://www.supremecourtcases.com/index2.php?option=com_content&itemid=5&do_pdf=1&id=21437
13. Farwell LA. Brain fingerprinting: A comprehensive tutorial review of detection of concealed information with event-related brain potentials. Cognit Neurodyn. 2012;6:115-54.
14. Jain DC, Pawar VP. The brain fingerprinting through digital electroencephalography signal technique. Int J Comput Sci Eng. 2011;3(3):1085-90.
15. Nandy A. Principles of Forensic Medicine including Toxicology, 3rd ed. Kolkata: New Central Book Agency (p) Ltd; 2010. p. 324.
16. Selvi and others vs. State of Karnataka and another (May 5, 2010)

section 2

TOXICOLOGY

Section Outline

- General Consideration of Toxicology
- Medicolegal Aspect of Toxicology
- Corrosive Poisons
- Inorganic Irritants: Non-metallic Poisons
- Inorganic Irritants: Metallic Poisons
- Organic Irritants of Plants and Vegetables Origin
- Organic Irritants of Animal Origin
- Mechanical Irritants
- Somniferous Poisons
- Alcohol and Alcoholism
- Agricultural Poisons
- Cardiac Poisons
- Deliriants and Psychotropic Poisons
- Spinal Poisons
- Peripheral Nerve Poison
- Asphyxiants (Toxic Gases)
- Paracetamol and Salicylates
- Food Poisoning
- Substance Abuse
- Weapons of Mass Destruction

CHAPTER 33

General Consideration of Toxicology

AJ Patowary, Putul Mahanta

LEARNING PLAN

- Learn what toxicology and poison is
- Know the nature, action, fate and diagnosis of poison
- Learn the factors modifying action of poison
- Classification of poison
- Know the general lines of treatment

WHAT IS TOXICOLOGY?

Toxicology is a branch of medical science that deals with the study of symptoms, mechanisms, treatments and detection of poison, especially in the poisoning cases. The Greek word "**toxicos**" means poisonous and "**logos**" means "the study of" or "**the science of**". Combining these two Greek words, we get the word toxicology.

Toxicology can also be defined as the branch of medical science dealing with properties, actions, toxicity, fatal dose, detection, estimation and treatment of poisons. Shortly, it the science that studies poisons in all its aspects. It has many categories as follows:

- Forensic Toxicology
- Clinical Toxicology
- Industrial Toxicology
- Environmental Toxicology.

Forensic toxicology deals with the medical and legal aspects of the harmful effects of chemicals on human beings.

DEFINITION OF POISON

A Poison can be defined as any substance which, when introduced into a living body by any route or comes in contact with the body, produces ill health, disease or death. In law, the real difference between a medicine and a poison is determined by the intent with which it is given or administered.

NATURE OF POISONING IN INDIA[1-4]

In India, poisoning usually occurs by the following modes:

Homicidal Poisoning

Criteria are of ideal homicidal poison:

- Should be easily available
- Should be cheap
- Should be tasteless or have a good taste
- Should be colorless and soluble
- Fatal dose should be small
- The symptoms produced should simulate a pathological disease
- There should be a time gap between administration and appearance of symptoms.
- Should not be easily detectable during postmortem and subsequent examinations.

Suicidal Poisoning

Criteria are of ideal suicidal poison:

- Should be easily available and cheap
- Should have a good taste or should be tasteless
- The effects should be sure
- Death should be, as far as, possible painless and peaceful.

Accidental Poisoning

Criteria are of ideal accidental poison:

- Ignorance, e.g. medicine-ignorance regarding dose, way of intake, etc.
- Carelessness, e.g. in storing poison
- Misbelieve, e.g. love philtre, aphrodisiac, fairing of complexion
- Industrial toxicity, while manufacturing and storing, viz iron ore containing arsenic during smelting liberates AsH_3, careless storing of methyl isocyanates.

Cattle and Animal Poisoning

It is common especially in rural areas. The main motive is destruction of cattle and animal of an enemy.

Stupefying Poisoning

Done in places where there is a confluence of unknown peoples. Legally it means making a person unconscious or semi-conscious, in the way of committing a crime.

ACTION OF POISON

Poisons act on the body in different ways. A poison may have:

1. **Local Action**: There are certain poisons which act only at the site of contact. These are known as locally acting poisons, e.g. corrosive mineral acids and alkalis.
2. **Remote Action**: These poisons act on selective areas after absorption and practically do not even have any local effect, e.g. opium, datura aconite.
3. **Both Local and Remote Action**: These poisons act locally and after being absorbed, they have action on a remote site, e.g. carbolic acid.

Fate of Poisons in the Body

After intake of the poison, the natural defense mechanism of the body tries to get rid of the poison from the body and that can be done by the following ways:

- By the way of vomiting, purging and through respiratory exhaled air
- By sweating, through milk or bile
- Through urine, e.g. carbolic acid, etc.
- By biotransformation: metabolism of poison takes place in the body partly or completely mainly in the liver
- Deposited in issue, e.g. lead, arsenic, etc.

Diagnosis of Poison

In Living

- History of taking something
- Uniformity of same type of symptoms in multiple persons points to particular poison
- Rapid recovery or death
- Previously healthy, no history of similar illness
- Detection of poison, circumstantial evidence, color, smell, etc.

Table 33.1 Poisons imparting color on post-mortem lividity

Poisoning	Color of postmortem lividity
Carbon monoxide	Cherry pink
Cyanide	Brick red
Hydrogen sulfide	Greenish blue
Phosphorus	Brown
Nitrobenzene, aniline, potassium chloride	Brownish red

- Baffling signs and symptom
- Laboratory examination.

In Dead Body

- Finding of peculiar color of postmortem lividity as shown in **Table 33.1**
- Deep cyanosis
- Staining over the body, clothing
- Odor of the poison, e.g. garlicky kerosene-like smell in Organo-phosphates, phenolic smell in carbolic acid, etc.
- Evidence of deep congestion of internal organs
- Laboratory examination including viscera and body fluid analysis for detection of poison.

Factors Modifying Action of Poison[1-8]

Quantity: The natural assumption is that a large dose of a poison will produce death more rapidly by causing severe symptoms than a smaller dose, but, in some cases, the ill effects are extenuated by vomiting excited by a large dose, e.g. copper sulfate. Moreover, action of poison varies with the quantity, e.g. arsenic, when administered in a very heavy dose (more than 1 gm), it will produce death without causing irritant symptoms, while in smaller dose it acts like an irritant.

Form of poison

a. **Physical State**
   i. Poison in gaseous form is more lethal than liquids and then comes the solid form.
   ii. Solid in finer molecular state acts better than coarse state.
   iii. Concentrated poison acts more severely than diluted ones.

b. **Chemical Combination:** The action of poison depends upon solubility and insolubility resulting from chemical combination, e.g. silver nitrate ($AgNO_3$) and hydrochloric acid (HCl), when taken separately, acts in severe way, whereas, the combined form an insoluble salt, viz innocuous. In the same way, strong acid and alkalis, when administered together, are rendered harmless by their neutralizing effect. Similarly, ingested opium is oxidized to oxydimorphine (which is inert) in stomach with potassium permanganate ($KMnO_4$) solution.

c. **Mechanical Combination**: The action of a poison may be changed much if combined mechanically with inert substances, e.g. a small dose of concentrated mineral acid diluted with water, may be taken orally without adverse effect.

Mode of Administration: Rapidity of poisoning depends on the way it is administered. A poison acts most rapidly when it is inhaled in gaseous form. Then comes, in order of merit, is introduction through IV or Intra-arterial route or injection by SC or IM route or application over a wound or application over serous or cellular surface or ingestion or introduction through rectal route or through unbroken skin.

Condition of the Body

a. **Age**: Ordinarily, poisons have a greater effect over the extremes of ages, but certain poisons, like belladonna, are better tolerated by children than by adults.

b. **Idiosyncrasy**: It means abnormal body response to a drug or substance. An individual may show toxic manifestation to a drug, even in normal dose.

c. **Tolerance**: By long continued use of certain drug, viz. opium and its preparation, tobacco, alcohol, strychnine, cocaine and arsenic, people acquire a tolerance towards a very large dose, which under ordinary circumstances, might have proved fatal.

Table 33.2 Toxicity rating of poison

Fatal dose	Rating	
Less than 5 mg/kg	6	Super toxic
5–50 mg/kg	5	Extremely toxic
51–500 mg/kg	4	Very toxic
501 mg/kg-5 g/kg	3	Moderately toxic
5.1–15 g/kg	2	Slightly toxic
More than 15 g/kg	1	Practically non-toxic

d. **Diseased Condition**: Certain drugs are tolerated better during certain diseases, viz. opium alkaloids in tetanus, barbiturate in delirium tremens and strychnine in paralysis. Similarly, digitalis or nicotine, even if given in similar dose in a person suffering from cardiac disease, may prove fatal.

5. **Synergistic Effect**: Effect of a poison may be enhanced in presence of another poison, e.g. alcohol with barbiturate.

Toxicity Rating of Poison (TRP)

The TRP has been developed to assess the nature of a poison by a physician while face a case of poisoning. Higher the toxicity rating for a given poison, the more would be its potency. It is based on the mortality and is applicable for acute exposure of a single poisonous substance. The toxicity rating of different poison is given in **Table 33.2**.

CLASSIFICATION OF POISONS[5,7]

Corrosive Poisons

i. **Strong Acids**:
  a. **Inorganic Acids**: Sulfuric acid, nitric acid and hydrochloric acid.
  b. **Organic Acids**: Carbolic, oxalic and acetic acids.

ii. **Alkalis**: Carbonates of sodium, potassium, bicarbonates and ammonia.

iii. **Metallic Salts**: Zinc chloride, potassium cyanide, ferric chloride, etc.

Irritants Poisons

i. **Inorganic Irritants**
  a. Non-metallic poisons: Phosphorous, chlorine, bromine, iodine, fluorine, etc.
  b. Metallic poisons: Arsenic, copper, lead, mercury, iron, zinc, antimony, etc.

ii. **Organic Irritants**
  a. Vegetable irritants: Castor seeds, croton seeds, abrus precatorius (rati), semicarpus, plumbago, etc.
  b. Animal irritants: Snake venom, insect bites, e.g. scorpions, spiders, poisonous insects, stings of wasps, bees, hornets and cantharides, etc.

iii. **Mechanical Irritants**: Powered glass, diamond dust, hairs, nails, dried sponge, etc.

Systemic Poisons

i. **Cerebral Poisons** (Affecting the brain)
  a. Somniferous and narcotics (Sleep-inducing): Opium and its alkaloids, e.g. morphine.
  b. Inebriants (which elevates mood): Alcohol, chloroform, ether, etc.
  c. Deliriants (causing delirium): Alkaloids of datura and cannabis Indica, cocaine, etc.

ii. **Spinal Poisons**
  a. Spinal stimulating poison: Nux vomica and its alkaloids like strychnine.
  b. Spinal depressant: Gelsemium.

iii. **Peripheral Nerve Poison**: Conium and Curare.

iv. **Cardiac Poisons**: Aconite, digitalis, oleander, etc.

v. **Asphyxiant Poisons**: Carbon dioxide, carbon monoxide, hydrogen sulfide, coal gas, war gases, hydrocyanic acid, sewer gas, etc.

vi. **Nephrotoxic Poison**: Mercury.

vii. **Hepatotoxic Poison**: Phosphorus.

Miscellaneous

Botulism poisoning (food poisoning) is the example of miscellaneous poisoning.

General Line of Treatment[1-6]

The general principle of treatment of poisoning is based on the following principles:

1. Evaluation and stabilization
2. Decontamination
3. Diagnostic testing
4. Antidotes.

Evaluation and Stabilization

The basic steps are:

i. Control the life-threatening problems.
ii. Maintain ABCD:
   - **A** Maintenance of **airway**: Patency of the airway is to be maintained; any foreign body, aspirate or secretions are to be cleared, intubated if required.
   - **B** Maintenance of **breathing**: Maintain the breathing; oxygen inhalation should be started immediately whenever necessary; put the patient in ventilator if spontaneous breathing is impaired.
   - **C** Maintenance of **circulation**: Put a proper sized cannula as soon as possible and start IV fluid to maintain the line so that all the IV medications can be introduced at ease.
   - **D** Prevention of **depression** of CNS: Level of consciousness to be assessed and do as is necessary to prevent depression of central nervous system.
iii. Correction of: Hypothermia, hyperthermia, acid-base imbalance, electrolyte imbalance, convulsion and agitation.

DECONTAMINATION

- Removal of unabsorbed poison
- Removal of the absorbed poison.

Removal of the Patient from Poisoned Environment

i. **Inhaled Poison:** Patient should be removed to fresh air, clothing should be loosened, clear airway should be ensured, artificial respiration should be started and administration of O_2 with mixture of CO_2 (95% and 5%) should be started.
ii. **Injected Poison:** For IM/IV injections, an elastic bandage is to be applied over the injection site to prevent the lymphatic drainage of the poison.
iii. **Contact Poisons:** For removal of the unabsorbed poison:
   a. **Eyes:** Wash with normal saline or tap water at least for 15 minutes.
   b. **Skin:** Remove all the contaminated cloth, rinse it thoroughly with cold water or saline but do not use neutralizing solution.
   c. **Ingestion:** In a case of ingestion the line of treatment is as follows:

Emetics

Indications

- Conscious patient
- Ingestion of toxic substance within 3–6 hours.

Different Preparations

I. **Syrup of Ipecacuanha** (Pediatric Ipecacuanha Emetic Mixture BP or Ipecac syrup USP): It's dose:
   - 6–12 months: 5–10 mL preceded or followed by 120–240 mL of water
   - 1 to 12 years: 15 mL preceded or followed by 120–240 mL of water
   - Over 12 years: 15–30 mL followed immediately by 240 ml of water
   - Can be repeated after 1/2 hour, if vomiting does not occur.
II. **Apomorphine**: The dose:
   - Adult: 6 mg
   - Child: 1–2 mg
   - Given subcutaneously
   - Contraindicated if chance of CNS depression is there.

Salt solutions, copper sulfate, large amount of water, tickling the posterior pharyngeal wall, etc. should not be used to induce emesis because of their high risk-benefit ratio.

Contraindications

- Unconscious or comatose patients
- Absent gag reflex
- Ingestion of corrosive or volatile poison
- Pregnancy.

Cathartics and Whole Bowel Irrigation

I. **Cathartics:** Saline or osmotic cathartics can be used to decontaminate the gut. The administration of cathartics alone has no role in management of poisoning cases.

II. **Whole Bowel Irrigation (WBI):** An isotonic solution may be useful to empty the bowel for iron, lithium, ingested button batteries, ingested illicit drug packets and overdose of sustained release or enteric-coated drugs, etc.

In WBI, the intestine can be cleaned by the oral administration of large amounts of polyethylene glycol electrolyte solution.

Gastric Lavage

Indications

1. History of poison ingestion with symptoms.
2. Ingestion of toxic substance within 1/2-1 hour.

Contraindications

1. Ingestion of a corrosive substance such as a strong acid or alkali.
2. Ingestion of a hydrocarbon with high aspiration potential.
3. Unless intubated, in the patients with loss of airway protective reflexes, such as in a patient with a depressed state of consciousness.
4. Patients who are at risk of hemorrhage or gastrointestinal perforation due to pathology, recent surgery or other medical condition, that could be further compromised by the use of gastric lavage.

Complications

1. Aspiration pneumonia
2. Laryngospasm
3. Hypoxia and hypercapnia
4. Mechanical injury to the throat, esophagus and stomach
5. Fluid and electrolyte imbalance
6. Combative patients may be at greater risk of complications.

Material Used

1. Ewald tube (**Figure 33.1**)
2. Lavacuator (**Figure 33.2**)
3. Ryle's tube for children (**Figure 33.3**)
4. Boas tube.

Procedure

1. Should be done by an experienced staff, not to be tried outside a health care center.
2. Procedure should be explained to the patient properly.
3. Endotracheal intubation (with endotracheal tube with a calf) should precede

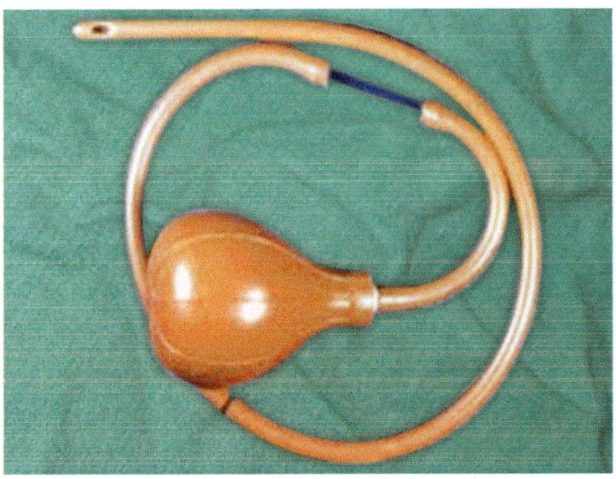

Figure 33.1 Ewald tube (Gastric lavage tube)

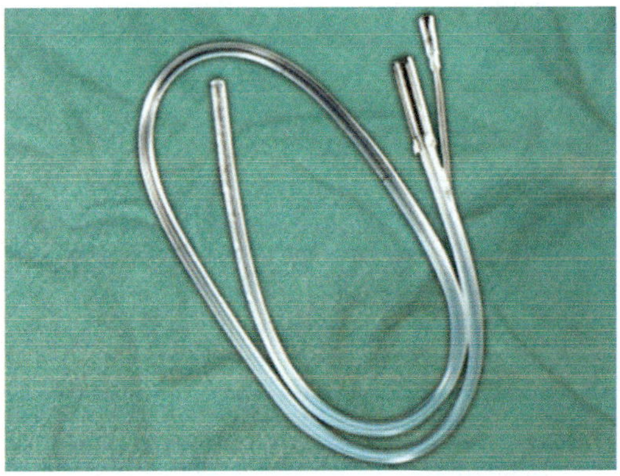

Figure 33.2 Lavacuator

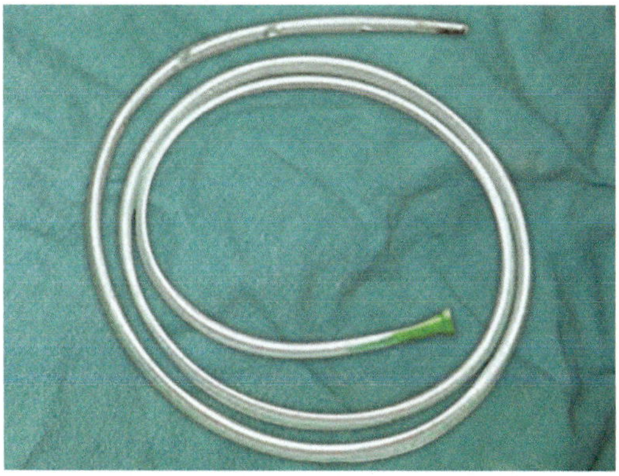

Figure 33.3 Ryle's tube

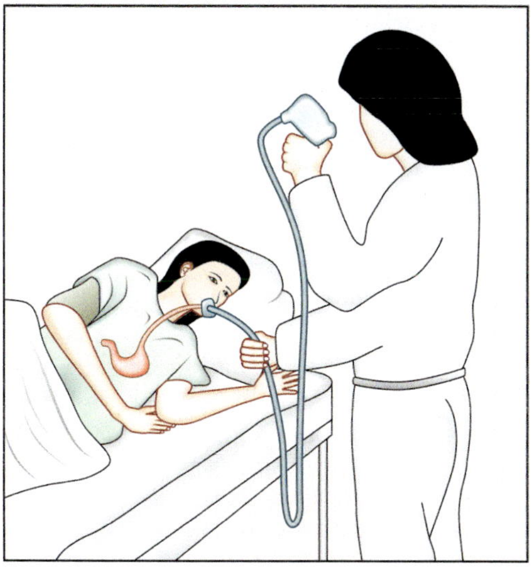

Figure 33.4 Position of the patient at the time of gastric lavage

gastric lavage in the comatose/unconscious patient without a gag reflex.

4. The patient should be placed in the left lateral, head down position (20 tilt on the table). The length of tube to be inserted is measured and marked before insertion (**Figure 33.4**).
5. A mouth gag is placed between teeth to prevent biting of the tube.
6. A large bore 36–40 French or 30 English gauge tube (external diameter approximately 12–13.3 mm) should be used in adults; and 24–28 French gauge (diameter 7.8–9.3 mm) tube in children.
7. The inserting end of tube is to be lubricated properly.
8. In an adult, 200–300 mL of warm normal saline (0.9%) or water should be used. In a child, 10 mL/kg body weight of warm normal saline (0.9%) should be given. It should be continued till a clear solution is returned.

The first stomach wash should be preserved for toxicological analysis.

Precautions

1. Large volume of fluid is to be avoided to prevent entering of the gastric content into duodenum.
2. Anesthetic gel/ointment should not be used.
3. Always preserve the **first wash fluid for toxicological** analysis.

Activated Charcoal

It 1831, in front of his colleagues at the French Academy of Medicine, Professor Touery drank a lethal dose of strychnine and lived to tell the story. He had mixed the deadly poison with activated charcoal.

That's why activated charcoal is as a powerful emergency decontaminant in the gastrointestinal tract. It is considered to be the most effective single agent available. It is used when a person swallows or absorbs almost any toxic substance.

Properties

1. Activated charcoal itself is a fine, black powder that is odorless, tasteless and non-toxic.
2. Activated charcoal works by adsorbing chemicals, thus reducing their toxicity (poisonous nature), through the entire length of the stomach and small and large intestines.
3. Activated charcoal is estimated to reduce absorption of poison up to 60%.
4. Activated charcoal is often given after the gastric lavage. Gastric lavage is only effective immediately after swallowing a toxic substance (within about ½ to 1 hour) and does not have effect on the poisons beyond the stomach as activated charcoal does.

Elimination of the Absorbed Poison

- Forced diuresis
- Dialysis
- Hemofiltration
- Plasma perfusion, etc.

Clinical Diagnosis

In most situations, the management of a victim of poisoning depends a lot upon the clinical diagnosis. However, in situations where laboratory diagnosis is not available, doctors must be ready to treat the victim based on clinical diagnosis. Poisoning should be suspected in all cases of sudden, severe and unexpected illness.

The doctors should investigate such situations by ensuring from clinical features, as quickly and thoroughly as possible. Signs and symptoms with different related poisons are narrated in **Table 33.3**.

Signs and Symptoms[1]

Toxidrome (Tables 33.4 to 33.9)[1,8]

A **toxidrome** is a syndrome caused by a dangerous level of toxins in the body. The term was coined in 1970 by Mofenson and Greensher.[9]

It is the association of several clinically recognizable features, signs, symptoms, phenomena or characteristics which often occur together, so that the presence of one feature alerts the physician to the presence of the others. Presence of the group of signs and symptoms will point towards the probable poisons, and thus, it helps in identification of the poison as well as starting the line of treatment for a particular group of poison. Apart from these, the routine laboratory tests as well as the different tests for the detection of a specific poison are of helpful.

Diagnostic Tests

i. Routine Blood and other body fluid can give some information about the state of the patient.
ii. All the body fluid and excreta of the patient can give information about the poisoning.

Analytical Techniques[1,2,6]

Details mentioned in chapter on Forensic Science Laboratory.

Different analytical techniques used for detection of poisons in biological samples give more accurate results than any other tests for the purpose. The most commonly used analytical techniques used in this field are:

Table 33.3 Few signs and the probable poisons

Agitation	Anticholinergic, hypoglycemia, phencyclidine, sympathomimetic, withdrawal from ethanol and sedative-hypnotics
Alopecia	Alkylating agents, radiation, selenium, thallium
Ataxia	Benzodiazepines, carbamazepine, carbon monoxide, ethanol, hypoglycemia, lithium, mercury, nitrous oxide, phenytoin
Blindness or decreased visual acuity	Caustics (direct), cocaine, cisplatin, mercury, methanol, quinine, thallium
Constipation	Anticholinergic, botulism, lead, opioids, thallium (severe)
Diaphoresis	Amphetamines, cholinergic, hypoglycemia, opioid withdrawal, salicylates, serotonin syndrome, sympathomimetic, withdrawal from ethanol and sedative-hypnotics
Diarrhea	Arsenic and other metals, boric acid (blue-green), botanical irritants, cathartics, cholinergic, colchicines, iron, lithium, opioid withdrawal, radiation
Gum discoloration	Arsenic, bismuth, hypervitaminosis A, lead, mercury
Miosis	Cholinergics, clonidine, opioids, phencyclidine, phenothiazines
Mydriasis	Anticholinergic, botulism, opioid withdrawal, sympathomimetic

i. **Qualitative Assays:** This qualitative assay includes different color tests for detection of the poisons.
ii. **Spectrophotometry:** This includes different colorimeters and autoanalyzers.
iii. **Chromatography:** Which includes the thin layer chromatograph (TLC), gas liquid chromatography (GLC), high performance liquid chromatography (HPLC), gas chromatography and mass spectrometry (GCMS), which can be used depending up on the poison for qualitative as well as quantitative assessment of the poisons.
iv. **Competitive Binding and Immunological Tests:** Which includes radioimmunoassay (RIA), enzyme immunoassay (EIA), etc.

Table 33.4 Cholinergic toxidrome

Syndrome	Signs and symptoms	Poisons	Antidote
Cholinergic sludge	Salivation	Carbamate	Atropine
	Lacrimation	Organophosphates	Pralidoxime for organophosphates
	Urination	Physostigmine	
	Diarrhea	Pilocarpine	
	GI cramps		
	Emesis		
	Wheezing		
	Diaphoresis		
	Bronchorrhea		
	Bradycardia		
	Miosis		

Table 33.5 The anticholinergic toxidrome

Syndrome	**Signs and symptoms**	**Poisons**	**Antidote**
Anticholinergic	Mydriasis	Antihistamines	Physostigmine (do not use in cyclic antidepressant overdose as will worsen conduction disturbances)
Hot as a hare	Blurred vision	Atropine	
Dry as a bone	Fever	Baclofen	
Red as a beet	Dry skin	Benztropine	
Mad as a hatter	Flushing	Tricyclic	
Blind as a bat	Ileus	Antidepressants	
	Urinary retention	Phenothiazines	
	Tachycardia	Propantheline	
	Hypertension	Scopolamine	
	Psychosis		
	Coma		
	Seizures		
	Myoclonus		

Table 33.6 Hallucinogenic sympathomimetic toxidrome

Syndrome	Signs and symptoms	Poisons	Antidote
Hallucinogenic	Disorientation	Amphetamine	Benzodiazepines
	Hallucinations	Cocaine	
	Hyperactive bowel	Pseudoephedrine	
	Panic	Phencyclidine	
	Seizure	Ephedrine	
	Tachycardia		
	Hypertension		
	Tachypnea		

Table 33.7 Sedative/hypnotic toxidrome

Syndrome	Signs and symptoms	Poisons	Antidote
Sedative/hypnotic	Stupor and coma	Anticonvulsants	Naloxone
	Confusion	Antipsychotics	Flumazenil
	Slurred speech	Barbiturates	Urinary alkanization for Phenobarbital
	Apnea	Benzodiazepines	
		Ethanol	
		Meprobamate	
		Opiates	

Table 33.8 Opiate toxidrome

Syndrome	Signs and Symptoms	Poisons	Antidote
Narcotic	Altered mental status	Dextromethorphan	Naloxone
	Slow shallow breaths	Opiates	
	Meiosis	Pentazocine	
	Bradycardia	Propoxyphene	
	Hypotension		
	Hypothermia		
	Decreased bowel sounds	Opiates	

Table 33.9 Serotonergic syndrome

Syndrome	Signs and symptoms	Poisons	Antidote
Serotonergic	Irritability	Fluoxetine	Benzodiazepine
	Hyperreflexia	Meperidine	
	Flushing	Paroxetine	
	Diarrhoea	Trazodone	
	Diaphoresis	Clomipramine	
	Fever		
	Trismus		
	Tremor		
	Myoclonus		

Poison Research Center/Poison Laboratory/Poison Information Center

Poison Information Center

The concept was first adopted in the Netherland in 1949. The main objective of the center is to provide information regarding poisons through a call center. In India, the first such center was established in the year 1994, in the form of National Poison Information Center at AIIMS, New Delhi. At present, a total of four poison information centers are there, which include The National Institute of Occupational Health, Ahmedabad, and Poison Information Centers at Government General Hospital, Chennai and Amrita Institute of Medical Sciences, Cochin.

Poison Control Center

The only WHO accredited poison control center in India is at Amrita Institute of Medical Science and Research, Cochin, Kerala, which came into existence in July 2003. The center has its full-fledged Poison Information Center as well as Analytical Toxicological Laboratory.

ANTIDOTE THERAPY

An antidote is a remedy to counteract the effect of a poison.

Mode of Action of the Antidotes

i. Inert complex formation, e.g. chelating agent for heavy metals.
ii. Accelerated detoxification, e.g. thiosulfate accelerates conversion of cyanide to non-toxic thiocyanate.
iii. Reduced toxic conversion, e.g. ethanol inhibits metabolism of methanol.
iv. Receptor site competition, e.g. naloxone antagonist effect of opiates at stereo-specific opioid receptor sites.
v. Receptor site blockade, e.g. atropine blocking effect of ACh at muscarinic receptors.
vi. Toxic effect bypass, e.g. use of 100% oxygen in cyanide poisoning.

Types of Antidotes

Physical or Mechanical Antidotes

They prevent the action of the poison mechanically, without destroying or inactivating the poison.

i. **Demulcents**: Egg albumin, starch, barley or milk, which have a soothing effect and form a protective layer on the mucous membrane of stomach. Sucralfate suspension can be used to protect the gastric mucosa.
ii. **Adsorbents**: Adsorb the poisons in to their surface, so that the poison cannot come in contact with the stomach wall, viz. activated charcoal, etc.
iii. **Diluents**: Water, milk or similar drinks that dilute the poison and delay its absorption.
iv. **Bulky food**: Boiled rice, boiled vegetables, etc. act by getting admixed with the poison and thereby allow small amount of the poison to come in contact with the gut mucosa.

Chemical Antidotes

Inactivate poisons by undergoing chemical reaction with them.

1. **Weak Alkalis**: In poisoning by acids. Carbonate alkalis are to be avoided as they produce CO_2 and inflate the stomach, may even lead to rupture.
2. **Weak Vegetable Acids**: In poisoning by alkalis, e.g. citric acid, acetic acid, etc.
3. **Potassium Permanganate**: Is a strong oxidizing agent. Dilute solution of $KMnO_4$ is used 1:10,000 dilution in poisoning by strychnine, nicotine, aluminum phosphide, opium, phosphorous, hydrocyanic acid, cyanides, morphine, atropine, etc. It can be used in gastric lavage fluid also.

Physiological Antidotes

Produce sign and symptoms just the opposite to those of the poison, thus counteracting the effect of the poisons, e.g. Atropine in organophosphate poisoning.

Universal Antidotes

Combination of physical and chemical antidotes used when exact nature of the poison is not known.

i. Activated charcoal: 2 parts
ii. Magnesium oxide: 1 part
iii. Tannic acid: 1 part.

Chelation Therapy for Toxic Metals

1. The objective is to administer a non-toxic compound that binds metal ions more strongly than cell macromolecules and forms a water-soluble compound which can be excreted.
2. Chelate are coordination compound in which the central atom (usually a metal) is covalently bonded to two or more other atoms.
3. Heterocyclic rings are formed with the metal atom as part of each ring.
4. A key concern is the risk of enhancing toxicity by forming complexes that favor absorption and/or distribution of the metal ion to tissues.
5. Risk of trace element depletion is there if chelating agents are given for prolonged periods.

Chelation therapy is applied to treat

1. Poisoning with metal ions.
2. In disease conditions like metal storage diseases, notably Wilson's disease (genetic ceruloplasmin deficiency) and hemochromatosis.
3. Sometimes it can be used to aid for elimination of metallic radionuclides.
4. Treatment will be most effective if given while the metal ion is still in the extracellular compartment.

Hemodialysis sometimes may be essential to remove the chelate if renal function is impaired, although chelator such as DMSA probably chelate metal ions in the gut, facilitating fecal elimination.

They can reduce absorption of the poisons from gastrointestinal tract by chelation with the poisons. It is important to maintain constant excess of chelating agent to minimize dissociation of the chelate.

Some of the Antidotes and their Uses

Activated Charcoal

Properties

1. Activated charcoal itself is a fine, black powder that is odorless, tasteless and non-toxic.
2. Activated charcoal works by adsorbing chemicals, thus reducing their toxicity (poisonous nature), through the entire length of the stomach and small and large intestines.
3. Activated charcoal is estimated to reduce absorption of poisonous substances up to 60%.
4. Activated charcoal is often given after the gastric lavage. Gastric lavage is only effective immediately after swallowing a toxic substance (within about ½ to 1 hour) and does not have effects on the poison that reached beyond the stomach as activated charcoal does.
5. Very effective in many other drugs, but not effective in iron, lithium, alcohols and glycol. The efficacies of activated charcoal on different poisons are narrated in **Table 33.10**.

Dose

- Up to one year: 1 gm/kg
- 1–12 years: 25–50 gm
- Over 12 years: 50–100 gm.

Activated charcoal usually mixed in 200 mL of water and is administered orally or instilled via a nasogastric tube, after emesis or gastric lavage.

Contraindications

1. Impaired consciousness.
2. Gastrointestinal bleeding.
3. Gastrointestinal perforation.

In absence of activated charcoal, any charcoal prepared by burning and then by grinding, egg albumin or bread toast can be used as substitute.

Table 33.10 Efficacy of activated charcoal on different poisons

Well adsorbed	Moderately adsorbed	Poorly adsorbed
Amphetamines	Antidiabetics	Alcohols
Antidepressants	Kerosene	Carbamates
Antiepileptic	Paracetamol	Corrosives
Antihistamines	Phenol	Cyanide
Atropine	Salicylates	Ethylene glycol
Barbiturates		Heavy Metals
Benzodiazepines		Hydrocarbons
Beta-blockers		Organophosphates
Digitalis		
NSAIDs		
Opiates		
Strychnine		
Phenothiazines		

Table 33.11 Atropine and its uses as physiological antidote

Antidote	Atropine
Indications	Organophosphates, carbamates, pilocarpine, physostigmine
Available as	Atropa injection. 0.6 mg/mL, 2 mL ampoules; Tropine injection. 0.6 mg/mL, 1 mL ampoules
Dose	2–4 mg, IV at 10–15 minutes, till the signs of atropinization children: 0.05 mg/kg, IV at 10–15 minutes

Multiple-dose activated charcoal (MDAC) therapy (repeated administration of oral activated charcoal) enhances elimination of poisons by disturbing the entero-enteric and in some cases, the entero-hepatic circulation.

Initial dose: 50–100 gm, then 12.5 gm/hour until recovery or the plasma drug concentration comes down to the normal therapeutic or non-toxic range.

Atropine

1. It is a physiological antidote.
2. It counteracts the action of organophosphates poisons.
3. Atropine if given alone has less effect as the muscarinic effects are only neutralized, the nicotinic effects remain. So, it should be given along with the oxime. Delayed neurological symptoms like muscular weakness, may be present if given alone.
4. Atropine and its uses as physiological antidote are mentioned in **Table 33.11**.

Precautions

1. May contain benzyl alcohol or chlorobutanol as preservative and may lead to toxicity of these at high dose. Preservative free atropine should be used if higher dose is required.
2. Half lives of atropine in children bellow 2 years and adults above 60 years, is longer; so, dose should be adjusted accordingly.

Adverse Effects

Atrial arrhythmias, A-V dissociation, ventricular ectopic, photophobia, raised intraocular pressure, hyperpyrexia, hallucinations, delirium.

Pralidoxime (2-PAM)

Mode of Action

Competes for the phosphate moiety of the organophosphates and release them from acetyl cholinesterase enzyme, thereby reactivating the enzyme.

Table 33.12 Pralidoxime as an antidote	
Antidote	**Pralidoxime**
Indication	Organophosphates
Available preparations	PAM tablet, 500 mg for oral use PAM-A injection. 500 mg in 20 mL for IV use
Dose	**Adult:** 1–2 gm in 100–150 mL of normal saline over 30 minutes period. Can be repeated every 6-12 hours for 24–48 hours. **Children:** 20–40 mg/kg, in 100–150 mL of normal saline infusion. Repeated every 6–12 hours, for 24–48 hours and to be given along with atropine

Table 33.13 BAL as a chelating agent	
Chelating agent	**British Anti Lewisite (BAL)**
Indications	Arsenic, mercury, bismuth, copper, antimony and nickel
Available preparation	BAL (Knoll Pharma), 2 mL ampoule, 100 mg/mL, in arachis oil
Doses	3 mg/kg, 4 hourly, on day 1 and 2 3 mg/kg, 6 hourly, on day 3 3 mg/kg, 12 hourly, next 10 days. It should be given as deep IM

Once the organophosphates are bound to the ChE receptor sites and remain there for 48 hours, the reversal becomes impossible. The condition is known as the aging of the enzyme. So, oximes should be stated within 48 hours of the ingestion of the poison. Pralidoxime as an antidote in poison treatment is narrated in **Table 33.12**.

WHO Recommendation

Initial bolus dose of 30 mg/kg, followed by infusion of 8 mg/kg/hour is necessary for maintaining the plasma concentration of at least 4 mg/L for pralidoxime to be effective.

Adverse Effects

Rapid administration can cause tachycardia, laryngospasm or even cardiac or respiratory arrest; apart from drowsiness, vertigo, headache and muscular weakness.

British Anti Lewisite (BAL)

Synonyms: Dimercaprol; 2, 3-dimercaptopropanol

British anti-lewisite has been in use in the medical community for more than 60 years. It is most commonly used chelator (remove a heavy metal from the body) in the treatment of poisoning from arsenic, mercury, lead and gold. It is also well-known for its role in World War II as an antidote to the chemical warfare agent Lewisite. Although other chelators with less toxicity has now been developed, BAL maintains a prominent role in the treatment of various medical conditions. BAL as a chelator is narrated in **Table 33.13**.

Side Effects

- Pain at the injection site
- Hypertension and tachycardia
- Abdominal pain, nausea and vomiting
- Headaches
- Burning sensation of the lips
- Excessive salivation
- Rhinorrhea and tearing
- Fever
- Muscle pain, muscle spasms and a feeling of chest constriction
- Profuse sweating.

Contraindications

1. Poisonings due to iron, cadmium, tellurium, selenium, vanadium and uranium.
2. Elemental mercury vapours, because it can further increase the metal in the brain.
3. Should not be given in case of acute renal failure (anuria) or extensive hepatic insufficiency and should be used with special care in hypertensive patients.

Table 33.14 DMSA as chelating agent	
Chelating agent	**DMSA (Succimer)**
Indication	Lead, mercury, arsenic
Contraindication	Pre-existing kidney or liver disease and pregnancy
Dose	10 g/kg 8 hourly for 5 days, orally

Table 33.15 Ethylenediaminetetraacetic acid chelating agent	
Chelating agent	**EDTA**
Indication	Lead, mercury, zinc, cadmium, copper, manganese poisoning
Contraindication	Pre-existing kidney or liver disease, pregnancy and raised ICP
Dose	25–30 mg/kg in 250–500 mL of 5% dextrose or normal saline infusion IV, 12 hourly for 5 days

Dimercaptosuccinic Acid

DMSA is less toxic than BAL, and it is sometimes substituted for BAL when the patient's condition improves. It is also used when intolerance to BAL develops. DMSA as a chelator is narrated in **Table 33.14**.

Side Effects

1. Nausea
2. Vomiting
3. Diarrhea
4. Rhinitis and cough
5. Rash.

Contraindications

They are contraindicated in pre-existing kidney or liver disease and pregnancy. Hydration is essential. DMSA is not used in conjunction with ETDA or D-penicillamine.

Ethylenediaminetetraacetic Acid (EDTA), Edetate Disodium

The EDTA is one of the oldest chelating agents, coming into prominence in the 1950s. It has an affinity for lead. It is often used as a second-line of treatment in combination with BAL and given by IV infusion. The clinical uses are mentioned in **Table 33.15**

Side Effects

i. Common side effects: Gastrointestinal upset and headache.
ii. More serious side effects: Seizures, numbness or tingling in the hands and feet, irregular heartbeat, skin rashes, fever or chills and blood in the urine (Ferner 2001).

Contraindications

1. EDTA is contraindicated in pregnancy
2. If there is kidney disease
3. It can also interact with insulin and cardiae medicines.

Dimercaptopropane Sulfonate (DMPS)

2, 3-Dimercapto-1-propanesulfonic acid (**DMPS**) and its sodium salt known as **unithiol** are chelating agents that form complexes with various heavy metals. They are related to Dimercaprol, which is another chelating agent. It is another analogue of BAL. DMPS was found to have some protective effect, prolonging the survival time,[10] but shown to be less effective and have more side effects than DMSA.

The DMPS is the drug of choice in Europe and Asia; however, the FDA has not approved DMPS for chelating purposes in the US. It does, however, appear on the FDA list of drugs that appear to be safe. In the US, DMPS is distributed to pharmacists in bulk form for compounding and dispensing in oral and injection forms (FDA 1999; Marcus 2001). The indications and doses are mentioned in **Table 33.16**.

Table 33.16 DMPA as chelating agent

Antidote	DMPS
Indication	Arsenic and mercury poisoning
Dose	5 mg/kg IV in 6 divided doze

Table 33.17 Penicillamine chelating agent

Antidote	D-penicillamine
Indication	Copper (Wilson's disease), arsenic, mercury (alternative to BAL), chronic lead poisoning. Also used to reduce cysteine excretion in cystinuria and patients with severe, active rheumatoid arthritis unresponsive to conventional therapy
Available as	Artin, cilamin 150 mg, 200 mg and 250 mg capsules
Dose	Children: 30 mg/kg/day Adult: 1–2 g daily in divided dose, orally, 1 hour before food

Penicillamine (D-Penicillamine)

Synonyms: Cuprimine

Penicillamine is 3-mercapto-D-valine. It is a white or practically white, crystalline powder, freely soluble in water, slightly soluble in alcohol and insoluble in ether, acetone, benzene, and carbon tetrachloride. Although its configuration is D, it is levorotatory as usually measured and is an oral chelating agent used to treat heavy-metal toxicity. The indications, available preparations and doses are mentioned in **Table 33.17**.

Side Effects

i. Gastrointestinal intolerance.
ii. Bone marrow suppression, anorexia, vomiting and diarrhea are the most common side effects, occurring in 20–30% of the patients treated with penicillamine.[11,12]
iii. Itchy skin (wheals).
iv. Aplastic anemia (idiosyncratic).[13]
v. Fever.
vi. Nephropathy,[11] membranous glomerulonephritis.
vii. Hepatotoxicity.[13]
viii. Antibody-mediated myasthenia gravis[11] and Lambert-Eaton myasthenic syndrome, which may persist even after its withdrawal.
ix. Drug-induced systemic lupus erythematosus.[14]
x. Besides, people allergic to penicillin may have hypersensitivity to penicillamine.[15]

Contraindications

1. Patient who are allergy to penicillin
2. Possible interaction with other drugs (immunosuppressant, digoxin)
3. Severe blood disorders
4. Renal insufficiency
5. Pregnancy.

Table 33.18 Desferrioxamine as chelating agent

Antidote	Desferrioxamine
Indication	Acute iron poisoning, iron overload, aluminium overload, transfusion siderosis, diagnosis of aluminium overload and diagnosis of iron storage disease and certain anemia
Available preparation	Desfereal 500 mg vials
Dose	0.5–1 g IM followed by 500 mg every 4 hourly for two doses, then 400 mg 4–12 hourly (maximum 6 g/day). In severe life-threatening poisoning or patient with shock should receive 15 mg/kg/hour in laevulose solution IV, with a maximum daily dose up to 360 mg/kg or up to 6 g total[16]

Desferrioxamine

Desferrioxamine is used to chelate iron, especially in acute iron poisoning in small children and administered by injection or intravenously. The indications, different preparations of Desferrioxamine and its doses are mentioned in **Table 33.18**.

Adverse Effects

i. Common side effects: Blurred vision, wheezing, rapid heartbeat, seizures, itching, skin rash, bluish skin and redness and pain at the injection site.
ii. Less common side effects: Gastrointestinal discomfort, fever, cramping and bruising.

Contraindications

Known sensitivity or allergy to any ingredient or who are allergies to certain foods or dyes, other medicines currently being taken, pregnancy or breastfeeding and kidney disease.

REFERENCES

1. Pillay VV. Comprehensive Medical Toxicology, 2nd ed. Hyderabad: Paras Publishing; 2008. pp. 8-39.
2. Pillay VV. Text Book of Forensic Medicine and Toxicology, 16th ed. Hyderabad: Paras Publishing; 2011. pp. 402-22.
3. Mathiharan K, Patnaik Amrit K (Eds). Modi's Medical Jurisprudence and Toxicology, 23rd ed. New Delhi: LexisNexis; 2006. pp. 31-43.
4. Krishan V. Textbook of Forensic Medicine and Toxicology: Principle and Practice, 5th ed. New Delhi: Elsevier; 2011. pp. 429-53.
5. Nandi A. Principles of Forensic Medicine, 1st ed. Calcutta: New Central Book Agency (P) Ltd; 1995. pp. 456-70.
6. Dikshit PC. Text Book of Forensic Medicine and Toxicology, 1st ed. New Delhi: Peepee Publisers and Distributors (P) Ltd; 2007. pp. 438-60.
7. Reddy KSN. Toxicology: general considerations. In: The Essentials of Forensic Medicine and Toxicology, 31st ed. Hyderabad: K. Suguana Devi; 2012. pp. 464-84.
8. James DH. Colour Atlas of Human Poisoning and Envenoming. New York: CRC Press; 2006. pp. 55-6.
9. Mofenson HC, Greensher J. The nontoxic ingestion. Ped Clin N Am. 1970;17(3):583-90.
10. Aposhian HV, Aposhian MM. Meso-2, 3-dimercaptosuccinic acid: Chemical, pharmacological and toxicological properties of an orally effective metal chelating agent. Ann Rev Pharmacol Toxicol. 1990;30(1):279-306.
11. Camp AV. Penicillamine in the treatment of rheumatoid arthritis. Proc Royal Soc Med. 1977;70(2):67-9.
12. Grasedyck K. D-penicillamine—side effects, pathogenesis and decreasing the risks. Zeitschrift fur Rheumatologie. 1988;1(47 Suppl):17-9.
13. Fishel B, Tishler M, Caspi D, Yaron M. Fatal aplastic anaemia and liver toxicity caused by D-penicillamine treatment of rheumatoid arthritis. Ann Rheumat Dis. 1989;48(7):609-10.
14. Chalmers A, Thompson D, Stein HE, Reid G, Patterson AC. Systemic lupus erythematous during penicillamine therapy for rheumatoid arthritis. Ann Intern Med. 1982;97(5):659-63.
15. Parker CW, Shapiro J, Kern M, Eisen HN. Hypersensitivity to penicillenic acid derivatives in human beings with penicillin allergy. J Exp Med. 1962;115(4):821-38.
16. Schiavone FM. Metals: Iron intoxication. In: Viccellio P (Ed), Handbook of Medical Toxicology, 1st ed. Boston: Little Brown and Company; 1993. pp. 294-302.

CHAPTER 34

Medicolegal Aspect of Toxicology

Putul Mahanta

LEARNING PLAN

- Brief overview of poisoning
- Role of a registered medical practitioner in dealing with poisoning cases
- Laws relating to poison in India

This chapter deals with the duties of registered medical practitioner to make their duties professionally and legally effective and empiric. Doctor should have the knowledge regarding first aid, life-saving measures, diagnosis and treatment and autopsy procedures in case of death, besides preservation of various biological samples for chemical analysis which may be helpful for the treatment as well as for investigative purpose. The medical professional should have the basic of legal knowledge while dealing with poisoning cases as ignorance on the part of the doctor's duties cannot be the defense in the court.

BRIEF STATISTICAL REVIEW OF THE POISONING CASES

Both suicidal and homicidal cases of poisoning are more common in India than in Western countries owing to the easy availability of poisonous substances on account of non-stringent application of the laws of the land. Accidental poisoning is also on the rise because of greater use of chemicals for agro industry and domestic purposes. Accidental cases of bites by venomous snakes are frequent in India. It is estimated that annually about 2 lakh people are bitten, of whom around 16,000 die.[1]

Suicidal cases are reaching a greater magnitude because of tension and worry in today's fast life. Because of overuse of organophosphorus compounds as insecticides, pesticides, industrial chemicals and drugs in agro industry, the pattern of misuse of poisonous substances keeps changing in our country.

Poisoning, both accidental and intentional, is a significant contributor to mortality and morbidity throughout the world. According to WHO, three million acute poisoning cases, with 220,000 deaths occur annually; of these, 90% of fatal poisoning occur in developing countries, particularly among agricultural workers.

Acute poisoning forms one of the commonest causes of emergency hospital admissions. Pattern of poisoning in a region depends upon a variety of factors, such as availability of poisons, socioeconomic status of population, religious and cultural influences and availability of drugs.

The exact incidence of poisoning in India is uncertain due to lack of data at central level, as most cases are not reported. Moreover, mortality data is a poor indicator of the incidence of poisoning. It has been estimated that about 5–6 people per lakh population die due to the wrath of poisoning every year. There are more than 4000 species of medicinal plants growing as herbs, shrubs and trees in India, many of which are poisonous when administered in large doses. In India, the common poisons are insecticides, pesticides such as organophosphorus, chlorinated hydro- carbons, aluminum phosphide, carbamates and pyrethroid.

The commonest agent used for poisoning in India and other developing countries is pesticides; the reasons being agriculture based economics, poverty and easy availability of highly toxic pesticides. Occupational poisoning due to pesticides is also common in developing countries, due to unsafe practices, illiteracy, ignorance and lack of protective measures. In India, organophosphates form the largest bulk of pesticide poisoning.[2]

An epidemiological study of poisoning cases reported to the National Poisons Information Centre, AIIMS, New Delhi, was conducted. In this study, the age range was from less than 1 to 70 years, with the highest incidence in the range of 14–40 years, with males outnumbering females. The most common mode of poisoning was suicidal, followed by accidental.[3] Poisoning, a major cause of morbidity among children, may be accidental or deliberate.[4]

As the poisoning cases are increasing day by day, the doctors at private or at government set up are facing a huge number of those cases in various stages. Hence, the doctors on duty should be equipped with the proper infrastructure to manage them to save the life of these patients.

There are so many legal obligations with the treatment procedures which cannot be undermined. In all such cases of poisoning, what should a doctor do both empirically as well as legally in managing such cases? The following points must be kept in mind while dealing with these cases either at private set up or in government hospital.

ROLE OF A DOCTOR IN DEALING WITH POISONING CASE

Though every doctor has a right to choose a patient, i.e. he can refuse to treat any patient, as per the Supreme Court Ruling (Parmananda Katara vs. Union of India); no doctor shall refuse to treat a patient in emergency.

Following are the few steps to remember in part of doctor duties while dealing with the poisoning case:

i. Assessment of condition of the patient.
ii. Removal of source from exposure if applicable. Stop further poisoning by isolating the patient to the hospital with due formalities.
iii. The first and the foremost duty is to resuscitate as well as treat the patient. Without wasting any further time, the doctor should try to save the life of the patient by efficiently treating him or her. In conscious and serious patient, who is dying, dying declaration is to be obtained without delay as per the laid down rules.
iv. Removal of unabsorbed poison, viz. induced vomiting, emesis, stomach wash, bowel wash, etc. depending on type of poison and time interval between exposure and attention.
v. Control of circulating poison by means of diuresis, ion exchange resin, etc.
vi. Antagonize the effects by using non-specific antidote, specific antidote, symptomatic, supportive and preventive drugs.
vii. Follow-up with the effects of treatment.
viii. Psychological counseling of the patient, who survives suicidal poisoning, prevention of further recurrence.
ix. Discharge and follow up in outpatient department (OPD).

Other Formalities

i. Note the particulars of the patient, i.e. full name, age, sex, address, date and time, brought by whom, identification marks, history of the case, etc.

ii. In suicidal or accidental poisoning, doctors in private set up is not bound to inform police.

iii. In all cases of definite or suspected homicidal poisoning, doctor must inform to the nearby police under section 39 CrPC. Assist the police to determine the manner of death.

iv. Maintain details of written records of treatment in all cases of poisoning. This is useful to the doctor in the court as well. A private medical officer is not bound to supply information on their own to police or magistrate if he/she is sure that his/her patient is suffering from suicidal or accidental poisoning, because this is not included in section **39** CrPC. But he/she has to give information about the case if he/she is summoned U/S **175** CrPC. If the medical officer conceals any information, he/she is liable for prosecution U/S **202** IPC. If he/she supplies false information, he/she can be prosecuted U/S **193** IPC.

v. Doctors in Government Hospitals are to report every case of poisoning irrespective of suicidal, homicidal or accidental to the nearby police station.
He is not liable for giving notice in cases where the case has already been registered with police officer by somebody else U/S **40** CrPC.
Though section 39 CrPC excludes **309** IPC, doctors are not investigators, so how can they judge that the case is suicidal, homicidal or accidental? So, they should report all the cases of poisoning to the police and they are competent to judge by investigation. Nowhere in law, discrimination is made between a private and government practitioner, so it is same as 39 CrPC starts as public to give information.

vi. The treating physician can call one doctor to consult the case. The patient should be removed to the hospital, so that no one except hospital nurse can administer the medication and nourishment. If the patient cannot be removed to hospital and if he can afford the expenses, employment of two trained nurses to take charge of the patient in his house and also preparation and administration of food and medicine by them for day and night will be a safeguard against further administration of poison. If that is not possible, the only alternative left for a medical practitioner is to take some near relative of friend in his confidence and inform them about his suspicion.

vii. In every case of suspected poisoning, a doctor, whether in private practice or government job, must preserve all the samples, like vomited matter, stomach wash contents and urine or feces passed that are likely to contain poison in his presence; and suspected food or medicinal articles should be collected in separate wide mouthed glass bottles with glass stoppers tightly fitted. These samples should be properly labeled and preserved and transferred for chemical examination. The treating doctor should also preserve any other evidence of suspected poisoning like bottle, cup, glass, syringes and piece of paper used for wrapping and dispensing the poison. If he fails to do the same or deliberately omits any information, it will lead to sanction u/s **201** IPC for disappearance of evidence.

viii. In a case of death, do not issue the death certificate instead advice autopsy. Police have to be informed for further investigation.

ix. If the public eateries like canteen, cafe and hotel are sourced in a case of food poisoning, public health authorities should be notified.
In conclusion, doctor in cases of poisoning should not refuse to treat the case due to fear of legality or others. They should treat the patient efficiently and adhere to the other legal duties like removal of the patient from the source of poisoning, proper collection of the biological samples for chemical

analysis, reporting the matter to police or magistrate as an where required, recording of dying declaration if needed, handing over the body, if the person dies, to the nearby police for autopsy for confirmation or for further investigation without issuing death certificate. By performing such duties, both clinical and legal, the doctor not only helps the patient but also helps the society by not omitting his duty bound responsibilities.

OPINION ON POISONING CASES

The medical practitioner should be very cautious in giving his or her opinion about the poisoning case. On simple suspicion, he or she should never give a verbal or a written opinion until and unless he or she is sure about the case from symptomology, history of the case and from final toxicological analysis report.

Poisoning report can be done after starting of treatment and having response. The report should never be pending, should give the primary opinion as done by clinicians like death was due to some irritant/corrosive poison or death was due to organophosphorus compound (if found at autopsy). However, exact nature of the poison can be opined after receipt of report of chemical analysis that will be helpful in future trial and help the next of keen of deceased.

LAWS RELATING TO POISON IN INDIA

Poison Act (Act 1 of 1904)

This law was promulgated for restriction of sale of all poisons in certain local areas and importation, possession and sale of white arsenic as well as making licensing mandatory.

The Poison Act, 1919

The Poisons Act, 1919, was enacted by the Government of India with a view to regulate possession for sale and sale of substances specified as poisons.

It is an Act to consolidate and amend the law regulating the importation, possession and sale of poisons. The Act was amended in 1958 and repeated in 1960.

Dangerous Drug Act (Act II of 1930)

The Act was promulgated with an idea to regulate import and sale of narcotics, especially those derived from opium, Indian hemp and coca leaves and this Act was passed to regulate contraband traffic.

Drug Act (Act 23 of 1940)

This Act was passed with an idea to control the quality, strength and purity of drugs and with a view to regulate the importation, manufacture and sale of drugs, such as:

i. Patent medicines
ii. Vaccine, sera, toxins and such other biological products
iii. Vitamins and hormones
iv. Other drugs which are intended for internal or external administration to human being or animals.

This Act was amended in 1955 to bring insecticide, pesticide and contraceptives under its purview. The Act was further amended in 1962 to be known as **Drug and Cosmetic Act, 1940**, to include cosmetics under its purview, and the Act was last amended in 1964 to include Ayurvedic and Unani medicines under its control.

The Drugs and Cosmetic Act, 1940

In the year 1937, a Bill was brought in by the Central Legislative Assembly to give effect to the recommendations of the Drugs Enquiry Committee for the regulation of the import of drugs into British India. With that, the Drugs and Cosmetics Bill was introduced in the Central Legislative Assembly.

Therefore, it is an Act to regulate the import, manufacture, distribution and sale of all kinds of drugs and cosmetics and this Act may be called the **Drugs and Cosmetics Act, 1940**.

One of the important features of this Act is to control the quality, purity and strength of drugs. The patent medicine should display on the label of the bottle, either the actual formula or a list of ingredients present within the medicine. Indian pharmaceutical Good Manufacturing Practice (GMP) guidelines are given in Drugs and cosmetics Act 1940. Rules are given for pharmaceuticals, and schedules are there to comply with those rules. This Act was amended in 1964.

The Drugs and Cosmetics Rules, 1945

This was framed under the Drugs Act, 1940, to regulate the importation of drugs, the functions and procedures of the Central Drugs Laboratory, the appointment of licensing authorities, and the manufacture, distribution and sale of drugs. The drugs and cosmetics rules 1945 have classified drugs into different schedules as follows (**Table 34.1**):

Supply of any drug against prescription must be recorded at the time of supply in a prescription register specially maintained for the purpose.

The Drugs (Control) Act, 1950

The drugs control Act, 1950, is an act to provide for the control of the sale, supply and distribution of drugs, the issue of cash memo for sale, marking of prices and exhibiting list of prices and stocks.

The Drugs and Magic Remedies (Objectionable Advertisements) Act, 1954

An Act to control the advertisement of drugs in certain cases, to prohibit the advertisement for certain purposes of remedies alleged to possess magic qualities and to provide for matters connected therewith.

An advertisement of the magic remedies is completely prohibited on the following:

i. For procuring abortion or prevention of conception
ii. Increase of sexual potency
iii. Correction of menstrual disorders
iv. Treatment of venereal disease

The Insecticides Act, 1968

An Act to regulate the import, manufacture, sale, transport, distribution and use of insecticides with a view to prevent risk to human beings or animals and for matters connected therewith.

It is to be noted that for the purpose of the Act, the term insecticide refers to all substances which are used for destroying any kind of pest in the agricultural, industrial or domestic scenario.

Section 29 of the Act lays down penal provisions for violation of any of the specified guidelines with reference to import, manufacture, sale or exhibition of insecticides.

Insecticides Rules, 1971

The Insecticides Rules, 1971, outlines the procedure for registration of insecticides, as well

Table 34.1 Different schedules of Drugs and Cosmetics Rules, 1945

Schedules	Medicinal substances/products
Schedules C	Biological and special products
Schedules E	List of poisons
Schedules F	Vaccines and sera
Schedules G	Hormone preparations
Schedules H	Drugs (poisons to be sold only on prescription of a registered medical practitioner)
Schedules J	List of diseases for the cure of which no drug should be advertised
Schedules L	Antibiotics, antihistamines and other recent chemotherapeutic agents

as for procuring licenses for their manufacture or sale.

Section 10C of the Rules specifies that "no person shall manufacture, store or expose for sale any insecticide in the same building where any articles consumable by human beings or animals are manufactured, stored or exposed for sale".

The label should also contain in a prominent place, a **diamond-shaped square** the **upper half (triangle)** of which must contain the **following information (Figure 34.1)**:

i. Insecticides belonging to **Category I** *(extremely toxic)* should have the **symbol of a skull and cross-bones** and the word **POISON** printed in **red color.** The following **statements** should also appear on the label **outside the diamond square**:
   a. Keep out of reach of children.
   b. If swallowed, or if symptoms of poisoning occur, call physician immediately.
ii. Insecticides belonging to **Category II** *(highly toxic)* should have the word **POISON** printed in **red color (yellow).** The following **statement** should appear outside: ***Keep out*** **of** ***reach*** **of** ***children.***
iii. Insecticides belonging to **Category III** *(moderately toxic)* should bear the word **DANGER** printed in **black color (blue).** The following statement should appear outside: ***Keep out*** **of** ***reach*** **of** ***children.***
iv. Insecticides belonging to **Category IV** *(slightly toxic)* should bear the word **CAUTION** printed in **black color (green).** The following **statement** should appear outside: ***Keep out*** **of** ***reach*** **of** ***children.***

The **lower half (triangle)** of the **diamond square** on the label should be **colored** as follows **(Figure 34.1)**:

i. **Category I insecticides: Red.** [Word **POISON** printed in **red color, symbol of a skull** and **cross-bones**].
ii. **Category II insecticides: Yellow.** [Word **POISON** printed in **red color].**
iii. **Category III insecticides: Blue.** [Word **DANGER** printed in **black color].**
iv. **Category IV insecticides: Green.** [Word **CAUTION** printed in **black color.**

Chapter VIII of the Insecticides Rules, 1971, details provisions regarding clothing, equipment, and other facilities for workers handling insecticides. **Periodic medical examination** has been made **mandatory**, which also includes blood checks or any other relevant investigations.

The Narcotic Drugs and Psychotropic Substance Act, 1985 (NDPS Act)

An Act to consolidate and amend the law relating to narcotic drugs to make rigorous provisions for the control and regulations of operations relating to narcotic drugs and psychotropic substances and for matters connected therewith.

NDPS Act was enacted in India, and subsequently amended in 1988, to implement the provisions of the convention on psychotropic substances (1971) and the convention against illicit Traffic in Narcotic Drugs and Psychotropic Substances (1988), both held in Vienna.

The minimum punishment for any offence committed under this Act is 10 years rigorous imprisonment and fine of ₹ 1 lakh, while the maximum punishment is for 20 years rigorous imprisonment and fine of ₹ 2 lakh. Provision of punishment for repeat offences is

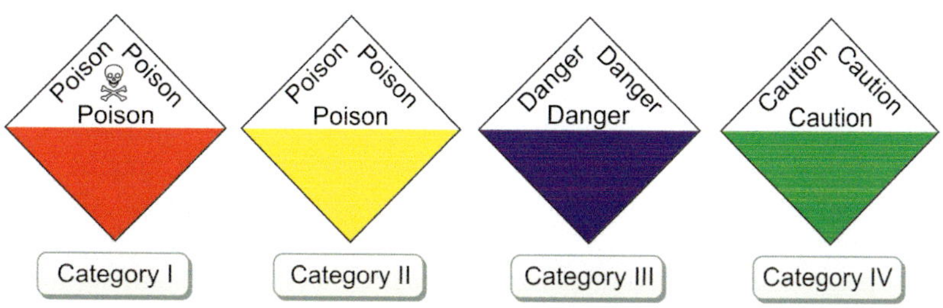

Figure 34.1 Different symbols used in labeling in insecticide preparation

Table 34.2 Substances and their Quantity (seized under NDPS Act)

Substances	Minimum quantity to be seized
Heroin, smack, brown sugar	Equal to or more than 250 mg
Hashish or Charas	5 g
Opium	5 g
Cocaine	125 mg
Ganja	500 g

the death penalty. Under NDPS Act, cultivation of poppy, cannabis and coca plants needs licence.

To constitute an offence under this act, the minimum quantity as quoted in the definition (seized) should be as follows (**Table 34.2**):

Some Other Relevant Acts and Rules

i. The Prevention of Food Adulteration Act, 1954
ii. The Prevention of Food Adulteration Rules 1955

POISONS AND RELATED INDIAN PENAL CODES

Suicide

The tragedy of self-inflicted death has always attracted the attention of the medicolegal fraternity. Attempted suicide is often manipulative and impulsive and undertaken to get rid of an intolerable situation. Drug ingestion is the commonest form. Most persons are psychologically disturbed.[5] Attempted suicide could not be taken as a lighter entity, for it may prove as equally dangerous as suicide itself and sometimes more than that because of so many residual temporary or permanent disabilities.[6]

As per **Section 309 IPC**, whoever attempt to commit suicide and does any act towards the commission of such offence shall be punished with simple imprisonment for a term which may extend to 1 year, or with fine, or with both. In many countries, attempt to commit suicide is regarded more as a manifestation of diseases condition of mind deserving a treatment and care rather than as an offence to be visited with punishment.[7]

Section 299 IPC (culpable homicide): Causing death of a person by an act, with the intention of causing such bodily injury and is likely to cause death, or with the knowledge that he is likely, by such an act to cause death.

Section 272 IPC: Punishment for adulterating food or drink intended for sale, so as to make the same noxious, may extend up to 6 months imprisonment of either term and or fine up to 1000 rupees.

Section 273 IPC: Punishment for selling noxious food or drink may be imprisonment of either description for a period of 6 months and or fine up to 1000 rupees.

Section 274 IPC: Punishment for adulteration of drugs in any form with any change in its effect knowing that it will be sold and used as unadulterated drug, may be imprisonment of either description for a period of 6 months and or fine.

Section 275 IPC: Punishment for knowingly selling adulterated drugs with fewer efficacies or altered action serving it for use as unadulterated may be imprisonment of either description for 6 months and or fine.

Section 276 IPC: Punishment for selling a drug as a different drug or preparation may be imprisonment of either description which may extend upto 6 months and or fine.

State Amendment: It may be mentioned that in the State of West Bengal, the punishment for these offences described under Sections 272 to 276 IPC may be up to imprisonment for life with or without fine.

Section 277 IPC: Punishment for fouling water of public spring or reservoir may be imprisonment of either description which may extend up to a period of 3 months and or fine.

Section 278 IPC: Punishment for voluntarily making atmosphere noxious to health is fine which may extend up to 500 rupees.

Section 284 IPC: Punishment for negligent conduct with respect to poisonous substance may be imprisonment of either description which may extend up to 6 months and or fine which may extend up to 1000 rupees.

Section 348 IPC: Punishment for causing hurt by means of poison or any stupefying, intoxicating or unwholesome drug or any other thing with the intent to commit an offence shall be imprisonment of either description for a term which may extend to 10 years with or without fine.

Section 336 IPC: Act endangering life or personal safety of others.

Section 337 IPC: Causing hurt by act endangering life or personal safety of other.

Section 338 IPC: Causing grievous hurt by act endangering life or personal safety of other.

REFERENCES

1. Gargi J, Rai H, Chanana A, Rai G, Singh K, Garg S. Role of doctor in poisoning—a review. J Punjab Acad Forensic Med Tox. 2008;8(2):34. ISSN 0972-5687.
2. Reddy NKS. The Essentials of Forensic Medicine and Toxicology, 31st ed. Hyderabad: K. Suguna Devi; 2012. p. 467.
3. Srivastava A, Peshin SS, Kaleekal T, Gupta SK. An epidemiological study of poisoning cases reported to the National Poisons Information Centre, All India Institute of Medical Sciences, New Delhi. Hum Exp Toxicol. 2005;24(6):279-85.
4. Jose A, Sivanandam S, Matthai J. Poisoning in children from an educationally and economically advanced urban area of South India. Asian J Epidemiol. 2012;5(4):123-9.
5. Mahanta P. Parasuicide: a case report. J Punjab Acad Forensic Med Tox. 2009;9:106-8.
6. Arun M, Palimar V. Parasuicide: A forensic viewpoint. Medico-Legal Update. 2008;8(1):1-6.
7. Ramchhoddas R, Thakore DK. Ratanlal and Dhirajlal's the IPC; Singh C editor. 28th ed. New Delhi: Wadhwa and Company; 1997. p. 434.

CHAPTER 35

Corrosive Poisons

Putul Mahanta

LEARNING PLAN

- Know the different types of corrosive poisons
- Learn different aspect of various corrosive poisons
- Identify the postmortem changes
- Understand the medicolegal importance of corrosive poisons

DEFINITION

Corrosive poisons are substance that causes burning of tissues when applied. Corrosive poisoning may results from ingestion, topical exposure or inhalation of corrosive compounds that causes tissue burning as a result of chemical reaction. An average home contains various cleaning products which are responsible for a large number of accidental or intentional poisoning. The incidence is about 2–5%, morbidity is more than 50% and mortality about 13%. About 80% of corrosive poisoning occurs in children less than five years of age. Adult exposure has more mortality and morbidity due to large volume of exposure with possible co-ingestion.

Different Corrosive Poisons

Corrosive poisons include various inorganic and organic acids, alkalis, metallic as well as non-metallic compounds as shown in **Table 35.1**.

INORGANIC ACIDS

Sulfuric Acid

Synonym: Oil of vitriol; battery acid.

Properties

Pure sulfuric acid (H_2SO_4) is colorless, heavy, oily, odorless, non-fuming hygroscopic liquid, which emits no fume when exposed to air. When mixed with water, it is reduced in volume and evolves much heat, thus the charring effect. Commercial H_2SO_4 is usually brown or dark in color, due to presence of impurities viz., $PbSO_4$, HNO_3 and lower oxides of N_2.

Uses

Sulfuric acids has many commercial uses, viz. wet battery manufacturing, industrial chemical

Table 35.1 Various corrosive compounds	
Inorganic acids	Sulfuric acid, Nitric acid, Hydrochloric acids
Organic acids	Acetic acid, Carbolic acids, Oxalic acids
Alkali	Sodium hydroxide, Potassium hydroxide, etc.
Metallic salts	Ferric chloride, Zinc chloride, Potassium cyanide, Chromate, etc.
Non-metal compounds	Iodine, Potassium permanganate, Hydrogen peroxide, etc.

(95–98% solution), fertilizer manufacturing (sulfate), drain cleaner (8–10%) and in chemical laboratories. In forensic laboratory, it is used as an ingredient in **diatom test**.

Fatal Dose: 5–10 mL of pure acid is enough to cause death in a human being, but recovery has been recorded to have occurred after ingestion of 120 mL.

Fatal Period: Average fatal period is from 12–24 hours.

Mode of Action

It has a local chemical action of corroding and destroying the tissues with which it comes in contact with and produces coagulation necrosis, by precipitating tissue protein. Sulfuric acid has no remote action.

Clinical Features

After ingestion, immediately there is a severe burning pain in mouth, throat and esophagus and in the stomach with retching, eructation, nausea and vomiting. The initial vomited material is food material which is highly acidic in nature, followed by slimy mucus, mixed with altered blood, which is brownish or blackish in color.

Local corrosive burnt areas are seen around lips with evidence of chemical burns, with dribbling marks over chin, even over the chest, may even sometimes be found over nose and over dorsum of hand. Death, if occurs within 24 hours, is due to circulatory failure and shock, and if within few days, it is due to superadded infection due to sloughing of the corroded membrane and if it is after several months, it is mostly due to malnutrition, due to total cicatrization of mucous membrane of stomach and small intestine.

Diagnosis

i. **Litmus test**: The pH of the saliva can be tested with a litmus paper to determine whether the chemical ingested is acid or an alkali.
ii. **Fresh stains** in clothing may be tested by adding a few drops of sodium carbonate. Production of bubble is an indicative of an acidic stain.

Management

i. Stomach-tube or emetics should not be used. However, a Levin tube may be passed within half an hour of ingestion.
ii. Antacids may reduce the chances of perforation.
iii. The acid should be immediately neutralized or diluted in situ, by administration a pint of water or milk with 4 tablespoonful of calcium or magnesium oxide or aluminum hydroxide or calcined magnesia (CO_3 and HCO_3 should never be used as it will liberate huge amount of CO_2 gas which may cause rupture of stomach).
iv. Demulcents, viz. barley water, olive oil and molten butter may be given.
v. Corticosteroids by injection to combat the circulatory failure and by oral route prevent cicatrization.

Postmortem Findings

Evidence of brownish coloration (marks of chemical burn), running vertically down from the angles of the mouth may be present.

Lips, tongue and mucous membrane of mouth will be seen to be grossly corroded with evidence of sub-mucosal hemorrhage. Tongue will be swollen, practically converted to a shapeless mass with a white coating, resembling soaked parchment, which ultimately turns brownish or blackish.

The wall of esophagus will be fragile with evidence of longitudinal corrosion along the whole length. The stomach will be blackish, corroded, may be converted into a shapeless mass with evidence of multiple perforations, and may contain inside, some blackish grumous mass.

There may be evidence of corrosion and blackening seen in other organs around the stomach, including under surface of liver, etc. Similarly, changes may be seen in the small intestine. If death is delayed, fatty degenerative changes in various organs, including liver, is seen.

Medicolegal Importance

i. **Suicide**: It is one of the very common poisons for committing suicide.
ii. **Vitriolage:** Throwing of sulfuric acid or other corrosive substances on another person is known as vitriolage. Because of jealousy, a person may throw corrosive to disfigure the clothes or the face. This may sometimes result in blindness. Death may result from shock or toxemia. Sometimes juice of marking nut or Calotropis is used to disfigure the face.
iii. Accidental poisoning though rare may occur and is due to mistaken for glycerin or castor oil or some other substances.

Nitric Acid (HNO_3)

Synonyms: Aqua forties or red spirit of niter

Properties

Nitric acid is a clear, colorless fluid, which gives off colorless fumes when exposed to air and has a peculiar choking odor. It is a strong oxidant which can dissolve all metal except antimony and platinum. When saturated with red oxide of N_2, N_2O_3, it gives a brown fume and is known as fuming HNO_3.

Uses

Commercial uses: Commonly used by goldsmiths and in industries, also used in fertilizers. Nitric acid is used for manufacturing picric acid and nitro-cellulose; both are used as an explosive. **Medicolegal uses** of nitric acid are suicidal and vitriolage.

Fatal Dose: 10–15 mL

Fatal Period: 12–24 hours.

Clinical Features

Almost same as sulfuric acid, except the following special features:

i. Reacts with protein to form a xanthoproteic compound, which has an intense yellow coloration.
ii. Oliguria with presence of cast and albumin.
iii. Because it has a fuming character, it involves upper respiratory tract, with yellowish color change and corrosion.

Treatment: Same as for sulfuric acid.

Postmortem Findings

Almost same as that of sulfuric acid, except for deep yellow coloration of mucous membrane due to xanthoproteic reaction on the tissue.

Hydrochloric Acid (HCl)

Synonyms: Muriatic acid, spirit of salts

Properties

Pure hydrochloric acid is a colorless gas, which is extremely soluble in water and one volume of water dissolves 480 volume of gas at 0°C. Commercial acid, commonly known as muriatic acid, is a yellowish liquid which fumes strongly and may yield dense white vapors, when mixed with NH_3 (Ammonia).

Uses

Hydrochloric acid is commonly used as cleaning agent of ceramic surfaces and for preparation of Chlorine.

Medical Uses: (i) In achlorhydria as treatment, (ii) In hemoglobin estimation, and (iii) In chemical and biochemical laboratory.

Oxalic Acid

Synonyms: Acid of sugar, salts of sorrel

Properties

It is colorless, odorless, transparent prismatic shiny crystal with a sour, slightly bitter taste. It is an organic acid and is intensely poisonous. It is soluble in 10 parts of cold water, and when heated at 82°C (180°F) it volatilizes.

Source

It is commonly obtained from sugar, by oxidation with Nitric Acid (HNO_3) and is commercially manufactured from pine saw dust, being oxidized by fusion with caustic alkalis.

Uses

i. As bleaching and cleaning agent used commonly for cleaning of glasses and metals.
ii. Manufacturing straw hats.
iii. To polish floor and for removal of ink stain or iron-mould from clothing.
iv. In industry: Ceramic, leather, pharmaceutical and rubber industry.

Criminal Use

Because of its ink staining removing property, it is used by forgers to remove writings from papers and documents.

Mode of Action

Local Action: It is a dual acting poison, which acts locally as corrosive.

Systemic Action: After absorption, it exerts its systemic activity by precipitation of ionized Ca^{++} in plasma, resulting hypocalcemia and insoluble calcium oxalate is precipitated in the liver, kidney, heart, lungs and blood and excreted in the urine, which is called **oxaluria.** Sometimes, after taking a huge dose, the patient may succumb within few minutes without showing much of the local effects.

Differential Diagnosis (Table 35.2)

Fatal Dose: 15–25 g

Fatal Period: 1–2 hours.

Clinical Features

Immediately after intake, there is intense sour taste with severe burning pain in the mouth, throat and stomach, which gradually spreads all over the abdomen. There is retching, nausea and vomiting. The vomited matter is highly acidic, may be mixed with food contents and later on will be just shredded mucus with altered blood, may have a coffee-ground appearance and this vomiting continues till death. Diarrhea is unusual but tenesmus is present.

Table 35.2 Differentiating points between oxalic acid, $MgSO_4$ and $ZnSO_4$

Differentiating point	Oxalic acid	Magnesium sulfate	Zinc sulfate
Taste	Sour	Nauseating and bitter	Metallic, bitter
Reaction	Strongly acidic	Neutral	Weakly acidic
Application of heat	Sublimes	Fixed	Fixed
Effect on stains (iron and ink, etc.)	Disappears	No change	No change

Initially there is oliguria or anuria, and if the patient survives for a few days, it will be replaced by diuresis. For first two days, urine shows presence of excess of albumin, hyaline cast and crystals of calcium-oxalate.

On absorption, oxalic acid combines with ionized Ca^{++} of the body, which is being predicted as Ca-oxalate and is excreted through kidney, resulting in development of features of hypocalcemia, manifested by tetany, convulsion, lock-jaw and is said to have an effect on parathyroid metabolism.

There is severe prostration with cold, clammy sweaty limbs and hurried respiration; gradually, the patient passes into coma which ultimately ends in death. Cramps, generalized convulsion and delirium may precede death.

Management

Stomach wash with plain water is not recommended as oxalic acid is freely soluble in water, and facilitates rapid absorption. Therefore, stomach washing is done by a fluid mixed with Ca, in the form of chalk, calcined magnesia or calcium lactate, which reacts with oxalic acid to form calcium oxalate crystals. It is said that 1 g of chalk neutralizes 1.5 g of oxalic acid.

i. Frequent administration of milk and saccharated lime solution is considered to be the best way of treatment.
ii. Alkalis and their carbonates should never be administered, as they unite with oxalic acid to form poisonous salts.
iii. Antidote is calcium gluconate which is given as 10% calcium gluconate, 10 mL, intravenously.
iv. Twenty five percent glucose should be given intravenously.
v. For acidosis, $NaHCO_3$ should be given.
vi. Some books have recommended use of 100 unit of Parathyroid Hormone, which helps in metabolism of calcium.
vii. Dialysis or exchange transfusion for renal failure.
viii. Affected skin or eyes should be washed copiously with water.

Postmortem Findings

With concentrated form, marked signs of corrosion will be seen in mouth, throat, esophagus and stomach. Mucous membrane of those places is seen to be whitish or ashy-white, shriveled, corroded and can be easily detached from the underlying tissues. They are sometimes found corroded, corrugated and show longitudinal corrosion.

All will show evidence of sub-mucosal hemorrhage. Stomach becomes very friable and on opening, contains dark brown grumous liquid due to formation of acid hematin. The mucous membrane will be corroded and can be easily separated from the sub mucosal layer, where the sub-mucosal blood vessel will appear like a black network due to intravascular formation of acid hematin.

Perforation of stomach is very rare. Shiny crystals of oxalic acid may be seen embedded in the inflamed and edematous mucous membrane of the stomach. When a person dies after intake of a heavy dose, there may not be any typical appearance in the stomach which may even look pale.

Upper part of small intestine may show similar changes that of stomach. If the acid has been taken in a very dilute form, there will be just sign of irritation with redness, congestion and inflammation of mucous membrane. Kidneys will be enlarged, inflamed and on section may show scattered hemorrhages and on histopathological examination, tubules will be seen to be loaded with octahedral crystals of Ca-oxalate with evidence of acute tubular necrosis.

Medicolegal Importance

i. **Accidental**: It is common because it is commonly being mistaken with $ZnSO_4$ and $MgSO_4$ from which it is to be differentiated.
ii. **Homicidal**: Not common for its intense sour taste and a burning sensation in the mouth, unless the taste in masked.
iii. **Suicidal**: Though a few cases are on record, it is not very common.

Carbolic Acid

Synonyms: Phenol or hydroxybenzene

Properties

Carbolic acid is a hydroxybenzene, obtained by fractional distillation of coal tar, but is commercially prepared from acetylene by synthesis.

In its pure form it appears as short, colorless prismatic needle-shaped crystals in masses, which have a burning sweetish taste, which are very hygroscopic, draws water from the atmosphere and becomes liquid and the color is changed to pinkish or brownish with peculiar, pungent, disagreeable odor containing several impurities, chiefly cresol. It is neither acidic, nor alkaline and it is rather amphoteric. Even though it is not acidic, it is called acid, because it forms carbonates, when acted upon by strong alkalis or bases.

Lysol is a 50% solution of cresol in saponified vegetable oil. Phenol is about eight times more toxic than Lysol. Dettol is a chlorinated phenol with turpineol.

Carbolism is a term used to denote carbolic acid poisoning.

Carbolemia means presence of carbolic acid in the blood.

Ochronosis means pigmentation of the cornea and various cartilages by the hydroquinone and pyrocatechol.

Carboluria mean color change as seen in voided urine in carbolic acid poisoning. Normal color of urine, on standing, changes to olive green color. This is due to further oxidation of metabolites of carbolic acid, namely, hydroxyquinone and pyrocatechol.

Commercial Uses

i. **Antiseptic and disinfectant**: Especially for sterilizing floor, walls, furnishings, glassware and instruments. Carbolic acid comes into composition of various antiseptic lotions, namely, cresol, Lysol, etc. It is popularly accepted to be a snake-repellent, though it has no basis.
ii. **Medical uses**: Previously, it was used as an antiseptic lotion for wound-dressing, especially dog-bite wounds, and even for cauterizing appendicular stump after appendectomy operation. It can also been used as "Face peel" in plastic surgery.
iii. **Pharmaceuticals**: It is a pharmacopeal product and is dispensed in the name of guttae for treatment of otitis externa.
iv. **Preservative**: Phenol is a commonly used preservative in injectable medications, e.g. glucagons, pethidine, neostigmine, guanidine and epinephrine.

Mode of Action

Carbolic acid is also a dual-acting poison.

Local Action: Locally it act as a mild corrosive and acts by coagulating tissue protein without coming into its composition, hence remaining free and thus having deep penetrating power. It has got local anesthetic effect over peripheral nerve. It causes extensive capillary damage and clotting in peripheral vessels. On intact skin, it causes burning sensation followed by tingling, numbness and anesthesia; forms white opaque eschar, which falls off in a few days, leaving brown stain which persists for a long time. When evaporation is prevented, even a weaker solution will cause necrosis and sloughing of the area. On mucus membrane, it causes irritation, inflammation, necrosis and sloughing.

Systemic Action: On absorption, it acts as a central nervous system depressant.

Absorption

It is readily absorbed from the GIT, respiratory tract, rectum, vagina, serous cavities and wounds and through infact the skin.

Fatal Dose: 2 g crystals; 25–50 mL of household phenol

Fatal Period: 3–4 hours on an average, may even be within 20 minutes.

Clinical Features

a. **Local**: When it comes in contact with skin, initially it produces burning sensation followed by tingling and numbness and loss of sensation due to its anesthetic action on peripheral sensory nerves. White opaque eschar, which falls off in a few days leaving a brown stain is seen, if the patient survives. Tissue necrosis may also be present.
b. **After ingestion**: Intense burning sensation in the mouth going down to throat to stomach with occasional vomiting. Vomiting is less intense due to local anesthetic effect on the nerves of stomach. Gangrenous changes of stomach and intestines may also be present.

It is rapidly absorbed in the bloodstream and neurological manifestations, namely, giddiness and insensibility, which gradually passes into coma. The face is usually cyanosed; pupils are contracted to pinpoint with cold and clammy skin with subnormal temperature.

Pulse is weak, and thready. Blood pressure is low, respiration slow, labored and stertorous. Initially, there is respiratory alkalosis with succeeding severe acidosis. The exhaled air smells strongly of carbolic acid.

There may be muscular spasm, convulsion and lockjaw, though rare. Anuria or oliguria is also present. When urine is voided, it is normal in color, on standing and on exposure to air, it becomes dark to olive green in color due to further oxidation of **hydroxyquinone** and **pyrocatechol**, which are oxidation products of carbolic acid. Deaths usually result from failure of respiratory center.

Management

Emetic fails to induce vomiting due to local anesthetic effect on gastric and mucous membrane. As such, soft stomach tube is passed with caution and stomach is thoroughly washed with luke-warm water or 10% glycerin in water. Mg or Na sulfate, saccharated lime or animal charcoal may be added to this. Stomach wash should be continued till smell of carbolic acid is perceivable. Some amount of castor oil or olive oil should be left in the stomach after stomach wash.

Intravenous infusion of normal saline or $NaHCO_3$ helps to combat acidosis and circulatory depression. Hemodialysis is useful for renal failure. Other symptomatic treatments should be given.

Postmortem Findings

Dark-brownish marks of corrosion will be seen at the angles of mouth. Mucous membrane of lip, mouth and throat will be ashy grey, hardened, congested and corroded, which can be easily peeled off showing gross, congested submucosa, from which strong smell of carbolic acid comes. Same changes will be seen in the upper-part of small intestine. All other viscera will be congested. Kidneys will be enlarged with cortical hemorrhages.

Medicolegal Importance

i. Previously it was a very popular poison for suicide, but nowadays it is not common.
ii. Accidental poisoning are common, more so as it is absorbed even from unbroken skin.
iii. Homicidal use of carbolic acid is very uncommon, because of its peculiar smell, though a few cases of infanticide have been recorded.

ACID THROWING

Synonyms: Acid attack, vitriolage

Acid throwing, also called an acid attack[1] or **vitriolage**, is a form of violent assault.[2] It is defined as the act of throwing acid onto the body of a person "with the intention of injuring or disfiguring [them] out of jealousy or revenge".[3]

Literally, it means throwing of oil of vitriol, i.e. H_2SO_4, on one's body or face maliciously in order to disfigure or blind him or her. The motive is usually revenge or jealousy. But, legally it means throwing of any corrosive, in the face or body of other persons that include any corrosive acids or even juice of semecarpus anacardium.

Perpetrators of these attacks throw acid at their victims, usually at their faces, burning them, and damaging skin tissue, often exposing and sometimes dissolving the bones.[4] The long-term consequences of these attacks include blindness and permanent scarring of the face and body.[5-7]

These attacks are most common in Cambodia,[8] Afghanistan,[9] India,[10] Bangladesh[5,6] Pakistan[5] and other nearby countries.[7] Globally, at least 1500 people in 20 countries are attacked in this way yearly, 80% of whom are female and somewhere between 40% and 70% under 18 years of age.[7,11]

In India, it is regarded as a grievous hurt. Death may occur from shock or toxemia if extensive area is involved. The burns are mainly painless and are penetrating that devitalizes the tissues and predispose to infection.

In **acid bath murder** case, concentrated sulfuric acids were being used to dissolve a human body, after causing murder.

CORROSIVE ALKALIS

Properties

It gives rise to OH^- ion in aqueous medium and reacts with acid to produce salt and water. Like mineral acids, the strong solution of alkalis also act as corrosive, but in dilute forms they act as an irritants. Concentrated corrosive alkalis are more dangerous than acid.

The **chief alkaline corrosives** are:

i. Ammonia: Gaseous ammonia dissolved in water, forms solution of ammonia known as "Sprits of Hartshorne", a colorless strongly alkaline pungent liquid.
ii. Potassium hydroxide or caustic soda.
iii. Sodium hydroxide or caustic soda.
iv. Calcium hydroxide.
v. Ammonium carbonate.
vi. Sodium carbonate or washing soda.

A mixture of caustic soda and washing soda is known as 'Lye' used for washing purposes.

Sources: Industries, laboratories.

Uses

i. As chemical
ii. As bleaching agents
iii. In industries
iv. Also in medicines.

Action

It causes irritation of the skin and corrodes mucous membrane. The caustic action of alkalis is due to its rapid absorption of water from the tissues. They combine with fats to form alkaline soap and with protein to form alkali proteinates, thus producing soft necrotic areas on contact with tissues. The action of corrosive alkali is slower than other corrosive like acid, but long sustained. Intense stimulation by alkalis on absorption may cause reflex loss of vascular tone and cardiac inhabitation.

Fatal Dose: Ammonia-30 mL, potassium or sodium hydroxide-5 g, potassium carbonate-15 gm, sodium carbonate-30 g

Fatal Period: Inhalation of ammonia vapor may cause death within four minutes from edematous glottis. Death more than a week or more is basically because of bronchopneumonia, exhaustion, etc.

Clinical Features

Local: The affected part will get burnt and discolored due to concentrated caustic alkaline solution. The extent of injuries will depend upon the duration of contact as the alkali penetrates skin slowly.

Ingestion: There is burning sensation in the mouth, throat and abdomen. Beside this there is a sensation of caustic, soapy and nauseous taste in the mouth. With concentrated solution, there will be excoriation and ulceration of mucous membrane of mouth, tongue and stomach; often it is reddish brown in appearance. This is due to hemorrhage. There is vomiting and products of vomitus contains altered blood, and it is alkaline in nature. There is loose motion and the stool may contain blood and excessive mucous. Dysphasia and dyspnea may be present.

The abdominal pain may assume colic and is tender on pressure. There may be delayed gastric or esophageal perforation after 2-4 days, even after initial recovery. Skin becomes cold and clammy, pulse-quick, weak and feeble. Eyes shrunken, pupils dilated. Later, shock, collapse and death will ensue.

Concentrated alkalis coming in contact with eyes may cause conjunctival edema, corneal dysfunction, leading to blindness of any degree.

Death may occur immediately from vagal inhibition or edema of the glottis, within 12–24 hours from shock or pulmonary edema, or later on from pneumonia or bronchopneumonia.

Management

i. Stomach wash and emetics should not be tried because of danger of perforation.
ii. Should try to neutralize the alkali by weak vegetable acids, viz. 3–5% of acetic acid (Vinegar), citric acid (lemon or orange juice), 0.5% hydrochloric acid, etc. along with water.
iii. Demulcent should be given to protect the stomach wall, viz. milk, lemon, barley, white of egg, etc.
iv. Sedatives can be used if pain is intolerable and if there is convulsion.
v. Supportive treatment for respiration and to combat shock if necessary.

Postmortem Findings

Marks of corrosion are found over lips, mucous membrane of mouth, lips, tongue and esophagus. They are found softened, swollen and edematous and inflamed with an evidence of shredding off at places, presenting deep chocolate or dark brown color.

Stomach looks congested and black-brownish in color, contains thick, dark slimy fluid, strongly alkaline in reaction. The walls are intensely inflamed with patchy areas of sub-mucosal hemorrhage. Perforation of stomach is rare.

Mucous membrane of respiratory passage will show inflammation, congestion and edema. All viscera are congested. Lungs may show bronchopneumonia and on section bronchiolitis may be seen.

Medicolegal Importance

Accidental poisoning from caustic alkalis is common for mistakenly taking it as ginger beer, medicines, lemonades, etc. Children can swallow cleaning agents left carelessly inside the house. Leakage in ammonia vapor in industries may cause fatal accident due to inhalation. Ammonia is usually not used for homicidal purpose for its strong odors. But it may be thrown on the face for revenge to disfigure. Otherwise homicidal and suicidal uses are rare.

AMMONIA

Ammonia or **azane** is a chemical compound of nitrogen and hydrogen and the formula is NH_3. It is a colorless gas with a characteristic pungent smell.

Properties

It is a gas, which when dissolved in water, forms strong liquid ammonia, popularly known as liquor common forties or aquq ammonia. It contains 32.5% of NH_3. It is a colorless liquid and strongly alkaline, having a very pungent, irritating characteristics odor.

Common Use: It is commercially used as refrigerant. In fertilizer industry for manufacture of NH_4SO_4.

Clinical Features of Poisoning

Taste is acrid and soapy, and vomitus is strongly alkaline and does not effervesce on contact with cement. Severe burning taste in the mouth is felt. Vomited matter initially is thick and slimy, later on contains dark altered blood. Unlike corrosive acid poisoning, purgation is a frequent, and as ammoniacal vapor is irritant to respiratory system and when inhaled, produces congestion, watering of eyes, running nose, salivation, sneezing, edema glottis and pulmonary edema. It may even produce corneal ulcer, iridocyclities, etc.

Fatal Dose: 30 mL of ammonia

Fatal Period: Usually 24 hours, but inhalation may cause death within four minutes.

Management

i. In mild cases, stomach tube can be used cautiously.
ii. To neutralize alkaline poisons, vegetable acid, like lemon or orange juice, vinegar, mixed with large quantity of water is used.
iii. Rest is symptomatic.

REFERENCES

1. BBC News. 2010-03-21. Archived from the original news on 25 March 2010. [cited on 2012-04-35].
2. Karmakar RN. Forensic Medicine and Toxicology, 1st ed. Kolkata: Academic Publishers; 2006. p. 56.
3. Krishan V. Textbook of Forensic Medicine and Toxicology: Principles and Practice, 5th ed. India: Elsevier; 2011. p. 462.
4. Swanson J. Acid attacks: Bangladesh's efforts to stop the violence. Harvard Health Policy Review 3 (Spring 2002). [cited 2012 June 18th]: p. 3.
5. Bandyopadhyay M, Khan MR. Loss of face: violence against women in South Asia. In: Lenore Manderson, Linda Rae Bennett (eds), Violence against Women in Asian Societies. Routledge; 2003. ISBN 978-0-7007-1741-5.
6. CNN.com—Bangladesh combats an acid onslaught against women—November 11, 2000" Archived from the original on September 22, 2007. [cited on 2009-03-13].
7. Bahl T, Syed MH. Encyclopaedia of the Muslim World. Anmol Publications Pvt. Ltd. 2004. ISBN 978-81-261-1419-1.
8. Mydans S. Vengeance Destroys Faces, and Souls, in Cambodia. The New York Times. Retrieved 2008-08-29.
9. Chavis EM. Meena. Heroine of Afghanistan. St Martin's Press; 2003. ISBN 978-0-312-30689-2.
10. Whalen AC. Mother Earth and the Gene Machines. Vantage Press; 2006. ISBN 978-0-535-15359-8.
11. Defacing Women: Acid Attacks on Film. Acid Survivors Trust International.

CHAPTER 36

Inorganic Irritants: Non-metallic Poisons

Putul Mahanta

LEARNING PLAN

- Know regarding the inorganic irritant non-metallic poisons
- Identify the postmortem changes
- Understand the medicolegal importance

INORGANIC IRRITANT POISONS

Inorganic irritant poisons are those which, by their specific action, set up an inflammatory reaction in the gastrointestinal tract. The examples of non-metallic inorganic irritant poisons are:

i. Iodine
ii. Phosphorus
iii. Chlorine
iv. Bromine
v. Fluorine, etc.

IODINE

Iodine is a naturally occurring chemical. For good health, small amounts are needed. However, large amount of it can cause harm. Children are especially sensitive to the effects of toxic dose of iodine.

Features

Iodine is a bluish-black, bright, solid, soft and scaly crystals. Although it is less reactive than the elements in group of fluorine, chlorine and bromine, etc. It still forms compounds with many other elements.

Though iodine is a non-metal, it displays some metallic properties. While dissolved in chloroform, carbon tetrachloride or carbon disulfide, it gives purple colored solutions. It is hardly soluble in water, giving a yellow solution.

Uses of Iodine

i. In medicine, in both radioactive and non-radioactive forms. Iodide and thyroxin, which contains iodine, are used inside the body.
ii. A solution containing potassium iodide and iodine in alcohol is used to disinfect external wounds.

iii. Elemental iodine is also used as a disinfectant.
iv. Iodine is added to edible salt to prevent thyroid disease.
v. Iodine's other uses include catalysts, animal feeds, printing inks, dyes and silver iodide in photography.

Mechanism of Action

Iodine is absorbed rapidly from gastrointestinal tract. Small doses are usually changed to iodide and iodate in the bowel. Large doses are absorbed unchanged and reacts with proteins of the body. Iodine is a protoplasmic poison fixing protein and causing necrosis. Strong iodine solution on local application causes an intense irritation. When its vapor is inhaled, it causes irritation of respiratory passages.

Fatal Dose: 2–4 g of iodine; 30–60 mL of tincture.

Fatal Period: 24 hours.

Clinical Features

Acute Poisoning

Local Features: Causes irritation, inflammation and necrosis with yellowish-brown staining of skin.

Inhalation: Inhalation causes irritation of respiratory tract, rhinorrhea and coughing, shortness of breath, pulmonary and glottic edema.

Ingestion: In the solid form when taken it act as corrosive. Symptoms include burning pain in the mouth and esophagus, metallic taste in mouth, thirst, salivation, abdominal pain, vomiting, diarrhea, delirium, fever, shock and stupor. There is nephritis, renal failure, oliguria and circulatory collapse. The mucous membranes are stained brown by iodine. Urine is red-brown in color and contains albumin. Seizures are also commonly observed.

Management

i. Local: Wash with plenty of water or alcohol (20%).
ii. For eye exposure, irrigation should be carried out with running clean water.
iii. When ingested, patient should receive gastric lavage, activated charcoal.
iv. Keep the person hydrated with enough fluids; milk, cornstarch and flour mixed with water will be an effective diet.
v. But, if the person is suffering from vomiting, then avoid giving him foods.
vi. Sodium bicarbonate for metabolic acidosis.
vii. 1–5% solution of sodium thiosulfate will convert tincture of iodine to harmless iodide.
viii. Hemodialysis followed by continuous venovenous hemodiafiltration.[1]
ix. Breathing support.
x. Symptomatic.

Autopsy Findings

i. Clothes, skin, lips, hand, etc., will be stained yellowish brown.
ii. Mucosa of mouth, esophagus, stomach and intestine will be yellowish-brown.
iii. The mucosa of the stomach and intestine will be inflamed, excoriated.
iv. Heart, liver and kidneys may show fatty degeneration.
v. Iodine-like smell will be present.
vi. All visceras will be congested.

Chronic Poisoning

The condition is called **iodism**. The person may appear to be nervous. The eyeballs of this patient might protrude, appearing to be too big. One of the signs is abnormal sensitivity in the retina. A person suffering from this poison might have clear distant vision, but his near vision will be weak. There is conjunctivitis, rhinorrhea and stomatitis.

There is loss of appetite, insomnia, lymphadenopathy and emaciation. In the skin, there is erythema, urticaria and acne, which are known as **ioderma**.

Management

i. Further iodine exposure should be stopped.
ii. Increase intake of sodium chloride as NaCl will compete with iodine at the level of renal tubules to promote excretion of iodide.

Medicolegal Importance

i. It rarely causes poisoning.
ii. Mainly accidental poisoning is seen due to overdose and idiosyncrasy.
iii. Iodinated radiologic contrast media sometimes causes anaphylactic reaction.

PHOSPHORUS

Types of Phosphorus

Elemental phosphorus exists in two major forms. They are:
i. White or yellow phosphorus
ii. Red phosphorus

The white variety of phosphorus becomes yellow on exposure to light. Hence, it is also known as yellow phosphorus. On exposure to air, it slowly gets oxidized and emits white fumes of phosphorus trioxide. They are poisonous.

Red phosphorus, on the other hand, is not poisonous, but commercial red variety may contain poisonous white phosphorus as impurity. The difference between white and red phosphorus are mentioned in **Table 36.1**.

Uses

White phosphorus is used in preparation of:
i. Insecticide and rodenticide
ii. Fertilizers
iii. Pyrotechnics (fireworks)
iv. Gun powder
v. Cleaning agents
vi. Alloys
vii. Water softening[2] for washing cloth with detergent.

Red phosphorus is used in preparation of:
i. Strike plate of match box
ii. Synthesis of drugs
iii. Flame retardant
iv. Smoke and obscurant devices also sometimes employ the properties of red phosphorous.

Fatal Dose: 50–100 mg of white phosphorus is deadly toxic.

Fatal Period: 2–8 days.

Mechanism of Action

White phosphorus acts as a protoplasmic poison and affects the oxidation at the cellular level. They are hepatotoxic, nephrotoxic, cardiotoxic and act as a strong irritant to skin and mucosa.

Absorption, Metabolism and Excretion

Phosphorus is absorbed rapidly when stomach contains fatty food. On absorption, phosphorus is distributed to all organs where it retained and metabolized to hypophosphate and it is excreted through urine. A very small part of it excreted unchanged through feces and expired air.

Clinical Features

The vast majority of phosphorus compounds are consumed as fertilizers. Other applications include the role of organophosphorus compounds in detergents, pesticides, nerve agents and matches.[3]

Table 36.1 Difference between white/yellow and red phosphorus

Properties	White or yellow phosphorus	Red phosphorus
Color and appearance	Waxy, white crystalline translucent soft cylinders. On exposure to air, it becomes yellow	Violet red amorphous mass
Taste and odor	Garlicky odor and taste	Odorless, tasteless
Brightness in dark	Luminous	Not luminous
Exposure to air	Phosphorescing vapor (white fumes of phosphorous trioxide)	Stable in air
Toxicity	Highly poisonous	Non-poisonous

Fulminating Poisoning: This is seen when more than 1 g is taken. The victim suffers from shock and cardiovascular collapse and dies within 12 hours.

Those who survive more than 12 hours are restless, delirious and may complain of thirst, severe vomiting and retching.

Acute Poisoning

There appear three stages extending over a period of 8–10 days.

First Stage: Due to local acute irritation of gastrointestinal tract, symptoms occur within a few minutes to few hours and last from eight hours to three days.

The intoxication is characterized initially by nausea, throat and stomach pain, vomiting, diarrhea and an odor of garlic on breath and excreta. Vomitus and stool may be luminous in the dark. Fumes may evolve from the stools, which is called **smoky stool syndrome**. Physical contact with the vomitus and feces of the patient is avoided.

Second Stage: If patient survives, the acuteness of symptoms may subside. This symptom-free period lasts for 2–3 days.

Third Stage: After a few days of apparent recovery, the symptoms of first stage reappear with increased severity and with renal and hepatic dysfunction.

There is enlarged and tender liver, jaundice, pruritus and encephalopathy. Renal failure is manifested by oliguria, hematuria, albuminuria and sometimes anuria.

Involvement of central nervous system causes convulsions, delirium and coma. In a case of survival, symptoms may last for a long time. Death may be due to shock, hepatic failure or renal failure or due to central nervous system damage.

Management

i. Gastric lavage with 1: 5000 solution of potassium permanganate. It oxidizes phosphorus into less toxic phosphoric acid and phosphate.
ii. Oils and fats are to be avoided, as they dissolve phosphorus and promote its absorption.
iii. Bowel should be evacuated with magnesium sulfate.
iv. IV glucose or plasma with vitamin K and noradrenaline is useful in protecting liver and combating shock, etc.
v. Hemodialysis or peritoneal dialysis may be required.

Autopsy Findings[4]

i. Petechial hemorrhages may be noted over skin
ii. Jaundice
iii. Garlicky odor
iv. Gastric mucosa is yellowish or greenish-white in color and softened
v. Gastric contents emits garlicky odor and luminous in dark
vi. Liver shows necrobiosis. Liver is enlarged, doughy in consistency, uniformly yellow and contains many hemorrhagic areas in parenchyma
vii. Heart, kidneys and voluntary muscle fibers shows fatty degeneration
viii On microscopy, hepatocellular necrosis and cholestasis are seen.

Chronic Poisoning

The main contact of the patients with the poison is inhalation of fumes while working in the factory over years. The chronic intoxication is initially characterized by nausea, vomiting, diarrhea, emaciation and abdominal pain. There is wasting, loss of weight and weakness of muscle. The patient develops anemia and jaundice.

Phossy Jaw or Glass Jaw

It develops in the lower jaw of the person who has caries of the tooth. The patient complains of pain with the tooth (and lower jaw) with swelling of the gums. There is loosening of teeth, sloughing of gums followed by necrosis, sequestration and osteomyelitis of mandible. There may be multiple sinuses discharging foul smelling pus.

Management

i. Periodic checkup of teeth of worker working in the match factory should be done.
ii. If caries of teeth is detected, it should be filled up or extracted if needed.
iii. Oils and fats are to be condemned.
iv. Turpentine vapors should be saturated in the working room.
v. Personnel cleanness should be advised.

Medicolegal Importance

i. Accidental poisoning is seen with the children due to chewing of phosphorus containing paste, though it's poisoning is rare in India.
ii. Liquid form of phosphorus is more harmful than the solid form. Suicidal and homicidal uses are rarely seen.

REFERENCES

1. Kanakiriya S, De Chazal I, Nath KA, Haugen EN, Albright RC, Juncos LA. Iodine toxicity treated with hemodialysis and continuous hemodiafiltration. Am J kidney Dis. 2003;41:702-8.
2. Hammond CR. The elements. In: Handbook of Chemistry and Physics, 81st ed. CRC Press; 2000. ISBN 0-8493-0481-4.
3. Diskowski H, Hofmann T. Phosphorus. In: Ullmann's Encyclopedia of Industrial Chemistry. Wiley-VCH, Weinheim; 2005.
4. Fernandez OU, Conizares LL. Acute hepatotoxicity from ingestion of yellow phosphorus containing fireworks. J clin Gastroenterol. 1995;21:139-42.

CHAPTER 37

Inorganic Irritants: Metallic Poisons

Putul Mahanta

LEARNING PLAN

- Learn the metallic poisons, viz. arsenic, lead, mercury, copper, silver, gold, thallium and iron
- Know the mechanism of action, clinical features, diagnosis and management
- Identify the postmortem changes
- Understand their medicolegal importance

METALLIC POISON

Many metals and their salts cause poisoning. They pose a significant threat to human health through environmental as well as occupational hazards. The metals may enter the body by: ingestion, inhalation and absorption through the skin or mucous membranes. These metals poisoning can be acute or chronic and may be caused by the followings: arsenic, lead, mercury, copper, silver, gold, thallium, iron, cadmium, iron, etc. Metals are then stored in the various soft tissues of the body. Once absorbed, they compete with other ions and bind to proteins, leading to impaired enzymatic activities resulting in damage to many organs throughout the body.

ARSENIC (As)

Arsenic is the most common source of acute heavy-metal poisoning and is second only to lead in the incidence of chronic toxicity (**Figure 37.1**).

Properties

Technically, it is not a true metal but semi-metal. Arsenic is not soluble and is not absorbed from the alimentary canal. Intrinsically, it is not poisonous. On exposure to air, it get oxidized and is converted to trioxide of arsenic or arsenious acid or arsenious oxide or white arsenic, which is most poisonous substance.

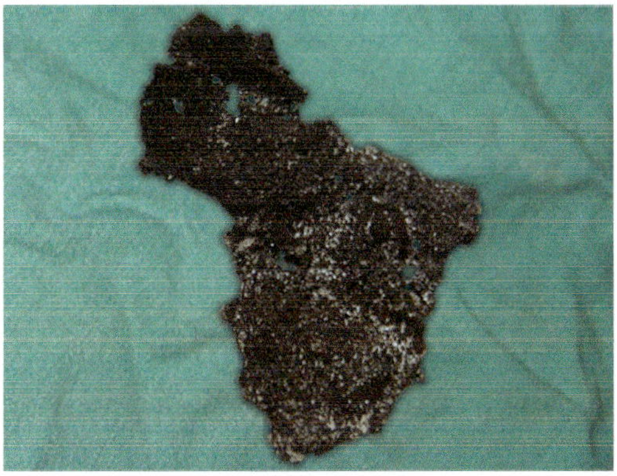

Figure 37.1 Arsenic

Inorganic Compounds

i. **Arsenious oxide** or **arsenic trioxide** (Common names: *Sankhya, somakhar, senkobish* or white arsenic): This form is most commonly used for homicidal purposes. It is obtained in white porcelainous form or white crystalline power. They are tasteless, colorless and odorless, having a high specific gravity of 3.669. It is very sparingly soluble in water, but moderately soluble in boiling water, to which it imparts faint acidic reaction, as such is known an arsenious acid. It dissolves in boiling milk, but precipitates on standing and curdles the milk. Even with its high specific gravity, when it is placed in a liquid medium, it floats over to the surface and forms a scum over it.
ii. **Arsenite-copper acetoarsenite** (Paris green) and **copper arsenite** (Scheele's green): They are green colored powder or crystal and used previously for coloring toys and wallpapers, but nowadays, it is being used for insecticidal and larvicidal purposes.
iii. **Arsenic trichloride**: They are highly poisonous, pungent liquid and are highly irritant to the eyes.
iv. **Sulfides**: There are two varieties: (i) Arsenic disulfide (Manseel or red arsenic). (ii) Arsenic trisulfide (Orpiment, *hartal* or yellow arsenic). They are usually non-poisonous because of non-absorbability; but in commercial grade, it contain fair amount of white arsenic as impurity and, as such, become poisonous.
v. **Arsine** (arsenuated hydrogen): This is accidentally produced when iron pyrite is charged with nascent hydrogen in blast furnaces. Iron pyrite contains fair amount of arsenic as impurity.

Organic Compounds (Used in Medical Idiom)

i. Cacodylic acid (methyl arsenic acid)
ii. Atoxyl (sodium para-amino phenyl arsonate)
iii. Stovarsol (3-acetyl-amino-4-phynol arsenide)
iv. Arsphenamine
v. Neo-arsphenamine.

These compounds were previously used as medicine for syphilis, eosinophilia, etc.

Common Use

i. White arsenic is used in calico-printing
ii. As mordant of dye or as rat-killer
iii. Manufacture of fly-paper, fly- powder
iv. As weeds killer, timber preservatives and sheep dip
v. Used in taxidermy and hide-preservation
vi. Used in tanning industry and for removal of hairs from the hide
v ii. Used as insecticide and larvicidal agent
viii. Sulfides are usually used for manufacture of paints
ix. Various preparations of arsenic are used as cheaper variety of depilatory agents.

Abuses

a. **For fairing of complexion**: Previously, ladies used to take little of it for this purpose.
b. **Love-philter**: In earlier days, when polygamy was in practice, there was an unhealthy competition amongst the wife to gain attraction of the husband and for that purpose, as a magic powder, white arsenic was being administered to the husband.
c. **Aphrodisiac purpose**: Little amount of arsenic causes a sense of well-being. As such, people of North-West Frontier Province and the adjoining areas which are hilly, with rough terrain, take little amount of arsenic daily to keep themselves fit. The person who takes arsenic daily is known as arsenophagists. It was also used to increase sexual desire.

Mechanism of Action

It has both local and remote action. Locally, they act as an irritant. It can penetrate the unbroken skin. It causes vasodilatation, hyper pigmentation and hyperkeratosis on the skin.

On absorption, it disturbs the metabolism by reversibly combining with sulfhydryl radicals of the enzymes in the tissue. It blocks Krebs cycle and interrupts oxidative phosphorylation causing depletion of ATP and thereby death of cells. It causes gastrointestinal capillary dilatation. Arsenic replaces phosphorus in the bone where it may remain for years. It gets deposited on hair as well. It is also a protoplasmic poison, causing capillary dilatation.

Fatal Dose: 180–200 mg

Fatal Period: Normally between 12–48 hours, but may be within 2 hours or even instantaneously.

Acute Arsenic Poisoning

A. **Fulminating type**: When the fatal dose is very high, i.e. more than 1 gm, the person will die within a very short time, without showing usual gastrointestinal manifestation. Here, patient complaints of giddiness, precordial distress, tenderness of muscles, fornication, become delirious. During autopsy, even the stomach may not show congestion.
B. **Gastrointestinal type**: This is the common type of manifestation that appears within half an hour after ingestion.

Clinical Features

There is burning pain with gritty sensation in the mouth, which goes down to the throat and stomach. A sense of constriction round the neck and difficulty in swallowing is seen. Excessive salivation, intense thirst, nausea and serious vomiting may follow this, which may be the constant symptom. The vomitus initially contains normal food matter and later it contains mucous with streaks of blood which can be colorless or dark brown (red sulfides) or yellow (yellow sulfides). Rarely, vomiting may be absent altogether.

Vomiting is followed by diarrhea, accompanied by tenesmus with pain and irritation round the anus. Initially it is dark-colored and bloody; but later it becomes colorless, odorless and rice watery, but invariably contains mucus with streaks of blood. Stool passes out involuntarily and frequently and, in the later part, the stool may look to be rice-watery.

Urine is suppressed, and sometimes, there may be anuria. The urine contains albumin, RBC and cast. There will be muscle cramps and patient shows signs of shock with cold and clammy skin, fall of blood pressure, eyes are sunken, cheeks are hollowed, respiration becomes labored.

In the latter part, hypoxic convulsion may precede coma and death, but brain remains clear till coma sets in. There is delayed loss of hair and skin eruptions.

Differential Diagnosis

The condition should be differentiated from cholera. The various points are narrated in **Table 37.1**.

Management

1. Emetics can be given.
2. Gastric lavage: The stomach should be washed with plain water and with a large amount of warm milk. Gastric lavage with 10% sodium thiosulfate is also useful.
3. Chemical antidote, i.e. **hydrated ferric oxide**, prepared just before administration by mixing 45 mL of liquor ferric, Perchlor and 5 g of magnesium oxide in ½ tumbler of water.
   This hydrated ferric oxide reacts with the free arsenic present in the stomach, to form ferric arsenite, which is insoluble and inert.
4. **Butter** and **greasy substances** to be given to prevent absorption.
5. Arsenic acts in the body, by inactivating sulfhydryl group of enzymes, which is essential for tissue metabolism; this hampers the metabolic process and also acts as a potent capillary poison thus causing gross capillary dilatation. To combat the effect of already absorbed poison in the system,

Table 37.1 Points of difference between acute arsenic poisoning and cholera

Symptoms	Arsenic	Cholera
Pain in the throat	Usually present before vomiting	Absent
Purging	Followed vomiting	Precedes vomiting
Vomited matter	Contains mucous, bile and streaks of blood	Whey-like or watery
Pain-abdomen	Present	Absent (painless diarrhea)
Stool	High-colored, bloody with fetid smell mixed with streaks of blood and mucous, discharged with straining with tenesmus and later part it is rice-watery, with streaks of blood	Rice-watery
Voice	Not affected	Peculiar rough and whistling
Conjunctivae	Inflamed	Not affected
Consciousness	Remains clear till end	Becomes cloudy after a few bouts of vomiting and diarrhea
Laboratory finding of stool	Reinsch test shows octa and tetrahedral crystals of **arsenic**	Shows presence of *Vibrio cholerae*

the following antidotes which either act by substrate competition or form chelate are used:

a. **BAL** (British anti-lewisite):
   Mode of action: BAL has two free SH radicals, and it acts by substrate competition and allures molecules of arsenic bound with 'SH' radicals in the system, to combine with free SH radical present in its chain to form a stable BAL arsenic compound, which is excreted through kidney.
   Administration: Recommended dose is 3–5 mg/kg body weight, by deep IM. over the gluteal region. It is given four hourly for two days, six hourly for one day and then 12 hourly, till required. It should never be given by IV route, as it may cause fat embolism.
b. Other **Chelating agents**, like **EDTA** (ethylenediaminetetraacetic acid): EDTA is given by IV at a dose of 5.25 mg/kg body weight to be dissolved in 500 mL glucose saline and given very slowly by IV drip, taking 1–2 hours to complete transfusion.
c. **Penicillamine**: It can be given orally or by parentally. The dose recommended being up to maximum 1 g/24 hours in four divided doses. Rest treatment is symptomatic.

Postmortem Findings

External Examination: Rigor mortis appears early and last longer because of low ATP level. The external appearance shows features of dehydration with sunken eyes, hollowed cheek and anxious facies. Sometimes yellowish discoloration over skin and mucous membrane may be seen.

Internal Examination: Mucous membrane of mouth, pharynx and esophagus is seen congested, inflamed and may rarely be ulcerated.

The most important features will be seen on opening the stomach, which, will be "**velvety stomach**" or "**crimson plus**", as it is popularly known due to reddish discoloration of mucous membrane. The mucus will be congested, eroded and edematous and some crystals of arsenic may be seen embedded in the mucosa.

Same changes are seen even when arsenic has been administered by other routes. The small intestine will be flabby, congested features will be more marked in the duodenum and jejunum. Large intestine is found congested with the presence of seromucoid exudates. The rectum will be inflamed; intestinal glands will be enlarged but not congested. Early fatty degenerative changes are seen in liver, kidney and spleen. Lung may show sub-pleural ecchymotic spots. The very **characteristic** feature is seen in the heart with **subendocardial hemorrhagic** spots.

In cases of arsenuated hydrogen poisoning, apart from these findings, inflammation of respiratory tract with evidence of hemolysis will be seen.

Preservation of Tissues for Chemical Analysis

i. Routine viscera
ii. Bone mainly long bone like femur
iii. Scalp hairs
iv. Teeth
v. Muscle
vi. Skin
vii. Nails

Subacute Arsenic Poisoning

This condition is usually seen in cases of slow poisoning, where the poison is administered in sub-lethal doses at repeated intervals and second dose is administered before all the poisons of the first dose are excreted out. The common clinical features are general loss of health with abdominal dyspepsia, occasional pain in the abdomen, vomiting and diarrhea, coated tongue. There is a feeling of depression. The patient sometimes feels cramps in the muscles.

Chronic Arsenic Poisoning

It occurs in persons who are exposed to arsenic in course of their work in various industries, including iron smelters, and it is commonly seen nowadays amongst general population, who gets affected by arsenic from polluted water taken from a shallow tube-well. The symptoms of chronic poisoning are insidious in onset and can be described in four different distinct stages as follows:

First Stage (stage of general loss of health and gastrointestinal upsets): There is loss of general health with loss of weight, malaise, loss of appetite, excessive salivation, colicky pain in the abdomen with alternative diarrhea and constipation. Vomiting with glaring mucus tinged with blood is also present. There may be inflamed gums, loss of tooth and coated furry tongue with periorbital edema and circumscribed edema around ankle.

Second Stage (stage of nasolacrimal and Bronchial inflammation): There is inflammation of the conjunctiva with watering from the eyes and nose, itching of the fauces with dry, husky cough, sometimes with blood-tinged spitting with features of bronchopneumonia.

Third Stage (stage of cutaneous involvement): There is cutaneous eruption that may be generalized or localized, with localized pigmentations, moreover the covered areas, known as '**rain drop pigmentation**'.

Epithelial hyperplasia with keratosis is seen mostly on sole or palms. Nails become brittle and show Aldrich Mees' lines, which are white transverse lines on nails.

Nails and hairs become brittle. Eczematous changes are seen over the flexor surface of arms and lower limbs called '**kissing eczema**'. Epithelioma may develop in 20% cases.

Fourth Stage (neurological involvement): There is peripheral neuropathy. This stage is manifested by headache, tingling and numbness of the extremities, hyperesthesia, marked tenderness and cramps of the muscles, arthralgia, gradual loss of knee and other jerks, with features like peripheral neuritis with foot and wrist drop, due to atrophy of extensor muscles.

Apart from these symptoms, there may be evidence of severe megaloblastic anemia due to bone marrow depression and interference with folic acid absorption.

Management

i. Removal of patient from source
ii. Administration of injection of BAL 1,100 mg IM, 6 hourly for 2–3 days, then once daily till it is required
iii. Injection of vitamin B1, B12, and B6 is given IM.

Postmortem Imbibitions of Arsenic

Postmortem imbibitions are seen when a body, especially is unconfined, is being interred in the soil, arsenic being carried by subsoil water imbibe into the tissues, following the direction of flow of subsoil water.

Diagnosis (Chemical Tests)

Reinsch's Test

This is a sensitive test and easy to perform and is sensitive to the extent of $1{:}10^6$–$1{:}7 \times 10^6$ if the solution is in concentration.

Procedure

Drop 1–2 copper strips in suspected solution previously acidified with pure HCL solution. It is then boiled for 5–10 minutes. Copper will be coated steel gray or black deposit of arsenic, if present. The copper is then removed, washed successively in distilled water, alcohol and ether, dried on filter paper, then heated by placing it in a small test-tube. The deposit, if due to arsenic, volatilizes to form a white deposit further up in the cooler portion of the tube. This white deposit is removed and seen under microscope, to show octa- and tetrahedral crystals of arsenic (**Figure 37.2**). A parallel control should be done to prove the purity of the arsenic.

Marsh's Test

This test is somewhat complicated but a very delicate and may detect arsenic even up to 1/1,000th of an mg concentration and requires a Woolf's bottle, generating hydrogen. Sample containing arsenic is put and hydrogen, being converted to AsH_3, burns with a bluish or greenish violet or purple tinge. When a porcelain dish put over the flame, a blackish-brown metallic stain deposit is seen, which is readily soluble in cold HCl, if deposit is treated with concentrated HNO_3, then $AgNO_3$ is added, brick red coloration is seen.

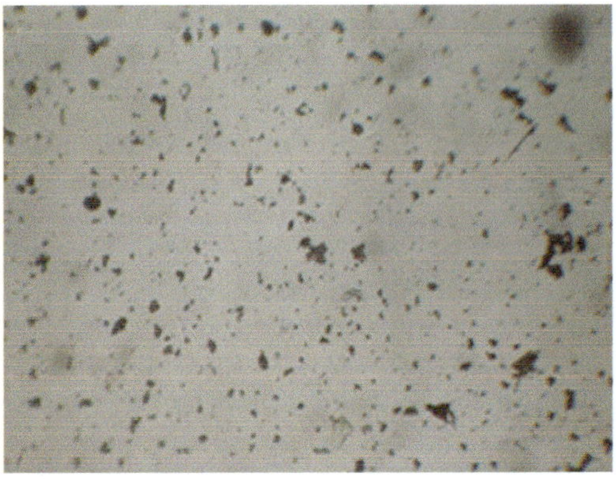

Figure 37.2 Octa and tetrahedral crystals of arsenic

Neutron Activation Analysis (NAA)

This test is done for detection of minute amount, even at the concentration of one monogram.

Sensitivity: One monogram.

Principle: Normally, metallic atom is non-radioactive and stable until there is alteration in the structure. Whenever the neutrality of the atomic structure is hampered, it becomes unstable and starts emanating some rays, like α, β or γ rays and are known as radioactive atom, having a half life depending on the element. In NAA, the tissue to be examined is first made grease free and dried and put in atomic reactor, where it is bombarded with slow-moving neutrons (known as neutron flux). These neutrons either get themselves implanted in the neutron or remove the neutron from the atom and the average of atom becomes unstable and becomes radioactive and it starts emanating rays, which are passed through Scintillation counter and multichannel detectors, by which both qualitative and quantitative assessment of the metal is possible.

Alternate Method: The best analytical method for detection of arsenic in biological samples is atomic absorption spectroscopy.

Medicolegal Importance

a. **Homicide:** Arsenic was one of the most favorite homicidal poisons which fulfil almost all the criteria of a homicidal poison except one, that it is detectable long time after death, even from decomposed bodies, nails, hairs and bones and even from the burnt ashes.
b. **Suicidal:** Though it was a common suicidal poison, nowadays its use is uncommon.

c. **Accidental**: Previously, mostly due to abuses of arsenic and water pollution, this was very commonly seen. Accidental poisoning is also seen amongst user of tube well water.
d. **Criminal** (other) **uses**:
   i. Different compounds of arsenic are used as an abortifacient, to be applied locally.
   ii. Arsenic disulfide also used for manufacturing crude bombs, in combination with sulfur and potassium nitrate.

LEAD (Pb)

Synonym: *Sisha*

Properties

Lead is a heavy, soft, steel-gray metal (**Figure 37.3**) that gives toxic fumes on melting. In its pure metallic form, it is non-poisonous. But, all lead compounds are poisonous. Lead compounds, being acted upon by intestinal enzymes and secretions and on absorption, act as poison.

Toxic Compounds

Most of the poisoning due to lead is either due to lead acetate, monoxide, tetroxide or lead-tetraethyl. The toxic compounds of lead are mentioned in **Table 37.2**.

Commercial Uses

i. Lead, as a metal has got the highest commercial use, starting from its use in electrical industry to ordnance factories (bullets) and in the plumbing industry
ii. Previously, it was used for manufacture of water-pipes
iii. Used for manufacture of wines, toys, cosmetics, ceramics, paints, etc.
iv. Used by married Hindu women as vermilion.

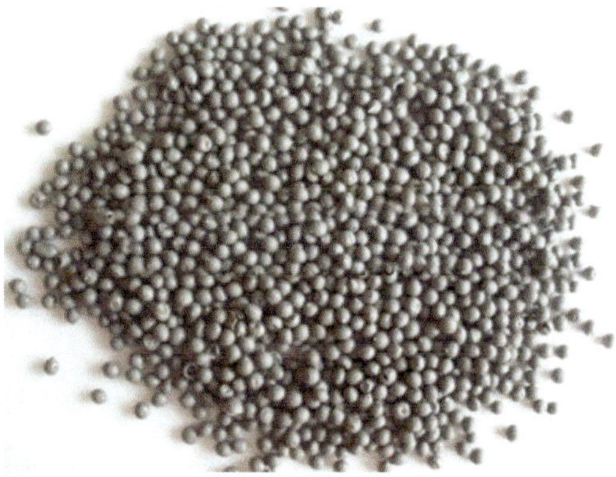

Figure 37.3 Lead metal granules

Table 37.2 Toxic compounds of lead

Compound	Common name	Properties
Lead acetate	Sugar of lead or salt of Saturn	White acicular crystals having sweetish astringent taste and used to sweeten wines in older days and also in therapeutics **(Figure 37.4)**
Lead sub-acetate	White lead or Safeeda	White acicular crystals having an astringent sweetish taste. Medically, used in preparation of Goulard's solution, which is used as an astringent lotion for sprain of joints
Lead carbonate	Chrome yellow	White crystalline powder, insoluble in water and is used in oil painting **(Figure 37.5A)**
Lead chromate	Litharge	Bright yellow, insoluble powder, commonly used in manufacture of chrome yellow paint and used to color sweetmeats and cheap variety of tobacco **(Figure 37.5B)**
Lead oxide	Red lead or metia sindur	Pale red or orange, scaly mass, and is essential for glazing of pottery and enamel ware; and it was medically used as a constituent of diachylon paste
Lead tetroxide	Galena	Orange-red or scarlet-red crystalline powder, adherent to the wall of the container, mostly used for pigment manufacture and still being used as sindur by married ladies in Hindu as vermilion **(Figure 37.6A)**
Lead sulfides	Or surma	Natural principal ore of lead, blackish, shiny and is used for manufacture of paints and eyeliner (surma) for the eyes of Muslims **(Figure 37.6B)**
Lead tetraethyl	-	Heavy, oily liquid used as an anti-knock agent being mixed with petrol

Fatal Dose: Average fatal dose (soluble lead):20 g

i. Lead acetate: 20 g
ii. Lead carbonate: 40 g
iii. Lead tetraethyl: 100 mg/kg (one drop of lead tetraethyl may produce serious symptoms)

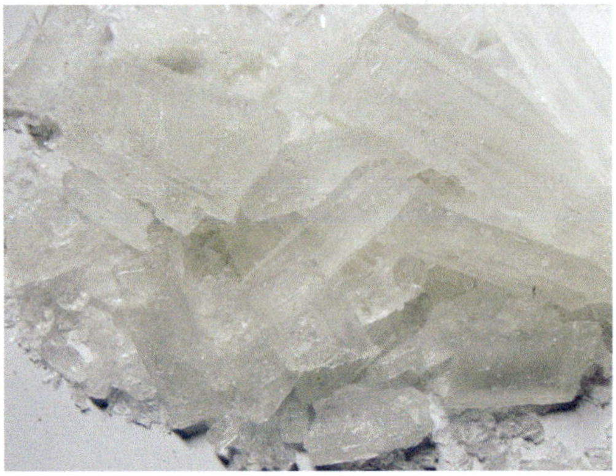

Figure 37.4 Lead acetate

Fatal Period: 2–3 days.

Mechanism of Action

The toxic compounds of lead combines with sulfhydryl groups and inhibits cell metabolism[1] and also inhibit tissue enzyme system; causes degenerative changes in the extensor group of muscles of the extremities and also the nerves; prevent maturation of the RBC. It also causes hemolysis of the mature red cells. Lead depresses the bone marrow and affects erythropoiesis, thus causing basophilic stippling of the red cells.

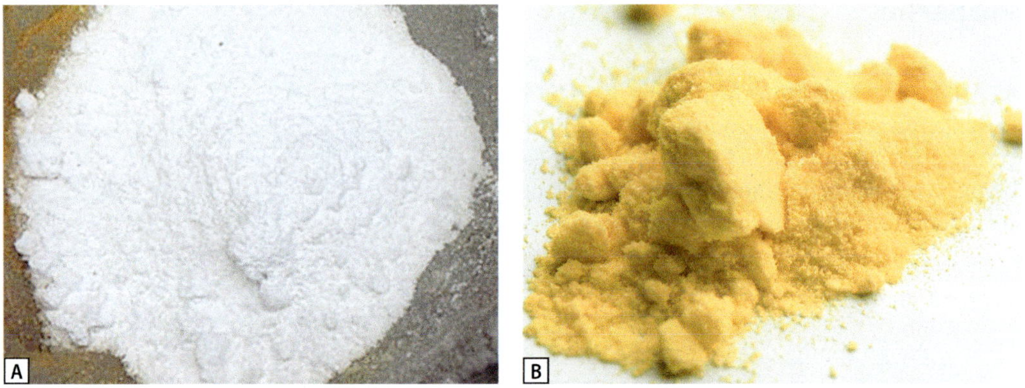

Figures 37.5A and B (A) Lead carbonate; (B) Lead chromate

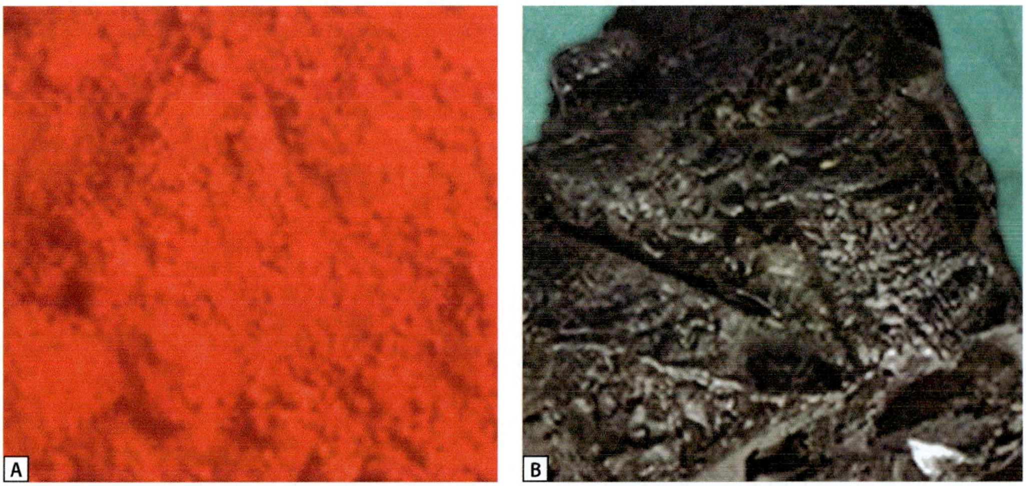

Figures 37.6A and B (A) Lead tetroxide; (B) Lead sulfide

Pharmacokinetics

It is absorbed from all routes, viz. skin, mucosa, inhalation and oral route. On absorption as phosphate and carbonate, it is stored in bones and also in the liver and kidney. It has a cumulative action. It is excreted in urine and bile.

Acute Lead Poisoning

i. Sweetish taste in mouth with metallic, astringent after taste, with dryness of the throat and excess salivation.
ii. Vomiting follows this. Vomitus will be whitish and will show streaks of blood.
iii. Pain abdomen comes in paroxysm and is relieved by pressure over abdomen.
iv. Constipation is common, though, in some cases, loose motion may be seen. Fecal matter will be black in color (due to formation of lead sulfide).
v. Urine is scanty.
vi. Typical neurological signs are pain, muscle weakness, paresthesia, and, rarely, symptoms associated with encephalitis.[2] Other neurological symptoms like drowsiness, insomnia, headache and vertigo, muscular cramps and convulsions, numbness and occasional paralysis are also present. Neurological features are more evident in cases of poisoning by lead tetraethyl.
vii. Convulsion and coma.

Management

i. Removal from thc source of lead.
ii. Emetics should be given to remove the unabsorbed lead from the stomach.
iii. Stomach should be washed with plain water or with 1% magnesium or sodium sulfate. Then saturated solution of magnesium sulfate is given to remove lead from the intestine.
iv. For people who have significantly high blood-lead levels or who have symptoms of poisoning, chelating therapy should be given. Lead has got chemical antidote. Of the antidotes, **EDTA** is said to be the most effective and is given as 5 mL ampoule containing 20% EDTA dissolved in a bottle of glucose saline and transfused IV slowly, twice daily for 5 days.
v. Whole bowel irrigation, cathartics, endoscopy or even surgical removal may be used to eliminate lead or lead containing substances from the gut to prevent further exposure, if detected on X-ray of abdomen.
vi. Lead containing bullets, etc. may also present a threat of further exposure and may need to be surgically removed.
vii. If lead encephalopathy is present, anticonvulsants are given to control seizures and to treat edematous brain corticosteroids and mannitol is used.
viii. To mobilize lead from blood stream and skeleton:
    a. $CaNa_2$ is given by slow IV route in a dose of 10–15 mg/kg body weight, twice in the 1st day. If the therapy is tolerated, it should be repeated with the same dose for next 4 days.
    b. High dose of vitamin B_6 and diet rich in calcium, iron and zinc is also recommended.

Postmortem Findings

Findings are not very characteristic. There is evidence of inflammation and corrosion of mucous membrane of gastrointestinal tract with deposition of whitish substances on the mucous membrane of stomach which can be easily detected on X-ray.

Chronic Lead Poisoning

Synonyms: Plumbism or saturnism.

People who survive of acute poisoning often go on to display symptoms of chronic poisoning.

Chronic poisoning usually presents with symptoms affecting multiple systems,[3] but is associated with symptoms with three main systems: gastrointestinal, neuromuscular and neurological. Plumbism is seen amongst the following people:

i. People working in industry handling lead and its salts
ii. People working with lead smelters
iii. Painters and glaziers using lead-based paints
iv. People working with glass blowing industries
v. Plumbers
vi. Compositors and typesetters
vii. Card players (white lead is used to glaze the cards)
viii. Women using lead tetroxide as vermilion
ix. People taking clarified butter or ghee in lead-lined container
x. Having a lead non-jacketed bullet inside the body of soldiers for a long time.

Clinical Features

i. **Facial pallor**: Facial pallor is a peculiar finding seen amongst chronic lead poisoning cases, where pallor appears exclusively in face, which might be due to selective vasoconstriction of facial vessels and partly due to anemia and is one of the earliest signs.
ii. **Colic** and **constipation** (dry belly ache): There is paroxysmal, spasmodic pain around umbilicus, relieved by pressure, with anorexia and severe constipation.
iii. **Lead line**: Bluish-black line (**Burtonian line**) is seen at the junction of gum and teeth, especially upper jaw, in persons having caries or dirty tooth due to sub-epithelial formation of lead sulfide granules following reaction of H_2S from decomposing food particles and lead within a week of exposure. A similar blue line is seen in cases of poisoning by mercury, copper, bismuth iron and silver.
iv. **Anemia:** This is due to impairment in the synthesis of heme from protoporphyrin and of porphobilinogen and alpha-aminolevulinic acid. Severe hypochromic anemia with reticulocytosis is seen; anisocytosis and poikilocytosis with punctate basophilia. Basophilic stippling means the presence of many dark-blue colored, pin-head sized spots in the cytoplasm of RBC. This is due to condensation of iron containing ribonucleic acid near the mitochondria of RBC, which is a constant and earliest finding in a case of lead poisoning, and when a slide is examined under ultraviolet light, 75–100% red cells look fluorescent. These are stained with basic dyes and so the name.
v. **Lead Palsy:** Typical extensor palsy, resulting into wrist and foot drop with claw hand is seen. This is rather a late and rare phenomenon. Here, tibialis anterior muscle is not affected due to reason not known.
vi. **Lead Encephalopathy**: It is noticed rarely, but seen almost in all the cases of Plumbism. This is more common with tetraethyl lead and not seen in adults.
vii. **Cardiovascular** and **Renal System**: Atherosclerotic changes leading to hypertension is observed with permanent arteriolar degeneration. Hypertensive cardiopathy is also seen.
Chronic atherosclerotic and interstitial nephritis is usually seen. Urine examination shows presence of albumin with increase of coproporphyrin III, and alpha levulinic acid in blood.
viii. **Reproductive System**: Menstrual derangements, viz. amenorrhea, dysmenorrhea, menorrhagia, miscarriage, stillbirth and sterility of both sexes are common. Abortion may also occur in pregnant women between 3 and 6 months.

Diagnosis

i. Clinical history.
ii. Brief clinical examination.
iii. **Blood examination**
Normal lead level: 0–50 μg/dL.
Mild toxicity: Blood lead: 50–60 μg/dL.
Moderate toxicity: Blood lead: 60–100 μg/dL.
Severe toxicity: Blood lead: >100 μg/dL.
iv. **Chemical test**
Hydrochloric acid, when mixed with lead salts, will produce white precipitate, which dissolves on boiling and reappears on cooling.

v. **Laboratory test**
   a. Porphyrinuria, mainly due to coproporphyrin III, is a valuable screening test. In the blood, levels above 0.07 mg% and in the urine 0.15–0.3 mg/L are diagnostic.
   b. Basophilic stippling.
   c. X-ray evidence of radiopaque bands (lead lines) at metaphysis of the long bones and flecks of lead paints on abdominal X-rays are diagnostic.

Management

i. Sodium bicarbonate 20–30 g daily in 4–5 divided doses is given to promote urinary excretion by transforming insoluble **tribasic lead phosphate** into soluble **dibasic** form.
ii. Magnesium sulfate or sodium sulfate in usual dose eliminates unabsorbed lead salt, transforming it into insoluble lead sulfate, through feces.
iii. EDTA is the chelating agent of choice given IV over a period of 1 hour in the dose of 5 mL of 20% solution in 250–500 mL normal saline or 5% glucose, twice daily for 5 days. EDTA transforms lead salts into a soluble, stable, less toxic calcium salts and excreted through urine.
iv. Cases of impaired renal function, BAL, 4 mg/kg of body weight is given, 4 hourly in deep IM for 3–5 days is better to use as it causes excretion of lead through bile. But it should be given earlier to EDTA, because EDTA releases the absorbed tissue lead and may increase the symptoms of poisoning.
v. Penicillamine 300–500 mg, 4–5 times daily, helps excretion of circulatory lead, but is less effective than EDTA.
vi. DMSA or DMPS are considered to be more effective than EDTA and give in usual dose.
vii. Low calcium diet.
viii. Symptomatic treatment.

Medicolegal Importance

i. Homicidal use is very rare.
ii. Suicide by lead is also not common.
iii. Accidental poisoning is, by far, the commonest, when soluble lead compounds are being used as an adulterant. Accidental poisoning is commonly seen amongst people handing with lead, i.e. plumbers and typesetters. Accidental inhalation of lead tetraethyl is also seen with laborers of petroleum dealers. Users of lead tetra-oxide may also get poisoned as it reacts with oil over scalp hairs, which may get absorbed even from intact skin as lead oleate.
iv. As abortifacient, lead can cause tonic contractions of uterus and may cause degenerative changes of the embryonic cells. Lead can be used in the abortion sticks.
v. As cattle poison, lead alone or mixed with arsenic trioxide is being used.

MERCURY (Hg)

Synonym: Quicksilver or *para*.

Properties

It is a liquid metal, bright silvery in appearance (**Figure 37.7**) and is volatile at room temperature and is not poisonous if swallowed for it is not absorbed. But if it is rubbed over the skin, some portion may be absorbed in the form of oxide and if injected intravenous or intra-arterial way, it may produce death due to embolism. They exist in three forms— metallic, mercurous, and mercuric. The compounds of mercury

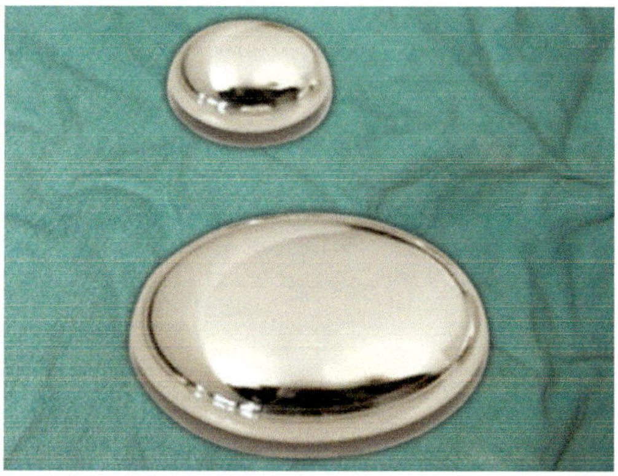

Figure 37.7 Mercury

are poisonous. Two series of compounds which are as follows:

A. **Mercuric compounds**: Soluble and intensely poisonous and are listed in **Table 37.3**.
B. **Mercurous compound**: They are less soluble and less active. Mercurous chloride (HgCl): White, fibers compound (Ayurvedic call it *Rasakarpoor*).

Organic Compounds

i. Mercurochrome 220 iridescent, green scales, readily dissolves in water or spirit.
ii. Novasurol: Double salt of sodium, mercury chlorophenyl oxyacetate with di-ethyl barbituric acid. It is a very powerful diuretic.
iii. Mersalyl: Previously used as diuretic.
iv. Mercury fulminates: Previously used as priming mixtures in firearm cartridge.

Common Use

i. As a metal, used to manufacture barometers and thermometers and as electric conductors. Mercury sulfides are used for manufacture of mirrors. Mercury fulminate was previously used as priming mixture for cartridges.
ii. Mercuric cyanide is used as fungicide and as fumigant.
iii. Mercuric chloride was used as antiseptic and disinfectant. It is used in manufacture of 'felt hat' and also for treating fur by 'furriers'.
iv. Mercurochrome is even being used as antiseptic lotion.
v. Previously 'gray powder' was used by fingerprint experts while taking fingerprints, but it is not used now.

Fatal dose

Mercuric chloride: 0.5–1 g/70 kg
Mercurous chloride: 1.5–2 g/70 kg

Fatal Period: Death may occur within few hours, but commonly delayed up to 3–5 days.

Acute Poisoning

Clinical Features

i. Usually symptoms appear very early, rarely delayed beyond for half an hour. There is an acid, metallic, styptic taste in the mouth with severe burning sensation, which goes down to the stomach, with a feeling of constriction around the throat with difficulty in breathing.
ii. It is followed by nausea and vomiting. The vomitus contains mucus initially, food material with altered blood and shreds of gastric mucosa followed by purging, which is bloody with tenesmus.
iii. There may be cough, dyspnea, fever, headache, chill and rigor (metal fume fever) and blurring vision.
iv. There occurs oliguria and urine may contain albumin, blood and casts.
v. There are features of shock, characterized by weak and thready pulse, fall of blood pressure and sometimes fine tremors and convulsion and insensibility precedes death.
vi. Death is usually due to hepatorenal failure and gangrenous colitis may occur sometimes if the patient survives for a few days.

Management

1. Stomach which is washed immediately, great care should be taken as the stomach

Table 37.3 Various mercuric compounds and their properties

Compound	Properties
Mercuric oxide (HgO)	Brick-red crystalline powder (**Figure 37.8A**)
Mercuric chloride ($HgCl_2$)	Corrosive sublimate-dirty white, heavy, crystals, having styptic metallic taste (**Figure 37.8B**)
Mercuric iodide (HgI_2)	Also known as red iodide of mercury or mercury bin iodide, scarlet red crystals or powder (**Figure 37.9A**)
Mercuric sulphides or red sulfides of mercury (HgS)	*China sindur* and in *Ayurbeda Rasasindur*. It is the principle mineral ore of mercury and is sometimes used in industry as pigment and in mirror manufacturing industry (**Figure 37.9B**)
Mercuric cyanide	White prismatic crystals, mostly used as fungicide

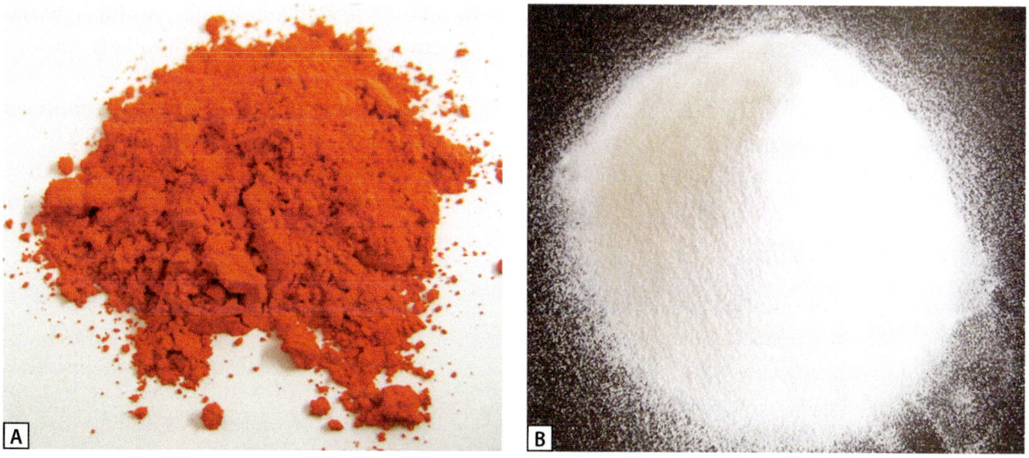

Figures 37.8A and B (A) Mercuric oxides; (B) Mercuric chloride

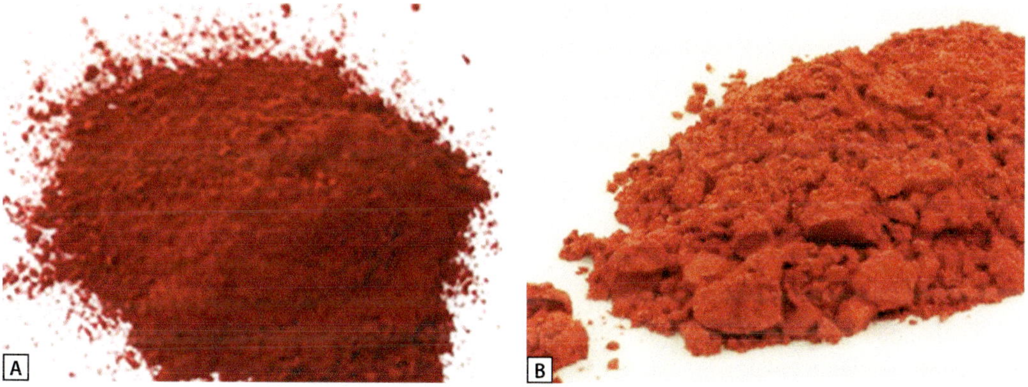

Figures 37.9A and B (A) Mercuric iodide; (B) Mercuric sulfide

is very friable. It should be initially washed with plain water and initial return kept for chemical examination. Then it should be washed with egg albumin, milk or animal charcoal to precipitate mercury and taken out immediately, otherwise it will be re-absorbed.

2. After this it should be washed with chemical antidote, viz. 250 mL of 5–10% solution of **sodium formaldehyde sulfoxylate**. It is a strong reducing agent and reduces mercury chloride ($HgCl_2$) to metallic mercury. A further 200 mL solution should be left inside the stomach as mercury is re-excreted and absorbed from the stomach.
3. 1:1000 solution of sulfoxylate twice daily should be used as retention enema and high colonic lavage, when there is possibility of gangrenous colitis.
4. Systemic administration of BAL as a chelator in the dose of 2.5 mg/kg body weight to be injected deep IM, 4 hourly for 2 days, 6 hourly for 1 day and then 12 hourly till required. While it is indicated in elemental and inorganic mercury poisoning, it is contraindicated in organic mercury poisoning as it leads to increased neurotoxicity.
5. Alternatively, chelating agent namely EDTA in the dose of 5.25 mg/kg body weight to be dissolved in 500 mL of glucose saline to be transfused by slow IV drip or penicillamine 20-30 mg/kg body weight up to maximum 1 gm/24 hours by oral route may be given in divided doses.

6. Peritoneal or hemodialysis helps excretion of absorbed poison.
7. Maintain fluid and electrolyte balance.
8. Demulcents can also be helpful.
9. Symptomatic treatment.
10. Calcium disodium versenate is not helpful.

Postmortem Findings

i. Mucous membrane of lips, mouth and tongue show typical appearance of being swollen with grayish-white coating which easily peelable, showing evidence of corrosion is underneath.
ii. Similar change seen in esophagus, and stomach will show evidence of coagulated albumin mixed with mucous and streaks of blood. Mucous membrane of stomach is corroded and covered with **ashy-gray layer,** which shows furrows running across.
iii. Evidence of corrosion is present in stomach and perforation of stomach, seen in rare cases. Cecum and colon may show evidence of gangrenous colitis.
iv. Liver is congested and heart may show fatty degeneration. The heart may also show subendocardial hemorrhage. Kidneys show tubular necrosis.

Chronic Poisoning

Synonyms: Hydrargyria or mercurialism

Chronic poisoning may occur due to:
i. People dealing with mercury in factories because of continuous accidental absorption.
ii. After effect on acute exposure.
iii. Injudicious medical use mercury and its compounds.

Clinical Features

They may show either of the following changes:
i. **Changes with eyes**: This is the first clinical sign of chronic mercury poisoning, manifested by a brownish or malt brown glow from the anterior lens capsule, when the eye is examined with slit-lamp. This is known as "**Mercuria lentis**".
ii. Excessive salivation with painful inflamed gums with occasional blue-black lines on the gum.
iii. There is metallic taste in mouth, anorexia, insomnia, headache, lassitude, etc.
iv. Neurological toxicity: Tremors known as "**Hatters' shake** or **Mercurial tremor** or **glass-blower's shakes**" which are course tremors more than that seen in thyrotoxicosis is seen. The muscles of fingers are affected initially, later on, the muscles of the tongue, resulting in development of stammering. The tremors then spread to extremities and are usually intentional tremor. It is one of the most important characteristic and consistent features of chronic mercury poisoning.

Diagnosis

Reinsch Test: Dissolve suspect sample in a hydrochloric acid solution. Insert a copper strip into the solution. The appearance of a silvery coating on the copper may indicate mercury. In the deposits, if seen under microscope, spherical globules of mercury **(Figure 37.10)** are seen.

Management

i. Affected person should be removed from the source of exposure.
ii. BAL or other chelating agent as per recommended doses.
iii. Oral hygiene should be maintained.
iv. Demulcent drinks and saline purgatives are given.

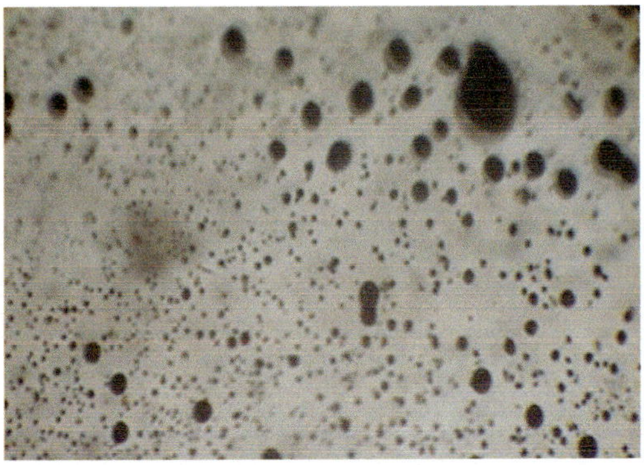

Figure 37.10 Black spherical globules of mercury

Medicolegal Importance

i. **Suicidal poisoning**: Suicide with mercuric chloride is not common, but a few cases were reported.
ii. **Homicidal poisoning**: Mercuric chloride is rarely used as a homicidal agent, for its styptic metallic taste and burning sensation after intake, but few cases were reported.
iii. **Accidental poisoning**: Occupational exposure to inorganic mercury may occur in factories like mercury mines, thermometer factories, etc. Mercurial vapor may produce accidental poisoning even at a concentration of 0.5 mg/cu m of air. Case is on record where a person died by rubbing ointment containing mercury over his body repeatedly.

COPPER (Cu)

Pure metallic copper is not poisonous; in fact it is a normal constituent of the human body. Many salts of copper are poisonous **(Figure 37.11)**.

Copper sulfate (**Figure 37.12**) is available as blue crystals (**blue vitriol**). When heated to 220°–240° C, it becomes anhydrous and becomes white which is highly hygroscopic, draws water from the atmosphere and again becomes blue.

Toxic Compounds

The salts of copper are presented in **Table 37.4**. Most of the copper salts have got a bitter, metallic, styptic taste.

Copper subacetate is available as blue minute crystals and occurs naturally when metallic copper is treated with an organic acid. It is a bluish salt formed by action of vegetable acids on improperly tinned cooking utensils.

Copper sulfate is soluble in water or liquid with pH < 5.5, hence food with pH < 5.5 stored in copper utensils or cooked in copper vessels will cause poisoning, whereas, copper subacetate is mostly soluble in fatty media.

Common Use

i. Copper as a metal has got numerous common uses:
   a. Industries
   b. Household appliances
   c. Manufacture of electrical goods, including wires
   d. Manufacture of vessels
   e. Manufacture of various alloys; a very hard alloy is cupro-nickel, which is used as jacket in bullet manufacturing.
ii. Of the salts, copper sulfate has got various uses for:
   a. Manufacture of pigments, to use as insect repellent by book binders
   b. In the bakeries to increase fermentation and to make the bread whiter
   c. To preserve the fruits and vegetables and to bring rich green coloration.
iii. Copper subacetate is mostly used in the art industries, as pigment.
iv. Copper arsenite and copper aceto-arsenic are being used as insecticides and pesticides.

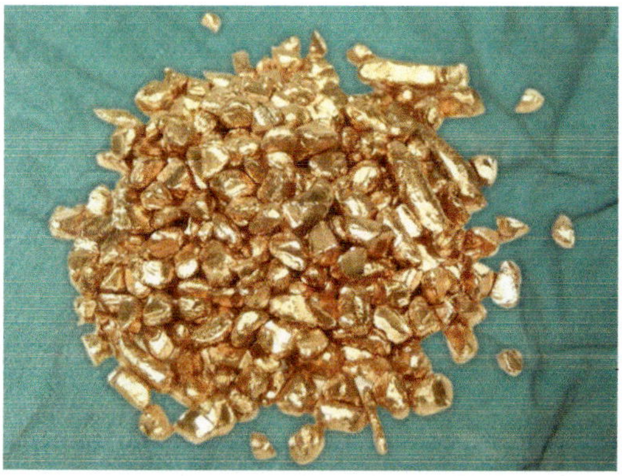

Figure 37.11 Copper metals

Figure 37.12 Copper sulfates (blue vitriol)

Table 37.4 Various salt of copper

Chemical name	Common name	Properties
Copper sulfate	Blue vitriol	Crystalline blue crystals, is most common source of poisoning (**Figure 37.12**)
Copper subacetate	Verdigris or zangal	Crystalline blue crystals
Copper arsenite	Scheele's green	Crystalline green powder
Copper aceto-arsenite	Paris green	Crystalline green powder
Copper carbonate	Mountain's green	Crystalline green powder

Medical Use

i. Copper sulfate solution is used for removal of granulation tissues.
ii. One percent copper sulfate solution is used as a chemical antidote in acute phosphorous poisoning.
iii. Copper sulfate also comes into composition of '**Fehling-I**' solution for determination of free sugar in urine.

Fatal Dose

i. Copper sulfate: As crystal 30 g and concentrated solution 10 ml.
ii. Copper subacetate: 15 g.

Fatal Period: 1–3 days (average).

Mechanism of Action: They are powerful inhibitors of enzymes.

Acute Poisoning

Clinical Features

i. Symptoms usually appear within ½ an hour of intake. There is styptic, metallic taste followed by burning sensation in the mouth and pain which gradually goes down to the stomach.
ii. There is excessive salivation.
iii. Followed by nausea and vomiting. Vomitus will be bluish green in color. Due to this coloration, sometimes, it is mistaken as bilious vomiting.
To differentiate this, sodium hydroxide solution is added. In a case of copper sulfate, color will change to deep blue, whereas color will remain same in a case of bilious vomiting.
iv. Diarrhea with tenesmus and straining, but in some cases, there may be constipation.
v. There is oliguria and hematuria with presence of albumin in the urine.
vi. Severe frontal headache with features of shock and circulatory failure is there.
vii. There may be myalgia, acidosis, pancreatitis, delirium and coma. In a case of death within 24 hours, it is due to shock and if the patient survives for few days, jaundice appears and patient usually dies of hepatorenal syndrome.

Management

i. Usually, emetic is not needed because copper sulfate itself is an emetic.
ii. Stomach should be washed with 1% solution of potassium ferrocyanide, which acts as a chemical antidote and reacts with copper sulfate to form insoluble cupric ferrocyanide.
Demulcent like drinks, viz. milk, egg albumin convert it into insoluble cupric albuminate, which is to be removed by stomach wash.
iii. Injection BAL should be given deep IM route, in the usual dose of 3–4 mg/kg body weight 4 hourly, then 12 hourly, or alternately, EDTA or penicillamine can be given.
iv. Glucose, vitamin C and B complex is to be given, both for purpose of maintenance of nutrition, as well as for protection of liver.
v. Hydrocortisone may also be needed sometimes.

Postmortem Findings

i. Yellowish discoloration of skin and conjunctivae is present. If the patient dies within few hours of intake, there may not be any evidence of yellowish discoloration of the mucous membrane of lips, mouth (including tongue). If the patient has survived for few days, yellowish discoloration of skin and mucous membrane will be seen due to jaundice.

ii. Greenish or bluish stomach contents; hepatic and renal necroses are the diagnostic findings. Greenish-bluish froth appears at mouth and nostrils.
iii. On opening the stomach, mucous membrane shows greenish or greenish bluish color, which will be grossly corroded and congested.
iv. Pale looking friable hepatomegaly is the typical change in case of survival for a durable period. On autopsy, liver-section will feel soapy to touch.

Microscopically, it will show features of fatty degenerative changes with centrilobular necrosis. Discrete discoloration and corrosion will be seen in the small intestine and the lower part of the large intestine may show evidence of gangrenous changes, may even be with perforation. Kidneys will be enlarged and congested and will show microscopically extensive degenerative changes in proximal tubules with evidence of deposition of copper in it.

Chronic Poisoning

Chronic poisoning is seen usually with people engaged in manufactures of copper products, especially amongst the copper smelter and copper welders and may sometimes be seen amongst the people who take oily food from copper vessels, contaminated with verdigris.

Clinical Features

i. Metallic taste in the mouth with purple or greenish layer appearing in the gum is seen. They show evidence of loss of general health.
ii. There may be nausea, dyspepsia, vomiting and diarrhea with evidence of jaundice.
iii. The urine and perspiration may become green and the hair takes a coppery hue (**green hair discoloration**).
iv. There may be dermatitis or eczematous changes seen amongst the people, coming in contact with copper dust.
v. As per **Mallory**, chronic copper poisoning result in syndrome (symptoms complex) known under different names, namely hemochromatosis, pigment cirrhosis or bronze diabetes.

Treatment

i. Removal of the patient from the chronic source of exposure.
ii. Injection BAL or other chelating agents in recommended doses should be started.
iii. Vitamin B complex, vitamin C should be given parenterally along with glucose.

Medicolegal Importance

1. **Homicide**
   Use of $CuSO_4$ as homicidal substance is very rare because of the following grounds:
   i. Specific bluish color
   ii. Strong metallic taste
   iii. High fatal dose (30 g)
   iv. Self-emetic in nature.
2. **Suicide**
   It is very common for the following reasons:
   i. Easy availability
   ii. Cheap price
   iii. People's belief of certainty of action.
3. **Accidental**: Acute accidental poisoning occurs mostly in children who being attracted with the colors and glaze of the copper sulfate, may chew them and get poisoned.
4. **Abortifacient**: It is introduced into the vaginal orifice in the form of paste staining abortion sticks.

SILVER (Ag)

Properties

Silver is a metallic chemical element with the chemical symbol Ag and found in free (native) as well as in combined state. It is a soft, white, lustrous transition metal; it has the highest electrical conductivity of any element and the highest thermal conductivity of any metal.

Native silver usually occurs associated with copper and gold.

Uses

i. As silver copper alloys in coins and ornaments.
ii. Silver amalgam (silvered mercury) was used in filling teeth.
iii. Silver leaves are used in Ayurvedic and Unani medicines.
iv. In preparation of silver salts used in silvering of mirror, photography and medicines.
v. Among the compounds of silver, silver nitrate is used widely in industry and in medicines as antiseptic or caustic properties.

When silver comes in contact with organic substances like skin, clothes, etc., it produces burning sensation like that of caustic and reduced to metallic silver, which is white like the moon (luna) hence it is called **Lunar Caustic**.

Management

i. In silver nitrate poisoning, stomach should be washed with sodium chloride solution to form non-toxic silver chloride
ii. Gastric lavage or emesis can be tried
iii. BAL injection may be given in usual recommended dose.

Postmortem Findings

All the visceras will be congested. Mouth, lips, mucous membrane of stomach; lungs are corroded, stained with grey white to black color.

GOLD (Au)

Properties

Gold is a yellow, soft and heavy metal. Gold and silver are called noble metals since they are not attacked by atmospheric oxygen. However, silver gets stained when exposed to air containing traces of H_2S. Gold is malleable, pliable and is a good conductor of heat and electricity. Pure gold is soft. Gold is quite inert. It does not react with oxygen, water and acids but dissolves in aqua regia.

Death can occur from the use of its salts.

Uses

i. It is alloyed with Ag or Cu for making jewellery.
ii. The salts are used in medicine in the treatment of rheumatoid arthritis and in industry.

Clinical Features

Idiosyncrasy is quite common. Besides this, the toxic reactions are like diarrhea, vomiting, albuminuria, exfoliating dermatitis; aplastic anemia and, occasionally, agranulocytosis are seen.

Treatment

i. BAL is an effective antidote.
ii. Can be treated by administration of sodium thiosulfate, either orally or by injection.

Postmortem Findings

Hepatic necrosis, necrosis of renal tubular epithelium, peripheral neuropathy and blood dyscrasias are the common findings.

THALLIUM (Tl)

Properties

In its pure form, thallium is odorless and tasteless **(Figure 37.13)**. Thallous sulfate, which is soluble colorless crystalline solid, is the most commonly used compounds. This soft gray post-transition metal, which is not found free in nature, but found in trace amounts in the earth's crust.

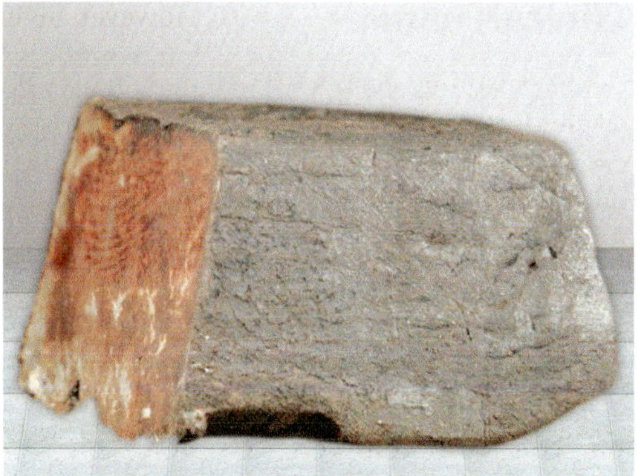

Figure 37.13 Thallium metal

Toxic Compounds of Thallium

i. Thallous sulfate
ii. Thallous acetate
iii. Thallous iodide
iv. Thallous nitrate
v. Thallous carbonate.

Fatal Dose: 12 mg/kg body weight.

Fatal Period: 24–30 hours.

Uses

i. Industrially, it is used in dying and special glass manufacture.
ii. Therapeutically it had been advocated for certain medical treatment like in ringworm in the form of thallium acetate.
iii. Thallium is used mostly in manufacturing electronic devices, switches and closures, primarily for the semiconductor industry.

Source

i. Eating food contaminated with thallium may be a major source of exposure for most of the cases.
ii. Breathing workplace air in industries that use thallium.
iii. Living near hazardous waste sites containing thallium and its compound.
iv. Touching or for children, eating soil contaminated with thallium.
v. Breathing low levels in air and water.

Clinical Feature

Thallium and its compounds are extremely toxic and should be handled with great care. There are numerous recorded cases of fatal thallium poisoning.[3]

Contact with skin is dangerous, and adequate ventilation should be provided when melting this metal. Thallium (I) compounds have a high aqueous solubility and are readily absorbed through the skin. Exposure to them should not exceed 0.1 mg per m^2 of skin in an 8-hour time weighted average (40 hours work week). Thallium is a suspected human carcinogen.[4]

Acute poisoning resulting from swallowing the substance is characterized by stimulation of heart followed by depression, which causes death from cardiac failure.

A powerful poison, if repeated in small doses, has a cumulative effect and may result chronic poisoning injuring the endocrine glands. Besides this, peripheral neuritis, alopecia, general malaise, headache, drowsiness, depression is its other symptoms.

Treatment

i. Stomach is emptied either by stomach tube or by emetics.
ii. Purgative such as magnesium sulfate should be given.
iii. Intravenous injection of potassium iodide, sodium thiosulfate cause gradual elimination of thallium from system.
iv. One of the main methods of removing thallium (both radioactive and normal) from humans is to use Prussian blue, a material which absorbs thallium.[5] Up to 20 g per day of Prussian blue is fed by mouth to the person, and it passes through their digestive system and comes out in the stool. Hemodialysis and hemoperfusion are also used to remove thallium from the blood serum. At a later stage of the treatment, additional potassium is used to mobilize thallium from the tissue.[6,7]
v. Fluids, especially milk, should be given by mouth and the patient should be kept warm.

Postmortem Findings

Autopsy findings are not significant. However, there may be alopecia, stomatitis, tubular necrosis, pulmonary edema, cerebral edema and fatty degeneration of the liver.

Medicolegal Importance

i. Thallium has been used as a homicidal agent.
ii. For a long time, thallium compounds were easily available as rat poison. This fact and that it is water soluble and nearly tasteless, led to frequent intoxications caused by accident or criminal intent.[8]

IRON (Fe)

Iron is the most widely used and available metal. Iron, one of the most abundant metals on Earth, is essential to most life forms and to normal human physiology.

On the other hand, excess amounts of iron can result in toxicity and even death. In children, death has occurred from ingesting 200 mg of iron.[9] They have caused number of deaths, especially among children. At home, the source of iron poisoning is from various iron preparation.

Toxic Iron Salts

i. Commonest salts are ferrous sulfate or iron sulfate.
ii. Ferric chloride or perchloride of iron.

What is the Risk of Iron Toxicity?

There is considerable potential for iron toxicity because very little iron is excreted from the body. Thus, iron can accumulate in body tissues and organs when normal storage sites are full. For example, people with hemochromatosis are at risk of developing iron toxicity because of their high iron stores.

Clinical Features

Acute poisoning occurs when a person, usually a child, swallows a large number of iron-containing preparations. These children may not be able or willing to tell you what and how much they swallowed. Intentional overdose can occur among adults, but it is rare.

Symptoms of iron poisoning usually become evident within 6 hours after an excessive amount of iron:

i. Severe vomiting
ii. Diarrhea
iii. Abdominal pain
iv. Dehydration and lethargy if not treated adequately
v. A child's vomit or stool may be bloody as iron corrodes the intestinal lining and is a direct irritant to the stomach mucosa
vi. If severe poisoning is inadequately treated, shock and death can occur.

Treatment

i. Often, after supportive care, the gastrointestinal symptoms appear to improve 6-24 hours after their onset
ii. Gastric lavage with sodium bicarbonate to convert ferrous sulfate to ferrous carbonate should be tried
iii. Emetics should be given
iv. Intake of bland fluids is necessary
v. Penicillamine may be used
vi. BAL is strictly contradicted
vii. Desferrioxamine is given as continuous IV infusion in normal saline at 15 mg/kg/hour.

Each 100 mg of Desferrioxamine binds to 9 mg of elemental iron producing ferrioxamine complex and are excreted by kidneys.

Postmortem Findings

i. The stomach may contain coffee ground material as there is hemorrhagic gastritis.
ii. The intestine show varying degree of vascular engorgement and edema and contents are black colored.

iii. Liver shows degenerative changes with necrosis.
iv. Kidney shows cloudy swelling with necrosis.
v. Small irregular hemorrhagic spots may be present on the surface of heart, lungs, thymus and aorta.

Medicolegal Importance

- Accidental poisoning is common
- Homicidal is rare.

METAL FUME FEVER

Synonyms: Brass chills, brazier disease, Foundry fever, Monday fever, smelter shakes, and Welder's ague.

Occupations Affected

i. Welding
ii. Galvanizing
iii. Smelting
iv. Metal refining
v. Electroplating
vi. Alloy making
vii. Ship breaking, etc.

Metals Involved

The syndrome is caused by inhalation of fumes of the following metals:

i. Zinc
ii. Copper
iii. Magnesium
iv. Iron
v. Chromium
vi. Cadmium
vii. Nickel
viii. Manganese
ix. Mercury
x. Cobalt
xi. Lead
xii. Antimony
xiii. Selenium
xiv. Beryllium
xv. Vanadium
xvi. Silver and aluminum.

Clinical Features

The syndrome resembles that of flu, beginning at 4 to 6 hours after exposure to fumes, and is characterized by chills, fever, myalgia, cough, dyspnea, fatigue, metallic taste, salivation, thirst, sweating, etc.

There is tachycardia, tachypnea, leukocytosis, cyanosis and reduced pulmonary function. Resolution of symptoms occurs 36 hours after stoppage of exposure.

Treatment should be of symptomatic and non-specific.

REFERENCES

1. Loomis TA. The basis of antidotal therapy. In: Klaassen CD, Watkins JB Iii, Essentials of Toxicology, 2nd ed. Lea and Febiger: Philadelphia; 1974. pp. 129-44.
2. Pearce JM. Burton's line in lead poisoning. Europ Neurol. 2007;57(2):118-9.
3. Fatal thallium poisoning. [cited 17th Feb 2013] Available from: URL:http://www.nj.com/news/index.ssf/2011/02/thallium_is_favored_method_of.html
4. Biology of Thallium. WebElemnts. Retrieved 2008-11-11.
5. Yang Y, Faustino P, Progar J, Brownell C, Sadrieh N, May J, et al. Quantitative determination of thallium binding to ferric hexacyanoferrate: Prussian blue. Int J Pharmacol. 2008;373(1–2):187-94.
6. Prussian blue fact sheet from the Centers for Disease Control and Prevention. [cited 17th Feb 2013]; Available from: URL: http://www.bt.cdc.gov/radiation/prussianblue.asp
7. Malbrain ML, Lambrecht GL, Zandijk E, Demedts PA, Neels HM, Lambert W, et al. Treatment of severe thallium intoxication. Clin Toxicol. 1997;37(1):97-100.
8. Emsley J. Thallium, The Elements of Murder: A History of Poison. Oxford University Press. 2006. pp. 326–7.
9. Corbett JV. Accidental poisoning with iron supplements. MCN Am J Matern Child Nurs. 1995;20:234.

CHAPTER 38

Organic Irritants of Plants and Vegetables Origin

Putul Mahanta

LEARNING PLAN

- Learn organic irritants of plants and vegetable origin, viz. abrus, castor, croton, capsicum, calotropis, marking nut, plumbago, colocynth, ergot on rye
- Know the mechanism of action, clinical features, diagnosis and management
- Identify the postmortem changes
- Understand their medicolegal importance

Plants cannot move to escape their predators, so they must have other means of protecting themselves from herbivorous animals. Some plants have physical defenses such as thorns; but, by far the most common protection is chemical.[1] Those organic chemicals can be grouped as: Gastrointestinal irritants (abrus, castor, capsicum, etc.), cardiotoxic poisons (aconite, oleander, tobacco, etc.), neurotoxic poisons (datura, cannabis, opium, etc.), hepatotoxic poisons (neem, akee) and dermal irritants (mango, St John's wort or Hypericum perforatum).

There are several species in India which are poisonous or injurious to human body in some way or the other. Human fatalities caused by poisonous plants, especially resulting from accidental ingestion, are rare in the US.[2]

List of some important plants containing poisonous parts that pose a serious risk of illness, injury or death to humans or animals are narrated in **Table 38.1**.

TOXIC PRINCIPLE IN PLANT

Plants are made up of simple to complex natural plant derived compounds often referred to as toxic principles in plant. These toxic principles in plants comprise of the following:

1. Toxalbumin (Phytotoxin)
2. Alkaloids
3. Gossypol
4. Glycosides
5. Minerals
6. Proteins
7. Amino acids
8. Plant acid
9. Resins and resinoids
10. Unclassified toxins and plants causing mechanical injury, etc.

Table 38.1 Poisonous parts of plants

All parts	Leaves	Fruits	Seeds	Stem or bark	Root
Nerium odorum	Tobacco	*Capsicum annum*	Abrus	Cinchona bark	Aconite
Cerbera thevetia	Conium maculatum	*Colocynth*	Castor	*Plumbago rosea*	*Plumbago*
Calatropis	Curare	*Strychnos nux vomica*	*Croton*		*Colocynth*
	Digitalis		*Datura*		Jalap
	Oleander		Semicarpus anacardium		

Table 38.2 Different toxic principles containing toxic ingredient (active principle)

Toxic principle	Active principle
Alkaloids	Atropine, strychnine, nicotine, curarine, ergotamine, morphine, etc.
Toxalbumin	Abrin, Ricin, crotin, etc.
Glycosides	Nerin, thevetin, cerebrin, digoxin, calotropin, etc.
Resins	Cannabinol
Juice or oil	Semicarpol
Plant acids	Insoluble calcium oxalates, soluble oxalates, isocupressic acid, quinines, tannic acid, triterpene acids, etc.

Various toxic principles present in the plant that contains different active ingredient (principle) are shown in **Table 38.2**.

ABRUS

Botanical Name: *Abrus precatorius.*

Common Name: Rati, gunja, jequirity, crab's eye, rosary pea, 'John Crow' bead, precatory bean, Indian licorice, akar saga, giddee giddee, jumbie bead and weather plant.

Features

Abrus is a genus of flowering plants in the pea family, Fabaceae. It contains, 13–18 species, but is best known for a single species, jequirity (***Abrus precatorius***). The plant is a slender, perennial climber that rolls around trees, shrubs and hedges. It is a leguminous plant with long, pinnate-leafleted leaves (**Figure 38.1**).

The plant is best known for its seeds, which are used as pearls and in percussion instruments and are toxic due to the presence of the active principle, i.e. the abrin.

The highly toxic seeds of that species are used to make jewelery.[3-5] The attractive seeds are about the size of a ladybug, glossy red with one black dot (**Figure 38.2**), which contains abrin that is related to ricin and very potent.

Toxic Part of the Plant

All part of the plant, i.e. seed, root and leaves are toxic. The seeds have been used as beads in jewellry and are very attractive to children and are dangerous; inhaled dust is toxic and pinpricks can be fatal.

Active Principle

Abrin.

Mechanism of Action

Abrins inhibit protein synthesis by inactivating the ribosomes. The B-chain binds to cell surface receptors and the toxin receptor complex is taken into the cell; the A-chain has endonuclease activity and extremely low concentrations will inhibit protein synthesis, thereby causing cell death.

Clinical Features

Local Manifestation: When abrin is injected into the skin, there is inflammatory reaction followed by tissue necrosis.

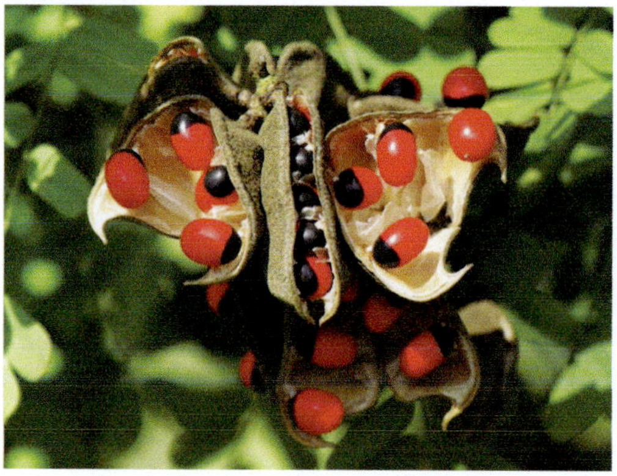

Figure 38.1 *Abrus precatorius* plant

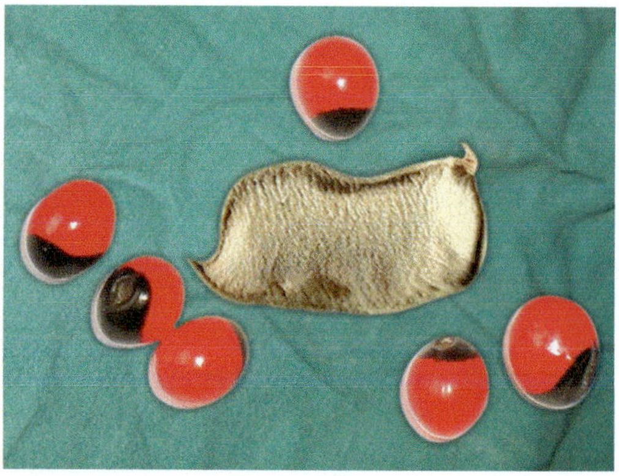

Figure 38.2 Seeds of *Abrus precatorius* plant

Ingestion: When ingested, there will be nausea, vomiting, fainting, vertigo and dyspnea. There is hemorrhagic gastritis which will be followed by liver failure. Convulsion may precede death from cardiac failure. **Ocular exposure** causes itching, redness, conjunctivitis and swelling.

Fatal Dose: Ingesting a single (crushed) seed can kill an adult human. Intact or boiled or cooked seed when swallowed do not cause poisoning.

Fatal Period: Usually after several (3–5) days.

Management

i. Stomach tube
ii. Activated charcoal
iii. Purgative to clear bowel
iv. Sodium bicarbonate 10 g orally/day to maintain alkaline urine and to prevent agglutination of RBC and to prevent blocking of renal tubules with hemoglobin G
v. Diazepam can be used to control the convulsion.

Autopsy Findings

Needle prick mark, fragments of the needle along with Sui may be found in the skin along with edema, inflammation, local necrosis and ecchymosis at the site of injection. Stomach mucosa found to be edematous with patchy hemorrhages. Visceras will be congested. Petechial hemorrhages under the pleura, pericardium and peritoneum may be seen.

Medicolegal Importance

i. Poisoning in India are mainly accidental with the children
ii. Used as cattle poison
iii. Can be used to kill human by Sui prepared with abrin
iv. For malingering to produce conjunctivitis powdered seeds are used
v. Seeds are used as an abortifacient.

CASTOR

Botanical Name: *Ricinus communis.*

Meaning: 'Ricinus' means tick (the skin of the castor beans looks like a tick) and 'communis' means common.

Common Name: Castor, arandi, castor bean plant, true castor oil plant, hand of Christ.

Medicinal Uses

The ancient Egyptians were associated with the 'castor oil plants' and made extended use of castor oil and other parts of the plant in the therapeutics collected in the Ebers Papyrus. It was drunk as a remedy for constipation and was also rubbed on the head to cure headaches or to promote growth of hair of a woman.

In these cases, it is used on its own but it also gets mixed with some other items. With yeast and water, it would cure roundworm. With red lead, it was capable of curing herpes on the face.

The leaves mixed with honey and 'clay from a statue' applied as a poultice would treat a 'flow of matter' from eyes.

Features

Ricinus communis is a large, full-bodied annual or recurrent woody herb, up to 3 m tall. Leaves are alternate, up to 40 cm long, simple, palmately seven to nine lobed, serrate with toothed margins (**Figure 38.3**). The plant grows all over India.

Fruit of castor oil plant is a three lobed capsule with a soft, spiny exterior. It has three seeds per capsule which are smooth, flattened, oval, shiny, greyish brown mottled with reddish brown or white with yellow brown or grey marking or wholly black or red that are 10 mm long and 6 to 7 mm wide, each resembling a female tick (**Figure 38.4**).

Unbroken and cooked seeds are not poisonous when swallowed. Seeds are rich in purgative oil that is pale yellow with a faint odor and acrid taste. In the South east, the plant is commonly planted not only as an ornamental but also in vegetable gardens to repel moles.

Active Principle

Whole plant is poisonous, mostly the seed containing toxalbumin ricin (the active principle) a water soluble glycoprotein which is also a powerful allergen. The poisonous principle is a phytotoxin called ricin.

Mechanism of Action

One of the main toxic proteins is 'ricin', named by Stillmark in 1888. Ricin can agglutinate RBC. Agglutination is also due to another toxin that is present, called RCA (Ricinus communis agglutinin). Ricin is a potent cytotoxin but a weak hemagglutinin, whereas RCA is a weak cytotoxin and a powerful hemagglutinin. Poisoning by **ingestion** of the castor bean is due to **ricin**, not RCA, because RCA does not penetrate the intestinal wall, and does not affect RBCs unless

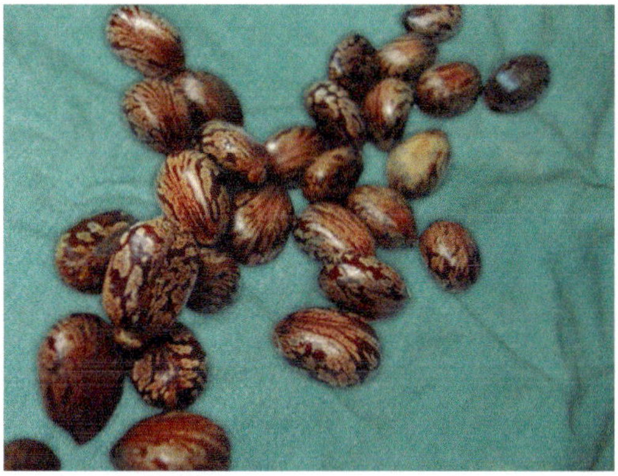

Figure 38.4 Castor oil seeds

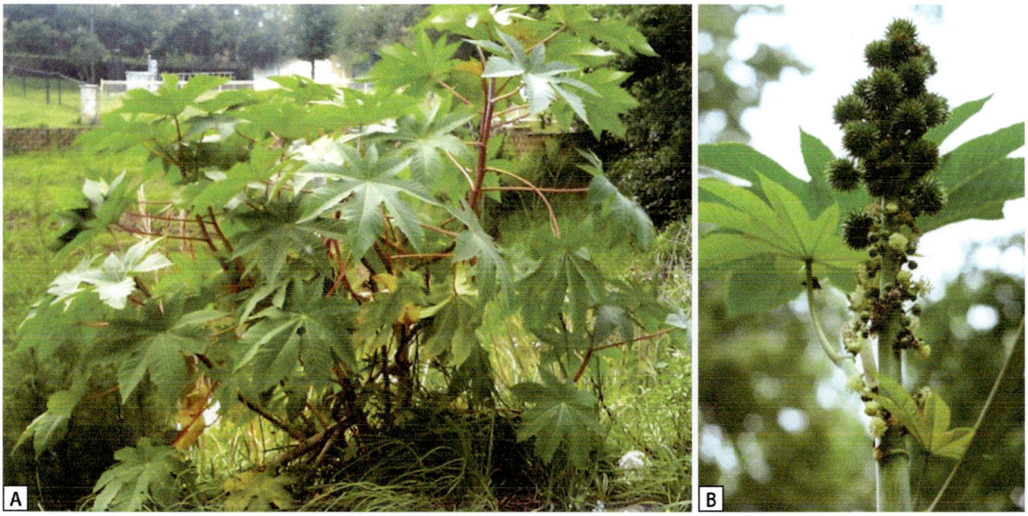

Figures 38.3A and B Castor oil plants

given intravenously. If RCA is injected into the blood, it will cause the red blood cells to agglutinate and burst by hemolysis.

Clinical Features

Animals (Horses) are most often poisoned when feed grains have become contaminated with the castor bean seeds; however, human can also be affected. Toxicity is seen most often in spring and summer. But, though ricin is extremely poisonous, it actually does little harm.

Depending upon the amount consumed, symptoms appear several hours to several days after consumption of the toxin. The clinical picture, clinical signs, symptoms and pathological manifestations in intoxicated victims depend on the route of exposure.[6]

When **inhaled** as a small particle aerosol, ricin produces symptoms within 8 hours. Respiratory distress, fever, cough, dyspnea, nausea and chest tightness are followed by profuse sweating, the development of pulmonary edema, cyanosis, hypotension and finally respiratory failure and circulatory collapse. Time to death ranges from 38–72 hours, depending on the dose received.

Ricin is extremely emetic, if ingested. **Ingestion** of ricin causes gastrointestinal features and gastrointestinal hemorrhage with necrosis of liver, spleen and kidneys. Violent purgation in the form of straining and bloody diarrhea is the classical sign. Other signs are dullness, abdominal pain, weakness, trembling and in-coordination.

Intramuscular route causes severe localized pain. There is necrosis of muscle and the regional lymph nodes with moderate involvement of visceral organs. Transient leukocytosis appears to be a constant feature in humans, whether intoxication is via injection or oral route. Leukocyte counts are 2–5 fold higher than the normal value.

Children are usually more sensitive than adults to fluid loss secondary to vomiting and diarrhea and get severely dehydrated and die. If death has not occurred within 3–5 days, the patient usually survives.

Fatal Dose: 5–10 seeds.

Fatal Period: 3–5 days.

Diagnosis

i. Like other possible toxic condition on the unlawful battlefield, epidemiological findings will likely play a major role in diagnosing.
ii. The notice of multiple cases of very severe pulmonary distress in a population of previously healthy young soldiers, linked with a history of their having been at the same place and time during climatic circumstances suitable for biological warfare assault, would be indicative of ricin intoxication.
iii. The differential diagnoses of aerosol exposure to ricin would include staphylococcal enterotoxin B, exposure to pyrolysis by products of organofluorine polymers[7] or other organohalides, oxides of nitrogen and phosgene. Laboratory findings are nonspecific but similar to other pulmonary irritants that cause pulmonary edema. Enzyme-linked immunosorbent assays in blood or other body fluids[8] or immunohistochemical techniques may be useful in confirming ricin intoxication but identification in body fluids or tissues is difficult.

Management

With no antidote, management totally relies on symptomatic support and the use of respiratory and circulatory support, kidney dialysis, etc. Usually after 3–5 days, symptoms decrease though death may take about the same time to occur.

Treatment depends on the route of exposure. Gastrointestinal intoxication is best managed by vigorous gastric decontamination with activated charcoal, followed by use of cathartics such as magnesium citrate. Fluid replacement of gastrointestinal fluid losses is important.

Patients with pulmonary intoxication are managed by appropriate treatment for pulmonary edema and respiratory support. In transdermal exposures, treatment would be mainly supportive.

Autopsy Findings

Crushed seeds may be found inside the stomach with congested, inflamed mucosa with occasional erosions and submucosal hemorrhage. It causes hemorrhagic inflammation of the gastrointestinal tract irrespective of route of administration. Heart is dilated. Petechial hemorrhage is present over the pleura, pericardium and renal capsule. There may be hemorrhages in the internal organs.

Medicolegal Importance

i. Accidental poisoning is common with the children from eating the seeds
ii. For homicidal purpose powdered seeds are used, though rare
iii. Used to procure criminal abortion and as cattle poison
iv. When applied to eye, it may cause conjunctivitis.

CROTON

Botanical Name: *Croton tiglium.*

Common Name: Croton.

Features

Croton is a decorative, often grown in tropical grounds and as a houseplant for its colorful foliage (**Figure 38.5**). The 10–15 cm (4–6 inches) leaves vary from linear and lance shaped to oval and lobed, depending upon the variety.

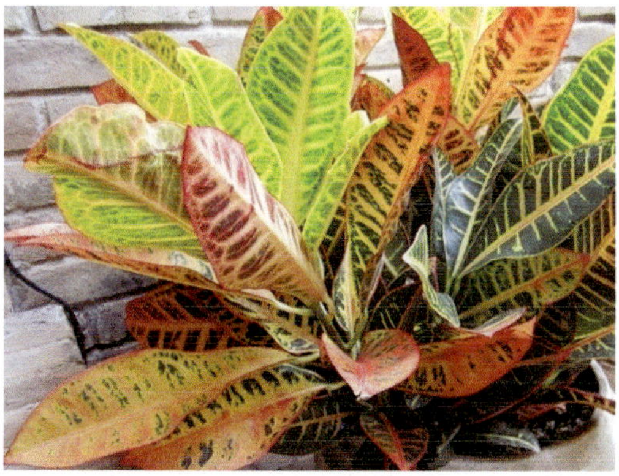

Figure 38.5 Croton plant

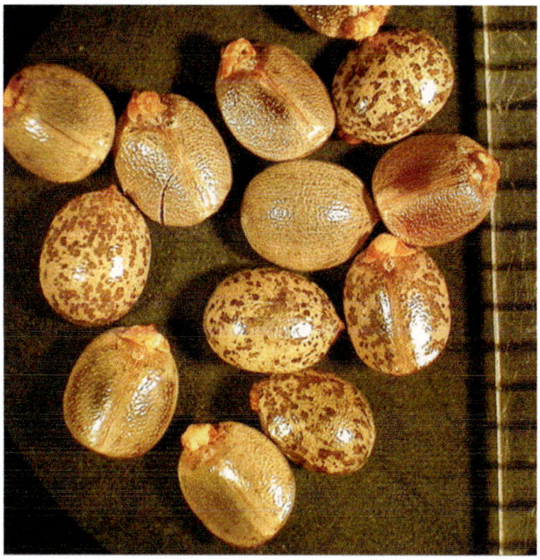

Figure 38.6 Croton seeds

Medicinal Uses

Previously croton oil was used in herbal medicine as a violent purgative, is extracted from its seeds. Nowadays, it is considered unsafe as it is violently purgative and irritating and it is no longer listed in the pharmacopeias of many countries. It is also suspected of being a co-carcinogen. Luckily, its taste is so dreadful, accidental poisonings are rare.

The croton seeds (*jamalgota* or naepala) are oval, having dark brown with longitudinal lines (**Figure 38.6**).

Toxic Part of the Plant

Every part of the plant is poisonous, especially the sap. Even dried plant materials retain their poisonous properties.

Active Principle

A seed contains crotin, the active principle, a toxalbumin is not expressed with the oil, Crotonoside, a glycoside, which is less poisonous is also present. The oil contains a powerful vesicating resin composed of cortonoleic acid, methyl crotonic acid and several other fatty acids.

Clinical Features

The list of signs and symptoms mentioned in various sources for croton poisoning includes the following:

i. Skin rash, skin irritation, redness and itching for skin exposure
ii. Abdominal pain
iii. Nausea
iv. Vomiting
v. Diarrhea
vi. Burning sensation from mouth to stomach
vii. Salivation
viii. Circulatory collapse and death.

Fatal Dose: 4–5 seeds.

Fatal Period: 6 hours to 3 days.

Management

The list of treatments mentioned in various sources for croton poisoning includes the following:

i. Decontamination
ii. Gastric lavage to wash stomach
iii. Demulcent drink
iv. Supportive or symptomatic measures.

Autopsy Findings

i. There is congestion, inflammation and erosion of the mucosa of stomach and intestine
ii. Congested visceras.

Medicolegal Importance

i. Accidental poisoning results from ingestion of croton oil by mistake or by eating seeds or inhaling their dust.
ii. Suicidal and homicidal use is rare.
iii. Its root and oil are used internally as an abortifacient.
iv. Oil is used in arrow poison.

CAPSICUM

Common Name: Chilli, red pepper, *mirch.*

Varieties of Species

Capsicum annum: Less hot.

Capsicum frutescenes: Hotter than *Capsicum annum*

Features

Capsicum annum plant is seasonal and, in the absence of winter frosts, can survive several seasons. The single flowers are an off-white or purplish in color, while the stem is densely branched and up to 60 cm.

Toxic parts of the plant are fruits and seeds. The fruit is a berry and may be green, yellow or red when ripe (**Figure 38.7**).

Active Principle

Capsaicin and capsicin.

Clinical Features

Most commonly reported poisoning is due to plant exposure; related to the mace product containing capsaicin. Capsaicin is an alkaloid that is a mucosal irritant causing severe burning pain, local irritation and edema; produces lacrimation, airway swelling and bronchospasm if inhaled.

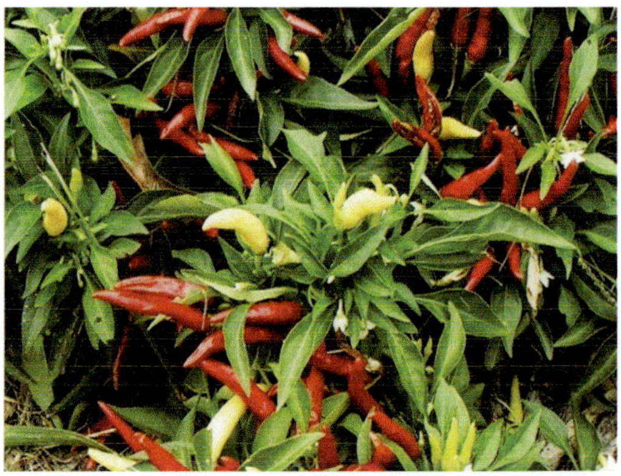

Figure 38.7 *Capsicum annum*

Most of the exposures are not dangerous; however, fatal airway edema or bronchospasm may occur which may lead to death.

Chronic poisoning to capsaicin depletes neurotransmitters leading to reduction in sensation and consequent alleviation of pain.

Other less serious side effects have also been reported infrequently. They are: Stomach upset, heartburn, diarrhea or burning sensation in the mouth or throat or with skin contact.

Management

i. Irrigation of exposed areas with vinegar (5% acetic acid) may provide some symptomatic relief.
ii. Supportive care.
iii. Bronchodilator.

Autopsy Findings

i. Congestion, inflammation and erosion of the mucosa of stomach and intestine.
ii. Stomach may contain remnants of seeds and fruit.
iii. Congested visceras.

Medicolegal Importance

i. Mainly accidental poisoning.
ii. Suicide and homicide are rare.
iii. Chili powder used for torture, extortion, kidnapping, self-defense by women as pepper spray, child abuse, etc.

CALOTROPIS

Common Name: Madar, akdo, common weeds.

Varieties

Calotropis plants are of two types: (i) *Calotropis gigantea* and (ii) *Calotropis procera.*

Features

Calotropis gigantea has purple flowers and *Calotropis procera* has white flowers (**Figure 38.8**).

Calotropis is a genus of flowering plants and are commonly known as **milkweeds** because of the latex they produce.

Calotropis species are considered common weeds in some parts of the world. The flowers are odorous and are often used in making floral tassels. Fibers of these plants are called madar or mader.

Medicinal Uses

The plant is known as *aak* in Ayurveda and was used in cases of cutaneous diseases, intestinal worms, cough, ascites, asthma, bronchitis, dyspepsia, paralysis, swellings.

The milky exudation from the plant act as a corrosive poison and the latex is said to have mercury-like effects on the human body and is sometimes referred to as vegetable mercury. Root bark has a Digitalis-like effect on the

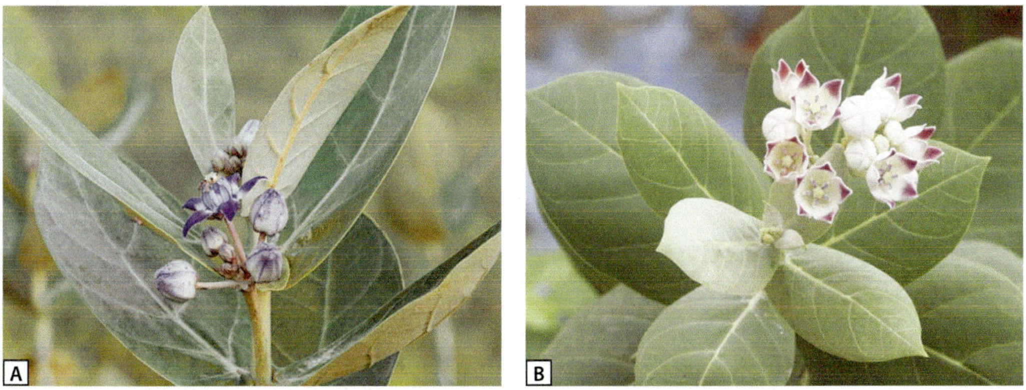

Figures 38.8A and B (A) *Calotropis gigantea;* and (B) *Calotropis procera*

heart, but was earlier used as a substitute of ipecacuanha.

Toxic Principles

i. Calotoxin
ii. Calotropin (cardiac glycosides)
iii. Calactin
iv. Uscharin.

Toxicity

Calotropis are poisonous plants and calotropin is an active principle in the latex, which is more toxic than strychnine. Calotropin is similar in structure to two cardiac glycosides which are responsible for the cytotoxicity. Extracts of the flowers of *Calotropis procera* have strong cytotoxic activity in the patients of colorectal cancer. They are harmful to the eyes.

Clinical Features

Dermal Exposure: Causes irritation, redness and vesication and erosion.

Ocular Exposure: Conjunctivitis like features.

Ingestion: Nausea, vomiting, burning sensation in the mouth and stomach with pain, diarrhea, convulsion, delirium and circulatory collapse and death.

Management

i. Stomach wash
ii. Demulcents with supportive treatment.

Autopsy Findings

i. Froth at mouth and nostril
ii. Congestion, inflammation and erosion of the mucosa of stomach and intestine
iii. Vesication, inflammation and redness at the site of contact
iv. Congested visceras.

Medicolegal Importance

i. Mainly accidental poisoning. Suicide and homicide are rare
ii. Used in folk medicine and for fabricating wounds
iii. Cattle poison
iv. Root of *Calotropis procera* is poisonous like cobra venom.

MARKING NUT

Botanical Name: *Semicarpus anacardium.*

Common Name: Marking nut, bhilawa, biba, dhobi nut tree, Indian marking nut tree, Malacca bean, marany nut, marsh nut, oriental cashew nut, varnish tree.

Synonyms: Anacardium orientale.

Features

Marking Nut is a moderate sized broad-leafed tree. Leaves are 7–24 inches long, 2–12 inches wide, simple oblong, rounded at the tip. Leaf base is rounded, heart-shaped or narrowed into the stalk and leathery in texture (**Figure 38.9**).

Fruit is a stone fruit one-inch long, oblong, smooth and shining, black when ripe with fleshy cup (**Figure 38.10**).

Common Use

i. Stem yields an acrid, viscid juice from which a varnish is prepared.
ii. Nut yields a powerful and bitter substance that is used everywhere in India as an alternative for marking ink for clothes by washermen, hence it is frequently called **Dhobi Nut.** They give a black color to cotton fabrics, but before application, it should be mixed with limewater as a fixator.
iii. Fruits are also used as a dye.
iv. Largely employed in Indian medicine.
v. The fleshy cups on which the nuts rest and the kernels of the nuts are consumed.

Medicinal Uses

i. Fruit is said to be useful in leukoderma, scaly skin, allergic, dermatitis, poisonous bites, leprosy, cough, asthma and dyspepsia.

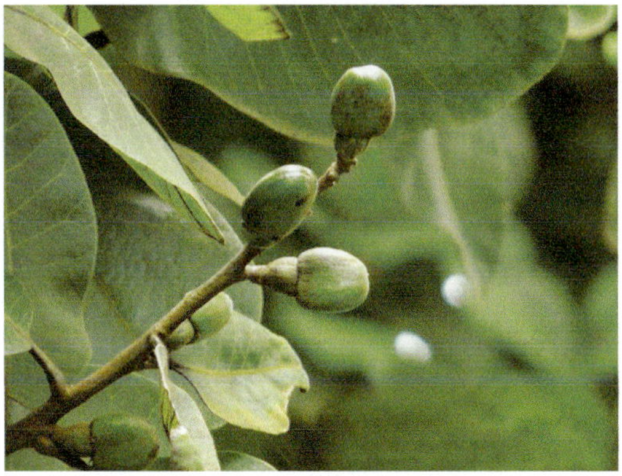

Figure 38.9 Marking nut tree

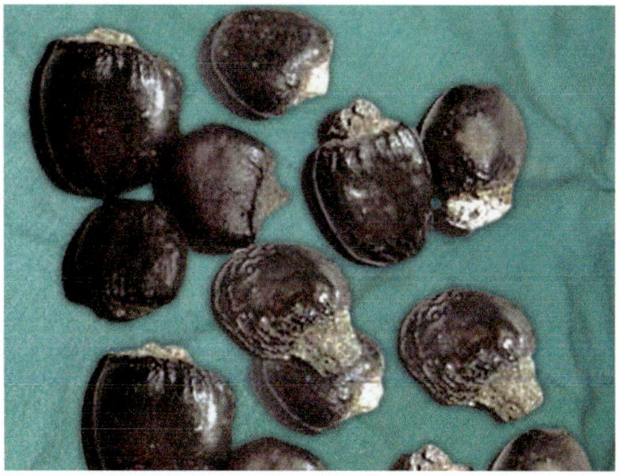

Figure 38.10 Nut of *Semicarpus anacardium*

ii. It is extremely beneficial in the diseases like piles, colitis, diarrhea, dyspepsia, ascites, tumors and worms.
iii. The topical application of its oil on swollen joints and traumatic wounds effectively controls the pain.

Active Principle

i. Semicarpol (0.1%)
ii. Bhilawanol (15–17%).

Clinical Features

Local Application: The juice induces irritation in the skin, painful blisters, itchy and eczematous eruption of adjacent skin, which look like bruise. Later on, ulcer is produced from these lesions.

Oral Ingestion: In large doses, it produces blisters on throat and severe gastrointestinal irritation, dyspnea, tachycardia, hypotension, cyanosis, areflexia, delirium, coma and death.

Fatal Dose: 5–10 g.

Fatal Period: 12–24 hours.

Management

i. Stomach wash
ii. Demulcents drinks
iii. Affected part should be washed with lukewarm water containing antiseptic solution
iv. Supportive treatment.

Autopsy Findings

i. Blisters at mouth, throat and stomach
ii. Congestion, inflammation and erosion of the mucosa of stomach and intestine
iii. Blister, inflammation and ulcer at the site of contact
iv. Congested visceras.

Medicolegal Importance

i. Mainly accidental poisoning
ii. Suicide and homicide is rare
iii. Used for fabricating wounds
iv. For criminal abortion.

PLUMBAGO

Varieties

There are two varieties of Plumbago plants. They are: (i) *Plumbago Indica* and (ii) *Plumbago Zeylanica*.

Features

i. ***Plumbago Indica*** (Indian leadwort, scarlet leadwort): ***Plumbago rosea*** (synonym) also called as lal chitra is a species of the flowering plant in the family Plumbaginaceae. Growing up to 2 m tall, it is a spreading evergreen shrub with oval leaves and racemes of deep pink or scarlet flowers in winter (**Figure 38.11**).

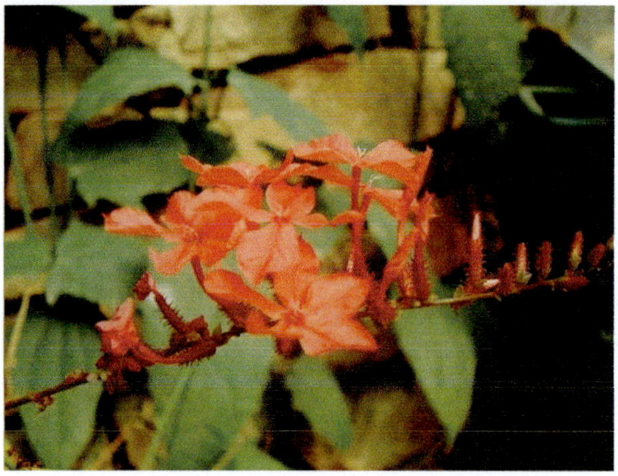

Figure 38.11 *Plumbago rosea*

ii. ***Plumbago zeylanica***: Chitra (synonym) bears white flowers. Toxic part of the plant is the root.

Active Principle

Plumbagin.

Medicinal Use

It is used as gastric stimulant and appetizer. Root is said to increase the digestive power and promote appetite. It has marked antiseptic properties. An embrocation made from bruised root mixed with a little bland oil is used as a rubefacient in rheumatism, paralytic affections, in enlarged glands, buboes, etc.

Clinical Features

Local application to skin causes irritation and inflammation. Locally plumbagin is a vesicant.

Ingestion causes pain abdomen, vomiting, diarrhea and shock. In large doses, it is acronarcotic poison. It has a specific action on the uterus. It can cause abortion. It is suggested that the action is probably due to the direct effect of the drug on the muscles.

It stimulates the central nervous system in small doses, while with larger doses paralysis sets in leading ultimately to death from respiratory failure. The blood pressure shows a slight fall. Plumbagin is a powerful irritant. In small doses, the drug is a diaphoretic.

Management

i. Stomach wash
ii. Demulcents drinks
iii. Affected part should be washed with lukewarm water containing antiseptic solution
iv. Supportive treatment.

Autopsy findings are same with marking nut poisoning.

Medicolegal Importance

i. Mainly accidental poisoning
ii. Suicide and homicide are rare
iii. Root paste is used for criminal abortion.

COLOCYNTH

Botanical Name: *Citrullus colocynthus.* Synonyms: *Cucumis colocynthis* L; *Colocynthis vulgaris* schrad.

Common Name: Colocynth, Indrayani, bitter apple, bitter gourd (English); bitter cucumber, desert gourd, chicotin (French), amaro (Italian), hanzal (Arabic), etc.

Features

It resembles a common watermelon vine, but bears small, hard fruits with a bitter pulp. Its fruit is lemon sized, yellowish and green mottled, spongy and extremely bitter. Colocynth capsule is yellowish-brown and spherical (**Figure 38.12**). Leaves are very similar to watermelon leaves, are palmed, angular with 3–7 divided lobes.

Colocynth seeds are gray yellowish and oval in shape, about 7.5 mm long, 5 mm broad and 1.5 mm thick (**Figure 38.13**). Toxic parts of the plant are fruit, root and leaves. Ripe fruit root and leaves are poisonous. Drying does not modify or reduce the toxicity of the plant.

Active Principle

Colocynthin (glycoside) is the active principle. It is a powerful hepatic stimulant and is a hydragogue cathartic and used strongly as laxative.

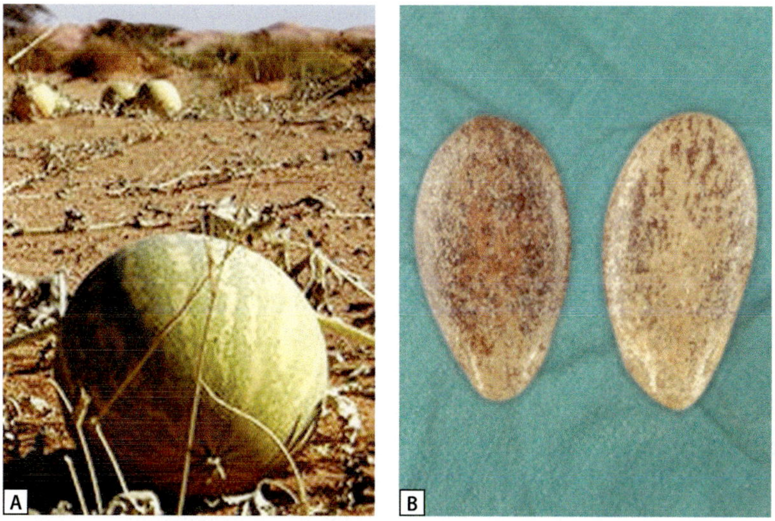

Figures 38.12A and B Colocynth capsule with seed

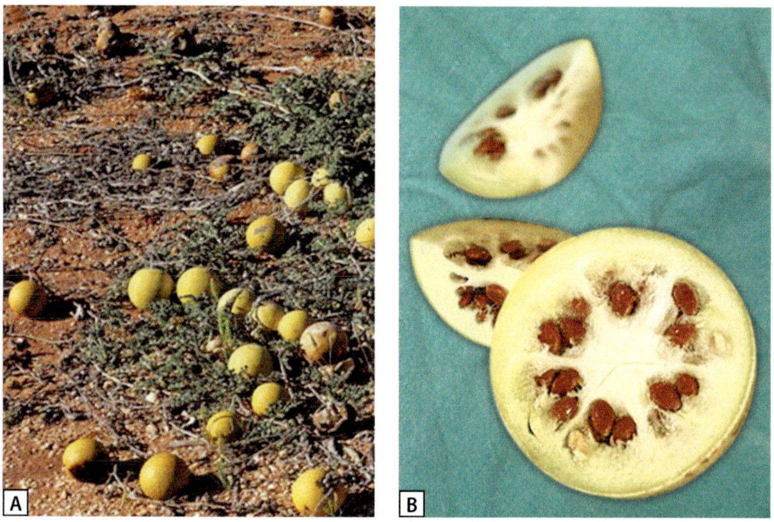

Figures 38.13A and B Dissected Colocynth capsule with seeds

Medicinal Uses

The ripe fruit is used as a medicine. Colocynthis is a debatable herbal treatment for a variety of conditions, primarily intestinal or menstrual in nature. The treatment comes from the fruit of the gourd-like colocynth plant. Ailments typically treated with colocynthis are: Constipation; liver and gallbladder problems; diarrhea; colic and painful menstruation. Others use to treat nerve and joint problems, such as sciatica, rheumatism and facial neuralgia.

Clinical Features

Colocynthin strongly irritates the gastrointestinal mucosa leading to violent cramping pain, vomiting, watery diarrhea, bleeding and dangerous inflammation of the bowel and shock. Death results from ½ teaspoonful of the powder. Management is mainly symptomatic.

Management

No specific antidote. Symptomatic care only. Adsorbents, i.e. activated vegetable charcoal;

tranquillizers or barbiturates if necessary; emollients, gastrointestinal demulcents, aluminum hydroxide gel should be tried.

Autopsy Findings

Features are of acute gastroenteritis; pulmonary edema; generalized congestion; petechiae or hemorrhages visible on the gastric mucosa and on renal capsule and kidneys. There is congestion, inflammation and erosion of the mucosa of stomach and intestine.

Medicolegal Importance

i. Mainly accidental poisoning
ii. Suicide and homicide are rare
iii. It is used to procure for criminal abortion.

ERGOT ON RYE

Ergot on Rye (**Figure 38.14**) is a plant disease that is caused by the fungus ***Claviceps purpurea***. The so-called **ergot** that replaces the grain of the rye is a dark, slight pinkish **sclerotium** (**Figure 38.15**), from which the sexual stage, of the lifecycle will form after over wintering. Thus, ergot is the over wintering stage and also the part of the life cycle containing the alkaloids.

The fungus grows on rye and related plants, produces alkaloids that can cause chronic poisoning (**ergotism**) in humans and other mammals who consume grains contaminated with its fruiting structure, i.e. sclerotium.

While the ergot is far different in appearance than the true grain, its occurrence was so common that it was thought to be part of the rye plant, until the 1850's, when the true nature of the ergot was understood.

In this ergot stage, the fungus that contains a storehouse of alkaloids has been useful for pharmaceutical drugs as well as **mycotoxins** that can be fatal when consumed. This species was also the original source from which LSD was first isolated. It is believed that symptoms of ergotism have been recorded since the Middle Ages and possibly even as far back as ancient Greece.

Alkaloids of Ergot

i. Ergotamine
ii. Ergotoxin
iii. Ergometrine
iv. Dihydroergotamine.

Current Uses of Ergot

There are some medicinal productions that have been extracted from Ergot. Some of the common examples are: (i) **Ergotamine**, which is prescribed for various causes of headaches, including migraine. (ii) **Ergonovine** is used to control postpartum hemorrhage and cause contraction of the uterus. (iii) **LSD**, which was

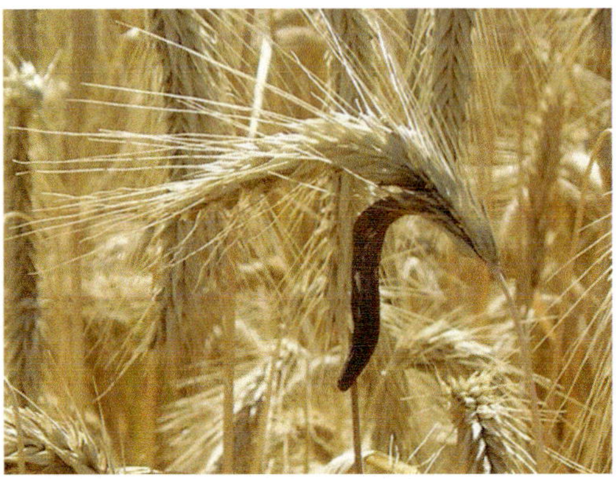

Figure 38.14 Ergot (sclerotia) on rye. Ergot replaces grain of rye

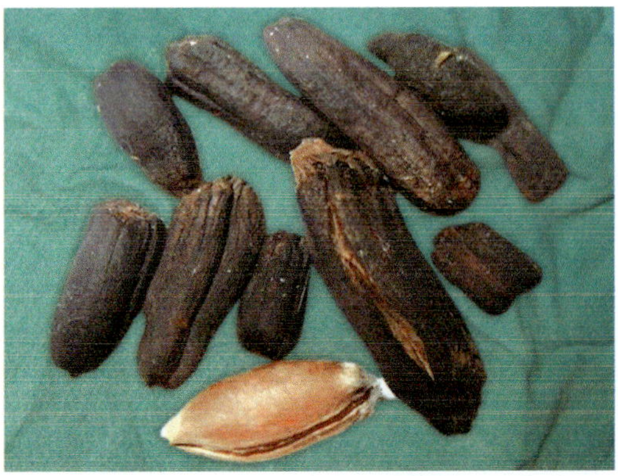

Figure 38.15 Ergot (sclerotia)

initially prescribed for psychiatric disorders, but is eventually made illegal due to its abuse.

Clinical Feature

Poisoning attributed to Ergot of Rye is referred to as **ergotism**. Although this fungus is recognized as one species, there are two sets of symptoms that can be found in cases where serious poisoning has occurred: **convulsive** and **gangrenous ergotism**.

Convulsive Ergotism: This set is characterized by nervous dysfunction, where the victim is twisting and distorting their body in pain, trembling and shaking and torticollis, a more or less fixed twisting of the neck, which seems to simulate convulsions or fits. This may be accompanied by muscle spasms, confusions, delusions and hallucinations, as well as a number of other symptoms.

Gangrenous Ergotism: Here the victim may lose parts of their extremities, such as toes, fingers, ear lobes or, in more serious cases, arms and legs may be lost. This type of ergotism causes gangrene to occur by constricting the blood vessels leading to the extremities. Because of the decrease in blood flow, infections occur in the extremities, accompanied by burning pain. Once gangrene has occurred, the fingers, toes, etc. become mummified, and will eventually fall off as a result of infection. If the infected extremities are not removed, infection can spread further up the extremity that has been infected. Gangrenous ergotism is common in grazing, farm animals.

Management

i. Stomach wash with activated charcoal
ii. Hypertension or cerebral or cardiac ischemia is controlled by IV nitroglycerine
iii. For peripheral ischemia, oral prazosin, captopril
iv. Diazepam to treat convulsion
v. Hypercoagulable state by heparin or dextran.

Medicolegal Importance

i. Mainly accidental poisoning due to consumption of contaminated grains
ii. It is used to procure for abortion.

REFERENCES

1. Keddy PA. Plants and Vegetation: Origins, Processes, Consequences. Cambridge, UK: Cambridge University Press; 2007. p. 666.
2. Krenzelok EP, Mrvos R. Friends and foes in the plant world: A profile of plant ingestions and fatalities. Clin Toxicol (Phila). 2011;49(3):142-9.
3. Lord MJ, Hartley MR (Eds). Toxic Plant Proteins. 2010; Springer. p. 134. ISBN 9783842121760.
4. Lewis RA. Lewis Dictionary of Toxicology. 1998; CRC Press. pp. 3-4. ISBN 9781566702232.
5. Allen, ON, Allen EK. The Leguminosae: A Source Book of Characteristics, Uses and Nodulation. University of Wisconsin Press. 1981; p. 4. ISBN 9780299084004.
6. Olsnes S, Sandvig K, Eiklid K, Pihl A. Properties and action mechanism of the toxic lectin modeccin: Interaction with cell lines resistant to modeccin, abrin, and ricin. J Supramol Struct. 1978;9:15-25.
7. Patocka J, Bajgar J. Toxicology of perfluoroisobuten. ASA Newsletter. 1998;16-8.
8. Poli MA, Rivera VR, Hewetson JF, Merril GA. Detection of ricin by colorimetric and chemiluminescence ELISA. Toxicon. 1994;32:1371-7.

CHAPTER 39

Organic Irritants of Animal Origin

TK Bose, Shouvanik Adhya, Putul Mahanta

LEARNING PLAN

- Know about the classification of snakes
- Learn the anatomy and identification of poisonous and non-poisonous snakes
- Know about the snake venom, features and management of snake bite
- Identify the postmortem finding in a case of death due to snake bite
- Know about other significant bites and stings in Indian scenario

ORGANIC IRRITANTS OF ANIMAL ORIGIN

Irritants are those chemicals which causes over-excitement of cells by its action. Truly, there are very few agents which have only these isolated effects. In most of the organic irritants of animal origin, the principle actions are enzymatic remote action than local irritation. There are thousands of animal irritants, but only the major ones having clinical significance are being discussed, of which the most important one is snake which kills more than 50,000 persons per year in our country.

SNAKES

In many parts of the South East Asian region, snakebite is an important medical emergency and cause of hospital admission. It results in the death or chronic disability of many active younger people, especially those involved in farming and plantation work. However, the true scale of mortality and acute and chronic morbidity from snakebite remains uncertain because of inadequate reporting in almost every part of the region.

To remedy this deficiency, it is strongly recommended[1] that snakebite should be made a specific notifiable disease in all countries of the South East Asian region.

Recent estimates indicate somewhere between 1.2 and 5.5 million snakebites worldwide each year, with 421,000–1,841,000 envenomations and 20,000–94,000 deaths.[2] Such wide range of estimate is due to problematic data collection in the developing world, the region's most affected by venomous snakes.

The Indian subcontinent is home to over 230 species of snakes, of whom, about 50 are venomous. However, only four are considered to be of major clinical significance as they contribute most to snake bite related deaths every year.[3]

Classification of Snakes[4]

The following snake families belong to the venomous snakes:

1. **Viperidae** includes sub family Viperinae, e.g. true viper (Russell's viper, Saw scaled viper); sub family Crotalinae, e.g. pit viper (Rattle snake).
2. Atractaspididae, e.g. Stiletto snake.
3. Elapidae includes sub family elapinae, e.g. cobra, mamba, krait, coral snake; sub family Hydrophiinae, e.g. sea snakes.
4. Colubridae (includes numerous sub families both poisonous and non-poisonous), e.g. African boom slang, twig snake.
5. Hydrophiidae— musculotoxic.

THE BIG FOUR (IN INDIA)[5,6]

Common Cobra (Naja Naja)

They are about 2–2.5 meter long, blackish or dark brown snake as shown in **Figure 39.1**, which can spread their neck into a fan shaped hood. The hood is dorsally marked by a monocellate (monocle) or binocellate (spectacle) patch. Each ventral scale of the tail is divided into two parts. The head is small with round pupils. 3rd supra-labial shield touches eye and nasal shield. A tiny triangular cuneate scale is present between the 4th and 5th infralabile scales.

Common Krait (Bungarus Caeruleus)

They are 1–2 meter long with a black or steel gray shiny body with whitish arches or half rings on dorsal surface (**Figure 39.2**). The ventral scales of the tail are not divided but the dorsal surface is marked by a mid-dorsal row of larger hexagonal scales (**Figure 39.3**). The 4th infralabial scale is the largest.

Russell's Viper (Vipera Russelli/Daboia Russelli)

This is 1.5–2 meter long, brownish, stout snake (**Figures 39.4** and **39.5**). The head is triangular, with a 'V' shaped mark (apex pointing forward), covered with small scales and the neck is prominent. Pupils are vertical and slit-like. The tail tapers abruptly. There are three rows of chained dark spots over dorsal surface.

Saw-Scaled Viper (Echis Carinata)

Common names: Carpet vipers

This is a small snake, about half a meter long, usually brown in color (**Figure 39.6**), with serrated scales. The head is triangular, covered with small scales. The body is fairly slender and cylindrical. A characteristic it is whitish, arrow or crowfoot shaped mark is present on the head. The pupils are vertical. There is a wavy white line along the entire length of each flank; while diamond shaped markings (25–30) extend over back.

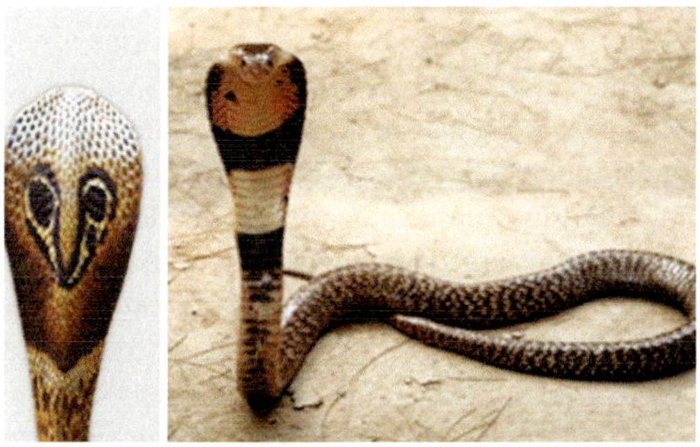

Figure 39.1 Common spectacled cobras (Naja naja) (*Courtesy*: Professor Sanjoy Das)

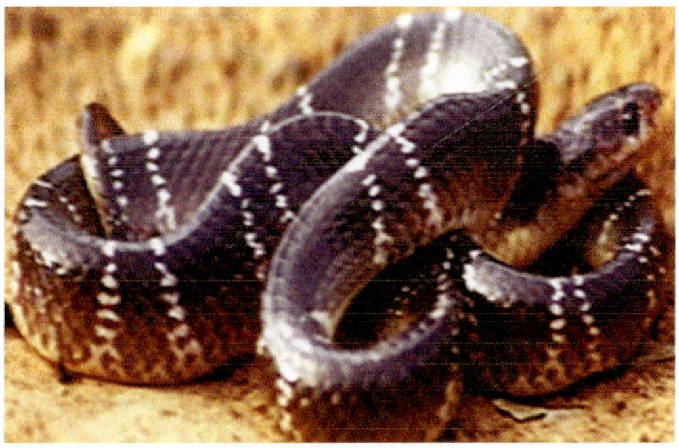

Figure 39.2 Common krait (Bungarus caeruleus) (*Courtesy*: www.indianreptiles.com)

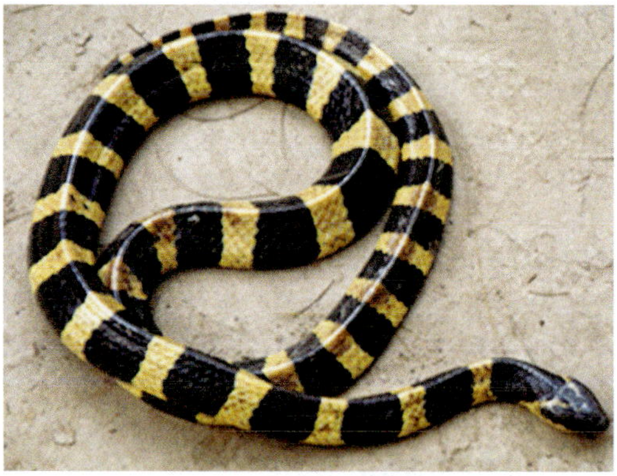

Figure 39.3 Banded krait
(*Courtesy*: Professor Sanjoy Das)

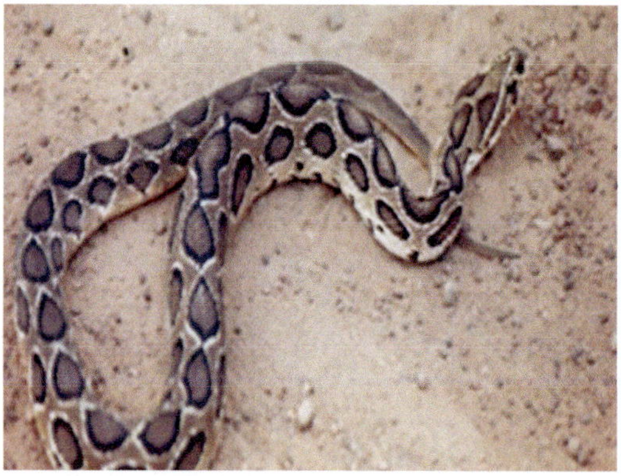

Figure 39.4 Russell's viper (Daboia russelli)
(*Courtesy*: www.indianreptiles.com)

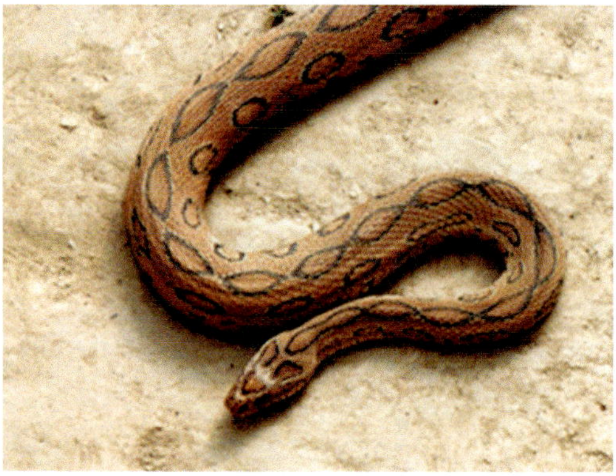

Figure 39.5 Russell's viper
(*Courtesy*: Professor Sanjoy Das)

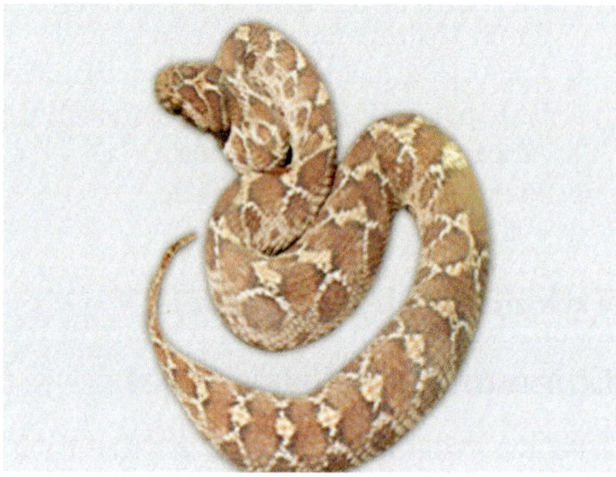

Figure 39.6 Saw-scaled vipers
(Echis carinata)

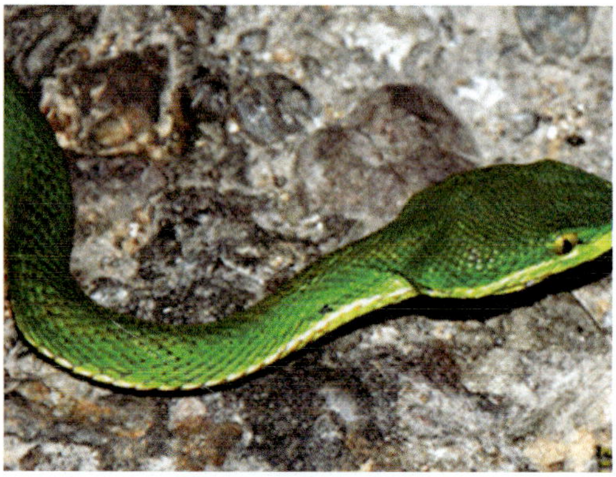

Figure 39.7 Green viper
(*Courtesy*: Professor Sanjoy Das)

An another venomous species of viper, i.e. Green viper found in North-Central Africa and China (**Figure 39.7**).

They display a characteristic threat, rubbing sections of their body together to produce a "sizzling" warning sound. The dorsal scales are mostly keeled.

RELEVANT ANATOMY

Venom Delivery Apparatus[4,6]

This includes a pair of poison glands, their ducts, fangs and muscles (**Figure 39.8**). Poison glands are modified to parotid salivary glands, situated one on either inner side of maxilla, below and behind eyes. Each gland is encapsulated with fibrous tissue and mostly covered with a constrictor muscle, its stretching during biting squeezes poison from gland into ducts. That duct leads to the base of a fang to enter its groove or canal.

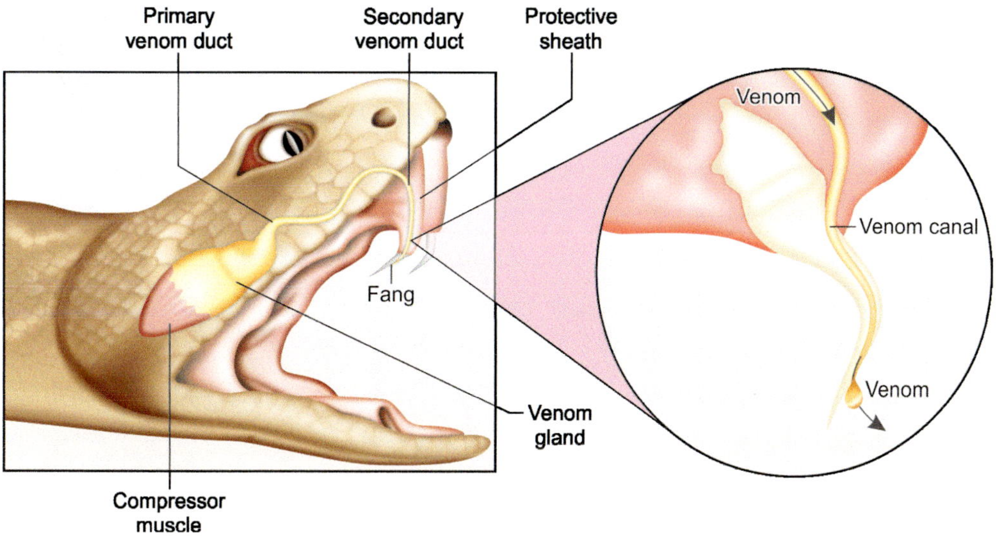

Figure 39.8 Snake fangs and venom

Fangs are sharply pointed and enlarged maxillary teeth, may be grooved or canalized, with opening at tip for passage of venom. Fangs may be fixed as in Elapidae, or movable as in Viperidae (fangs can be folded back when mouth is closed and will be erected when snake strikes).

IDENTIFICATION OF POISONOUS AND NON-POISONOUS SNAKES[7]

The placement and size of the scales, plates and shields help in the recognition of poisonous and non-poisonous snakes which are narrated in **Table 39.1** and **Figure 39.9.**

The usual features of both the poisonous and non-poisonous snakes are as follows:

1. Ventral side of a snake to be looked to ascertain the scale pattern. If the distributions of scales are small and uniform, or if they are transversely long and some of the rows of small scales of the back are visible on the ventral side, it is non-poisonous.
2. The scale pattern on the ventral side, if shows transversely arranged plates and no small scales of the back reach the ventral side, then it may be poisonous or non-poisonous. For confirmation, scale pattern on the top of the head need to be studied; if the head is covered with small scales, it should be one of the deadly poisonous snakes such as a viper.
3. If the head is covered with large scales or plates, it may be non-poisonous or one of poisonous snakes, like a pit-viper, a cobra, king cobra or a coral snake. Therefore, to confirm side of the face need to be studied:
   i. If a pit bigger than the nostril is present between the nostril and the eye, then it is a pit-viper.
   ii. If no pit is present, but the third upper labial (supralabial) scale touches the nasal scale and the eye, it is a cobra, king cobra or a coral snake, Naja Naja (cobra).
   iii. If none of the two above characters is present, then look for the following two characters: (A) The middle row of scales on the back enlarged and (B). The fourth scale on the lower lip (infralabial) along the margin of the lower jaw is the largest, then it is a Krait. If the features mentioned above (i, ii and iii) are absent, then it's non-poisonous.

Table 39.1 Identification of poisonous and nonpoisonous snakes

Structures	Characters	Nature	Snakes
1. Tail	Flat and laterally compressed	Poisonous hydrophis, enhydrina	Sea snakes
	Pointed and cylindrical or tapering	Poisonous or non-poisonous further examination for confirmation is needed	Land snakes
2. Belly scales or ventrals	Small, continuous with dorsal	Non-poisonous	Pythons
	Narrow belly scales	Non-poisonous	-
	Ventrals not fully broad to cover belly	Non-poisonous	Pit less vipers
	Ventrals broad, fully covering belly	Poisonous or non-poisonous. Further examination for confirmation is needed	Vipera russelli
3. Head scales, subcaudal	• Head scales small with triangular head No loreal pit	Poisonous	Echis carinata
	– Loreal pit	Poisonous	Pit vipers
	– Subcaudals single	Poisonous	-
	• Head scales small. A loreal pit present between nostril and eye	Poisonous	Krait, Bungaurus
	• Head with large shields. No loreal pit	Poisonous or non-poisonous. Further examination for confirmation is needed	Cobra, Naja
4. Vertebrals, 4th infra-labial, 3rd supralabial	• Vertebrals enlarged, hexagonal 4th infralabial largest	Poisonous	Coral snakes
	• Vertebrals not enlarged, 3rd supralabial touches eye and nostril	Poisonous	
	– Neck with a hood and spectacle mark	Poisonous	
	– Hood absent. Coral spots on belly	Poisonous	
	• If no such characters	Non-poisonous	

Snake Venom[4,5]

It is actually modified saliva which exhibit toxic and enzymatic properties. The functions of snake venom are prey acquisition, digestion and defense. Fresh snake venom is an aqueous, viscous, amber colored liquid. That composition is highly variable among species. Most of the dry weight of venom is constituted by proteins, comprising a variety of enzymes, non-enzymatic polypeptide toxins and non-toxic proteins. Non-protein ingredients are carbohydrates, metals (often in form of glycoprotein metalloprotein enzymes), lipids, free amino acids, nucleotides and biogenic amines (histamine, serotonin).

Snake venom enzymes can be divided into five major groups

1. Enzymes acting on glycosyl compounds, e.g. hyaluronidase, which depolimerizes hyaluronic acid leading to the formation of gaps and fissures in skin and underlying tissues, facilitating penetration of venom.
2. Enzymes acting on phosphate esters, e.g. 5′-nucleotidase is present in sea snake venom.
3. Enzyme acting on carboxylic ester bonds, e.g. phospholipase A_2 present in all snake venom, hydrolyses soluble or membrane bound phospholipids leading to lysis of RBC or muscle necrosis or blockade of neurotransmitter release. Acetylcholine esterase is exclusively found in elapidae venom.
4. Enzymes acting on peptide bonds, e.g. Peptidases and proteases in Viperidae venom interfering with coagulation or causing vessel wall damage as hemorrhagins or kininogenases, which releases hypotensive peptide bradykinins.

Clotting enzymes (pro-coagulants) are found in viperidae venom, such as

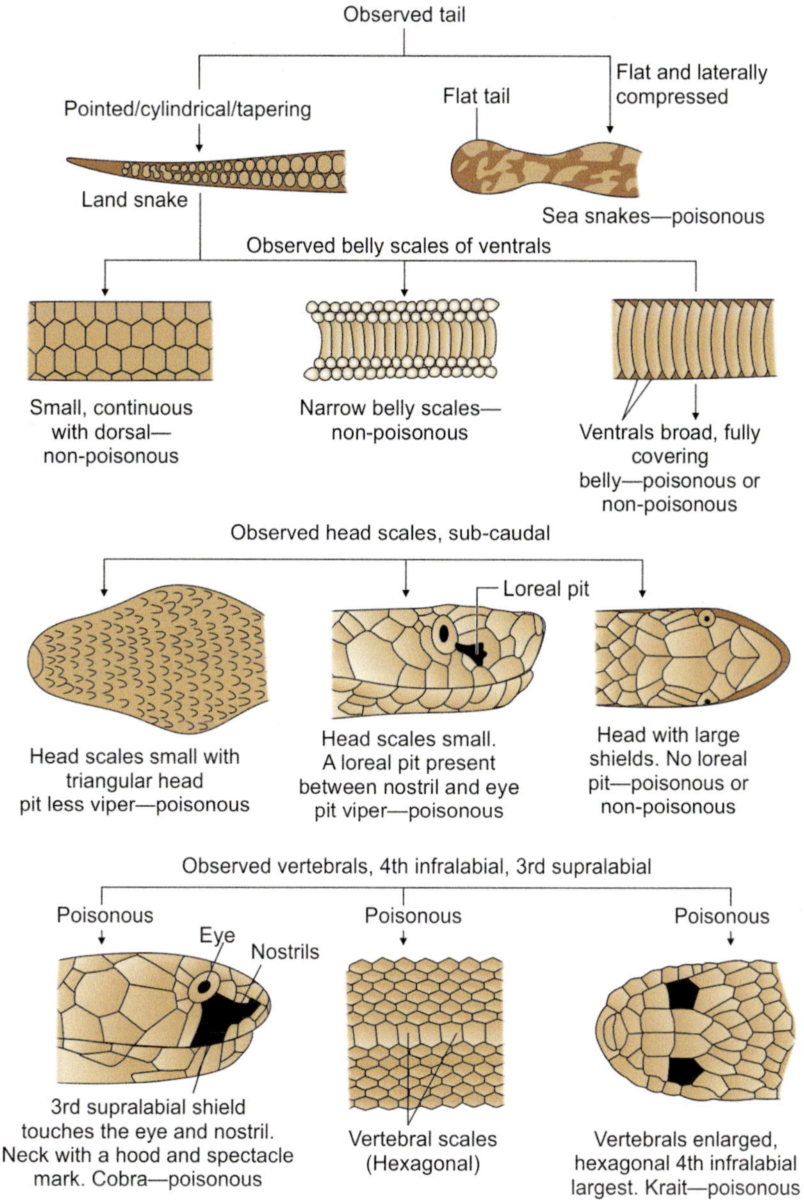

Figure 39.9 Key features for identification of snakes

thrombin like enzymes (convert fibrinogen to fibrin), or enzymes convert prothrombin to thrombin, or Factor X or Factor V activator. As a reaction following massive formation of fibrin, the endogenous fibrinolytic system is rapidly activated and clots are dissolved. Ultimately, there is incoagulability of blood due to consumption coagulopathy.

5. L-amino acid oxidases-no involvement in envenomations.

Polypeptide Toxins

They are mainly neurotoxins (found in elapid venom), affect the peripheral, but not the central nervous system; postsynaptic alpha neuro-toxins—curare like (as in cobra venom), bind to acetylcholine receptors on motor end plate. Toxins affecting presynaptic membrane are of two distinct types. One type is beta neurotoxins—phospholipase A_2 (as in krait venom), prevent release of acetylcholine at neuromuscular junction. The other type of toxin blocks ion channels, causing increase of neurotransmitter release.

SNAKE BITE

Clinical Features[5,8,9]

A significant proportion of cases are bites by non-poisonous snakes. Due to psychological shock, patient may present with sweating, palpitation, tachycardia, hypotension, giddiness, syncope, etc.

It is also common that there is absence of serious envenomations in spite of being bitten by poisonous snakes. Reasons may be dry bite (biting without injecting venom); body part protected by heavy clothing or shoes, leakage of venom outside the bite site, superficial bites, etc.

Fang Marks[5]

Typically there are 2 puncture wounds with a gap of varying (8 mm–4 cm) distance. But there may be a single puncture in case of sideswipe or multiple marks made by fangs along with other teeth as shown in **Figure 39.10**.

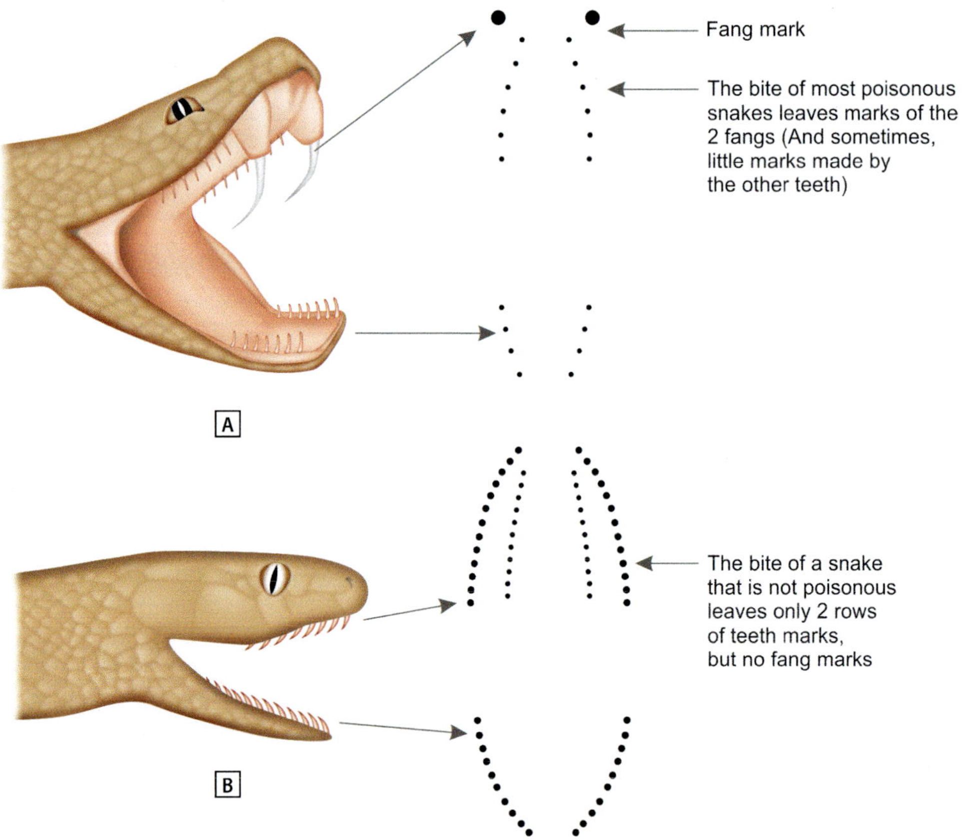

Figures 39.10A and B Diagramatic representation of fang mark, (A) Venomous snake; (B) Non-venomous snake

General Signs and Symptoms of Viperine Envenomations

1. Swelling and local pain. Tender enlargement of local lymph nodes is seen, as large molecular weight viper venom molecules enter the system via the lymphatic system. There is persistent bleeding from the bite site. Blister formation initially around bite area, then entire limb (**Figure 39.11**). There may be extensive necrosis of local tissue (**Figure 39.12**).
2. Raised intracompartmental pressure in affected limb.
3. Epistaxis and bleeding from gingival sulci and other orifices.
4. Emesis and acute abdominal tenderness suggesting gastrointestinal or retroperitoneal bleeding.
5. Hypotension resulting from hypovolemia or direct vasodilatation. There is low back pain, indicative of an early renal failure or retroperitoneal bleeding.
6. The skin and mucous membranes may show evidence of petechiae, purpuras and ecchymoses.
7. The passing of reddish or dark-brown urine or declining or no urine output.
8. Lateralizing neurological symptoms and asymmetric pupils indicating intracranial hemorrhage.
9. Muscle pain indicating rhabdomyolysis.
10. Parotid swelling, conjunctival edema, subconjunctival hemorrhage (**Figure 39.13**).
11. Intravascular hemolysis, acute renal failure, disseminated intravascular coagulation. DIC results in renal tubular and cortical necrosis.

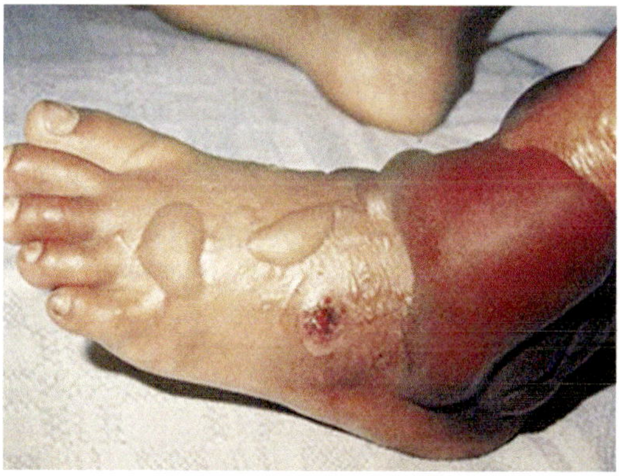

Figure 39.11 Blister formation

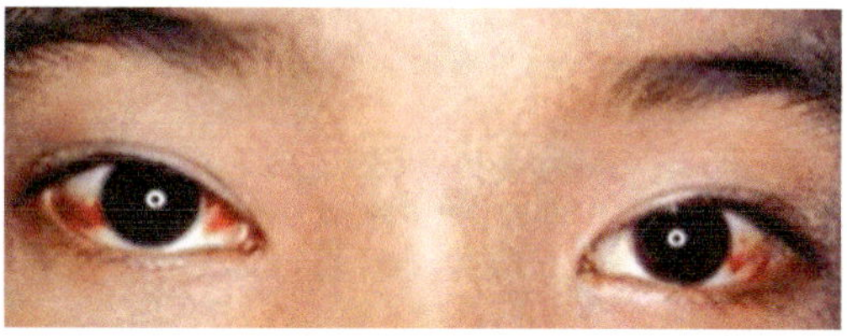

Figure 39.13 Subconjunctival hemorrhages

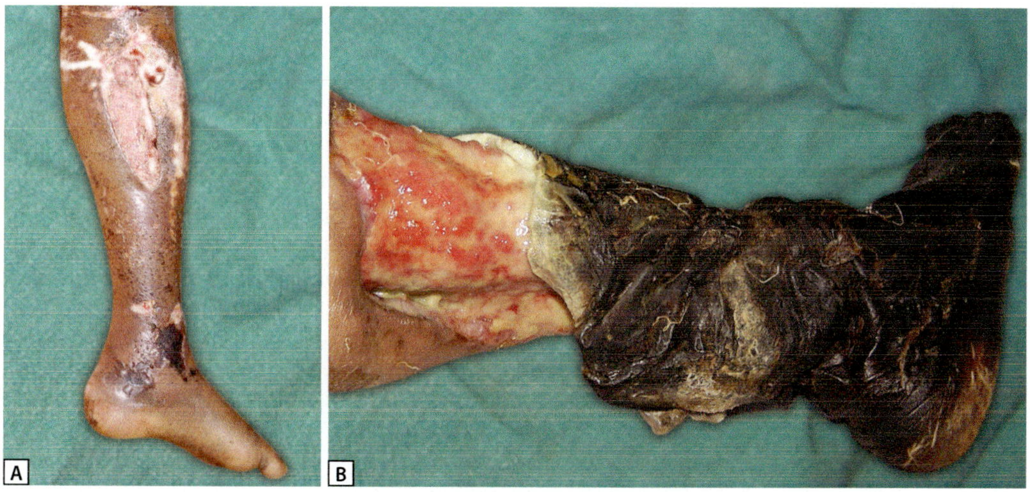

Figures 39.12A and B Tissue necrosis

12. Cardiotoxicity with wide variety of ECG abnormality.
13. Some neurological features may be there in case of Russell's viper bite.

General Signs and Symptoms of Elapid Envenomations

1. Swelling and local pain (Cobra).
2. Local necrosis and/or blistering (Cobra). Local effects are absent in krait bite.
3. Neurotoxic symptoms appear early (15–30 min) in cobra bite; they are often delayed upto several hours in krait bite.
4. Descending paralysis, initially of muscles innervated by the cranial nerves, commencing with poses, diplopia or ophthalmoplegia. The patient complains of difficulty in focusing and the eyelids feel heavy. There may be bilateral ptosis due to paralysis of neuromuscular junction (**Figure 39.14**).
5. Paralysis of jaw and tongue may lead to upper airway obstruction and aspiration of pooled secretions because of the patient's inability to swallow.
6. Numbness around the lips and mouth, progressing to pooling of secretions, bulbar paralysis and respiratory failure.

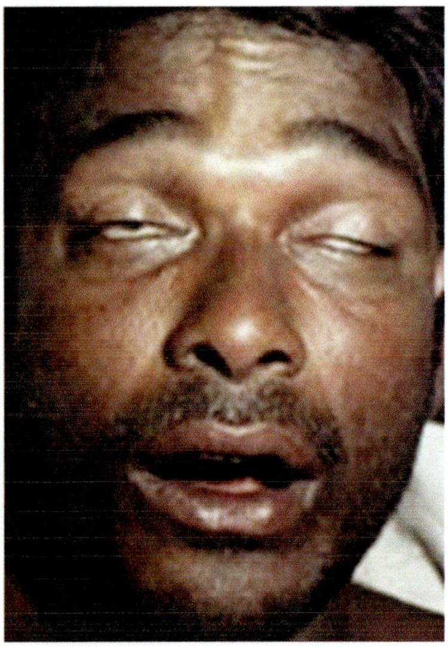

Figure 39.14 Bilateral ptosis

7. Hypoxia due to inadequate ventilation can cause cyanosis, altered sensorium and coma.
8. Paradoxical respiration, as a result of the intercostal muscles becoming paralyzed, is a frequent sign.
9. Stomach pain indicating submucosal hemorrhages.

Sea snake bites produce minimal local effect. The prominent finding is myalgia, stiffness and tenderness of muscles. This is due to rhabdomyolysis, which leads to hyperkalemia, myoglobinemia, myoglobinuria, acute renal failure. Trismus is an early feature. Neurotoxic features like cobra are also found.

MANAGEMENT OF SNAKE BITE[3,9,10]

Of primary importance is the need to recommend the most effective first aid for victims, to enable them to reach the nearest medical facility in the best possible condition. The first aid being currently recommended is based around the mnemonic:

"Do it RIGHT"

It consists of the following:

1. R = Reassure the patient. 70% of all snakebites are from non-venomous species. Only 50% of bites caused by venomous species, actually envenomate the patient.
2. I = Immobilize in the same way as a fractured limb. Use bandages or cloth to hold the splints, not to block the blood supply or apply pressure. Do not apply any compression in the form of tight ligatures, they do not work and can be dangerous!
3. G and H = Get to hospital immediately. Traditional remedies have **no proven** benefit in treating snake bite.
4. T = Tell the doctor of any systemic symptoms such as ptosis that manifest on the way to the hospital.

Traditional Methods to be Discarded

Tourniquets

The use of tight tourniquets made of rope, belt, string or cloth have been traditionally used to stop venom flow into the body following snakebite. However, they have the following drawbacks and problems:

i. Ischemia, necrosis and amputation of extremities.
ii. Chance of neurotoxic blockade during release.
iii. Risk of embolism if used in viper bites. Procoagulant enzymes will cause clotting in distal blood. In addition, the effect of the venom in causing vasodilatation presents the danger of massive hypotension when the tourniquet is released.

Cutting and Suction

i. Cutting a victim with incoagulable blood, increases the risk of severe bleeding and infection.
ii. Suction devices are of no use, but can increase chance of necrosis.

Washing the Wound

Washing may increase the flow of venom through lymphatic.

Electrical Therapy and Cryotherapy

Those methods are of no benefit, can enhance necrotic effect of the venom.

Newer Methods Considered Inapplicable in the Indian Context

Pressure Immobilization Method (Sutherland wrap): Use of pressure bandage and splints are not as useful as there is risk of local tissue damage in viperine and cobra bites. But it is well accepted that patient should be put at rest and bitten extremity should not be moved.

Snake Bite Treatment Protocol[3,5,9,10]

Patient Assessment Phase

On Arrival

1. Deal with any life, threatening symptoms on presentation, i.e. airway, breathing and circulation.
2. If there is evidence of a bite, where the skin has been broken, give tetanus toxoid.
3. Routine use of antibiotic is not necessary, although it should be considered if there is evidence of cellulitis or necrosis.

Diagnosis Phase (General Principles)

1. Where possible identify the snake responsible.
2. All patients will be kept under observation for a minimum of 24 hours.
3. Determine the exact time of the bite. This can give indications as to the progression of any symptoms.

Diagnosis Phase: Investigations

1. 20 Minute Whole Blood Clotting Test (20WBCT) is considered the most reliable test of coagulation and can be carried out at the bedside without specialist training.
2. A few milliliters of fresh venous blood is placed in a new, clean and dry glass vessel and left at ambient temperature for 20 minutes. The glass vessel should be left undisturbed for 20 minutes and then gently tilted, not shaken. If the blood is still liquid, then the patient has incoagulable blood. The vessel must not have been washed with detergent as this will inhibit the contact element of the clotting mechanism.
3. The test should be carried out every 30 minutes from admission for three hours and then hourly after that. If incoagulable blood is discovered, the 6 hourly cycles will then be adopted to test for the requirement for repeat doses of anti-snake venom (ASV).

Table 39.2 Comparison of features among various snake bites

Feature	Cobras	Kraits	Russell's viper	Saw scaled viper
Local pain/tissue damage	Yes	No	Yes	Yes
Ptosis/neurological signs	Yes	Yes	Yes	No
Hemostatic abnormalities	No	No	Yes	Yes
Renal complications	No	No	Yes	No

Other Useful Tests Depending on Availability

1. Hemoglobin/PCV/Platelet count/PT/APTT/FDP/D-Dimer
2. Peripheral smear
3. Urine tests for proteinuria/RBC/hemoglobinuria/myoglobinuria
4. Biochemistry for serum creatinine/urea/potassium
5. Oxygen saturation pulse rate/blood pressure/respiratory rate/postural blood pressure
6. ECG/X-ray/CT/ultrasound (The use of X-ray and ultrasound are of unproven benefit, apart from identification of bleeding in viperine bites).

Diagnosis Phase: Symptoms (Table 39.2)

Late-onset Envenoming

The patient should be kept under close observation for at least 24 hours. Many species, particularly the Krait, is known for taking long time for symptoms to manifest.

ANTI-SNAKE VENOM (ASV) SERUM POLYVALENT

In India, it is available in purified form; enzyme refined and concentrated equine globulins in lyophilized vials with 10 mL ampoule of distilled water. After reconstitution, each mL neutralizes **(Figure 39.15)**:[11]

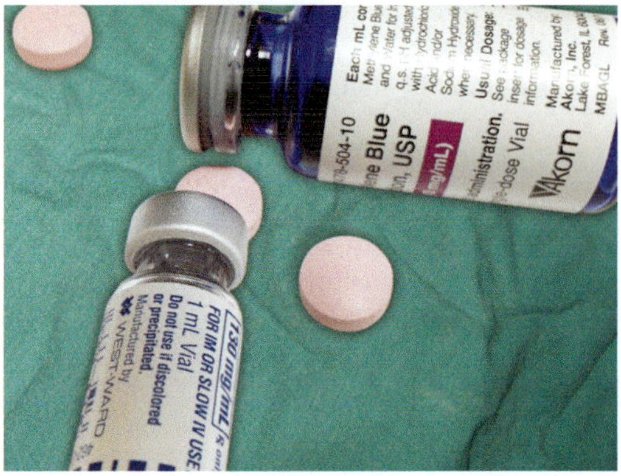

Figure 39.15 Anti-snake venom serum

1. 0.6 mg of standard cobra (Naja naja) venom.
2. 0.6 mg of standard Russell's viper (Vipera russelli) venom
3. 0.45 mg of standard Saw scaled viper (Echis carinatus) venom
4. 0.45 mg of standard Krait (Bungarus caeruleus) venom

There are known species such as the Hump-nosed pit viper (Hypnale Hypnale), where polyvalent ASV is known to be ineffective.

ASV Administration Criteria

The ASV is a scarce, costly commodity and should only be administered when there are definite signs of envenomations. Unbound, free flowing venom can only be neutralized when it is in the blood stream or tissue fluid. Also, ASV carries risk of anaphylactic reactions and should not, therefore, be used unnecessarily.

Table 39.3 Indications of ASV therapy
Systemic envenomations
1. Evidence of coagulopathy
2. Evidence of neurotoxicity
Local envenomations (Severe current)
1. Local swelling involving more than half of the bitten limb
2. Rapid extension of swelling

Primary Determinants (Table 39.3)

Systemic Envenomations

1. **Evidence of Coagulopathy**: Primarily detected by 20WBCT or visible spontaneous systemic bleeding, gums bleeding, etc.
2. **Evidence of Neurotoxicity**: Ptosis, external ophthalmoplegia, muscle paralysis, inability to lift the head, etc.

Local Envenomations (Severe Current)

1. **Severe Current**: Local swelling involves more than half of the bitten limb in the absence of a tourniquet.
2. Rapid extension of swelling, e.g. beyond wrist or ankle within a few hours of the bite on the hands or feet.

Prevention of ASV Reactions

Prophylactic Regimes: Two regimens are normally recommended:

1. 100 mg of hydrocortisone and H_1 antihistamine IV, 5 minutes before ASV administration should be given; or
2. 0.25–0.3 mg adrenaline 1:1000 given subcutaneously.

ASV Administration

Dosage: ASV is recommended to be administered in the following initial dose:

1. Neurotoxic/anti-hemostatic 8–10 vials.
2. Children receive the same ASV dosage as adults.
3. Pregnant women are treated in exactly the same way as other victims with the same dosage of ASV.

ASV can be Administered in Two Ways:

1. **Intravenous Injection**: Reconstituted or liquid ASV is administered by slow intravenous injection (2 mL/min). Each vial is 10 mL of reconstituted ASV.
2. **Infusion**: Liquid or reconstituted ASV is diluted in 5–10 mL/kg body weight of isotonic saline or glucose.
   a. All ASV to be administered over 1 hour at constant speed.
   b. The patient should be closely monitored for 2 hours.

Local administration of ASV, near bite site, is ineffective, painful and raises the intra-compartmental pressure, particularly in the digits. It should not be used. Victims often arrive late after the bite, often after several days, usually with acute renal failure.

Should the Clinician Administer ASV?

Perform a 20WBCT. If coagulopathy is present, administer ASV. If no coagulopathy is evident, treat renal failure by refereeing to nephrologists to carry out dialysis, etc.

In the case of neurotoxic envenoming where the victim is evidencing symptoms such as ptosis, respiratory failure, etc. it is better to administer 1 dose of 8–10 vials of ASV to ensure that no unbound venom is present. But at this stage, it is likely that all the venom is bound and respiratory support or normal recovery will be the outcome.

ASV Reactions

Anaphylaxis is a life-threatening emergency, for which adrenaline should always be immediately available. The patient should be monitored closely and at the first sign of any of the following: Urticaria, itching, fever, shaking chills, nausea, vomiting, diarrhea, abdominal cramps, tachycardia, hypotension, bronchospasm and angioedema.

a. ASV will be discontinued.
b. 0.5 mg of 1:1000 adrenalines will be given IM.

If after 10–15 minutes, the patient's condition has not improved or is worsening, a second dose of 0.5 mg of adrenalin 1:1000 IM is given. This can be repeated for a third time. If there is hypotension or hemodynamic instability, IV fluids should be given.

Once the patient has recovered, ASV can be restarted slowly for 10–15 minutes, and patient should be closely monitored. Then the normal drip rate should be resumed.

Late serum sickness reactions can be easily treated with oral steroid such as prednisolone, 5 mg 6 hourly and oral H_1 antihistamines.

Neurotoxic Envenomations

Neostigmine is an anticholinesterase that prolongs the life of acetylcholine and can, therefore, reverse respiratory failure and neurotoxic symptoms. It is particularly effective for postsynaptic neurotoxins such as those of the cobra venom.

Initially, neostigmine test is to be administered, 1.5–2.0 mg of neostigmine IM, together with 0.6 mg of atropine IV. Patient is closely observed for 1 hour and following points are noted.

a. Single breath count.
b. mm of Iris uncovered (Amount covered by the descending eyelid).
c. Inter incisor distance (Measured distance between upper and lower incisors).
d. Length of time upward gaze can be maintained.
e. FEV_1 or FVC (If available).

If the victim responds to the neostigmine test, then continue with 0.5 mg of neostigmine IM half hourly plus 0.6 mg of atropine IV over an 8-hour period by continuous infusion.

Recovery Phase

If an adequate dose of appropriate antivenom has been administered, the following responses may be seen:

1. Spontaneous systemic bleeding such as gum bleeding usually stops within 15–30 minutes.
2. Blood coagulability is usually restored within 6 hours. Principal test is 20WBCT.
3. Post-synaptic neurotoxic envenoming such as the Cobra may begin to improve as early as 30 minutes after antivenom, but can take several hours.
4. Presynaptic neurotoxic envenoming such as the Krait usually takes a considerable time to improve reflecting the need for body to generate new acetylcholine emitters.
5. Active hemolysis and rhabdomyolysis may cease within a few hours and urine returns to normal color.
6. In shocked patients, blood pressure may increase after 30 minutes.

Repeat Doses: Antihemostatic

The same full dose of ASV can be repeated every 6 hours until coagulation has been restored (up to 30 vials). After that, transfusion of fresh frozen plasma or clotting factors may be considered.

Repeat Doses: Neurotoxic

The same full dose of ASV can be repeated once after 1–2 hours (up to 20 vials). In case of worsening of respiratory insufficiency, mechanical ventilation is required.

Treatment of Other Symptoms

Pain

Snakebite can often cause severe pain at the bite site. This can be treated with analgesic such as paracetamol (adult dose of 500–1000 mg 4–6 hourly and pediatric dose 10 mg/kg every 4–6 hourly orally).

Aspirin and non-steroidal anti-inflammatory drugs (NSAIDs), as they can cause bleeding, should be avoided. This can be particularly dangerous in a patient already having coagulopathy.

If available, mild opiates such as Tramadol, 50 mg can be used orally for relief of severe pain. In cases of severe pain at a tertiary center, Tramadol can be given IV.

For Hypotension

Hypotension can have a number of causes, particularly loss of circulating volume due to hemorrhaging and vasodilatation due to the action of the venom or direct effects on the heart. Treatment is by means of plasma expanders.

In cases where generalized capillary permeability has been established, a vasoconstrictor such as dopamine can be used.

Surgical Intervention

In case of tissue necrosis, surgical debridement is necessary.

Intracompartmental syndrome is suspected if the followings are present:

- Pain on passive stretching
- Pain out of proportion
- Pulselessness
- Pallor
- Paresthesia
- Paralysis.

Significant swelling in the limb can lead to the conclusion that the intracompartmental pressure is above 40 mm of mercury, causing blood vessels to collapse and lead to ischemia. So, fasciotomy is indicated. Intracompartmental pressure should be measured with Stryker intracompartmental pressure monitoring equipment.

Renal Failure

Renal failure is a common complication of Russell's viper bite. The contributing factors are intravascular hemolysis, DIC, direct nephrotoxicity and hypotension and rhabdomyolysis.

The following are indicator:

1. Declining or no urine output.
2. Blood Testing:
   i. Serum creatinine > 5 mg/dL or rise of > 1 mg/day.
   ii. Urea > 200 mg/dL
   iii. Potassium > 5.6 mmol/L, Confirm hyperkalemia with EKG.
3. Evidence of uremia or metabolic acidosis.

Declining renal parameters require referral to specialist nephrologists with access to dialysis equipment. Peritoneal dialysis could be performed but hemodialysis is preferable in cases of hypotension or hyperkalemia.

Autopsy Findings

External

One of the important sign of snake bite is the fang marks (**Figure 39.16**), but fang marks may not be easily found in all cases.

Usual finding in obvious cases are local swelling, blister and necrosis (**Figure 39.17**).

Internal

There is subcutaneous bleeding under bite marks, pulmonary edema or petechial hemorrhages in different organs depending on species involved.

There may be punctate hemorrhages in brain stem in certain cases and can be the only sign in a case of sudden death following bite by brown snake.

Death after a brown snake (genus pseudonaja) bite is often sudden and unexpected. Cerebral hemorrhage was confirmed at autopsy in a study in Australia in three patients bitten by tiger snakes and in one bitten by a brown snake.[12]

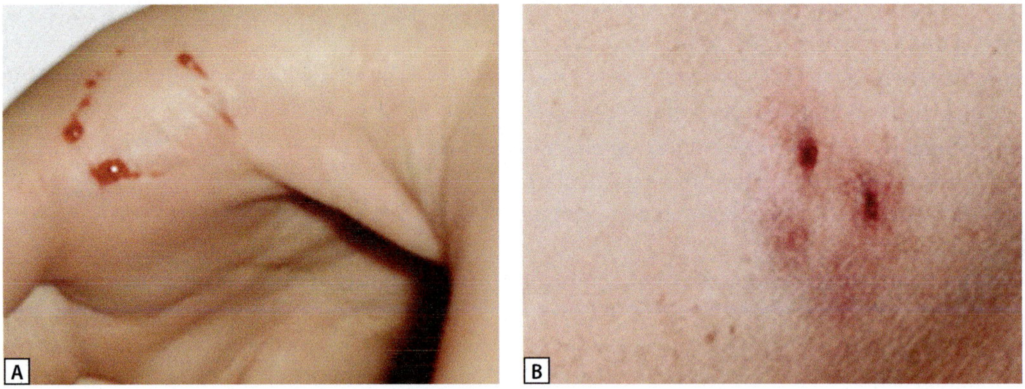

Figures 39.16A and B Fang mark

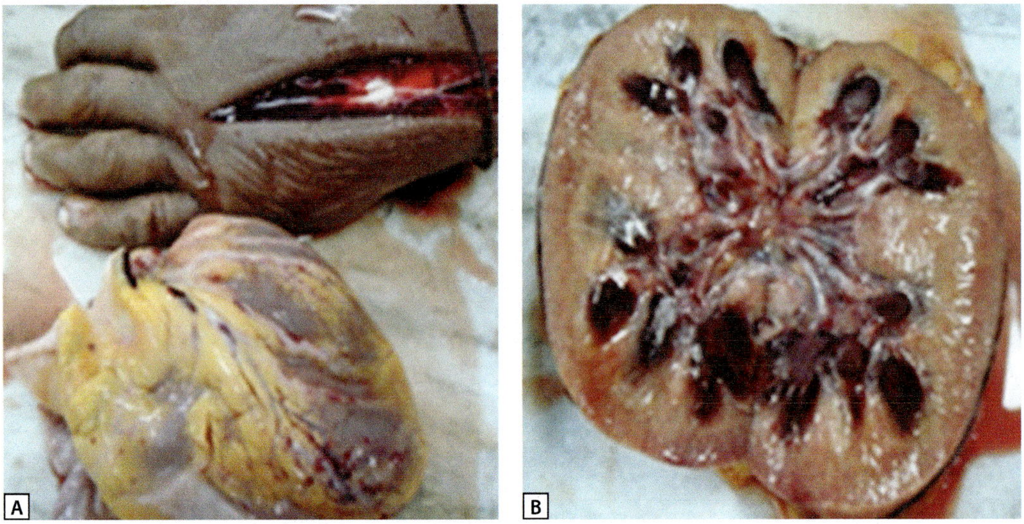

Figures 39.17A and B Subcutaneous bleeding under bite marks, petechial hemorrhages in heart and kidney

In a study of fatal bites by Naja in India, the macroscopic examination of the kidneys showed bilateral congestion and bilateral subcapsular pinpoint hemorrhage. Longitudinal section of the kidneys reported congestion of the cortex and medulla along with pinpoint cortical hemorrhages.[13]

OTHER SIGNIFICANT BITES AND STINGS IN INDIAN SCENARIO

Wasp and Bee Sting[5]

All those insects, including ants belong, to the order hymenoptera.

Sting: A stinger or sting is a sharp organ found in various animals that delivers venom, usually piercing the skin of another animal (**Figures 39.18 and 39.19**). Stings are usually located at the rear of the animal. Animals with stings include bees, wasps (including hornets, yellow jackets), scorpions and some groups of ants, e.g. fire ants.

Unlike most other stings, honey bee workers' stings are strongly barbed **(Figure 39.20)**, and lodge in skin of victim upon use, tearing free from the honeybee's body, leading to the bee's death within minutes. The stinger continues to inject venom after the bee departs and should be removed without squeezing it.

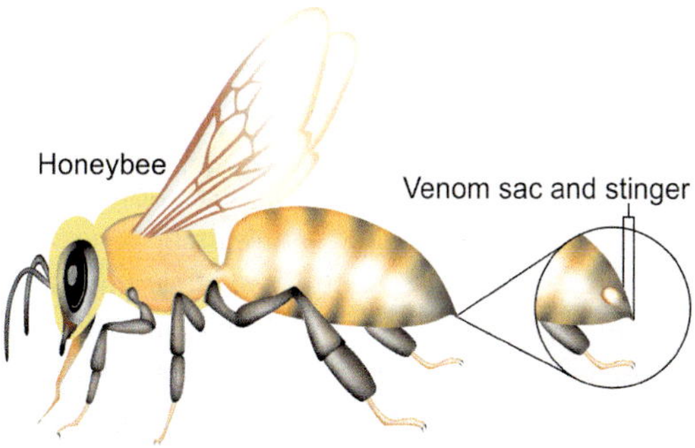

Figure 39.18 Honeybee (Apis mellifera)
(*Courtesy*: www.adameducation.com/adam_images.aspx)

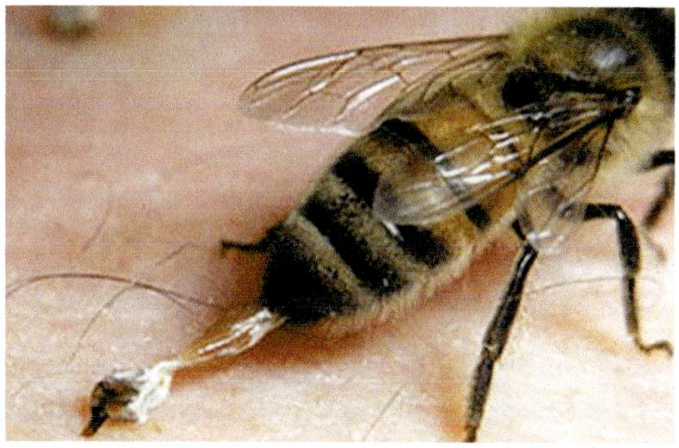

Figure 39.19 Honeybee's sting and sac embedded in skin
(*Courtesy:* http://www.hiltonpond.org)

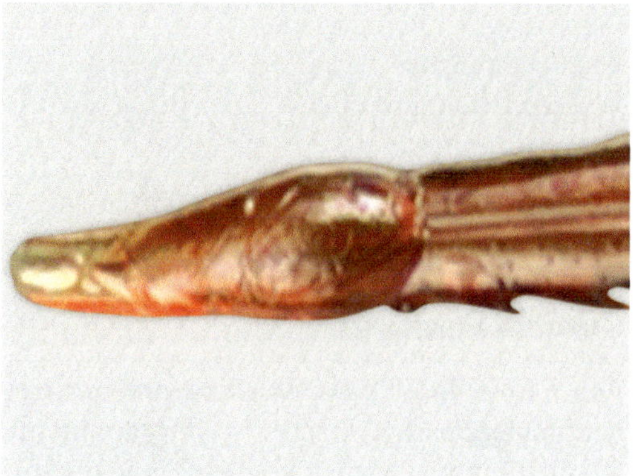

Figure 39.20 Barbed property of honeybee sting
(*Courtesy*: Rik Littlefield)

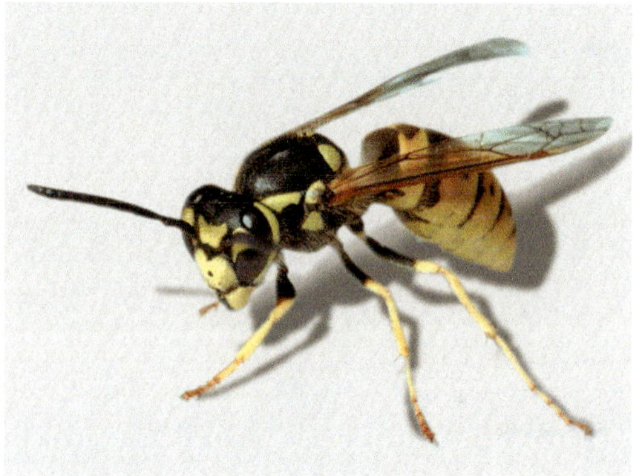

Figure 39.21 Hornet (a type of wasp)
(*Courtesy*: http://commandpestcontrol.com)

A wasp (**Figure 39.21**) stinger is not barbed and the wasp can therefore insert the stinger into the target several times and at different sites. The wasp survives the process.

Hymenoptera venom is a mixture of amines (histamine, serotonin, acetylcholine), enzymes like hyaluronidase, phospholipase A, etc., and peptides like kinin in wasps; apamin, mast cell degranulating peptide in bees.

Clinical Features

Local Finding: In non-sensitized individual, a single sting develops pain, redness, swelling, irritation which are short lasting.

Systemic Findings: Anaphylaxis may occur in sensitive individuals. In severe cases (multiple stings/vital location), urticaria, angioedema, laryngeal edema, hypotension, coma may occur.

Instead of anaphylaxis, massive envenomations can occur in case of multiple stings, characterized by vasodilatation, hypotension, seizures in early stage and subsequently hepatic failure, disseminated intra vascular coagulation, etc.

Management

1. Embedded sting should be removed by scrapping with blade, should not be grasped with forceps as that may push more venom into the affected site (**Figure 39.22**).
2. Local infiltration with adrenaline 1:1000, local cold compress, antihistamines can be given.
3. Patient with multiple stings should be observed for at least 6 hours for abnormality of coagulation profile, hematological parameters, liver and renal function, evidence of rhabdomyolysis, etc.

4. For anaphylaxis parenteral adrenaline, antihistamines, corticosteroid and bronchodilator have to be administered. Continuous airway and cardiac monitoring are required.

Scorpion Stings[5]

Most common Indian varieties of scorpionare Palamnaeus (Heterometrus) swammerdami (black, as shown in **Figure 39.23**) and Mesobuthus (Hottentotta) tamulus (red) **(Figure 39.24)**. The red one is more lethal.

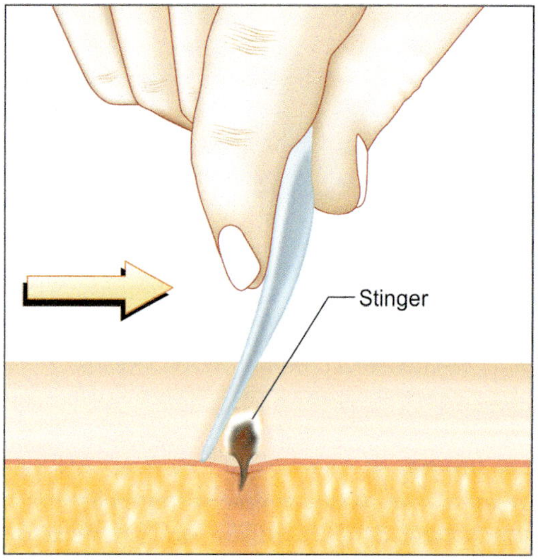

Figure 39.22 Removing bee stings
(*Courtesy*: http://www.adameducation.com/adam_images.aspx)

Scorpion venom contains phospholipase A, hyaluronidase, acetyl cholinesterase, serotonin and neurotoxins. Those venoms affects sodium channels with prolongation of action potentials, also causes spontaneous depolarization of both sympathetic and parasympathetic nervous system. Characteristic features of *M. tamulus* sting are hypersecretion of rennin and aldosterone, hyperkalemia and reduced insulin secretion.

Venom

The venom is clear, colorless fluid and contains following toxic components:
- Phospholipase
- Acetylcholinesterase
- Hyaluronidase
- Serotonin
- Neurotoxin.

Clinical Features

Apart from local pain, swelling and regional lymphadenopathy, signs of autonomic stimulation may occur. Other systemic findings are pulmonary edema, hyperglycemia, allergic reaction and abnormality in cardiac rhythm.

Management

i. Patient with cardiac disease/hypertension, elderly victims or under five children should be hospitalized.

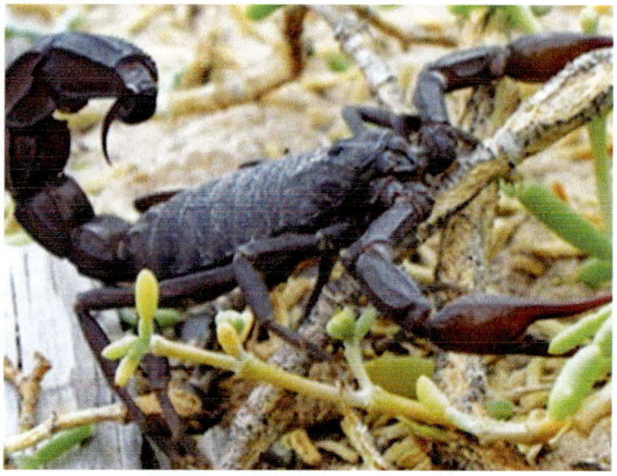

Figure 39.23 Indian black scorpion
(*Courtesy*: http://www.walkthroughindia.com/wildlife)

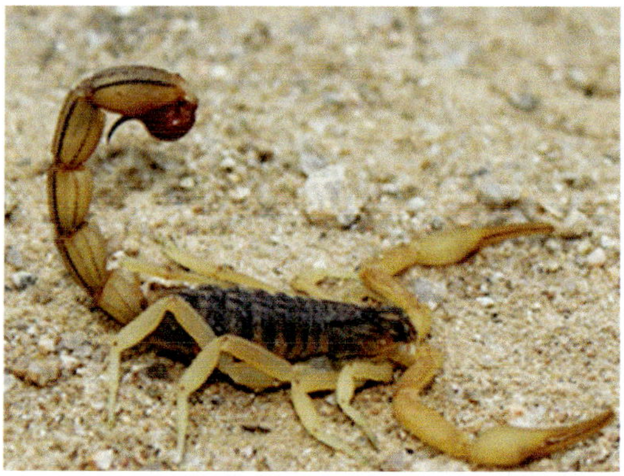

Figure 39.24 Scorpion
(*Courtesy*: Professor. Sanjoy Das)

ii. During transport, affected limb should be immobilized.
iii. Symptomatic treatment for pain, allergic reaction, hypertension (with nifedipine) or hypotension, cardiac dysrhythmias, hyperglycemia, etc.
iv. Prazocin hydrochloride is claimed to have an antagonistic role to scorpion venom. Recently in India, specific antivenom against *M. tamulus* is introduced.

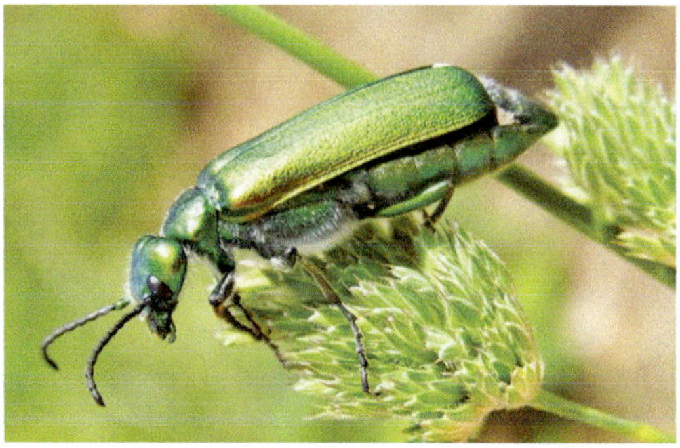

Figure 39.25 Lytta vesicatoria (Cantharides-Spanish fly) (*Courtesy*: http://apps.who.int/classifications/icd10/browse/2010/en#/T63.0)

CANTHARIDES

The toxic manifestations are due to this type of insect is not because of bites or stings, but as a result of ingestion of dried, powdered insects (Lytta vesicatoria-Blister beetle/Spanish fly) believing it as an aphrodisiac **(Figure 39.25)**.

The active principle **Cantharidin** may cause urinary tract irritation, painful, frequent micturation, hematuria and priapism. Treatment is usually symptomatic.

REFERENCES

1. The Clinical Management of Snake Bites in the South East Asian Region. World Health Organization, Regional office for South East Asia, Updated on Oct 5, 2005.
2. Auerbach PS, Norris RL. Disorders caused by venomous snakebites and marine animal exposures. In: Longo DL, Fauci AS, Kasper DL, Hauser SL, Jameson JL, Loscalzo J (Eds). Harrison's Principles of Internal Medicine, 18th ed. Vol. 2, USA: McGraw Hill Medical; 2012. p. 3566.
3. Bambery P. Snake bites and arthropod envenomation. In: Shah SN (Ed). API Textbook of Medicine, 8th ed. Vol. 2. Mumbai, India: Association of Physicians; 2008. pp. 1517-20.
4. Mebs D. Venomous and Poisonous Animals: A Handbook for Biologist, Toxicologists and Toxicologist, Physicians and Pharmacist. Stuttgart Germany: Medpharm-Scientific Publishers CRC press; 2002. pp. 239-51.
5. Pillay VV. Modern Medical Toxicology, 4th ed. India: Jaypee Brothers Medical Publishers (P) Ltd; 2013. pp. 149-55.
6. Biobasics: Snakes. Biology Today. India. April 2010. p. 6.
7. Identification of poisonous and non-poisonous snakes. [cited 2013 25th March]; Available from: URL:http://www.2classnotes.com/digital_notes.asp?
8. Wikipedia. [Cited 2013 25th March]; Available from: URL:http://apps.who.int/classifications/icd10/browse/2010/en#/T63.0
9. Indian National Snakebite Protocols 2007. First aid and snakebite prevention, snakebite treatment, Support Concepts. [Cited 2013 25th March]; Available from: URL:http://www.scribd.com/doc/13591739/Snake-Bite-Protocol-2007-India
10. Warrell DA. Guidelines for the management of snake-bites © World Health Organization 2010, Regional Office for South-East Asia. [Cited 2013 25th March]; Available from: URL:http://www.toxinology.org/resources/protocols/WHO- SEARO%20Snakebite%20Guidelines%202010%20copy.pdf
11. Tripathi KD. Essentials of Medical Pharmacology, 6th ed. India: Jaypee Brothers Medical Publishers (P) Ltd; 2008. pp. 887-8.
12. CSL Limited, Parkville, Vic. Deaths from snake bite in Australia (1981-1991). Med J Aust. 1992;157 (11-12):740-6.
13. Mukhopadhyay PP, Ghosh S, Ghosh TK. Pattern of Renal Pathology in Fatal Envenomation by Indian Cobra (Naja naja). J Indian Acad Forensic Med. 2010;32(2):132-3.

CHAPTER 40

Mechanical Irritants

Sunit Kr Joshi, Putul Mahanta

LEARNING PLAN

- Identify different mechanical irritant, viz glass and diamond powder, needles and pins, chopped animal hairs, etc.
- Evaluate clinical features, management of its poisoning
- Know the autopsy findings in a case of death
- Know the medicolegal importance

MECHANICAL IRRITANT

Mechanical irritants do not produce toxic effect like corrosives, metallic, non-metallic and organic irritants, cerebral and spinal poison, etc. as they are not absorbed into the circulation from gastrointestinal tract but cause mechanical obstruction in gastrointestinal tract leading to partial or complete intestinal obstruction, which may, sometimes, lead to death. These substances do not possess any poisonous quality like chemicals, but occasionally, symptoms like those of poisoning, e.g. dehydration, acute pain and even death, in consequence of their mechanical qualities only are observed. They have, therefore, been excluded from toxicological analysis system following medicolegal work on a case of poisoning. It would be wrong to pass these cases without thorough and detailed clinical study and postmortem examination.

They usually cause irritation of gastrointestinal tract, and also perforation and obstruction due to their rough edges or sharp points. Their efficacy as fatal agents per se are questionable, but they have been used as homicidal agents from very ancient period of time. Some common mechanical poisons are powdered glass, diamond powder, pins, needles, nails and chopped animal and vegetable hairs. Examples of mechanical irritant are:

- Powdered glass or broken pieces (**Figures 40.1** and **40.2**)
- Diamond powder (**Figures 40.3** and **40.4**)
- Needles and pins (**Figures 40.5** and **40.6**)
- Chopped animal hair
- Vegetable hair
- Nails, etc.

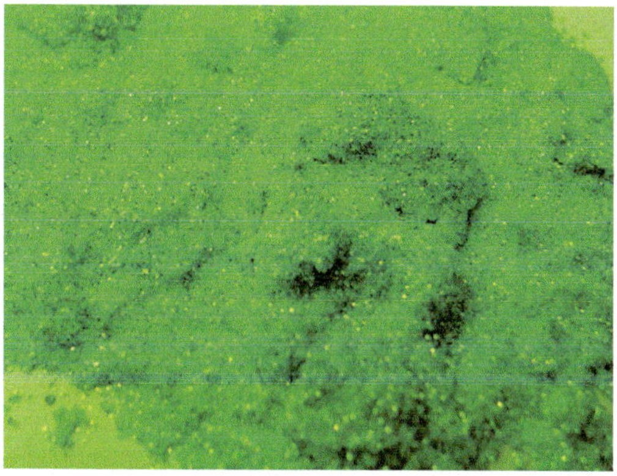

Figure 40.1 Showing powdered green glass

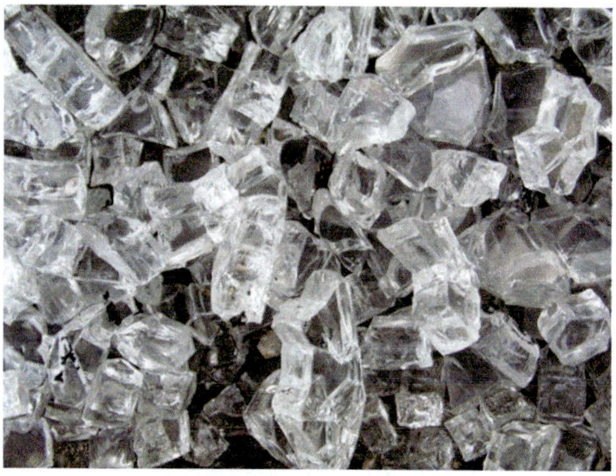

Figure 40.2 Broken pieces of glass

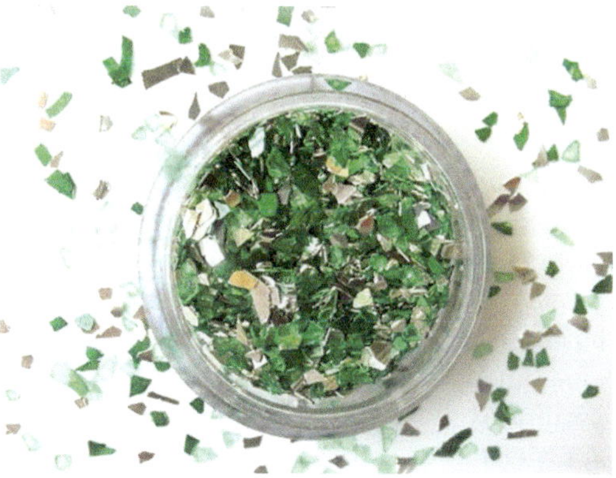

Figure 40.3 Pieces of sapphire diamond

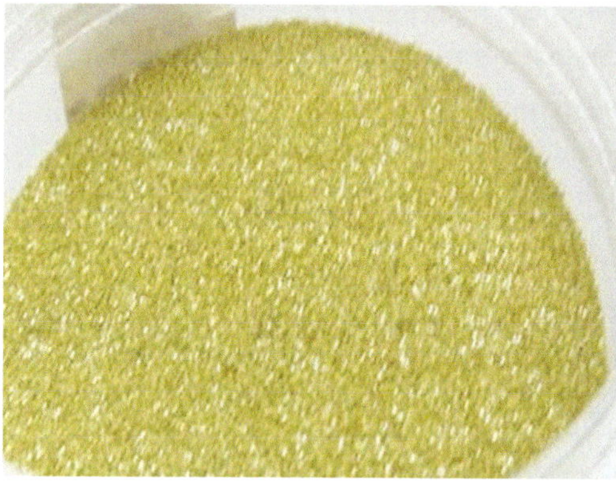

Figure 40.4 Powdered diamonds

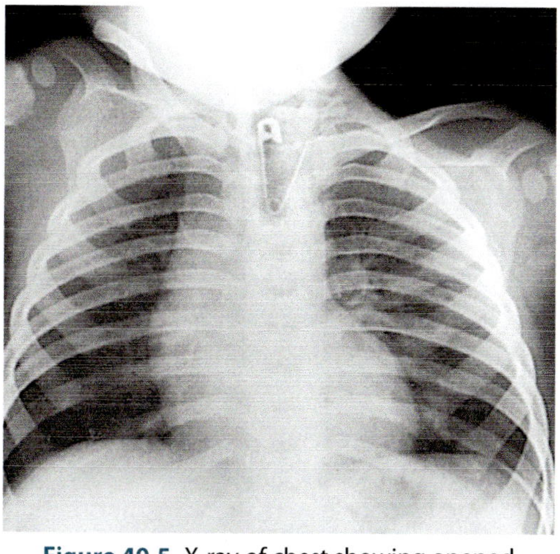

Figure 40.5 X-ray of chest showing opened up safety pin in the esophagus

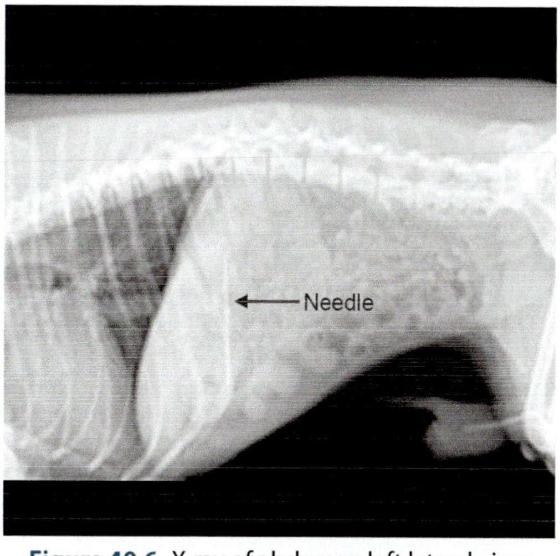

Figure 40.6 X-ray of abdomen left lateral view showing presence of needle in stomach

Powdered Glass or Broken Pieces

Clinical Features

There is acute and severe burning pain in throat and stomach area. Nausea and vomiting may follow. The sharp ends of glass may cause severe erosion of the esophagus, stomach and intestine, leading to severe bleeding or perforation, but, in all cases, it is not usual. Generally, constipation occurs, but diarrhea may also be seen with blood. If death occurs in any such case, then it occurs due to injury to mucous membrane and internal hemorrhage.

Fatal Dose: Uncertain and depends on the physical character of the substance. Even large doses are sometimes not fatal.

Fatal Period: Uncertain death may occur in hours to a few days.

Management

Give bulky food like bananas, rice or *isabgol*. After that, purgative may be given. Antacids may be given later to sooth gastric or esophageal mucosa. If sharp ends are present, one may have to resort to surgery to remove the pieces.

Postmortem Findings

Erosions are widely seen in mouth, pharynx, esophagus, stomach and intestine, depending on the level of involvement of gastrointestinal tract. The mucosal membranes are congested and inflamed. Peritonitis is usually uncommon except in cases of perforation of gastrointestinal tract. Signs of intestinal hemorrhage and inflammation are more common.

Medicolegal Importance

Powdered glass is given for homicidal purposes by mixing it in food like rice or vegetables or in some drinks, since it is believed to be very effective mechanical irritant poison. Usually, though given for over a long period for the expected "slow poisoning effect", the victims withstand the exposure, most of the time without any alarming sign and many of such victims are killed subsequently by some other means, a postmortem examination reveals.

Powdered glass is rarely used for suicidal purposes. It may be used for killing cattle. Many artists show eating of glass in circuses and public shows.

Diamond Powder

The **diamond** is not a poison in any true sense of the word, but its incomparable hardness enables it, unlike ordinary stones, to retain very acute angles. When every other stone is pounded, that extreme sharpness of edge is lost; their fragments become blunt and rounded.

Diamond alone preserves its trenchant qualities. Wherefore, if it chances to enter the stomach together with food, the peristaltic motion needful to digestion brings it into contact with the coats of the stomach and the bowels, where it sticks, and by the action of fresh food forcing it further inwards, after some time, **perforates** the organs leading to **hemorrhage** and **peritonitis**. This eventually causes death. Any other sort of stone or glass mingled with the food has not the power to attach to the organs, but passes onward with the victuals.[1]

Management

In case of short duration of poisoning detected early: Bulky food, demulcent drinks are helpful to the patient; but in case of late diagnosis, colonic lavage may be helpful. In case of long duration of poisoning, there is no definitive treatment.

Needles and Pins

A severe burning pain and irritation occurs in esophagus and stomach when these are consumed orally. There may be perforation, which may even cause death or impaction over a mucosal wall.

Management

Bulky food and laxatives are usually given. Sometimes, surgery is required to remove pins and needles as they are impacted in mucosal wall. X-ray helps in locating the exact site of impaction.

Medicolegal Importance

Needles and pins may be ingested accidently, usually by children. Suicidal and homicidal cases are seen very rarely.

Chopped Animal Hairs

In contrary to general belief that chopped animal hairs are poisonous, it is not true in real. Pieces of chopped animal hairs can be mixed with food, which when ingested may cause irritation of stomach and intestine, which may further cause diarrhea and vomiting.

Sometimes, chopped animal hairs are used to cause ill health rather than to produce fatality.

Vegetable Hairs

These are fine, short hairs derived from leaves and stalks of certain plants and are called stinging hairs. They cause mechanical irritation once it comes in contact with mucosa or skin. Sometimes, these hairs may contain short bulbs which contain irritant fluid containing histamine and acetylcholine[2] and produce poisonous effect after absorption through mucosa of small and large intestine.

Management

Thorough washing of the area with drinking water should be done and later on by antiseptic and anti-inflammatory lotions, where the juice comes in to contact. If these vegetable hairs are ingested, give bulky food followed by laxatives.

Medicolegal Importance

Some cases have been reported where these hair have been applied to produce irritation to fellow passengers with a view to divert attention to rob the person.

REFERENCES

1. Freitas RA Jr. Nanomedicine, Volume IIA: Biocompatibility, Georgetown, Texas; Landes Biosciences, 2003.
2. Sharma RK. Irritant poisons-mechanical poisons. In: Concise Textbook of Forensic Medicine and Toxicology. New Delhi (INDIA), Elsevier, a division of Reed Elsevier India Private limited. p. 254.

CHAPTER 41

Somniferous Poisons

Putul Mahanta

LEARNING PLAN

- Identify different alkaloids
- Learn about opium alkaloids, mechanism of action, clinical features and management
- Identify the postmortem findings
- Learn about heroin, codeine, thebaine and papaverine
- Understand the medicolegal importance

The term somniferous means 'sleep inducing', which is exactly what narcosis means. Therefore, a somniferous poison can also be referred to as a narcotic. There are many drugs that produce same effects, but somniferous group includes only opiates that are derived from opium. Those that have similar pharmacologic actions to the natural opium alkaloids, but are not derived from opium are often called opioids.

In medicine, the term opiate describes any of the narcotic opioid alkaloids found as natural products in the opium poppy plant.[1]

WHAT ARE ALKALOIDS?

Alkaloids are a group of complex content that has a nitrogenous base and is found in several plants. They have the strong physiological actions, hence they have a toxicological interest, and they are widely used in medicine. Chemically, it behaves like an alkali but they are not true alkalies, but they react with acids, forming salts and water. Some of the important **alkaloids** are atropine, morphine, strychnine, cocaine, etc.

OPIUM OR AFIM

Opium is one of the important narcotics. The word '**opium**' is Greek for '**juice**'. It is the inspissated milky-white exudates or air-dried latex of unripe poppy capsule of the species **Papaver somniferum** (white poppy), which belongs to the family Papaveraceae, a herb that is grow up to 0.3–1.5 meter in height (**Figure 41.1**). These milky-white exudates are obtained by longitudinal (vertical) incision of unripe poppy capsule (**Figure 41.2**). On drying, this yields opium.

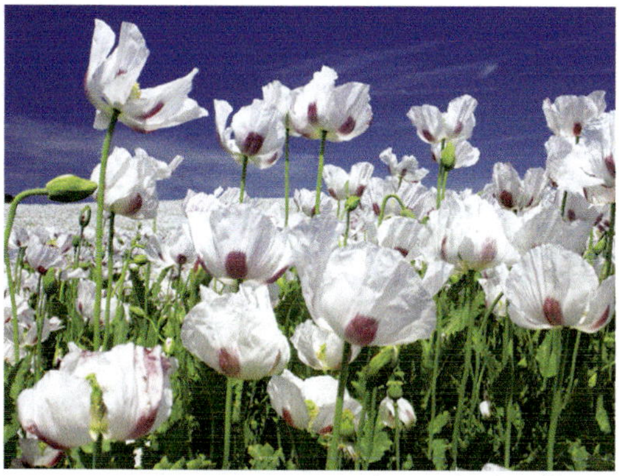
Figure 41.1 Poppy plants with fruit capsule and flower

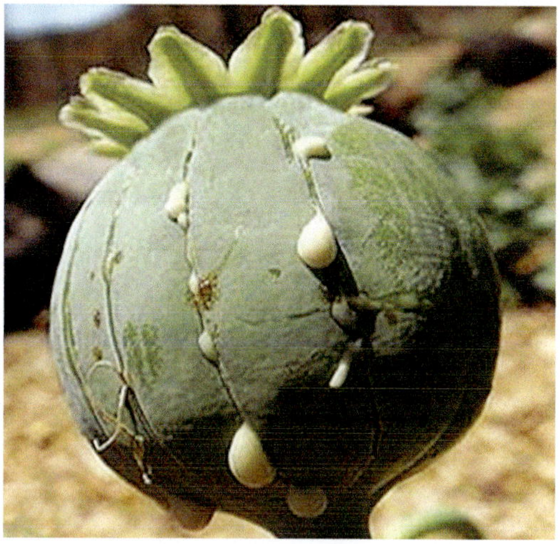
Figure 41.2 Incised unripe poppy capsule

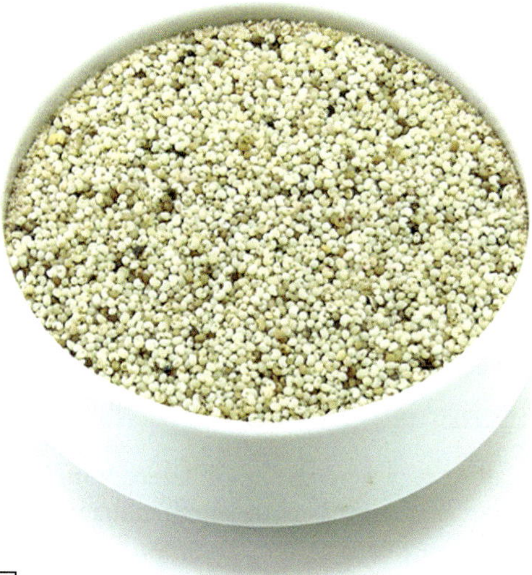
A

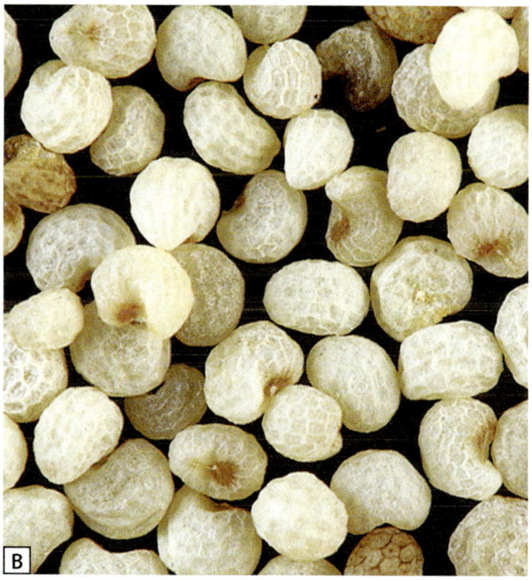
B

Figures 41.3A and B White poppy seeds, with close-up view

The crude opium is dark brownish in color, bitter in taste, having a peculiar vegetables odor and is sticky. The poppy capsule contains **poppy seeds** known as **khas-khas/posto/afu (Figure 41.3)**, which are innocuous and is an edible product. When pressed, oil known as **poppy seed oil**, comes out, which is largely used for culinary and lighting purposes.

Contrary to popular belief, poppy seeds which are used widely for culinary purposes do contain traces of morphine and codeine. Eating a large quantity of these seeds can lead to positive screening for both the alkaloids.[2] Poppy seeds have long been used as a folk remedy to aid sleeping, promote fertility and wealth, and even to provide supposed magical powers of invisibility.[3]

The **ripe** and **dried poppy capsule (Figure 41.4)** and poppy seeds are not toxic. Dried poppy capsule is also sold in the market, popularly known as '**Post ka Doda**' and is being purchased by those people who cannot afford purchasing

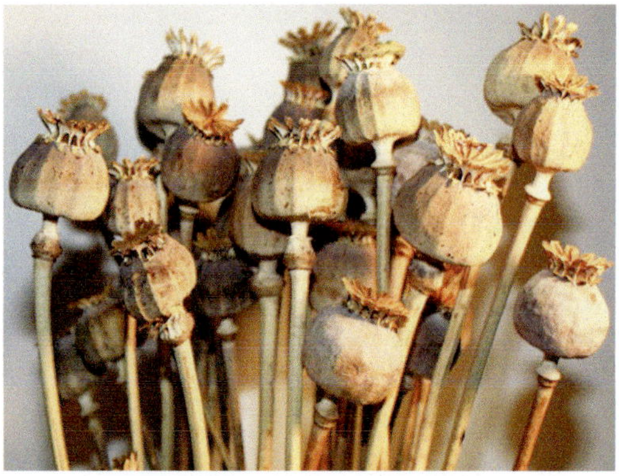

Figure 41.4 Dry poppy capsule

crude opium. The dried capsule still contains about 0.3% of crude opium inside. They make a decoction of it, and take it.

Classifications of Opium Alkaloids

Crude opium contains as many as 25 alkaloids, of which morphine is the principal one. The various natural opium alkaloids and their derivatives are given in **Table 41.1**.

The production of opium itself has basically not changed since ancient times. However, through selective breeding of the papaver somniferum plant, the content of the Phenanthrene alkaloids morphine, codeine, and, to a lesser extent, thebaine, has been greatly increased. In modern times, much of the thebaine, which often serves as the raw material for the synthesis for hydrocodone, hydromorphine and other semi-synthetic opiates, originates from extracting papaver orientale or papaver bracteatum.

Opium, for illegal use, is often converted into heroin, which is less bulky, making it easier to smuggle, and which multiplies its potency to approximately twice that of morphine. In India, thousands of small land owners are licensed to grow opium. From the seeds to the refined paste and medicinal alkaloids, production is controlled by **Central Narcotics Bureau**, a branch of the Ministry of Finance.

Most of the raw opium paste produced in Ghazipur and Neemuch is exported to the US, UK, France and Japan, generating an estimated revenue ₹ 300 million per year; a tidy profit for India's foreign exchange starved coffers. The morphine content of opium is standardized in the Government. Opium factory at Ghazipur is about 10%.

Pharmacokinetics

Well absorbed from GIT, nasal mucosa, pulmonary mucosa and from SC and IV routes. It has extensive hepatic metabolism and undergo conjugation with glucuronic acid and hydrolysis, and oxidation occurs. The unchanged and unconjugated morphine are excreted by the colon and in conjugated form as morphine-3-glucoronite by the kidneys. A small amount is excreted by milk. Heroin is reduced to morphine by the liver.

Mechanism of Action

Opiates act on specific opioids receptors found in periventricular and periaqeductal areas. The most important receptors are:

μ (mu) receptors: Cortical, mediate supraspinal analgesia, euphoria and respiratory depression.

κ (Kappa) receptors: Spinal, mediate spinal analgesia, CNS depression and miosis.

Table 41.1 Alkaloids of opium

Natural opium alkaloids	Semi-synthetics	Synthetics
a. *Phenanthrene group:* Alkaloids, having sedative and analgesic properties, viz. morphine (about 10%), codeine (about 0.2%), thebaine (about 0.3%) b. *Benzyl-Isoquinoline group:* Mostly smooth muscle relaxants, viz. papaverine (about 1%), narcotine narceine, etc.	Heroin (Diacetylmorphine), Benzylmorphine, Hydromorphine, Dehydromorphine, Oxymorphine, Hydrocodone bitartrate, Oxycodone, etc.	Pethidine Hydroxypethidine Methadone Isomethadone Normethadone Levorphanol tartrate meperidine, fentanyl, etc.

δ (delta) receptors: Mediate analgesia, psychotomimetic effects as hallucination and delusion.

Drugs act on **opiate receptors**, may be:
Agonists (most opiate mainly act on mu and kappa receptors).

Antagonists, which again can be of, (A) **Agonist-antagonist** (act mainly on kappa and sigma receptors, e.g. nalbuphine, nalorphine) and (B) **Pure antagonist** which block all receptors, e.g. naloxone, nalmefene, naltrexone, etc. **Opioid** referred to those agonists and antagonists which have morphine like activity, but are not derived from opium.

Fatal Dose and Fatal Period

These doses are absolutely variable and may cause death with lesser dose and recovery with a higher dose. Therapeutic and fatal dose of various alkaloids are mentioned in **Table 41.2**. Average **fatal period** is about 12–24 hours.

Elimination and Detection

They are eliminated as morphine, in the urine and feces. A small amount is secreted through the bile in to the stomach and intestine even when administered hypodermically and is reabsorbed. Some amount of poison is secreted in the bile, saliva and milk and is with possibility of fatal poisoning in infants sucking breast milk from mother. Elimination is very slow; some amount is oxidized to oxydimorphine, which is found in the urine. Opium is said to withstand putrefaction, even in presence of decomposing bacteria. The plasma half-lives of these drugs range from 2.5–3 hours for morphine, >22 hour for methadone and even longer for levomethadyl acetate.

Criminal Uses

1. **Suicidal Agent**: Opium is one of the most popular suicidal agents, because of its painless way of producing death. If it is mixed with mustard oil, it makes the poison difficult to eliminate, thus increases absorption.
2. **Homicidal Agent**: For its color and taste, opium can rarely be used as a homicidal agent, but it can be used as a homicidal agent when its taste is masked by mixing it with some other agent and when it is administered to an infant.
3. **Accidental**: It can occur, especially in case of children.
4. **Cattle Poisoning**: Rarely used. It is also used for doping race horses.
5. **Aphrodisiac**: To increase libido.
6. Infanticide.
7. Used in euthanasia.
8. Drug abuse.
9. Doping for horse race.

Table 41.2 Therapeutic and fatal dose of various alkaloids

Alkaloids	Therapeutic dose in mg	Average fatal dose in mg
Crude opium	–	500
Morphine	10–15	200–250*, 80–100
Pethidine	50–150	About 1000
Codeine	10–60*	800*
Methadone	5–10	100
Heroin	–	50
Pantazocine	30–60	300
Propoxyphene	100–150*	1000*
Diphenoxylate	10–20*	200*

* Orally; others are parenteral route

Clinical Features

Acute Opium Poisoning

Appear, within half hour after intake. Can be divided into three different stages, but if the dose consumed is very high, the stages may be overlap and the person may die even within 45 minutes.

Stage of Excitement or Euphoria: This stage is very short lasting and may be altogether absent if the dose is very high. There is increase in the sense of well-being and mental activities. Patient feels freeness from anxiety and some sort of restlessness and sometimes it may be associated with visual hallucinations. There may be excessive excitement and the patient may even become violent.

Stage of Stupor: The nerve centers are depressed, which sometimes comes on very suddenly. The symptoms are headache, nausea and vomiting (stimulation of CTZ in medulla), giddiness, lethargic condition, drowsiness and an uncontrollable desire to sleep, from which the patient may be roused by external stimulation. The pupil starts contracting (stimulant effect on papillary constrictor center). Face and lips are cyanosed and an itching sensation is felt all over the skin. The pulse and respiration are still normal.

Stage of Narcosis: Gradually, the patient passes into deep coma, from which he cannot be roused. Marked insensibility to pain, with muscle relaxed and reflexes lost. All secretions are suspended, except the sweat, which makes the skin cool and clammy. The face is pale, lips are livid and cyanosed and due to muscle relaxation, the jaw drops.

Pupils are Contracted Pinpoint, not reacting to light reflex, might be due to depression of supranuclear inhibition of papillary constrictor, tone but prior to death, there may be dilatation of the pupil known as **pre-mortal dilation.** Conjunctivae are congested, BP falls, pulse weak and thready, respiration is slow, labored stertorous, **Cheyne Stoke's type** and the rate may even be as low as 4–6 per minute. Recovery is still possible if prompt and proper treatment is undertaken. Otherwise, lividity increases, pulse becomes slower, more irregular and imperceptible, convulsive twisting may occur in group of muscles and pupils may become widely dilated, just prior to death. Sometimes, tetanoid convulsions and hyperpyrexia may be noted. Death is due to respiration failure or sometimes due to heart failure. The **classical triad** for opioid poisoning is **miosis** or **pinpoint pupil, coma** and **respiratory depression.**

Differential Diagnosis

Differential diagnosis of opium poisoning is shown in **Table 41.3**.

Tests for Morphine

Marquis Test: One drop from a mixture of 3 mL of concentrated sulfuric acid and three drops of formalin is dropped to a blotting paper soaked with the extract of the suspected material. If the suspected material contains opium, there will be resultant changes of color, which will be first purple then violet and finally blue.

Other important tests are: Deniges's test, Husemann's test, etc.

Management

Its guideline is improvement in the rate of respiration and dilatation of pupils. Best result of it is obtained if the treatment is started in 1st or 2nd stage.

1. Stomach wash should be given with plain water and to be followed by 0.02% aqueous solution of potassium permanganate. This washing should be continued till normal pink color retained (returning fluid will be at first rusty brown in color). After washing is completed, ½ pint of potassium permanganate solution should be left in the stomach, to neutralize any re-excreted morphine.
2. If patient is conscious, to induce vomiting, kitchen room emetics (powdered mustard) can be tried. However, for ingested poison, **Syrup of Ipecacuanha** is the best emetics, followed by the subcutaneous injection of **Apomorphine**.

Table 41.3 Differential diagnosis of opium poisoning

Diseases	Poisonings
Cerebrovascular accident: Hypertensive elderly patients with dilated pupils, full pulse and evidence of paralysis	*Carbolic acid poisoning:* Brownish patches on lips and mouth with strong, characteristic odor, green coloration of urine and pin-point contracted pupils
Uremic coma: Patients with renal disease with presence of albumin, casts in the urine, with a typical urinous odor emanated by the patient	*Alcoholic coma:* Manifested by congested face, injected eyes, dilated pupil, with strong odor of alcohol in exhaled air
Diabetic coma: Gradual, in a known patient suffering from diabetes on anti-diabetic drugs with history of skipping medicine. The respiration is slow and deep, ocular tension is low, exhaled air will give the sweet smell of acetone. Urine contains sugar and aceto-acetic acid. Papillary changes are non-descript	*Barbiturate poisoning:* Pupils are dilated, history of taking tablets with greater respiration rate, with loss of reflexes, with fall of blood pressure
Hypoglycemic coma: Diabetic patient on drug, with history of having skipped lunch, but has taken medicine, gradual development of weakness with features like vasovagal attack. Gradually passes to coma. Pupils little contracted, blood sugar or urine sugar alarmingly low	*Datura poisoning:* Pupils dilated, rise in body temperature with dry skin, flushes of face, delirium, carpology, etc.
Epileptic coma: Follows an epileptic fit. Pupils dilated, coma is less profound	Carbon monoxide poisoning
Others: Hysterical coma (Commonly seen in young female), cerebral malaria, meningitis	

3. To inactivate the already absorbed poison, **physiological antidote** is necessary. Atropine is the physiological antidote, but it cannot be used because both morphine and atropine have the same depressant effect on respiratory center.
4. Most recent antidote is **Nalmefene**, a naltrexone derivative. It has got pure opiate antagonistic effects. Routes: IV (common), IM and SC dose begin with 0.1 mg, and if withdrawal reaction does not occur, administer 0.5 mg, followed by 1 mg in 2–5 minutes if necessary.
   Antidotes not used today are nalorphine and levallorphan. Because they are (i) weak competitive antagonists and (ii) have undesirable kappa receptor agonist properties (producing dysphoria).
5. **Naloxone hydrochloride** given IM, IV (common), sublingually, or even instilled down an endotracheal tube. Since repeated doses may be required, naloxone infusion may be better. Dose is 1.2 mg for adult and 0.4 mg for children. It can be repeated. A total of 75 mg in 24 hours can be given.

Postmortem Findings

External: Not very characteristics. Many a times, mark of needle prick or tattooing is seen in case of intravenous drug users.

Signs of asphyxia are very pronounced, with deep cyanosis in the face and finger nails, etc. Froth may be seen in the mouth and nostrils, blood may be dark and fluid. Postmortem staining is well-marked and cyanotic.

Internal: If the patient has consumed crude opium, on opening the stomach, brownish small lumps may be seen adhering to the mucous membrane. On opening the chest, the typical smell of opium is detected, but it disappears if putrefaction has set in.

Combination of edema of the lungs and intense, lividity of face almost approaching to blackness are the "**hallmark**" of diagnostic findings.

Cerebral edema is seen. Enlargement of liver with enlarged hepatic lymph nodes are found in chronic users and chemical analysis of them give positive result for morphine.[4,5]

HEROIN (DIACETYLMORPHINE)

The name heroin comes from '**heroisch**', the German word for hero. Heroin was originally sold as a painkiller in the 19th century, by the chemical company Bayer, until doctors realized its highly addictive quality. Bayer even marketed heroin as a "**cure**" for morphine addiction and cough medicine for children. It is now known that heroin, along with most opiates, are converted by the human liver into the morphine with varying degrees of concentration in the bloodstream. Pure heroin is a white powder, but street heroin comes as a brownish-white powder that can be smoked, snorted or dissolved and injected.

Heroin (diacetylmorphine), also known as diamorphine or, especially in older literature, as morphine diacetate, is an opioid drug synthesized from morphine, which is a derivative of the opium poppy. It is the 3, 6-diacetyl ester of morphine and functions as a morphine prodrug (meaning that it is metabolically converted to morphine inside the body).[6] The white crystalline form, considered "**pure heroin**", is usually the hydrochloride salt, diacetylmorphine hydrochloride. When heroin is supplied illegally, though, it is often adulterated to a freebase form, dulling the sheen and consistency to a matte white powder.[7] Currently, over 80% of the world supply of opium and its derivatives, including heroin, is thought to be produced in Afghanistan.[8]

As with other opioids, diacetylmorphine is used as both an analgesic and a recreational drug. Frequent and regular administration is associated with tolerance and physical dependence, which may develop into addiction. Internationally, diacetylmorphine is controlled under schedules I and IV of the single convention on narcotic drugs.[9] It is illegal to manufacture, possess or sell diacetylmorphine without a license in almost every country.

Under the chemical name diamorphine, diacetylmorphine is a legally prescribed controlled drug in the UK and is supplied in tablet or injectable form for the same indications as morphine is. It is available for prescription to long-term users in the Netherlands, UK, Switzerland, Germany and Denmark, alongside psycho-social care,[10,11] and a similar program is being campaigned for by liberal political parties in Norway.

CODEINE (3 METHYLMORPHINE)

Codeine or 3-methylmorphine is an opiate used for its analgesic, anti-tussive and anti-diarrheal properties. Codeine is the second-most predominant alkaloid in opium, at up to 3%; it is much more prevalent in the Iranian poppy (Papaver bractreatum), and codeine is extracted from this species in some places, although the morphine methylation process is still much more common. It is considered the prototype of the weak to midrange opioids. The codeine content of opium is related inversely to the morphine content, but only in a general way. The opiums of the principal exporting countries have approximately the following percentages of codeine: Balkans 1.25%; Turkey 1.25%; Iran 3.4%; India 3.0%. The highest percentages of codeine obtained by the United Nations Secretariat (averaging about 4.3%) were found in opium samples that came from North-Eastern Asia (Korea, Northern China).

Codeine is used to manufacture dihydrocodeine, hydrocodone and others. It may also be used to manufacture the drugs ordinarily made by conversion of thebaine.

THEBAINE AND PAPAVERINE

Thebaine is the most poisonous opium alkaloid and is scarcely used medically. It is even omitted from some of the preparations of mixed opium alkaloids, which are used as soluble substitutes for opium. However, it is converted into several other narcotics which have medical use: hydrocodone (dihydrocodeinone), acetyldihydrocodeinone and oxycodone (dihydro-hydroxycodeinone).

Papaverine has a considerable medical use, so much so that supplies available from opium have sometimes run short. It is then manufactured.

REFERENCES

1. Opiate–Definitions from Dictionary.com. [cited 2006 May 5]; Available from: URL:http://www.Dictionary.reference.com
2. Selavka CM. Poppy seed investigation as a contributing factor to opiate-positive urinalysis results. The Pacific perspective. J Forensic Sci. 1991;36:685-96.
3. Cunningham S. Cunningham's Encyclopedia of Magical Herbs. Llewellyn. 2004.p.211.
4. Pillay VV. Comprehensive Medical Toxicology. 2nd ed. Hyderabad. Paras Publishing. 2008.p.533-51.
5. Pillay VV. Text Book of Forensic Medicine and Toxicology. 16th ed. Hyderabad. Paras Publishing. 2011.p. 485-90.
6. Sawynok J. The therapeutic use of heroin. A review of the pharmacological literature. Can J Physiol Pharmacol. 1986;64(1):1-6.
7. Basic Facts about Heroin. [cited 2006 May 5]; Available from: URL:http://www.Alcoholism.about.com
8. Afghanistan opium survey. 2004. [cited 2006 May 5]; Available from: URL:http://www.United Nations Office on Drugs and Crime.about.com
9. Yellow List. List of Narcotic drugs Under International Control" (PDF). International Narcotics Control Board. 2004 Dec; [cited 2006 May 5]; Available from: URL:http://www.incb.org/incb/yellow_list.html
10. Europe. German parliament Approves Heroin Maintenances. [cited 2006 May 5]; Available from: URL:http://www.StoptheDrugWar.org
11. Europe. Denmark parliament Approves Heroin Maintenances Pilot Project. [cited 2006 May 5]; Available from: URL:http://www.StoptheDrugWar.org

CHAPTER 42

Alcohol and Alcoholism

Gunajit Das, Putul Mahanta

LEARNING PLAN

- Know what alcohol is
- Identify different aspects of ethyl alcohol
- Learn about acute alcohol intoxication and its management
- Understand alcoholism and chronic alcohol poisoning
- Learn about drunkenness, its examination and reporting
- Know about postmortem alcohol estimation
- Understand medicolegal aspects of alcohol intoxication
- Learn about the agencies working for curbing alcoholism
- Know about methyl alcohol

Hundreds of thousands of years ago, man presumably became aware that a strange metamorphosis occurred when honey, fruits, berries, cereals and other plant materials were mixed with water and left in the warmth of the Sun.[1] The record of alcohol is a colorful chapter in the history of mankind; the details are of more than intrinsic interest, for they illuminate the development of the cultural drinking patterns, drinking attitudes and habits and the wise and unwise uses of alcoholic beverages, which have now become matters of great medical, social and toxicological significance.

HISTORICAL PERSPECTIVE

Existence of the purposely fermented beverages dates back to even 10,000 BC, substantiated by the discovery of late Stone Age beer glass jug. The name originates from the Arabic, **alcuhl**, which means fine metallic powder. Greek loves wine, so they had a "God of wine" called Dyonisus and Romans called it Bacchus. Beer was a very important Egyptian drink. Throughout the first 1000 years of church history, Christians consumed alcoholic beverages as a common part of everyday life. They held that both the

Bible and Christian tradition taught that alcohol is a gift of god. The word whisky was derived from Gaelic *uisge beatha* meaning 'water of life'. In India, alcoholic beverages in Indus valley civilization appeared in the Chalcolithic era between 3000 and 2000 BC. *Sura* and *suma* were two main drinks popular in ancient Hindu civilization. *Sura* was more popular, used to be drunk by warriors. *Sura* is considered to be a favorite drink of Indra, the king of all gods and goddesses. The Hindu Ayurvedic text also describe about the use of alcohol. Even the two Hindu epics, Ramayana and Mahabharata, mention the use of alcohol.[2-4]

INTRODUCTION

Alcohol is a colorless volatile flammable liquid, synthesized or obtained by fermentation of sugars and starches and widely used, either in pure or denatured form, as a solvent and in drugs, cleaning solutions, explosives, intoxicating beverages as well as preservative solutions.[5] In terms of toxicology, alcohol is an inebriant, cerebral neurotoxic poison. Chemically, these are (hydroxy) derivative of (aliphatic) hydrocarbons routinely divided into three categories (**Table 42.1**).

The following representation (**Table 42.2**) gives us an idea about the toxicity of different types of Monohydroxy alcohol.[6] Commonly the word alcohol refers to ethyl alcohol or ethanol.

ETHYL ALCOHOL (ETHANOL)

i. Pure or anhydrous ethyl alcohol (molecular weight: 46.06844 g/mol) is a clear colorless, flammable liquid with pleasant faint fruity odor and a sweetish burning taste. It absorbs water rapidly from air. Its boiling point is 78.5°C, freezing point is –130°C and its density at 15.56°C (60°F) is 0.798. It is readily miscible with water in any proportion. It is also lipid soluble.[1]
ii. The common term alcohol means a watery solution containing 95% of ethanol.
iii. Absolute alcohol contains 99.95% of ethanol.
iv. Rectified spirit contains 90% by volume of ethyl alcohol.
v. Industrial methylated spirit or denatured alcohol is a mixture of 95% ethyl alcohol and wood naphtha.
vi. Proof spirit contains 49.24% by weight of absolute alcohol or 57.10% by volume ethyl alcohol.

Mechanism of Production

Alcohol is produced by fermentation of sugar by yeast. Yeasts are living microorganisms which die in concentrations of alcohol greater than 15%. Therefore, strong alcoholic beverages need to be produced by two stage method, fermentation followed by distillation.

Table 42.1 Chemical categories of alcohol

1.	Monohydroxy alcohols	With 1 hydroxyl (OH) group, e.g. ethyl alcohol (ethanol), methyl alcohol (methanol), isopropyl alcohol (isopropanol), isobutyl alcohol, etc.
2.	Dihydroxy alcohol	Possesses two OH groups and referred to as glycols, e.g. ethylene glycol, propylene glycol, etc.
3.	Trihydroxy alcohol	They are not really alcohol but derivatives of alcohol, e.g. glycerol or glycerin

Table 42.2 Different types of toxicity of monohydroxy alcohol

Ethyl alcohol	Toxic
Methyl alcohol	More toxic than ethyl alcohol
Isopropyl alcohol	Three times more toxic than methyl alcohol
Isobutyl alcohol	One and a half times more toxic than isopropyl alcohol
Amyl alcohol	Six times more toxic than isobutyl alcohol

$$C_6H_{12}O_6 \rightarrow 2(CH_3\text{-}CH_2\text{-}OH) + 2CO_2$$
$$(\text{Yeasts} + \text{sugar} + \text{water} = CO_2 + \text{ethanol})$$

As yeast cannot ferment starch, starch has to be converted to maltose for further processing.

$$\text{Starch} \xrightarrow[\text{Convertase}]{} \text{Maltose}$$

Types of Alcoholic Beverages

Standard Type Alcoholic Beverages

1. **Malted Liquors**: Fermented liquids without distillation with low alcohol concentration made from fermentation of germinating cereals (malts) mostly barley:
   - Light Beers: 4–6% (Lager and Pilsener)
   - Strong Beers: 6–8% (Ale and Stout)
2. **Wines**: Fermented liquids without distillation prepared from fermentation of natural sugars like grapes, apples and other fruits and have different varieties:
   - Light and without distillation: 10–15% (Claret, Cider)
   - Fortified: Distilled beverages added from outside: 15–20% (Port, Sherry)
   - Effervescent wine, bottled before completion of the process of fermentation: 12–16% (Champagne)
3. **Spirits**: 40–55% v/v (range), 42.8% v/v or 37% w/w (standard)
   (**Whisky**—distilled grain, **Rum**—distilled molasses, **Gin**—any sugar source, **Brandy**—distilled wine or grapes, **Vodka**—any of grain, rye, wheat, potatoes, grapes, sugar beet or molasses).

Unlike beers and wines, the alcohol content of most distilled alcoholic beverages is expressed in degrees of proof. This term probably developed from the 17th Century English custom of estimating alcohol content by moistening gunpowder with beverage and applying a flame to the mixture. The lowest alcohol concentration which would allow ignition, a concentration of about 57% by volume, was considered to be "proof spirits". British and Canadian regulations are still based on this yardstick; a concentration of 57.35% alcohol is considered to be "proof spirits", while other concentrations are described as "over" or "under" proof. In the US, however, regulations are based on a proof value, which is exactly double the alcohol concentration by volume. Thus a 100% proof whiskey contains 50% alcohol by volume.[1]

Some Indigenous Beverages

- Mexico: Teqila
- Japan: Sake
- France: Eau De Brandy/Fruit Brandy
- India: Arrack, Fenny, Toddy, Gudamba, Khopri, Lattha, Nanatang, etc.

Country Liquor

These alcoholic beverages are made from any cheap raw materials available locally, e.g. sugarcane, rice, jaggery, coarse grain, coconut, etc. Generally produced in distilleries and sold from authorized outlet. Different names are used in different parts of the country, e.g. arrack, tari, fenny, etc. Controlling system (a government body) monitors alcohol content (around 40%) and also other quality.

Illicit Liquor

Besides licensed distilleries, a number of small production units operate secretly and produces local drink where quality control is not maintained. In this type, the alcohol content may be as high as 50–60%. Adulteration is frequent, seen with common adulterant being the methylated spirit. Many tribes in India produce alcoholic drink for domestic use.

Standard Drink

One Drink Equals

- 340 mL (12 oz) of beer
- 115 mL (4 oz) of non-fortified wine
- 43 mL (1.5 oz) of proof spirit such as whisky, gin, vodka, etc.

One standard drink contains approximately 10–15 g of ethanol. These alcoholic beverages also contain additional congeners to enhance taste, strength, etc. and might contribute to the adverse effect to the body.

Absorption

Alcohol itself is absorbed rapidly through all mucous membranes. The vapors of alcohol may be absorbed through the lung. When consumed as an alcoholic beverage, about 20% is absorbed from the stomach and the rest 80% from the small intestine, mostly in the proximal part. The rate of absorption is greatly influenced by:

a. The alcohol concentration, e.g. higher the concentration of alcohol up to a maximum of 40% by volume, the more rapid is its absorption.
b. The nature and concentration of other chemicals in the beverage.
c. Presence or absence of food in the stomach, e.g. absence of food increases the absorption and presence delays it.
d. The emptying time of stomach, e.g. absorption is slowed when the emptying of the stomach is delayed. This may occur because of presence of food in the stomach, emotional tension, or nausea. Occasionally, a very large dose of alcohol in high concentration may produce pyloric spasm resulting in delayed emptying.
e. The condition of the gastric mucosa, e.g. gastric sclerosis delays the absorption.

Distribution

Once absorbed, alcohol is distributed rapidly throughout the body by the bloodstream, and the concentration quickly reaches equilibrium, with a ratio dependent upon the water content of the tissues. Generally, women have a higher peak ethanol concentration than men if exposed to the same amount of ethanol, due to their lower body water content and the lower level of alcohol dehydrogenase in gastric mucosal cells. Alcohol readily crosses placenta and exposes the fetus. It also crosses blood brain barrier readily.

The distribution makes it possible to calculate blood-alcohol levels by measuring the alcohol content of expired air or of the urine.

- Blood : Urine = 1 : 1.31
- Blood : Exhaled air = 1 : 2100
- Blood : Saliva = 1 : 1.12
- Bood : Cisternal fluid = 1 : 1.16
- Blood : Brain/liver = 1 : 0.85

Metabolism and Elimination

Metabolism of alcohol takes place in liver. Three pathways which are responsible:

1. Alcohol dehydrogenase pathway (in cell cytosol).
2. Microsomal ethanol oxidizing system (MEOS, located in endoplasmic reticulum).
3. Peroxidase—catalase system (in hepatic peroxisome). Less significant.

Alcohol liberates about 7 calories per gram. More than 90% of the ingested ethanol is oxidized to acetaldehyde by liver and gastric mucosal cells; 5–10% is excreted unchanged by kidneys, lungs and sweat. Oxidation of ethanol to acetaldehyde occurs predominantly in the liver by alcohol dehydrogenase (ADH). In addition, hepatic cytochrome P450, principally the isoform 2E1 (CYP2E1) in endoplasmic reticulum and catalase in peroxisome, are also able to catalyze the oxidation of ethanol to acetaldehyde. The acetaldehyde formed is further converted to acetate via the action of aldehyde dehydrogenase (ALDH) present in liver mitochondria. The average rate of ethanol metabolism in adults is 100 to 125 mg/kg/h in occasional drinkers, and can be up to 175 mg/kg/h in chronic drinkers. For medium-sized adults, the blood ethanol level drops at an average rate of 15–20 mg/dL/h.[7]

Alcohol metabolism follows zero order kinetics. Ethanol excretion by lung obeys Henry's law, i.e. ratio between the concentration of ethanol in alveolar air and the blood is constant (1:2100).

Step - I

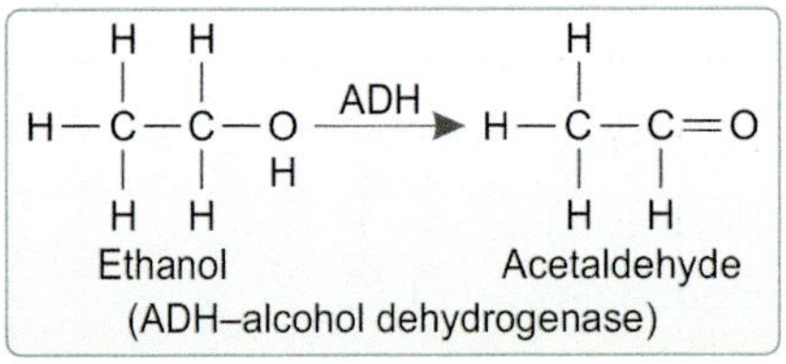

Step - II

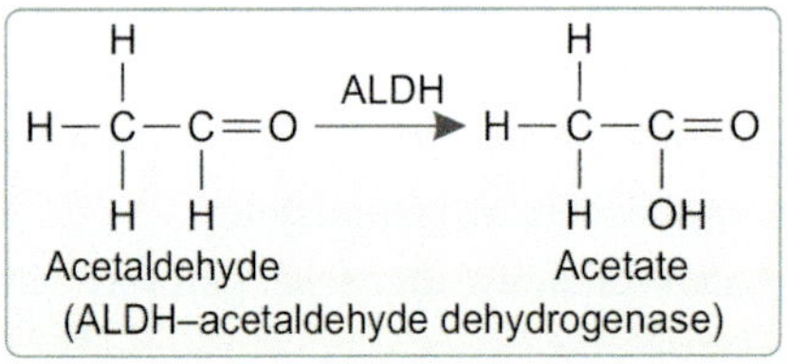

Mode of Action of Ethanol

Two Theories of Mode of Action of Ethanol

i. According to the first theory, ethanol acts by enhancing gama aminobutyric acid (GABA) function through interaction with $GABA_a$ receptor and associated chloride channel postulated by Charness, Simon and Greenberg.
ii. The second theory has to do with N-methyl-d-aspartate (NMDA) ligand gated glutamate receptor, NMDA receptors mediated neurotoxicity by increasing permeability to calcium and regulated neuronal long-term potentiation postulated by Hu and Ticku.

Tolerance

Repeated use of alcohol contributes to acquire tolerance. Mechanism involving in tolerance are mainly three types:

1. **Metabolic** or **Pharmacokinetic Tolerance**: Seen after 1–2 weeks of daily use, with up to 30% increase in hepatic metabolism.
2. **Cellular** or **Pharmacodynamics Tolerance**: Develop through neurochemical changes that maintain relatively normal physiologic functioning despite presence of alcohol. Subsequent decrease in blood level produces symptoms of withdrawal.
3. **Learned** or **Behavior Tolerance**: Individual learns to adapt their behavior that they can function better than expected under influence of alcohol.

Dependence

i. During acute intoxication, there is raised GABA and diminished NDMA receptor activity and opposite happened during withdrawal.
ii. Pleasurable activities of drinking are due to increase level of dopamine in the brain especially in the ventral tegmentum.
iii. Also due to raised serotonin level, increases release of stress hormones and release of endorphin.
iv. Hence, during abstinence blood level of these neurochemical also fall resulting in craving, dependence, relapse.

Fatal Dose

i. Adult: 6 g of ethanol/kg body weight
ii. Children: 3 g of ethanol/kg body weight
iii. Addict can tolerate bigger doses.

Fatal Period

i. 12–24 hours
ii. May be delayed for 4–6 days.

Effects of Ethanol Consumption

Central Nervous System (Stimulates First then Depresses)

i. Alcohol exerts its stimulant effect in the form of euphoric exaltation, impulsive behavior, unwarranted self-confidence and daring act.
ii. Due to release of lower center from higher center.
iii. Thereafter, depresses the highest evolutionary centers, i.e. center regulating conduct, memory, judgment, insight, concentration and self-criticism.
iv. In increased concentration, the motor centers, such as vital centers in medulla, are finally depressed.

v. Disturbed sleep, snoring, exacerbation of sleep apnea.
vi. Prolonged use causes peripheral neuropathy.
vii. Affect efficient muscular activity.
viii. Increases auditory threshold, decreases visual acuity.
ix. 1% alcoholics develop cerebellar degeneration or atrophy.
x. A very few alcoholics develop Wernicke's (ophthalmoparesis, ataxia and encephalopathy) and Korsakoff's (retrograde and antegrade amnesia) syndrome.

Cerebrovascular System

i. Small doses—Cutaneous vasodilatation, flushing.
ii. Medium dose—Tachycardia and mild rise in BP.
iii. Large dose—Vasodilatation due to direct vascular smooth muscle dilation and vasomotor center depression (clinical implication).

Respiratory System

i. Stimulation of respiration by irritation of pharyngeal and buccal mucosa.
ii. Central action causes depression.

Blood

i. Moderate drinking increases HDL (cholesterol level)
ii. Decrease in LDL oxidation.

Gastrointestinal System

i. Stimulate GI acid, dissolves mucosal lining, hemorrhagic lesions
ii. Chronic use: Pancreatitis, diabetes or reactive hypoglycemia, hepatic cellular damage, fibrosis and scarring, cirrhosis and hepatitis, nutritional deficiency.

Kidney

Diuresis—Increased water ingestion and inhibition of ADH, renal damage in chronic use.

Uterus

Relaxation of uterine muscles.

Endocrine

i. Low dose—Adrenaline release and hyperglycemia
ii. High dose—Hypoglycemia.

Sexual

Not a true aphrodisiac. Provokes the desire but takes away the performance.

Acute Alcohol Intoxication

Acute alcohol intoxication or poisoning may result from heavy and deliberate drinking alcoholic beverages:

i. In small dose, but short intervals.
ii. Excessively high dose at a time.
iii. Alcoholic vapor inhalation for long time.

Signs and Symptoms

Stage of Excitement: (BAC*—0.05%-0.15%, 50-150 mg %)

a. Sense of wellbeing
b. Euphoria
c. Increased confidence
d. Excitement

Stage of In-coordination: (BAC—0.15-0.25%, 50-250 mg%)

a. Muscle in-coordination
b. Increased reaction time
c. Disordered sense perception
d. Slurring of speech
e. Unsteady gait
f. Flushed face.

Stage of Stupor and Coma: (BAC > 0.3-0.5%, 300-500 mg)

Gradually becomes drowsy and goes to coma.

***BAC**: Blood alcohol concentration.

Blood Alcohol Concentration and Behavior

The concentration of alcohol in the blood—not simply the amount swallowed—is generally related to the over-all attitude or behavior of an individual. This may be alliteratively indicated, as Joseph E Bogen suggested as follows:

i. At a blood alcohol content less than 0.03%, it may be said, the individual is **Dull** and **Dignified**
ii. At 0.05%, he is **Dashing** and **Debonair**

iii. At 0.10%, he may become **Dangerous** and **Devilish**
iv. At 0.20%, he is likely to be **Dizzy** and **Disturbing**
v. At 0.30%, he may be **Disgusting** and **Disheveled**
vi. At 0.40%, he is **Delirious** and **Disoriented**
vii. At 0.50%, he is surely **Drunk**
viii. At 0.60%, he is **Dead Drunk**
ix. At 0.70%, the chances are that he is **Dead.**

The above stages apply only to how he may appear to others and not necessarily correspond at all with the mood which the individual feels inwardly. Subjective effects of alcohol are often at variance with the objective behavioral manifestations.

Barbiturate and paraldehyde poisoning, cardiovascular accidents, hypoglycemia, schizophrenia and head injury should always be excluded before coming to a conclusion of alcohol intoxication at the first instance.

Management

Acute alcohol poisoning is a medical emergency due to the risk of death from respiratory depression and/or inhalation of vomit if emesis occurs while the patient is unconscious and unresponsive. Emergency treatment for acute alcohol poisoning strives to stabilize the patient and maintain a patent airway and respiration, while waiting for the alcohol to metabolize.[8]

Also

i. Protect vital signs by monitoring ABCs, or airway, breathing and circulation; that is, if the person is thought to be at risk for severe respiratory depression, consider an endotracheal tube to protect the airway and assist with breathing.
ii. Protect the airway from aspirating stomach contents that could cause aspiration pneumonia.
iii. Treat hypoglycemia (low blood sugar) with 50 mL of 50% dextrose solution and saline flush, as ethanol induced hypoglycemia is unresponsive to glucagon.
iv. Administer vitamin thiamine to prevent Wernicke-Korsakoff syndrome, which can cause a seizure (more usually a treatment for chronic alcoholism, but in the acute context, usually co-administered to ensure maximal benefit).
v. Check urea and electrolytes to guide fluid replacement.
vi. Apply hemodialysis if the blood concentration is dangerously high (> 400 mg%), and especially if there is metabolic acidosis.
vii. Provide oxygen therapy as needed via nasal cannula or non-rebreather mask.

Additional medication may be indicated for treatment of nausea, tremor and anxiety.

Prognosis

A normal liver detoxifies the blood of alcohol over a period of time that depends on the initial level and the patient's overall physical condition. An abnormal liver will take longer but still succeed, provided the alcohol does not cause liver failure.[9] People who have been drinking heavily for several days or weeks may have withdrawal symptoms after the acute intoxication has subsided.[10] A person who consumes a dangerous amount of alcohol persistently can develop memory blackouts and idiosyncratic intoxication or pathological drunkenness symptoms.[11] Long-term persistent consumption of excessive amounts of alcohol can cause liver damage and have other deleterious health effects.

Postmortem Appearance in Case of Death[12]

i. Rigor mortis may lasis for unusually long period.
ii. Retarded decomposition in some cases.
iii. Alcoholic odor in the stomach, lung and brain before decomposition sets in.
iv. Red, intensely congested and inflamed gastric mucosa. In some cases, gastric mucosa may remain pale.
v. Blood appears fluid and dark.
vi. Visceras usually found congested.

Alcoholism and Chronic Alcohol Poisoning

The chronic excessive consumption of alcohol has become an increasingly important problem and has received growing attention from physicians, physiologists, biochemists, sociologists, clergymen, educators, police officials, lawyers, legislators and statisticians. From this point of interest has come an enormous literature on the subject. The useful definition of the true alcoholic lies in the concept that he is a person:

i. Who has a compulsion to drink, or an inability to stop drinking once he has begun, and
ii. Whose drinking has become a serious problem, either to himself or to society, or both.

Keller defined alcoholism as "a chronic disease, or disorder of behavior, characterized by the repeated drinking of alcoholic beverages to an extent that exceeds customary dietary use or ordinary compliance with the social drinking customs of the community, and that interferes with the individual's health, interpersonal relations or economic functioning".

Findings may be:

i. Loss of appetite
ii. Vomiting
iii. Nutritional deficiency
iv. Disordered hepatic function
v. Cognitive defects
vi. Cirrhosis of liver
vii. Magnesium depletion
viii. Impaired mental function
ix. Neurological damages.

Clinical Syndromes:

i. Common abstinence syndrome (6–8 hours)
ii. Alcoholic hallucinosis/confusional insanity (24–36 hours)
iii. Rum fits/seizures (7–48 hours)
iv. Alcoholic ketoacidosis (24–72 hours)
v. Delirium tremens (3–5 days)
vi. Wernicke-Korsakoff syndrome.

Management

Management should be aimed at minimizing the effect of alcohol withdrawal in those patients who already have developed a physical dependence on alcohol. Management is done in three ways:

1. Psychological support
2. Managing the withdrawal symptoms
3. Aversion therapy.

Psychotherapy

Psychotherapy in the form of a group than single individual is more preferable. Alcohol anonymous (an independent voluntary organization) plays an important role for those who actually want to get rid of the problem of alcoholism.

Managing the Withdrawal Symptoms

i. Sudden withdrawal undesirable, gradually weaned
ii. Paraldehyde 10 cc IM/rectally/orally
iii. Chlorpromazine 50–100 mg IM/orally
iv. Chlordiazepoxide 25–50 mg orally/IV
v. Diazepam 2–10 mg orally/IV
vi. Phenobarbitone for seizures.

Aversion Therapy

1. **Disulfiram** (Tetraethylthiuram): Single daily dose of 0.5 g, can be continued, antiabuse drug nowadays not used frequently. Disulfiram causes a reaction of flushing, sweating, nausea and tachycardia when the patient ingests alcohol. It is most effective when medication compliance can be monitored. Contraindications are use of alcohol-containing preparations, metronidazole, severe cardiac disease and unwillingness to completely abstain from alcohol.
2. Anti-craving drug like acamprosate, opioid antagonist likes naltrexone.
3. Conditioned reflex treatment.
4. Vitamin B_1, B_6, B_{12} supplementation.
5. Diet and rehabilitation.

Postmortem Findings in Case of Death

i. Deep reddish-brown colored and hypertrophied or atrophied gastric mucosa with patches of congestion or effusion.
ii. Fatty changes in liver/cirrhosis.
iii. Fatty degeneration and dilated heart/cardiomyopathy.
iv. Granular degeneration in kidneys.
v. Postmortem blood alcohol concentration > 0.2% suggest alcohol ingestion before death.

DRUNKENNESS

It is a condition produced in a person, who has taken alcohol in a quantity sufficient to cause him to lose control of his faculties to such an extent that he is unable to execute safely the occupation or profession in which he was engaged at the material time.[13]

Examination of an Alleged Case of Drunkenness and its Reporting

Examination of an alleged case of drunkenness should be carried out keeping in mind the different provisions of the Law (IPC, CrPC and other relevant Acts) so as to avoid any complications afterwards as there is every possibility of misinterpretation of findings if the things are not done in a proper way.

The alleged person may be brought or sent for examination by investigative, administrative or judicial authority. The individual may be either under detention or under formal arrest. Section 53 CrPC will apply if the individual in question is already under arrest.

Procedure

i. Examination of the relevant papers sent along with the alleged individual and then registration of the case putting all details including name, age, identification mark, occupation and address in the register maintained for that purpose in the medical establishment, so that in future correspondence can be made with ease with any authority regarding the case.
ii. The individual should be explained properly the purpose and procedure of the examination, so that it becomes easier for the physician to solve any dispute relating to the consent for examination.

Consent

There is every possibility that it becomes difficult to take the consent of the individual if he is already in an inebriated or unconscious state. In such condition, the primary responsibility of the doctor will be to save the patient by giving treatment by admitting to the hospital after collecting the requisite urine and blood sample and also after recording all clinical details. No findings should be divulged to any authority, unless it is extremely necessary, till the individual becomes normal and sober and understands properly the whole procedure. At this moment, if the individual gives consent, the report with the findings already recorded can be submitted to the authority. Else, the findings do not constitute a report of examination of an alleged drunkenness case; rather it becomes just a medical record of admission of the individual to be accessible with limitation as prescribed under different legal provisions relating to medical records of any individual.

For arrested person brought for examination, Section 53 of CrPC allows application of reasonable force if consent is denied by such person for completion of the examination process.

Procedure Proper

1. History: A detailed history should be taken to exclude any pre-existing disease which may mimic drunkenness.
2. General behavior, state of dress, speech, response to verbal commands, etc.
3. Memory and mental alertness, ability to write and read, time taken in different tasks of reading and writing.

4. **Physical examination**
   a. Pulse: Resting pulse, usually rapid, full and bounding.
   b. Blood pressure: Increase in systolic blood pressure.
   c. Temperature: Raised (peripheral).
   d. Skin: May be dry or moist and flushed or pale depending on the amount consumed and the blood alcohol level.
   e. Mouth: General state of mouth teeth and tongue should be noted in respect to the dryness, furred or bitten.
   f. Eyes: Red and swollen eyelids, congested conjunctiva, initially dilated and then constricted pupil, difficulty in convergence, positive strabismus, positive nystagmus (a strong proof of drunkenness).
   g. Reflexes: Sluggish knee and ankle reflexes.
   h. Gait: Staggering gait, disturbances in gait while making a turn.
   i. Muscle coordination: Finger-nose test, coin picking test.
5. **Laboratory tests**
   a. **Breath analysis of alcohol**: 60–100 mL of breath is received into a dry balloon and analyzed by breath analyzer. Amount of alcohol in 2100 mL of alveolar air = amount of alcohol in 1 mL of blood. Test to be repeated after 20 minutes.

      Mechanism of operation: Alcohol absorbs radiations in the infrared region of spectrum and amount of infrared light absorbed by vapor is proportional to the concentration of alcohol in that vapor.

      Procedure: The person is asked to blow into a plastic balloon through a glass tube containing crystalline bichromate—sulfuric acid mixture.

      Causes of false positive result: Alcohol may remain in the mouth up to 20–30 minutes after a small peg, hyperventilation, physical exercise, emesis, regurgitation.
   b. **Blood analysis**: Skin is cleaned with 1:1000 mercuric chloride and 10 mL of blood is collected in a glass vial containing 10 g NaF (sodium fluoride) or 30 g of potassium oxalate. After collecting sample, analysis should be performed within a week. Whole blood alcohol concentration is 12–20% lesser than serum or plasma concentration. Tests are based on the presence of any volatile reducing substance. Basic principle is reduction of potassium bichromate by the test substances. Method used are (i) Kozelka and Hine test (macro test), and (ii) Cavett test (micro test).
   c. **Urine analysis**: Two samples should collected, 1st as soon as following the incident after complete emptying the bladder, 2nd after a period of 25–30 minutes.

      Preservative: 30 mg phenyl mercuric nitrate to every 10 mL of urine. Concentration of alcohol in urine is 20% higher than blood when collected at same time.

      Disadvantage: (i) Maximum concentration in urine reaches 20–25 minutes later than the blood, and (ii) After the maximum concentration of alcohol in blood has been reached, the urine alcohol concentration will be higher by 20–30%.
   d. **Saliva analysis**: Wash mouth thoroughly with water. Chew a small square of paraffin. 5 cc in a test tube in 10 mg sodium fluoride.
6. **Final opinion**

   The medical officer has to come to a conclusion as to the state of drunkenness of the individual in the following format, any one of which only is applicable depending on the findings:
   i. The individual has not consumed alcohol.
   ii. The individual has consumed alcohol but not under its influence.

iii. The individual has consumed alcohol and is under its influence but he can take care of himself as well as others.

iv. The individual has consumed alcohol and is under its influence, but he cannot take care of himself as well as others.

PROFORMA FOR EXAMINATION OF A CASE OF DRUNKENNESS

Hospital No: **Reg. No:** **Dated:**

Reference:

A. Personal Information

1. Name:
2. Age: years. Sex: M/F. Occupation: Service/business/cultivation/others
3. Guardian's name:
4. Address:
5. Accompanying person:
6. Consent:
7. Accompanying police constable:
8. Identification marks:
   i. ii.
9. Date and time of examination: Time: AM/PM
10. Time and place of incident: AM/PM. Place:
11. Place of examination:
12. Time completed:

B. History:

C. Physical Examination

13. General appearance:

Contd...

Contd...

14. Vital data:
    Temperature: ______ F/C. Pulse: ______ /Min, Rapid/ bounding/ slow.
    Respiratory Rate: ______ / Min. BP ______ mm Hg;
    Weight: ______ kg. Height: ______ cm

15. General manners and behavior: Calm/ talkative/abusive/obscene/others ______

16. State of dress: Decent/soiled/disarrange/ ______

17. Speech: Normal/thick/slurred/over-precise/incoherent/ ______

18. Breath: Smell of alcohol present/absent/ ______

19. Stance: Stand up properly/swing/ ______ Romberg sign: Positive/negative

20. Gait: Normal/unsteady/staggering/ ______

21. Handwriting: ______

22. Skin: Dry/moist/flushed/pale/ ______

23. Eyes: Conjunctivas: Normal/congested, pupils: Dilated/constricted/pin point constriction, pupillary reflex: Normal/ sluggish/absent, convergence test: Can/cannot converse his/her eyes, nystagmus: Fine lateral nystagmus present/ absent

24. Reflexes: knee and ankle reflexes: Sluggish/delayed. Planter reflex: Extensor/flexor. Others: ______

25. Muscular coordination: Finger nose test: Can/cannot perform. Finger to finger test: Can/cannot perform, unbuttoning and buttoning: Can/cannot do; picking objects from floor: Can/cannot perform.

26. CNS examination: Memory and mental alertness: Memory of recent events: Intact/lost, orientation to time and place: Present/absent.

27. Respiratory system: ______

28. GIT: ______

D. Result of laboratory investigation: i. Blood: ______ **ii. Urine:** ______ **iii. Others if any:** ______

E. Opinion: After through physical examination and laboratory investigation of the person ______ I am /we are of the opinion that:

1. The individual has not consumed alcohol.
2. The examined individual has consumed alcohol but he is not under its influence.
3. The examined individual has consumed alcohol and he is under its influence.

Date: ______ **Place:** ______ **Signature with seal**

Postmortem Alcohol Estimation

The technical details and the procedure for measuring ethanol in different biological samples collected from the corpse are same as those used when analyzing specimens from living. However, the interpretation of the analytical results obtained from autopsy samples is confounded by problems such as the lack of homogeneity of blood samples, microbial alcohol production postmortem, alcohol diffusion from gastric residue and contaminated airways and the lack of or unreliability of information on the clinical condition of the person prior to death. On the other hand, autopsy offers opportunities for sampling body fluids and tissues not accessible or not readily available in the living. Different samples which can be used postmortem for alcohol analysis are:[14]

i. Blood from multiple vascular sites
ii. Vitreous humor of the eye
iii. Gastric contents
iv. Sequestrated hematomas
v. Bile
vi. Brain
vii. Skeletal muscle
viii. CSF.

Medicolegal Aspect of Alcohol Intoxication

i. Drunkenness and medical practice: It will constitute rash and negligent act under Section 304(A) IPC. It can also categorize as infamous conduct that may leads to erasure of name.
ii. Section 85 and Section 86 IPC deal with the act done by an intoxicated individual. The individual is not criminally responsible provided the intoxicating substance was consumed without his knowledge.
iii. Driving: Section 185 of Motor Vehicles Act, 1988, imprisonment up to 6 months, fine up to ₹ 2000.
iv. Contractual obligations/will—Indian Contract Act 1872.
v. Loses testamentary capacity—Indian Succession Act Section 59.
vi. Section 510 IPC: Misconduct by a drunken person in public is punishable with imprisonment up to 24 hours with fine.
vii. Section 185 of Motor Vehicles act 1988, (amended in 2000) fixes blood alcohol level at 30 mg per 100 mL.
viii. Section 203 Motor Vehicles Act 1988, (amended in 2000) mention procedure of breath test.
ix. Fine up to ₹ 2000, imprisonment up to 6 months or both.
x. If repeated within 3 years, fine up to ₹ 3000 and imprisonment up to 2 years or both.
xi. **Statutory limits for blood alcohol level are given in Table 42.3.**

Table 42.3 Statutory limits of blood alcohol level in different country

0 mg%	Bulgaria, Russia, Romania, Hungary, Turkey, Belgium
20 mg%	Sweden, Poland
30 mg%	India, Czechoslovakia
50 mg%	Finland, Greece, Australia, Netherlands, France
80 mg%	Denmark, Germany, UK, Switzerland, Spain, Canada
100 mg%	Ireland
80–150 mg%	USA

AGENCIES WORKING FOR CURBING ALCOHOLISM

Indian Alcohol Policy Alliance (IAPA) is a non-governmental organization (NGO), having registered office at Chennai, established and registered under the Indian Trust Act in 2004, to prevent alcohol related harm through evidence based policy intervention, advocacy and capacity building. IAPA is affiliated to the Global Alcohol Policy Alliance (GAPA, UK under Institute of Alcohol Studies) and is supported by FORUT—Campaign for development and solidarity. FORUT is a Norwegian development organization established in 1981 by three NGOs specialized in alcohol and drug prevention: IOGT Norway, Juvente and IOGT Junior Association.

IAPA aims to control alcohol use and reduce alcohol related harms. The laws related to ban on promotion and advertising of alcohol, alcohol taxation, restricting number of sale outlets, hours of operation, enforcing age limit, laws on drinking and driving, etc. would be advocated at state level through IAPA's network, under guidance of IAPA members in different states of India

METHYL ALCOHOL

Synonyms: methanol, wood naphtha, colonial spirit

i. Methyl alcohol is a clear, colorless, volatile liquid with characteristic odor and bitter taste produced by the destructive distillation of wood or molasses.
ii. It boils at 64.7°C.
iii. It mixes with water in all proportions.
iv. Burns with a pale blue non-luminous flame.

Uses

i. Antifreeze (10–50%)
ii. Denatured spirit (5–10%)
iii. Embalming fluid (20%)
iv. Leather dyes (30%)
v. Varnish and shellac (5%)
vi. Windshield washing fluid (35–95%).

Clinical Features (12–24 Hours)

i. Visual impairment
ii. Headache, vertigo, meningismus, nausea, vomiting, abdominal pain
iii. Flashes/snowstorm, blurred vision, photophobia
iv. Metabolic acidosis
v. Tachycardia, hypotension, convulsions
vi. Respiratory failure.

Diagnosis

i. High anion gap acidosis.
ii. Blood methanol > 50 mg/100 mL.
iii. Ophthalmologic examination—dilated pupil, sluggish light reaction.
iv. Fundoscopy: Hyperemic optic disc, retinal edema, optic atrophy, visual field impairment.

Management

i. Stomach wash—sodium bicarbonate, 500 mL retained.
ii. Ethanol 10% ethanol, 10 mg/kg, IV over 30 minutes. Followed by 1.5 mL/kg/h to maintain blood ethanol level 100 mg/100 mL.
iii. 1 mL/kg of 95% ethanol in fruit juice orally over 30 minutes. Maintain 0.17–0.28 mL/kg/h as 50% ethanol.
iv. 4 Methyl pyrazole/fomepizole.
v. Sodium bicarbonate IV 500–800 mg/kg 6 hourly.
vi. Hemodialysis.
vii. No hemoperfusion.

Postmortem Appearance

i. Cyanosis prominent
ii. Liver, kidney shows toxic damage
iii. Lungs edematous and emphysematous desquamation alveolar epithelium
iv. Eyes—retinal edema
v. Viscera preserved in saturated solution of sodium chloride.

REFERENCES

1. Leake CD, Silverman M. Alcoholic Beverages in Clinical Medicine. Chicago: Yearbook Medical Publishers; 1966. p. 9-124.
2. Dasgupta A. The Science of Drinking: How Alcohol Affects Your Body and Mind. Rowman and Littlefield Publishing, Inc: UK; 2011. pp. 3-4.
3. Hanson DJ. Preventing Alcohol Abuse: Alcohol, Culture and Control. Greenwood Publishing group (Praeger): London; 1995. pp. 25-70.
4. Heath D. International Handbook on Alcohol and Culture. Greenwood Publishing Group: London; 1995. pp. 128-141.
5. Alcohol Definition. [Cited 2013 April 13]; Available from: URL:http://www.thefreedictionary.com/alcohol
6. Rao NG. Textbook of Forensic Medicine and Toxicology, 2nd. New Delhi: Jaypee Brothers Medical Publishers (P) Ltd; 2010. pp. 501-16.
7. Barile FA. Clinical Toxicology-Principles and Mechanisms, CRC Press, 2005, p. 264.
8. Devi G, Castro VJ, Huitink J, Buitelaar D, Kosten T, O'Connor P. Management of Drug and Alcohol Withdrawal, The New Eng J Med. 2003;349(4):405-7.
9. Management of alcoholic hepatitis. Drug and Therapeutics Bulletin. 2003;41:49-52.
10. DeBellis R, Smith BS, Choi S, Malloy M. Management of delirium tremens. J Intensive Care Med. 2005;20:164-73.
11. Gelder M, Mayou R, Geddes J. Psychiatry. 3rd ed. New York: Oxford; 2005. p. 186.
12. Kannan K, Mathiharan K (Eds). A Textbook of Medical Jurisprudence and Toxicology, 24th ed. LexisNexis Butterworths Wadhwa: Nagpur; 2011. p. 177-188.
13. Reddy KSN. Medical Jurisprudence and Toxicology (Law Practice and Procedure). ALT Publications, Hyderabad, 2004 (reprint). p. 585.
14. Karch SB (Ed). Forensic Issues in Alcohol Testing. CRC Press, 2008, p. 65.

CHAPTER 43

Agricultural Poisons

Putul Mahanta, AJ Patowary, Anurupa Choudhury

LEARNING PLAN

- Learn about the classification of agricultural poisons
- Know details of organophosphates and organochlorines poisoning
- Learn about carbamates, pyrethrum, pyrethrins and pyrethroids, paraquat poisoning
- Identify the postmortem findings
- Understand the medicolegal importance

Pesticides are substances or mixtures of substances intended to prevent, destroy, repel or mitigate any pest.[1] Pesticides are unusual among environmental pollutants in that they are used deliberately for the purpose of killing some form of life.[2] Agricultural poison includes pesticides, herbicides, rodenticides, etc.

CLASSIFICATION

1. **Insecticide**: It kills and repels insects and related species, e.g. organophosphates, carbamates, organochlorines, pyrethroids, etc.
2. **Rodenticide**: It kills rodents like rat, mice, etc. Examples: Anticoagulant, phosphorous, cholecalciferol, bromethalin, strychnine, zinc phosphide, etc.
3. **Herbicide**: It kills weeds, e.g. acrolein, paraquat, diquat, atrazine, chlorphenoxy compound, etc.
4. **Fungicide**: It kills fungi and moulds, e.g. thiocarbamates, captan, captafol, sodium azide, etc.
5. **Nematicide**: It kills worms, e.g. ethylene dibromide, etc.
6. **Acaricide**: It kills mites ticks, and spiders, e.g. azobenzene, chlorobenzilate, kelthane, etc.
7. **Molluscicide**: It kills molluscs such as snails and slugs, e.g. metaldehyde.
8. **Miscellaneous**: Compounds of lead, copper, mercury, nicotine, hydrogen cyanide, methyl bromide, naphthalene, dinitrophenol, dinitrocresol, chlorphenson, chloralose, etc.

ORGANOPHOSPHATES

Acute poisoning by these agents is a major global problem, with thousands of deaths occurring every year.[3] Most of the organophosphates (OP) pesticides poisoning and subsequent death occur in developing countries following deliberate self-ingestion particularly in young, productive-age group, as highly toxic pesticides are readily available at the moment of stress due to family problem, failure in love and exam phobia.[4]

A host of such compounds have been introduced in Indian market since 1950 as agricultural insecticide, but a number of it proved toxic to human health. Historically, organophosphates have been used as toxic nerve agents by the military in war or for terrorist activities.

Chemically, these compounds are the esters of phosphoric acid or thiophosphoric acid. They are found as liquids, dusts or in granular form. Some are diluted in water. They are mixed with a solvent, usually aromax; it gives the kerosene-like smell in the body cavities, stomach contents, vomit, froth, etc.

Classification

They are of two groups[5]

i. **Alkyl phosphates**:
   a. Hexaethyl tetraphosphate (HETP)
   b. Tetraethyl pyrophosphate (TEPP)
   c. Octamethyl pyrophosphate (OMPA)
   d. Dime fox
   e. Isopestox
   f. Malathion sulfotep
   g. Demeton
   h. Trichlorfon

ii. **Aryl phosphates**:
   a. Parathion (nitrostigmine)
   b. Paraoxon
   c. Methyl parathion
   d. Chlorthion
   e. Diazinon, etc.

Uses of Organophosphates

- De-wormers applied to farm animals
- Fly sprays and vaporizing strips used in industrial, commercial and domestic premises
- Flea collars and treatment for pests
- Anti-lice shampoo.

Nowadays, organophosphates are used as ship dips, military nerve agents, pour-ons in cattle farms, preservatives for crop and store grains, domestically as fly strips, wood worm preservatives, pet flea preparation and treatment of human arthropod infestation (malathion), etc.[6,7]

Toxicokinetics

1. They are absorbed by any routes like inhalation, transdermal, mucosal, gastro-intestinal, transconjunctival, etc.
2. Metabolism occurs in liver. Detoxification occurs via Cytochrome p_{450} monooxygenase.
3. Some of the compounds, such as parathion, are stored as fat in the body and released slowly into the circulation; hence duration of exposure with the toxic substances is prolonged.
4. Metabolites are excreted in urine.

Mode of Action

Many organophosphates are potent nerve inhibitors, act by inhibiting the action of acetylcholinesterase (AChE) in nerve cells. Acetylcholinesterase is an enzyme present in human nervous system. Its job is to break down acetylcholine, which is a chemical that carries signals between the nerves and muscle. AChE hydrolyzes acetylcholine to choline and acetic acid.

Mechanism of Action

i. Inhibits enzyme acetylcholinesterase, thus hampers the hydrolysis of acetylcholine after completion of its function.
ii. Continuous accumulation of acetylcholine at synapses, resulting in continuous stimulation of the receptors leading to paralysis of the nerve and the muscle.
iii. Organophosphates bind to the active site and phosphorylate the serine moiety. Phosphorylated enzymes degrade very slowly, making acetylcholinesterase inactive.

iv. Once the acetylcholinesterase remains phosphorylated over a period of 24–48 hours, an alkyl group is lost from the conjugate, further complicating the situation as at this stage the enzyme can no longer hydrolyze and become permanently inactivated, the condition is known as aging of the enzyme.

Fatal Dose[8]

Toxicity Rating

1. Extremely toxic (LD_{50}:1–50 mg/kg).
2. Highly toxic (LD_{50}:51-500 mg/kg): Chlorpyrifos, demeton, diazinon, dichlorvos, dimethoate, disulfoton, ediphenphos, ethion, methyl parathion, etc.
3. Moderately toxic (LD_{50}:501–5000 mg/kg).
4. Slightly toxic (LD_{50}: more than 5000 mg/kg): Abate, acephate, coumaphos, famphur, malathion, phenthoate, temephos, etc.

Fatal period is about 24 hours if not treated; and in hospitalized, cases it may be delayed upto 2 weeks if treatments is proved ineffective.

Clinical Features

Depending upon the route of entry and amount of poison absorbed, the signs and symptoms appear within ½ to 2 hours.

Severity depends on the blood level of cholinesterase (ChE) as follows:

1. **Mild poisoning**: When ChE level is 20–50% of normal.
2. **Moderate poisoning**: When ChE level is 10–20% of normal.
3. **Severe poisoning**: When ChE level is less than 10% of normal.

As the ChE level drops below 30% of its normal value, the involuntary muscles and the secretory glands are first affected, then affected are the voluntary muscles and vital centers in the brain. The respiratory or gastrointestinal features depend upon route of entry.

The types and severity of ChE inhibition symptoms depend on:

- Toxicity of the pesticide
- Amount of pesticide involved in the exposure
- Route of exposure (inhalation is fastest, followed by ingestion, then dermal)
- Duration of exposure.

Some of the most commonly reported early symptoms include, in possible order of occurrence: Headache, nausea, dizziness, sweating, salivation, muscle twitching, weakness, tremors, in-coordination, vomiting, abdominal cramps, diarrhea and paralysis.

Acute Poisoning

The signs and symptoms of organophosphorus poisoning can be divided into three separate categories:

Nicotinic Manifestations

- Muscle weakness
- Fasciculation: Small, local contractions of muscles visible through the skin, representing a spontaneous discharge of a number of fibers innervated by a single motor nerve filament
- Cramps
- Areflexia: Absence of reflexes
- Paralysis
- Hypertension
- Tachycardia: Rapid heart rate, >100 beats/min
- Pallor
- Mydriasis.

CNS Manifestations

- Restlessness
- Headache
- Tremor
- Drowsiness
- Confusion
- Delirium
- Slurred speech
- Ataxia
- Convulsion.

Muscarinic Manifestations

It is better remembered as "**SLUDGE**" which includes: **S**alivation, **L**acrimation, **U**rination, **D**efecation, **G**I cramping and **E**mesis.

1. Increased contractions of smooth muscle: GI tract and ureters.
2. Increased secretions of gland cells: Lacrimal, sweat, salivary, gastric, intestinal, pancreatic.
3. Bradycardia, hypotension.
4. Bronchoconstriction with wheezing and dyspnea, cough, pulmonary edema.
5. Miosis: Constricted pupils.

A very rare sign is **chromodachryrrhea** (shedding of red tears) and is due to accumulation of porphyrin in the lachrymal glands. **Intermediate syndromes** sometimes occur 1–4 days after poisoning because of too long-lasting ChE inhibition and muscle necrosis usually due to inadequate treatment of the acute episode, like use of sub-therapeutic dose of oximes. Here, there is muscle weakness and paralysis characterized by motor cranial nerve palsies, weakness of neck flexors and proximal limb muscles and respiratory paresis. It does not respond to oxime or atropine. Death usually results from respiratory failure.

Delayed peripheral neuropathy occurs 1–5 weeks after exposure to certain compounds like parathion and malathion. It is due to nerve demyelination and is characterized by flaccid weakness and atrophy of distal limb muscles simulate to Guillain-Barre syndrome.

Chronic Poisoning

It mainly happens to agriculturalists and manifested by muscle cramps, weakness, gait disorders, paresthesia, drowsiness, confusion, irritability, anxiety, etc.

Diagnosis[4,8]

a. **Depression of ChE activity**: Sample: 10 mL of heparinized blood.
   Acetylcholine is found abundantly in nerves, muscles, glands and RBCs (true ChE) and plasma (pseudo ChE). ChE in RBC < 50%, indicates poisoning. [Mild: 20–50%, moderate: 10–20%, severe: <10%]
   Normal AChE in RBC **77–142** and in plasma is: **41–140**.
   However, false depression is also seen in pernicious anemia, hemoglobinopathies, antimalarial treatment, etc.
b. **Atropine test**: 1–2 mg (0.05 mg/kg) IV, if do not produce dryness of mouth, dry flashed skin, tachycardia in 5–20 minutes.
c. **P-nitrophenol test**: Metabolite of some organophosphates and is excreted in urine.
   Procedure: Steam distil 10 mL of urine, add sodium hydroxide and heat in water bath for 10 minutes. Yellow color indicates presence of P-nitrophenol.
d. Thin layer and paper chromatography.

Management

Decontamination

a. Contaminated clothes should be removed and exposed skin should be washed with soap and copious amount of water.
b. If eyes are contaminated, wash thoroughly with tap water or normal saline.
c. When it is ingested, stomach wash is done with 1:5000 potassium permanganate and then activated charcoal can be introduced to absorb the remaining poison.

Supportive Measures

a. Check airways, breathing and circulation.
b. Monitor arterial oxygen saturation, cardiac rhythms, BP, pulse rate.
c. Oxygenation/positive pressure ventilation if required.
d. Diazepam for convulsion can be used.

Antidotes

1. **Atropine**: It blocks muscarinic effects of the postganglionic parasympathetic activity and arrests CNS effects. It has no effect on muscle weakness or paralysis. **Dose**: 1–2 mg IV or IM in adult or 0.05 mg/kg in child, every 10–15 minutes until signs of atropinization occurs, i.e. drying up of tracheobronchial secretion (but not

papillary dilatation). Then dose should be adjusted to maintain the effect for at least 24 hours.

2. **Pralidoxime** or **Pyridine-2-aldoxime methiodide** or **2-PAM:** It acts by competing for the phosphate moiety of organophosphorus compound and releases it from the cholinesterase enzyme. Its action is marked at nicotinic sites, often improving muscle strength within 10–40 minutes. It also decreases muscarinic and CNS symptoms. Dose for adult: 1–2 g in 100–150 mL of 0.9% sodium chloride, given IV over 30 minutes. This can be repeated after 1 hour, and subsequently every 6–12 hours, for 24–48 hours up to a maximum dose of 12 g in 24-hour period. Dose for children: 20-40 mg/kg to a maximum of 1 g/dose given IV, and repeated every 6–12 hours. It should not be given in carbamate poisoning.
3. **Diazepam:** It reduces the risk of seizure-induced brain and cardiac damage. Dose for adult: 5-10 mg IV slowly every 15 minutes, up to maximum of 30 mg. Dose for children: 0.25-0.4 mg/kg IV slowly, every 5–10 minutes, up to a maximum of 10 mg.

Postmortem Findings

External

a. Characteristic garlicky or kerosene-like smell may be present. The kerosene-like smell is present due to presence of the aromax oil, the solvent used.
b. Frothing at the mouth and nostrils.
c. Cyanosis of extremities. It is usually found in lip, finger and nose of the victim.
d. Constricted pupils (pin-point pupil).

Internal

a. Generalized visceral congestion.
b. Garlicky or kerosene-like smell of stomach content.
c. Pulmonary and cerebral edema.
d. Signs of toxic myocarditis may be present. Microscopic examination of heart reveals dilation of pericardial blood vessels with hemorrhages in the surrounding tissues, interstitial edema of myocardium, inflammatory cells, hemosiderin-laden macrophages and fatty infiltration of the myocardium.[10]
e. Submucosal petechial hemorrhage is found in stomach. Excessive edema and sub-pleural petechial hemorrhage are present. Heart is soft and flabby. Brain is also congested and edematous.[9]

Medicolegal Importance

1. Accidental poisoning can occur with farmers while handling the poisons in the field.
2. Suicidal consumption is common.
3. Homicidal use is rare as it is difficult to mask the smell of insecticide.

ORGANOCHLORINES

Organochlorines are the compounds of chlorinated hydrocarbons. They are found as liquid, emulsion, dust or granules and used as insecticide, scabicide and pediculocide. Endrin is known as "**plant penicillin**" due to its broad spectrum of activity.

Chlorinated hydrocarbon (organochlorine) insecticides, solvents and fumigants are widely used around the world. This class comprises a variety of compounds containing carbon, hydrogen and chlorine. These compounds can be highly toxic, and the overwhelming majorities have been universally banned because of their unacceptably slow degradation and subsequent bioaccumulation and toxicity.[11] Among the more notable, dichlorodiphenyltrichloroethane (DDT) is an organochlorine pesticide, and its inventor Paul Muller won the Nobel Prize for Physiology or Medicine in 1948.[12] The toxicity of these agents varies according to their molecular size, volatility and effects on the CNS. In general, they cause either CNS depression or stimulation, depending upon the agent and dose.[13]

Classification

These compounds can be assorted into five groups, as follows:

1. Dichlorodiphenyltrichloroethane (DDT) and analogs, e.g. dicofol, methoxychlor.
2. Hexachlorocyclohexane, i.e. benzene hexachloride and isomers, e.g. lindane, gamma-hexachlorocyclohexane.
3. Cyclodienes and related compounds, e.g. endosulfan, chlordane, heptachlor, aldrin, dieldrin, endrin, isobenzan.
4. Chlordecone, kelevan and mirex.
5. Toxaphene and related compounds, e.g. toxaphene.

Absorption and Metabolism

They are absorbed through skin, orally and via inhalation. They are partially metabolized in liver and excreted in urine, feces and milk. They require long time to degrade, and so act as persistent organic pollutant.

1. Damaged skin facilitates absorption.
2. Gastrointestinal absorption enhanced by fat or solvents.
3. Most can be assessed in the lipid fraction of blood either as the based chemical or a metabolite.
4. Most are dechlorinated and excreted to some degree.
5. DDT and its isomers, hexachlorocyclohexane, dieldrin, heptachlor epoxide and mirex tend to get stored in body fat.
6. Lindane and endosulfan are generally well-absorbed across the skin and are metabolized more quickly.
7. DDT, mirex, dicofol, marlate and toxophene are less well absorbed across the skin.
8. Aerosols may be deposited in airways, coughed and swallowed.
9. Biliary is the chief route of excretion and chemical may be reabsorbed (enterohepatic circulation), slowing excretion.

Organochlorines are well absorbed orally and by inhalation. Transdermal absorption is variable. For example, DDT is poorly absorbed transdermally, whereas cyclodienes have significant transdermal absorption rates.[14] Cyclodienes have high absorption levels when taken orally, as in the case of food contamination with these pesticides.[15] Lindane is known to be absorbed after topical application, but oral ingestions are not rare.[16] Studies have shown that the young, malnourished and those with frequent application are at increased risk for toxicity.[17]

Organic chlorines (organochlorines) are strongly lipid soluble and sequester in body tissues with high lipid content, such as the brain and liver. Consequently, blood levels tend to be much lower than fatty tissue levels.[14] The lipophilic tendency of organochlorines accounts for prolonged systemic effects in overdose. The half-life of DDT has been measured in months or years, whereas other organic chlorines are metabolized faster, like lindane, with a half-life of 21 hours.[18]

Mode of Action

1. Organochlorines bind to sodium channels in neurons, increasing permeability to sodium. This increased permeability facilitates uncoordinated discharge of neurons.
2. Alter the metabolism of serotonin, norepinephrine and acetylcholine.
3. Cyclodienes and Lindane inhibit the GABA-mediated chloride channels in CNS.
4. This uncoordinated discharge can lead to CNS alterations including myoclonus and seizures.
5. Cyclodienes (dieldrin, heptachlor mirex and aldrin) may induce seizures for days after over exposure.
6. Thus, they inhibit the nerve impulse transmission and cause increase stimulation of CNS first and then depression.

Other Effects

1. High levels of organochlorine may cause myocardial instability, i.e. arrhythmias.
2. Organochlorines may cause increase microsomal activity and increase drug metabolism.

3. Hexachlorobenzene has been responsible for porphyria cutanea tarda.
4. Organochlorines may interact with endocrine receptors which may impact reproductive processes.

Fatal Dose[19]

DDT, lindane: 15–30 g
Aldrin, dieldrin: 2–6 g

Clinical Features

Acute Poisoning

a. Nausea, vomiting, paresthesia of the mouth and face, headache, vertigo, dizziness, mydriasis, agitation, confusion, incoordination, tremor, fever, pneumonitis, renal failure.
b. Severe symptoms: Myoclonic jerking, tonic-clonic seizures.
c. Cyclodienes may cause seizures without warning and may occur as late as 48 hours after exposure.
d. Severe organochlorine poisoning may lead to status epilepticus.

Chronic Poisoning

- Anorexia, loss of weight
- Weakness
- Tremor
- Ataxia
- Mental changes
- Oligospermia
- Increased tendency to leukemia
- Aplastic anemia
- Liver carcinoma.

Diagnosis

1. Some of the organochlorines are radio-paque and are seen in abdominal radiograph.
2. Detection of it in serum and urine by gas chromatography.

Management

a. Almost same as organophosphorus.
b. Cholestyramine enhances fecal excretion.
c. For **status epilepticus**: Cardiac monitoring should be initiated and phenobarbital can be used to control seizures.
d. The following are contraindicated:
   i. Oil-based cathartics
   ii. Adrenaline
   iii. Atropine.

Postmortem Findings: Same as organophosphorus poisoning death.

Medicolegal Importance

1. Accidental poisoning may occurs with farmers while spraying in the field.
2. Children are particularly vulnerable due to their surface area to body weight ratio. Literatures show that lindane, long used for scabies, are absorbed rapidly and levels peak about 6 hours of application. Levels of 24–28 ng/mL were seen after scabies treatment with lindane.
3. Suicidal poisoning is very common.
4. Homicidal is rare as it is difficult to mask the smell of the poisons.

CARBAMATES

The threat of using chemical compounds by terrorists as weapons of mass casualties has been a rising concern in recent years. Carbamates, a group of reversible acetylcholinesterase inhibitors, could be potentially involved in such toxic mass casualty events because they can cause cholinergic crisis that could lead to fatality, similar to that of organophosphate poisoning.[20] Carbamates are the derivative of carbonic acid and found as dusts or solution and are popular insecticides.

Toxicity Rating

1. Extremely or highly toxic: Carbaryl, carbofuran, methomyl, propoxur (Baygon)

2. Moderately or slightly toxic: Aldicarb, carbendazim, triallate.

Mode of Action

They are reversible acetylcholinesterase inhibitors, inhibiting acetylcholinesterase by carbamylating the serine moiety at the active site, instead of phosphorylation. It is a reversible type of binding, and so, symptoms are less severe and shorter duration.

Because of this action, there is accumulation of acetylcholine at muscarinic and nicotine receptors and in the CNS.

Clinical Features

1. Begins within 15 minutes to 2 hours.
2. They are similar to organophosphorus, except that their actions are reversible and CNS toxicity are limited.

Management

Similar to organophosphorus poisoning, but oximes are not used here. The medical management of carbamate poisoning consists of:

i. Decontamination.
ii. Specific antidotal treatment, that is, the anticholinergic compound atropine.
   The administration of oxime, acetyl cholinesterase reactivators, in carbamate poisoning is controversial because of the potential toxicity of oximes in conjunction with carbamate, especially in the case of the carbamate "carbaryl" poisoning. However, recent data suggest that this concern may be unwarranted.[20]
iii. Supportive measures.

Postmortem Findings

Same as organophosphate poisoning death.

Medicolegal Importance

1. Accidental poisoning may occurs.
2. Suicidal poisoning is very common.
3. Homicidal is rare, as it is difficult to mask the smell of the poisons.

PYRETHRUM, PYRETHRINS AND PYRETHROIDS

Pyrethrins are extracted from chrysanthemum plant and pyrethroids are their synthetic analogs (**Figure 43.1**). They are used as indoor insect repellents and insecticides. Human is resistant to them as they are rapidly metabolized and detoxified in body. A large amount is usually required to produce toxicity in human.

The type and severity of symptoms varies depending on the amount of chemical involved and the nature of the exposure. They are available as liquid, sprays, coils, dusts, powders and mats.

Clinical Features[19]

1. Skin contact: Dermatitis, blistering and erythema.
2. Eye contact: Irritation and lacrimation.
3. Inhalation: Rhinorrhea, sore throat, wheezing, coughing and dyspnea.
4. Ingestion: Nausea, vomiting, vertigo, hyperthermia, fasciculation, altered mental status, seizures, pulmonary edema and coma.

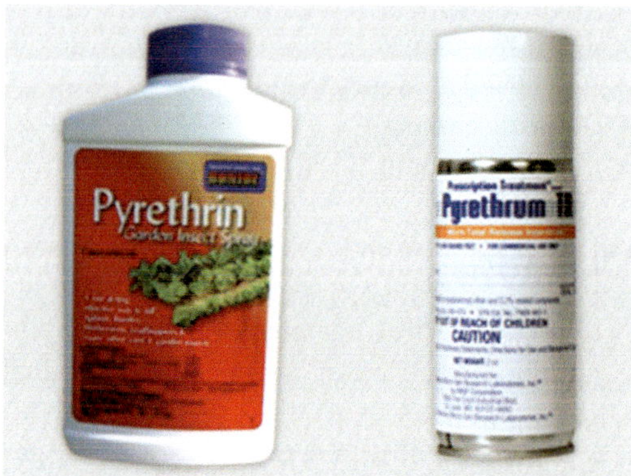

Figure 43.1 Different pyrethrum preparations

Management

Decontamination

Main aim of it is removal from source of exposure.

a. Contaminated clothes should be removed and exposed skin should be washed with soap and copious amount of water.
b. If eyes are contaminated, wash thoroughly with tap water or normal saline.
c. When it is ingested, stomach wash is done and then activated charcoal in the dose of 1 g/kg can be used.

Supportive Treatment

a. Oils and fat should be avoided.
b. Allergic reaction should be treated with Adrenaline 0.5–1 mL of 1:1000 solutions.
c. Atropine and oxime are contraindicated.
d. Oxygen administration, ventilator assistance should be given.

Postmortem Findings

a. Characteristic insect-repellent-like smell.
b. Frothing at mouth and nostrils.
c. Cyanosis of extremities. It is usually found in lip, finger and nose of the victim.
d. Generalized visceral congestion.
e. Pulmonary and cerebral edema.

Medicolegal Importance

1. Accidental poisoning may occur.
2. Suicidal poisoning is rare.

PARAQUAT POISONING

Paraquat (dipyridylium) is a highly toxic weed killer, once promoted by the US for use in Mexico to destroy marijuana plants. Researchers found that this herbicide was dangerous to workers who applied it to the plants. The health hazards can occur from swallowing or breathing in Paraquat.

Clinical Features

1. People get sick if paraquat touches a cut on their skin.
2. Breathing in paraquat may cause lung damage and can lead to a disease called "**paraquat lung**". There is difficulty in breathing, nasal bleeding, seizures and shortness of breath.
3. Paraquat, when ingested, causes damage to the mucosa of the mouth, esophagus, stomach or intestines. It may cause pain in the mouth, esophagus and stomach, diarrhea, vomiting, dysphasia and aphonia. Paraquat may also damage the kidneys, liver and esophagus. On oral ingestion, death can occur rapidly. Death may occur from shock and coma, from the perforation in the esophagus or from acute inflammation of the mediastinum, the area that surrounds the major blood vessels and airways in the middle of the chest.
4. Chronic exposure to Paraquat may cause pulmonary fibrosis, a stiffening of the lung tissue.

Diagnosis

Blood and urine tests can be done to determine the level of paraquat in the blood. The other tests that may be done include:

- Arterial blood gases (measures of oxygen, carbon dioxide and acid-base balance)
- BUN and creatinine (kidney function tests)
- Chem-20
- Chest X-ray
- Lung function tests
- Urinalysis and
- Urine toxicology screen.

Management

Decontamination

a. Contaminated clothes should be removed.
b. If the chemical touched the skin, wash the area with soap and water for 15 minutes,

without scrubbing hard, so as not to cause abrasions, which will allow greater absorption of the toxin.

c. If eyes are contaminated, wash thoroughly with tap water or normal saline.
d. When it is ingested, stomach wash is done and then activated charcoal in the dose of 1 g/kg be used.

Supportive Treatment

1. Oxygen administration, ventilator assistance should be given.
2. There is no specific treatment for paraquat poisoning. The goal is to relieve symptoms and treat complications (supportive care).
3. Hemoperfusion, which filters the blood through charcoal to remove paraquat from the lungs.

Postmortem Findings

a. Corrosion around lips, mouth, esophagus and stomach.
b. Lungs may be edematous, or there may be pulmonary fibrosis or stiffening of the lung tissue.
c. Signs of hepatic and renal failure (acute tubular necrosis).
d. Generalized visceral congestion.

Medicolegal Importance

1. Accidental poisoning may occurs.
2. Suicidal poisoning may also occur though rare.

HAZARDS OF PESTICIDES

1. **Human Health**
   a. Agriculturalists are exposed to it in day-to-day life, and there by common accidental poisoning.
   b. As it is easily available, it is the most common suicidal poisoning in India.
2. **To Ecosystem**
   a. Contamination of water and soil.
   b. By-products of chlorinated pesticides are leading causes of cancer.

REFERENCES

1. Nelson LS, Lewin NA, Howland MA, Hoffman RS, Goldfrank LR, Flomenbaum NE. Goldfrank's Toxicologic Emergencies: Part C-The Clinical Basis of Medical Toxicology, Section I-Case Studies, K–Pesticides. Chapter 104 - Pesticides: An Overview with a Focus on Principles and Rodenticide, 8th ed. McGraw-Hill; 2006. p. 1470.
2. Ernest H. Agricultural chemicals. In: A Textbook of Modern Toxicology, 3rd ed. New Jersey (US): 2004. p. 54.
3. Eddleston M, Buckley NA, Checketts H, Senarathna L, Mohamed F, et al. Speed of initial atropinisation in significant organophosphorus pesticide poisoning-a systematic comparison of recommended regimens. J Toxicol Clin Toxicol. 2004;42:865-75.
4. Karalliedde L, Eddleston M, Murray V. The global picture of organophosphate poisoning. In: Karalliedde L, Feldman F, Henry J, Marrs T (Eds), Organophosphates and Health. Imperial Press London; 2001. pp. 432-71.
5. Reddy KNS. The Essentials of Forensic Medicine and Toxicology: Agricultural Poisons, 28th ed. Hyderabad: K. Suguna Devi; 2004. pp. 457-65.
6. Davies R, Ghouse A, Tegweed F. Chronic exposure to organophosphates: Background and clinical picture. Adv Psychiatric Treatment. 2000;6:187-92.
7. Kasper DL, Braunwald E, Fauci AS, Hausar SL, Longo DL, Jameson JL. Principles of Internal Medicine, Vol-1, 16th ed. New York: McGraw-Hill; 2005. pp. 1292-4.
8. Pillay VV. Comprehensive Medical Toxicology: Hydrocarbons and Pesticides, 2nd ed. Hyderabad: Paras Medical Publisher; 2008. pp. 233-46.
9. Nandy A. Principles of Forensic Medicine including Toxicology, 2nd ed. Kolkata India: New Central Book agency (P) Ltd; 2001. pp. 439-94.

10. Chhabra ML, Sepaha GC, Jain SR, Bhagwat RP, Khandekar JD. ECG and necropsy, changes in organophosphorus compound (Malathion) poisoning. Indian J Med Sci. 1969;424-9.
11. Stockholm Convention. [cited 2013 Jan10]; Available from: URL:http://chm.pops.int/default.aspx
12. Paul Muller Biography. NobelPrize.org. [cited 2013 Jan10]; Available from: URL:http://www.nobelprize.org/nobel_prizes/medicine/laureates/1948/muller-bio.html
13. Bhalla M, Thami GP. Reversible neurotoxicity after an overdose of topical lindane in an infant. Pediatr Dermatol. 2004;21(5):597-9.
14. Reigart JR, Roberts JR (Eds). Recognition and Management of Pesticide Poisonings, 5th ed. Washington DC: Environmental Protection Agency; 1999.
15. Centers for Disease Control and Prevention. Acute convulsions associated with endrin poisoning in Pakistan. MMWR Morb Mortal Wkly Rep. 1984;33(49):687-8,693.
16. Centers for Disease Control and Prevention. Unintentional topical lindane ingestions-United States, 1998-2003. MMWR Morb Mortal Wkly Rep. 2005;54(21):533-5.
17. Pramanik AK, Hansen RC. Transcutaneous gamma benzene hexachloride absorption and toxicity in infants and children. Arch Dermatol. 1979;115(10):1224-5.
18. Mortensen ML. Management of acute childhood poisonings caused by selected insecticides and herbicides. Pediatr Clin North Am. 1986;33(2):421-45.
19. Pillay VV. Pesticides. In: Textbook of Forensic Medicine and Toxicology, 15th ed. Hyderabad: Paras Medical Publisher; 2010. pp. 546-59.
20. Rosman Y, Makarovsky I, Bentur Y, Shrot S, Dushnistky T, Krivoy A. Carbamate poisoning: treatment recommendations in the setting of a mass casualties event. Am J Emerg Med. 2009;27(9):1117-24.

CHAPTER 44

Cardiac Poisons

Putul Mahanta

LEARNING PLAN

- Learn the cardiac poisons, viz. digitalis, tobacco, oleander, aconite and hydrocyanic acid
- Know details of their poisoning ways and management
- Identify their diagnostic and autopsy findings
- Understand their medicolegal importance

These are the poisons having an action mainly on the heart, either directly or through the nerves. Digitalis, Oleander, Aconite and Tobacco are important in this group. Other examples are: hydrocyanic acid and its salts, quinine, quinidine, cinchonine, cinchonidine, etc. Many of the cardiac poisons are easily available, but comparatively incidence of the cardiac poisoning is less.

DIGITALIS (CARDIAC GLYCOSIDE)

In 1785, **Sir William Withering** described the use of the foxglove plant, ***Digitalis purpurea***, for the treatment of heart failure.[1] More than 200 years later, cardiac glycosides are still prescribed for patients with atrial fibrillation and heart failure or left ventricular dysfunction.

While the overall use of digitalis has declined, the number of patients admitted with digitalis toxicity has remained stable and the use of digitalis antibody fragments has increased.[2] In 2007, there were 2565 cases of cardiac glycoside exposures reported to US poison control centers; of these, 121 patients suffered major toxicity and 10 died.[3]

Digitalis purpurea

This is a poisonous plant (**Figure 44.1**). Its root, leaves and seeds contains over 30 cardiac and steroidal glycosides, of which digitoxin, digoxin, digitalin, digitalein and digitonin are the most important and have a cumulative action. Its main toxic effects are irritation of stomach, slowing of heart rate, leading to heart block, extra systoles and ventricular fibrillation.

Clinical Features of Poisoning

i. The patient develops nausea, vomiting, abdominal pain, diarrhea, depression, headache and giddiness.

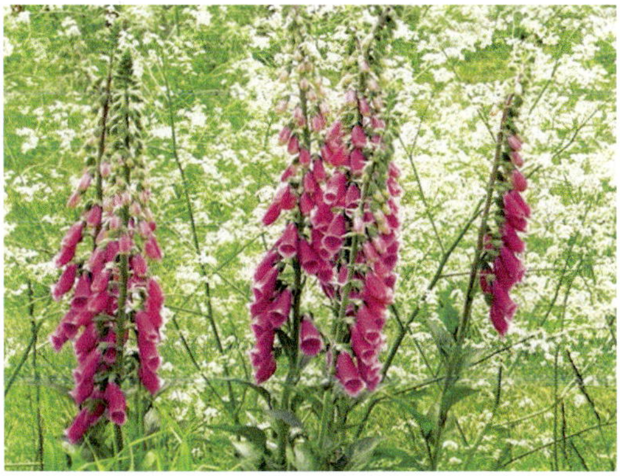

Figure 44.1 *Digitalis purpurea*

ii. Toxic effect on heart includes bradycardia (rate may fall to 20 per minute), heart block, extra systole and fibrillation.
iii. There is feeling of faintness and precordial compression.
iv. The respirations become slow and sighing.
v. The patient becomes drowsy and the condition may deepen into coma.
vi. Convulsions may precede death.

Fatal Dose and Fatal Period

Digitalin: 15–30 mg
Digitoxin: 4 mg

Fatal Period: Varies from half an hour to 24 hours.

Factors Predisposing to Digitalis Toxicity

Reduced tolerance of digoxin may be seen in the following conditions:

i. Advanced age
ii. Acute myocardial infarction/ischemia/ hypoxemia
iii. Magnesium depletion (**hypomagnesemia**)
iv. **Hypocalcemia** (Calcium synergizes with digitalis and precipitates its toxicity)
v. **Hypothyroidism** (Both **hyperthyroidism** and hypothyroidism enhance digitalis toxicity. Thyrotoxicosis patients are more prone to develop digitalis arrhythmias, and myxedema enhances responsiveness to digitalis. Myxedema patients eliminate digoxin more slowly)
vi. Renal insufficiency (Digoxin is mainly excreted by kidneys)
vii. Electrical cardioversion
viii. Digitalis toxicity causes hyperkalemia, but hypokalemia enhances digitalis toxicity (by increasing its binding to Na^+/K^+ ATPase.)
ix. The administration of the following drugs raises the serum concentration of digoxin: Quinidine, verapamil, procainamide, Amiodarone, etc.

Management

i. Withdrawal of the drug, followed by stomach wash with solution of tannic acid.
ii. If parts of plant are taken, then bowels should be evacuated.
iii. Atropine in dose of 0.6 mg should be given hypodermically to combat bradycardia.
iv. Potassium: Administer cautiously and by oral route, whenever possible, if hypokalemia is present. Potassium must not be employed in the presence of A-V block or hyperkalemia.
v. Specific antidotes such as **Phenytoin/ Beta blocker** or **Lidocaine** is effective in treatment of digitalis induced ventricular tachyarrhythmias.
vi. Trisodium EDTA may help to lower serum calcium.
v. ECG monitoring is necessary as a guide to treatment.
vi. Cardiac pacemaker: may be required in digitalis induced A-V block.
vii. Electrical conversion: It may be life-saving in digitalis-induced ventricular fibrillation.
viii. FAB fragments/digitalis antibodies: are potentially life savings in severe intoxication.
ix. Hemodialysis is not useful in digoxin toxicity.
x. The rest of the treatment is symptomatic.

Autopsy Findings

i. The postmortem findings are not very characteristic.

ii. Inflammations of gastric mucosa.
iii. Visceras are congested.
iv. Seeds that are reddish brown, remarkably small and somewhat angular in shape, with peculiar markings may be seen along with digitalis leaves in the stomach.

Medicolegal Importance

Accidental from an overdose of medicinal preparation or from eating leaves by mistake.

Homicide poisoning is recorded, and it is interesting to note that no suspicion of poisoning may arise in such cases. Rarely it may be used to stimulate the heart and result in death.

In addition to digitalis, other cardiac glycosides exist and have been associated with toxicity. These include: the xenobiotics ouabain and lanatoside C; various plants, including foxglove, dogbane, red squill, lily of the valley, oleander, yellow oleander and henbane; and bufadienolides (Cardioactive steroids found in the skin of toads belonging to the Bufonidae family).[4]

TOBACCO

Tobacco, which is known as **Tambakhu**, is prepared from the leaves of ***Nicotiana Tabacum*** (**Figure 44.2**).

Tobacco is an agricultural product processed from the leaves of plants in the genus Nicotiana. It can be consumed, used as a pesticide and, in the form of nicotine tartrate, used in some medicines (**Figure 44.3**).[5]

There are more than 70 species of tobacco in the plant genus Nicotiana. The word nicotiana (as well as nicotine) is in honor of Jean Nicot, French ambassador to Portugal, who in 1559, sent it as a medicine to the court of Catherine de Medici.[6]

The usage of tobacco is an activity that is practiced by some 1.1 billion people, and up to 1/3 of the adult population.[7] The World Health Organization (WHO) reports it to be the leading preventable cause of death worldwide and estimates that it currently causes 5.4 million deaths per year.[8] Rates of smoking have leveled off or declined in developed countries, but continue to rise in developing countries.

Active Principles

Nicotine and nornicotine are the active principles of this plant responsible for all the pharmacological activities. The dried leaves contain 1–9% of nicotine. Nicotine is a colorless, volatile, bitter and hygroscopic liquid.

Uses

The most common uses of tobacco are for cigarettes, cigars, pipe, chewing and snuff. The plant is used to obtain nicotine sulfate, for use in insecticides, and nicotine tartrate, which is used in some medicines.

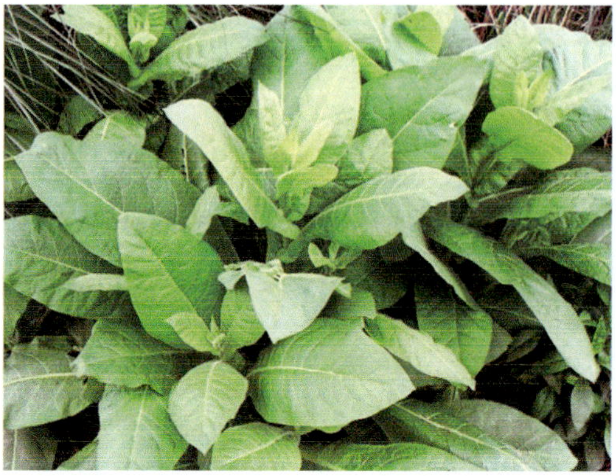

Figure 44.2 Raw tobacco (leaves of *Nicotiana Tabacum*)

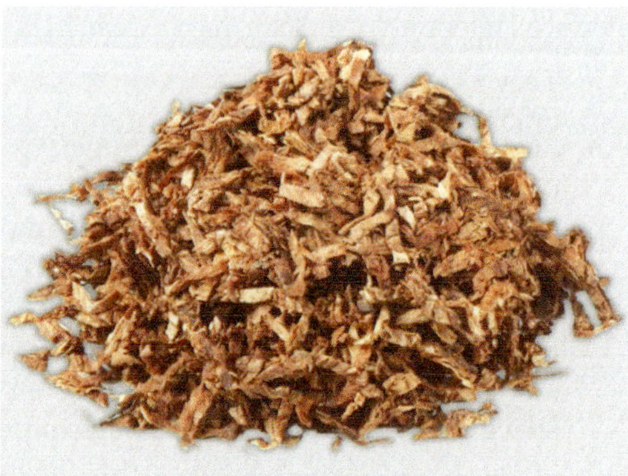

Figure 44.3 Tobacco

Mechanism of Action

Nicotine acts on nicotine receptors present in autonomic ganglia, adrenal medulla, central nervous system, spinal cord, neuromuscular junction and chemoreceptor of carotid and aortic bodies.

Pharmacokinetics

Because of the powerfully addictive properties of nicotine, tolerance and dependence develop. Absorption quantity, frequency and speed of tobacco consumption are believed to be directly related to biological strength of nicotine dependence, addiction and tolerance.[9,10] It is absorbed from skin, mucous membrane and lungs and metabolized in liver and excreted in urine. Small amounts are excreted in milk.

Fatal Dose and Fatal Period

Nicotine: 40–60 mg
Crude Tobacco: 15–30 g

Fatal period is about 5–15 minutes

Nicotine is a bitter-tasting compound that naturally occurs in large amounts in the leaves of tobacco plants. Nicotine poisoning results from too much ingestion of nicotine. Acute nicotine poisoning usually occurs in young children who accidentally chew on nicotine gum or patches.

Acute Poisoning

Clinical Features

i. The patient develop nausea, vomiting, abdominal pain, diarrhea and salivation.
ii. They also develop tachycardia followed by bradycardia.
iii. Many of them complain of anxiety and headache.
iv. Blurred vision, confusion followed by fasciculation, convulsions.
v. Finally paralysis and coma.

Chronic Poisoning

It is also known as nicotine addiction, which is common amongst smokers and tobacco chewers. They develop a psychological dependence that is manifested by recurrent craving for tobacco, tolerance, cough, impaired memory and amblyopia. The dependence is associated with withdrawal syndrome.

Withdrawal Symptoms

Smokers become psychologically dependent and will suffer from withdrawal symptoms, including changes in the body temperature, heart rate, digestion, muscle tone and appetite.

The **psychological symptoms** include: Insomnia, irritability, anxiety, sleep disturbances, nervousness, headaches, fatigue, nausea and cravings for tobacco that can last days, weeks, months, years or an entire lifetime.

Complications

- Frequent colds, smoker's throat
- Chronic bronchitis
- Thromboangiitis obliterans
- Tobacco amblyopia
- Diminished or extinguished sense of smell and taste
- Gastric ulcers
- Increase in heart rate and blood pressure
- Premature and more abundant face wrinkles
- Emphysema
- Heart disease
- Cancer of the mouth, larynx, pharynx, esophagus, lungs, pancreas, cervix, uterus and bladder.

Maternal smoking leads to increased risk of spontaneous abortion, fetal death and increased frequency of abruptio placentae or placenta previa and low-birth-weight baby.[11]

Cause of Death

Death is usually due to respiratory failure that is due to paralysis of CNS or paralysis of the endings of the respiratory nerves (myoneural junctions). Early death is due to stimulation of vagal cardiac ganglia.

Management

i. Gastric lavage should be done with activated charcoal, tannin or potassium permanganate.
ii. Colonic wash-out and a purge.
iii. Benzodiazepines for convulsions.
iv. Protect airway and give oxygen if needed.
v. Symptomatic treatment.

Autopsy Findings

- Tobacco smell may be present
- Signs of asphyxia are present
- Brownish stains/froth may be present at the mouth and nostrils
- Brownish discoloration of the esophagus and gastric mucosa
- Stomach may contain fragments of tobacco leaves and may smell of tobacco.

Medicolegal Importance

- Accidental poisoning may occur due to overdose
- Occupational hazard
- Malingering to induce illness
- Suicide or homicide is rare.

COMMON OLEANDER

Botanical Name: *Nerium Odorum*

Common Name: White Oleander (**Figure 44.4**), Kaner

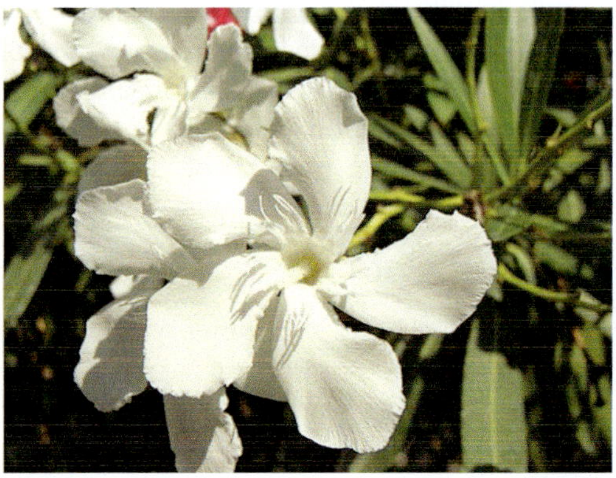

Figure 44.4 White oleanders

Active Principles

The plant grows wild in all parts of our country. All parts of the plant are toxic. The nectar yields poisonous honey. Important active principles are: Oleandrin, neriin, folinerin, rosagenin, etc.

Uses

i. Various parts of the plant find use in folk remedies for various ailments
ii. It is an abortifacient alkaloid, used to cause abortion.

Mechanism of Action

It has digoxin-like action and inhibits sodium-potassium ATPase, causing death from cardiac failure.

Fatal Dose and Fatal Period

i. 5–15 leaves
ii. 15–20 g of root

Fatal Period is about 20–36 hours.

Clinical Features

i. The patients develop nausea, vomiting, abdominal pain, profuse frothy salivation, followed by restlessness and diarrhea.
ii. Ingestion causes difficulty in swallowing and often locks jaw.
iii. Pulse is at first slow and weak, BP falls, respiratory rate increased, pupils dilated, muscular twitching and tetanic spasm.
iv. Ventricular tachycardia, breathlessness, fibrillation, AV blocks.
v. This is followed by exhaustion, delirium, drowsiness, coma and death occurs from heart failure.

Management

i. Decontamination in the usual way, i.e. stomach wash, cathartics, etc. Gastric lavage with activated charcoal.
ii. ECG monitoring.

iii. Correction of cardiac arrhythmias with antiarrhythmic drugs such as lidocaine and phenytoin.
iv. Atropine for AV block and sinus tachycardia
v. Correction of fluid and electrolyte disturbances.
vi. Symptomatic treatment.

Autopsy Findings

Findings are not significant. Signs of congestion of all visceras are present. Petechial hemorrhages over myocardium are seen. Nerium odorum resists heat and can be detected even from burnt remains of the dead body.

Medicolegal Importance

i. Because of the easy availability, it is commonly used as suicidal poison.
ii. Commonly seen in rural areas.
iii. Accidental poisoning may result from its misuse as folk remedy.
iv. The extract of this plant or a twig or root may be employed to procure illicit abortion.
v. Cattle poison.
vi. Common oleander resist decomposition and burning thus can be detected from decomposed bodies or ash.

YELLOW OLEANDER

Botanical Name: *Cascabela Thevetia*

Common Name: Yellow oleander, Lucky nut, Pila kaner, Exile

Other Common Name: Cook tree, Be-still tree, Dicky plant

They are large spreading shrub usually 2.5–3.5 m tall.

Flower: The sweetly perfumed flowers are funnel-shaped, bright yellow or peach colored, 5.5–7 cm long and 2.5–4 cm wide, grouped in clusters at the end of the branches. It is a large ornamental shrub like Nerium, but the leaves are oblong, and the flowers are tubular and yellowish.

Fruit: The fruits are angular, green when immature, ripening black, broader than long and somewhat triangular in outline, with a raised ridge around the middle, about 3–4.5 cm in diameter. The fruit is fleshy and soft like a plum and encloses a "stone" comprising two starchy kernels.

Active Principles

i. **Thevetin** is powerful cardiac poison.
ii. **Thevetoxin** is less toxic than thevetin and resembles the glycosides of digitalis in action.
iii. **Cerberin** has an action like strychnine.

Fatal Dose and Fatal Period

All parts of the plant are toxic if eaten, particularly the fruit and seed. The toxic doses are:

i. 8–10 seeds
ii. 15–20 g of root
iii. 5–10 leaves

Fatal Period is about 2–3 hours if powdered root is taken.

Clinical Features

i. Symptoms may include a burning sensation in the mouth, vomiting, diarrhea, headache, dizziness and a slow or irregular heartbeat. The sap may be an irritant and cause dermatitis or blistering.
ii. Numbness in mouth and tongue.
iii. Loss of muscle power.
iv. Ventricular tachycardia, fibrillation, AV blocks.
v. Tetanic convulsions are occasionally observed.
vi. Jaundice and renal failure[12] may occur.
vii. Death results from cardiac failure.

Management

i. Gastric lavage with multiple dose of activated charcoals is useful as it binds glycoside in the gut lumen and promotes elimination.[13]

ii. Atropine is said to be useful for bradyarrhythmias as intravenous boluses, with intravenous infusion of isoprenaline.
iii. Correction of cardiac arrhythmias, and fluid and electrolyte disturbances.

Autopsy Findings

- Signs of gastrointestinal irritation
- Congestion of all the visceras
- Generalized engorgement of veins
- Subendocardial and perivascular hemorrhage with focal myocardial edema
- Yellow oleander resists putrefaction and can be detected even years after death in exhumed putrefied bodies.

Medicolegal Importance

i. Because of its easy availability, suicidal poisoning is more common
ii. Its prevalence is more in rural areas
iii. Root and seeds are taken for criminal abortion
iv. Seeds are crushed and fed to the animal with corn or dread for cattle poisoning.

ACONITE

Common Name: Mitha Zahar, Bish, Bikh, Monk's Hood, Devil's Helmet

Botanical Names: *Aconitum napellus* is the European variety, *Aconitum columbianum* is the American variety and *Aconitum ferox* is the Indian variety.

Aconitine was the poison used by George Henry Lamson in 1881 to murder his brother-in-law in order to secure an inheritance. Lamson had learnt about aconitine as a medical student from Professor Robert Christison, who had taught that it was undetectable, but forensic science had improved since Lamson's student days.[14-16]

Aconitine was also made famous by its use in Oscar Wilde's 1891 story, Lord Arthur Savile's Crime. Aconite also plays a prominent role in James Joyce's Ulysses, in which the protagonist Leopold Bloom's father used pastilles of the chemical to commit suicide.

In 1953, aconitine was used by a Soviet biochemist and poison developer Grigory Mairanovsky in experiments with prisoners in the secret NKVD laboratory in Moscow. He admitted killing around 10 people using the poison.[14]

In 2009, Lakhvir Singh of Feltham, West London, used aconitine to poison the food of her ex-lover (who died as a result of the poisoning) and received a life sentence for the murder.[17]

Features

The green set of small leaves that surround the flower makes this plant look like a line-up of ballerinas (**Figure 44.5**).

The root of *Aconitum napellus* is conical (tapering), slightly arched, about 5–10 cm long and 1.5–2 cm thick, usually shriveled, brown with longitudinal wrinkles on its surface (**Figure 44.6**).

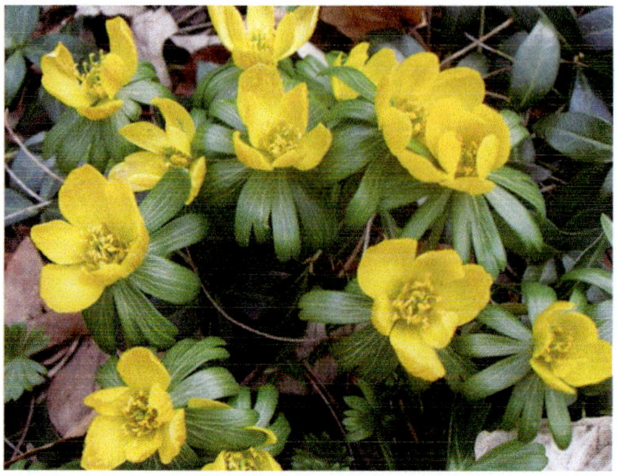

Figure 44.5 Aconite plant

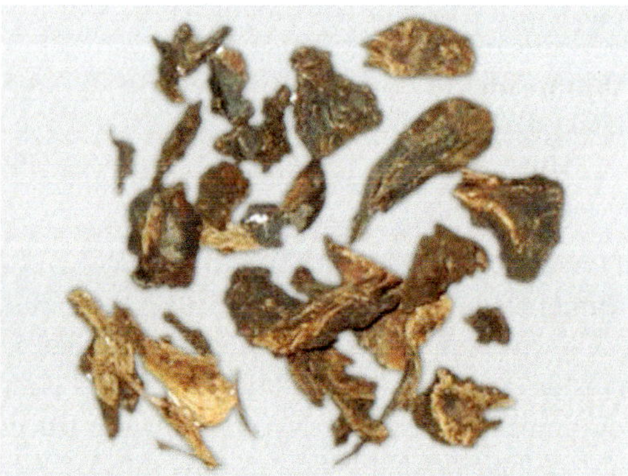

Figure 44.6 Dried root of *Aconitum napellus*

Active Principles

Main active principle is aconitine. Others alkaloids are mesoaconitine, hypoaconitine, pseudoaconitine, bikhaconitine, aconine, indacontine and picraconitine.

Aconitine (sometimes known as the Queen of Poisons; the King being arsenic) is a highly poisonous alkaloid derived from various aconite species.

Uses

It is a neurotoxin that opens TTX (**Tetrodotoxin**, also known as "tetrodox" and frequently abbreviated as **TTX**) sensitive Na^+ channels in the heart and other tissues[18] and is used for creating models of cardiac arrhythmia. Aconitine was previously used as an antipyretic and analgesic and still has some limited application in herbal medicine, although the narrow therapeutic index makes calculating appropriate dosage difficult.[19]

Mechanism of Action

Aconitine acts on nerve axons by opening sodium channels. It also inhibits complete depolarization of the membrane of myocardial tissue causing repetitive firing. It stimulates vagal medullary center. It stimulates and then depresses the myocardial muscles, smooth muscles, skeletal muscles, central nervous system and peripheral nerves.

Fatal Dose and Fatal Period

All parts of the plant are poisonous, but the root is more toxic.

Root: 1–2 g

Aconitine: 3–5 mg

250 mg of the **extract**,

25 drops of the **tincture**

Fatal period is about 2–6 hours.

Clinical Features

i. It is quickly absorbed from mucous membranes and skin.
ii. Contact with any preparation of aconite produces immediate tingling and numbness, which extends over the whole body.
iii. There is tingling and numbness in the lips, mouth, tongue and pharynx, followed by salivation, nausea, vomiting and diarrhea.
iv. The patient feels giddy, vision and speech are impaired, the limbs become weak, and he is unable to stand or walk.
v. Twitching of the muscles and convulsions may occur.
vi. The pulse is slow and irregular when collapse takes place.
vii. The pupils alternately contract and dilate but remain fully dilated in later stage (Hippus).
viii. Death ensues from cardiac arrhythmia or respiratory paralysis.

Management

There is no antidote, so only the symptoms can be treated,[20] traditionally with compounds such as atropine, strychnine or barakol, although it is unclear whether any of these are effective. Some other toxins, such as **Tetrodotoxin**, that bind to the same target site but have opposite effects, can reduce the effects of aconitine, but are so toxic themselves that death may result nonetheless.[21] The antidysrhythmic drug lidocaine, which is clinically used for treating unusual cardiac rhythms, also blocks these sodium channels, and there is a single report of a successful treatment of accidental aconitine poisoning using this drug.[22]

Autopsy Findings

Serum or urine concentrations of the chemical may be measured to confirm diagnosis in hospitalized poisoning victims, while post-mortem blood levels have been reported in at least five fatal cases.[23] No specific findings other than congestion of all visceras.

Medicolegal Importance

i. Aconite is often treated as an ideal homicidal poison because it is easily available, inexpensive, kills with very small doses, difficulty in detection by chemical analysis and can be mixed with food or drinks, but its actual use as homicidal poison is quite rare.

ii. The root is often used to procure abortion.
iii. It is also used as an arrow poison and cattle poison.
iv. Aconite is also used as suicidal poison.
v. Accidental poisoning may occurs when it is mistaken with horseradish. Cut-section of it appears pink, whereas in horseradish, it appears white.

HYDROCYANIC ACID

Common name: Hydrogen cyanide, prussic acid, cyanide poisoning

Appearance

Cyanide is found in all forms of matter. In the gaseous state, it is known as Hydrogen cyanide (HCN), and in the liquid form, hydrocyanic acid or prussic acid. Salts of cyanide occur as solids, white and crystalline.

i. **Gas Form**: **Hydrogen cyanide** is a colorless and extremely poisonous. HCN has a faint, bitter, almond-like smell that has been used as inhalation rodenticide and human poison. HCN is produced on an industrial scale and is a highly valuable precursor to many chemical compounds ranging from polymers to pharmaceuticals.
ii. **Liquid Form**: **Hydrocyanic acid** (prussic acid) is a solution of hydrogen cyanide in water, which is a colorless, volatile liquid having a typical odor.
iii. **Solid Form**: The salts of hydrogen cyanide are known as cyanides, such as potassium cyanide or sodium cyanide.

Hydrogen cyanide, prussic acid or cyanide are all terms relating to the same toxic substance. It is one of the most rapidly acting toxins which affect mammals. Cyanide is a lethal ingredient that has been used in rodent and vermin killers. The taste of cyanide is said to be bitter and burning in nature.

Source

Plants: Cyanide is present in the form of cyanogenic glycoside in the following plants:

• Wild black cherry	• Poison suckleya
• Johnson grass	• Sorghum
• Apricot	• Velvet grass
• Arrow grass	• White clover
• Peach	• Indian grass
• Apple seeds	

Burning: Following burning of woolen or silky cloth, plastic furniture and cigarette smoking.

Uses

i. **Industrial**: In metal processing, mining, plastics, artificial rubber and electroplating industries, it is used.
ii. Insecticides and rodenticide.
iii. **Medicinal**: (a) Synthetic amygdalin, laetrile, is used as a chemotherapeutic agent in the treatment of Cancer in certain parts of the world, although there is still a question mark regarding its efficacy. (b) Sodium nitroprusside is an effective antihypertensive agent, useful in hypertensive crises, as an IV infusion. Its use, however, is restricted as it is converted into cyanide in the body after metabolism and doses exceeding recommendations may lead to cyanide buildup and toxicity.
iv. Laboratory reagents.
v. Household uses as rodenticide and insecticides, silver polishes.
vi. **Warfare**: Cyanogen and its halides, e.g. chlorides, bromides, etc. have been used as chemical warfare agents, releasing HCN on application.

Pharmacokinetics

Hydrogen cyanide is rapidly absorbed and distributed following inhalation, oral or dermal exposure. Cyanide ion blocks oxidative respiration, causing failure of oxygen usage with tissue hypoxia leading to metabolic acidosis. Metabolism of cyanide occurs primarily through formation of thiocyanate, which is readily excreted in the urine. Small amounts of cyanide are excreted in breath and sweat.

Mechanism of Action

They interfere with **cellular respiration**. Cellular respiration is the set of the metabolic reactions and processes that take place in the cells to convert biochemical energy from nutrients into adenosine triphosphate (ATP) and then release waste products.

Specifically, cyanide prevents the cell from producing ATP by binding to one of the proteins involved in the electron transport chain.[24] This protein, cytochrome oxidase, contains several subunits and has substances containing iron groups. Cyanide reversibly inhibits ferric iron containing enzymes. Cyanide attaches to the iron of the prosthetic group of cytochrome oxidase, resulting in disturbance of the transport and utilization of oxygen in cells and causing a cytotoxic anoxia.

Fatal Dose

Hydrocyanic acid: 50–100 mg
Sodium or potassium cyanide: 200–300 mg
Bitter almonds: 50–80 numbers
Hydrogen cyanide: Inhalation of one part of 2000.

Fatal Period: Exposure to HCN gas: 2–10 minutes, sodium or potassium cyanide: 15–30 minutes.

Clinical Features

Acute Exposure

i. Hydrogen cyanide and its solutions may be fatal following exposure via all routes.
ii. The onset of signs and symptoms following exposure is rapid after inhalation and ingestion.
iii. Features are mostly non-specific and include: **CNS**: Headache, anxiety, dizziness, agitation, confusion, convulsions and coma. **GIT**: Nausea, vomiting, abdominal pain, numbness. **CVS**: Initially bradycardia, raised blood pressure, tachycardia and arrhythmias. **Respiratory System**: Dyspnea, tachypnea, followed by bradypnea.
iv. High concentrations may cause loss of consciousness, cardiac arrhythmias, coma and death.
v. Lactic acidosis is a key feature and correlates with the severity of cyanide intoxication.
vi. Profound neurological impairment manifest as Parkinsonism may develop and may persist on survival from severe intoxication.

Chronic Exposure

i. Long-term exposure to low levels of cyanide may lead to neurological effects.
ii. Hydrogen cyanide does not have any mutagenic properties and is not considered to be a carcinogen.
iii. Hydrogen cyanide is not considered to be a human reproductive or developmental toxicant.

Management

- Remove the patient from source of poisoning
- Gastric lavage with 5% sodium thiosulfate solution if ingested
- Amyl nitrate is the antidote if inhaled
- Sodium nitrate slowly IV
- Sodium thiosulfate is the accepted antidote for cyanide poisoning. It should be given as 25% solution IV. A combination treatment of sodium nitrite and sodium thiosulfate has given good results. The success of any form of therapy depends very largely upon the promptness of administration.

Mechanism of Action of Nitrites: Nitrate induces methemoglobinemia, which causes detachment of cyanide from the heme group of cytochrome oxidase, as methemoglobin has a higher binding affinity for cyanide. Cyanide combines with methemoglobin and form a non-toxic substance.

On the other hand, sodium thiosulfate serves up as a substrate for the enzyme rhodanese to catabolize cyanide to non-toxic thiocyanate, which is excreted in the urine.

Autopsy Findings

i. A diagnosis of prussic acid poisoning is made on clinical and/or postmortem findings. There may be a smell of bitter almonds.
ii. On postmortem examination, the blood may be bright red and clot poorly (the blood will return to a dark color a few hours after death).
iii. Cyanosis.
iv. Froth at mouth and nose.
v. Cherry red color or postmortem lividity.
vi. Congested visceras.
vii. Serosal surface may show hemorrhages.
viii. Stomach mucosa may show erosion and appear blackened due to formation of alkaline hematin.
ix. Muscles may be dark, and there may be hemorrhages in the trachea and lungs.
x. Hemorrhages will be evident on the surface of the heart.
xi. Samples for laboratory analysis include: Blood, viscera, stomach contents. Spleen is considered as best specimen due to presence of more RBCs.

Medicolegal Importance

i. Use of hydrocyanic acid and its salts for suicidal poisoning is not common. It is seen commonly with those persons who are employed in electroplating, chemistry, mining and metal heat treatment, etc.
ii. Homicidal poisoning is also rare.
iii. Accidental poisoning occasionally occurs.
iv. Cattle poisoning has been known to have occurred from eating kadvi jowar and plant.

REFERENCES

1. Eichhorn EJ, Gheorghiade M. Digoxin. Prog Cardiovasc Dis. 2002;44:251.
2. Hussain Z, Swindle J, Hauptman PJ. Digoxin use and digoxin toxicity in the post-DIG trial era. J Card Fail. 2006;12:343.
3. Bronstein AC, Spyker DA, Cantilena LR Jr, et al. Annual Report of the American Association of Poison Control Centers' National Poison Data System (NPDS): 25th Annual Report 2007. Clin Toxicol (Phila). 2008;46:927.
4. Brubacher JR, Lachmanen D, Ravikumar PR, Hoffman RS. Efficacy of digoxin specific Fab fragments (Digibind) in the treatment of toad venom poisoning. Toxicon. 1999;37:931.
5. Britannica Kids. Encyclopadia Britannica Kids. [cited 2012 Aug 15]; Available from: URL:http://student.britannica.com
6. Colonia 13 509 Heading: 1550–1575 Tobacco, Europe.
7. Gilman SL, Xun Z. Introduction. In: Smoke: A Global History of Smoking. Reaktion Books;2004. p. 26.
8. WHO Report on the global tobacco epidemic: Tobacco is the single most preventable cause of death in the world today. World Health Organization. 2008.
9. Tobacco Facts. Why is Tobacco So Addictive? [cited 2013 march 25]; Available from: URL:http//www.Tobaccofacts.org
10. Philip Morris Information Sheet. [cited 2013 march 25]; Available from: URL:http//www.Stanford.edu
11. Kintz P, Kieffer I, Messer J, Mangin P. Nicotine analysis in neonates hair for measuring gestational exposure to tobacco. J Forensic Sci. 1993;38:119-23.
12. Tsukada K, Akizuki S, Matsuoka Y, Irimajiri S. A case of aconitine poisoning accompanied by bidirectional ventricular tachycardia treated with lidocaine. Kokyu to Junkan. 2008;40(10):1003-6.
13. De Silva HA, Forsake MM, Pathmeswaran A, Alahakone DG, Ratnatilake GA, Gunatilake SB, et al. Multiple dose activated charcoal for treatment of yellow oleander poisoning: a single-blind, randomized, placebo-controlled that. Lancet. 2003;361:1935-8.
14. Macinnis P. It's true! You eat poison every day. In: It's True. Allen and Unwin. 2006; p. 80-1.

15. Macinnis P. Poisons: From hemlock to Botox and the killer bean of Calabar. Arcade Publishing. 2005. pp. 25-6.
16. Parry LA, Wright WH. Some Famous Medical Trials. Beard Books.2000. p. 103.
17. Wang SY, Wang GK. Voltage-gated sodium channels as primary targets of diverse lipid-soluble neurotoxins. Cellular Signal. 2003;15(2):151-9.
18. Rivera VR, Poli MA, Bignami GS. Prophylaxis and treatment with a monoclonal antibody of Tetrodotoxin poisoning in mice. Toxicon.1995;33(9):1231-7.
19. Octopus Envenomations at eMedicine.com
20. Roth L, Daunderer M, Kormann K. Giftpflanzen - Pflanzengifte. Nikol Verlag; 2006.
21. Ohno Y, Chiba S, Uchigasaki S, Uchima E, Nagamori H, Mizugaki M, et al. The influence of tetrodotoxin on the toxic effects of aconitine in vivo. Tohoku J Exp Med. 1992; 167(2):155-8.
22. Baselt R. Disposition of Toxic Drugs and Chemicals in Man, 8th ed. Biomedical Publications, Foster City, CA; 2008. pp. 25-7.
23. Samal KK, Sahu HK, Kar MK, Palit SK, Kar BC, Sahu CS. Yellow oleander (Cerbera Thevetia) poisoning with jaundice and renal failure. J Assoc Physicians India. 1989;232-3.
24. Nelson DL, Cox MM. Lehniger Principles of Biochemistry (3rd ed). New York: Worth Publishers.2000; pp. 668, 670-1, 676.

CHAPTER 45

Deliriants and Psychotropic Poisons

Putul Mahanta

LEARNING PLAN

- Learn about deliriant poisons, viz. datura, cannabis and cocaine
- Know their management
- Identify their diagnostic and autopsy findings
- Understand their medicolegal importance

Deliriant drugs act on the brain and induce delirium, i.e. altered consciousness with confusion, delusions, hallucinations and agitation. Deliriants are antagonists of the acetylcholine receptors. Important examples are datura, cannabis and cocaine.

DATURA (ANTICHOLINERGICS)

Common Name: Thorn apple, Jimson seed

Datura is a genus of nine species of vespertine flowering plants belonging to the family Solanaceae. Daturas are woody-stalked, leafy annuals and short-lived perennials which can reach up to 2 m in height, as shown in **Figure 45.1**. The flowers are erect or spreading, trumpet shaped, 5-20 cm long and 4-12 cm broad at the mouth; colors vary from white to yellow, pink and pale purple.

The fruit is a spiny capsule 4-10 cm long and 2-6 cm broad, splitting open when ripe to release the numerous seeds. The seeds disperse freely over pastures, fields and even wasteland locations (**Figure 45.2**).

Most parts of the plants contain toxic hallucinogens and it has a long history of causing delirious states and death.

The natural alkaloids of datura are atropine, hyoscyamine and hyoscine (scopolamine), which are found in all parts of the following plants:

1. ***Atropa belladonna***: Atropa belladonna or Atropa bella-donna, commonly known as belladonna, devil's berries, death cherries or deadly nightshade, is a perennial herbaceous plant in the family Solanacae, native to Europe, North Africa and Western Asia. The foliage and berries are extremely

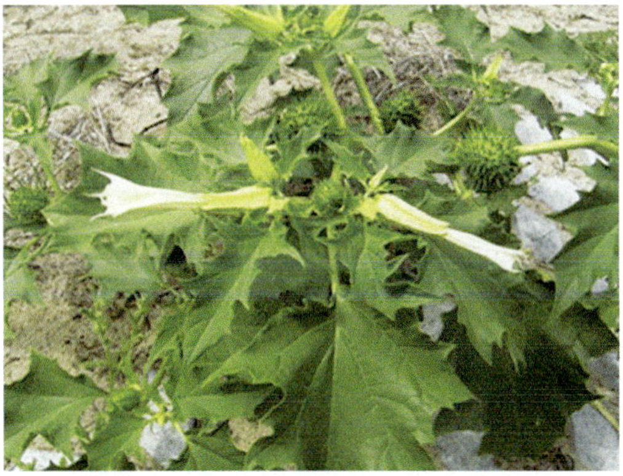

Figure 45.1 *Datura stramonium* plant

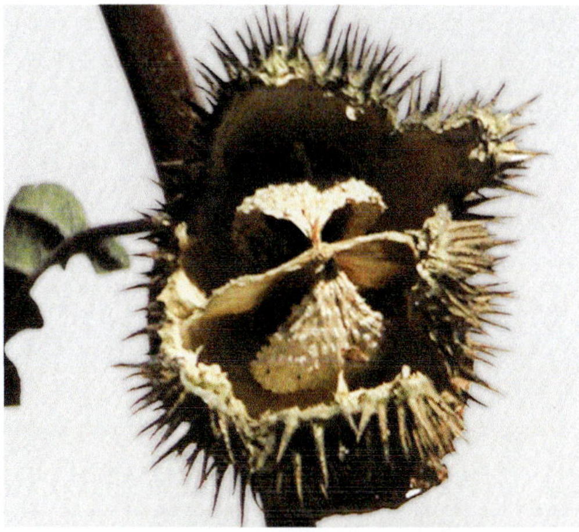

Figure 45.2 Dry fruit of datura

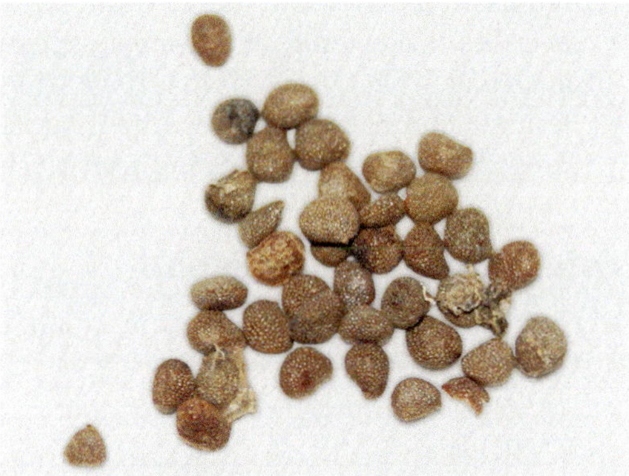

Figure 45.3 *Atropa belladonna* seeds

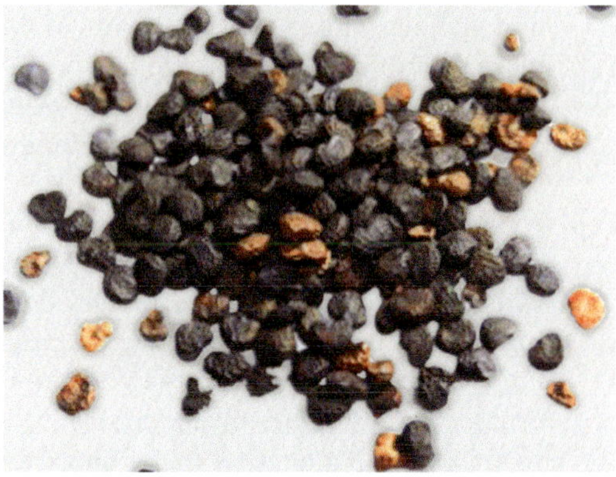

Figure 45.4 *Datura stramonium* seeds

toxic, containing tropane alkaloids. These toxins include **scopolamine** and **hyoscyamine** which cause a bizarre delirium and hallucinations.[1] Its seeds are small, brown mammilated and kidney shaped **Figure 45.3**.

2. ***Datura stramonium***: This variety grows in hilly areas. It is also known by the common names, viz. Jimson weed, devil's trumpet, devil's weed, thorn apple, tolguacha, Jamestown weed, stinkweed, locoweed, datura, prickly burr, devil's cucumber, hell's bells and moonflower[2] and, in South Africa, **malpitte** and **mad seeds.** It is a common weed in the Solanaceae (nightshade) family. It is an erect annual herb forming a bush up to 1–1.5 m tall.[3] The leaves are soft, irregularly undulated and toothed. The fragrant flowers are trumpet-shaped, white to creamy or violet. They rarely open completely.

   The egg-shaped seed capsule is walnut sized and either covered with spikes or bald. At maturity, it splits into four chambers, each with dozens of small black seeds. The seeds are black and kidney-shaped and mammilated as shown in **Figure 45.4**.

3. ***Datura fastuosa***: It is a plant belonging to the family Solanaceae. *Datura fastuosa* is also known as **thorn apple**. It has got two varieties, viz. *Datura alba* (**safed *Datura***), a white flowered plant, and *Datura niger* (**kala *Datura***).

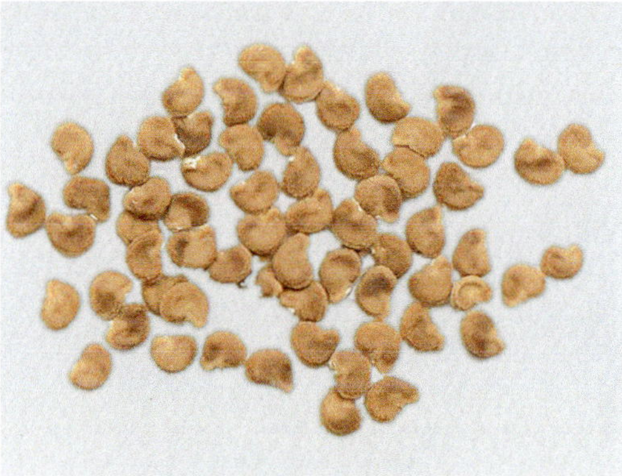

Figure 45.5 *Datura fastuosa* seeds

The plant grows to a height of 2–3 m having lush green leaves, bell-shaped flowers and globular thorny fruits. All parts of the plant, from flower to root, are poisonous. This variety grows in plain areas. Its seeds are large mammilated, brown and kidney-shaped as shown in **Figure 45.5**.

4. ***Hyoscyamus niger** and **Hyoscyamus muticus***: Commercial henbane, which consists of the dried leaves of *Hyoscyamus niger* and, sometimes, of *Hyoscyamus muticus*, of Egypt, yields three dangerous drugs, viz. atropine, hyoscyamine and scopolamine. Among the major suppliers of these leaves, are Hungary, Egypt and the US, all of which grow it commercially. In France, another species of henbane, *H. albus*, is used for the same. An average sized datura fruit contain 350–450 seeds.

Active Principle

Seed is the most toxic constituent and contains the following active principles: **Hyoscine** (scopolamine) 1.4%, **Hyoscyamine** and **dl-Hyoscyamine**, which are converted to **Atropine** during extraction process. Hyoscine and hyoscyamine both are pharmacopeal products. The functions of atropine and hyoscyamine are similar to each other but hyoscine is differing as follows:

a. It is depressant from the start and has no action of initial CNS stimulation,
b. It has milder peripheral effects and
c. Its fatal dose is 60 mg half of atropine and hyoscyamine, i.e. 120 mg.

Medical Uses

- As antispasmodic and as an antisecretory
- As antidepressants
- As antiparkinsonisms
- Due to its anodyne (analgesic) effects, it is also used locally in the form of belladonna plaster
- As antipsychotic
- Used in ophthalmic preparations as a cycloplegic and as a mydriatic. Atropine can be given to patients who have direct globe trauma
- As a life-saving drug in organophosphate poisoning
- Resuscitation in the treatment of bradycardia. Atropine is also useful in treating heart block.

Fatal Dose and Fatal Period

- In terms of seeds, it is about 100–125 number
- 10–100 mg of atropine
- For causing stupefaction, half of that, i.e. 50–60 seeds.

Fatal time is roughly within 24 hours.

Mechanism of Action

First stimulates the higher centers of brain, then the motor centers and, finally, causes depression and paralysis, especially of the vital centers in the medulla. Respiration is first stimulated, and then depressed, and the heart center is stimulated. It blocks the neurotransmitter acetylcholine, muscarinic receptor (M_1) antagonist.

The reason for most of these symptoms is atropine's effect on the parasympathetic nervous system. Atropine competitively inhibits the action of acetylcholine (ACh) at the acetylcholine receptor in the nerve synapse, thereby preventing the parasympathetic nervous system from sending out electrical nerve impulses. Since the parasympathetic nervous system regulates non-volitional or subconscious activities (such as sweating, breathing and heart rate) when it is prevented from sending out signals, the heartbeat and breathing become extremely irregular.

Clinical Features

Due to the potent combination of anticholinergic substances it contains, datura intoxication typically produces effects similar to that of an anticholinergic delirium: a complete inability to differentiate reality from fantasy (frank delirium, as contrasted to hallucination); hyperthermia; tachycardia; bizarre and possibly violent behavior and severe mydriasis, with resultant painful photophobia that can last several days. Pronounced amnesia is another commonly reported effect.

Clinical features can be well-described in classical phrase quoted by Morton Still '**blind as bat**, **hot as hare**, **dry as bone**, **red as beet** and **mad as wet hen**'.

Symptoms appear within half hours of intake, and if bitter taste not masked, vomiting may occur, when crushed seeds are given. The clinical features are best remembered as **D**s.

1. **D**ryness of mouth and throat, with burning sensation in the stomach.
2. **D**ysphasia, are the first symptoms the patient will complain of, followed by giddiness.
3. **D**runken (staggering) gait (ataxia) and in-coordination of the muscles.
4. **D**ry and hot skin because there is total suppression of sweat secretion, resulting in rise of body temperature. Peculiar flushed appearance of the skin, especially over the face.
5. **D**ermatitis (exfoliative) with rashes and exfoliation of skin may be seen all over the body sometimes.
6. **D**ilated pupils with resultant painful photophobia, with loss of accommodation reflex and near vision, with conjunctivae becoming red and congested that can last several days.
7. **D**istension of bladder (Retention of urine).
8. **D**rowsiness supervenes. Pulse is full and bounding initially; later on will be weak, thready and irregular.
9. **D**elirium—patient becomes restless, markedly excited and delirious, and this delirium has got a peculiar character, manifested by muttering, indistinct and inaudible words (**muttering delirium**). Patient may try to run away from bed and pick up the bed cloth (**Carpology**) and try to pullout imaginary threads from the fingertips. There may be associated hallucination of dreadful nature, related to visual and auditory type (mad as wet hen).
10. **D**eficit of recent memory—in non-fatal cases, while recovering, secondary delirium may occur and the patient will have anterograde amnesia and will not remember anything about his illness and will be surprised to find himself in hospital.
11. **D**eath — usually the patient, if not treated, pass off to stupor and coma and dies due to respiratory failure.

Management

1. Immediate stomach washes, initially with plain water and then with 2–4% solution of tannic acid, should be given.
2. Saline purgatives should be given by mouth, if patient is conscious
3. If patient is restless or violent, injection **chlorpromazine** (50–100 mg) by sub-cutaneous route can be given. Injection **diazepam** parentally may also help. In case of rise in temperature, repeated cold sponging will be of helpful.
4. Antidote, injections of **physostigmine** by IM or IV route at a dose of 0.5 mg, 1–2 hourly, usually relives both peripheral and cerebral symptom. Encouraging result will be seen just after one injection, manifested by contraction of pupil, moistening of skin and fall in body temperature and flushing.
5. Injection **pilocarpine nitrate** (dose 6–15 mg) by subcutaneous route relives patient rapidly of peripheral symptoms, but does not relieve the central effect.

6. **Injection Morphine** in the dose of 15 mg subcutaneous is considered to be physiological antidote, but is not given, due to its depressant action on the brain.

Postmortem Findings

- Autopsy findings are not very characteristic
- The stomach may show slight inflammation
- Presence of broken seeds in the stomach or in upper intestine will be seen
- Viscera will be found grossly congested
- The seed resist putrefaction for a long time.

Medicolegal Importance

1. **Suicide**: Due to easy availability, it is considered to be one of the most popular poisons for suicides, especially in rural areas.
2. **Homicide**: It is one of the popular agents for causing homicide also because of its availability and easy way of administration.
3. **Accident**: It is not very uncommon and it is seen amongst children, who may take it being attracted by its attractive color and flower, and also, it occurs when datura is mixed with country liquors to give a boost.
4. **Stupefaction**: It literally means making a person stupid. Legally, it means rendering a person unconscious or semi-conscious, to make him incapable of offering resistance in the way of committing a crime, mainly like child-lifting, committing rape or theft. This is done usually in a place where there is confluence of unknown people, like railway compartment, railway station, ferry ghat, mela, etc. where a person, being offered food by another person, takes it to lose consciousness, to regain consciousness in a hospital minus his belongings. Thus, datura is also known as railroad poison.

CANNABIS

Botanical Name: *Cannabis indica* or *sativa*

Common Name: Indian hemp

The plant belongs to the natural order Urticacae. The female plant is taller (from 4 to 6 m) and has got more dark and luxuriant foliage than the male (**Figure 45.6**). *Cannabis sativa* plant grows all over the country, but the cultivation is restricted by government.

Cannabis, also known as **marijuana** (sometimes spelled "marihuana")[4] among many other names, refers to any number of preparations of the cannabis plant intended for use as a psychoactive drug or for medicinal purposes. According to the United Nations, cannabis "is the most widely used illicit substance in the world".[5]

The typical herbal form of cannabis consists of the flowers and subtending leaves and stalks of mature pistillate female plants. The resinous form of the drug is known as **hashish** (or merely as 'hash').[6]

Documented instances of cannabis use go back as far as the 3rd millennium BC.[7] In modern times, the drug has been used for recreational, religious or spiritual and medicinal purposes. The UN estimated that in 2004, about 4% of the world's adult population (162 million people) use cannabis annually, and about 0.6% (22.5 million) uses it on a daily basis.[8] The possession, use or sale of cannabis preparations containing psychoactive cannabinoids became illegal in most parts of the world in the early 20th century,[9] and in India, it comes under preview of Narcotic drugs and psychotropic substances **(NDPS) Act.**

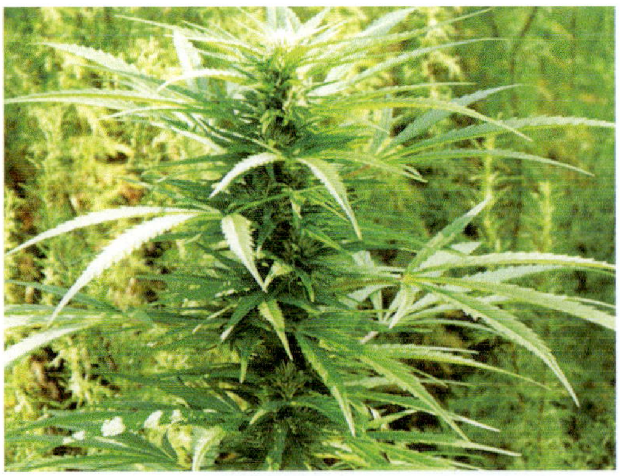

Figure 45.6 *Cannabis indica* or *sativa*

Forms in which Consumed

1. **Bhang** or **Siddhi**, **Sabji**: Consists of dried mature leaves and flower stems of cannabis and stalk of the plant, having greenish coloration with a peculiar but not unpleasant odor, which is almost tasteless and ground with water and mixed with fruit juice or milk. It is consumed in the form of decoction or the dried leaves are made into paste and taken in the form of bolus or may even be mixed with sweets as described.
2. **Ganja**: It is brownish, dried, flowery and fruity top of the female plant, having strong characteristic odor and it is smoked through pipe. It may also be smoked in a cigarette by throwing off ½ of tobacco and filling with ganja. In later term, it is known as Marijuana or Marihuana, which means 'Pleasurable feeling'.
3. **Charas** or **Hashish**: Hashish (also spelled hasheesh, hashisha or simply hash) is a concentrated resin produced from the flowers of the female cannabis plant. Hash can often be more potent than marijuana and can be smoked or chewed.[10]
4. **Sinsemilla**: Highly potent marijuana from female plants that are especially tended and kept seedless by preventing pollination in order to induce high resin content. This seedless marijuana is a popular form of cannabis in the US.
5. **Majun**: A sweet, prepared with bhang. It increases appetite and sexual desire.

Uses

- As an antiemetic in patients under chemotherapy to stop nausea and vomiting
- Stimulation of hunger in chemotherapy and AIDS patients
- Tentative role in the treatment of convulsions, anxiety, analgesic and as anti-inflammatory
- Lowered intraocular eye pressure (shown to be effective for treating glaucoma). However, in most of the countries of the world, includ-ing India, it is banned drug now.

Active Principle

The major psychoactive chemical compound in cannabis is Δ^9-tetrahydrocannabinol (commonly abbreviated as THC). Cannabis contains more than 400 different chemical compounds, including at least 66 other cannabinoids (cannabidiol (CBD), cannabinol (CBN) and tetrahydrocannabivarin (THCV), etc.) which can result in different effects from those of THC alone.[11]

Active principles are contained in its resin. Principle constitute of the resin are cannabinol, which has no action, and also inert, but on exposure to heat, it is partly converted to the very active isomeric **tetrahydrocannabinol** (THC). All parts of the plant, male or female, contain the active material, except stem, root and seeds. It is a CNS stimulant. It is a psychoactive drug. It is variously known as pot, grass, weed, hash, marijuana hashish or bhang. THC is metabolized in the liver and excreted in the urine and feces.

Fatal Dose and Fatal Period

1. **Charas**: 2 g/kg body weight
2. **Ganja**: 8 g/kg body weight
3. **Bhang**: 10 g/kg body weight—all in terms of Δ^9 THC

Death is most uncommon. Even, if occurs, may take several days.

Mechanism of Action

The high lipid-solubility of cannabinoids results in their persisting present in the body for long periods of time. Even after a single administration of THC, detectable levels of THC can be found in the body for weeks or longer (depending on the amount administered and the sensitivity of the assessment method). A number of investigators have suggested that this is an important factor in marijuana's effects, which is perhaps because cannabinoids may accumulate in the body, particularly in the lipid membranes of neurons.[12]

Until recently, little was known about the specific mechanisms of action of THC at the neuronal level. However, researchers have now confirmed that THC exerts its most prominent effects via its actions on two types of cannabinoid receptors, the CB_1 and the CB_2 receptors, both of which are G-Protein coupled receptors. The CB_1 receptor is found primarily in the brain as well as in some peripheral tissues, and the CB_2 receptor is found exclusively in peripheral tissues.[13]

THC appears to alter mood and cognition through its agonist actions on the CB_1 receptors, which inhibit a secondary messenger system (adenylate cyclase) in a dose-dependent manner. These actions can be blocked by the selective CB_1 receptor antagonist SR141716A (**rimonabant**), which interestingly has been shown in clinical trials to be an effective treatment for smoking cessation, weight loss and as a means of controlling or reducing metabolic syndrome risk factors.[14]

Cannabis is the most widely used illicit drug worldwide. As societies reconsider the legal status of cannabis, policy makers and clinicians require sound knowledge of the acute and chronic effects of cannabis.

Acute Poisoning

Clinical Features

Usually it is more pronounced in a case of inhalation than ingestion and seen in persons not accustomed to its use and also from over dosage. Appear soon if it is taken in the form of "Ganja or Charas' and within half hour after consumption of 'Bhang'. The symptoms are basically divided into two stages:

Stage of Inebriation and Release of Inhibition

Characterized by a sense of well-being, followed by excitement and visual hallucination, impulsive ideas, talkativeness, uncontrollable laughter and marked increase in appetite, particularly sweets, craving for sleep and purposeless muscular movement. There may be vomiting at this stage. The patient loses all perception of time, place and person and gradually the patient passes over to the stage of narcosis.

Stage of Narcosis

This stage is characterized by consciousness changing to a dream-like state, frightful hallucination, and delirium, sometimes development of a homicidal tendency or thanatophobia.

Patient becomes giddy, ataxic, feels tingling and numbness of skin and becomes deeply narcotized. Recovery usually occurs after a deep sleep, but with a heavy head. Death, if at all occurs, is due to respiratory failure.

Management

The main principle of treatment of acute poisoning are:

1. Decontamination: Stomach is evacuated if it is ingested.
2. Purgation to remove the toxic elements from intestine.
3. Maintenance of respiration and nutrition.
4. Fear of death should be controlled by IV, diazepam or haloperidol or other antipsychotic drugs.
5. Psychotherapy is also needed.

Chronic Poisoning

The drug-induced psychosis seen when cannabis is the main substance being abused is distinct phenomenologically from other psychosis. Chronic cannabis use is associated with psychiatric, respiratory, cardiovascular and bone effects. It also has oncogenic, teratogenic and mutagenic effects, all of which depend upon dose and duration of use.

One who takes the intoxicant repeatedly for a long time develops a feature by which they can be easily identified. There is general loss of health, emaciation with trembling, loss of sexual power and lower reproductive activities. Gynecomastia, the cheek becomes hollowed due to absorption of buckle pad of fat and eyes become bloodshot with very prominent conjunctival blood vessels. There is a definite degradation of mental faculties.

Psychiatric Toxicity

Cannabis has now been implicated in the etiology of many major long-term psychiatric conditions including depression, anxiety, psychosis, bipolar disorder and an amotivational state. In **amotivational syndrome**, the person is lethargic, apathetic and disinterested to work, with lack of concentration.

Cannabis Psychosis

Here the person develops a psychic disturbances preceded by the ingestion of a large dose of cannabis marked by "sudden onset of confusion, generally associated with delusion, hallucinations (usually visual) and emotional liability, amnesia, disorientation, depersonalization and paranoid symptoms".[15]

A condition like '**Run amok**,' which sometimes spelled as '**Run amuck**,' is to behave in a wild or unruly manner, is also associated with its chronic uses.

Running amok, sometimes referred to as simply **amok**[16] (also spelled **amuk**, from the Malay meaning "mad with uncontrollable rage") is a term for a killing spree perpetrated by an individual out of rage or resentment over perceived mistreatment.

Here the person develops a psychic disturbance marked by a period of depression, followed by violent behavior, culminating in homicide or suicide (Running amok).[17]

It is seen among chronic ganja smokers or even in a person, who is taking ganja for the first time. They suffer from some **hallucination** or **delusion of persecutory nature** or **sexual infidelity** and, due to this, the patient is overpowered by an irresistible impulse to destroy life and property and will go on killing persons against whom he has real or imaginary grudge and later on, kills anybody who comes in this way.

A person, committing a crime under this condition will not be held responsible in many countries, including India. If the abuse is continued for a considerable time, it may lead to behavioral problems, crime and even mental derangement.

Cardiovascular Toxicity

There is evidence of cardiovascular toxicity associated with chronic cannabis use. Cannabis has been linked in a dose-dependent manner with elevated rates of myocardial infarction and cardiac arrhythmias.

Respiratory Toxicity

There is evidence of respiratory toxicity associated with chronic cannabis use. Respiratory conditions linked with cannabis include reduced lung density, lung cysts and chronic bronchitis.

Others

It is known to affect bone metabolism. It has teratogenic effects on the developing brain, following perinatal exposure. Cannabis has been linked to cancers at eight sites, including children after in utero maternal exposure, and multiple molecular pathways to oncogenesis exist. Bhang or Siddhi, Sabji and Marijuana lead to neuronal atrophy.

Detection

THC and its major (inactive) metabolite can be quantitated in blood, urine, hair, oral fluid or sweat using chromatographic techniques, as part of a drug use testing program or a forensic investigation of a traffic or other criminal offense. The concentrations obtained from such analysis can often be helpful in distinguishing active use from passive exposure, prescription use from illicit use, elapsed time since use and extent or duration of use. These tests cannot, however, distinguish authorized cannabis smoking for medical purposes from unauthorized recreational smoking.[18]

Commercial cannabinoid **immunoassays**, often employed as the initial screening method when testing physiological specimens for marijuana presence, have different degrees of cross-reactivity with THC and its metabolites. Urine contains predominantly THC-COOH, while hair, oral fluid and sweat contain primarily THC. Blood may contain both substances, with the relative amounts dependent on the recency and extent of usage.[18,19]

The **Duquenois-Levine test** is commonly used as a screening test in the field, but it cannot definitively confirm the presence of marijuana, as a large range of substances have been shown to give false positives. Despite this, it is common in the US for prosecutors to seek plea bargains on the basis of positive D-L tests, claiming them definitive, or even to seek conviction without the use of gas chromatography confirmation, which can only be done in the laboratory.[20]

Medicolegal Importance

It is the commonest drug abuse, being abused by Sanyasis, Sadhoos, Western musicians, etc. Cannabis does not cause physiological dependence or addiction, but causes psychological dependence.

Postmortem Findings

Apart from the general findings of poisoning, no characteristic features of cannabis poisonous death is found.

COCAINE

It is an active alkaloid obtained from the leaves of plant *Erythroxylon coca* (**Figure 45.7**). It is produced as a salt, i.e. cocaine hydrochloride or as an alkaloid known as freebase or crack. An ester of benzoic acid and a base, containing 'N' is synthetic cocaine.

Preparation

Cocaine hydrochloride is a white powder (**Figure 45.8**), which is usually adulterated with other substances such as caffeine, amphetamine, etc. It is called speed ball, when it adulterated with heroin. It, in purest form, causes numbness of the tongue and mucous membrane. It is sparingly soluble in water, but readily dissolves in other solvents, viz. alcohol, ether, benzene, to which it imparts alkaline reaction.

People get addicted to it because it increases mental concentration (euphoric agent) and alertness, which reduces hunger and increases libido.

Routes of Administration

- Chewing, mainly the coca leaves
- Smoking (Pyrolysis)
- Snorting
- Intravenous injection
- Ingestion.

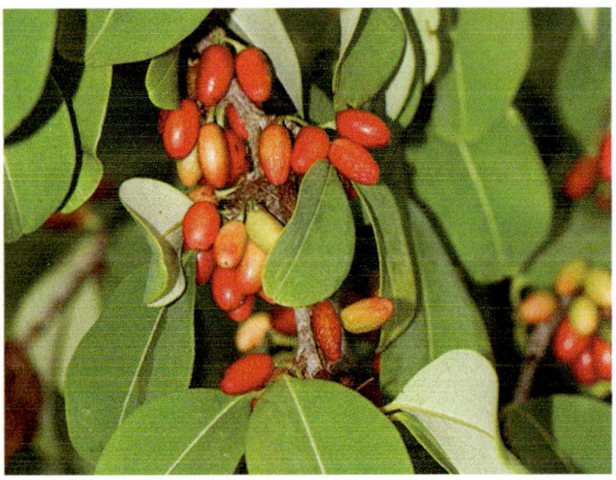

Figure 45.7 Plant *Erythroxylon coca*

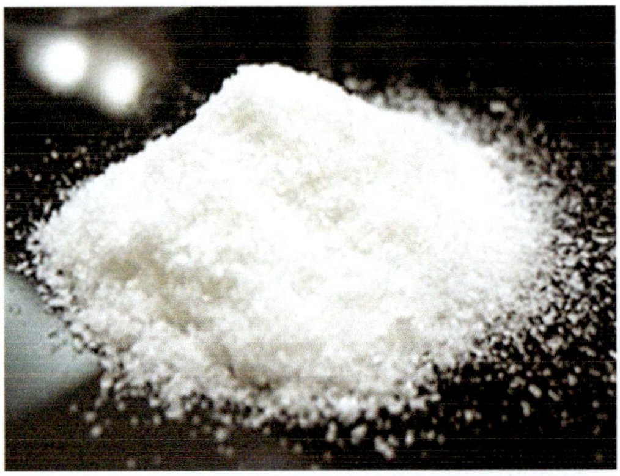

Figure 45.8 Cocaine powder

Medical Usage

As **cocaine HCl**, it is used as a local anesthetic agent in ophthalmic operation, but it often causes damage to the cornea. It was also used in dental practice and in minor surgery as local anesthetic agent. It causes paralysis of nerve endings by blocking of fast Na^+ channel. It also acts as a local vasoconstrictor.

Mechanism of Action

Cocaine modifies the action of dopamine in the brain. The dopamine rich areas of the brain are the ventral tegmental area, the nucleus accumbens and the caudate nucleus—these areas are collectively known as the brain's 'reward pathway'. Cocaine binds to dopamine reuptake transporters on the pre-synaptic membranes of dopaminergic neurons. This binding inhibits the removal of dopamine from the synaptic cleft and its subsequent degradation by monoamine oxidase in the nerve terminal. Dopamine remains in the synaptic cleft and is free to bind to its receptors on the postsynaptic membrane, producing further nerve impulses. This increased activation of the dopaminergic reward pathway leads to the feelings of euphoria and the 'high' associated with cocaine use.

Absorption, Metabolism and Excretion

Cocaine is well absorbed from oral, nasal and respiratory sites. With intravenous injection or inhalation, the onset is fast with level achieved in 3–5 minutes. The half-life is approximately one hour. It is metabolized by liver and the metabolites are excreted through urine.

Fatal Dose

Oral route 1.25 mg, hypodermic injection is 40 mg, but larger dose can be tolerated, for its habit-forming property. Fatal period may be very short, within few minutes to a few hours.

Acute Poisoning

Clinical Features

CNS Effect: A powerful CNS stimulant. In small doses, it gives a sense of well-being and euphoria with excitement, restlessness, tremor convulsion with increase in reflexes, followed by depression. There may be sudden rise of temperature with rigor. There is dryness of mouth, dysphasia, tingling and numbness of the tongue, gradually spreading all over the body. Pupils dilate.

CVS Effect: Sympathomimetic affects leads to hypertension, tachycardia and cardiac arrhythmia. Pulse becomes weak, irregular. Excessive vasoconstriction (vasospasm) leads to organ ischemia, viz. myocardial infarction, renal infarction, etc.

Respiratory Effect: Respiration becomes shallow and gasping with profuse perspiration, more over the forehead. There may be hallucination and person dies of respiratory failure.

Sympathomimetic Effects: Reactive dilated pupil (**reactive mydriasis**), diaphoresis with decreased other body secretions, which may cause further hyperthermia.

Management

Hyperthermia is managed by cold sponging. Convulsion can be treated by diazepam or lorazepam. Tachycardia can be managed by beta-blockers. Phenytoin is for cardiac arrhythmia. Better to avoid propranolol, which may precipitate severe hypertension. Labetalol for hypertension can also be given.

Postmortem Findings

Identification of chronic cocaine takers: Those who take cocaine by mouth, their tongue and teeth becomes black, perhaps due to the action of saliva and lime on cocaine; and if it is taken as a snuff, there is chronic ulceration of the nasal septum, with perforation sometimes.

Multiple scar marks are noticed at injected site in case of intravenous abusers.

Signs of asphyxia are evident. Infective endocarditis as sequelae to septic injection practice, hepatic necrosis in a case of coca paste smokers may present. Evidence of myocardial infarction may also be associated with certain cases.

Samples to be Preserved

- Blood
- Brain
- Skin from injection site
- Swab from nasal mucosa.

Cocainisim or Chronic Cocaine Poisoning

Clinical Features

Insomnia, defective memory, pale face, sunken eyes, dilated pupils, digestive disturbances, wasting and emaciation, impotence, derangement of special senses with certain features, viz. delusion of persecution, dreadful hallucination and melancholia. Sexual perversion, especially homosexuality, is a characteristic feature.

Cocaine Bug or Magnan's Syndrome

It is seen among the chronic takers, who develop a feelings as if grains of sand are lying under the skin or some small insect is creeping under the skin (cocaine bug), giving rise to intense itching.

Medicolegal Importance

It is a drug of abuse. Usually, **poisoning** is due to **accidental overdose** or **adulteration**. Rarely, it can be suicidal. Desire to procure the drug is overpowering, but they develop no tolerance. There is a tendency to develop psychological dependence, but no withdrawal symptom appears. When used in combination with heroin, morphine-like compounds, it develops tolerance rapidly. Prostitutes may place cocaine solution into vagina to produce local constriction, which may sometimes cause poisoning.

REFERENCES

1. Kuhn C, Swartzwelder S, Wilson W, Wilson LH, Foster J. Buzzed: The Straight Facts about the Most Used and Abused Drugs from Alcohol to Ecstasy. New York, WW Norton; 2008. p. 107.
2. "Datura Stramonium information from NPGS/GRIN". Retrieved 2008-02-05.
3. Stace C. New Flora of the British Isles. Cambridge University Press; 1997. p. 532.
4. Company Houghton Mifflin; American Heritage Dictionaries. Spanish Word Histories and Mysteries. Houghton Mifflin Harcourt. 2007-11-14. p. 142.
5. UNODC. World Drug Report 2010. United Nations Publication. p. 198. Retrieved 2010-07-19.
6. Matthew J. Atha (Independent Drug Monitoring Unit). Types of Cannabis available in the United Kingdom (UK).
7. Rudgley R. Lost Civilizations of the Stone Age. New York: Free Press; 1998.
8. United Nations Office on Drugs and Crime (PDF). Cannabis: Why We Should Care. 1. S.l.: United Nations. 14.2006.
9. Why is Marijuana illegal? Drugwarrant.com. Retrieved 12 May 2011.
10. Hashish. Definitions from Dictionary.com. dictionary.reference.com.
11. Fusar-Poli P, Crippa JA, Bhattacharyya S, et al. Distinct effects of {delta} 9-tetrahydrocannabinol and cannabidiol on neural activation during emotional processing. Arch Gen Psychiatry. 2009;66(1):95-105.
12. Hollister LE, et al. Health aspects of cannabis. Pharma Rev March. 1986;(38):1-20.
13. Wilson R, Nicoll A. Endocannabinoid signaling in the brain. Science. 2002;296 (5568):678-82.
14. Fernandez J, Allison B. Rimbonabant Sanofi-Synthelabo. Cur Opin Investigat Drugs. 2004;5:450–5.
15. Chopra GS, Smith JW. Psychotic reactions following cannabis use in East Indians. Arch Gen Psychiatry. 1974;30:24-7.

16. Carr JE, Tan EK. In search of the true amok: amok as viewed with the Malay culture. Am J Psychiatry. 1976;133(11):1295-9.
17. Carney MWP, Bacelle L, Robinson B. Psychosis after cannabis use. BMJ. 1984;288:1047.
18. Baselt R. Disposition of Toxic Drugs and Chemicals in Man, 8th ed. Foster City, CA: Biomedical Publications, 2008. pp. 1513–8.
19. Coulter C, Taruc M, Tuyay J, Moore C. Quantitation of tetrahydrocannabinol in hair using immunoassay and liquid chromatography with tandem mass spectrometric detection. Drug Test Anal. 2009;1:234-9.
20. AlterNet. Has the Most Common Marijuana Test Resulted in Tens of Thousands of Wrongful Convictions? 28 July 2010.

CHAPTER 46

Spinal Poisons

Putul Mahanta

LEARNING PLAN

- Learn the spinal poisons strychnine
- Know the details of strychnine poisoning and its management
- Identify the differences between strychnine and tetanus
- Learn about autopsy findings and its medicolegal important

SPINAL POISON

The actions of the spinal poisons are mainly noted on the spinal cord. It may be stimulant, like strychnine that may result in convulsion, or depressant, like gelsemium which may result in paralysis or loss of sensation.

STRYCHNINE

Common Name: Nux vomica, poison nut, snake-wood, semen strychnos, Quaker buttons, strychnine tree, ma qian zi, etc.

The **Strychnine tree** (*Strychnos nux-vomica L.*) is a deciduous tree native to India, Southeast Asia and a member of family Loganiaceae. It is a medium-sized tree, growing in open habitats. Its leaves are ovate and 5.1–8.9 cm in size[1] (**Figure 46.1**).

Fruits are globular. The seeds are round, disk shaped, concave on one side and convex on the other side as shown in **Figures 46.2A** and **B**.

The seeds are removed from the fruit when ripe. They are then cleaned, dried and sorted. The seeds are completely covered with hairs radiating from the center to the sides. The seeds are very hard, with a dark gray horny endosperm,

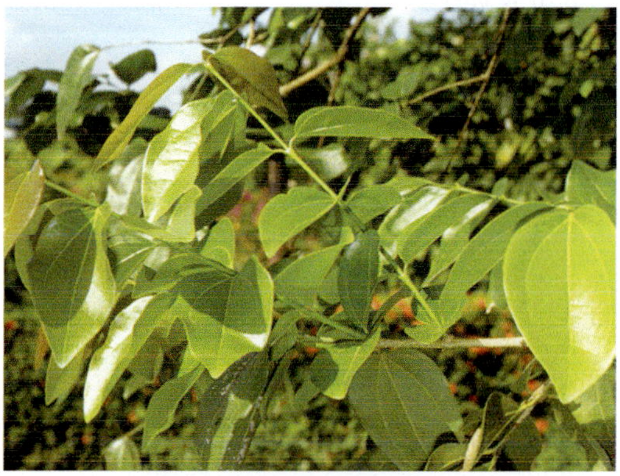

Figure 46.1 Strychnine tree

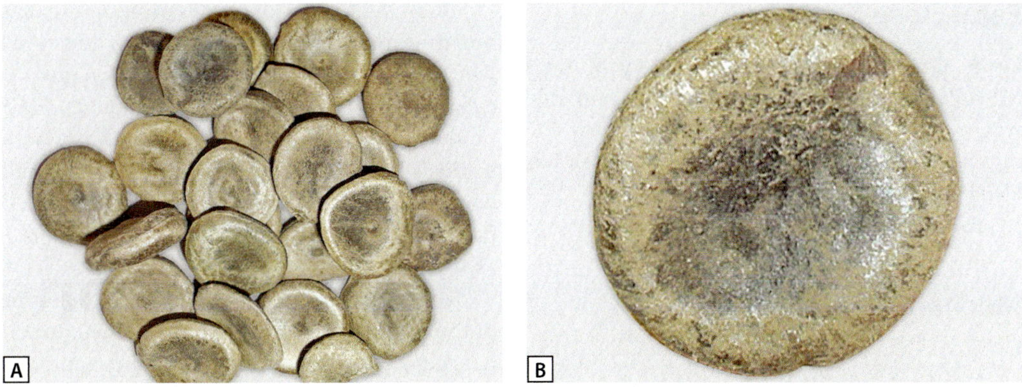

Figures 46.2A and B (A) Strychnos nux-vomica seed; (B) Strychnos nux-vomica seed (close-up view)

where the small embryo is housed, that gives off no odor but possess a very bitter taste. The plant is native to Southeast Asia and Australia, normally in tropical and subtropical areas.

Alkaloids

Strychnine is the main alkaloid found in the seeds of the plant Strychnos Nux-vomica, which is used in Homeopathic as well as Ayurvedic preparations. The seeds contain two principal alkaloids — Strychnine and Brucine — 1.5% each. Root, stem, bark and leaves contains brucine as a toxic principle and loganin as glycoside.

The seeds contain approximately 1.5% strychnine, and the dried blossoms contain 1.023%.[1] However, the tree's bark also contains brucine and other poisonous compounds.

Strychnine is an odorless white crystalline prism that melts at 275–285°C with decomposition. It is very bitter in taste and more powerful than brucine.

Medical Use

In herbal medicine, it is recommended for liver cancer, upset stomach, vomiting, abdominal pain, constipation, intestinal irritation, hangovers, heartburn, insomnia, certain heart diseases, circulatory problems, eye diseases, depression, migraines, nervous conditions, problems related to menopause and respiratory diseases in the elderly.

In folk medicine, it is used as a healing tonic and appetite stimulant. Strychnos nux-vomica is used in Chinese herbal medicine to unblock channels and obstructions, reduce swelling, and alleviate pain and to treat abscesses and yin-type ulcers. In traditional Chinese treatment of cancer, it can be used in combination with other herbs.

There are no uses in modern medicine, although it was widely used in medicine before World War II. The properties of nux-vomica are those of the alkaloid strychnine. The powder made from the strychnine seeds was used to alleviate indigestion. Mixtures of nux-vomica were also used as a stimulant on the gastrointestinal tract. In the mouth, it acts as a bitter dietary, increasing appetite by stimulating peristalsis. Strychnine also increases the flow of gastric juice. Brucine was used in pruritus and as a local anodyne in inflammations of the external ear.

Other Uses: Used as cattle poison, aphrodisiac agent, rodenticide, arrow poison for hunting, etc.

Pharmacokinetics

It is absorbed mainly from GIT and nasal mucosa, but not through skin. About 50% of the dose is distributed to all tissues within 5 minutes after absorption. It is metabolized in the liver to unknown metabolites. About 5–20% of the dose is excreted unchanged in the urine within 24 hours. Strychnine is eliminated with a half-life of about 12 hours.[2]

Fatal Dose

Seeds: One to two crushed seeds. Strychnine is a deadly poison and toxicity is mainly accidental with a lethal dose to humans is about 30–120 mg. Survival of substantially higher doses has also been reported.

Fatal period is 1–2 hours.

Mechanism of Action

It causes powerful stimulation of subcortical centers (thalamus, brainstem and spinal cord) by competitive inhibition of postsynaptic receptors of glycine (aminoacid), which is the major inhibitory neurotransmitter. Widespread inhibition in the spinal cord results in release of excitement. The action is particularly noted in the anterior horn cells.

Clinical Manifestations

Strychnine is rapidly absorbed as it reaches the intestines, after which it affects the central nervous system and the movements of respiratory system, causing a quicker and deeper breathing motion. Onset of symptoms appears after 15–30 minutes. it starts as restlessness, increased visual and auditory acuity, nausea, vomiting and muscle twitching, followed by sudden onset of generalized and extremely painful tonic fits in a completely conscious patient. These fit are characterized by sudden onset, generalized and tonic convulsions, and lasts for 0.5–2 minutes with 10–15 minutes intervals of complete relaxation in between fits. Retraction of jaw gives peculiar complexion called **risus sardonicus (Devil's laugh)**.

Body takes extensor position called **opisthotonus** position (antigravity position). During fits, there are apnea, bulging of eyes, cyanosis, bloody froth, dilated pupil, bradycardia, hypertension, hyperthermia, lactic acidosis and rhabdomyolysis. Patient is fully conscious. Patient cannot tolerate more than 2–3 fits and death occurs mainly from exhaustion or asphyxia during fits.

The heart is also slowed through excitation of the vagus center. The senses of smell, touch, hearing and vision are rendered more acute.

The most direct symptom caused by strychnine is violent convulsions due to a simultaneous stimulation of the motor or sensory ganglia of the spinal cord. Brucine closely resembles strychnine in its action, but is slightly less poisonous as it only causes paralysis of the peripheral motor nerves. It is said that the convulsive action of strychnine is absent in brucine.

Differential Diagnosis

Tetanus (basic differences between Strychnine poisoning and tetanus has mentioned in **Table 46.1**), head injury, meningitis, idiopathetic epilepsy and hysteria.

Management

Dark room, free from noise and disturbances is useful. A stomach pump should be used immediately, and potassium permanganate should be given to inactivate strychnine.

Convulsions may be controlled initially with diazepam 0.1–0.5 mg/kg IV slowly, and then phenobarbital IV should be given. Violent

Table 46.1 Differences between strychnine poisoning and tetanus

Differences	Strychnine poisoning	Tetanus
History of	Consumption of food	Injury
Onset	Sudden	Gradual
Convulsion	Generalized fits (all muscles) and complete relaxation in between fits	Start at lower jaw and tonic contractions with fixation of chest
Death	Rapid (1–2 hours)	More than 24 hours
Laboratory test	Positive for strychnine	Positive for bacteria

convulsions can be controlled with modern anesthetics, first by inhalation anesthesia followed by generalized anesthesia by interval and or muscle relaxation immediately by using curare, gallamine or pancuronium bromide. The convulsions may cause lactic acidosis and rhabdomyolysis.

Amyl nitrite is also useful owing to its rapid action during the convulsion, and in absence of respiration, 3–5 minutes may be hypodermically injected.

Antidote: There is no specific antidote. Mephenesin 20–30 mg IV and suxamethonium pancuronium 0.06–0.1 mg/kg IV Urethane in large doses is considered an antidote.

Acidifying the urine will increase excretion of strychnine. Supportive treatment: Maintain ABC and to treat acidosis and control myoglobinemia.

Postmortem Findings

Rigor mortis is rapid and persists for a longer time. Signs of asphyxia present. Extravasated blood may be found in the muscles. Froth at mouth. The stomach and duodenum show patches of extravasations of blood.

The spinal cord will also be congested. Microscopy shows multiple hemorrhages in anterior and posterior horns, with ring hemorrhages around the capillaries. Neurons may show chromatolysis.[3]

The Circumstances of Poisoning

It is sometimes used as homicidal in the form of alkaloid, or as powdered nux-vomica seeds, in spite of bitter taste. Suicide is rare because of the painful death. Accidental deaths are common.

REFERENCES

1. Arnold MD, Harry L. Poisonous Plants of Hawaii. Tokyo, Japan: Charles E. Tuttle Co. 1968; p. 20. ISBN 0804804745.
2. Strychnos Nux-vomica. American Cancer Society. Retrieved 3 Nov 2010.
3. Perper JA. Fatal strychnine poisoning a case report and review of the literature. J Forensic Sci. 1985;30:1 248-55.

CHAPTER 47

Peripheral Nerve Poison

Putul Mahanta, KK Bairagi

LEARNING PLAN

- Learn about peripheral nerve poisoning and management
- Identify the autopsy findings
- Understand their medicolegal importance

The actions of the peripheral nerve poisons are primarily noted on the end plates of the motor nerve terminals. The two important peripheral nerve poisons are: Curare and conium maculatum. The occurrence of these poisoning, however, is rare.

CURARE

Common Names: Curare, grieswurzel, pareira brava, vigne sauvage.

Curare is a dark resinous extract found from several tropical American woody plants, especially ***Chondrodendron tomentosum*** or certain species of **strychnos (Figure 47.1)**.

Medicinal Uses

1. Active ingredient D-tubocurarine, is used in medicine as skeletal muscle relaxant.
2. Brazilians consider the root as diuretic and use it internally in small quantities for madness and dropsy, and externally for bruises.
3. Also used for edema, fever and kidney stones.

Active Principles: D-tubocurarine

Mechanism of Action

Curare is an alkaloid, and acts as a neuromuscular blocking agent to produce paralysis in muscles. The action is seen on peripheral muscles. It blocks the postsynaptic nicotinic acetylcholine receptors at myoneural junction. Hence, it causes paralysis of skeletal muscle without affecting consciousness.

Fatal Dose: 30–60 mg.

Fatal Period: May be few hours.

Absorption, Metabolism and Excretion

It is slowly absorbed from gastrointestinal tract. On subcutaneous and intramuscular route, its absorption is rapid. Curarine is metabolized by liver and excreted through urine.

Clinical Features

It first affects the muscles of the toes, ears and eyes, then those of the neck, arms and legs and, finally, those involved in breathing. They cause flaccidity of muscle, headache, hypotension, vertigo, mydriasis, blurring of vision, hyperthermia, convulsions, etc.

With the fatal dose, death is caused due to respiratory paralysis. Curare must get into the blood system for it to work.

Management

i. Artificial respiration, such as mouth-to-mouth resuscitation, is useful in curare poisoning.
ii. In a study of 27 army volunteers who were paralyzed with curare, artificial respiration managed to keep an oxygen saturation of always above 85%,[1] a level at which there is no evidence of altered state of consciousness.[2] Yet, curare poisoning mimics the total locked-in syndrome in that there is paralysis of every voluntarily controlled muscle in the body (including the eyes), making it practically impossible for the victim to confirm consciousness while paralyzed.[3]
iii. Spontaneous breathing is resumed after the end of the duration of action of curare, which is generally between 30 minutes[4] to 8 hours,[5] depending on the variant of the toxin and dosage. The muscle paralysis can be reversed by administration of a cholinesterase inhibitor such as physostigmine, if available.[6]
iv. As the cardiac muscle is not affected by curare, cardiac resuscitation is unnecessary.
v. Atropine 0.6-1.2 mg, followed by 1-2 mg of physostigmine is given in a usual dose.

Autopsy Findings: There are those of asphyxia-like features with congested visceras.

Medicolegal Importance

i. Accidental poisoning is seen mainly.
ii. Used as arrow poison in hunting wild game.
iii. Homicidal use is rare.
iv. Anesthetic death may occur though rare.

CONIUM MACULATUM (FIGURE 47.2)

Common Name: Poison hemlock (hemlock - The Socrates poison), common hemlock, spotted hemlock, deadly hemlock, snake weed, wode whistle, California fern, herb bonnet, kill cow, muskrat weed bunk, etc.

Active Principles: Coniine and gamma-coniceine.

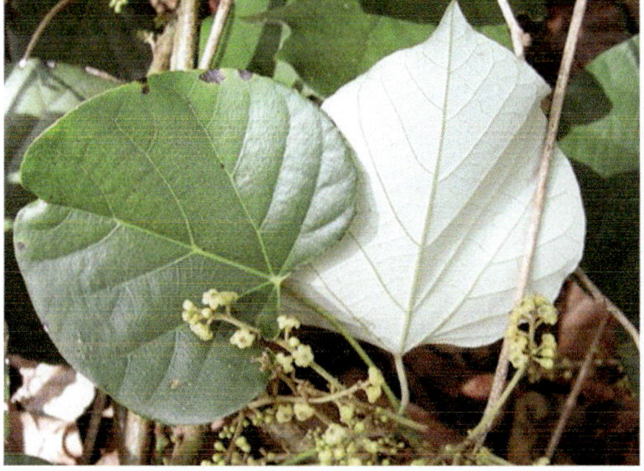

Figure 47.1 Curare plant

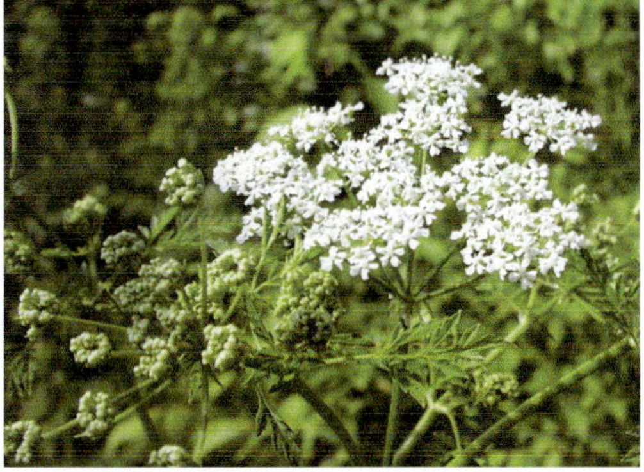

Figure 47.2 *Conium maculatum* plant

Medicinal Uses

1. Has been used as a sedative, antispasmodic
2. Also used by Greek and Persian physicians for a variety of problems, such as arthritis.

Mechanism of Action

It acts at neuromuscular junction as non-depolarizing blockers and causes flaccid paralysis and at autonomic ganglia, producing nicotinic effects such as salivation, mydriasis, tachycardia followed by bradycardia.

Fatal Dose: 60 mg of coniine.

Fatal Period: 1–3 hours

Clinical Features

The patient usually complains of nausea, vomiting, abdominal pain, salivation, tremors, sweating, convulsions, mydriasis, and tachycardia, followed by bradycardia. Overdoses can produce motor paralysis, hypotension and loss of speech, followed by depression of the respiratory function, and then death. The clinical feature appears immediately, hence demand emergent treatment.

Management

i. Airway maintenance and respiratory support.
ii. Gastrointestinal decontamination with activated charcoal.
iii. Benzodiazepines for convulsions.

Autopsy Findings

Signs are those of asphyxia. There may be mousy odor, when the poison is mixed with caustic potash and crushed in a mortar. The remains of the roots or leaves may be inside the stomach.

Medicolegal Importance

i. In older days, poison hemlock was used for execution. Socrates was executed by giving poison hemlock.
ii. Poisoning is rare in India. Most of the reported cases are accidental.
iii. It is also not a popular suicidal agent.

REFERENCES

1. Paradis NA. Cardiac Arrest: The Science and Practice of Resuscitation Medicine. Cambridge, UK: Cambridge University Press; 2007. p. 520.
2. McEvoy M. Oxymoron: Our Love-Hate Relationship with Oxygen. Albany Medical College. New York.
3. Damasio AR. The Feeling of What Happens: Body and Emotion in the Making of Consciousness. San Diego: Harcourt Brace; 1999. p. 357.
4. Rang HP. Pharmacology: For Therapeutic Dose of Tubocurarine by Shorter Limit. Edinburgh: Churchill Livingstone; 2003. p. 151.
5. The Alkaloids: A Review of Chemical Literature (Specialist Periodical Reports). For 20-fold paralytic dose of toxiferine ("calebas curare"). Cambridge: Royal Society of Chemistry; 1971. p. 330.
6. Morgan T III, Kalman B. Neuroimmunology in Clinical Practice. Wiley-Blackwell. 2007. p. 153.

CHAPTER 48

Asphyxiants (Toxic Gases)

YN Singha, Putul Mahanta

LEARNING PLAN

- Learn about different types of asphyxiants
- Know carbon dioxide, carbon monoxide, hydrogen sulfide and phosphine poisoning and thier management
- Identify their autopsy findings
- Understand the medicolegal importance

Asphyxiants are gases or vapors that can cause unconsciousness or death, by producing suffocation due to lack of oxygen. It is one of the major potential hazards for people working in a confined room where chemicals are used or stored. The chemical vapors can become so concentrated that it may reduce the normal oxygen level (about 21%) in the air to dangerous levels (<19%). Carbon monoxide (CO) works as asphyxiants by reducing the blood's ability to carry oxygen.

CLASSIFICATION OF ASPHYXIANTS OR TOXIC GASES

- Simple asphyxiants
- Respiratory irritants
- Systemic asphyxiants
- Volatile compounds.

Simple Asphyxiants

They remove oxygen (O_2) from surrounding air and bring about a reduction in the partial pressure of remaining available oxygen. There is alveolar displacement O_2, and they are non-irritating and have no direct mitochondrial toxicity. Examples are:

- Carbon dioxide
- Nitrogen
- Butane, Methane
- Noble gases like argon, helium
- Nitrous oxide.

Respiratory Irritants

They cause damage to the respiratory tract by neutralizing the mucosal barrier defenses. Examples are:

- Ammonia

- Chlorine
- Hydrogen sulfide
- Methyl isocyanates
- Sulfur dioxide.

Systemic Asphyxiants

They produce toxicity by systemic mechanisms, targeting different steps in the respiratory chain. Examples are:
- Carbon monoxide
- Cyanide
- Smoke.

Volatile Compounds

They act as anesthetic agents. The examples are:
- Aliphatic hydrocarbons
- Halogenated hydrocarbons
- Aromatic hydrocarbons.

CARBON DIOXIDE (CO_2)

Properties

- CO_2 is a colorless, odorless and heavy gas.
- Solid state of it is known as dry ice, which is used for industrial purposes.
- Atmosphere contains about 0.4% of CO_2.

Sources

- Mine explosions
- Deep wells, manholes, soil or cellar
- Respiration
- Decomposition of organic matter.

Action

In mild doses, stimulates breathing and is the chief physiological mechanism for control of respiration; an excess, however, conversely paralyses the same control mechanism.

Uses

- As fire extinguisher
- As respiratory stimulant in medicine
- Soft drinks aeration
- Gas welding.

Clinical Features

The normal concentration of CO_2 in air is 0.04%. According to the arterial oxygen concentration gradient, four stages have been described depending on oxygen saturation, as follows:

i. **Stage of Indifference**: Saturation up to 90% shows a decrease in night vision.

ii. **Stage of Compensation**: Saturation in between 82 and 90% shows compensatory increased rate of respiration, pulse and significant reduction in the performance ability, night vision and alertness.
Such a person may develop symptomatic conditions in coexisting diseases of cardiac, hematological and lung origin.

iii. **Stage of Disturbance**: Saturation in between 64 and 82%.
Failure of compensatory mechanisms leads to air hunger, fatigue, tunnel vision and dizziness. There is headache, nonchalance, euphoria and reduced visual acuity, along with hyperventilation, memory loss, confusion, cyanosis and poor judgment, all of which handicaps the person in his attempt to escape from his toxic surroundings.

iv. **Terminal or Critical Stage**: Saturation 60–70% or less. A cascading fall in judgment, comprehension and coordination abilities takes place in a matter of 3–5 minutes or less, leading to unconsciousness and coma rapidly. Death ensues when the oxygen levels go down to 6–8% or less.
Diagnosis: Assessment of arterial blood gases.

Management

i. Prompt removal to a safe environment.
ii. Airway care and removal of any obstructions.
iii. Artificial respiration with assisted ventilation.

Autopsy Findings

i. Cyanosis
ii. Prominent postmortem hypostasis
iii. Froth at nostrils and mouth
iv. Dilated pupils
v. Petechial hemorrhages
vi. Venous engorgement with pinkish-red and fluidic blood
vii. Congested organs and pulmonary edema
viii. Distended right chamber of heart.

Medicolegal Importance

Poisonings are mostly accidental, resulting from inadvertent carbon dioxide build-ups in a confined environment, e.g. mines, deep wells or burning house.

CARBON MONOXIDE (CO)

Properties

i. Colorless, odorless and lighter than air.
ii. It readily mixes with air to form a highly explosive, inflammable mixture.
iii. It results from the incomplete oxidation of carbon.
iv. It is also known as carbonic oxide, exhaust gas or flue gas.

Actions

i. Higher affinity for hemoglobin, 230–270 times greater than oxygen, bringing about a fall in the arterial oxygen content, forming carboxy-hemoglobin (COHb).
ii. It is further postulated that CO may also interfere with cellular respiration at the mitochondrial level by inactivating mitochondrial cytochrome oxidase.
iii. Causes brain lipid peroxidation, found in experimental animals, causing cellular toxicity. This occurs during the recovery stages, where peroxidation takes place, in turn producing reversible demyelination in the brain.
iv. Cardiac damage resulting in dysrhythmias is mainly because of reduced oxygen carrying capacity of the blood due to insult after CO toxicity, usually due to reduced oxygenation as a result of COHb formation and, partially, due to the binding of CO with myoglobin.[1]

Sources

i. Automobile exhaust gases
ii. Blast furnaces
iii. Fuel gas
iv. Tobacco smoke
v. Generated in explosions.

Maximum permissible concentration of CO for single exposure in air is 400 ppm; for chronic exposure it is 100 ppm. The usual fatal dose, expressed in terms of plasma concentration of COHb is 1–5% in adults, which may go up to 7%–8% in smokers.

Clinical Features

There may be variance according to the physical condition of the victim, health, oxygen demand and oxygen concentration of inspired air.

Acute Poisoning

Early features are often non-specific and manifestations get more profound with the severity of toxicity, which are tabulated below. The features of acute CO poisoning are mentioned in **Table 48.1**.

Thorough examination of the eyes may reveal that retinal hemorrhages occur frequently and usually, if not always, involves the nerve fiber layer near the disc.

The features are often mistaken or misdiagnosed and the differential diagnosis may include conditions ranging from alcoholism, cerebrovascular accidents and myocardial infarctions to less severe conditions including epilepsy.

Table 48.1 Clinical features of CO poisoning

Severity	Features
Mild (COHb <30%)	Headache, nausea, vomiting, giddiness, dyspnea
Moderate (30–40%)	Confusion, blurred vision, weakness, increased dyspnea and tachypnea, severe headache flushing, syncope, cyanosis, perspiration, prolonged reaction time, loss of judgment, muscular control, tinnitus drowsiness, etc.
Severe	Trismus, convulsions, muscle spasms, palpitations, hypotension, dysrhythmias, ischemia, pulmonary edema, coma and death

Other features include:

i. Sensorineural hearing loss
ii. Myocardial ischemia
iii. Muscle necrosis, rhabdomyolysis and compartment syndrome
iv. Bullae on the palms and soles, occasionally
v. Post CO syndrome of headache, nausea and weakness may persist for 2–3 weeks
vi. Sequelae may include dementia, amnesia, psychosis, Parkinsonism and paralysis along with personality changes such as irritability, aggressiveness, violence and moodiness.

Chronic Exposure

The chronic feature includes the following:

i. Headache, giddiness, confusion and intellectual deterioration
ii. Weakness, abdominal cramps, vomiting, nausea
iii. Paresthesia, muscle cramps
iv. Papilledema, scotomata, retinal hemorrhages
v. Hypertension, hyperthermia
vi. Red skin
vii. Palpitations, angina
viii. Increased RBC and WBC
ix. Albuminuria, glycosuria
x. Neurological and personality disorders as mentioned earlier.

Diagnosis

i. Determination of COHb level at the beginning and to be repeated every 2–3 hours till patient recovers.
ii. Monitor, ECG, CPK, urinalysis, arterial blood gases if symptomatic or if COHb is more than 20%.
iii. Bedsides, pulse oximetry may be done, but may not be reliable.

Management

i. Removal from site of vitiated environment
ii. Airway care
iii. Artificial respiration
iv. Administration of hyperbaric oxygen, to be inhaled at a pressure greater than 1 atmosphere absolute (ATA). 100% oxygen at ambient pressure reduces the half-life of COHb to 40 minutes; while at 2.5 ATA reduces it to 20 minutes. Hyperbaric oxygen is given with 30 minutes of 100% oxygen at 3ATA, followed by 60 minutes of 100% oxygen at 2ATA/until COHb of less than 10% is achieved.

Autopsy Findings

i. Pink to cherry red color of skin and mucosa
ii. Prominent postmortem hypostasis. The color of the lividity is pinkish
iii. Froth at nostrils and mouth
iv. Congested organs and pulmonary edema
v. Cutaneous blisters and bullae
vi. Cherry red color of viscera and blood
vii. Petechial hemorrhages
viii. Venous engorgement
ix. Color of blood is pinkish red and fluid
x. Petechial hemorrhages in white matter and putamen
xi. Necrosis of basal ganglia especially globus pallidus.

Medicolegal Importance

i. Mostly accidental in females. Death cases are usually domestic; and children and people with higher metabolic rates, e.g. pregnant women, elderly people and people with anemia, heart and lung diseases, are more prone to succumb.
ii. Suicidal use in man is popular in Western countries. Vehicular exhaust is used for this purpose.

HYDROGEN SULFIDE (H_2S)

Properties

i. Also known as dihydrogen monosulfide, dihydrogen sulfide, sulfur hydride or sulphuretted hydrogen. It is a colorless, heavy gas with a characteristic rotten egg smell.
ii. It rapidly paralyses olfactory nerve endings; thereby smell is not a dependable means of detection.
iii. It is a liquid at high pressure and low temperatures and is transported as liquid under its own vapor pressure.

Sources

Sewers, brewers vats, tanneries, cesspools and abandoned wells and excavations.

Actions

i. Irritation in the eyes, mucous membranes of the respiratory tracts, lungs
ii. Depresses the central nervous system
iii. Depresses the respiratory center.

Gets rapidly absorbed through the respiratory tract and changes to sulfate, thiosulfate, alkali and metallic sulfides and are excreted through the lungs, feces and kidneys.

Clinical Features

i. Eyes: Lacrimation and photophobia
ii. Pulmonary edema
iii. In mild toxicity there is vertigo, headache, muscle cramps and weakness
iv. In severe poisoning, there is initially respiratory stimulation then depression, bradycardia, cardiovascular collapse and coma, convulsion and death due to respiratory failure.

Fatal Dose and Period

Exposure to 1000 ppm causes loss of consciousness and death within an hour. When the concentration is doubled, it causes immediate death.

Management

i. Removal from exposure
ii. Oxygen inhalation
iii. Artificial and assisted respiration
iv. Maintenance of circulation.

Nitrites are antidotes in hydrogen sulfide poisoning. Methemoglobinemia, resultant of nitrites, attract H_2S, which has greater affinity for methemoglobin than cytochrome oxidase. Cytochrome oxidase thus freed is available for respiration.

Autopsy Findings

i. Greenish discoloration appears early, even before rigor mortis has passed off
ii. Congested viscera
iii. Petechial hemorrhages
iv. Degenerative changes.

Medicolegal Importance

Majority of cases are accidents from industrial and laboratory settings. Sewer cleaners have an occupational hazard in the sense that H_2S build-up in sewers may be potentially life threatening.

PHOSPHINE

Phosphine is a respiratory irritant and is generated from metallic phosphide.

It causes respiratory tract irritation, dyspnea, oppressive feeling in the chest and backache. In high concentrations, there may be pulmonary edema.

Management

i. Removal from site of exposure
ii. Respiratory assistance and continuity
iii. Oxygen therapy
iv. Symptomatic.

Autopsy Findings

i. Signs of respiratory tract irritation
ii. Signs of asphyxia
iii. Pulmonary congestion and edema.

Medicolegal Importance

Both acute and chronic exposure may take place, mostly in an industrial and commercial center accidentally.

REFERENCE

1. VV Pillay. Toxic Gases. In: Modern Medical Toxicology, 4th ed. New Delhi: Jaypee Brothers Medical Publishers (P) Ltd; 2013. p. 359.

CHAPTER 49

Paracetamol and Salicylates

YN Singha, Putul Mahanta

LEARNING PLAN

- Learn about paracetamol and salicylate poisoning and management
- Identify their diagnostic and autopsy findings
- Know the medicolegal importance of these poisoning

Salicylates and paracetamol fall under the class of analgesics and antipyretics. Antipyretics bring about fall in fever temperatures, whereas analgesics relieve pain. Anti-inflammatory drugs, obviously going by the name reduces inflammation.

There is nevertheless considerable overlap of all these characteristics in any given drug, and it is then classified according to the dominant property.

Analgesics and antipyretics of utmost import are salicylates and paracetamol and hence this book tries to inculcate knowledge of what these everyday drugs could cause when not used in temperance or without proper guidelines in the minds of the student.

SALICYLATES

These are derivatives of salicylic acid and include acetyl salicylic acid, sodium salicylates and methyl salicylates (**Figure 49.1**).

Salicylic acid (orthohydroxy benzoic acid) as such is highly irritant substance and can only be used externally. It was Hoffman from **Bayer** who first synthesized acetyl salicylate in 1897 and, along with **Heinrich Dreser**, made it fit for human consumption.

The name aspirin was coined in 1899, and since then, the drug has sustained in the service of humanity for so long in various ailments under different doses and schedules, apart from the original antipyretic and analgesic benefits.

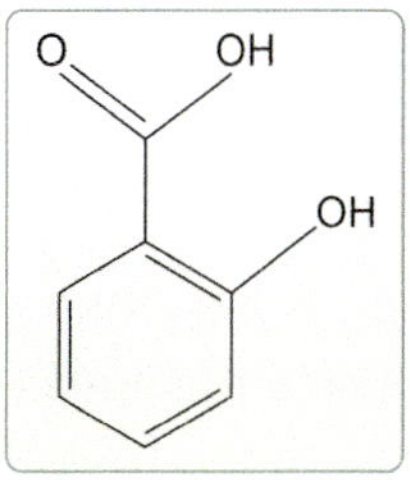

Figure 49.1 Chemical structure of salicylates

Appearance

Aspirin is an odorless, white, crystalline powder with an unpleasant salty taste. Sodium salicylates are again odorless, with white flaky crystals and salty taste. Methyl salicylates are liquid, colorless and aromatic with a sweetish taste.

They are available as tablets, capsules, powders, creams and liniments, syrups and injectable liquids.

Naturally salicin, a salicylate, is found in several plants, prominent among them being the willow tree, more famous for the manufacture of Cricket bats, marigolds, poplar trees, etc.

Uses

i. Aspirin and sodium salicylates used as:
   a. Antipyretic
   b. Analgesic
   c. Therapeutic use in rheumatoid arthritis
   d. Low doses are used in prevention of ischemic cerebrovascular events.
ii. Sodium aminosalicylate: Sometimes used as a second line therapy in tuberculosis.
iii. Bismuth subsalicylate: Indicated in the treatment of diarrhea and prophylaxis for traveler's diarrhea.
iv. A newer derivative, **mesalamine** (5-amino salicylate), is used in inflammatory bowel diseases for its local effects as a suppository. Benorylate an ester of aspirin and paracetamol (4-acetamidophenyl-o-acetyl salicylate) causes less gastric adversities.
v. **Locally acting**: Methyl salicylate oil, also known as "**oil of wintergreen**", is used as a topical liniment in musculoskeletal pain.

Pharmacokinetics

Reduction of fever by aspirin and its analogues is due to lowering of the elevated hypothalamic set point by reducing the level of PGE_2 in the thermoregulatory center, the production of which depends on the enzyme cyclooxygenase (COX).[1]

Hence, COX inhibitors are good antipyretics. This is the normal usage. In this present chapter, we are trying to zoom in on the adversities, which may follow due to an irrational use and toxic overdoses.

These are rapidly absorbed from the stomach and the small intestines. Methyl salicylates and salicylic acid are absorbed from the skin. These are then widely distributed in the body fluids and tissues, where after they are then metabolized in the liver.

They are broken down into salicylic acid, ether and ester glucoronide and gentisic acid. Excretion is mainly through the urine.

1. Salicylates stimulate the respiratory center in the brainstem, leading to hyperventilation and respiratory alkalosis.
2. Interferes with Krebs cycle, causes a reduction in ATP production and an increase in lactate production.
3. In minors, metabolic acidosis is the prominent feature; and such an effect in salicylate overdose invites serious consequences, often seen with pulmonary edema.
4. CNS depression may ensue in mixed overdose, especially with benzodiazepines, alcohol, barbiturates and tricyclic.
5. These are extreme gastric irritants, overdose often resulting in hemorrhagic gastritis. This is by far the most common toxic effect on note.

Clinical Features

Aspirin toxicity has potentially serious consequences, sometimes leading to significant morbidity and death.

Acute Poisoning

1. **Early:** Nausea, vomiting, tinnitus, hyperventilation resultant of respiratory alkalosis, vertigo. Confusion, irritability, disorientation, ataxia and inability to speak may be features of severe toxicity.
2. **Late:** Agitation, delirium, hearing loss, hallucinations and convulsions.

3. **Late Complications:** Thrombocytopenic purpurea, rhabdomyolysis, metabolic acidosis, cardiovascular depression, pulmonary edema, etc. GI bleeds, perforations are less common complications.

Salicylates are contraindicated in children, especially if they are suffering from chicken pox or influenza, for the possible development of **Reye's syndrome**, which can be life threatening, with acute hepatic failure and encephalopathy.[2]

Chronic Poisoning (Salicylism)

1. There is a slow onset of confusion, restlessness, lethargy and disorientation. Hallucinations, coma and convulsions may follow along with tinnitus and loss of hearing, vomiting and nausea, arrhythmias and the occasional rise in temperature.
2. Salicylism, may manifest as fever, Leukocytosis, hypotension, multi-organ failure and fever mimicking a septic condition, hence the term pseudo sepsis syndrome.
3. There may be thrombocytopenia, hypofibrinogenemia, increased fibrin degradation products, red blood cell fragmentation in patients with chronic salicylism.
4. Long-term use in the case of pregnant women is seen to be associated with stillbirths, ante- and postpartum bleeding, delayed labor and low birth weight.

The American academy of Pediatrics recommends cautious use of salicylates during breastfeeding.[2]

Acute toxic dose of Aspirin is generally taken to be 150 mg/kg of body mass. Moderate toxicity takes place at doses up to 300 mg/kg, severe toxicity occurs between 300 and 500 mg/kg, and a potentially lethal dose is greater than 500 mg/kg. Chronic toxicity may occur following doses of 100 mg/kg per day for two or more days.[3]

Diagnosis

Biochemical parameters such as electrolytes, liver and kidney function, urinalysis and complete blood count is measured and monitored, concurrent with serial measurements of salicylate and blood sugar levels.

Arterial blood gas titers will typically show respiratory alkalosis early in the course of toxicity due to excessive stimulation of the respiratory center, and is frequently the only finding in a mild case of toxicity.

An anion-gap metabolic acidosis occurs late in the course of the poisoning, especially if it is a moderate to severe overdose, due to the increase in protons in the blood.

Bedside Tests

i. **Ferric chloride test:** Few drops of 10% ferric chloride solution are added to 1 mL of urine. A purple color change indicates presence of salicylates. It is not specific, as similar results can be obtained in phenol, phenothiazine, phenylbutazone and oxyphenbutazone.

ii. **Trinder's test:** Trinder's reagent (40 g of mercuric chloride in 850 mL water with 120 mL of aqueous HCl and 40 g of hydrated ferric nitrate, diluted in a liter of distilled water) and sample evidence, viz. urine, vomitus, etc., 2 mL is mixed with 0.1 mL of this reagent and stirred for 5 seconds, a strong violet color indicates presence of salicylates.

iii. **Confirmatory tests:** Serum salicylate levels.

Management

All such patients should be conveyed to a hospital immediately for management and resuscitation.

Initial treatment of an acute toxicity includes resuscitation followed by gastric lavage, administering activated charcoal, which adsorbs the aspirin in the gastrointestinal tract. Stomach pumping is no longer routinely used in the treatment of poisonings, but is sometimes considered if the patient has ingested a potentially lethal amount. Emesis induction with syrup of ipecac is not recommended. Repeated doses of charcoal have been found to be of benefit in cases of aspirin toxicity.

Most clinical toxicologists administer additional charcoal if serum salicylate levels are found to be increasing.

Postmortem Findings

1. Occasional skin petechiae;
2. Gastric erosions, black altered blood may be present in the stomach;
3. Petechiae may be seen in the serous membranes;
4. There may be cerebral and pulmonary edema.

Medicolegal Importance

1. Most of the toxicities result from attempted suicides, a few may be accidental.
2. Fatalities due to aspirin induced anaphylaxis may not be ruled out without taking a proper medical and family history.

PARACETAMOL

Paracetamol toxicity follows excessive use or overdose of the drug paracetamol (acetaminophen). Chiefly causing liver injury, paracetamol toxicity is one of the most common causes of poisoning worldwide. In the US and the UK, it is found to be the major cause of acute liver failure (**Figure 49.2**).[4,5]

Individuals with paracetamol toxicity may be asymptomatic in the first 24 hours following overdose, while some others may present non-specific complaints such as abdominal pain and nausea. With progression, signs of liver failure develop which may include low blood sugar, low blood pH, bleeding and hepatic encephalopathy. Some cases spontaneously resolve, while untreated cases may even result in death.

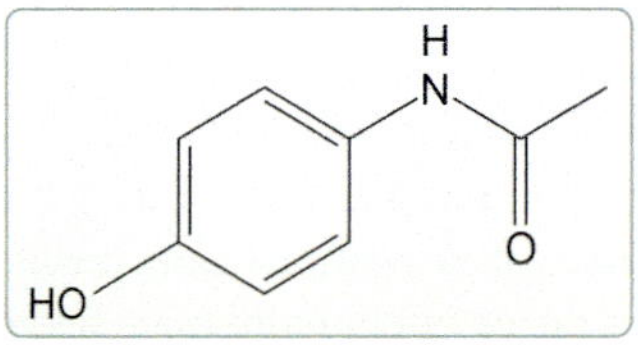

Figure 49.2 Chemical structure of paracetamol

Physical Appearance

- White in color
- Odorless
- Bitter in taste
- Crystalline shapes

Uses

- Antipyretic
- Analgesic

Pharmacokinetics

1. Rapidly absorbed from the alimentary tract, with peak levels in the serum attained within the hour. There may be delay in absorption in concurrence with other drugs or food.
2. Protein binding is around 5–20%; hence in overdose, half-life may be as long as 12 hours.
3. Metabolized in the liver by glucoronide conjugation, some part is oxidized to NAPQI by P450 mediation. A highly reactive intermediate hepatotoxicity results from one of the metabolites, N-acetyl-p-benzoquinoneimine (NAPQI; also known as N-acetylimidoquinone). NAPQI directly damages cells in the liver by depleting its natural antioxidant, Glutathione, which leads to liver failure. Risk factors for toxicity are excessive in chronic alcohol intake, fasting or anorexia nervosa and the use of certain drugs such as isoniazid.

Clinical Features

Acute Toxicity

1. Stage I: Within 24 hour, characterized by anorexia, nausea and retching, malaise and heavy sweating.
2. Stage II: 24–72 hour, less symptomatic, there may be right hypochondrial pain of a dull aching type. Liver assays may be abnormal.
3. Stage III: 72–96 hour, necrotic effects of acute toxic hepatitis sets in, featuring, coagulation

defects, jaundice and encephalopathy. There is re-emergence of nausea and vomiting, frequently, there are renal and myocardial damages. Death follows coma and is usually as a result of hepatic failure.

4. Stage IV: If the patient survives stage III, complete hepatic resolution is the rule, rather than an exception to it.

Chronic Toxicity

1. Uncommon.
2. Overdose more common in children, possibly due to miscalculation in dose schedule by ignorant guardians, characterized by anorexia, nausea, vomiting, lethargy, low body temperatures, hepatomegaly and oliguria.

Fatal Dose

1. Usually 20–25 g.
2. Children are seen to resist toxic effects better than adults.

Diagnosis

The most assured way for diagnosing paracetamol poisoning is a blood paracetamol level measurement. A drug monogram (developed in 1975, called the Rumack-Matthew monogram), calculates the risk of toxicity based on the serum concentration at given number of hours after ingestion. With a view to measure the risk of hepatotoxicity, paracetamol levels are traced along the monogram. Utilization of a timed serum paracetamol level plotting appears to be the best marker for liver injury.[6]

Clinical or biochemical evidence of liver damage may manifest in 1 to 4 days, although, in more extreme cases, it may be present in 12 hours. Right-hypochondrial tenderness can aid in diagnosis. Laboratory studies may show presence of hepatic necrosis with elevated AST, ALT, bilirubin and prolonged coagulation times, especially an elevated prothrombin time.[7] Following paracetamol poisoning, when AST and ALT exceed 1000 IU/L, paracetamol-induced hepatotoxicity can be expected.

Detection in Body Fluids

Paracetamol may be measured in blood, plasma or urine as a diagnostic tool in clinical poisoning situations or to assist the medicolegal investigation of suspicious deaths. Serum concentrations during treatment usually range from 2–20 mg/L, levels of 30–300 mg/L are often observed in poisonings. Postmortem blood levels have ranged from 50–400 mg/L in persons dying due to acute toxicity.

Management

- Stomach wash
- Activated charcoal
- Anti-emetic
- Supportive measures include, dextrose to counter hypoglycemia, vitamin K_I if Prothrombin time is elevated, fresh/frozen plasma in cases of overt bleeds, proton pump inhibitors and H_2 antagonists to counter upper GI bleeds
- Mannitol in cerebral edema
- Antibiotics
- Antidotal therapy:
    i. Methionine, a glutathione precursor, protects against paracetamol induced hepatic and renal damage, provided administration is done within 8–10 hours of ingestion at a dose of 2.5 g, 4 doses at 4 hourly intervals.
    ii. N-acetyl cysteine, a derivative of L-cysteine is naturally occurring and is the antidote of choice in most parts of the world; it gives maximum protection against hepatotoxicity when given within 10 hours of ingestion. It can be given both by the oral and IV routes according to the condition of the patient.[2]

Postmortem Findings

1. Enlarged liver, yellowish in color with centrilobular necrosis on microscopy.
2. Histological evidence of renal damage.
3. Cerebral and pulmonary edema.
4. Occasional sub-endocardial hemorrhages, focal degeneration and fatty changes.

Medicolegal Importance

1. Most cases come with a history of suicidal attempt.
2. Accidental cases may be seen in cases of inadvertent therapeutic overdose, more so in children.
3. Anaphylaxis is rare.

REFERENCES

1. Longo D, Fauci A, Kasper D, Hauser S, Jameson J, Loscalzo J. Harrison's Principles of Internal Medicine, 18th ed. New Delhi: McGraw Hill Medical; 2012. p. 989.
2. Pillay VV. Modern Medical Toxicology, 4th ed. New Delhi: Jaypee Brothers Medical Publishers (P) Ltd; 2013. pp. 422-513.
3. Temple AR. Acute and chronic effects of aspirin toxicity and their treatment. Arch Internal Med. 1981;141(3 Spec No):364-9.
4. Larson AM, Polson J, Fontana RJ, Davern TJ, Lalani E, Hynan LS, et al. Acute Liver Failure Study Group. Acetaminophen-induced acute liver failure: results of a United States multicenter, prospective study. Hepatology Baltimore, Md. 2005;42(6):1364-72.
5. Ryder SD, Beckingham IJ. Other causes of parenchymal liver disease. BMJ. 2001;22(7281):290-2.
6. Daly FF, Fountain JS, Murray L, Graudins A, Buckley NA. Guidelines for the management of paracetamol poisoning in Australia and New Zealand—explanation and elaboration. A consensus statement from clinical toxicologists consulting to the Australasian poisons information centres. March 2008.
7. Farrell, Susan E. Emedicine. Toxicity, Acetaminophen. Emedicine. October 3, 2007. [Cited 2013 March 25].

CHAPTER 50

Food Poisoning

Deepjyoti Kalita, Vijayamahantesh SN, Putul Mahanta

LEARNING PLAN

- What is food poisoning and what are the sources?
- Learn how to classify food poisoning
- Know about different etiological agents of food poisoning, e.g. bacteria, virus, fungi, plants, fish and other marine sources
- Understand about the pathogenesis and management of food poisoning
- Identify their diagnostic and autopsy findings
- Understand their medicolegal importannce

WHAT IS FOOD POISONING?

Food poisoning might be described as a food borne disease. Food that contains a toxin, chemical or infectious agent (like a bacterium, virus, parasite or prion) and cause symptoms in the body are considered food poisoning by most investigators. Those symptoms may be related only to the gastrointestinal tract, causing vomiting or diarrhea or may involve other organs such as the kidney, brain or muscle. Typically, most food-borne diseases result in vomiting and diarrhea that tend to be short lived and resolve on their own, but dehydration and electrolyte abnormalities may develop. According to the Center for Disease Control (CDC Atlanta) and Prevention, 76 million people become ill from food-related diseases each year, resulting in 325,000 hospitalizations and 5,000 deaths annually. People from 3rd world countries suffer frequently from food poisoning, and this is mainly attributable to lack of awareness, education, hygiene, sanitation, etc. in these countries.

Food poisoning can be of different sources

i. Microbes: Bacterial, viral, protozoal, fungal or parasitic origin
ii. Plants
iii. Fish
iv. Chemicals.

Classification of Food Poisoning

Based on symptoms and duration of onset

a. Nausea and vomiting within 6 hours (*Staphylococcus aureus, Bacillus cereus*).

b. Abdominal cramps and diarrhea within 8–16 hours (*Clostridium perfringens, Bacillus cereus*).
c. Fever, abdominal cramps and diarrhea within 16–48 hours (*Salmonella, Shigella, Vibrio parahemolyticus,* enteroinvasive *E. coli, Campylobacter jejuni*).
d. Abdominal cramps and watery diarrhea within 16–72 hours (Enterotoxigenic *E. coli, Vibrio cholerae* O1, *Vibrio cholerae* O139, *Vibrio parahemolyticus,* NAG vibrios, Norwalk virus).
e. Fever and abdominal cramps within 16–48 hours (*Yersinia enterocolitica*).
f. Bloody diarrhea without fever within 72–120 hours (Enterohemorrhagic *E. coli* O157:H7).
g. Nausea, vomiting, diarrhea and paralysis within 18–36 hours (*Clostridium botulinum*).

Based on pathogenesis

a. Food intoxications resulting from the ingestion of preformed bacterial toxins (*Staphylococcus aureus, Bacillus cereus, Clostridium botulinum* and *Clostridium perfringens*).
b. Food intoxications caused by non-invasive bacteria that secrete toxins while adhering to the intestinal wall (Enterotoxigenic *E. coli, Vibrio cholerae, Campylobacter jejuni*).
c. Food intoxications that follow an intracellular invasion of the intestinal epithelial cells (*Shigella, Salmonella).*
d. Diseases caused by bacteria that enter the bloodstream via the intestinal tract (*Salmonella typhi, Listeria monocytogenes*).

BACTERIA

Among the bacteria, the most important causes of food poisoning are: *Staphylococcus aureus, Salmonella, Shigella, Campylobacter, E coli* O157:H7, *Listeria monocytogenes* and *Clostridium botulinum.* Out of these **Botulism** (by *Clostridium botulinum*), is a condition of important forensic implication.

Botulism (Caused by *Clostridium botulinum*)

Clostridium botulinum is a sporulated anaerobic organism and responsible for one of the serious variant of microbial origin food poisoning. Out of 8 serotypes (A, B, C1, C2, D, E, F and G) A, B, E and F is the principal type responsible for human disease.

i. ***Clostridium botulinum*** releases a toxin called botulinum neurotoxin (BONT).
   a. This is considered most powerful toxin known and just 1–2 μg in pure crystalline form is enough to kill an adult human being.
   b. Toxin is exotoxin in nature and gets released more upon death/autolysis of the bacterial cell.
ii. Being a spore bearing agent, needs 121°C for 20 minutes to kill the pathogen. But the toxin is neutralized by boiling (at 100°C) suspected food for 10–15 minutes.
iii. **Pathogenicity**: Once spores contaminate food and anaerobiasis develops, spores germinate and vegetative bacilli multiply to release toxin. This toxin gets absorbed (from intestine or wound) via blood circulation, reaches cholinergic synapses, acts in the presynaptic membranes to stop acetylcholine release. This blockade at synapses and neuromuscular junction result in flaccid type of paralysis.
iv. **Three types of disease manifestation**

Food-borne

i. Most common end results from consumption of contaminated food, usually preserved food, where anaerobiasis is created, e.g. canned meat and meat product, vegetables, fish (canned).
ii. Rare but life-threatening paralytic disease.
iii. Incubation period: 12–36 hours.
iv. Clinical features: Vomiting, thirst, constipation, ocular paresis, dysphasia, dysarthria and dyspnea. First sign of illness is invariably constipation; diarrhea never a feature.

v. Descending, symmetric type flaccid paralysis first cranial nerves (diplopia, dysphasia, flaccid facial expression) progressing centripetally.
vi. Poor prognosis: 25–70% fatality, mainly due to respiratory paralysis.

Wound Botulism

Upon contamination of open wound with spores of *Clostridium botulinum*:

i. Extremely rare.
ii. Toxin produced at the site of wound is absorbed in blood and rest features are same as food-borne disease.

Infant Botulism

It is possibly due to contaminated honey feeding.

i. Rare, affects infants in the age group 3–20 weeks, often with start of mixed feeding.
ii. Disease is not due to preformed toxin (as above two types) but probably for spore-contaminated honey feeding, which results in establishment of *Clostridium botulinum* proliferation at the infant gut. Then botulinum toxin is absorbed from the gut.
iii. Disease manifests after a period of normal development, followed by constipation, weakness, lethargy and cranial palsies. Toxin and spores are excreted in the feces.

Diagnosis

Laboratory Diagnosis: To confirm clinical diagnosis.

i. **Demonstration of toxin**: Filtered extract from suspected food, vomitus, stool, wound swab etc., are injected intraperitoneally to 2–3 mice. One mouse (control) is protected with previous injection with antibody to botulinum toxin. Animal is watched for typical features of botulism within 24 hours of injection.
ii. **Demonstration of organisms**: By Gram staining and culture in media like Blood agar, Robertson's cooked meat, etc.

a. **Tensilon test**: To differentiate between botulism (negative result) and myasthenia gravis (positive result).
b. **Electromyography**: Brief, small, abundant motor unit action potential visualized.

Treatment

i. Prompt hospital admission and continuous monitoring is essential. In case of signs of bulbar palsy (diplopia, dysphasia, etc.) intubation/tracheotomy is life-saving.
ii. Respiratory support is very essential. Oral feeds contraindicated, unless gag reflex returns/intact.
iii. Gastric lavage or other methods of GI evacuation like catharsis/activated charcoal, etc. can make GI system free from spores and toxin.
iv. Trivalent (against common types, i.e. A, B and E) botulinum antitoxin can be injected IV. A pentavalent botulinum immunoglobulin (against type A, B, C, D and E) of human origin is available too. Availability of both in India is difficult.
v. Guanidine to improve flaccid paralysis. But side effects are high.
vi. Antibiotics indicated only in wound botulism, Penicillin G being the preferred agent.

Medicolegal Importance

i. Usually an accidental poisoning. But it has the potential for being used as homicidal agent or as agent of bioterrorism.
ii. Mostly occur as food-borne disease from eating improperly preserved home-canned food in the western world. Incidence in our country is very rare due to obvious food habit of ours.
iii. About 2% of reported cases are due to consumption of foods originating in commercial food processing units, 4% from restaurant purchased foods, but almost all the rest cases are due to faulty home-canning.
iv. Vegetables are the source in 70% cases, meat in 17% and fish in 13% cases.

Other Bacterial Agents

Staphylococcus aureus

Staphylococcus aureus is Gram-positive cocci that occur commonly in grape-like clusters. It is present ubiquitously in the environment. Only those strains that produce enterotoxin can cause food poisoning. Food is usually contaminated from infected food handler. The food handler with an active lesion or carriage can contaminate food.

Incriminated Food

Custard and cream-filled bakery food, ham, chicken, meat, milk, fish, salads, puddings, pie, etc.

Pathogenesis

If the food is stored for some time at room temperature, the organism may multiply in the food and produce toxin. The bacteria produce enterotoxin, while multiplying in food. *Staphylococcus aureus* is known to produce six serologically different types of enterotoxins (A, B, C, C2, D and E) that differ in toxicity. Most food poisoning is caused by enterotoxin A. Staphylococcal enterotoxins act as superantigens. The toxin acts on the receptors in the gut and sensory stimulus is carried to the vomiting center in the brain by vagus and sympathetic nerves.

Clinical Features

The onset is sudden and is characterized by vomiting and diarrhea, but no fever. The illness lasts usually less than 12 hours (most commonly much less than that). There are no complications, and treatment is usually not necessary.

Laboratory Diagnosis

The presence of a large number of *Staphylococcus aureus* organisms in a food may indicate poor handling or sanitation; however, it is not sufficient evidence to incriminate a food as the cause of food poisoning. Staphylococcal food poisoning can be diagnosed if they are isolated in large numbers from the food and their toxins (enterotoxin) are demonstrated in the food or the isolate. Dilutions of food may be placed on Baird-Parker agar or Mannitol Salt agar. Enterotoxin may be detected and identified by gel diffusion.

Bacillus cereus

Bacillus cereus is a Gram-positive aerobic spore bearing bacilli. It is found abundantly in environment and vegetation.

Incriminated Food

Commonly associated with **rice** and vegetables.

Pathogenesis

During the slow cooling, spores germinate and vegetative bacteria multiply, then they sporulated again. Sporulation is also associated with toxin production. The toxin is heat-stable and can easily withstand the brief high temperatures used to cook fried rice. The short-incubation form is most often associated with fried rice that has been cooked and then held at warm temperatures for several hours. Long-incubation food poisoning is frequently associated with meat or vegetable-containing foods after cooking. The short-incubation form is caused by a preformed heat-stable enterotoxin of molecular weight less than 5,000 Daltons. The long-incubation form of illness is mediated by a heat-labile enterotoxin (molecular weight of approximately 50,000 Daltons), which activates intestinal adenylate cyclase and causes intestinal fluid secretion.

Incubation Period

About 1–6 hours in short-incubation form, and 8–16 hours in long incubation form.

Clinical Features

Bacillus cereus causes two types of food-borne intoxications. The 'emetic-' or short-incubation type has an incubation period of 1–6 hours. It is characterized by nausea, vomiting and abdominal cramps and resembles *S. aureus* food poisoning in its symptoms and incubation period. Within 16 hours of eating contaminated fried rice, patients suffer a bout of vomiting that generally lasts for less than a day. The second type is manifested primarily by abdominal cramps and diarrhea with an incubation period of 8–16 hours. Diarrhea may be a small volume or profuse and watery. This type is referred to as the "long-incubation tppe" or diarrheal form of the disease, and it resembles food poisoning caused by *Clostridium perfringens.* In either type, the illness usually lasts less than 24 hours after onset.

Laboratory Diagnosis

The short-incubation form of the disease is diagnosed by the isolation of *B. cereus* from the incriminated food. The long-incubation or diarrheal form is diagnosed by isolation of the organism from stool and food. Isolation from stools alone is not sufficient because 14% of healthy adults have been reported to have transient gastrointestinal colonization with *B. cereus.*

Salmonella

Most often, food poisoning by *Salmonella* species occurs due to drinking of unpasteurized milk or eating of undercooked poultry and poultry products such as eggs. Any food prepared on the surfaces contaminated by raw chicken or turkey can also become tainted with *Salmonella.* Less often, the illness may stem from food contaminated by a food worker (see below for *Salmonella enteritidis* — the most important food-poisoning causing *salmonella*).

Enterotoxigenic E. coli (ETEC)

Enterotoxigenic *E coli* are Gram-negative enteric bacilli that are carried normally in the intestine of humans and animals. Some specific serotypes harbor plasmids that code for toxin production. The enterotoxin production is limited to following O serotypes: O6, O8, O15, O25, O63, O78, O148 and O159.

Incriminated Food

Infection is acquired by ingestion of food or water contaminated with ETEC. Contamination of water with human sewage may lead to contamination of foods. Infected food handlers may also contaminate foods. The infective dose is 10^6–10^{10} bacilli.

Pathogenesis

The bacteria colonize the GI tract by means of fimbriae to specific receptors on enterocytes of the proximal small intestine. Enterotoxins produced by ETEC include the LT (heat-labile) toxin and or the ST (heat-stable) toxin. LTs are similar to cholera toxin in structure and mode of action. They are holotoxin consisting of A subunit and B subunit. The B subunit of LTs binds to a specific ganglioside receptors (GM1) on the epithelial cells of small intestine and facilitates the entry of A subunit, where it activates adenylate cyclase. Stimulation of adenylate cyclase causes an increased production of cAMP, which leads to hyper-secretion of water and electrolytes into the lumen and inhibition of sodium reabsorption.

Incubation Period: 16–72 hours.

Clinical Features

Sudden onset of watery diarrhea associated with nausea, vomiting, abdominal cramping and bloating is commonly observed. This bacterium is responsible for majority of traveler's diarrhea. The disease is self-limiting and resolves in few days.

Laboratory Diagnosis

The sample of feces is cultured on McConkey's agar. The ETEC stains are indistinguishable from the resident enterotoxigenic coli by biochemical tests. These strains are differentiated from non-toxigenic enterotoxigenic coli present in the bowel by a variety of in vitro immunochemical, tissue culture or DNA hybridization tests designed to detect either the toxins or genes that encode for these toxins. With the availability of a gene probe method, foods can be analyzed directly for the presence of enterotoxigenic coli in about 3 days. LTs can be detected by Ligated rabbit ileal loop test, morphological changes in Chinese hamster ovary cells and Y1 adrenal cells, ELISA, immunodiffusion, coagglutination, etc.

Enterohemorrhagic E. coli (EHEC)

Enterohemorrhagic *E. coli* are Gram-negative enteric bacilli that are carried normally in the intestine of humans and animals. EHEC strains have been associated with many serogroups, including O4, O26, O45, O91, O111, O145 and O157. The most serotype is O157:H7.

Incriminated Food

Cattle appear to be the main source of infection; most cases being associated with the consumption of undercooked beef burgers and similar foods. This disease is often associated with ingestion of inadequately cooked hamburger meat, raw milk, cream and cheeses made from raw milk.

Pathogenesis

EHEC strains may produce one or more types of cytotoxin, which are collectively referred as Shiga-like toxins (SLT), since they are antigenically and functionally similar to Shiga toxin produced by *Shigella dysenteriae*. SLTs were previously known as verotoxin. The toxins provoke cell secretion and kill colonic epithelial cells.

Incubation Period: 72–120 hours.

Clinical Features

Initial symptoms may be diarrhea with abdominal cramps, which may turn into grossly bloody diarrhea in a few days. There is, however, no fever.

Laboratory Diagnosis

Laboratory diagnoses involve culturing the feces on McConkey's agar or on sorbitol McConkey's agar, where they do not ferment sorbitol. Strains can then be identified by serotyping using specific antisera. SLTs can be detected by ELISA and genes coding for them can be detected by DNA hybridization techniques.

Vibrio parahaemolyticus

They are straight or curved Gram-negative halophilic (salt loving) bacilli. In morphology and staining, it resembles *V. cholerae* and is actively motile in liquid cultures. It is commonly found in coastal seas, where it has been isolated from marine fauna such as crabs, shrimps, fishes and molluscs.

Incriminated Food

Infections are associated with consumption of uncooked or undercooked crabs, prawns, shrimps and other sea foods.

Pathogenesis

No enterotoxin has been demonstrated in the bacterium. The infection is thought to result from invasion of intestinal epithelium.

Incubation Period: 7–48 hours.

Clinical Features

The clinical infection is characterized by a sudden onset of acute gastroenteritis. Infection may also result in diarrhea, abdominal pain, vomiting and fever.

Laboratory Diagnosis

Homogenized food may be inoculated into TCBS agar or into double strength alkaline peptone water and incubated overnight at 37°C. This bacterium is positive for Kanagawa phenomenon, where isolates from human feces show hemolysis on blood agar.

Salmonella enteritidis

These are Gram-negative rod-shaped bacteria that are classified under family Enterobacteriaceae. Several animals act as reservoirs.

Incriminated Food

Most important sources are chicken and poultry. Chicken, duck, turkey and goose may be infected with *Salmonella*, which then find its way into its feces, eggs or flesh of dressed fowl. Milk and milk products, including ice creams, have been incriminated.

Pathogenesis

Organism penetrates and passes through the epithelial cells lining the terminal portion of the small intestine. Multiplication of bacteria in the lamina propria produces inflammatory mediators, recruits neutrophils and triggers inflammation. Release of LPS causes fever. Inflammation causes release of prostaglandins from epithelial cells. Prostaglandins cause electrolytes to flow into lumen of the intestine.

Water flows into lumen in response to osmotic imbalance, resulting in diarrhea.

Incubation Period: 12–36 hours.

Clinical Features

Sudden onset of abdominal pain, nausea, vomiting and diarrhea, this may be watery, greenish and foul smelling. This may be preceded by headache and chills. Other findings include prostration, muscular weakness and moderate fever. In most cases, the symptoms resolve in 2–3 days without any complications.

Laboratory Diagnosis

Homogenized food is cultured in selenite F broth and then sub-cultured on deoxycholate citrate agar. Plates are incubated at 37°C overnight and growth identified by biochemical tests and slide agglutination test.

Yersinia enterocolitica

It is a Gram-negative psychrophilic rod-shaped bacterium that is motile only at temperature below 30°C. *Yersinia enterocolitica* is widely distributed in environment and have been isolated frequently from soil, water and animals. The major animal reservoir for *Y. enterocolitica* strains that cause human illness is pigs, but may also found in many other animals including rodents, rabbits, sheep, cattle, horses, dogs, and cats. Serogroups that predominate in human illness are O: 3, O: 8, O: 9, and O: 5.

Incriminated Food

Infection is most often acquired by eating contaminated food, especially raw or under-cooked pork products. Drinking contaminated unpasteurized milk or untreated water can also transmit the infection.

Pathogenesis

This organism may survive and grow during refrigerated storage. Strains that cause human yersiniosis carry a plasmid that is associated with a number of virulence traits. Ingested bacteria adhere and invade M cells or epithelial cells. They exhibit resistance to complement and phagocytosis. They produce ST only at temperatures below 30ºC. The role of ST in the disease process remains uncertain.

Incubation Period: 4–7 days.

Clinical Features

Disease produced by *Y. enterocolitica* is a typical gastroenteritis characterized by fever, abdominal pain and diarrhea, which is often bloody. Illness generally lasts from 1 to 2 weeks, but chronic cases may persist for up to a year. Apart from gastroenteritis, it may also cause pseudoappendicitis, mesenteric lymphadenitis and terminal ileitis.

Laboratory Diagnosis

Suspected food is homogenized in phosphate-buffered saline and inoculated into selenite F broth and held at 4°C for 6 weeks. The broth is sub-cultured at weekly intervals on DCA or Yersinia selective agar plates. This is termed as cold enrichment technique.

Clostridium perfringens

It is a Gram-positive anaerobic spore bearing bacilli that is present abundantly in the environment, vegetation, sewage and animal feces.

Incriminated Food

Food-borne outbreaks of *Clostridium perfringens* involve meat products that are eaten 1–2 days after preparation. Meats that have been cooked, allowed to cool slowly, and then held for some time before eating are commonly incriminated. Fish pastes and cold chicken too have been incriminated.

Pathogenesis

Spores in food may survive cooking and then germinate when they are improperly stored.

When these vegetative cells form endospores in the intestine, they release enterotoxins. The bacterium is known to produce at least 12 different toxins. Food poisoning is mainly caused by Type A strains, which produces alpha and theta toxins. The toxins result in excessive fluid accumulation in the intestinal lumen.

Incubation period: 8–24 hours.

Clinical Features

Illness is characterized by acute abdominal pain, diarrhea and vomiting. Illness is self-limiting, and patient recovers in 18–24 hours.

Laboratory Diagnosis

Since the bacterium is present normally in the intestine, their isolation from feces may not be sufficient to implicate it. Similarly, isolation from food except in large numbers (>105/g) may not be significant. The homogenized food is diluted and plated on selective medium as well as Robertson cooked meat medium and incubated anaerobically. The isolated bacteria must be shown to produce enterotoxin.

VIRAL AGENTS

Various viruses are responsible for food poisoning; mainly:

i. Norovirus, calcivirus, hepatitis A virus (in the early stage), rotavirus, etc.
ii. Norovirus food poisoning manifests as severe gastroenteritis of very rapid onset. It is highly contagious and is responsible for outbreaks in ship, community and other facilities set-up for treating cases.

PROTOZOAL AGENTS

Cryptosporidium parvum and *Giardia lamblia* are capable of living in and causing gastrointestinal symptoms. Contaminated feces get into drinking water or water kept for cooking. Usually, these organisms get into domestic water supply and causes epidemic subsequently.

Protozoa produce cysts, and they are usually removed by filtration. Only few cysts are all that is required for causation of protozoal diseases. Giardia in stool sample can be demonstrated under light microscopy **(Figures 50.1A and B)**.

FUNGAL (MUSHROOM POISONING)

i. Less than 5% of world's mushroom is poisonous, and these fall under two genus: *Basidiomycetes* and *Ascomycetes*.
ii. Among the rest, many are edible and part of popular cuisine all over the world. Some are considered for their medicinal quality too.
iii. Important morphological parts in mushroom (**Figure 50.2**) include:
    a. **Pileus**: Cap-like broad structure at the top. Shape and color varies from species to species.
    b. **Gills** or **lamellae**: Seen in the under surface of pileus, fans out like a spoke of wheel. Lamellae contain a microscopic structure called **spores** in millions, and they are responsible for reproduction. Color of spore varies with species of mushroom. Lamellae

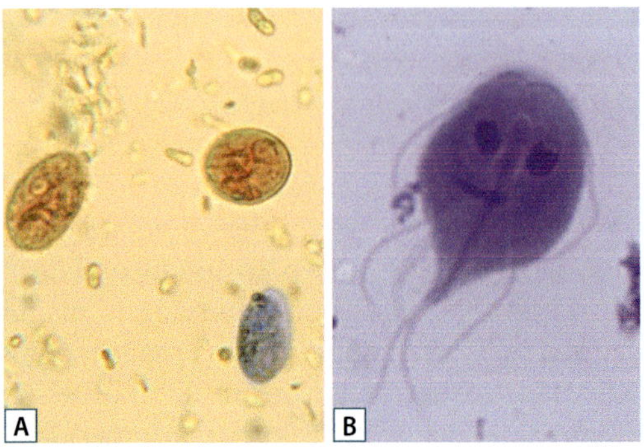

Figure 50.1A and B *Giardia* in stool sample under light microscopy, (A) Cyst; (B) Trophozoite

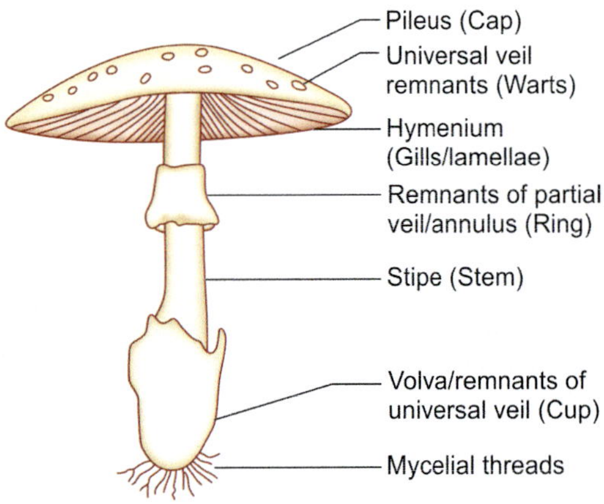

Figure 50.2 Various part of mushroom

may contain **pits**, which are under surface opening of hundreds of micro-tunnel expanding the breadth of pileus.

c. **Stipe**: Stem or stalk supporting the pileus.
d. **Annulus**: Rig-like structure at the junction of stipe and pileus.
e. **Veil** is the membrane covering lamellae often incompletely. Remnant of veil at the base of the stipe is known as **Volva**.
f. **Mycelium**: This is the underground, usually invisible, part of mushroom, a mass of filaments or hyphae, consisting the main vegetative portion.

Though there are no easy methods to identify the poisonous varieties of mushrooms, they are said to be having bitter astringent acid or salt taste, and on cut section and exposure, brown green or blue color develops over the surface. There are eight types of toxin producing or poisonous mushrooms, viz.

i. Cyclopeptide containing mushroom, e.g. *Amanita* species (*A. phalloides, A. virosa*); *Galerina* species (*G. autumnalis, G. marginata*), *Lepiota species* (*L. helviola, L. chlorophyllum*).
ii. Monomethyl hydrazine containing mushrooms, e.g. *Gyromitra* species (*G. esculenta*, G *californica*), *Lycoperdon* species (*L. marginatum, L. perlatum*).
iii. Muscarine containing mushrooms, e.g. *Clitocybe* species (*C. dealbata, C. cerussata*), *Inocybe* species (*I. lacera, I. napipes*).
iv. *Coprine* containing mushrooms, e.g. *Coprinus atramentarius.*
v. Ibotenic acid and Muscimol containing mushroom, e.g. *Amanita muscaria, A. pantherina.*
vi. Psilocybin containing mushrooms, e.g. *Psilocybe caerulipes, P. semilanceata.*
vii. Gastroenteritis inducing mushrooms, e.g. *Agaricus augustus, Boletus sensibilis, Chlorophyllum molybdites.*
viii. Orelline and Orellanine containing mushrooms, e.g. *Cortinarius orellanus.*

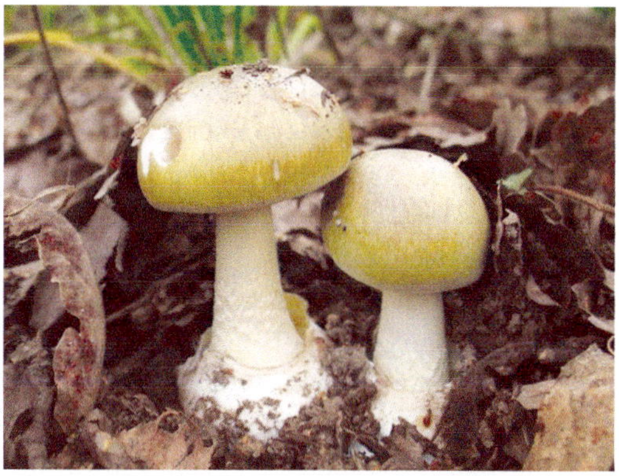

Figure 50.3 *Amanita phalloides*

Cyclopeptide Containing Mushrooms

i. Commonest species is *Amanita phalloides* (**Figure 50.3**), also known as death cap.
ii. Contains cyclopeptide toxins like amatoxin, phallotoxin and virotoxin. They target those organs with highest cell turnover, e.g. gastrointestinal epithelium, hepatocytes and kidney.

Clinical Features

Incubation Period: 6–24 hours.

Fatal Dose: 2–3 mushrooms.

The features are: Abdominal pain, diarrhea, vomiting initially for a day or about; followed by phase of remission, where patient feels well and cured, but soon (2–3 days after ingestion) fatal third phase ensues with hepatorenal failure and pancreas shut down. Raised liver enzymes, unconjugated hyperbilirubinemia and marked hypoglycemia are the hallmarks. Patient develops hepatic encephalopathy and coma, followed by death within 10 days of ingestion of so-called Death Cap. 2–3 mushrooms of *A. phalloides* is fatal.

Diagnosis

i. Above clinical and laboratory features
ii. Toxin may be detected in gastric aspirate, serum, urine, stool, liver and kidney biopsies.

Management

i. Restoration of fluid and electrolyte.
ii. IV glucose for hypoglycemia.
iii. FFP, packed RBC and vitamin K infusion in case of massive fluid loss/GI bleeding.
iv. Decontamination by activated charcoal, forced diuresis, etc.
v. Benzyl penicillin (3–10 lacs) displaces toxin from plasma protein binding site, leading to renal excretion.
vi. Silymarin extract, e.g. Silybinin to counter hepatotoxicity.
vii. Cimetidine may have hepatoprotective action against alpha amanitin as Cytochrome P450 inhibitor.
viii. Anti-phalloidin serum.

Autopsy Findings

a. Main target organ of this group of mushroom (Cyclopeptide containing) is liver, unlike other groups of mushrooms.
b. Liver findings: Steatosis, central zone necrosis, centrilobular hemorrhage.
c. Fatty degeneration is also seen. Inflammation of mucous membrane of alimentary tract is present.

PLANTS

Accidental contamination or deliberate adulteration of food by few plant products may cause food poisoning. Prominent among these are: Cyanogenic plants, fava beans, cycads, sweet pea and Mexican poppy.

Mexican Poppy or Argemone Mexicana or Prickly Poppy

i. A prickly robust herb bearing thistle-like leaves and yellowish flower. Plant can grow up to 4 feet in height.
ii. Seeds are similar to dark mustard: small, round and brownish black. Deliberate or accidental contamination is easy.
iii. Seeds are toxic part containing toxic principle, an alkaloid called sanguinarine or its derivative hydrosanguinarine.
iv. Argemone causes cell membrane destruction. Its principal action is over the small blood vessels, causing increase permeability and loss of fluid and protein from vascular compartment of the body. The hypovolemia will cause decrease blood flow to kidney and compensatory fluid and salt retention via (rennin angiotensin aldosterone system). If compensation is not sufficient, severe cases hypovolemia will persists and so also salt and water retention, leading to a marked anasarca. Finally pulmonary edema, right-sided heart failure, congestive hepatomegaly and effusion into other body cavities result.

Chronic consumption of food prepared with adulterated mustard or vegetable oil (with Argemone oil) leads to a condition called epidemic dropsy.

i. It is of slow onset with pitting pedal edema and limb pain.
ii. Diarrhea, pain abdomen, fever in the early stage.
iii. Glaucoma, retinal bleeding, disc edema seen.
iv. Erythematous skin with telangiectasias.
v. Cardiac failure, pulmonary edema, hepatomegaly, renal dysfunction, normocytic hypochromic anemia with raises ESR.

Management

i. Withdrawal of contaminated oil.
ii. Leg elevation, protein rich diet, vitamin supplement, antioxidant, calcium tabs.
iii. Corticosteroids, diuretics.
iv. Management of cardiac failure.
v. Glaucoma treatment: surgical usually.

Medicolegal Importance

i. There is no legitimate use of Argemone seed or oil in India. Here, mustard oil or other vegetable is adulterated with

Argemone oil very often. Sometime dark variety of mustard seed is mixed with Argemone seed.

ii. Since first reported case of epidemic dropsy in Calcutta (1877), number of cases has been reported as a type of periodic epidemic. It is reported from other countries, like South Africa, Mauritius, Myanmar, Fiji, Madagascar, also, especially where Indian population exists.

iii. In India, it is mainly a North-Indian syndrome, confined to states like West Bengal, Odisha, Bihar, MP, Gujarat, Maharashtra. almost all outbreaks are due to consumption of contaminated mustard or vegetable oil. Cases from South India are extremely rare as mustard oil is not popular there.

iv. Latest epidemic in Delhi on 1998: Not only the unsealed, open variety of mustard oil was contaminated, but oils sold in sealed branded containers (Tin, Bottle) were found to be contaminated with Argemone oil. In fact, other vegetable oil, vanaspati and ghee (clarified butter) were found to be contaminated.

CHEMICALS

This includes heavy metals, pesticides and food additive.

Food Additive: Antioxidants, flavoring agents, coloring agents, sweetening agents, thickening agents, preservatives, etc. Toxicity of a chemical called Monosodium Glutamate (MSG) is significant.

MSG (Monosodium Glutamate)

(Ajinomoto, Accent, Vetsin)

i. Flavoring agent in foods like Chinese dishes, sausage, canned soup, etc.
ii. Large quantity ingestion might result in Chinese restaurant syndrome (CRS).
iii. Burning sensation and numbness in face, trunk and upper limbs. Flushing, chest pain, headache, nausea, bronchospasm and angioedema may be seen.
iv. Convulsive attack in young children (shudder attack) is seen.
v. Self-limited condition.

Lathyrus Sativus

This is a staple food in certain parts of central India, a pulse which can grow in draught-like conditions. The active principle is b-oxalyl aminoalanine (**BOAA**), which is present as a free amino acid in the seeds. Consumption of these seeds in large quantities is known to cause paralysis.

Clinical Features

i. Pain in the back.
ii. Weakness of legs.
iii. Difficulty in sitting down and getting up.

In the later stages:

i. There is difficulty in walking without aid of a stick.
ii. There is spastic gait, characterized by walking on tip toes with legs crossing scissor wise.
iii. The knee jerks are increased.
iv. Ankle clonus is marked.
v. Babinski sign is present.
vi. Later, complete paraplegia occurs.

Prevention: Rich diet with exclusion of the pulse. Steeping the pulse in hot water and parboiling is said to remove most of the toxic substance.

Death is rare and autopsy of lateral columns of spinal cord show sclerosis.

POISONING BY FISH AND MARINE ORGANISMS

Poisoning by consumption of certain kinds of fish is referred as **Icthyotoxicosis**. This may be of various types and include:

1. **Ciguatoxin** is odorless and colorless and is present in some algae consumed by certain fish. Poisoning occurs when such fish is consumed by humans. In these conditions poisoning can occur in spite of proper storage and cooking of fish, and there is no

alteration in the smell or taste of the fish. Symptoms include diarrhea, vomiting, cramps, paresthesia, headache, blurred vision, ataxia and weakness. The reversal of hot-cold sensation is said to be feature of this type of fish poisoning. Treatment is supportive and symptoms resolve with amitriptyline.

2. **Scombrotoxin** is breakdown product of muscles of scombroid fish. Poisoning mainly results from improper preservation of the fish. There will be histamine-like symptoms, which may include pruritus, urticaria, dysphasia and headache. Cardiac arrhythmias can occur. Symptoms subside in few hours. Treatment involves supportive measures. Antihistamines are useful.
3. **Saxitoxin** is present in certain dinoflagellates concentrated by bivalve shellfish. Consumption of such fish results in vomiting, diarrhea, abdominal pain, ataxia and myalgia. Treatment is supportive.
4. **Tetrodotoxin** is present in liver, ovaries, kidneys and intestines of puffer fish. On ingestion there is vomiting, weakness, paresthesia, followed by ascending paralysis. In serious conditions, there is hypotension, bradycardia and fixed dilated pupils. Atropine is useful in treating such patients and neostigmine restores muscle strength.

Fatalities are uncommon and are of no or very little medicolegal significance. Almost all of them are accidental in nature, and autopsy findings are not adequately reported in the literature.

CHAPTER 51

Substance Abuse

Anku Moni Saikia, Putul Mahanta

LEARNING PLAN

- Learn about situational analysis of substance abuse
- Understand the various terminologies
- Learn commonly used substances of abuse and their effects
- Know the causes and risk factors
- Understand the medicolegal aspect of substance abuse
- Know about the management

BRIEF OVERVIEW OF SUBSTANCE ABUSE

Substance abuse forms an important public-health priority in terms of disease, disability and productivity. Harmful or hazardous use of psychoactive substances, including alcohol and illicit drugs, is called **substance abuse**.[1] The non-medical use of psychoactive drugs and alcohol has become an issue of grave concern in the world. Substance use is a serious problem, more so because it is gradually engulfing the younger segment of the population with serious health, social and economic impact. Strict legal restriction on production, supply and sale of psychoactive substances, education and counselling of the community and facilities for treatment and rehabilitation are the important measures to tackle this problem.

Substance abuse has been a menace throughout the world for many centuries. It is not a new phenomenon. Throughout the history, psychoactive substances have been found to be used commonly for a variety of purposes such as medicine or in rituals and ceremonies. However, this problem has catapulted to massive proportions throughout the world in recent times. More and more adolescents are drawn into this quagmire of substance use. There is enough evidence regarding the relationship of younger age of initiation with increased risk of dependence in later life. The World Health Report, 2002, identifies tobacco, alcohol and illicit drugs as three risk factors among the list of 20 leading risk factors for health. It also indicated that 8.9% of the total burden of disease arises from the use of psychoactive substances. Variety of health and social problems including

HIV/AIDS is attributable to substance use and dependence. The WHO estimates that, globally, 8.8% (4.9 million), 3.2% (1.8 millions) and 0.4% (0.2 million) of deaths are attributable to tobacco, alcohol and illicit drugs use, respectively. It is predicted that it will cause an estimated 10 million deaths each year by the 2020s or early 2030s, with 70% of these deaths occurring in developing countries.[2]

The South East Asian region is a part of the world which is greatly affected by this problem. A part of the notorious **Golden Triangle** (Myanmar, Thailand and Laos) falls within this region. India, Bangladesh and Nepal have become major trans-shipment points for hard drugs. In India, North Eastern region is observed to be heavily affected and this is due to easy drug trafficking across the international border with Myanmar and the Golden Triangle.

DEFINITIONS

The term '**Substance**' can refer to a drug of abuse, a medication or a toxin.[3] '**Substance use**' means "inappropriate consumption of medicines, drugs or other materials including prescription drugs, over-the counter drugs, alcohol and tobacco".[4]

The World Health Organization (WHO) defines '**substance abuse**' as "the harmful or hazardous use of psychoactive substances, including alcohol and **illicit drugs**". In DSM-IV, '**psychoactive substance abuse**' is defined as a "maladaptive pattern of use indicated by ... continued use despite knowledge of having a persistent or recurrent social, occupational, psychological or physical problem that is caused or exacerbated by the use (or by) recurrent use in situations in which it is physically hazardous".[1]

WHO expert committee introduced the term '**dependence**' to replace '**addiction**' and '**habituation**'. In DSM-IIIR, '**dependence**' is defined as "a cluster of cognitive, behavioral and physiologic symptoms that indicate a person has impaired control of psychoactive substance use and continues use of the substance despite adverse consequences.[1]

Dependence has both physical and psychological elements. In **physical dependence**, drug user becomes accustomed to a particular drug for functioning normally. When the person stops taking the drug abruptly, he experiences a variety of adverse effects, known as the 'withdrawal symptoms'. **Psychological dependence** refers to the experience of impaired control over the use of drug or substance. There is emotional distress if drug is withdrawn.

Tolerance: Tolerance as defined by either of the following: (a) A need for markedly increased amounts of the substance to achieve intoxication or the desired effect or (b) Markedly diminished effect with continued use of the same amount of the substance.

Substance Withdrawal: Withdrawal is characterized by maladaptive behavior and clinically significant distress or impairment in social, occupational or other important areas of functioning. The signs and symptoms of withdrawal vary with the class of drug, its dose and duration of use. Usually, the symptoms appear by 8–24 hours of stopping of the drug and last for a week or so. The same substance (or closely related substance) is needed to be used to relieve or avoid these symptoms.

Some drugs (alcohol, opiates and tranquilizers) produce significant physical withdrawal. Some drugs (cocaine, marijuana and ecstasy) produce more emotional and little physical withdrawal. Emotional symptoms are anxiety, restlessness, irritability, insomnia, headache, poor concentration, depression, social isolation, etc. The physical symptoms may include sweating, palpitation, difficulty in breathing, tremor, nausea, vomiting, diarrhea, muscle tension, tightness in the chest, etc. Alcohol and tranquilizers produce the most dangerous physical consequences like seizures, strokes or heart attack in high-risk patients.[5]

Hard Drugs: Hard drugs are more addictive, usually injectable and lead to severe psychological and also physical dependence, e.g. heroin, cocaine.

Soft Drugs: These drugs may produce psychological dependence but little or no physical dependence; hence their uses are relatively accepted in the society, e.g. sedatives, caffeine, cannabis, tranquilizers, amphetamines, alcohol, tobacco, hallucinogens, etc.

Substances of abuse can be divided into following groups:

- Ethanol
- Tranquilizers, sedatives and hypnotics like barbiturates, benzodiazepines, etc.
- Cannabis
- Opiates and other opioids.
- Hallucinogens like LSD, phencyclidine, etc.
- Tobacco
- Amphetamine and related drugs Hallucinogens like LSD, phencyclidine, etc.
- Cocaine
- Inhalants: Volatile solvents, aerosols, gases and nitrites.
- Miscellaneous including prescription medicines: Caffeine, analgesic, anabolic steroid, etc.

SOME COMMONLY ABUSED SUBSTANCES AND THEIR EFFECTS

Alcohol

It is a substance that depresses the central nervous system. One of the commonly consumed intoxicating substances in India, alcohol has traditionally been drunk in tribal societies. Gradually, it has won increasing social acceptance among other groups, urban males being the prime example. Easy availability is one of the important reasons of alcohol being widely used especially during festivals. Apart from acute and chronic intoxication, alcohol causes serious physical conditions like cirrhosis of liver, toxic psychosis, gastritis, pancreatitis, cardiac myopathy and peripheral neuropathy. Evidence is mounting that it is related to cancers of mouth, pharynx, larynx and esophagus. Alcohol is an important precipitating factor in suicide, accidents, social and family disorganization, crime, etc.

Sedatives and Hypnotics

This group includes sedative and hypnotics drugs like barbiturate, benzodiazepine (diazepam), chloral hydrate, glutethimide, meprobamate, etc. These drugs act as CNS depressants.

Cannabis

Cannabis (marijuana) is a generic term used to denote several psychoactive preparations obtained from the plant *Cannabis sativa* (Indian hemp). Cannabis has mind altering properties. It exerts diffuse depression of the CNS, as has been observed in alcohol and barbiturates. Besides sedation, it can also cause paradoxical excitement due to disinhibition.[6] The main products under this category are bhang, charas and ganja. Cannabis is, by far, the most widely cultivated, trafficked and abused drug in the world. It is a matter of great concern that the age of initiation of this drug is usually much lower than for other drugs.

Opiates and Other Opioids

Opiates are of natural origin derived from poppy (*Papaver somniferum*), for example morphine, codeine, thebaine. Synthetic alkaloids are known as **opioids** (e.g. buprenorphine). All of them are grouped as '**narcotics**'; '**narco**' means '**to deaden**' or '**benumb**'. The narcotics have the property of numbing and thus relieving pain. Widely used for therapeutic purposes, narcotics are commonly abused also. A significant number of children get addicted to this group of substances. Some anti-tussive preparations containing codeine is easily abused as over-the-counter drug. Perhaps this is the worst type of addiction. Opiates are both physically and psychologically addictive. Some psychological symptoms greatly outlast the physical symptoms and can last for months after cessation of use. High tolerance with rapid withdrawal develops in this group of drugs. Major withdrawal symptoms are tiredness, agitation, nausea, cramps, etc.

Hallucinogens

Lysergic acid diethylamide (LSD) is a potent hallucinogenic drug. It alters the perception of the individual. Abusers may see vivid colors and images, hear sounds and feel sensations that do not really exist. Increased body temperature, blood pressure and heart rate, sweating, sleeplessness, loss of appetite and tremors are some of its short-term effects.

Tobacco

Tobacco use is of grave public health concern that results in significant morbidity and mortality. Tobacco use is responsible for an estimated 5 million yearly deaths worldwide.[7] All forms of tobacco are addictive and even lethal. Conclusive scientific evidences confirm that smokers face significantly elevated risks of death from cancers (particularly lung cancer), heart and respiratory diseases, stroke and many other fatal conditions. Cigar, pipe, water pipe and bidi smokers suffer the same types of health consequences as cigarette smokers. The term '**smokeless tobacco**' is used to describe tobacco that is consumed without heating or burning at the time of use. Smokeless tobacco can be used orally or nasally. The oral mode of use of smokeless tobacco is widely prevalent in India; the different methods of consumption include chewing, sucking and keeping tobacco preparations inside the mouth.

Amphetamines and Related Drugs

This group of drugs acts as CNS stimulants. Stimulants are the substances that elevate mood, increase the sense of wellbeing and also energy and alertness. Widely used as prescription medicines throughout the world, these illicit substances have got extensive recreational use or abuse. Amphetamines are used in medical practice to treat obesity, mild depression, narcolepsy and certain behavioral disorders in children. Also known as '**superman**' drugs, they give tremendous self-confidence and energy; hence that are often used as performance enhancer. The use of this drug results in psychological dependence. This dependence may lead to psychosis. Its use is typically cyclical with alternate periods of heavy use (binger) and of no use (crash period). Irritability and depression may be experienced when use is discontinued. Nowadays, designer amphetamines (created to avoid regulations by existing drug laws) are extensively used by young party-goers (Rave Parties). **Ecstasy** is the most wellknown psychoactive drug in this group. It acts both as stimulant and hallucinogen. Sometimes, tablets of ecstasy in combination with some other substances may be lethal. It can cause extreme hyperthermia which damages brain, heart, kidney, etc.

Cocaine

Cocaine, as a pure alkaloid, is obtained from the leaves of the plant Erythroxylon Coca. Cocaine hydrochloride is sniffed, snorted, injected or smoked. Crack cocaine, the alkaloid free base, is sniffed. Cocaine is powerfully addictive stimulant that directly affects the brain. Cocaine was formerly used in medical practice as a potent anesthetic drug. Aggressive behavior, excitement, paranoid ideation and hallucinations may occur. Since cocaine has a reputation of enhancing sexual pleasure, its widespread use has led to increased spread of sexually transmitted diseases including HIV/AIDS. Psychological dependence with intense compulsive drug-seeking behavior is characteristic of even short-term use, but physical dependence is slight or absent. Because of its scarcity and higher cost, its use is relatively restricted till now.

Inhalants

Inhalants are volatile substances whose chemical vapors are inhaled to induce a rapid psychoactive action. Some categories of inhalants are: Volatile solvents, aerosols, gases and nitrites. Nearly all abused inhalants produce a pleasurable effect by depressing CNS. Most inhalants produce a rapid high that resemble alcohol intoxication with initial excitation, then drowsiness, lack of inhibition, light headedness and agitation. Because of easy availability, it is very popular among adolescents. Unlike alcohol and cannabis, intoxication usually lasts only for a few minutes, making abuse easier to conceal.[8] The highly concentrated chemicals in solvents or aerosol spray can lead to fatal heart failure within minutes of prolonged sniffing in otherwise healthy young person. This syndrome is known as '**sudden sniffing death**'.[9] The chronic use of inhalants may cause irreversible damage to the brain, kidneys and lungs.

Different ways of inhalant use are:

i. Inhaling fumes from a container (**sniffing** or **snoring**).
ii. Spraying aerosols directly into the nose or mouth.
iii. Inhaling fumes from substance inside a plastic or paper bag (**bagging**).
iv. From an inhalant soaked rag stuffed in the mouth (**huffing**).
v. Inhaling from balloons filled with nitrous oxide.

Found in a range of cheap and readily available household, office, industrial and automotive products, inhalants include substances such as hair spray, shoe polish, glue, gasoline, lighter fluid, spray paints and other aerosol sprays (**Figure 51.1**). In India, **Dendrite**, an adhesive, and **Eraz-ex**, a whitener, are commonly used inhalant products. **Iodex**, a pain relief balm, is reported to be eaten as a bread-spread.

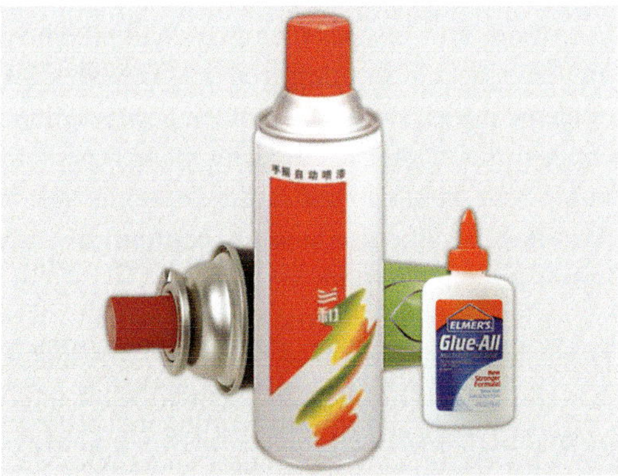

Figure 51.1 Containers of gas, glue, and aerosol

Miscellaneous Including Prescription Medications

The practice of over-the-counter drugs is a common phenomenon in a country like India. These drugs are increasingly being abused and used for non-medical purposes. Commonly abused prescription drugs include painkillers, sedatives and stimulants. The use of these substances is seen more among the teenagers.

Steroids are prescribed for some medical conditions, but are abused to increase muscle mass and to improve athletic performances. Oral and injectable formulations of different steroids are often used simultaneously. Because detection of different steroids in the body fluids is difficult and expensive, the history from the person is more useful for diagnosing abuse.

Distribution, Causes and Risk Factors

i. **Age**: Most vulnerable age group is between 16–35 years. The average age of drug users has decreased considerably in recent years.
ii. **Sex**: Women are less likely to be substance abuser compared to males.
iii. **Locality**: Predominantly an urban problem, most prevalent among slum dwellers.

A combination of various factors, like genetic, environment and behavior, influences a person's addiction risk, making it an incredibly complicated issue. As such, study of all these factors from biology to family is important to unravel the complexities of the addicted brain. Twin studies and researches indicate that drug abuse disorders tend to run in families. The children, who grow up in a family of illicit drug use, first see their parents using drugs. This put them at a higher risk for developing an addiction later in their life, explaining both environmental and genetic reasons.[10]

Rapid changes in political alignment, social and psychological maladjustment, changes in social norms and values, reduced family and community binding and togetherness, disturbed home environment, illiteracy, poverty, unemployment, juvenile delinquency, stressful life and inability to cope with the stress have been the root causes of substance use.

Adolescence is the critical period for initiation of this harmful behavior. This is a period of curiosity and experimentation. Adolescents are afflicted with many health and behavioral problems. Encouragement by peer groups, the lure of popularity, easy availability of many such substances makes a teenager an easy prey.

Drug-related Harms

A wide range of harms is associated with substance use: physical, psychological, social, financial and legal. These can be experienced by not only the individual users, but also by their family, friends, colleagues and the society as a whole. Social and economic consequences of substance abuse arising out of financial loss, family dysfunction, greater demands for medical and other treatment facilities is a matter of concern.

Drug-related harms or problems can be classified into two categories: **Health problems** and **behavioral** and **social problems.** The effects may be of manifold:

i. Injury, disease or death following accident, violence, overdose, HIV/AIDS, hepatitis B, hepatitis C, cancers, etc.
ii. Crime like theft, corruption, murder, suicide, prostitution, etc.
iii. Family and community problems (disharmony, unrest).
iv. Economic loss (loss of productivity, absenteeism).

Blood-borne infections and overdose are the most common and serious causes of mortality and morbidity related to drug use. It is estimated that more than 5% of all HIV infections are related to injecting drugs with infected needles.[11] The risk also stems from engaging in risky behavior as a result of intoxication.

In India, the most commonly abused drugs (apart from alcohol and tobacco) are found to be cannabis, opiates, sedatives and tranquilizers. Multiple drug use has become more common nowadays. Because of drug-drug interaction, such practices often pose significantly higher risks compared to use of a single drug.

Abused individuals are likely to have more psychological symptoms than physical symptoms. Changes in sleeping and eating habits, less interest in dressing and grooming, mood changes, anger, sneaky behavior, poor family relationship, not keeping up with old friend and activities, problems at schools or workplaces, unlawful activities are some of the features of drug abuse. These features do not always implicate a person using drug, but are common among drug users.

A strong relationship exists between the abuse of drugs and occurrence of various accidents and the acts of criminal behavior. Schizophrenia is associated with an increased risk of violent crime. This association was attenuated by adjustment for substance abuse suggesting a mediating effect.[12] Sudden death due to massive overdose can occur in either a body packer or a body stuffer, if one or more of the ingested packages burst within the gastrointestinal tract.[13]

Modes of Trafficking

'**Body packer**' and '**body stuffer**' are two common exercises for illegal drugs smuggling by the smugglers. The practice of swallowing balloons, condoms or plastic packets filled with illegal drugs for the purpose of smuggling is called '**body packing**' and the individual who does this is referred as '**mule**'.[14] This must be differentiated from '**body stuffing**', in which an individual, who is on the verge of becoming arrested for possession of illegal drugs, swallows his illicit contraband to conceal the evidence.[15] Toxicity in such persons may occur from rupture of the container inside the intestine, like the famous '**condom of time bomb**' case in Pakistan.

A 94-year-old woman was caught with 10.45 lbs marijuana at the airport of Nogales, Arizona, USA (**Figure 51.2**).[16] The incidence has proved that the drug trafficker has no limit of age and place; they can do anything to support their habits.[10]

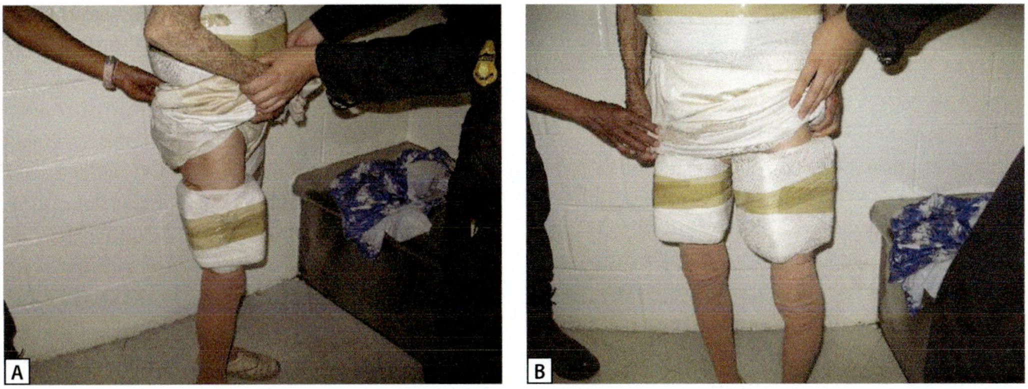

Figures 51.2A and B An old lady caught in airport checkpoint with packed drugs

Investigation of Drug-abuse Death

The pathological probe of a drug-abuse death need not be considered a burdensome task. The doctor must be aware that it is a medicolegal investigation and proceed with the examination in a scientific and medicolegal manner, having verified all the circumstances, documents to ascertain the evidences. This approach should be a multidisciplinary approach requiring coordination of all information with proper authorities.

Addicts often die from complication, like accidents while under the influence of drugs, or may commit suicide or homicide or other sexual offences, which may result in death, necessitating the help of professional expert in the field of investigation. The brief features to be looked during autopsy are mentioned in **Table 51.1**.

Table 51.1 Brief features to be looked during autopsy

General observation	External	Internal
i. Check dead person's clothes and the belongings for drugs	Wasting, signs of asphyxia and self neglect, froth in the mouth and nostrils, black tongue and teeth with ulceration of nasal septum, marked postmortem staining	Diffuse subcutaneous scaring in the skin, generalized visceral congestion
ii. Check for needle, syringe and tourniquet	Body may be tattooed to hide scars known as railroad tracks	Gastrointestinal tract may contain pills or capsules or packet containing drugs
iii. Photographs of the scene are to be taken and to search for any drugs	Stains at tips of fingers and teeth, needle track scars, fibrosed veins, recent injection sites may show zones of inflammation	Hepatosplenomegaly with congested visceras, valvular heart diseases, infective endocarditis, etc
iv. Body is to be looked for any caches of drugs that may be in orifices, etc.	Regional lymph nodes may be enlarged	Multiple spleen infarctions with secondary mixed bacterial infection and abscesses in chronic cocaine abusers
v. Specific precautions are to be taken for prevention of infectious diseases like, HIV, hepatitis B, during the time of examination	Look for the perforation of nasal septum. Froth may be at mouth and nose. Vaginal swabs are to be taken for laboratory examination	Focal areas of necrosis in brain due to hypoxia. Viscera, blood, urine, etc., are mandatory to preserve for chemical analysis

Legal Issues of Substance Abuse

Most of the countries have designed legislation to criminalize certain types of drug use. These drugs are often called "illegal drugs", but generally what are illegal are their unlicensed production, distribution and possession. These drugs are also called "**controlled substances**". Even for simple possession, legal punishment can be quite severe, including the capital sentence. Laws vary across countries, and even within them, and have fluctuated widely throughout history. Attempts by government-sponsored drug control policy to interdict drug supply and eliminate drug abuse have been largely unsuccessful. In spite of the huge efforts by the US, drug supply and purity has reached an all-time high, with the vast majority of resources spent on interdiction and law enforcement instead of public health.[17]

In the US, the number of non-violent drug offenders in prison exceeds by 100,000, the total incarcerated population in the EU, despite the fact that the EU has 100 million more citizens.

India has braced itself to face the menace of drug trafficking both at the national and international levels. Legal aspect of drug abuse in India involves two main areas: **Licensing Laws Regulating Production** and supply of drugs and **legislation for offences** committed under intoxication circumstances. Several measures, involving innovative changes in enforcement, legal and judicial systems, have been brought into effect. **The Drugs and Cosmetics Act 1940** was legislated to regulate the import, manufacture, distribution and sale of drugs and cosmetics. The Narcotic Drugs and Psychotropic Substances (**NDPS**) Act, 1985, was enacted with stringent provisions to curb this menace. The Act envisages a minimum term of 10 years imprisonment expendable to 20 years and fine of ₹ 1 lakh, expendable up to ₹ 2 lakhs for the offenders. The Act has been further amended by making provisions for the forfeiture of assets derived from illicit drugs trafficking. India has bilateral agreements on drug trafficking with 13 countries, including Pakistan and Burma. Prior to 1999, extradition between India and the US occurred under the auspices of a 1931 treaty signed by the US and the UK, which was made applicable to India in 1942. However, a new extradition treaty between India and the US entered in to force in July 1999. A Mutual Legal Assistance Treaty was signed by India and the US in October 2001. India also is signatory to the following treaties and conventions:[18] 1961 UN Convention on Narcotic Drugs, 1971 UN Convention on Psychotropic Substances, 1988 UN Convention against Illicit Traffic in Narcotic Drugs and Psychotropic Substances and 2000 Transnational Crime Convention.

Management

Treatment cannot take place unless the individual comes forward for treatment and is cooperative. He must come to learn with the possibility of a life without drugs. Unfortunately, drug takers, as a rule, have little or no motivation to undergo treatment. Alcoholics tend to deny that their consumption is abnormal; others openly defend their habits. Long-term treatment is not only a medical problem, but needs the cooperation of psychologists and sociologists. There is a high relapse rate with all treatment methods.[19]

Though drug addiction may be considered as a social problem, the first step in its management is medical care, which includes:

i. Identification of drug addicts and their motivation for detoxication
ii. Detoxication (requires hospitalization)
iii. Post-detoxication counseling and follow-up (based on clinic and home visits) and
iv. Rehabilitation.

Simultaneously with medical treatment, changes in environment (home, school, college, social circles) are important. The patient must affect a complete break with his group; otherwise the chances of relapse are 100%. Psychotherapy has a valuable place in the management of the addict.[19]

Efforts must be made to identify the abusers and potential abusers, the factors influencing them and effective measures to stop it. The addicted victims should be best treated or detoxicated in hospital (drug de-addiction centers). These centers should be easily assessable for all them with the facility of ICU and modern laboratory. Drug dependence and drug abuse is a disease and not a character defect. A person being treated for this condition requires the same respect as a person with any other medical condition.

The rehabilitation of former drug user, regardless of age, is in most cases a long and difficult process. Relapses are very frequent. Success of the treatment necessitates the adoption of mature and realistic attitude by the local community and the avoidance of panic, moral condemnation and discrimination. Facilities for vocational training and sometimes the provision of sheltered work opportunities are useful in rehabilitation and help to prevent relapse. Generally speaking, facilities for the registration, diagnosis, treatment, after-care, etc., of drug dependent individuals and groups should be regarded as indispensable integrated parts of the health and social services structure of any community in which drug dependence exists. It is suggested that when there is evidence of significant "alienation" among a group, especially of younger persons, it should be regarded as indication of possible presence of actual or potential drug takers and should lead to an analysis of the situation and to such preventive or remedial action as may be indicated.[20]

Substance use is not simply as an individual behavior, but shaped by different environmental factors, including the economic, social and physical. So, preventive efforts must be focused not only on the individual, but also on the community and society.

Strong family support, social rehabilitation and training for gainful employment are the most important components after weaning the addicts away from drug dependency to prevent relapses.

Furthermore, drug abuse is not a matter of moral weakness or faulty willpower. It is a vicious cycle that actually causes changes in the brain, leading to stronger impulses to use. Without left untreated, substance abuse may destroy family and take lives. With the right support and treatment, the road to recovery is possible.[10]

REFERENCES

1. WHO. Lexicon of alcohol and drug terms. Geneva; World Health Organization; 1994.
2. World Health Organization: The World Health Report: Reducing Risks, Promoting Healthy Life. Geneva: World Health organization; 2002.
3. American Psychiatric Association. Diagnostic and Statistical Manual of Mental Disorders Text Revision; DSM-IV-TR (4thed). Washington DC: American Psychiatric Association; 2000.
4. Miller-Keane, O'Toole MT. Miller-Keane Encyclopaedia and Dictionary of Medicine, Nursing and Allied Health, 7th ed. Pennsylvania: Saunder's Elsevier; 2005. Substance use.
5. Addiction and Recovery information for Individuals, Families and Health Professionals (internet). Addiction and Recovery.org. (Updated 2013 March 23; [cited 2013 April 17]; Available from: URL:http// www.AddictionAnd Recovery.org
6. Lal R (ed.). Substance Use Disorder: A Manual for Physicians. New Delhi; Drug Dependence Treatment Centre AIIMS, 2005.
7. NIDA. Drugs, Brain, and Behaviour-the Science of Addiction (Internet). National Institute of Drug abuse; U.S Department of Health and Human Services,2007 (Revised on 2010), [cited 2013 April 21]; Available from: URL:http//www.drugabuse.gov
8. Volkow NW: Inhalant abuse: Danger under the kitchen sinks. NIDA Notes. 2005; 20(3).
9. NIDA. Research Report Series, Inhalant abuse (internet) National Institute of Drug Abuse; US dept of Health and Human Science; 1999 May (Revised on 2012 July), [cited 2013 April 17]; Available from: URL:http//www.drugabuse.gov
10. Mahanta P. Substance abuse and its medico-legal considerations. J Clin Pathol Forensic Med (internet). 2011;2(2):7-12. [Cited 2013 April 17]; Available from: URL:http://www.academicjournals.org/JCPFM ISSN 2141-2405 @2011

11. United Nations Office for Drug Control and Crime Prevention. Drug Abuse and HIV/AIDS: A devastating combination. United States National Library of Medicine; 2010. [Cited 2013 April 17]; Available from: URL:http://sis.nlm.nih.gov/hiv/substanceabuse.html
12. Fazel S, Langstrom N, Hjern A, Grann M, Lichtenstein P. Schizophrenia, substance abuse and violent crime. JAMA. 2009;301(19):2016-23.
13. Introna FJR, Smialek JE. The "mini-packer" syndrome: Fatal ingestion of drug containers in Baltimore, Maryland. Am J Forensic Med Pathol. 1989;10:21-4.
14. Margaret M, McCarron MD, Wood JD. The cocaine 'Body Packer' syndrome. JAMA. 1983;250:1417-20.
15. Robert JR, Price D, Goldfrank L, Hartnett L. The body stuffer syndrome: A clandestine form of drug overdose. Am J Emerg Med. 1986;4:21-7.
16. Shortarmguy. Old Lady Smuggler (Internet). Shortarmguy. [Cited 2013 March 11]; Available from: URL:http://www.shortarmguy.blogspot.com/2010/06/old-ladysmuggler.html
17. Copeman M. Drug supply and drug abuse. CMAJ. 2003;168(9):1113.
18. Drug Abuse in India (Internet). Azad India Foundation 2010. [Cited 2013 March 11]; Available from: URL:http://www.azadindia.org/socialissues/Drug-Abuse-in-India.html
19. World Bank. World Development Report 1993, Investing in Health. New York: Oxford University Press (published for the World Bank 1993).
20. WHO Expert Committee on Drug Dependence. WHO technical report series 836; 1993. Geneva: World Health Organisation. Report no 28.

CHAPTER 52

Weapons of Mass Destruction

Raktim Pratim Tamuli, Putul Mahanta, Yogender Malik

LEARNING PLAN

- Know about the weapon of mass destruction (WMD)
- Understand different types of WMD
- Know the role of medicolegal expert in mass disaster

WEAPON OF MASS DESTRUCTION

A **weapon of mass destruction** (**WMD**) is a weapon that can kill and bring significant harm to a large number of humans and/or cause great damage to man-made structures, natural structures or the biosphere in general **(Figure 52.1)**. The scope and application of the term has evolved and been disputed, often more politically than technically. Coined in reference to aerial bombing with chemical explosives, it has come to distinguish large-scale weaponry of other technologies, such as chemical, biological, radiological or nuclear.[1]

The term chemical, biological, radiological, and nuclear (CBRN) is a replacement for the cold-war term nuclear, biological and chemical (NBC), which had replaced the term atomic, biological and chemical (ABC) that was used in the 50s. The addition of the R (for radiological) is a consequence of the "new" threat of a radiological weapon (also known as "dirty bombs"). In the new millennium, the term CBRNe has been introduced as an extension of CBRN — the e in this term representing the enhanced (improvised) explosives threat.[2]

The first recorded use of the term "weapon of mass destruction" was by Cosmo Gordon Lang, Archbishop of Canterbury, in 1937 in reference to the aerial bombardment of Guernica, Spain.[3]

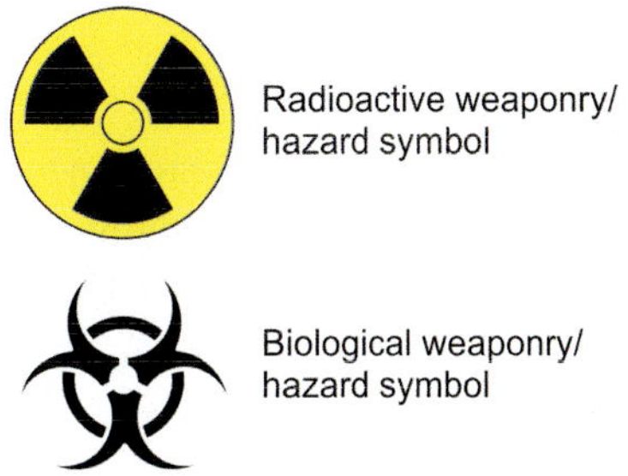

Figure 52.1 Hazard symbols used worldwide

CHEMICAL WARFARE OR WEAPON

Chemical Warfare (**CW**) involves using toxic properties of chemical substances as weapons. These do not fall under the term conventional weapons, which are primarily effective due to their destructive potential. CW does not depend upon explosive force to achieve an objective. Rather it depends upon the unique properties of the chemical agent weaponized. A lethal agent is designed to injure or incapacitate the enemy or deny unhindered use of a particular area of terrain. Defoliants are used to quickly kill vegetation and deny its use for cover and concealment. It can also be used against agriculture and livestock to promote hunger and starvation. With proper protective equipment, training and decontamination measures, the primary effects of chemical weapons can be overcome.[4]

Classes of CW Agents[5,6]

Nerve Agent

Agents

The common nerve agents are: Tabun (GA), Sarin (GB), Soman (GD), Cycloserine (GF) and VX gas.

Schrader synthesized the first nerve agent Tabun (GA), in late 1936; Sarin was introduced in 1937 and Soman in 1944.

Mode of Action

They inactivate enzyme acetylcholinesterase, preventing the breakdown of the neurotransmitter acetylcholine in the victim's synapses and causing both muscarinic and nicotinic effects.

Clinical Features

Miosis (pinpoint pupils), blurred or dim vision, headache, nausea, vomiting, diarrhea, copious secretions/sweating, muscle twitching or fasciculation, dyspnea, seizures, loss of consciousness.

Rate of Action

Vapors: seconds to minutes; Skin: 2–18 hours.

Persistency

VX is persistent and a contact hazard; other agents are non-persistent and present mostly inhalation hazard.

Asphyxiant/Blood Agent

Agents

Most common agents are— arsines, cyanogens chloride, hydrogen cyanide, etc.

Mode of Action

Arsine: Causes intravascular hemolysis that may lead to renal failure.

Cyanogen chloride/hydrogen cyanide: Cyanide directly prevents cells from using oxygen. The cells then use anaerobic respiration, creating excess lactic acid and metabolic acidosis.

Clinical Features

Possible cherry-red skin, cyanosis, confusion, nausea, patients may gasp for air, seizures prior to death, metabolic acidosis.

Rate of Action

Onset is sudden, non-persistent, and it has an inhalation hazard.

Vesicant/Blistering Agent

Agents

Sulfur mustard, nitrogen mustard, lewisite (L) and phosgene oxime (CX).

Mode of Action

Agents are acid-forming compounds that damages skin and respiratory system, resulting burns and respiratory problems.

Clinical Features

Severe skin, eye and mucosal pain and irritation, skin erythema with large fluid blisters that heal slowly and may become infected, tearing, conjunctivitis, corneal damage, mild respiratory distress to marked airway damage.

Rate of Action

Mustards: Vapors: 4–6 hours, eyes and lungs affected more rapidly; Skin: 2–48 hours.
Lewisite: Immediate.

Persistency

Persistent and a contact hazard.

Chocking/Pulmonary Agent

Agents

The common agents are chlorine, hydrogen chloride, nitrogen oxides, phosgene, etc.

Mode of Action

The mode of action is same to blister agents in that the compounds are acids or acid-forming, but action is more pronounced in respiratory system, flooding it and resulting in suffocation; survivors often suffer chronic breathing problems.

Clinical Features

There is airway irritation, eye and skin irritation, dyspnea, cough, sore throat, chest tightness, wheezing, bronchospasm.

Rate of Action

It acts immediately and may extends up to 3 hours. Its action is non-persistent and has an inhalation hazard.

Lesser CW Agents

i. Lacrimators/tear gases.
ii. Sternutators or nasal irritants.

Tear Gases

Tear gas, formally known as a **lachrymatory agent** or lachrymator (from lacrima meaning "tear" in Latin), is a possibly lethal chemical weapon that stimulates the corneal nerves in the eyes to cause tears, pain and even leads to blindness. Common lachrymators include CS (Ortho-chlorobenzylidene malononitrile), CR (dibenzoxazepine), CN (phenacyl chloride), nonivamide, bromoacetone, xylyl bromide and syn-propanethial-S-oxide (from onions).

First used in 1914, xylyl bromide was a popular tearing agent since it was easily brewed. Tear gas works by irritating mucous membranes in the eyes, nose, mouth and lungs, and causes crying, sneezing, coughing, difficulty in breathing, pain in the eyes, temporary blindness, etc. Lachrymators are thought to act by attacking sulfhydryl functional groups in enzymes.

Lachrymatory agents are commonly used as riot control and CW agents. During World War I, more toxic lachrymatory agents were used. Certain lachrymatory agents are often used by police to force compliance, most notably tear gas.

Sternutators

These are organic compounds of arsenic dispersed by heat or detonation in the form of very fine, particulate clouds or smokes. In Latin "sternuto" means sneezing. Commonly used compounds are: diphenylchlorarsine (DA), chlorodihydrophenarsazine (DM), diphenyl-cyanoarsine (DC).

Examples of CW

Use of CW began with the **First World War** (1914–1918), during which more than one lac people died and about 1.2 million seriously affected due to the use of phosgene, chlorine and nitrogen mustard.

During the **Second World War** (1939–1945), the Germans used a number of nerve agents like tabun (GA), sarine (GB) and soman (GD), together referred as "G" military agents causing organophosphorus poisoning.

Agent Orange

US Military force used **Agent Orange**, a combination of Herbicide Orange (HO) and Agent LNX as a part of its CW program in Operation Ranch Hand during the Vietnam War (1961–1971) killing 4 lacs people and creating birth defects in 5 lacs children.

Pepper Spray

Recently, much has been talked about the use of less toxic agents like *Pepper Spray* (derived from red chili or capsicum which contains active principle *capsaicin*) over lacrimators or tear gases for controlling riots. It can also be used as a self-protecting agent especially by women for protecting themselves from unwanted situations.

BIOLOGICAL WEAPONS (POOR MAN'S WMD)

Introduction[7]

Biological warfare (BW) also known as **germ warfare** is the use of biological toxins or infectious agents such as bacteria, viruses and fungi with intent to kill or incapacitate humans, animals or plants as an act of war. Biological weapons are toxic materials produced from pathogenic organisms (usually microbes) or artificially manufactured toxic substances that are used to intentionally interfere with the biological processes of a host. These substances work to kill or incapacitate the host. Biological weapons may be used to target living organisms such as humans, animals or vegetation. They may also be used to contaminate non-living substances such as air, water and soil.

History

Rudimentary forms of BW have been practiced over and over again throughout history. Many examples are recorded from antiquity. During the 6th century BC, the Assyrians poisoned enemy wells with a fungus that would render the enemy delirious.

Historical accounts from medieval Europe detail the use of infected animal carcasses, by Mongols, Turks and other groups, to infect enemy water supplies. Before the bubonic plague epidemic known as the 'black death,' Mongol and Turkish armies were reported to have catapulted disease-laden corpses into besieged cities.[8]

The last known incident of using plague corpses for BW purposes occurred in 1710, when Russian forces attacked the Swedes by flinging plague-infected corpses over the city walls of Reval (Tallinn). The British army, at least once, attempted to use smallpox as a weapon, when they gave contaminated blankets to the Lenape during Pontiac's War (1763–1766). It is suspected, but not confirmed, that BW was used against Native Americans at other times as well.

In response to suspected BW development in Nazi Germany, the US, the UK and Canada initiated a BW development program in 1941 that resulted in the weaponization of anthrax, brucellosis and botulism toxin. But fear of the German program turned out to be vastly exaggerated.[9]

A large outbreak of *Salmonella* in a small town along the Columbia River in Oregon in 1984 caused gastroenteritis in 751 people when a religious sect wanted to poison a whole community to influence an upcoming local election. Bacteria were found in a number of salad bars in various restaurants in a manner that could not be traced back to a naturally occurring outbreak, and the sect was eventually identified as culprit due to the testimony of an insider. Recently, in a short span of time, i.e. from September to November 2001, 23 cases of bio-terrorism occurred in the US, mostly involving postal workers, where letters contaminated with anthrax were handled or opened.

Types[10]

There are a variety of microorganisms that can be used as biological weapons. Agents are commonly chosen because they are highly toxic, easily obtainable and inexpensive to produce, easily transferable from person to person, can be dispersed in aerosol form or have no known vaccine. While it is possible to develop biological weapons from microbes, typically a bacterium, finding a means of distributing the substances is difficult. One possible way is through aerosols. This can be ineffective as the materials often get clogged while spraying. Biological agents distributed by air may also be destroyed by UV light or rain may wash them away. Another method of distribution may be to attach the toxins to a bomb, so that they may be released upon explosion. The problem with this is that the microbes will, most likely, be destroyed by the explosion as well.

The BW agents can be classified as in **Table 52.1**.

The different microbes used as BW agents and there features are mentioned in **Table 52.2**.

Table 52.1 Different BW agents

Agents	Examples
Bacteria	Anthrax, plague, brucellosis, cholera, *Clostridium perfringens* toxin, staphenterotoxin B, melioidosis, tularemia
Virus	Congo Crimean hemorrhagic fever, Ebola hemorrhagic fever, smallpox, Rift Valley fever, Venezuelan equine encephalitis
Fungus	Trichothecene mycotoxin
Rickettsia	Q fever
Miscellaneous	Saxitoxin (derived from paralytic shellfish), Ricin (cytotoxin derived from caster bean mesh)

Table 52.2 Different microbes used as BW agents and their features

Microbes	Natural environment	Target host	Mode of contraction	Diseases or symptoms
Anthrax bacillus anthracis	Soil	Human, domestic animals	Open wounds, inhalation	Pulmonary anthrax septicemia, flu-like symptoms
Clostridium botulinum	Soil	Human	Contaminated food or water	Inhalation
Clostridium perfringen	Intestines of humans and other animals, soil	Human, domestic animals	Open wounds	Gas gangrene, severe abdominal cramps, diarrhea
RICIN protein toxin	Extracted from castor bean plants	Human	Contaminated food or water, inhalation, injection	Severe abdominal pain, watery and bloody diarrhea, vomiting, weakness, fever, cough, and pulmonary edema
Smallpox	Eradicated from nature. Now obtained from laboratory stockpiles	Human	Direct contact with bodily fluids or contaminated objects, inhalation	Persistent fever, vomiting, rash on tongue and in mouth, rash and bumps on skin
Francisella tularensis (Rabbit fever)	Birds, reptiles, invertebrates, fish, etc.	Human, animals	Bite of an infected animal, by contact with blood or fine dust from the animal's body, by the ingestion of infected animal products	Painful sore at the site of the infection and a swelling of the lymph node infected person has a fever with headache, vomiting, body pains, and general weakness. Infection of the eye
Brucella B. melitensis (goats and sheep), *B. suis* (swine), and *B. abortus* (cattle)	Unsterilized milk or meat of infected animals	Human, domestic animals	Ingestion of contaminated food or by direct entrance of brucellae through abrasions of the skin or through the mucous membrane of the eyes	Inconstant fevers, sweating, weakness, anemia, headaches, depression, and muscular and bodily pain. triad of undulant fever: sweating with characteristic wet hay smell, migratory arthalgia and myalgia
Rickettsiaceae	Arthropods like ticks and lice	Human	Bite of arthropods	Acute, self-limiting fevers

Advantages[11]

1. A single microbial biological weapon can, because it reproduces in the host, theoretically produce the desired detrimental outcome in a target host. That is, a single smallpox virus or plague bacillus, if deposited in the right place in the host, can grow and produce a disease.
2. Biological toxins are among the most toxic agents known. For example, the quantity of botox (Botulinum Toxin) in the dot of an 'i' is, when delivered properly, enough to kill about 10 people.
3. Most biological agents are relatively easy and inexpensive to grow. Their cultivations do not require large factories and can utilize common commercial equipment, such as that used in making cheese. While viral agents are more difficult to cultivate than bacterial agents, both can be cultivated by individuals with limited scientific training.
4. Large quantities of biological weapons can, in most cases, be produced in a short period (a few days to a few weeks) at small facilities scattered over a large area.
5. Nondetection by routine scrutiny systems.
6. Destruction of enemy without any infrastructure damage.
7. Perpetrators can escape long before biological weapons cause casualties.
8. Biological weapons are typically invisible in aerosol clouds and not easy to detect until humans become ill.

Disadvantages[11]

1. **Difficulty of protecting the workers at all stages of production, transportation, loading of delivery systems and final delivery**: Untrained and inexperienced personnel, ignorant of routine precautions necessary to prevent contamination with the agents, are accident prone. Immunization of these personnel will not be effective in all cases.
2. **Difficulty in maintaining quality control and sufficient containment during growth and harvesting of agents**: Primitive conditions increase chances for the accidental release of the biological weapons into the surrounding environment (as happened in Russia with anthrax).
3. **Effective delivery problems**: Most biological materials, including spores, are destroyed by exposure to UV light and drying. Agents released in the air may disperse in unexpected ways due to the vulgarities of wind patterns. Dispersal patterns may be ineffectual. Rain may wash the agents out of the air before they reach their target.
4. **Poor storage survival**: Many biological weapons must be stored under special conditions to maintain efficacy. Further, they are often difficult to maintain in a weapons delivery state (e.g. loaded and ready to be fired in a rocket).
5. **Difficult to control once released**: One's own troops may be infected under the chaos of a war. In theory, it may be possible to protect your own population against a BW you plan to use by vaccination or the prophylactic administration of antibiotics, but the chance that your enemy will discover what you are doing is high.

Characteristics of Ideal Biological Weapon[11]

1. Highly infectious; requiring only a few organisms to cause the desired effect (e.g. smallpox) or highly effective; requiring a small quantity of material to cause the desired effect (e.g. botox).
2. Efficiently dispersible, usually in the air; contagious or effective on contact.
3. Readily grown and produced in large quantities.
4. Stable in storage; preferably in a ready-to-deliver state.
5. Resistant enough to environmental conditions so as to remain infectious or operational long enough to affect the majority of the target, but not so persistent as to affect the occupying army.
6. Resistant to treatment, e.g. antibiotics, antibodies, pharmaceutical drugs, etc.

RADIOLOGICAL WEAPON

A **radiological weapon** or **radiological dispersion device (RDD)** is any weapon that is designed to spread radioactive material with the intent to kill and cause disruption.

One version, known as a dirty bomb, is not a true nuclear weapon and does not yield the same explosive power. It uses conventional explosives to spread radioactive material, most commonly the spent fuels from nuclear power plants or radioactive medical waste.

Another version is the salted bomb, a true nuclear weapon designed to produce larger amounts of nuclear fallout than a regular nuclear weapon.[12]

Autopsy on a Radioactive Body

Before conducting the autopsy, the autopsy surgeon must enquire about[13]

1. The dose given to the patient.
2. Type and activity of radiation.
3. The interval since the last dose, and
4. Residual radioactivity in the body.

The following procedure should be followed when an autopsy is to be performed on bodies containing high levels of liquid radioactivity[14,15]

1. Supervision by an individual knowledgeable in radiation (radiation safety officer from a local licensed facility).
2. External exposure monitoring of personnel (whole body and hand).
3. Pre-selection of tools.
4. Anticipated supplies in room.
5. Secured area access.
6. Personnel time limits (rotation of personnel).
7. Bioassay of personnel at conclusion of procedure (to assure radioactivity was not inhaled, absorbed or ingested).
8. Surveys of personnel with portable instrumentation upon exit from procedure area.
9. Survey and decontamination of area and all equipments.
10. Disposal of contaminated waste items as radioactive.
11. Use of personal protective equipments:
    i. Double gloves
    ii. Face mask
    iii. Eye (splash) protection
    iv. Surgical hats
    v. Plastic gowns
    vi. Plastic shoe covers or rubber boots
    vii. Lead aprons (where they might reasonably reduce exposure levels).

Removal of highly radioactive organs is dependent upon anticipated disposition of the body. If a full autopsy will be performed, removal of the organs is encouraged to limit pathological exposure. If there will only be embalming, removal of organs could reduce exposure. Embalming should not be performed within 48 hours of the administration of I^{131} for therapy, unless there are extenuating circumstances.[16]

Cremation of bodies containing radionuclides will contaminate the crematorium and, in most cases, will leave contaminated ashes. Removal and handling of the ashes must be performed with appropriate personal protective equipments. No radiation hazard would exist if a crematorium were to handle a total of up to 200 mCi (miliicurie) ^{131}I or 2000 mCi of all other radionuclides annually.[14]

Instruments and clothing that must be decontaminated (versus becoming radioactive waste) can generally be cleaned by repeated soaking in water with regular detergents. Some items, as determined by the radiation safety professional, may need to be held for decay of the radionuclide. Items to be disposed as radioactive waste must be bagged and properly marked with radionuclide, date and amount of radioactivity. If the half-life is short, the material can be held for decay and disposed as non-radioactive. If the half-life is long, a radiation-safety professional should determine the most appropriate way to dispose of the materials.[17]

NUCLEAR WEAPON

A **nuclear weapon** is an explosive device that derives its destructive force from nuclear reactions, either fission or a combination

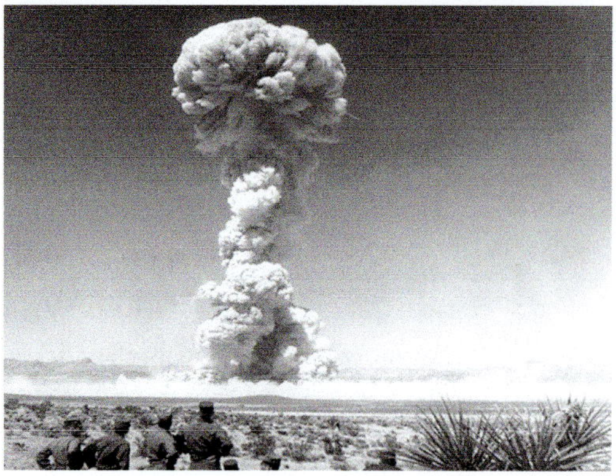

Figure 52.2 Nuclear explosion

of fission and fusion. Both reactions release vast quantities of energy from relatively small amounts of matter **(Figure 52.2)**.

Only two nuclear weapons have been used in the course of warfare, both by the US near the end of World War II. On 6 August, 1945, a Uranium gun type fission bomb, code named "Little Boy", was detonated over the Japanese city of Hiroshima. Three days later, on 9 August, a Plutonium implosion type fission bomb, code-named "Fat Man", was exploded over Nagasaki, Japan. These two bombings resulted in the deaths of approximately 200,000 people, mostly civilians, from acute injuries sustained from the explosions. The role of the bombings in Japan's surrender, and their ethical status, remain the subject of scholarly and popular debate.[18]

MASS DISASTER MANAGEMENT (FOCUS ON ROLE OF MEDICO-LEGAL EXPERT)

Disaster strikes without warning is indiscriminate in its choice of victims and has the potential of overcoming even the most prepared of systems. So, we need to plan to effectively manage such incidents. All the planning in the world will not prevent tragedy from occurring, whether it is by natural causes or manmade, still the only way to prepare for rare, uncommon and unrepetitive events is to think about them, to attempt to generalize the problems they cause and to try to develop a system that can respond to the known but can improvise and also respond to the unknown and not previously experienced as well.[19]

Mass disasters are mainly divided in manmade and natural disasters. In these, there is loss of life and property and resources in managing such incidents are strained and stretched. Although generally contemplated as a second-tier response consideration, after the management of living victims, the appropriate handling, identification and disposition of the deceased nevertheless have specific importance.[19]

The management of dead bodies involves a series of activities that begins with the search for corpses, in situ identification of the body, transfer to the facility that serves as a morgue, delivery of the body to family members and assistance from the State for final disposal of the body in accordance with the wishes of the family and the religious and cultural norms of the community.[20]

In medicolegal work, the objectives are to:[20]

1. Legally determine or pronounce death.
2. Recover the remains of the dead.
3. Establish identity of the dead.
4. Estimate the time of death.
5. Determine the cause of death.
6. Explain the possible circumstances of death.
7. Prepare the remains for final disposal, and
8. Study the event to assist in prevention in the future.

Keeping in mind the objectives of medico-legal work and as integral part of mass disaster management team member, the medicologist should either set a temporary morgue at the site of disaster or should choose a permanent morgue. These are mass fatality incident morgue, which means the facility where the confirmed identification of the remains is established, where a medicolegal autopsy is performed, where detailed death incident reports are filled out and where all elements of aftercare are completed.[21]

REFERENCES

1. Weapons of Mass Destruction. [Cited 2013 Feb 9]. Available from: URL:http://en.wikipedia.org/wiki/Weapon_of_mass_destruction
2. CBRNe. [cited 2013 Feb 9]. Available from: URL:http://ib-consultancy.eu/cbrne/
3. Archbishop Appeal, Times (London), 28th December 1937. p. 9.
4. Chemical Warfare. [Cited 2013 Feb 9]. Available from: URL:http://en.wikipedia.org/wiki/Chemical_warfare
5. Gray C. Another Bloody Century: Future Warfare. Phoenix. 2007. p. 269. ISBN 0-304-36734-6
6. Vij K. Textbook of Forensic Medicine and Toxicology, 4th ed. Noida: Elsevier; 2009. pp. 36-7.
7. Biological Warfare. [Cited 2013 Feb 9]. Available from: URL:http://en.wikipedia.org/wiki/Biological_warfare
8. Wheelis M. Biological warfare at the 1346 siege of Caffa. Emerg Infect Dis (Center for Disease Control). 2002.
9. Covert, Norman M. Biological Warfare of Fort Detrick, Maryland, 4th edn. 2000.
10. Agarwal R, Shukla SK, Dharmani S, Gandhi A. Biological warfare – an emerging threat. J Assoc Physicians India. 2004;52:734.
11. BiologicalWeapon.[cited2013Feb9].Availablefrom:URL:http://www.file:///D:/BW/101biologicalweapons.html
12. Radiological Weapon. [cited 2013 Feb 9]. Available from: URL:http://en.wikipedia.org/wiki/Radiological_weapon
13. Mathiharan K, Patnaik AK (Eds). Modi's Textbook of Medical Jurisprudences and Toxicology, 23rd ed. Nagpur, LexisNexis Butterworths Wadhwa; 2009. pp. 664-5.
14. National Council on Radiation Protection Measurement. Precautions in the management of patients who have received therapeutic amounts of radionuclides. Bathesda, NCRP Report No. 37, 1970.
15. Waters LB. Handbook of Autopsy Practice, 4th ed. Humana Press, Totowa, USA; 2009. pp. 107-10
16. Greaves CD, Tindale WB. Radioiodine therapy: Care of the helpless patient and handling of the radioactive corpse. J Radiol Protection. 2001;21:381-92.
17. US Nuclear Regulatory Commission. Code of Federal Regulations, Title 10, Part 20. US Government Printing Office, Washington DC, 1997.
18. Nuclear Weapon. [Cited 2013 Feb 10]. Available from: URL:http://www.en.wikipedia.org/wiki/Nuclear_weapon
19. Gregory R Ciottone, Philip D Anderson, et al. Disaster Medicine. 3rd ed. 2006. pp. 23, 25 and 280.
20. Disaster Manuals and Guidelines on Disasters Series, No. 5: Management of Dead Bodies in Disaster Situations. Washington, DC: Pan American Health Organization; 2004. p. 190.
21. Jensen RA. Mass Fatality and Casualty Incidents: A Field Guide. CRC Press. 1999.

section 3

ANNEXURES

Section Outline

- Proforma for Age Certification
- Proforma for Injury Certificate
- Proforma for Examination of a Sex Crime (Victim)
- Proforma for Examination of an Accused of Sexual Offence
- Proforma for Examination of a Sodomy Case
- Requisition for Radiological Investigation
- Letter for Permission for Analysis of Viscera, Blood, etc. at State Forensic Science Laboratory
- Viscera Labeling Form
- Final Opinion Form after Chemical Analysis of Viscera or Histopathological Examination of Tissue
- Dead Body Disposal Certificate after Autopsy
- First Information Report
- Form for Despatching Viscera/Body Fluids for Chemical Examination
- Examination of a Case of Drunkenness
- Fetal and Perinatal Autopsy—A Holistic Approach

ANNEXURE 1

PROFORMA FOR AGE CERTIFICATION

No. FM/SC: ______ Date and Time: ______

Ref: ______ PSCaseNo: ______ U/S: ______

1. **Name:** ______ 2. **Sex:** ______
3. **Address:** ______
4. **Religion:** ______
5. **Marital Status:** ______ 6. **Age** (as told by the person): ______
7. **Occupation:** ______
8. **Accompanying** and **identifying Police:** No. ______ 9. **Name:** ______

   Signature: ______ **Date:** ______
10. **Male/Female attendant:**

    Name: ______

    Signature: ______ Date: ______
11. **Consent** for examination (Informed consent): ______ Date: ______
12. **Date of Examination:** ______ Place: ______ Time: ______
13. **Marks of Identification:** A. ______ B. ______
14. **Physical Examination:**

    I. Height: ______ cm II. Weight: ______ kg

    III. Chest girth: ______ cm IV. Abdomen girth: ______ cm

    V. **Teeth:**

	Right	Left
Upper	8 (S) 7 6 5 4 3 2 1	1 2 3 4 5 6 7 (S) 8
Lower	8 (S) 7 6 5 4 3 2 1	1 2 3 4 5 6 7 (S) 8

Contd...

Contd...

Temporary: ______ Permanent: ______ Total: ______

Space for third molar teeth: ______

VI. **Hair**: (Should be looked for color, length and shape)
A. Scalp: ______
B. Axillary: ______
C. Pubic: ______
D. Body: ______
E. Beard and Moustaches: ______

VII. **Breast**: ______

15. **Genital organs**: ______

16. **Report of radiological investigations**: Skiagram No. ______ Date: ______

17. **Opinion**: On the basis of physical examination and radiological investigations done on:.

I am/we are of the opinion that

Date and Time: ______

Signature and seal of the examining doctor

ANNEXURE 2

PROFORMA FOR INJURY CERTIFICATE

Medicolegal registration no: ______ **Date:** ______

Reference: ______

Name: ______ **Age:** ______ month/years; Sex: M/F ______

Son/daughter/wife of: ______

Resident of: ______

Date and time of arrival: ______

Date and time of admission: ______

Date and time of examination: ______

Consent for examination: ______

Brought by/identified by Mr/Mrs: ______

Constable No: ______

Police Station: ______

Place of incident: ______

Identification marks:

1. ______
2. ______

Place of examination: ______

Brief history:

______

Contd...

Contd...

1	2	3	4	5	6	7	8
Sl. no.	Type of injury, i.e. whether abrasion, laceration, incised, bruise, burn, etc.	Size of each injury in cm, i.e. length, breadth and depth, along with color of wound	On what part of the body inflicted	Nature of injuries whether simple or grievous	By what kind of weapon inflicted or how caused blunt/sharp force, fire, etc.	Age of injury	Remarks (whether X-rayed, admitted under observation, where referred for further examination, or report ort treatment or any other relevant information)

Station: Date:

Opinion:

Signature and seal of the examining doctor

ANNEXURE 3

PROFORMA FOR EXAMINATION OF A SEX CRIME (VICTIM)

No. FM/SC: ______ Date: ______

Ref: ______ PSCaseNo: ______ U/S: ______

1. **Name:** ______ 2. **Sex:** ______
3. **Address:** ______
4. **Religion:** ______
5. **Marital Status:** ______ 6. **Age** (as told by the person): ______
7. **Occupation:** ______
8. **Accompanying** and **identifying Police**: No. ______ 9. **Name:** ______

   Signature: ______ **Date:** ______

10. **Male (in a case of male victim)/Female (in a case of female victive) attendant**:

    Name: ______

    Signature: ______ Date: ______

11. **Consent** for examination (Informed consent): ______ Date: ______
12. **Date of Examination**: ______ Place: ______ Time: ______
13. **Marks of Identification**: A. ______ B. ______
14. **Case History**:: From Police: ______ From Person: ______
15. **Physical Examination:**

    I. Height: ______ cm II. Weight: ______ kg

    III. Chest girth: ______ cm IV. Abdomen girth: ______ cm

    V. **Teeth:**

	8 (S) 7 6 5 4 3 2 1	1 2 3 4 5 6 7 (S) 8	
Right			Left
	8 (S) 7 6 5 4 3 2 1	1 2 3 4 5 6 7 (S) 8	

Contd...

Contd...

Temporary: ______ Permanent: ______ Total: ______

Space for third molar teeth: ______

VI. **Hair**: A. Scalp: ______

B. Axillary: ______

C. Pubic: ______

VII. **Breast**: ______

16. **Menstrual History:** Menarche: ______ Cycle: ______ Last Menstrual Period: ______
17. Genital Examination:
    A. Genital organs: ______
    B. Vulva: ______
    C. Hymen: ______
    D. Vagina: ______
    E. Cervix: ______
    F. Uterus: ______
    G. Evidence of venereal disease: ______
    H. Vaginal swabs collected from: ______
18. Injury on the body: ______
19. Wearing garments: Evidence of struggle: ______ Evidence of stain: ______
20. Mental condition at the time of examination: ______
21. Cooperation and behavior: ______
22. Intelligence and memory: ______
23. Gait: ______
24. **Report of radiological investigations**: Skiagram No. ______ Date: ______
25. Result of laboratory investigation: ______
26. **Opinion**: On the basis of physical examination and radiological investigations done on:.

    ______

    I am/we are of the opinion that

    ______

Date and Time: ______ **Signature and seal of the examining doctor**

ANNEXURE **4**

PROFORMA FOR EXAMINATION OF AN ACCUSED OF SEXUAL OFFENCE

No. FM/SC: ____ Date: ____

Ref: ____ PS Case No: ____ U/S: ____

1. **Name:** ____ 2. **Sex:** ____

3. **Address:** ____

4. **Religion:** ____

5. **Marital Status:** ____ 6. **Age** (as told by the person): ____

7. **Occupation:** ____

8. **Accompanying** and **identifying Police**: No. ____ 9. **Name:** ____

Signature: ____ **Date:** ____

10. **Male/Female attendant:**

Name: ____

Signature: ____ Date: ____

11. **Consent** for examination (Informed consent): ____

12. **Date of Examination:** ____ Place: ____ Time: ____

13. **Marks of Identification:** A. ____ B. ____

14. **Case History:**: From Police: ____ From Person: ____

15. **Physical Examination:**

I. Height: ____ cm II. Weight ____ kg

III. Chest girth: ____ cm IV. Abdomen girth: ____ cm

V. **Teeth:**

	Right	Left
Upper	8 (S) 7 6 5 4 3 2 1	1 2 3 4 5 6 7 (S) 8
Lower	8 (S) 7 6 5 4 3 2 1	1 2 3 4 5 6 7 (S) 8

Contd...

Contd...

Temporary: ______ Permanent: ______ Total: ______

Space for third molar teeth: ______

VI. **Hair**: A. Scalp: ______

B. Axillary: ______

C. Pubic: ______

D. Body: ______

E. Beard and Moustaches: ______

VII. **Breast**: ______

17. Genital Examination:

A. Genital organs: ______

B. Penis

a. Length: In flaccid condition: ______ cm During erection: ______ cm

b. Circumference: In flaccid condition: ______ cm During erection: ______ cm

c. Prepuce: ______

d. Frenulum: ______

e. Glans: ______

f. Smegma: ______

C. Scrotum: ______

D. Testis: ______

E. Evidence of venereal disease: ______

F. Penile swabs collected from: ______

18. Injury on the body: ______

19. Wearing garments: A. Evidence of struggle: ______ B. Evidence of stain: ______

20. Mental condition at the time of examination: ______

21. Cooperation and behavior: ______

22. Intelligence and memory: ______

Contd...

Contd...

23. Gait:

24. Report of radiological investigations: Skiagram No. Date:

25. Result of laboratory investigation:

26. **Opinion**: On the basis of physical examination and radiological investigations done on:

I am/we are of the opinion that

Date and Time: **Signature and seal of the examining doctor**

ANNEXURE 5

PROFORMA FOR EXAMINATION OF A SODOMY CASE

No. FM/SC: ______ Date: ______

Ref: ______ PS Case No: ______ U/S: ______

1. **Name:** ______ 2. **Sex:** ______
3. **Address:** ______
4. **Religion:** ______
5. **Marital Status:** ______ 6. **Age** (as told by the person): ______
7. **Occupation:** ______
8. **Accompanying** and **identifying Police:** No. ______ 9. **Name:** ______

   Signature: ______ **Date:** ______
10. **Male/Female attendant:**

    Name: ______

    Signature: ______ Date: ______
11. **Consent** for examination (Informed consent): ______
12. **Date of Examination:** ______ Place: ______ Time: ______
13. **Marks of Identification:** A. ______ B. ______
14. **Case History::** From Police: ______ From Person: ______
15. **Physical Examination:**

    I. Height: ______ cm II. Weight ______ kg

    III. Chest girth: ______ cm IV. Abdomen girth: ______ cm

    V. **Teeth:**

	8 (S) 7 6 5 4 3 2 1	1 2 3 4 5 6 7 (S) 8	
Right			Left
	8 (S) 7 6 5 4 3 2 1	1 2 3 4 5 6 7 (S) 8	

Contd...

Contd...

Temporary: ______ Permanent: ______ Total: ______

Space for third molar teeth: ______

VI. **Hair**: A. Scalp: ______

B. Axillary: ______

C. Pubic: ______

D. Body: ______

E. Beard and Moustaches: ______

VII. **Breast**: ______

17. Genital Examination:

A. Genital organs: ______

B. Penis:

a. Length: In flaccid condition: ______ cm During erection: ______ cm

b. Circumference: In flaccid condition: ______ cm During erection: ______ cm

c. Prepuce: ______

d. Frenulum: ______

e. Glans: ______

f. Smegma: ______

C. Scrotum and testis: ______

D. Anus and anal canal: ______

E. Oral cavity: ______

F. Evidence of venereal disease: ______

G. Anal/oral swabs collected from: ______

18. Injury on the body: ______

19. Wearing garments: A. Evidence of struggle: ______ B. Evidence of stain: ______

20. Mental condition at the time of examination: ______

21. Cooperation and behavior: ______

Contd...

Contd...

22. Intelligence and memory:
23. Gait:
24. Report of radiological investigations: Skiagram No. Date:
25. Result of laboratory investigation:
26. **Opinion**: On the basis of physical examination and radiological investigations done on:

    I am/we are of the opinion that

Date and Time: **Signature and seal of the examining doctor**

ANNEXURE 6

REQUISITION FOR RADIOLOGICAL INVESTIGATION

FM/SC/No: ____________ Date: ____________

Ref: ____________ PS: ____________ Case No: ____________ U/S: ____________

Name of the Victim/Accused: ____________ Sex: Male/Female

Part to be investigated	For
1. AP view of *Wrist Joint.*	Appearance of centers of ossification and union of bones with epiphyses
2. AP view of *Elbow Joint.*	
3. Lateral view of *Elbow Joint.*	
4. AP view of *Shoulder Joint* including medial end of clavicle.	
5. AP view of *Pelvic Bones* including *Iliac Crest* and *Ischial Tuberosity.*	
6. Lateral view of the *Shoulder Joint* keeping the shoulder joint in extended position.	Osteoporotic changes of glenoid margins
7. Lateral view of *Head and Face* with neck in extended position, keeping the mouth partly open.	Calcification of root of all permanent teeth and obliteration of cranial sutures
8. AP view of the *Head* keeping the neck in flexed position,	Obliteration of cranial sutures
9. Lateral view of *Chest.*	Union of sternal segments and xiphisternum
10. USG of *Lower Abdomen.*	Diagnosis/duration of Pregnancy
11. Others, specify: ____________	

Identification marks:

1. ____________
2. ____________

Identified by police officer/constable no: ____________ Name: ____________

Accompanied by: ____________ Relationship: ____________

Received:

1.
2.

Signature of medical officer on duty

ANNEXURE 7

LETTER FOR PERMISSION FOR ANALYSIS OF VISCERA, BLOOD, ETC. AT STATE FORENSIC SCIENCE LABORATORY

To

The Chief Judicial Magistrate,

Subject: Permission for analysis of viscera/blood/body fluid at State Forensic Science Laboratory

Ref:

Case No. Date:

Postmortem Registration/Sex Crime Registration No.

Date:

Name of deceased: Age: Sex:

Sir,

I have the honor to inform you that analysis of viscera/blood/body fluid is essential in connection with the above mentioned cases. So, necessary permission may be granted for analysis of the preserved material in the State Forensic Science Laboratory,

Yours faithfully

Signature of Medical Officer

Date: **Name and seal**

ANNEXURE 8

VISCERA LABELING FORM

Ref:

Case No.

PMR No. Date:

Name: Age: Sex

Viscera preserved: Stomach with its contents, portion of small intestine, lung, liver, brain, kidney, others

Preservative used: Rectified spirit/SS Common salt/

Date:

Signature of Medical Officer on duty

Name and Seal

ANNEXURE 9

FINAL OPINION FORM AFTER CHEMICAL ANALYSIS OF VISCERA OR HISTOPATHOLOGICAL EXAMINATION OF TISSUE

To

The Officer in Charge of: ______ PS: ______

Ref. No.: ______

PMR No.: ______ Date: ______

Sir,

On the basis of the postmortem findings and chemical examination report of viscera/histopathological examination of the sample of tissue of deceased

Chemical examination report of viscera/histopathological examination of the sample of tissue of deceased: ....

I am of the opinion that

______

Please refer to viscera analysis report/histopathological examination report No

______

which read as

______

Date: ______

Signature of the Medical Officer

With Seal

ANNEXURE 10

DEAD BODY DISPOSAL CERTIFICATE AFTER AUTOPSY

TO WHOM IT MAY CONCERN

This is to certify that, autopsy examination on the dead body of ______

SO/DO/WO/CO ______ of ______

Brought by ______ PS/OP vide case No ______

and escorted by constable No: ______ Name: ______

is handed over to the escorting police/relative of the deceased after completion of autopsy.

Optional: The body has been embalmed and is safe to be carried by air/train/road and will remain so for next ______ hours/days.

Received by:

1. Constable No: ______ Name and Signature: ______
2. Relationship: ______ Name and Signature: ______

Date and Time: ______

Signature of Medical Officer

Name and Seal

ANNEXURE 11

FIRST INFORMATION REPORT

FIRST INFORMATION OF COGNIZABLE CRIME REPORTED UNDER SECTION 154

Criminal Procedure Code, at police station:

Subdivision: District:

No Date and hour of occurrence:

Date and hour when reported	Place of occurrence and distance and direction from police station and jurisdiction number	Date of dispatch from police station

[NB: FIRST INFORMATION MUST BE AUTHENTICATED BY THE SIGNATURE, MARK OR THUMB-IMPRESSION AND ATTESTED BY THE SIGNATURE OF THE OFFICER RECORDING IT]

Name and residence of informant and complainant	Name and residence of accused	Brief description of offence with section and of property carried off, if any	Steps taken regarding investigation, explanation of delay in recording information	Result of the cause
1	2	3	4	5

FIRST INFORMATION TO BE RECORDED BELOW]

Note: The signature, seal or mark of information should be affixed at foot of the information.

Signature:

Designation:

Date and Time:

ANNEXURE 12

FORM FOR DESPATCHING VISCERA/ BODY FLUIDS FOR CHEMICAL EXAMINATION

From

The Department of Forensic Medicine and Toxicology

To,

The Director

Description of viscera forwarded for examination:

Mode of packing	Seal	Sd/-
Weight of parcel		**Medical officer**
Mode of Despatch, Escorting police, examination office	Date of despatch	**Date of receipt in chemical**

Contd...

Contd...

Information furnished by police

Reference:

Case No:

Name: Age: Sex:

Address:

Case history:

Signature of Medical Officer

Name:

Date:

ANNEXURE 13

EXAMINATION OF A CASE OF DRUNKENNESS

Hospital No: ________ Reg. No: ________ Date: ________

Reference: ________

A. Personal Information:

1. Name: ________
2. Age: ____ yrs Sex: ____ Occupation: Service/Business/Cultivation/Others
3 Guardian's Name: ________
4. Address: ________
5. Accompanying person: ________
6. Consent: ________
7. Accompanying Police Constable: ________
8. Identification Marks:
   i. ________
   ii. ________
9. Date and time of examination: ____ / ____ / ____ Time: ____ am/pm
10. Time and place of incident: ________ am/pm. Place: ________
11. Place of examination: ________
12. Time completed: ________

B. History: ________

C. Physical Examination:

13. General appearance: ________

14. Vital data: Temperature: ____ Pulse: ____ /min, Rapid/bounding/slow Respiratory rate: ____ /min BP: ____ mm of Hg; Weight: ____ kg Height: ____ cm

Contd...

Contd...

14. General manners and behavior: Calm/talkative/abusive/obscene/others:
15. State of dress: Decent/soiled/disarranged:
16. Speech: Normal/thick/slurred/over-precise/incoherent:
17. Breath: Smell of alcohol present/absent:
18. Stance: Stand up properly/swing: Romberg sign: Positive/negative
19. Gait: Normal/unsteady/staggering:
20. Handwriting:
21. Skin: Dry/moist/flushed/pale/
22. Eyes: Conjunctivae: Normal/congested, Pupils: Dilated/constricted/Pin-point constriction. Pupillary reflex: Normal/Sluggish/Absent. Convergence Test: Can/cannot converse his/her eyes. Nystagmus: Fine lateral nystagmus present/absent
23. Reflexes: Knee and ankle reflexes: Sluggish/delayed. Planter reflex: Extensor or flexor. Others:
24. Muscular coordination: Finger Nose Test: Can/cannot perform. Finger to finger test: Can/cannot perform. Unbuttoning and buttoning: Can/cannot do. Picking objects from floor: Can/cannot perform
25. CNS Examination: Memory and mental alertness: Memory of recent events: Intact or lost. Orientation to time and place: Present/absent
26. Respiratory System:
27. GIT:

D. Result of laboratory investigation:

i. Blood:

ii. Urine:

iii. Others if any:

E. Opinion: After thorough physical examination and laboratory investigation of the person ________ I am/we are of the opinion that (Wichever is applicable):

i. The individual has not consumed alcohol.

ii. The examined individual has consumed alcohol but he is not under its influence.

iii. The examined individual has consumed alcohol and he is under its influence.

Date: Place:

Signature with Seal

ANNEXURE 14

Fetal and Perinatal Autopsy—A Holistic Approach

Manish Nigam

Autopsy of any conceptus after 8th week of gestational age, till early neonatal age, i.e. within 2 weeks of birth and stillbirths, are included under fetal and perinatal autopsy. A fetal autopsy is one that is performed on a fetus dying in utero or born dead. For a fetal autopsy to satisfy the autopsy requirement of the American Board of Pathology, the criteria must include—autopsy consent signed for a complete autopsy. This is not the same as an anatomic disposal. The fetus must be intact and the Examination of the placenta must be part of the autopsy report.

PRE-REQUISITE

A prior detailed maternal, present and past obstetrics, medical and surgical history is obtained together with the relevant investigations and scans. If the fetus was live born, then knowledge regarding its neonatal course, resuscitative measures, birth weight and state of the infant at birth is obtained. Detailed photography, whole body roentgenographic examination, bacteriology, virology, metabolic studies and chromosomal analysis is performed in each case, according to the requirement. In case of maceration, an assessment of interval since intrauterine death and delivery by the degree of maceration and infection screen is carried out.

Consent is of paramount importance in pathological fetal autopsies as opposed to medicolegal autopsy and is taken from the next of the kin. Consent should deal sensitively and comprehensively with issues regarding retention of organs and tissues, storage and disposal of body. Further consent is required to specify the extent to which the autopsy can be conducted and whether the parents wish to limit the autopsy to a particular organ or system, for purposes other than diagnosis like teaching and research and for any ancillary investigations. Written consent is required for diagnosis on all tissues or fluid specimens, and is likely to require separate permission for non-diagnostic usage.

PRECAUTIONS

Caution through genetic counseling is required before performing fetal autopsy, as they may lead to unrealistic expectations from the parents, who may be expecting some diagnosis that was not answered prenatally, and miraculous treatment. Psychological counseling is required to understand the frame of mind of the parents, who may be seeking compensation for malpractice. Furthermore, post-autopsy genetic counseling should be done and parents be advised for karyotyping and/or cytogenetics in order to plan further. During autopsy, one must be careful, that the complete fetus is obtained and not deformed or in parts, as may occur during an attempt at delivery of the fetus, for instance decapitation injury during delivery of a hydrops fetus. If not informed antenatally to the parents, this may reflect as an outcome of a crude or butchered autopsy.

Fetal autopsy are considered as an unnecessary burden to the already existing heavy workload of medicolegal autopsy in Indian setting. However, a meticulous autopsy opens up avenues in scientific and research field in addition to providing information to the parents that may alter the risk factor in subsequent pregnancies. In addition, guilt and blame are often present in the families; a fetal autopsy provides some clue to parents.

One should understand that the information of fetal or neonatal demise is a difficult time for all the parents and to consider the issue of a postmortem examination is even more painful, but working with the hope that proper counseling will help them to understand the reasons for undertaking it and will solve the questions such as, what it involves, and why it may be important. One should also encourage asking any number of questions, by parents or relatives, in any matter related to autopsy, with any of the staff involved in it.

CASE REPORTS

As per case report observation at Shri Aurobindo Institute of Medical Sciences (SAIMS), the autopsy surgeon had not only provided concordant results with the prenatal findings in almost all the cases, but also had provided relevant additional information in about 30% of cases. In their department, they overcome across various cases of rare lethal anomalies like CHAOS (Congenital High Airway Obstruction Syndrome) where there is complete or near complete intrinsic obstruction of fetal airway in the form of laryngeal atresia, laryngeal or tracheal web, subglottic stenosis and the case was confirmed by putting guidewire in upper airway (**Figures 1A and B**).

Umbilical cord stricture along with its torsion and kinking 2–3 cm from the umbilicus, which resulted in sudden and unexplained mid-trimester fetal death, which may be an acute event due to rotation of the fetus around the torsion causing vascular compromise and fetal demise or chronic event presenting as intrauterine growth retardation (IUD) (**Figure 2**).

Confirming meconium peritonitis, subsequent to intestinal perforation and excessive muco-liths in a fetus leading to a sudden development of septate abdominal cystic mass in a previously normal fetus, and causing death of the fetus and later on associating it with cystic fibrosis and/or maternal TORCH syndrome in an unexplained IUD, was one

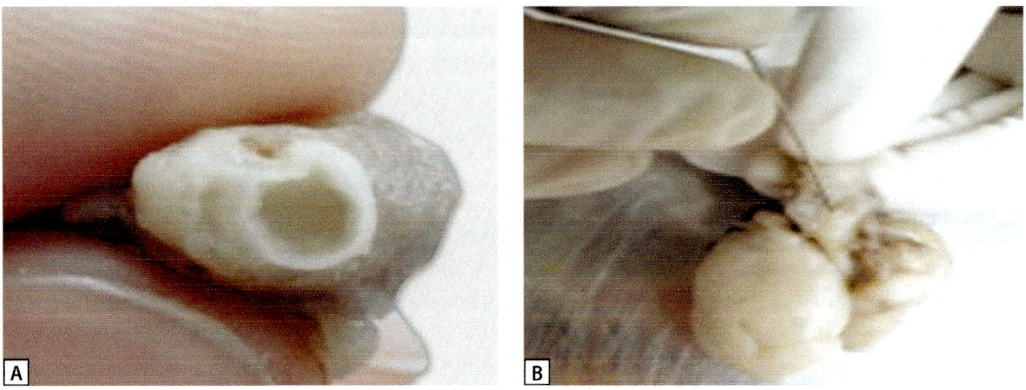

Figures 1A and B (A) Congenital high airway obstruction; (B) CHAOS – Confirmed by guidewire

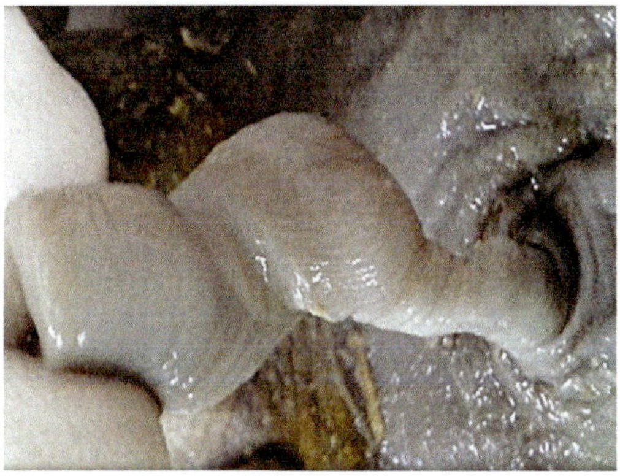

Figure 2 Umbilical stricture and twist

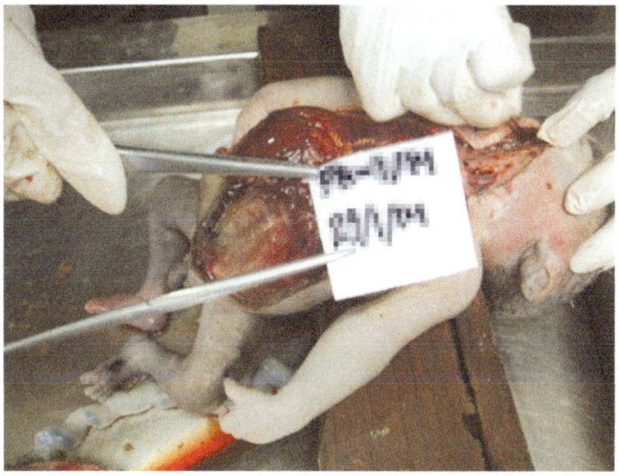

Figure 3 Meconium peritonitis

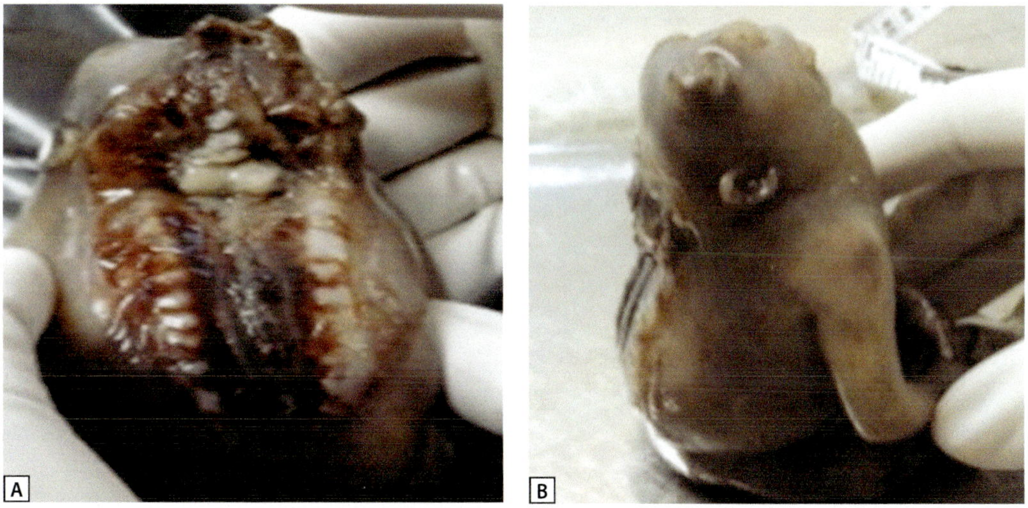

Figures 4A and B (A) and (B) Inencephaly and anencephaly with absence of fetal calvaria and rachischisis

of our achievements. Few of such cases were supported by genetic analysis (**Figure 3**).

Fetus with neural tube defects like inencephaly and anencephaly causing absence of fetal calvaria and brain tissue along with rachischisis, which is a type of complete spina bifida and leads to a fatal outcome, are another set of more common cases that we have come across (**Figures 4 A and B**).

CONCLUSION

The main causes of congenital malformations are structural heart disease, chromosomal abnormalities and central nervous system defects. Most of the cases referred belong to the cases with unexplained death in mid-trimester. Nowadays mid-trimester target scans are very commonly performed by various sonologists, but still many causes remain unexplained due to lack of fetal autopsies.

The benefits of fetal autopsy can only be emphasized by aforementioned examples, where a detailed autopsy allows, to detect the anomaly, diagnose the exact location, the extent of the anomaly, and associated features, which is either not possible or difficult to diagnose through routine antenatal investigations. A fetal autopsy helps to confirm, modify or refute clinical diagnosis, helps in education, causes of diseases, allows evaluation of new diagnostic and therapeutic technique, provides epidemiologic data, and provides new information on disease manifestations. Legally, it helps monitor public health issues, explains sudden unexpected and unexplained deaths, can clarify concerns that may otherwise lead to malpractice lawsuits.

BIBLIOGRAPHY

1. Sheaff M, Hopster D. Post Mortem Technique Handbook. Springer- Verlag London Limited. 2005.
2. Enid G-B, Diane D-S. Handbook of Pediatric Autopsy Pathology. New Jersey: Humana Press Inc. 2005.
3. Cho HJ, Kim YM, Lee HY, Won H-S. A case of congenital high airway obstruction syndrome caused by complete tracheal obstruction with associated anomalies. Korean J Obstet Gynecol. 2012;55(2):115-8.
4. Sun W-C, Zhai H-B, Wang Z-H. Intrauterine death in a fetus with umbilical cord stricture: a case report. J Pak Med Stu. 2013;3(2):85-6.

Index

Page numbers followed by *f* refer to figure and *t* refer to table

A

A. pantherina 709
Abdomen 384
Abdominal
  cavity, opening of 205, 207, 208*f*
  examination 385
    breasts 385
    cervix 385
    uterus 385
    vagina 385
  injuries 293
  pain 586
  wall linea nigra 380*f*
Abortion
  and MTP Act 387
  artificial 390
  classification of 388, 388*f*
  definition of 387
  evidences of 394
  incidence of 387
  incomplete 389
  induced *See also Abortion, artificial*
  inevitable 389
  missed 390
  natural 388
  place of 391
  precautions of 390
  spontaneous 388
Abrasion 219
  age of 222, 222*t*
  mechanism of 219, 219*f*
  multiple ligature marks with 351*f*
  over front of chest 221*f*
  tag 220*f*
  types of 220
Abrus 589
  features 589
    active principle 589
    management 590
    toxic part of plant 589
  precatorius plant 590*f*
    seeds of 590*f*
Absence of
  axillary 77
  pubic hair 77
Absorbed poison
  signs 534
  symptoms 534
Abuse, substance 713
Academic autopsy 200
Accident
  meaning of 51
  poisoning 528, 581
  prevention 304
Accountability and transparency, principle of 63
Acetic acid 93
Acid
  phosphatase isoenzyme test 479
  phosphatase test 479
  throwing 558
Aconite 664
  autopsy findings 665
  features 664
  management 665
  plant 664*f*
  uses 665
Act 1 of 1904 *See Laws relating to poison in India Poison Act*
Act 23 of 1940 *See Laws relating to poison in India Drug Act*
Act endangering life 336
Act II of 1930 *See Laws relating to poison in India dangerous Drug Act*
Active sodomy *See Assailant, examination of*
Acts, different 33
Actual road accidents, mean force calculation in 299*f*
Acute
  alcohol
    intoxication 637
      signs 637
      symptoms 637
  arsenic poisoning 569
    management 569
  lead poisoning 575
    management 575
    postmortem findings 575
  opium poisoning 628
  poisoning 661
  SDH 284
  starvation 367, 368
  subdural hemorrhages 284*f*
  toxicity 698
Adenine paired thiamine 172*f*
Admissions in psychiatric hospitals 452*f*
Adult long bones of European origin, Karl Pearson formula for 125*t*
Affecting injury, physical factors 217
Afim *See also Opium*
Ag *See Silver*
Agaricus augustus 709
Age
  determination of 78, 166
  estimation, radiological examination for 83
Agent orange 725
Agonal artefacts 462
Agricultural poisons 647
AIDS/HIV safety kit 493*f*
Airbags of car 303*f*
Alcohol 632, 639, 715
  intoxication, medicolegal aspect of 644
Alcoholic beverages, types of 634
Alkaloids 683
  of ergot 600

Alleged victim of custodial torture 506
Aluminum dust *See Gray powder*
Amanita
  muscaria 709
  phalloides 709
  phalloides 709*f*
  species 709
Ammonia 560
  clinical features of poisoning 560
  management 561
  properties 560
Amphetamines and related drugs 716
Anemia 315, 576
Anemic anoxia 340
Anencephaly 401*f*
Anesthesia
  and rape 422
  used in surgical procedure, types of 362
Anesthetic
  deaths, classification of 362
  procedures and death 361
Animal hair, cross section of 106*f*
Anoxic anoxia 340
Antemortem
  and postmortem data, comparison between 157*t*
  burn 315*f*
    tissues, microscopic findings of 317*f*
  radiograph 157*f*, 160*f*
  scalds 319*f*
  separations of head 291*f*
Anteriorly proclined upper teeth 154*f*
Anthropometry 90
  principle 91
Anticholinergics *See Datura*
Antidotes
  accelerated detoxification 537
  adsorbents 537
  bulky food 537
  chemical 537
    potassium permanganate 537
    weak alkalis 537
    weak vegetable acids 537
  demulcents 537
  diluents 537
  inert complex formation 537
  mechanical 537
  mode of action of 537
  physical 537
  receptor site
    blockade 537
    competition 537
  reduced toxic conversion 537
  therapy 537
  toxic effect bypass 537
  types of 537
  uses 538
Antipyretic 696
Anti-snake venom serum 612*f*
  polyvalent 612
Anus, dilated 434*f*
Anxiety, disorders of 448
Apis mellifera *See Honeybee*
Apparent death *See Suspended animation*
Applied force, duration of 217
Arborescent marks 324
Areola, hyperpigmentation of 380*f*
Argemone mexicana *See also Mexican poppy*
Armor-piercing bullet 258
Arrest 497
Arsenic 567, 567*f*
  abuses 568
    aphrodisiac purpose 568
    love-philter 568
  common use 568
  organic compounds 568
  properties 567
  trichloride 568
  trioxide *See also Arsenious oxide*
Arsenious oxide 568
Arsenite-copper acetoarsenite 568
Arsine 568
Artefact
  acquired autopsy 467
  definition 462
  in toxicological analysis 467
  induced
    in firearm wounds 465
    time of handling of cadaver 466
  medicolegal importance 467
  of animal 465
  of brain 463
  of decomposition 464
  of embalming 466
  of emergency intervention 464
  of environment 467
  of exhumation 467
  of hair 464
  of insect bites 465
  of liver 463
  of postmortem hemorrhage 463
  related to
    changes after death 462
    postmortem lividity 463
    rigor mortis 462
  to burns 467
  types of 462
Artificial insemination 376
  donor 376
    legal precautions of 376
  types 376
Aryl phosphates 648
AS *See Arsenic*
Ascomycetes 708
Asphyxia 344
  begets asphyxia 341
  classical signs of 341
  classification of 342, 342*f*
  congestion, classical signs of 341
  cyanosis, classical signs of 341
  deaths 340
  definition of 340
  fluidity of blood, classical signs of 341
  mechanical, classification of 343
  non-mechanical, classification of 342
  petechial hemorrhages, classical signs of 342
  pharyngeal hemorrhage, classical signs of 342
Asphyxiant 724
  classification of 689
Aspirin 696
Assailant
  examination of 434
  position of 266
ASV administration criteria 612
Atropa belladonna 670
  seeds 671*f*
Atropine 539
  adverse effects 539
  precautions 539
Attendance in court, procedure of 17
AU *See Gold*
Auditory hallucination 442
Automatism 457
Autopsy 4, 199
  definition 199
  examination 203, 364
    clothing external 203
    external 203
  findings 659
  incision 209
  medicolegal 200
  types of 200

Avulsion laceration 229*f*
Axonal injury *See Neuronal injury, diffuse*
  diffuse 281

B

Bacillus cereus 701, 702, 704
  incriminated food 704
Bacteria 702
Bailable offences 328
Balling 251
Ballistics, external 240
Banded krait 604
Barbed property of honeybee sting 617*f*
Barberio test 479
Barr body 75*f*, 475
Basidiomycetes 708
Battered baby syndrome 404
  definition 404
  features 404
Bee stings, removing 618*f*
Belt, ligature materials 343*f*
Benzodiazepine 362
Bertillon system *See Anthropometry*
Bhang 675
Bhilawanol 597
Bicondylar width of femur 122*f*
Bilateral ptosis 610*f*
Billiard ball ricochet effect 251
Biological
  factors affecting injury 217
  weapons 726
Biomedical waste
  authorization, duties of 58
  collection of 57
  definition
    disposal of 58
    duties of 58
    segregation of 56
    storage of 57
    treatment of 58
  disposal of 58
    liquid waste, disposal of 58
    solid waste, disposal of 58
  duration, storage of 57
  duties of 58
  emphasis on sharps, segregation of 56
  ethical aspect, management of 55
  handling of 55
  importance, management of 54
  management of 55
  objectives, treatment of 58
  responsibility for segregation 56
  segregation of 56
  significance, segregation of 56
  site
    disposal of 58
    treatment of 58
  solution, segregation of 57
  storage of 57
  treatment of 58
Bipolar mood disorder 446
  mania 446
Birth in helmeted head 383
Birthmark *See Mongolian spot*
Bite mark 161*f*
  analysis 161
  description of 162
  evidence 162
  matched with dental cast of suspect 162*f*
  measurement of 163*f*
  on breast 424*f*
  on nipples 424*f*
  over cheek 161*f*
  over human leg 161*f*
  over leg 161*f*
Black
  and smokeless powder, differences between 246*t*
  eye 227, 273*f*
  powder 245
  spherical globules of mercury 580*f*
Bladder 212
  changes in 401
Blade of knife, cross-section of 237
Bleeding *See also Hemorrhage*
Blister formation 609*f*
Bloated features in decomposition 193
Blood 175, 470, 637
  agent *See Asphyxiant*
  alcohol
    behavior 637
    concentration 637
    management 638, 639
    psychotherapy 639
  clot 175
  evaluation of 472
  grouping 476
    absorption-elution 477
    absorption-inhibition 476
    mixed agglutination 476
  profile, changes in 196
  samples, precautions during collection of 366
  sources 474
  spatter stains 472
  stain 474
    age of 474
  stained knife crime scene 483*f*
  stains
    classes of 472
    on floor 471*f*
    on wall direction 472*f*
Blue vitriol *See also Copper sulfates*
Blunt
  pointed 329
  weapon 329
Body
  fluids 212
  hairs, no singeing of 319*f*
  surface
    bluish discolorations, clothing 203
    clothing 203
    female breast, clothing 204
    neck, clothing 204
    petechial hemorrhages, clothing 203
    postmortem color changes, clothing 203
    rigor mortis, clothing 204
Bolam test 44
Boletus sensibilis 709
Bone 111, 213
  for calculation of stature of Indian, multiplication factors for different 126*t*
  marrow, changes in 196
  of foot 80
  of head, injury to 274
Bony pattern 155
Bore of
  rifled firearm *See also Caliber*
  shotgun 253*f*
Borrowed servant doctrine 52
Botulinum neurotoxin 702
Botulinum toxin 728
Botulism 702
Boyde's method 150
Brain 271
  box *See Calvaria*
  consists 271
  death 178
    agonal period 180
    antecedent cause 181
    beating heart donor 180
    cause of death 180
    form for medical certificate 181

immediate cause 181
organ transplantation 180
persistent vegetative state 180
stupor 180
suspended animation 180
dissection of 210*f*
function, permanent cessation of 185
higher functions of 447
injury 279
parts of 178*f*, 271
Brainstem
death 178
diagnosis of 179
tests 179
apnea test 179
Braxton Hick's contraction 381
Breast
action 242
changes 379, 384
Breech loaders 244
Brentamine fast blue test 479
Breslau's test 400
British anti lewisite 540
contraindications 540
side effects 540
British Association for Forensic Odontology 166
Broken pieces *See also Powdered glass*
Bruise *See Conjunctiva*
Bruise
counter pressure 227
doughnut 227
kicking 227
love bite 227
of scalp 272
patterned intradermal 226
subcutaneous 226
Bruising, types of 226
Brush
abrasion *See also Graze*
burn 220, 221*f*
Bullet
emboli 265, 267
entry wound on skull
outer table 263*f*
with beveling in inner table 263*f*
exit wound on skull with external beveling 263*f*
fracture 275
in fluid filled viscera, effect of 266
nose, types of 256*f*
presence of unexpected 265
shaped 255*t*, 256*f*
striking skull without entry wound 264
wipe soiling 259
wound on skull 276*f*
Bungarus caeruleus 612
Bungarus caeruleus *See Common krait*
Burn 307, 309
age of victim 313
classification of 310
full thickness 314*f*
injuries
case of 273
depth of 311
site of 313
over forearm, second degree 311*f*
over leg with deposition of yellowish slough 318*f*
sex of victim 313
surface 324
to lightning, surface 326*f*
Burnt bodies of an aircraft accident 70*f*
Burtonian line 576
Butorphenol—opioid 362
Butyric acid 93

C

Cadaveric lividity 187
definition 188
Cadaveric spasm 191
Calcification deciduous teeth 147*t*
Calcivirus 708
Caliber 253*f*
of non-rifled weapon 244
Calligraphy *See Handwriting*
Calotropis 595
features 595
gigantean 595*f*
medicinal uses 595
procera 595*f*
toxic principles 596
calactin 596
calotropin 596
uscharin 596
varieties 595
Calvaria 271
Campylobacter jejuni 702
Cannabis 674, 715
indica 674*f*
psychosis 677
Cannelure 255
Cantharides 619
Cantharides-spanish fly *See Lytta vesicatoria*
Capsicum 594
annum 594*f*
autopsy findings 595
management 595
medicolegal importance 595
varieties of species 594
Caput succedaneum, changes in 401
Carbamates 653
management 654
medicolegal importance 654
Carbolic acid 557
commercial uses 557
absorption 557
antiseptic 557
clinical features 558
medical uses 557
pharmaceuticals 557
preservative 557
management 558
medicolegal importance 558
postmortem findings 558
properties 557
Carbon
dating 111
dioxide 690
monoxide 691
Cardiac
glycosides *See Calotropis toxic principles calotropin*
poisons 658
tamponade 184*f*
sudden death 184
Cardiovascular
and renal system 576
toxicity 677
Carpal bones 85
Cartridge of rifled firearm 255*f*
parts of 255*f*
Carunculae myrtiformes 385
Caste 72
Castor 590
autopsy findings 593
management 592
medicinal uses 590
medicolegal importance 593
oil plants 591*f*
oil seeds 591*f*
Catalytic tests 472
Cathartics 532
and whole bowel irrigation 532

Cattle and animal poisoning 528
Caucasoid, shape of 73*f*
Causing hurt by act endangering life 336
Cavett test 641
Cecum, rupture of 294
Cell injury, principles of 218
Cellular death *See also Molecular death*
Cellular death, early signs 186
Centers of ossification
  for fibula 127*t*
  for scapula 128*t*
  observed by Galstaun in Indian subjects 84*t*
Central nervous system 636
Cephalic index 117
  in various races 117*t*
Cerebral
  anoxia 344
  compression 282
  concussion 280
  contusion 280
  edema 279, 281
  hemorrhage 281
  irritation 282
  laceration 281
  poisons 214
Cerebrovascular system 637
Certain medicolegal term 383
Certificate, injury 337
Cervical factors 375
Cervix 381
Chadwick's sign *See also Jacquemier's sign*
Charas 675
Charcoal activated 533, 538
  contraindications 538
  dose 538
  properties 533, 538
Charting of teeth 150
  Gustafson's method 151, 152
    attrition 151
    cementum apposition 151
    periodontosis 151
    root resorption 152
    secondary dentine 151
  Haderup system 150
  modified FDI system 151
Cheapest method to extract confession practiced in Germany 500*f*
Cheiloscopy *See Lip prints*
Chelation therapy
  for toxic metals 538
  to treat 538
Chemical
  injuries 219
  warfare 724
Chest
  injuries of traumatic asphyxia 355*f*
  injuries on 291
  shape of 399
Chief judicial magistrate 12
Chilblains 320
Child
  abuse 163
  for pornographic purposes, use of (section 13) 420
Chlorophyllum molybdites 709
Chlorthion 648
Choke, various degree of 244*t*
Choking 244
  to obstruction of air passages from
    blood 355*f*
    foreign bodies 354*f*
Chop wound 234, 235*f*
  definition 234
  features 234
  medicolegal importance 235
Chopped animal hairs 623
Chronic
  alcohol poisoning 639
  arsenic poisoning 571
    diagnosis 572
    management 571
    Marsh's test 572
    medicolegal importance 572
      accidental 573
      homicide 572
      suicidal 572
    procedure 572
    Reinsch's test 572
  cocaine poisoning *See also Cocainisim*
  lead poisoning 575
  poisoning 580, 661, 697
    cause of death 661
    changes with eyes 580
    complications 661
    diagnosis 580
    management 580, 662
    medicolegal importance 581
    withdrawal symptoms 661
  SDH 285
  starvation 367, 368
  toxicity 699
Chronology of eruption 146, 149
Church abhors blood 4
Ciguatoxin 711
Circulation, changes in 401
Civil
  courts 10
  responsibilities of insane 459
Clavicle 84, 128
  age 128
  sex 128
  stature 129
Cleft palate 100*f*
Clinical autopsy *See also Academic autopsy*
Clitocybe species 709
Close range 249
Closing incisions 209*f*
Clostridium
  botulinum 702, 703
  perfringens 702, 707
    incriminated food 707
Cloth to kill newborn 403*f*
Cloth, injury marks over 236*f*
CNS manifestations 649
CO_2 *See also Carbon dioxide*
Cobra *See Naja naja*
Cobras, common spectacled 603*f*
Cocaine 678, 716
  bug 680
  powder 678*f*
Cocainisim 680
Codeine 630
Cognizable offence 17, 329
Cold *See also Low temperature, injuries to*
  stiffening 191
  water drowning 356
Colic 576
Colocynth 598
  capsule with seed 599*f*
  management 599
  medicinal uses 599
  medicolegal importance 600
Colubridae African boom slang 603
Coma, causes of 183*t*
Combined asphyxia 344
Comminuted fracture 274, 274*f*
Commit
  culpable homicide, attempt to 335
  suicide, attempt to 335
Common
  cobra 603
  krait 603
  oleander 662
    uses 662
Commotio cerebri 280

Community agreement, principle of 63
Competency to plead trial, restoration of 458
Complete abortion 389
Complete cessation of circulatory function 186
Completion illusions 443
Compliance, principle of 63
Complication of MTP 393
Component
- I-dorsal plateau 137*t*
- III-symphyseal rim 137*t*
- II-ventral rampart 137*t*
- of consent 36

Composite negligence 53
Compoundable offences 329
Computer-assisted skull identification video superimposition 99
Concealed
- firearm wounds 266
- punctured wounds 273
- sex 76

Concept of adult
- majority 38
- minority 38

Concerned police station 338
Concussion of cord 296
Condition of gastrointestinal 196
Confirmatory test 473
Congested
- brains 349*f*
- lungs 183*f*, 348*f*
- membrane 184*f*

Conium maculatum 687
- plant 687*f*

Conjunctiva 225
Consciousness
- amnesia, disorders of 447
- disorders of 447
- loss of 344
- lucid interval, disorders of 447
- narcolepsy, disorders of 447
- somnambulism, disorders of 447

Consent 34, 40
- and age 36
- and medicolegal cases 40
- criteria for 36
- for abortion 39
- for sterilization 39
- importance of 34
- of abortion 391
- of female patients 38
- of spouse 38
- scope of 38
- types of 35

Considering public health matter 490
Constipation 576
Constituents of DNA 172
Constitutes rape 420
Constitution of India grants 491
Consumer Protection Act 54, 166
Consumer redressal forum 53, 54*f*
Contact injury 322
- electrical mark 322
- types of 322

Contact poisons 531
- eyes 531
- ingestion 531
- skin 531

Contact shot 260
Contrecoup
- fracture 277
- injury of brain 278*f*

Contributory
- factors in crashes 304
- negligence 52
  - advantages of 52

Control of HIV, some legislations for 491
Contusion 223
- age of 224, 225*t*
- collar 259
- formation, mechanism of 223*f*
- mechanism of 223
- medicolegal importance 228
- multiple ligature marks with 351*f*
- of muscles of neck 352*f*

Cooling
- factors modifying rate of 187
- of body 187

Copper 581
- acute poisoning 582
- chronic poisoning 583
  - medicolegal importance 583
  - treatment 583
- common 581
- management 582
- medical use 582
- metals 581*f*
- sulfates 581*f*
- toxic compounds 581

Coprinus atramentarius 709
Coral snake 603
Cornea, opacity of 186
Corneal reflex, loss of 186
Coroner's inquest 10
Corporate negligence 53
Corpus
- delicti 70
- luteum 382

Corrosive alkalis 559
- action 559
- clinical features 559
- management 560
- medicolegal importance 560
- postmortem findings 560
- properties 559
- uses 559
  - bleaching agents 559
  - chemical 559
  - in industries 559
  - medicines 559

Corrosive poisons 530, 552
- alkalis 530
- definition 552
- metallic salts 530
- strong
  - acids 530
  - inorganic acids 530
  - organic acids 530

Cortical
- bone, microscopic findings of 112*f*
- brain death 178

Cortinarius orellanus 709
Cosmetic
- incision 206
- summary of 209

Cotton fibers 106
- microscopic pictures of 106*f*

Counter pressure bruises over bony prominences 227*f*
Country liquor 634
Country-made firearms 251
Coup 278*f*
Court case 489
Court of
- law, attendance in 378
- magistrates *See also Magistrate's court*

Court's views in favor of doctors 46
Courts 10
- of law and powers 10

Cranial
- index *See also Cephalic index*
- sutures, use of 118

Cranium, opening 205, 209, 209*f*
Creatine phosphokinase 479
Crescentic hymen 410
Cribriform 410

Crime scene 481, 481*f*
collection of evidence 483
evidence to proper agency 484
examination of 482
final survey of 484
identification of evidence 482
investigating police officer 482
investigation 481, 485
must for 484
maintaining chain of evidence 484
preserving evidence 483
purpose 481
Criminal abortion 89, 392
complications of 394*t*
general methods for 393
IPC 312 393
IPC 314 393
IPC 315 393
IPC 316 393
legal
bearing for 392
status of 393
local violence methods for 393
methods for inducing 392
motives for 392
violence methods for 393
Criminal
and civil negligence, differences between 43*t*
courts 11
importance 477
liability of mentally ill offenders 454
negligence 46
examples of 48
procedure
code 1973 8
1973, code of 506
responsibility 86, 454
concept of Act 454
Croton 593
active principle 593
autopsy findings 594
features 593
management 594
medicinal uses 593
medicolegal importance 594
plant 593*f*
seeds 593*f*
toxic part of plant 593
CRPC, Indian 174, 176, 200, 201
Crush
fracture 277
hair root to blunt force impact 229*f*
laceration of
leg 229*f*
pelvis 229*f*
Crystal test 473
CSF, changes in 196
Cu *See also Copper*
Culpable homicide 332
Cultural prohibitions 504
Curare 686
plant 687*f*
Curbing alcoholism, agencies for 644
Curling's ulcer 316
Current
intensity of 321
type of 321
voltage, intensity of 321
Custodial death 214
investigations 506
Custodial torture and deaths 496
Cut fracture 276, 277*f*
Cut injury 273
CW agents, classes of 724
CW, examples of 725
Cyclopeptide containing mushrooms 709
Cytological detection of spermatozoa 426
Cytosine bonded with guanine 172*f*

D

Daboia russelli *See Russell's viper*
Dangerous weapon 329
Dark red scabs 222*f*
Data for injury certificate 337
Date rape 418
Datura 670
alba 671
fastuosa 671
seeds 672*f*
niger 671
stramonium 671
plant 671*f*
seeds 671*f*
Davidson body 475*f*
Dead
body disposal certificate after autopsy 751
born 398
baby with signs of maceration 398*f*
definition 398
postmortem findings 398
person, methods of identification of 71
victim in state of rigor mortis 189*f*
Death
asphyxia, modes of 337
certificate 180
circumstances of 69
coma, modes of 337
during police action 498
in burn injuries
cause of 314
immediate causes 314
in cut throat injury, causes of 291
in drowning, causes of 356
in hanging, causes of 344
in strangulation, causes of 351
manner of 182, 183, 184, 190, 336
mechanism of 182, 336, 337
modes of 182, 183, 184, 337
of abortion, evidences after 394
of child after birth 403
precipitate labor 403
of infant
accidental causes 402
cause of 401, 402*f*
natural causes 402
of mother 403
signs of 185*t*
syncope, modes of 337
to ascertain PMI, changes after 196*t*
to general anesthesia, causes of 363
types of 177
Declaration of
code of medical ethics in India 26
Geneva 25
Decomposition and decay, factors affecting 192*t*
Deep
cyanosis of lips 346*f*
dermal burns 313*f*
Defense
in medical negligence 53
wound 234
on palmer aspect of hand 234*f*
Degenerated atrophied root without sheath fallen by itself 108*f*
Delhi High Court ruling on Section 377 IPC 435
Deliriants and psychotropic poisons 670
Delivery 378, 383
signs of 378, 384

Delusion
  depending on content, types of 443
  disorders 441
  of grandeur 444*f*
  of guilt and unworthiness 443
  of infidelity 443
  of influence or control 443
  of love 443
  of persecution 443
  of poverty 443
  of reference 444
Dementia 446
  pre-senile 446
  pugilistica 289
  secondary 446
  senile 446
  types of 446
Dentaire international, federation 150
Dental
  age, radiographic estimation of 153
  cast 163*f*
  examination for age estimation 83
  identification 153
    comparative method of 157
    factors of 154
    in mass disaster 160*f*
    methods 157
  impression 163*f*
  profiling 167
    case of 167*f*
  prosthesis 155, 156*f*
  records 153*f*
    management of 145
    storage of 145
  restorations 156*f*
Dentition, mixed 147, 147*f*
Denture labeling 166, 167*f*
Depressed
  comminuted fracture 274
  fractures 274, 274*f*
Depth of burn, calculation of 312
Dermal nitrate test 267
Desferrioxamine 542
  adverse effects 542
  contraindications 542
Detention 497
  in reformatories 13
Devastator bullets 258
DFSA *See Drug-facilitated sexual assault*
Diacetylmorphine *See Heroin*
Diamond powder 622
  management 622
Diaphanous test 186
Diarrhea 586
Diatom test 359
Dies of brainstem compression 282
Digital forensics 168
Digitalis 658
  purpurea 658, 659*f*
  toxicity 659
Dihydroergotamine 600
Dimercaptopropane sulfonate 541
Dimercaptosuccinic acid 541
  side effects 541
    contraindications 541
    cough 541
    diarrhea 541
    nausea 541
    rash 541
    rhinitis 541
    vomiting 541
Diminished responsibility 457
Discharge of
  projectile, mechanism of 258
  rifled firearm, effect of 260*f*
Disciplinary enquiry, procedure of 24
Discrimination, employment and 490
Dislocation of cervical vertebrae *See Fracture*
Disorders of body functions, responsibility in 460
Disulfiram 639
Divorce 378
DMPS *See also Dimercaptopropane sulfonate*
DNA
  bands to solve paternity 176*f*
  base pair sequence in 172
  chromosome 172
  extractions from sample 173*f*
  fingerprinting 173
    for forensic purpose, methods of 173
    methods applied in 173
  identification 167
  introduction to 171
  profiling 76
    usefulness of 175, 176*t*
    various application of 175*t*
  restriction enzyme 173
  structure 172*f*
  typing 477
    in forensic investigation, uses of 175
Doctor
  and media 26
  in general, duties of 25
  in poisoning case, role of 545
  negligent, law for holding 47
  to each other, duties of 25
  to sick, duties of 25
  witness in court, duty of 20
Doctrine of
  calculated risk 49
  common knowledge 50
  error of judgment 49
  loco parentis 39
  res ipsa loquitur 45
  respondent superior 51
Documentary evidence in relation to medical practice 14
Domestic violence 163
Dorsal demi-face 137*t*
Doughnut bruise over back of chest 227*f*
Dowry death 334
D-penicillamine *See Penicillamine*
Dried blood stains over knife 472*f*
Dried root of aconitum napellus 664*f*
Drink 421
  spiking 421
Drowning 356
  definition 356
  event of 356
  fatal period 357
  postmortem appearance 357
  tests for 359
  treatment 357
  types of 356
Drug 421
  abuse death, investigation of 719
  and Cosmetic Act, 1940 492
  facilitated sexual assault 421
  for criminal abortion, internal use of 392
  intoxication *See Poisoning*
  related harms 718
Drunkenness 640
  and cerebral concussion, differences between 289*t*
  case of 41, 640
  reporting 640
    blood analysis 641
    consent 640
    procedure 640
      proper 640
    saliva analysis 641
    urine analysis 641

Dry
drowning 356
fruit of datura 671*f*
poppy capsule 626
Dumdum bullet 257
Dupertuis 125*t*
Dupuytren's
classification 310
ulcer 315, 316
Dyed hairs 108*f*
Dying declaration and dying deposition, differences between 16*t*
Dynapar—NSAIDs 362

E

Ear
bleeding to ruptured tympanic membrane 326*f*
prints 97
Early signs 186
Echis carinata *See Saw-scaled viper*
Echis carinatus venom 612
Edetate disodium 541
EDH
fate of 283
over occipitoparietal areas 283
EDTA *See Ethylenediaminetetraacetic acid*
Elapid envenomations
signs of 610
symptoms of 610
Electrical injuries 320
intensity of current 321
types of 322, 232
Electron microscopy-energy dispersive X-ray spectrometry 268
Eliptical shaped
incised wound 231*f*
stab wound 237*f*
Emaciated body to starvation 368*f*
Emasculation *See Penis, excision of*
Embryo 78
Endocrine 637
Endogenous toxicant 183
Enlarged sebaceous glands 380
Enterohemorrhagic *E coli* 705
incriminated food 706
Enterotoxigenic *E coli* 705
incriminated food 705
Entry and exit wound, differences between 263*t*
Entry wound
in rifled firearm 260
of bullet imprint abrasion of muzzle end 261*f*
on hand 322*f*
and exit wound on foot 322*f*
Environment protection agency of USA 55
Ergometrine 600
Ergot 600*f*
current uses of 600
on rye 600
replaces grain of rye 600
Ergotamine 600
Ergotoxin 600
Erotomanic type *See also Delusion of love*
Eruption of deciduous teeth 147*t*
Erythema, slough places 315*f*
Essence of crime *See Corpus delicti*
Essentiality, principle of 63
Ethanol *See Ethyl alcohol*
consumption, effects of 636
mode of action of 636
Ethical aspects of medical practice 24
Ethics and medical research 60
Ethyl alcohol 633
introduction 633
Ethylenediaminetetraacetic acid 541
Eugenic grounds of abortion 390
Euthanasia 32, 65
cons 66
definition 65
history 65
medicolegal importance 67
physician sentiment 66
pros 66
types of 66
Every man's fundamental right 41
Evidence
collection of 164*t*
from victim, collection of 163
Ewald tube 532*f*
Executive magistrates 12
Exemplar prints 92
Exit wound 262
of bullet 262*f*
of shotgun 250
on foot 322*f*
Exogenous toxins 183
Explosive bullet 257
Extensive charring all over body 315*f*
External and internal wad, differences between 247*t*
Extra-axial hemorrhage 282
Extradural hemorrhage 283*f*
Eye, changes in 186
Eyes, clothing 203

F

Fabricated
abortion 394
wound 233
Face, external injuries on 271
Facial
pallor 576
skeleton 271
Faint
ligature marks with fingertip bruises 351*f*
transverse ligature marks with finger tip bruises 352*f*
Fang mark 616*f*
Fatal
dose 659
period 344, 368, 659
factors influencing 368
Fatty acids 93
Fe *See Iron*
Feigned mental illness 449
Female
feticide 406
genitalia 212
humerus 129*f*
pseudohermaphroditism 78
radius 131*f*
sacrum 138*f*
sterility, causes of 375
sternum 132*f*
Femur 84, 122
age 122
bone length 124
index 124
indices in various races 124*t*
length of 126*f*
lower end of 80
of both sex 122*f*
ossification centers 122
race 124
radiographic changes 122
sex 122
stature 124
structural appearances 124
Ferric chloride 586
test 697
Ferrous sulfate 586

Fetal 212
- heart sounds 382
- skeletons in X-ray of abdomen 382*f*

Feticide 397
Fetus 78
- age of 79
- age-related changes in 81*t*

Fibers 105
Fibula 85, 127
- age 127
- sex 127
- stature 127

Fimbriated hymen 410
Finger pad bruises 226
- over legs 226*f*

Fingerprint
- development of 94*f*
- in decomposed bodies 94
- lifting of 94, 94*f*
- mutilation of 95
- system 91
  - classification 92
  - definition 91
  - individuality of fingerprints 93
  - latent prints 92
  - mode of production 93
  - patent prints 93
  - plastic prints 93
  - principle of use 91

Fire, direction of 251, 266
Firearm
- classification of 242
- general make up of 241
- injuries 240
  - terminologies 240
- parts of 241*f*

Firing, distance of 266
First Class Judicial Magistrate 12
First degree burns 311*f*
First DNA fingerprints 172*f*
First information report 752
Fissured 274
- fracture 274*f*

Fissures 434*f*
Fitness to stand trial 458
Flaccidity of eyeball 186
Flameless atomic absorption spectrometry 268
Flash burn injury, types of 322, 323
Flaying laceration 301*f*
Floatation test *See also Hydrostatic test*
Fluorosis stains 159*f*
Fodere's test 399
Food
- and vomitus particles in air passage 355*f*
- borne 702
- poisoning 701
  - classification of 701

Footprint 96
- in mud 483*f*
- types of 96*f*

Force
- application, direction of 217
- degree of 217
- enforced, degree of 224

Forceful fist 272
Forensic
- anthropology 111
- ballistics 240
- DNA typing 171
- entomology 196
- medicine 3, 6
  - future of 6
  - history of 3
  - in India, phylogenesis of 5
  - introduction of 3
- odontologist 160
  - role of 159
- odontology 83, 142
  - definition 143
  - dental records 144
  - dentition 145
  - maintenance of dental records 145
  - organizations in field of 166
  - patient record 144
  - recent advances in 166
- of patient records 145
- or legal medicine 3
- osteology 76, 111
- pathologist 200
- psychiatry 440
  - practice
    - abreaction, terms in 444
    - affect, terms in 444
    - aggression, terms in 445
    - agitation, terms in 445
    - ambivalence, terms in 445
    - aphasia, terms in 445
    - compulsion, terms in 445
    - coprolalia, terms in 445
    - enuresis, terms in 445
    - euphoria, terms in 445
    - hypersomnia, terms in 445
    - insight, terms in 445
    - terms in 444
- science 517
  - brain mapping 521
  - chromatography 520
  - electrophoresis 520
  - in India 516
  - laboratory 516
    - organizational set up of 519
  - microscopy 520
  - narco analysis 521
  - neutron activation analysis 521
  - photography 520
  - polygraph 522
    - DNA profiling 523
    - in test 522
    - pre-test interview 522
  - spectrophotometry and colorimetry 521
- serology 470
- significance 142

Formic acid 93
Fracture 344
- hyoid bone 352*f*
- la signaturea 275*f*
- of middle fossa 279
- of posterior fossa 279
- of skull 274
  - mechanism of 278, 278
- on anterior fossa 278

Frangible bullet 257
Freezing of cadaver 467
French chalk *See also Lead carbonate*
Frigidity 374
- causes 374
- medicolegal importance 374
- types 374

Frontal lobes 282
Frost nip 320
Frostbite 320
Fungal 708

G

Gait 109
Galerina species 709
Gallbladders, distended 370*f*
Galstaun 123*t*, 127*t*, 128*t*, 130*t*, 135*t*
Gamma hydroxybutyric acid 421
Gang rape 418
Ganja 675
Gastric lavage 532
- complications 532
- contraindications 532

indications 532
material used 532
precautions 533
procedure 532
tube *See Ewald tube*
Gastrointestinal
system 637
tract
kidney 212
liver 212
spleen 212
ulceration 315
Gel documentation 173*f*
Generic names of drugs, use of 28
Gestational period 383
Getting registered, procedure of 27
Gettler's test 359
Ghaffir guns 243
GHB *See Gamma hydroxybutyric acid*
Ghon's technique 210
Giardia in stool 708
Glass jaw 565
Glass, broken pieces of 621*f*
Glass-blower's shakes 580
Gold 584
clinical features 584
postmortem findings 584
properties 584
treatment 584
uses 584
Gonadal biopsy 75
Goodell's sign 381
Gordon's classification of death 340
Granulation tissue formations over-hand extensive burn injuries 318*f*
Gravid uterus containing product of conceptus 388*f*
Gray powder 94
Graze 220
Great vessels, dissection of 211
Green viper 604
Grievous injury 219
Growth in individual bones 115
Gun
ballistics 240, 241
barrel, back spatters on 248*f*
itself, type of 251
Gunshot
injuries, patterns of 268
wound imaging 267
wounds in bone 262
Gustatory hallucination 442
Gutter fracture 275
Gyromitra species 709

H

H_2S *See Hydrogen sulfide*
Habitual sodomist, sign of 433
Hadden's formulae for stature from long bones 125*t*
Haddon counter measures, strategies for 305*t*
Hair 105, 213
growth, changes in 196
Hallucination, types of 442
Hallucinogens 716
Hand
guns 253
rest *See also Hand guns*
Handwriting 109
Hanging 343
definition 343
ligature material 343
mechanism of neck constriction 344
sequence of events in hanging 344
Hangman's fracture 296
Haptic hallucination 442
Hard blunt weapon 329
Harelip 100*f*
Hashish *See also Charas*
Hatters' shake 580
Haversian
canal 112
system 112
Hazard
of pesticides 656
symbols used worldwide 723*f*
HCl *See Hydrochloric acid*
Head
anatomical review of 270
contact range injuries to 248
external injuries on 271
injury 183, 271, 288
tilted opposite to knot 345*f*
Healed areas of burn around knee joint 318*f*
Healing of
abrasion 221
incised wound 232*t*
Health care, discrimination in 490
Hearsay evidence 13
Heat
fracture 277
hematoma 317
intensity of 314
rupture 316, 316*f*
Heavy metal poisons 214
Hebra's classification 311
Hegar's sign 381
Helsinki
code 61
declaration 62
Hemorrhage 223
Hepatitis virus 708
Heroin 630
Hickey *See Love bite*
High court 11
High temperature heat
cramps 309
exhaustion 309
autopsy findings 309
treatment 309
hyperpyrexia 309
stroke 308
Hine test See Kozelka test
Hinge fracture 276, 276*f*
Hip bone 84
HIV
positive patient's disclosure to interested parties 489
status of positive individuals in death certificate 491
HNO_3 *See Nitric acid*
Homicidal *See Antemortem separations of head*
cut throat 233, 233*f*, 291*f*
poisoning 528, 581
Homicide 332, 337
classification of 332, 332*f*
Honeybee 617*f*
sting 617*f*
Hormonal analysis 75
Human
and animal hair, difference between 106, 107*t*
blood biconcave 475*f*
cross section of 106*f*
experimentation 60
types of 60
hair 105, 109*f*
anatomy of 105*f*
cortex 105
crushed end indicative of blunt force impact 109*f*
cut by sharp cutting weapon 109*f*
cuticle 105
medicolegal questions 107
medulla 105
pulled by force 109*f*
life, security of 48
mandible 119, 120*f*
adults 121
age from mandible 120

birth 121
female 120*f*
old age 122
old male 120*f*
race 120
sex 119
stature 119
remains, identification of 160
rights 31, 496
skeleton recovered on bank of river 112*f*
spermatozoa 478*f*
Humanitarian grounds of abortion 390
Humerus 84, 129
age 130
bone length 129
brachial index 130
humerofemoral index 130
index 129
intermembral index 130
ossification centers 130
race 129
sex 129
stature 129
Hydrated ferric oxide 569
Hydrochloric acid 554
properties 554
uses 555
Hydrocution drowning 356
Hydrocyanic acid 666
appearance 666
source 666
uses 666
Hydrogen sulfide 693
Hydrostatic test 399
Hymen 410
congenital absence of 411
intact 410*f*
rupture of 411
types of 410
Hyoid bone 133
Hyoscyamus muticus 672
Hyoscyamus niger 672
Hypnogogic 442
Hypnopompic hallucinations 442
Hypnotism 460
crime 460
hypnosis 460
Hypochondrial delusion 443
Hypoproteinemia 315
Hypothermia
causes 319
of death 319
classification 319
Hypovolemic shock 314

I

Icard's test 186
ICMR guidelines for human research, 1995 62
Ideal biological weapon, characteristics of 728
Identification, types of 69
Illegal detention 452
Illegitimate pregnancy infanticide 396
Illicit liquor 634
Illusion 443
affect 443
types of 443
Immediate signs 185
Immersion
foot *See also Trench foot*
syndrome 356
Immoral traffic, prevention of 491
Imperforate hymen 410
Implications, legal 59
Implied consent 35
Impotence
case of 372
causes of 372
frigidity 372
sterility 372
types of 372
Impression scene of crime, persistence of 95
Imprint abrasion 221, 221*f*
Imprisonment 498
Impulse control disorder 448
dipsomania 448
kleptomania 448
mutilomania 448
pyromania 448
sexual impulses 448
types of 448
In birth certificate 14
Incarceration 498
Incendiary bullets 258
Incest 432
Incestual rape 419
Incised
split laceration 272*f*
wound 230
age 231
medicolegal importance 232
over face 231*f*
over plantar aspect of foot 231*f*
Incision
closing of 209
in front 208*f*
on back *See also Positioning body*
on mid-axillary line, extension of 4th 207*f*
Incisors, shaped 72*f*
Indecent assault 413
Indented fracture *See also Pond*
Indian
Evidence Act
1872 8, 506
1869 8
legal system 8
Medical Council 2002 26, 60
ethics 2002 26, 60
etiquette 2002 26, 60
professional conduct 2002 26, 60
regulations, 2002 26, 60
Medical Register 22
maintenance of 22
Penal Code 216
1860 8
Police Act 506
Indications of artificial insemination 376
Indices from humerus in various races 130*t*
Induction of MTP, methods for 391
Infant
born alive 399
botulism 703
death during birth 402
cord prolapse 402
prolonged labor 402
death syndrome
autopsy findings, sudden 406
definition, sudden 405
etiology, sudden 406
risk factors, sudden 406
sudden 405
periods of 79*t*
skull, case of 275
Infanticide 89, 396
definition 396
motive for 396
Infantile hymen 410
Infertility *See also Sterility*, types of
secondary 374
Informed consent 35, 488
exception to 35
Inhalants 716
Inhalation of irrespirable gases 355
Inhaled poisons 214
Inheritance infanticide
Injected poisons 214, 531

Injection of liquid paraffin into terminal phalanx 95*f*
Injuries
  assault, legal issues of 330
  biophysics of 217
  blasting, miscellaneous 219
  electrical, miscellaneous 219
  grievous hurt, legal issues of 330
  hurt, legal issues of 330
  legal issues of 330
  lightning, miscellaneous 219
  mechanical 216
    injuries, types of 218
  medical classification, types of 218
  miscellaneous 219
  production, mechanism of 298
  radiation, miscellaneous 219
  thermal
    application of
      cold, types of 219
      heat, types of 219
    injuries, types of 219
    local application of heat, types of 219
  types of 218
Inocybe species 709
Inorganic
  acids 552
  compounds 568
  irritant poisons 562
    absorption 564
    excretion 564
    excretion acute poisoning 565
      autopsy findings 565
      management 565
    excretion chronic poisoning 565
      management 566
      phossy jaw 565
    iodine 562
    iodine acute poisoning 563
      autopsy findings 563
      management 563
    iodine chronic poisoning 563
      management 563
    iodine
      clinical features 563
      features 562
      mechanism of action 563
      medicolegal importance 564
    medicolegal importance 566
    metabolism 564
    phosphorus 564
  irritants
    metallic poisons 567
    non-metallic poisons 562
Inquest 9
  definition 9
  types of 9
Inquiry by magistrate into cause of death 202
Insane person *See also Suicide of child*, abetment of
Insanity in Indian perspective 456
Insecticide preparation, symbols in labeling in 549*f*
Institutional arrangement, principle of 63
Intermediate range 249
  shot 261
Intermittent uterine contractions 381, 384
Internal
  ballistics 240
  injuries, associated 238
  wad *See also Powder wad*
International Code of Medical Ethics 25
Intersex state 76
  gonadal
    agenesis 76
    dysgenesis 76
  types of 76
Interstitial system 112
Intoxication 457
Intra axial hemorrhage 282
  classification 284
  extradural 282
  medicolegal importance 283, 285
  subdural 283
Intracranial injuries
  age of 288
  complications of 287
Intradermal bruise, patterned 226*f*
Intraventricular hemorrhage 286
Involuntary active euthanasia 66
Iodine, uses of 562
IPC 313 393
Iron 586
  medicolegal importance 587
  postmortem findings 586
  sulfate 586
  toxicity, risk of 586
  treatment 586
Irritants poisons 530

J

Jacketed bullets 256
Jacquemier's sign 380
Jefferson fracture 296
Jigsaw fit 105
Judges, types of 11
Judicial
  punishment 88
  responsibility of insane offenders 454
Justifiable 390
Juvenile magistrates 12

K

Kaiserling method 511
Kaiserling's solution 511
Kala datura *See also Datura niger*
Keloid
  formations with contractures 318*f*
  scars types of 102*f*
Kennedy phenomenon 265
Kevorkian sign 186
Kidnapping 89
Kidney 637
  changes in 401
Kinetic energy 217
Klinefelter's syndrome 76, 76, 637
Kozelka test 641
Krait venom 612

L

Labia 384
Laceration 228
  and incised wound, differences between 232*t*
  avulsion 229
  crush 229
  cut 230
  in inner part of lips 354*f*
  medicolegal importance 230
  over lips 354*f*
  split 228
  stretch 228
  tear 229
  types of 228
Langer's lines 236
Lanugo hair 107
Late signs 191
Latent lip prints 168
Lathyrus sativus, chemicals 711
Lavacuator 532*f*
Law 40

Lawful homicide 332
  excusable 332
  justifiable 332
Laws
  against torture 499
  relating to poison in India 547
    Dangerous Drug Act 547
    Drug Act 547
    Drugs (control) Act, 1950 548
    Drugs and
      Cosmetic Act, 1940 547
      Cosmetics Rules, 1945 548
      Magic Remedies (objectionable advertisements) Act, 1954 548
    Insecticides
      Act, 1968 548
      Rules, 1971 548
    Narcotic Drugs 549
    Poison Act 547
      1919 547
    Psychotropic Substance Act, 1985 540
Lax sphincter 434*f*
LDH isoenzyme method 479
Lead 573
  acetate 574*f*
  carbonate 94, 574*f*
  chromate 574*f*
  commercial uses 573
  encephalopathy 576
  line 576
  metal granules 573*f*
  palsy 576
  pellet 242*f*
  properties 573
  shot 242*f*
  slug 242
  sulfide 574*f*
  tetroxide 574*f*
  toxic compounds 573
Left arm, injuries over 507*f*
Legal
  abortion *See also Justifiable*
  responsibility 288
  restrictions, evasion of 33
Legitimacy 378
Legitimacy 386
Lepiota species 709
Lesser CW agents 725
Letuli's technique 210
Lie detector *See Forensic science polygraph*
Life
  imprisonment 12
  of abortion, evidences during 394
Ligature material
  cloth 343*f*
  examination of 344
  nylon rope 343*f*
Ligature strangulation 290*f*
Lightning 323
  strike, complications to 325*t*
Lilliputian hallucinations 442
Limbs, injuries on 294
Linea
  albicantes, scars types of 102*f*
  nigra 380
Linear
  abrasion 220*f*
  fracture 274
  lightning burn 324*f*
    injury 324
Linen
  fibers 105
  microscopic pictures of 106*f*
Lip
  laceration 346*f*
  print 97, 97*f*
    definition 97
Listeria monocytogenes 702
Liver, rupture of 294
Living person, methods of identification of 71
Long barrel 243
Love bite 165*f*, 227*f*
Low temperature
  hypothermia, injuries to 319
  injuries to 319
Lower limb, ant bite marks on 466*f*
Lucid interval in head injury cases 289
Lycoperdon species 709
Lytta vesicatoria 619*f*

M

Macro test 641
Maggots 213
Magistrate
  and police inquest, differences between 10*t*
  court 12
  inquest 9, 10
Magnan's syndrome *See also Cocaine bug*
Magnesium sulfate 577
Magnus 186
Majun 675
Male
  and female
    differentiating points between 75*t*
    femur, differences between 122*t*
  genitalia 212
  humerus 129*f*
  impotence 372
  infants weigh 79
  pseudohermaphroditism 78
  radius 131*f*
  sacrum 138*f*
  sterility, causes of 374
  sternum 132*f*
Malingering 449
Malocclusion 156*f*
Malpractice, civil cases in 166
Mammalian blood of camel type oval and non-nucleated RBCs 475*f*
Mandible 119
  adult 121*f*
  age-related changes of 121*t*
  birth 121*f*
  male and female differences in 120*t*
  old-aged person 121*f*
Manual strangulation with imprint abrasions and bruises 222*f*
Marbling on chest 192*f*
Marine organisms 711
Marking nut 596
  tree 597*f*
Marks left on bullet 252
Marriage contract 89
Mass disaster
  case of 160*f*
  management 730
Mass fatality incidences 160
Master-servant rule 51
Material, ligature 343*f*
Maternity disputes *See also DNA bands to solve paternity*
Maturation, disturbance in 86
Maturity of fetus, signs of 398
Maxilla, arch of 114*f*
MCI
  and medical record 34
  composition of 21
  constitution of 21
  duration of 22
  functions of 22

McNaghten rule 456
    1843 454
Medical
    abortion 391
    civil negligence 42
    Council of India 21, 22
        structure of 21
    education, maintenance of quality of 22
    ethics 21, 24
        code of 26
    etiquette 24
    evidence 13
        types 13
            documentary evidence 13
            dying declaration 14
            dying deposition 15
            medical certificates 14
            oral evidence 13
    examination of sexcrime accused 430
        legal procedure for 431
    insanity vs legal insanity 457
    law 21
    maloccurrence 50
    negligence 42
        classification of 42
        instances of 44
    practice, legal aspects of 33
    practitioner, duties of registered 29
    professionals in tackling torture menace, role of 505
    research combined with professional care 62
    termination of pregnancy 390
    Waste Tracking Act 55
Medicolegal
    aspect of
        injury 328
        offence 328
    autopsy
        objectives of 200, 201*t*
        of HIV infected case 492
    importance 370, 373, 376
        injury, terms of 216
        lesion, terms of 216
        of age 86
        of examination of blood 477
        of fiber 108
        of hair 108
        of people living with HIV/AIDS 487
        of powder marks 260
        of virginity 412
        of wad 247
        terms of 216
        trauma, terms of 216
        wound, terms of 216
    issues of brain death 179
    queries of infanticide 397
    questions
        in case of drowning 359
        related to hanging 349
Medullary
    cavity 122
        reaches anatomical neck 123*f*
    index of hair 106
Memory 110
Meninges, anatomy of 271*f*
Mens rea *See Mental element, different degrees of*
Mental
    element, different degrees of 455
    Health Act 1987 450
        objectives of 450
    health
        disorders, classification of 441
        problems, marriage and 459
    ill, restraining of 453
    illness
        causes of 450
        diagnosis of 450
    retardation 442, 448
        some old terms for 448
    state time of offence 454
Mercurial tremor *See also Hatters' shake*
Mercuric
    chloride 579*f*
    compounds 578
    iodide 579*f*
    oxides 579*f*
    sulfide 579*f*
Mercurous compound 578
Mercury 577, 577*f*
    properties 577
Mercy killing *See Euthanasia*
Metacarpals 85
Metal fume fever 587
    alloy making 587
    electroplating 587
    galvanizing 587
    involved 587
        antimony 587
        beryllium 587
        cadmium 587
        chromium 587
        cobalt 587
        copper 587
        iron 587
        lead 587
        magnesium 587
        manganese 587
        mercury 587
        nickel 587
        selenium 587
        silver and aluminum 587
        vanadium 587
        zinc 587
    occupations affected 587
    refining 587
    smelting 587
    welding 587
Metal jacket
    bullet, full 256
    round, total 256
Metallic poison 567
Metatarsal bone 85
Methyl alcohol 645
    management 645
    uses 645
        antifreeze 645
        denatured spirit 645
        embalming fluid 645
        leather dyes 645
        shellac 645
        varnish 645
        windshield washing fluid 645
Methyl parathion 648
Metropolitan Magistrate *See also First Class Judicial Magistrate*
Mexican poppy 710
Micro test 641
Microperforate hymen *See also Cribriform*
Microscopic examination 74
Midazolam 362
Middle
    ear changes 401
    meningeal artery 282
Missile 267
Molecular death 177
Molestation *See Indecent assault*
Mongolian spot 100*f*
Mongoloid, shape of 73*f*
Monosodium glutamate 711
Monster baby *See also Anencephaly*
Montgomery's tubercles, appearance of 380

Mood affective disorders 441
Morphine, tests for 628
Morphological examination 74
Motor vehicle injury control, strategies for 305*t*
Motorcycle accident, causes of 304
Motorcyclists, injuries of 303
MSG, chemicals 711
MTP *See Medical termination of pregnancy*
Mucous membrane of
  lips 580
  mouth 580
  tongue 580
Multiple
  bruises 354*f*
  ligature marks 347
Mummification 194
  definition 194
Mummified
  body 195*f*
  human legs 195*f*
Munchausen's syndrome 405
  by proxy 405
    treatment 405
Murder 333
  attempt to 335
  distinguished from culpable homicide 334
Muscle 213
  primary flaccidity of 187
  relaxant used for intubation 363
Muscular
  condition 190
  contraction in rigor mortis 190*f*
Museum
  arrangement of specimen 510*f*
  basic techniques 510
  construction of jar 512
  different specimen 510*f*
  division of 510*f*
  fixation 510
  glass jar 512*f*
    specimen 513*f*
  labeling of specimen 513
  mounting of specimen 513
  preparation 510
  preservation 510
  reception 510
  specimens 511
  techniques bones 514
  techniques gross staining 513
    calcium 513
    fat 513
    hematoxylin and eosin stains 513
    iron 513
    myocardial infarction 513
  techniques photography 514
Mushroom
  bullet 257
  part of 708
  poisoning *See Fungal*
Mutilated bodies *See also Sex from decomposed*
Muzzle
  end and effects, discharging components from 259*t*
  end, discharging components from 259*f*
  loader 243
  marks of gun 226*f*
MWTA *See Medical Waste Tracking Act*

N

NAA *See Neutron activation analysis*
Nag vibrios 702
Nail 213
  scratch abrasions 351*f*, 352*f*
Naja naja 605
Naja naja See *Common cobra*
  venom 612
Naked-eye 473
Narcotic Drugs and Psychotropic Substances Act 12
Nasal aperture, shape of 73*f*
Natural
  causes of abortion 389*t*
  orifices, clothing 203
Nature of
  explosive 251
  poisoning in India 527
NDPS Act *See Narcotic Drugs and Psychotropic Substances Act*
Neck, injury to 290
Needle puncture wound 236
Negligence
  by medical professionals 47
  causing death by 334
  essential elements of 43
Negroid, shape of 73*f*
Neonaticide 397
Nerve agent 724
Neurogenic shock 314
Neuronal injury, diffuse 281
Neurosis 449
Neurotoxic 614
  envenomations 614
Neutron activation analysis 268, 572
New bullet, example of 266
Newborn by cloth, smothering of 353*f*
NHRC guidelines 506
Nicotiana tabacum, leaves of 660
Nicotinic manifestations 649
Nipple, hyperpigmentation of 380*f*
Nitric acid 554
  clinical features 554
  postmortem findings 554
  properties 554
  uses 554
Nitrostigmine 648
Non-bailable offences 328
Non-closure of anterior fontanelle 118*f*
Non-cognizable offence 17, 329
Non-displaced comminuted fracture 274
Non-exploitation, principle of 63
Non-mammalian blood nucleated RBCs 475
Non-nucleated RBCs 475*f*
Non-poisonous snakes, identification of 605
Non-traumatic intracerebral hemorrhage 286
Non-venomous snake 608*f*
Non-voluntary active euthanasia 66
Norovirus 708
  food poisoning 708
Norwalk virus 702
Nose print 97
Novus actus interveniens 50
Nterior ethmoidal artery 282
Nuclear
  explosion 730*f*
  sexing *See Sex chromatin test*
  weapon 729
Number of teeth 154
Numbering
  permanent teeth, systems of 152*f*
  teeth, systems of 151*t*
Nursing home under MHA-1987 *See also Admissions in psychiatric hospitals*
Nut of semicarpus anacardium 597*f*

O

Oblique ligature marks around neck 347*f*
Obsessive-compulsive disorder 447

compulsion 448
obsession 447
Occipital lobes 282
Occupational stigmata 104
permanent 104
recent and temporary 104
OCTA and tetrahedral crystals of arsenic 572*f*
Offence 17
attending court 18
classification of 328
conduct money 18
oath taking 18
perjury 18
types of 17
Old
bullet, example of 265
hymenal tear 425*f*
Olfactory hallucination 442
Opiates 715
Opium 624
alkaloids, classifications of 626
criminal uses 627
fatal
dose 627
period 627
Oral
evidence 13
pathology 155
Orbits, shape of 73*f*
Organ transplantation 32, 180
Organic
irritants of animal origin 602
psychiatric disorders 441
Organizational set up of FSL 519*t*
Organochlorines 651
absorption 652
acute poisoning 653
chronic poisoning 653
classification 652
fatal dose 653
management 653
medicolegal importance 653
metabolism 652
Organophosphates 647
classification 648
alkyl phosphates 648
demeton 648
dime fox 648
hexaethyl tetraphosphate 648
isopestox 648
malathion sulfotep 648
octamethyl pyrophosphate 648
tetraethyl pyrophosphate 648
uses of 648
Organs
brain, dissection of different 210
dissection of different 210
gastrointestinal tract, dissection of different 212
genitalia, dissection of different 212
heart, dissection of 211
lungs, dissection of 211
spinal cord, dissection of 211
Orthodontic brackets 159*f*
Ossification
centers
appearance of 80, 83
for sternum 133*f*
fusion of 83
lower end of femur 80*f*
of femur 123*f*
of sternum 80*f*
of bones of foot 140*f*
of clavicle 129*t*
of femur 123*t*
of hipbone 135*t*
of humerus 130*t*
of small bones of hand 140*f*
of tibia 127*t*
of ulna 132*t*
Osteometric board 114*f*
Osteons *See Haversian system*
Ovulation disorders 375
Oxalic acid 555
clinical features 555
criminal use 555
management 556
medicolegal importance 556
accidental 556
homicidal 556
suicidal 556
mode of action 555
properties 555
source 555
uses 555

P

P. semilanceata 709
Pachymeningitis hemorrhagica interna 285
Palatoprints 97
Palm prints 96
Palmar sign 381
Palmer aspect of hand 161*f*
Pancreas, Rupture of 294
Papaverine 630
Paracetamol 695, 698
chemical structure of 698
Paraffin test 267
Paraoxon 648
Paraphilias
exhibitionism 437
fetishism 436
frotteurism 437
lust murder 436
masochism 436
masturbation 437
necrophilia 436
sadism 435
transvestism 436
undinism 437
voyeurism 437
Paraquat poisoning 655
Parasuicidal mutilation 234
Parathion 648
Pareidolic illusions 443
Parous cervix 384*f*
with slit like external os 385*f*, 386*f*
Passive euthanasia 66
Patella 85
Patent and copyrights 31
Paternity 378, 386
Pathological intracerebral hemorrhage *See Non-traumatic intracerebral hemorrhage*
Patient time of gastric lavage, position of 533*f*
Pb *See Lead*
PC and PNDT Act 1996, objective of 406
PCPNDT Act
2003 406
features of 407
Pelvic bones, male and female 134*f*
Pelvis and hipbone 134
age 134
ossification centers 134
race 136
sex 134
Penetrating
fracture 275
wound, description of 236*t*
Penetrative sexual assault (section 3) 419
Penicillamine 542, 570
side effects 542
Penis, excision of 330*f*
Pentazocine (fortwin)—opioid 362
Pepper spray 725

Perception
  disturbances of 442
  hallucination, disturbances of 442
Perchloride of iron 586
Perforating
  fracture 275*f*
  wound 236
Perinatal autopsy 212
Periorbital hematoma 273
Periorbital hematoma *See also Black eye*
Peripheral nerve poison 686
Permanent teeth 148
  bicuspids 149
  calcification of 149*t*
  canines 149
  emergence of 149
  eruption of 149*t*
  in each jaw, set of 147*f*, 149*f*
  incisors 148
  molars 149
  premolars 149
Pernio *See Chilblains*
Persistent vegetative state 180
Personal
  effects on cadaver 196
  safety of others 336
  safety of others *See also Act endangering life*
PET bottles *See Polyethylene terephthalate bottles*
Phalanga 501
  of hand 85
Phantom pregnancy 383
Phobia 449
  acrophobia 449
  agoraphobias 449
  claustrophobia 449
  mysophobia 449
  nyctophobia 449
  types of 449
  xenophobia 449
Phosphine 693
Phosphorus
  types of 564
  uses of 564
Physical exhibits encountered, types of 517
Physician
  assisted suicide 66
  in case of consultation, duties of 30
  in firearm injuries, role of 268
  to patients, duties of 29
Physiological antidotes 537
Pistol and revolver, features of semi-automatic 253*t*
Pit viper 603
Plain arch 92*f*
Plant 710
  erythroxylon coca 678*f*
  management 710
  medicolegal importance 710
Plastic bullet 257
Plead See also Fitness to stand trial
Plumbago 597
  indica 597
  rosea 597, 598*f*
  varieties 597
  zeylanica 598
Podogram *See also Footprints*
Point blank shot *See also Contact shot*
Pointed weapon 329
Poison
  action of 528
  control center 537
  definition of 527
  diagnosis of 528
  elimination of absorbed 534
  environment, removal of patient from 531
  factors modifying action of 529
  in dead body, diagnosis of 529
  in living, diagnosis of 528
  information center 537
  laboratory 537
  local action of 528
  remote action of 528
  research center 537
Poisoning 213*t*
  by fish 711
  cases
    opinion of 547
    review of 544
  clinical features of 658
Poisonous snakes, identification of 605
Poisons
  classification of 530
  different corrosive 552
  in body, fate of 528
  inorganic irritants 530
  metallic poisons 530
  miscellaneous 530
  non-metallic poisons 530
  of decontamination 531
    emetics 531
  organic irritants 530
    animal irritants 530
    mechanical irritants 530
    vegetable irritants 530
Police
  custody 497
  inquest 9, 10
Polydactyl types, different 100*f*
Polyethylene terephthalate bottles 512
Polymerase chain reaction 174, 174*f*
Polypeptide toxins 607
Pond 275
Poor man's WMD *See also Biological weapons*
Poppy plants with fruit capsule and flower 625*f*
Pornographic material involving child, storage of (section 15) 420
Poroscopy 95, 96*f*
Positional torture 502
Positioning body 206*f*
Posterior flap, reflection of 206, 207*f*
Postgraduate medical education 22
Posthumous child 383
Postmortem alcohol estimation 644
  bile 644
  blood from multiple vascular sites 644
  brain 644
  CSF 644
  gastric contents 644
  sequestrated hematomas 644
  skeletal muscle 644
  vitreous humor of eye 644
Postmortem
  artefacts 462
  bruise 225
  caloricity 187
  dental profiling 157
  findings 345, 351, 399
  imbibitions of arsenic 572
  incisions over
    contused area 225*f*
    hypostasis area 225*f*
  interval 195
  lividity and
    antemortem bruise, differences between 189*t*
    congestion, differences between 189*t*
  lividity
    differentiation from 225
    on back 188*f*
  predation by aquatic animals 468*f*
  radiograph 157*f*, 160*f*

Post-traumatic
  amnesia 288
  automatism 288
  encephalopathy in boxers 288
Potency test 373
Powder wad 246
Powdered
  diamonds 621*f*
  glass 622
    management 622
    medicolegal importance 622
    postmortem findings 622
Pralidoxime 539
  adverse effects 540
  mode of action 539
  WHO recommendation 540
Preanesthetic medication 362
Precaution and risk minimization, principle of 63
Pregnancy 378
  in dead, signs of 382
  in living women, diagnosis of 379
  of abortion, duration of 391
  signs of 378
Premature ejaculation 372
Pre-requisite for doing pcpndt 407
Preservatives used for common visceras 214
Pressure abrasion 221
  around neck 221*f*
Presumptive
  signs 379
  tests 472
Prickly poppy 710
Primary infertility 374
Privacy and confidentiality, principle of 63
Private parts, injuries to 295
Privileged communications 30
Probable signs 380
Product liability 53
Professional
  competence, principle of 63
  misconduct 32
  negligence 42
  secrecy 30
Proforma for examination of
  accused of sexual offence 741
  drunkenness 642
  sex crime 739
  sexcrime victim 428
  sodomy case 744
Proforma for injury certificate 339
Prognosis of burns, factors affecting 311
Projectiles, secondary 249
Prostate specific antigen 479
Protection of Children from Sexual Offences Act, 2012 419
Protozoal agents 708
Protruded tongue bitten by teeth 345*f*
Pseudocyesis 383
Pseudogunshot wounds 265
Pseudohermaphroditism 78
Psilocybe caerulipes 709
Psychiatric
  disorders of medicolegal importance 445
    schizophrenia 445
  toxicity 677
Psychoactive substance 441
Psychological autopsy 200
Psychosis 449
Pubic
  hair gets darker 82
  symphysis
    component 136
    phase 135
    stages of 135*f*
Public
  domain, principle of 63
  interest and of distributive justice, principle of maximization of 63
Pugilistic attitude 190, 316
Pulmonary
  agent 725
  edema 314
Pulvertaft 511
Punch drunk 289
Puncture wound 235
  by blunt objects 238
  versus instruments, shape of 238*f*
Punishment
  appeal against 60
  authorized by law in India 12
  for culpable homicide not amounting to murder 334
  for murder by life convict 334
  for rape 415
  for voluntarily causing
    grievous hurt 331
    hurt 330
Pupils 186
Purpose of torture 501
Putrefaction
  factors modifying rate of 193
  in water 193
Pyrethrins 654
Pyrethroids 654
Pyrethrum 654
  management 655
    decontamination 655
    medicolegal importance 655
    supportive treatment 655

Q

Questions by court 20

R

Rabbit punch 296
Race
  clothing, determination of 72
  complexion, determination of 72
  determination of 72
    using femur, hands fit under femur 124*f*
  differentiating points between 74
  eye color, determination of 72
  from sacrum, determination of 139*t*
  from teeth, determinant of 158*t*
  hair, determination of 72
  teeth, determination of 72
Racial variation from
  interspinous 138*t*
  morphological changes 137*t*
Radius 84, 131
  age 131
  sex 131
Rail-track bruises 226
Railway spine 296
Range of
  entry 258*f*
  exit wound 258*f*
  firing 247, 258*f*
  track 258*f*
Rape 88, 378, 415, 421, 503
  375 IPC 415
  376 IPC 415
  376a, IPC 417
  376b, IPC 417
  376c, IPC 417
  376d, IPC 417
  376e, IPC 418
  by husband upon his wife during separation 417
  criminal law 422
  evidence of 427
  punishment for causing death 417

substitution of new sections for sections 375, 376, 376a, 376b, 376c and 376d 415
trauma syndrome 427
types of 418
victim
blaming 422
different objectives 422
examination of 422
procedures 422
step of examination 423
consent 423
paper documents 423
proper 424
proper clothes 424
proper general physical examination 424
proper genitals 424
proper signs of violence 424
Rattle snake 603
Raw tobacco 660
Recapture of mentally ill 453
Recent delivery in
dead, signs of 385
living, signs of 384
Recent hymenal tears 425*f*
Recognition of foreign medical degrees 23
Recovered skull with piece of stone between teeth of both jaws 143*f*
Referral of patient, procedure of 30
Regional injuries 270
Registered medical practitioner 26
Registration number, display of 31
Relation between osteons and age 113
Religion 72
of caste
Hindu
females 72
males 72
Muslim females 72
Religious and social attitudes of autopsy 4
Remote
action of poison 528
delivery in
dead, signs of 385
living, signs of 385
Renal failure 315
Report, injury 337
Reproductive system 576
Res ipsa loquitur 46
examples of 45
Respiratory toxicity 677
Restriction fragments length polymorphism method 173
Retinal vessels 186
Retrograde amnesia 288
Revolver 253
and different parts 254*f*
Rh system 477
Rifle
bore 253
firearm 222
atypical entry wound 264
bullet graze or slap 264
cartridge of 253
casualties with blank cartridges 265
close shot 261
depending on
firing mechanism 252
length of barrel 252
muzzle velocity 252
distant shot 262
or shotgun injuries 258
ricochet bullet 264
single entrance and multiple exits 263
types of 252
uses of 252
wound 259
general features of 254*f*
Rifling 252
in barrel 252*f*
marks 267
Right
and duties of attending physician in consultation 30
and privileges of registered medical practitioners 26
of consultant during consultation 30
to refuse
consent 41
treatment 41
Rigor mortis 188
and cadaveric spasm, differences between 191*t*
definition 188
factors affecting 190
mechanism of 189
Rigorous imprisonment 13
Ring fracture 275, 276*f*
Road traffic
accident 298
airbags injury 302
injuries 297
definition 297
pattern of 299
to pedestrians 299
other safety features 303
primary impact injuries 299
run over injury 301
safety devices seat belts 303
seat belt injuries 302
secondary impact injuries 300
whiplash injury 302
Rodent bite-marks 466*f*
Rokitansky's technique 210
Rotavirus 708
Routine visceras to be preserved in case poisoning 213*t*
RTA reconstruction 304
Rubber bullet 257
Rugoscopy 97
Rule
for doing mtp 391
of five 312*t*
of haase 79
of nine 312*f*
of palm 312*f*
Run over by vehicle 301*f*
Rupture of hymen, causes of 412
Russell's viper 603, 604
bite 610
venom 612
Ryle's tube 533*f*

S

Sabji *See also Bhang*
Sac embedded in skin 617*f*
Sacrum 138
age 138
race 139
sex 138
Safed datura *See also Datura alba*
Safety devices 303
Salicylates 695
chemical structure of 695*f*
Salicylism 697
Saliva 480
Salmonella 702, 705
enteritidis 706
incriminated food 706
typhi 702
Salt 93
of copper, various 582*t*
Samples for DNA extraction, collection of 175
Sapphire diamond, pieces of 621*f*
Sativa *See also Cannabis indica*

Saw scaled viper 603
Saxitoxin 712
Scald 318
Scalp 270
  anatomy of 271*f*
  hairs, clothing 203
  incision 206*f*
    on back, extension of 206*f*
Scapula 84, 128
  age 128
  ossification center of 128*f*
Scar 100, 102*f*
  age of 101
  characters 101
  examination 100
  growth 101
  medicolegal importance 101
  surgical 102*f*
  types of 102*f*
  vaccination 102*f*
Schizophrenia 441, 446
Schizotypal disorders 441
Sclerotia *See Ergot*
Scombrotoxin 712
Scoptophilia *See also Araphilias voyeurism*
Scorpion 618*f*
  Indian black 618*f*
  stings 618
Scraping of epidermis in grazed abrasion 220*f*
SDH
  fate of 285
  secondary 285
Sea snakes 603
Second class judicial magistrate 12
Secondary relaxation, period of 191
Secret remedies 31
Secretors 477
Section 354 IPC *See Indecent assault*
Section 354a, IPC *See Sexual harassment*
Self-inflicted 232
Self-inflicted injury 233
Semen 477
  chemical examination 479
  collection of material 478
  microscopic examination 478
  physical examination 478
Semi-automatic pistol 253, 254*f*
Semicarpol 597
Semi-jacketed bullet 257, 257*f*
Semilunar hymen *See also Crescentic hymen*
Seminal fluid 437
Semi-smokeless powder 246
Septate hymen 410, 410*f*
Septic abortion 390
Septicemia 314
Sequelae of burns *See Keloid formations with contractures*
Serum salicylate levels 697
Sessions court 11
Severe vomiting 586
Severely attrited teeth 156*f*
Severity of burn injury 313
Sex 107
  chromatin test 74
  determination 73, 166
  differences from
    clavicle 128*t*
    fibula 127*t*
    humerus 129*t*
    radius 131*t*
    sacrum 139*t*
    sternum 133*t*
    tibia 126*t*
  differences in
    pelvis 134*t*
    skull and mandible 116*t*
  from decomposed 76
  from skeleton 76
  identification of 73
  of individual, determination of 74
Sexing from bones, Krogman accuracy of 113*t*
Sex-linked offences 413
Sexual
  asphyxia 350
  assault
    aggravated 419
      penetrative 419
    section 7 419
  characters, secondary 82
  harassment 413
    and punishment 413
    of child (section 11) 419
  intercourse 88
    by person in authority 417
    causes of 412
  natural offences 412, 414
  offences 412
    and perversions 409
    classification of 412, 412*f*
  paraphilias 435
  perversions 413, 435
  problems 375
  torture, other 503
  torture, other *See also Rape*
  unnatural offences 413
Shaken baby syndrome 405
  features 405
Sharp weapon 329
Sharpey's fibers 118
Shigella 702
Shoe
  foot *See also Bruise kicking*
  print crime scene 483*f*
Short barrel 253
Short rifled *See also Short barrel*
Shot, size of 250
Shotgun
  cartridge 245*f*
  choke of 244*f*
  firearms *See also Smooth bored*
  types of 243
  uses of 244
  wound, factors altering 247
Shoulder rest *See Long barrel*
Siddhi *See also Bhang*
Sigmoid sinuses 282
Signature fracture 275*f*
Silk fibers 105
Silk, microscopic pictures of 106*f*
Silver 583
Silver
  management 584
  postmortem findings 584
  properties 583
  uses 584
Simple
  asphyxiants 689
  imprisonment 13
Sinsemilla 675
Sixth degree burns over right leg including thigh 311*f*
Skeletal
  growth, disturbance in 86
  remains
    age from bone 112
    bone 111
    cause of death 115
    examination of 111
    human or animal 112
    manner of separation 115
    nature of death 115
    personal identity 115
    race from bone 114
    sex from bone 113
    single or multiple individual 112
    stature from bone 114
    time since death 115

Skilled witness 16
Skin 317*f*
changes in 186
pigmentation of 380
Skull 116, 271
age 117
closure of fontanelles 118
fusion of bone 118
of fusion 118
cranial sutures 119
frontal suture 119
metopic suture 119
suture closure 118
basal suture 118
circummeatal suture 118
lapsed union 118
precocious closure 118
premature closure 118
vault sutures 118
anatomy of 271*f*
base of 278
caucasian (white) 117
cephalic index 117
mongoloid (yellow) 117
negro (black) 117
race 117
sex 116
stature 116
Smallpox 728
Smokeless powders 246
Smooth
bore firearm
injury 247
types of 243*f*
bored 242
rectal mucosa membrane 434*f*
Snake 602
bite 608
bite *See Injected poisons*
fang marks 608
management of 610
treatment protocol 611
classification of 603
cobra 603
fangs 605
identification of 607
krait 603
mamba 603
venom 606
Social grounds of abortion 390
Society, loss to 46
Sodium
salicylates 696
sulfate *See also Magnesium sulfate*
Sodomy examination of victim 433
Soft blunt weapon 329
Solitary imprisonment 13
Somatic death signs 185
Somniferous poisons 624
Souvenir bullet 258
Spark burn injury, types of 322, 323
Special museum techniques 513
Species origin 476
Specimen
preparation table 511*f*
to collected from
rape victim 426
sexcrime accused 430
Speech
circumstantiality, disorders of 444
delusion, disorders of 443
derailment, disorders of 443
disorders of 443
echolalia, disorders of 444
flight of ideas, disorders of 444
formal thought disorder, disorders of 444
loosening of association, disorders of 443
word salad, disorders of 444
Speed of
impact versus fatalities 301*t*
weapon's approach 237
Spermatozoa in post-coital vaginal slide 426*f*
Spinal
cord, injuries to 295
poison 214, 682
Spleen, rupture of 294
Split laceration 229*f*
Sporting gun 243
parts of 243*f*
Spouse rape 418
Spurious 383
Srinivasan method of identity 97
Stab wound
classification of 235
effects of stabbing 237
features of 236
length 236
penetrating 235
to back of chest 235*f*
Stack's method 150
Stagnant anoxia 340
Stains
disease 103
on teeth 158*f*
resembling blood 474
Standard of judgment 43
Staphylococcus aureus 701, 702, 704
incriminated food 704
Starvation
causes of 369
death 367
causes of 369
definition 367
types of 367
State Medical
Council, functions of 23
Register, maintenance of 23
Static test 399
Stature 90
from fibula, multiplication factors for calculation of 127*t*
from humerus, multiplication factors for calculation of 130*t*
from tibia, methods for calculation of 127*t*
from ulna, multiplication factors for calculation of 132*f*
of dismembered body 90
Statutory
provisions 38
rape 420
safeguards 506
Stellate shaped entry wound in contact shot 261*f*
Sterility 374
causes of 374
types of 374
Sterilization 375
medicolegal importance 375
methods 375
types 375
compulsory sterilization 375
voluntary sterilization 375
Sternal end See Clavicle
Sternum 80, 132
age 132
appearance of ossification of 133*t*
fusion of ossification of 133*t*
sex 132
sternal index 132
Sternutators 725
Stiletto snake 603
Stillbirth, causes of 397
Stillborn 397
baby 397*f*
definition 397
postmortem findings 398
Stimulates first depresses 636

Stomach
of burnt victim Dupuytren's ulcer late complication 315*f*
wash 597
Strangulation 351
definition 351
types of 351
Strychnine 682
Strychnine tree 682
Strychnos nux-vomica seed 683
Stupefying poisoning 528
Subacute arsenic poisoning 571
Subacute sdh 285
Subarachnoid hemorrhage 285, 286*f*
causes 286
injuries of brain 287
intracerebral 286
intraventricular 286
medicolegal importance 287
natural causes 286
traumatic causes 285
Subconjunctival hemorrhage 225, 346*f*, 609*f*
Subdural hemorrhage, causes of 283, 283*t*
Substance abuse 713
legal issues of 720
Successional permanent teeth 148
Sudden death, causes of 184, 185*t*
Suffocation 353
burking 356
choking 354
definition 353
smothering 353
traumatic asphyxia 354
Suffused and swollen face, dilated pupil with 345*f*
Suicidal
and homicidal cut throat injuries 292*t*
cut throat 232, 233*f*
gunshot wounds 273
incised wound *See also Self-inflicted*
notes in case of suicidal hanging 350*f*
poisoning 528
tentative incisions over wrist 233*f*
Suicide 337, 550, 583, 568
of child, abetment of 334
abetment of 335
Sulfuric acid 552
diagnosis 553
fresh stains 553
litmus test 553
management 553
postmortem findings 553
vitriolage 554
properties 552
uses 552
Super fecundation 383
Superadded permanent teeth 148
Superfetation 383
Superficial dermal burns 313*f*
Superimposition 98*f*
Superior sagittal sinus 282
Suppositious child 383
Supreme court 11
Surgical abortion 392
Surrogate mother 376
Suspended animation 195
Sutura frontalis persistens 119
Sutural separation *See also Suture fracture*
Suture
closure of vault of skull 118*f*
fracture 277, 277*f*
Symphyseal surface 137*t*
Syncope
asthenia, causes of 182
hemorrhage, causes of 182
vasovagal shock, causes of 182
Syndrome
battered baby 404
behavioral 441
definition, battered baby 404
features, battered baby 404
immersion 356
Klinefelter's 76, 76, 637
Synesthesia 442
Systemic
asphyxiant poisons 530
asphyxiants 690
cardiac poisons 530
cerebral poisons 530
hepatotoxic poison 530
nephrotoxic poison 530
peripheral nerve poison 530
poisons 530
somniferous and narcotics 530
spinal poisons 530

T

Taboos such dietary codes 504
Tactile hallucination 442
Takayama test crystals of hemochromogen 473*f*
Talons cusp 159*f*
X-ray 159*f*
Tandem or piggy-back bullet 257
Tangential passage of bullet 267*f*
Tardieu's spots 183
Tarsal
bones 85
phalanges 85
Tattoo mark 102, 102*f*
complications 103
erasures 103
medicolegal importance 103
Tear gases 725
Tear laceration of left ear 230*f*
Tear-gas cartridge gunshot wounds 265
Techniques
in museum 509
of fingerprints 93
Teeth
and gum chronic toxicity 169*t*
palmer notation, charting of 150
universal system, charting of 150
Teichmann test crystals of hematin hydrochloride 473*f*
Temporary
and permanent teeth, differences between 148*t*
guardianship 40
teeth 147
emergence of 146
Tented arch 92*f*
Terminal ballistics 241
Test firing 267*f*
Testamentary capacity 459
Tetraethylthiuram *See Disulfiram*
Tetrodotoxin 712
Thallium 584
medicolegal importance 586
metal 585*f*
postmortem findings 586
properties 584
source 585
treatment 585
uses 585
Thallous
acetate 585
carbonate 585
iodide 585
nitrate 585
sulfate 585

Thanatology 177
changes after death 184
manner of death 182
mechanism of death 182
modes of death 182, 183, 184
asphyxia 182
causes of syncope 182
coma 183
syncope 182, 183, 184
sudden death 184
Thebaine 630
Therapeutic 390
grounds of abortion 390
misadventure 50
privilege 35
Thermal injuries 307
classification of 307, 308*f*
to high temperature 308
Thickened coronaries 183*f*
Third-party artefact 464
Thoracic
cavity, opening of 205, 208*f*
visceras of stillborn baby 400*f*
Thorax, opening of 208
Thought
circumstantiality, disorders of 444
delusion, disorders of 443
derailment, disorders of 443
disorders of 443
echolalia, disorders of 444
flight of ideas, disorders of 444
formal thought disorder, disorders of 444
loosening of association 443
word salad, disorders of 444
Threatened abortion 389
Three methylmorphine *See Codeine*
Ti *See Thallium*
Tibia 85, 126
age 126
race 126
sex 126
stature 126
upper end of 80
with fibula gross features 112*f*
Time since death *See also Postmortem interval*
Tissue
biomechanical properties of 217
for chemical analysis, preservation of 571
necrosis 609*f*
resistance of 321
Tobacco 660, 660*f*, 716
active principles 660
stains 159*f*
uses 660
Tooth
anatomy of 145
development 146
loss 155
representation of 146*f*
Torture 498
chair, probably most gruesome method 501*f*
history of 499
methods practiced in
Germany 500*f*
Spain 500*f*
murder 505
ethics 505
pharmacological 504
physical 501
abnormal stretching 502
beatings on soles of feet 501*f*
burning and scalding 503
crushing injuries 502
electric shocks 503
immediate signs and symptoms 501
prolonged handcuffing 502
repeated beatings 501
suspension for long hours 502
trauma to eyes 503
psychological 504
forced breach of religious 504
mock execution 504
near asphyxiation 504
prolonged sleep deprivation 504
prolonged solitary confinement 504*f*
sensory bombardment 504
sexual humiliation 504
use of animals 504
types of 501
Totality of responsibility, principle of 63
Toxemia 314
Toxic
compounds of thallium 585
gases *See Asphyxiant*
gases, classification of 689
iron salts 586
principle in plant 588
alkaloids 588
amino acids 588
glycosides 588
gossypol 588
minerals 588
organic irritants of plants 588
phytotoxin 588
plant acid 588
proteins 588
resins and resinoids 588
toxalbumin 588
vegetables origin 588
Toxicity 596
rating 649, 653
of poison 530
Toxicokinetics 648
Toxicology 6, 527
general consideration of 527
medicolegal aspect of 544
Toxidrome 534
Traffic rules 304
Tramadol—synthetic opioids 362
Tram-line 226
Transfixing wound *See also Perforating wound*
Transition ballistics 240
Translucency of root 153
Transmission, modes of 488
Transportation of biomedical waste 57
definition 57
documentation system 58
timing of transportation 58
type of vehicle 57
Transportational of pedestrian injuries, dynamics of 300*f*
Trauma to ears 503
Traumatic
brain lesions 280*t*
types of 280
intracerebral hemorrhage 286
neurasthenia 296
swelling of dorsal aspect of left hand 507*f*
Trench foot 320
Trichlorfon 648
Tricks of manner and habit 110
Trinder's test 697
Tripod of life 177
Troubles in sex determination 76
True hermaphroditism 77
example of 78*f*
Tumbling bullet 264

Turner's syndrome 77, 77*f*
Twig snake 603
Two sets of teeth 148
Typical appearance of cigarette burn 503*f*
Typical case of child abuse 165*f*

U

Ulna 84, 131
  age 131
  sex 131
  stature 131
Umbilical cord, changes in 401
Unconscious patient 38
Undergraduate medical education 22
Unethical
  acts 31
  conduct, exposure of 28
Union of cranial sutures 119*f*
Universal antidotes 538
Unlawful homicide 332
Unnatural sexual offences 433
  bestiality 434
  buccal coitus 434
  sodomy 433
  tribadism or lesbianism 434
Unrestrained front seat occupants in head on crashes, movement of 302*f*
Unusual effect of rifled firearm 263
Unwilling partner, signs in 434
Upper jaw hard palate 73*f*
  caucasoid 73*f*
  mongoloid 73*f*
  negroid 73*f*
Urea 93
Ureters 212
Urinary
  bladder, rupture of 294
  disturbances 380
  tract 196
Uterine
  factors 375
  souffle 381
Uterus 381, 384, 637
  changes in 382
  fundal height of 381*f*

V

Vacuum-aspiration abortions 392*f*
  amniotic sac 392*f*
  embryo 392*f*
  speculum 392*f*
  uterine lining 392*f*
Vagal shock 344, 356
Vagina 384
  changes in 380
Vaginal fluids 480
Variation in humerus length against different races 130*t*
Various dental works 154*f*
Vegetable hairs 623
Vehicle occupants, injuries to 301
Venereal infection, signs of 426
Venom 605, 618
  delivery apparatus 604
Venomous snake 608*f*
Venous congestion 344
Ventral demi-face 137*t*
Vertebrae 139
Vertebral artery trauma, mechanism of 289
Vertebrobasilar artery injury 289
Vibrio
  cholerae 702
  parahaemolyticus 702, 706
    incriminated food 706
Vicious cycle of asphyxia 341*f*
Violent
  asphyxial deaths 290
  or unnatural death 336
Vipera russelli 603
Viperine envenomations
  signs 609
  symptoms of 609
Viral agents 708
Virchow's technique 210
Virgin breasts 409*f*
Virginity 409
  breast signs 409
  genital signs 409
  signs of 409
Virtual museums 515
Viscera
  examination technique 210
  labeling form 749
  preservation of 364
  preservatives for 214*t*
Visual
  examination *See Naked-eye*
  hallucination 442
Vitriolage, case of 273
Volatile compounds 690
Voluntarily causing grievous hurt 330
  by dangerous weapons 331
  by use of acids 331
  on provocation 336
Voluntarily causing hurt 330
  by dangerous weapons or means 330
  on provocation 335
Voluntarily throwing or attempting to throw acid 331
Voluntariness
  of consent 36
  principle of 63
Voluntary active euthanasia 66
Voyeurism (354c, IPC) 414

W

Wad, functions of 247
Washerwoman's feet 358*f*
Waste management, biomedical 54
Weapon *See also Chemical warfare*
Weapon 329
  advantages, biological 728
  disadvantages, biological 728
  identification of 267
  introduction, biological 726
  of mass destruction 723
  penetrating 329
  radiological 729
  types of 329
    biological 726
Welding of shot *See Balling*
Well-organized museum, functions of 509
Wet blood stains 175
Wet specimen *See Parous cervixes* with slit like external OS
  of fimbriated hymen 411*f*
Whiplash injury 295
White
  poppy seeds, with close-up view 625*f*
  powders 94
Whole
  bowel irrigation 532
  brain death 179
  liquid blood 175
Wilson's classification 310
  deep 310
  dermo-epidermal 310
  epidermal 310

Witness 16
    types of 16
Wound
    botulism 703
    different ranges of fire, features
        of entrance 262*t*
    disease 103
    distant 250
    shape of 237
    track depth 237
Wredin's test 401

Y

Yawning bullet 264
Yellow oleander 663
    active principles 663
Yersinia enterocolitica 702, 707
    incriminated food 707

Z

Zsigmondy palmer system 151